MOSBY'S ESSENTIAL SCIENCES for Therapeutic Massage

Anatomy, Physiology, Biomechanics, and Pathology

SEVENTH EDITION

MOSBY'S ESSENTIAL SCIENCES for Therapeutic Massage

Anatomy, Physiology, Biomechanics, and Pathology

Sandy Fritz, MS, BCTMB, CMBE

Founder, Owner, Director, and Head Instructor, Health Enrichment Center, School of Therapeutic Massage and Bodywork, Lapeer, Michigan

Luke Allen Fritz, BAS (Massage Therapy), LMT

Instructor, Health Enrichment Center, School of Therapeutic Massage and Bodywork, Lapeer, Michigan

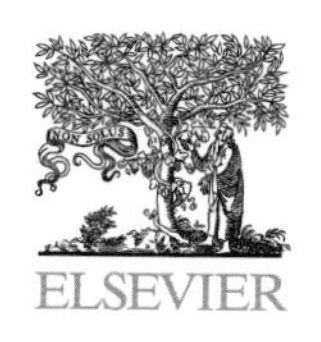

ELSEVIER

ELSEVIER
3251 Riverport Lane
St. Louis, Missouri 63043

MOSBY'S ESSENTIAL SCIENCES FOR THERAPEUTIC MASSAGE, SEVENTH EDITION ISBN: 978-0-443-11706-0

Publishing Director: Kristin Wilhelm
Content Strategist: Melissa Rawe
Senior Content Development Manager: Lisa Newton
Senior Content Development Specialist: Laura Goodrich
Publishing Services Manager: Deepthi Unni
Senior Project Manager: Kamatchi Madhavan
Book Designer: Maggie Reid

Printed in India

Last digit is the print number: 9 8 7 6 5 4 3 2 1

Contents in Brief

Dedication

This edition of *Mosby's Essential Science for Therapeutic Massage* is dedicated to my peers who began the journey of massage education with me in the late 1970s and early 1980s. A lot has changed, and much has stayed the same. We have had to change without losing the essence of massage therapy practice. Those I think about as I write this dedication have endured. You know who you are, and so will others, because you have been committed to quality massage education for more than 30 years.

This textbook is also dedicated to the massage therapy teachers in the classroom now who are becoming future leaders. The time will come when you will be the elders.

Sandy Fritz, MS, BCTMB, CMBE
Luke Allen Fritz, BAS (Massage Therapy), LMT

Acknowledgments

This text was reviewed, revised, and written by teachers seeking a more efficient and gentle way to help students understand and use this information. Credit and appreciation are given to the authors of the reference texts and research papers consulted in the development of this textbook. Without their efforts, this book could never have been written. Thanks also go to those who reviewed the manuscript. Their dedicated attention adds to the quality of this text.

Special thanks go to all of the individuals on my support team, past and present, at Elsevier. It truly has been a team effort.

Reviewers

Damien A. Archambeau, LMT, BCTMB, AAS, CLT-ALM, NCBTMB Approved CE Provider
Corporate Controller, Director of Student and Career Services, Instructor
TruMantra Education Group
New York, New York

Michele D. Clearman-Warner, LMT
Bachelor of Arts in English
Master of Pastoral Studies
License in Massage Therapy
Wellness Coaching Certification
Capri College
Davenport, Iowa

Jimmy Gialelis, LMT, BCTMB
Owner, Chief Officer
Advanced Massage Arts and Education
Tempe, Arizona

Michelle McConnell, LMT, CKTP, BCTMB
Massage Theory Educator
City Pointe Beauty Academy
Webb City, Missouri

Kendra McKellar
Business Management Degree
Licensed Massage Therapist and Instructor
Licensed Esthetician and Instructor
Licensed Nail Technician and Instructor
Director of Indiana Academy of Massage
Indiana Academy of Massage
Zionsville, Indiana

REVIEWERS TO PREVIOUS EDITIONS

Sandra K. Anderson, BA, LMT, NCTMB
Damien A. Archambeau, LMT, BCTMB, ERYT, YACEP
Jennifer P. Bell, BA, LMT
Celia Bucci, MA, LMT
April Christopher, RN, RVT
Teresa Cowan, MP, DA
Laura Weir Danso, MS, LMT
Angelica De Geer, BA, BFA, CA, LMT
Gautam J. Desai, DO, FACOFP, CPI
Rovin Devine, RMT, CLT
Rachel Minniefield Ersing, DC, MBA, LMT, CLT, CCT
Lisa Erawoc, LMT, Certified Aromatherapist
Marjorie Foley, LMT Certified Paralegal
Luke Allen Fritz, BAS (Massage Therapy), LMT
Bruce Froelich, JD, NCTMB
Jimmy Gialelis, LMT, BCTMB
Julie Goodwin, BA, LMT
Jarrod Harrall, DO
Christopher V. Jones, LMT, NCTMB
Joseph C. Muscolino, BA
Joseph E. Muscolino, DC
James R. Nieland, BS, DC
James O'Hara, MS, MA
Kevin Pierce, MBA, NCBTMB
Roberta L. Pohlman, PhD
Diana M. Reeder, BSHA, CCMA, CBCS
Monica J. Reno, AAS, LMT
Dawn M. Saunders, BS, LMT, RMTI
Shannon Saunders, LMT, AAS Therapeutic Massage
Jeffrey A. Simancek, BS, CMT, NCBTMB
Michael M. Steeves, BS, RN
Renee Stenbjorn, CMT (Virginia), LMT (Oregon and Washington, DC), BS, MPA
Aaron Swanson, PT, DPT, CSCS
Deanna L. Sylvester, BS, LMT
Melissa C. Wheeler
Jeffery B. Wood, LMT, COTA/L, BS

Preface

Mosby's Essential Sciences for Therapeutic Massage, Seventh edition, presents comprehensive science essentials—anatomy, physiology, biomechanics, and pathology—with a focus on clinical application for a specific audience: future massage professionals.

Mosby's Essential Sciences for Therapeutic Massage is a solid, Western-based scientific text focused specifically on the massage curriculum.

ABOUT THIS EDITION

The textbook and Evolve site have comprehensive imbedded review content for the MBLEx exam. At the end of each chapter is a series of multiple-choice questions for discussion and review. The more exposure the reader has to the critical thinking process involved in navigating multiple-choice type questions, the more confident they will be with the MBLEx or other licensing exam.

At the end of each chapter is a critical thinking scenario that combines the content of the chapter into a real-life situation with a massage therapy client. A series of questions are posed to stimulate a critical thinking process and encourage literature research and interpretation. The authors' responses to these questions are found on the Evolve site.

The text is heavily illustrated in full color to provide the best visual representation of anatomy and physiology concepts. In addition to anatomy and physiology, the book includes sections on pathologic conditions with suggestions for referral protocols and indications and contraindications for therapeutic massage. The text is clinically relevant, enabling the student to see how the content applies to real massage therapy practice.

The massage therapy community tends to view the body in a holistic manner. To support this view, two themes are woven through this text:

Dynamic balance or homeostasis

Critical thinking, including data collection, analysis, and reasoning. This theme honors both the scientific model of cause and effect and the larger picture of intention, intuition, possibilities, and the feelings of the people involved.

This textbook presents objective facts and information about human beings as they currently exist. Information is not static but dynamic, and like life, it is ever-changing. Teachers and students are encouraged to question and explore the information to make it their own.

Practices from ancient indigenous, culture-based healing systems often form the basis for massage methodology. Unique to this textbook is the inclusion of relevant information from cultural healing systems. This indigenous wisdom is related directly to body structure and function and does not represent any particular spiritual discipline. The content highlights the language and conceptual similarities and differences related to understanding the human experience.

The information presented in this textbook has been selected to best serve the beginning and intermediate students of therapeutic massage and to reflect the current competencies of the profession. Decisions were made as to what to include based on the Massage Therapy Body of Knowledge (mtbok.org), Entry Level Analysis Project (elapmassage.org), Federation of State Massage Therapy Boards Job Task Analysis and MBLEx Content Outline, and the National Certification Board for Therapeutic Massage and Bodywork job task analysis and content outline for the Board Certification Exam, current research, and the guidance of several expert reviewers who analyzed the manuscript content.

Also unique to this science text for massage therapy are a variety of features that make the sciences relevant to the practice of massage therapy. The features include *Mentoring Tips*, *Practical Application*, and *Focus on Professionalism*.

This text is designed for a 500- to 1500-hour curriculum (approximately 15–30 credits). A more generalized approach will need to be taken with the shorter curriculums, while additional class time will allow for a more in-depth integration process. Since the text is student friendly and self-directed, much of the work can be assigned in a self-study format.

A conversational tone has been used whenever possible, supported by metaphors and practical applications relating specifically to massage therapy.

ORGANIZATION

The text is divided into four sections/units. Fundamentals, Systems of Control, Kinesiology and Biomechanics, and Remaining Body Systems.

There is no single correct way to use this book. The sections do not need to be presented in any specific order.

Section I sets the stage for learning by providing an overview of the Body as a Whole, Mechanisms of Health and Disease, and Terminology: Scientific, Medical, Social, and Cultural Communication.

Section II describes the importance of the nervous system and endocrine system and supports the current research findings that massage therapy benefits are primarily related to these systems of control.

Section III is unique in that the content includes anatomy and physiology of bones, joints, and muscles but also expands on the importance of the connective tissue network of the myofascial structure. In addition, this unit prepares the student for the ability to assess and address biomechanical function and dysfunction.

Section IV completes the science studies by presorting and targeting relevant content of eight body systems that are affected by massage therapy in a general and indirect way based on homeostatic regulation of the systems of control or supporting musculoskeletal function.

Pathology and indications and contraindications for massage are included for each body system.

Each chapter is divided into short content segments that support recommendations for study in 15- to 30-minute time periods. Each section has objectives, activities, and a summary.

WHO WILL BENEFIT FROM THIS BOOK?

The format of this text has been designed to address the various learning approaches of therapeutic massage students. Throughout the text are activities that assist the student in transferring new information from short-term to long-term memory and in developing clinical reasoning skills. These activities do not have only one correct answer. Instead, they are designed for the student to use what is familiar from past experiences as a vehicle to transport the new or unfamiliar information to a level of understanding through a gentle and effective learning process. This enhances the student's ability to utilize creative problem-solving skills. Because there is seldom only one correct way to do anything, developing a process to determine the most effective decision at the time is important. This may seem uncomfortable for some at first, but an example is often provided to give the student direction within the activities.

Understanding is the learning goal of this text. Memorization is not the goal. Instead, the activities identify fundamental material and ask the student to manipulate it in a personal way to enhance the learning process.

Indications and contraindications for clinical massage practice have also been included. The word *indication* in the context of this book is defined as when treatment is appropriate and beneficial. The word *contraindication* encompasses both avoidance and cautions for the application of treatment. This practical feature allows the student to take the knowledge from the classroom straight into actual massage therapy practice. The result is a user-friendly text that relates to daily professional application for the massage therapist.

Sandy Fritz, MS, BCTMB, CMBE
Luke Allen Fritz, BAS (Massage Therapy), LMT

Anatomy, Physiology, Biomechanics, and Pathology—Comprehensive and Specifically Designed for the Massage Therapy Student

Welcome to the Seventh Edition!

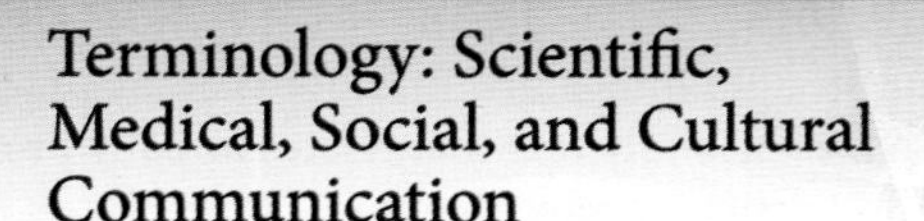

https://evolve.elsevier.com/Fritz/essential/

CHAPTER OBJECTIVES

After completing this chapter, the learner will be able to:

1. Identify the importance of terminology essential for the practice of therapeutic massage.
2. Use medical terminology to interpret the meanings of anatomical and physiological terms.
3. Define terms used to describe regions of the body and surface anatomy.
4. Define terms used to describe the positions of the body and the parts of the body in relation to other body parts.
5. Define *kinesiology*, body planes, and terms of movement.
6. Describe and use quality of life terminology.
7. Explore terminology used in Indigenous and cultural-based healing systems.
8. Use a charting method that incorporates a clinical reasoning/problem-solving model.

CHAPTER OUTLINE

Key Terms

activities of daily living (ADLs): Normal activities we carry out each day. They include self-care, such as eating, bathing, dressing, grooming, going to work, housekeeping duties, and leisure activities.
acupuncture: The practice of inserting needles at specific points on meridians, or channels. This stimulates or sedates energy flow to regulate or alter body function. A branch of Chinese medicine, acupuncture is the art and science of manipulating the flow of Qi, the basic life force; and of xue, the blood, body fluids, and nourishing essences.
biomechanics: The principles and methods of mechanics applied to the structure and function of the human body.
charting/documentation: The process of keeping a written record of a client or patient. The most effective charting methods follow clinical reasoning, which emphasizes a problem-solving approach. Many systems of charting are used, but they all have similar components based on the problem-oriented medical record (POMR) and SOAP (subjective, objective, analysis/assessment, and plan).
combining vowel: A vowel added between two roots or a root and a suffix to make the pronunciation of the word
kinematics: **(kin-i-MAT-ics)** A branch of mechanics tha the aspects of time, space, and mass in a moving sy
kinesiology: **(ki-ne-ze-OL-o-je)** The study of moven combines the fields of anatomy, physiology, physic geometry and relates them to human movement.
kinetics: **(ki-NET-ics)** The forces that cause moveme system.
mechanics: The branch of physics that deals with th forces and the motion produced by their actions.
medical terminology: Terms used to describe the h medical treatments and conditions, and processes care in a science-based manner.
motion: A change in position with respect to some r frame or starting point.
prefix: A word element added to the start of a root t the meaning of the word.
quality of life: Individuals' perceptions of their positi the context of the culture and value systems in wh live and in relation to their goals, expectations, sta concerns.
root: A word element that contains the basic meaning

suffix: A word element added to the end of a root to change the meaning of the word.
terminology: A vocabulary used by people involved in a specialized activity or field of work. Also, the study of the meaning of words used in a language.
word elements: The parts of a word: the prefix, root, and suffix.

LEARNING HOW TO LEARN

This chapter is about learning a language. As you encounter each new word, translate it into an example that you understand. For example, the definition of terminology is a vocabulary used by people involved in a specialized activity or field of work; also, the study of the meaning of words used in a language. How would you explain this definition to yourself? Maybe you would describe terminology as the words used to describe a unique language people use to understand one another at work or when talking to one another about a task. The learning happens as you try to figure out how to say the same thing differently.

Especially when learning the definition of words, you must review the material over and over again. You need to see the material at least four times—ideally at least six times. Each time you review the same information, you need to do it uniquely. Examples are flashcards, singing the terms and definitions, listening to someone else read them to you, writing the terms and definitions, listening to music while reviewing, and reading the terms and definitions aloud. This book offers activities to help you with new types of review methods.

You also need to review the material over several days, and then once every week or so to keep yourself from forgetting it. The adage "Use it or lose it" is especially true when it comes to terminology! Remember to take your "brain breaks"—study for about 30 minutes, then take a short break. Mindless tasks are productive during brain breaks. Water the plants, take out the trash, or do some dishes.

We need to be able to communicate using terms that are meaningful and understandable. Consider these definitions:

- A *word* is a speech sound or series of speech sounds that symbolize and communicate a meaning.
- A *term* is a word or an expression that has a precise meaning peculiar to a science, art, profession, or subject.
- A *vocabulary* is made up of the words used or understood by a particular person or group; it also includes technical terms used in a particular field, subject, science, or art.
- *Communication* is the exchange of information.
- *Terminology* is a vocabulary used by people involved in a specialized activity or field of work; it is also the study of the meaning of words used in a language. *Terminology* is a language of communication, with a system of words used to name things in a particular discipline.

For example, the title of this textbook is *Mosby's Essential Sciences for Therapeutic Massage*. The words in this title have a meaning relevant to your massage therapy studies. The word *essential* means "relevant and necessary." Something is relevant if it is pertinent, connected, and applicable to a given purpose. Our purpose is the study of therapeutic massage. *Science* refers to a system of acquiring knowledge through observation and

Box 3.1 **Branches of Science**

Physics is the science that deals with matter and energy and their interactions. Matter makes up physical objects. It deals with the fundamental particles of which the universe is made and the interactions between those particles, the objects composed of them (e.g., nuclei, atoms, molecules), and energy.

Chemistry is the science that deals with the composition, structure, and properties of substances and with the transformations that they undergo. We learned a little bit about chemistry in Chapter 1.

Biology is the science of living organisms and vital processes. It describes the characteristics, classification, and behaviors of organisms; how species come into existence; and the interactions of species with one another and with the environment. We started learning about biology in Chapter 1, and Chapter 2 was all about biology. Much of the information in this textbook is based on biology.

Earth science or geoscience is the study of the planet Earth. Eventually, we will even cover a little bit about earth sciences in this book.

experimentation to describe and explain natural phenomena. The word *science* comes from the Latin *scientia*, meaning knowledge. Science can be any systematic field of study or the knowledge gained from it. Knowledge is an understanding gained through experience or study by learning facts and information, resulting in the ability to do something. Because the word in the title is *sciences*, it means more than one science (Box 3.1). *Therapeutic* refers to the capability to restore and maintain health.

According to the Model Practice Act developed by the Federation of State Massage Therapy Boards, massage therapy is a healthcare profession:

> *(A) The practice of Massage Therapy means the manual application of a system of structured touch to the soft tissues of the human body, including but not limited to: (1) Assessment, evaluation, or treatment; (2) Pressure, friction, stroking, rocking, gliding, kneading, percussion or vibration; (3) Active or passive stretching of the body within the normal anatomical range of movement; (4) Use of manual methods or mechanical or electrical devices or tools that mimic or enhance the action of human hands; (5) Use of hot or cold applications; (6) Use of hydrotherapy; and (7) Client education (Section 104. Practice of Massage Therapy).*

As defined by the Massage Therapy Body of Knowledge (MTBOK) massage therapy is a healthcare and wellness profession involving the manipulation of soft tissue. In 2013 the Entry Level Analysis Projects (ELAP), which was sponsored by the Coalition of National Massage Therapy Organizations, defined bodywork and massage as follows:

Bodywork—A broad term that refers to many forms, methods, and styles, including massage, that positively influence the body through various methods that may or may not include soft tissue deformation, energy manipulation, movement reeducation, and postural reeducation.

Massage—The ethical and professional application of structured, therapeutic touch to benefit soft tissue health, movement, posture, and neurological patterns. *Healthcare-oriented*

ALL CHAPTERS HAVE BEEN REVISED AND UPDATED to reflect changes in curriculum standards and to include new research.

CHAPTERS ARE DIVIDED INTO 15- TO 30-MINUTE TEACHING AND STUDY SECTIONS with objectives that relate directly to chapter and section objectives with a dedicated section summary.

KEY TERMS are identified, defined, and have pronunciation guidance when helpful at the beginning of each chapter, providing the terminology reinforcement necessary to fully understand anatomy and physiology and their relationship to massage.

LEARNING HOW TO LEARN boxes at the beginning of each chapter prepare students for optimizing their learning experience.

ACTIVITY 10.2—cont'd

Scapular Elevation

Assesses for strength and endurance in the isolation position and tension or shortening in the scapular depression pattern

Muscles Involved

Trapezius (upper fibers)
Levator scapulae
Rhomboideus major and rhomboideus minor

Range of Motion

0 to 40 degrees

Position of Client

Seated, with legs over the side of the table and arms relaxed

Isolation and Assessment

Client lifts shoulders toward ears, as in shrugging, while examiner applies resistance to push the shoulders down.

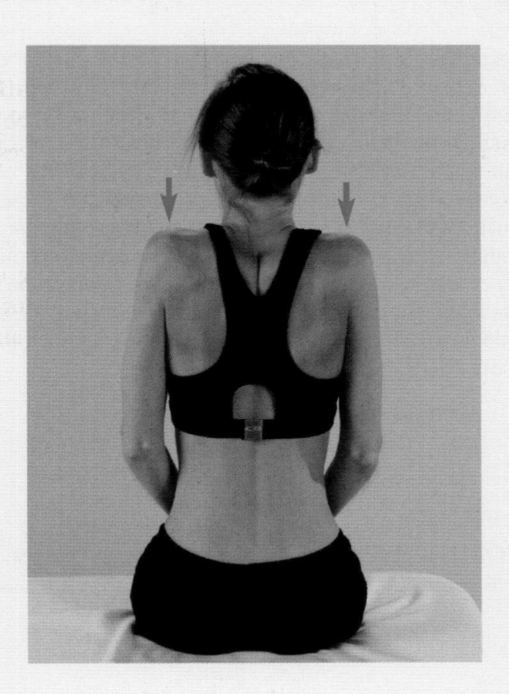

Scapular Upward Rotation With Abduction

Assesses for strength and endurance in the isolation position and tension or shortening in the scapular downward rotation pattern

Muscles Involved

Upper and lower trapezius
Anterior serratus
Pectoralis minor

Range of Motion

Reliable values are not available.

Position of Client

Seated, with legs over the side of the table, arms resting at the sides

Isolation and Assessment

Client flexes shoulder forward to 120 degrees with no rotation or horizontal movement while examiner applies resistance to arm just above the elbow to push it down.

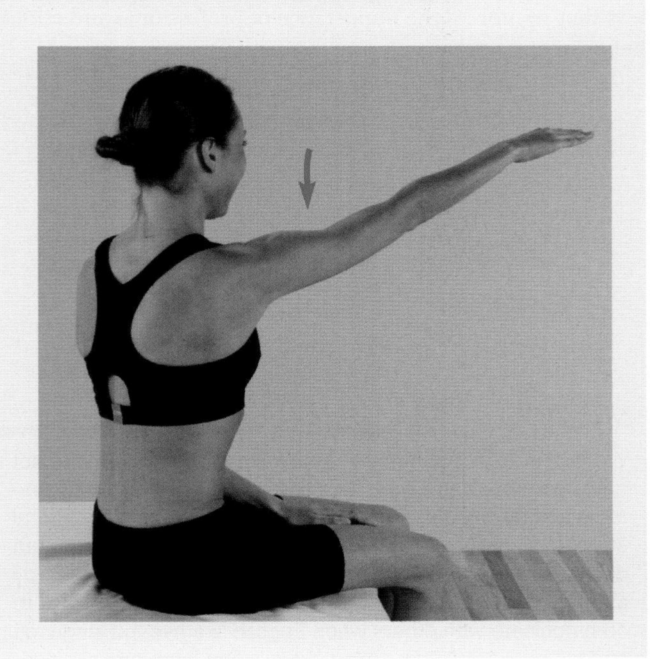

ASSESSMENT PROCEDURES feature full-color photos of clients being assessed for range of motion and muscle function.

Practical Application

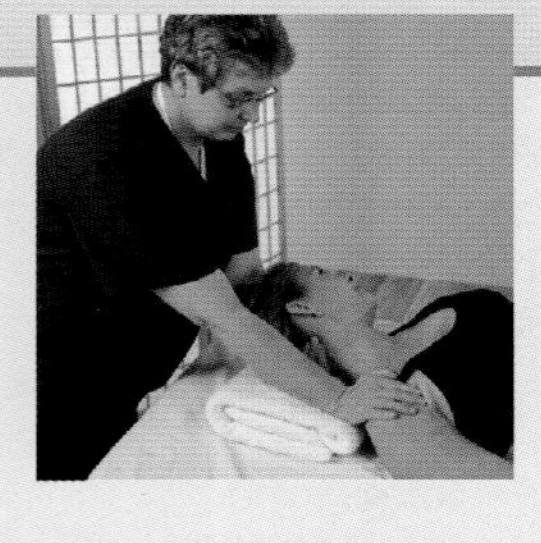

Quality of life terminology can serve as a useful tool for obtaining and documenting a client's history, and for assessment, as you develop the client's initial database. The terminology also helps frame questions during the history-taking process and for developing outcome-based goals for the massage. For example, the energy and fatigue content from domain I can be used as part of the subjective aspect of gathering data from the client (see Box 3.2).

PRACTICAL APPLICATION boxes throughout the text highlight and reinforce anatomy and physiology, pathology, and biomechanics concepts specifically for massage therapy.

FOCUS ON PROFESSIONALISM feature throughout the text that reinforces the importance of professional and ethical behavior.

FOCUS ON PROFESSIONALISM

Massage therapy clients are becoming educated. They no longer consider massage to be just something you do to pamper yourself. Clients expect benefits. They want to relax, feel less stressed, feel less pain, and move more effectively. Clients expect massage to enhance their quality of life. Measures of the benefits of massage are related to aspects of quality of life. If a client finds movement painful, her quality of life is diminished. If a client is stressed and anxious, his quality of life is reduced. Relating massage to outcome goals and describing it as a means to enhance quality of life activities makes sense to clients and helps people understand the value of massage therapy.

MENTORING TIP

We live in a global society. Many different cultures interact daily. Communication can be a challenge. Many different systems and beliefs about health and illness are found in cultural structures. As health professionals, we need to learn about different cultures and understand the use of massage therapy as part of a variety of healing traditions. We have to learn to communicate with others when English is a second language and we may not speak an individual's first language. Be curious and respectful of cultural diversity. Learn from others and be willing to share your culture as well.

MENTORING TIPS feature from the experiences of the author to promote introspection and classroom discussion.

INDICATIONS/CONTRAINDICATIONS FOR THERAPEUTIC MASSAGE boxes prepare students for when to continue with a massage or refer a client to another professional.

INDICATIONS/CONTRAINDICATIONS for Therapeutic Massage

Therapeutic massage in a supervised setting can be supportive during rehabilitation. The benefits of massage therapy are effective in managing the discomfort caused when the functioning portions of the body must work harder to compensate for nonfunctioning areas. In addition, stress management is an important part of the long-term management of these conditions. Because anticoagulants are commonly used to prevent further CVAs or TIAs, care must be taken when using soft tissue methods so that bruising does not occur during therapy. Careful attention should be paid to any symptom of thrombosis, and the type of massage application chosen should not place heavy pressure over vulnerable vessels to prevent the rare but possible mobilization of an embolism.

ACTIVITIES THROUGHOUT offer students the opportunity to review and test their skills.

A FOCUS ON CRITICAL THINKING AND CLINICAL REASONING Each chapter will feature a critical thinking and clinical reasoning application of the content related to massage therapy practice. A client scenario will be presented with recommendations for additional research, often using MedlinePlus or PubMed. Relevant questions based on the chapter content outline are provided to guide discussion. The author's decision-making process related to the scenario and questions is on the EVOLVE site.

A SELF-STUDY DESIGN This textbook is developed to be a self-teaching tool. A classroom teacher has limited time to present the information. View this textbook as a teacher and expand your comprehension of the ESSENTIAL SCIENCES needed for successful massage therapy practice.

QUICK CONTENT REVIEW IN QUESTION FORM is a Student EVOLVE Resource that reinforces key concepts in the chapter and allows the learners to quiz themselves as a review and learning strategy.

WORKBOOK Sections are available in an e-format on EVOLVE.

LICENSING REVIEW QUESTIONS reinforce content and provide practice for the licensing exam.

8 PRACTICE EXAMS FOR THE MBLEx are located on the EVOLVE site.

SCIENTIFIC ANIMATIONS accessed on the EVOLVE site reinforce textbook content.

Contents

CHAPTER 1

The Body as a Whole

https://evolve.elsevier.com/Fritz/essential/

CHAPTER OBJECTIVES

After completing this chapter, the learner will be able to:

1. Define the terms *anatomy* and *physiology*.
2. List and describe the characteristics of life.
3. List and discuss the levels of organization in the body.
4. Explain the importance of understanding the relationships among the structures and functions of the body as a whole.
5. Use valid criteria to evaluate the plausibility of massage therapy effects and to support evidence-informed professional practice.

CHAPTER OUTLINE

KEY TERMS

active transport: The transport of substances into or out of a cell using energy.

adenosine triphosphate (ATP): (ah-DEN-o-seen tri-FOS-fate) A compound that stores energy in the muscles. When ATP is broken down during catabolic reactions, it releases energy.

anabolism: (ah-NAB-o-lizm) Chemical processes in the body that join simple compounds to form more complex compounds of carbohydrates, lipids, proteins, and nucleic acids. The processes require energy supplied by adenosine triphosphate.

anatomy: (ah-NAT-o-mee) The study of the structures of the body and the relationships of its parts.

apical surface: (AY-pi-kuhl) The surface of an epithelial cell that is exposed to the external environment.

atom: The smallest particle of an element that retains and exhibits the properties of that element. Atoms are made up of protons, neutrons, and electrons.

atrophy: (AT-ro-fe) A decrease in the size of a body part or organ caused by a decrease in the size of the cells.

basal surface: (BA-sal) The tissue surface that faces the inside of the body.

basement membrane: A permeable membrane that attaches epithelial tissues to the underlying connective tissues.

biological plausibility: The theory that a therapy is sufficiently biologically plausible (i.e., scientifically plausible) when the biological rationale fits reasonably within the current understanding of anatomy and physiology, even if proof of its efficacy is lacking—it makes "biological sense." Plausibility is not proof of the validity of a method, and because biological knowledge is ever expanding, a lack of biological plausibility does not necessarily disprove a theory about the effect.

carbohydrates: (kar-bo-HY-drates) Sugars, starches, and cellulose composed of carbon, hydrogen, and oxygen.

cardiac muscle fibers: (KAR-de-ak) Smaller, striated, involuntary muscle fibers (cells) in the heart that contract to pump blood.

catabolism: (kah-TAB-o-lizm) Chemical processes in the body that release energy as complex compounds are broken down into simpler ones.

causation: An event that is the result of the occurrence of another event. Also referred to as *cause and effect*.

cell: The basic structural unit of a living organism. A cell contains a nucleus and cytoplasm and is surrounded by a membrane.

clinical plausibility: An approach considered plausible because it is supported by clinical data from epidemiological studies, case reports, case series, and small, formal open or controlled clinical trials.

collagen: (KOL-ah-jen) A protein substance composed of small fibrils that combine to create the connective tissue of fasciae, tendons, and ligaments. Collagen constitutes approximately one-fourth of the protein in the body.

collagenous fibers: (ko-LAJ-uh-nuhs) Strong fibers with little capacity for stretch. They have a high degree of tensile strength, which allows them to withstand longitudinal stress.

compounds: Substances made up of different kinds of atoms.

connective tissue: The most abundant type of tissue in the body. It supports and holds together the body and its parts, protects the body from foreign matter, and is organized to transport substances throughout the body.

correlation: A relationship between two or more events that appear to be related but are not.

cytoplasm: (SI-to-plasm) Material enclosed by the cell membrane.

cytoskeleton: (SI-to-skel-e-ton) A framework of proteins inside the cell that provides flexibility and strength.

cytosol: (SI-to-sol) The fluid that surrounds the nucleus or organelles inside the cell membrane.

deoxyribonucleic acid (DNA): (dee-OX-see-RYE-bo-noo-KLE-ik) Genetic material of the cell that carries the chemical "blueprint" of the body.

developmental anatomy: The way anatomy changes over the life cycle.

diffusion: (di-FU-zhun) The movement of ions and molecules from an area of higher concentration to one of lower concentration.

elastic fibers: Connective tissue fibers that are extensible and elastic. They are made of a protein called elastin, which returns to its original length after being stretched.

element: (EL-a-ment) A substance that contains only a single kind of atom.

endocytosis: (EN-do-sy-TO-sis) The process by which a cell engulfs particles located outside its cell membrane and brings them into itself by forming vesicles.

endoplasmic reticulum: (EN-do-PLAS-mic re-TIC-u-lum) A network of intracellular membranes, in the form of tubes, that is connected to the nuclear membrane.

energy: The capacity to work; *work* is movement or a change in the physical structure of matter.

enzymes: (EN-zīms) Proteins that speed up chemical reactions but are not consumed or altered in the process.

epithelial tissues: (ep-i-THEE-lee-al) A specialized group of tissues that cover and protect the surface of the body and its parts, line body cavities, and form glands. Epithelial tissue is usually found in areas that move substances into and out of the body during secretion, absorption, and excretion.

exocytosis: (EX-o-sy-TO-sis) The movement of substances out of a cell.

evidence-informed practice: Massage therapy supported by the best information available to inform the clinical reasoning process by which the massage therapist develops and implements therapeutic massage care plans for clients.

fascia: (FAY-sh[ē]ə) A sheath, sheet, or any number of other dissectible aggregations of connective tissue that forms beneath the skin to attach, enclose, and separate muscles and other internal organs.

fascial system: (FAY-sh(ē-)əl) A network of interacting, interrelated, interdependent tissues that form a complex whole, all collaborating to perform a movement. The fascial system consists of a three-dimensional continuum of soft collagen that contains loose and dense fibrous connective tissues that permeate the body.

filtration: (fil-TRAY-shun) Occurs when hydrostatic pressure forces water across a semipermeable membrane.

gross anatomy: The study of body structures visible to the naked eye.

high-energy bonds: Covalent bonds created in specific organic substrates in the presence of enzymes.

homeostasis: (ho-me-o-STA-sis) The relatively constant state of the internal environment of the body maintained by adaptive responses. Specific control and feedback mechanisms are responsible for adjusting body systems to maintain this state.

hypertrophy: (hye-PER-tro-fe) An increase in the size of a cell, which results in an increase in the size of a body part or organ.

impermeable: (im-PER-me-abl) The quality of not permitting entry of a substance.

inorganic compounds: Chemical structures that do not have carbon and hydrogen atoms as the primary structure.

interphase: (IN-ter-faze) The period during which a cell grows and carries on its internal activities but is not yet dividing.

ion pumps: Carriers that transport charged particles into or out of a cell using energy.

lipids: (LIP-idz) Organic compounds that have carbon, hydrogen, and oxygen atoms but in a different proportion from that of carbohydrates.

lysosome: (LY-so-som) A cell organelle that is part of the intracellular digestive system.

matrix (extracellular matrix): (MAY-triks) The basic substance between the cells of a tissue. Also called the *extracellular matrix*. Matrix is composed of an amorphous ground substance consisting of molecules that expand when water molecules and electrolytes bind to them. Fibers make up the other component of the matrix.

meiosis: (my-O-sis) A type of cell division in which each daughter cell receives half the normal number of chromosomes from the parent cell, forming two reproductive cells.

membrane: A thin, sheetlike layer of tissue that covers a cell, an organ, or some other structure; that lines a tube or a cavity; or that divides or separates one part from another.

metabolism: (me-TAB-o-lizm) Chemical processes in the body that convert food and air into energy to support growth, distribute nutrients, and eliminate waste.

metabolites: (me-TAB-o-lyts) Molecules synthesized or broken down inside the body by chemical reactions.

microvilli: (MY-kro-VIL-li) Small projections of the cell membrane that increase the surface area of the cell.

mitochondria: (MY-to-KON-dre-a) Rod- or oval-shaped cell organelles that provide energy for cellular activity.

mitosis: (my-TOE-sis) Cell division in which the cell duplicates its DNA and divides into two identical daughter cells.

molecule: (MOL-e-kyool) A combination of two or more atoms. A molecule is the smallest portion of a substance that can exist separately without losing the physical and chemical properties of that substance.

muscle tissue: A specialized form of tissue that contracts and shortens to provide movement, maintain posture, and produce heat.

nervous tissue: A specialized tissue that coordinates and regulates body activity. It can develop more excitability and conductivity than other types of tissue.

nutrients: Essential elements and molecules obtained from the diet that are required by the body for normal body functioning.

organelles: (or-gan-ELLZ) The basic components of a cell that perform specific functions within the cell.

organic compounds: Substances that have carbon and hydrogen as part of their basic structure.

osmosis: (oz-MO-sis) The diffusion of water from a region of lower concentration of solution to a region of higher concentration of solution across the semipermeable membrane of a cell.

passive transport: Transportation of a substance across the cell membrane without the use of energy.

phagocytosis: (FA-go-sy-TO-sis) The process of endocytosis that is followed by digestion of the vesicle's contents by enzymes present in the cytoplasm.

phospholipid bilayer: (FOS-fo-LIP-id) A cell membrane made up of lipids, carbohydrates, and proteins.

physiology: (fiz-ee-OL-o-jee) The study of the processes and functions of the body involved in supporting life.

proteins: (PRO-teens) Substances formed from amino acids.

regional anatomy: The study of the structures of a particular area of the body.

reticular fibers: (rə-TIK-u-lar) Delicate, connective tissue fibers that occur in networks and support small structures, such as capillaries, nerve fibers, and the basement membrane. Reticular fibers are made of a specialized type of collagen called *reticulin*.

ribonucleic acid (RNA): (RYE-bo-noo-KLEE-ik) A type of nucleic acid. It is transcribed (copied) from DNA by enzymes. RNA carries information from DNA to ribosomes, where it is read and translated so that cells can make the proteins necessary for body functions.

selectively permeable: (PER-me-uh-bl) A membrane allows the passage of some molecules or ions and inhibits the passage of others.

semipermeable: (SEM-ee-per-me-uh-bl) A membrane that only allows certain types of particles to move through it under certain conditions.

skeletal muscle fibers: Muscle fibers made up of large, cross-striated cells that make up the muscles connected to the skeleton; these muscle fibers are under voluntary control of the nervous system.

smooth muscle fibers: Muscle fibers that are neither striated nor voluntary. These muscle cells help regulate blood flow through the cardiovascular system, propel food through the digestive tract, and squeeze secretions from glands.

surface anatomy: The study of internal organs and structures as they can be recognized and related to external features.

systemic anatomy: The study of the structure of a particular body system.

tissue: (TISH-yoo) A group of similar cells that work together to perform a common function.

LEARNING HOW TO LEARN

You will find this feature at the beginning of each chapter. The information and suggestions will help you learn the skills you will need to become your own best teacher, both in school and in your profession. Lifelong learning is necessary to be a successful massage therapist, and these skills will support and enhance your efforts to achieve your career goals.

Study Tips

Learning is best accomplished in manageable chunks. The chunks of information in these chapters entail 15 to 30 minutes of reading, doing activities, and reviewing. At the end of each learning chunk, it is important to take a 5- to 10-minute break to give your brain, eyes, and ears a rest. When you study, plan to spend 30 to 90 minutes, and divide these sessions into 15- to 30-minute segments, implementing brain breaks as you go along.

Here is an example of a 30-minute study period:

- Reading, doing activities, and reviewing: 15 minutes
- Brain break: 5 minutes
- Reading, doing activities, and reviewing: 10 minutes
- End of the study period

A 60-minute study period could be scheduled this way:

- Reading, doing activities, and reviewing: 30 minutes
- Brain break: 10 minutes
- Reading, doing activities, and reviewing: 20 minutes
- End of the study period

A 90-minute study period might look like this:

- Reading, doing activities, and reviewing: 30 minutes
- First brain break: 10 minutes
- Reading, doing activities, and reviewing: 30 minutes
- Second brain break: 10 minutes
- Review of content studied: 10 minutes
- End of the study period

The textbook design is based on the 15-minute reading period. The chapter outline is a general guide for study periods. For example, starting with the section Anatomy and Physiology and reading up to (but not including) the section Characteristics of Life makes up one reading period. Reading from the section Characteristics of Life to the section Organization of the Body's Structure is another 15-minute segment. The section Organization of the Body's Structure to the section Biological Plausibility, Clinical Plausibility, and Evidence-Informed Massage Practice is yet another 15-minute reading segment. In the forthcoming chapters, the main topics in the chapter outline can serve as a guide for developing a study segment plan. You expand the 15-minute reading with the various activities provided.

Elsevier eBook on VitalSource supports the electronic version of this book and has the ability to read the book aloud. There are multiple ways to use the electronic version. You can follow along in the paper book while the book is being read. You can listen to the content multiple times while performing other tasks. The voice used to read can be changed, and the speed can be made slower or faster. All these variations support comprehension.

The best way to give the brain a break is by moving the body. Get up and stretch, go outside for a short walk, and do some breathing activities (e.g., singing or blowing bubbles). Have a drink of water, brush your teeth, wash your face with cool water, fold some laundry, do the dishes, or make your bed. Do something that does not require too much thinking.

An effective study schedule for a day would be a 30-minute period, a 60-minute period, and a 90-minute period, all separated by at least 1 hour or longer. Whether you have the 90-minute period in the morning, afternoon, or evening depends on your family and work schedule and whether you are more alert and focused in the morning or the evening.

Okay, now that you have some guidelines to follow while studying, take a 5- or 10-minute break. Stay focused and get back to studying as soon as the break is over.

The science aspect of your massage therapy studies is as important as the mechanics of giving a massage. The content in this textbook provides information that you can use to make decisions as you work with each person you touch. The more familiar we are with the body and its functions, the better we are able to use the methods of therapeutic massage that will most benefit our clients. It is the scientific information that supports your ability to use critical thinking and clinical reasoning during the practice of massage (Box 1.1).

This textbook will provide the information and support the thinking skills you will need to become an excellent massage therapist. It covers all the information found in general anatomy and physiology textbooks. However, the scientific information presented in *Mosby's Essential Sciences for Therapeutic Massage: Anatomy, Physiology, Biomechanics, and Pathology*, is based on its relevance to your future practice as a massage therapist. This means that some of the body's structures, such as the nervous system, bones, joints, and muscles, are covered in more detail than other structures, such as the urinary system.

There are no shortcuts to becoming a great massage therapist. How well you understand the workings of the human body will determine your ability to serve your future clients. One of the most important skills you will learn is *where* to find information based on the many *what* and *how* questions you will find yourself asking.

You can learn this information in a practical way so that you can formulate and ask intelligent questions related to the practice of massage therapy. You do not have to memorize everything—instead, question everything and investigate the available resources to find an answer to your question.

This first chapter provides information about the body as a whole because massage professionals deal with the wholeness of each client they serve.

Box 1.1 Critical Thinking, the Scientific Method, and Clinical Reasoning

Massage is mindful, not mindless. Excellent massage therapists have two things in common:

- They use critical thinking.
- They apply critical thinking to clinical reasoning.

In general, critical thinking and clinical reasoning are similar concepts: **Critical thinking** is a process of systematic thought that is analyzed and assessed for clarity, accuracy, relevance, and logic. It is the rational examination of ideas, opinions, assumptions, beliefs, conclusions, statements, and actions to identify bias, error, limitations, omissions, and data accuracy that have the potential to create flawed information. Thinking and communicating are closely related processes.

Critical thinking is similar to the scientific method. The **scientific method** is an objective, consistent, and self-checking process used to identify causes, effects, and relationships between intervention and outcome without opinion, bias, or flawed concepts. The basic steps of the scientific method are as follows:

1. *Make observations:* Through observations, you will be able to identify a question to research.
2. *Develop a research question:* Often the question is related to a problem to solve. A question will help you form a hypothesis, which will focus your study.
3. *Research the topic:* Conduct background research to learn as much as you can about the topics involved in the research question.
4. *Formulate a hypothesis:* A hypothesis is what you think will occur. A simple way to create the hypothesis is by using an "if, then" statement. For example: "If I do X, then Y will happen."
5. *Design and perform an experiment to test the hypothesis:* The experiment will somehow determine whether doing X will actually cause Y to happen. A basic experiment has variables, which are factors you can measure. The two main variables are the independent variable (the one you control or change) and the dependent variable (the one you measure to see whether it is affected when you change the independent variable). So the independent variable is X and the defendant variable is Y. During the experiment, X is done to see what happens to Y. Then X is changed to W to see what happens to Y.
6. *Record and analyze the data from the experiment:* Record all the steps and the outcomes from the experiment. Also record anything unusual or unexpected. Once you have the data, analyze the results so that you understand what it all means.
7. *Determine whether you accept or reject the hypothesis:* Do the results support the hypothesis, or do they not? There is no "right" or "wrong." Information is important; it is good to know whether X really does cause Y—and just as helpful to know whether X does not cause Y. Unexpected results may lead to a new research question.
8. *Draw a conclusion and report the results of the experiment:* Record the finding and discuss its relevance.

Clinical reasoning is using critical thinking in a therapeutic setting. Clinical reasoning is both a process and a set of skills. Using the clinical reasoning process teaches us how to be critical thinkers. A critical thinker considers what is important in a situation, imagines and explores alternatives, considers ethical principles, and makes informed decisions. Even though the clinical reasoning process involves a series of steps, the process can be used in many creative and intuitive ways. In the professional setting, we need to use an active, organized, cognitive process to examine our thinking carefully, as well as the thinking of others. The steps in the process are as follows:

1. Recognize the nature of the client's reason for massage. Then, clearly define the outcome.
2. Collect and analyze information about the client and the expected outcome of the massage. Collect the facts and do research.
3. Evaluate information specific to the individual client and brainstorm potential interventions. Generate possibilities.
4. Draw conclusions and make decisions.
   a. Develop and implement an intervention plan.
   b. Analyze the results and adapt the plan as needed.

This process is then written down so that others understand what you are doing and why you are doing it.

ANATOMY AND PHYSIOLOGY AND CHARACTERISTICS OF LIFE

SECTION OBJECTIVES

Chapter objectives covered in this section:

1. Define the terms *anatomy* and *physiology*.
2. List and describe the characteristics of life.

Using the information presented in this section, the learner will be able to:

- Define the term *anatomy*.
- Define the term *physiology*.
- List five categories of anatomical study.
- Describe two physiological fields of study.
- Relate the traditional Chinese medicine theory of yin and yang to the Western theory of structure and function.
- Define 13 characteristics of life.

Anatomy and physiology are two distinct yet interrelated biological studies that combine to present the operation of the body as a whole organism. **Anatomy** is the scientific study of the structures of the body and the relationship among its parts. **Physiology** is the scientific study of the processes and functions of the body that support life.

The word *anatomy* means to "cut apart." Anatomy is a broad field with many subdivisions, each of which is a comprehensive study in itself. These categories are examples of the divisions and subdivisions:

- **Developmental anatomy**: How anatomy changes over the life cycle
- **Gross anatomy**: The study of body structures large enough to be visible to the naked eye
- **Regional anatomy**: The study of all the structures of a particular area
- **Systemic anatomy**: The study of the body divided into the systems that contribute to the same function
- **Surface anatomy**: The study of the internal organs and structures as they are recognized from and related to the overlying skin surface

The term *physiology* is a combination of two Greek words: *physis*, which means "nature," and *logos*, which means "science." Physiology, the study of the way the body works, can be categorized into two main divisions:

- *Systemic physiology:* The study of body systems (e.g., cardiophysiology)
- *Pathophysiology:* The study of disease and the functional changes in the body during the course of an illness

Structure and Function

Structure (anatomy) and function (physiology) cannot be separated, any more than a person can be separated into body, mind, and spirit. Structure and function form a continuum; structure guides function, and function can modify structure.

The concepts of anatomy and physiology are examples of the duality of wholeness. *Duality* means two opposite states, both of which are parts of unity and wholeness. Opposite aspects of the whole become the foundation for understanding the interplay between structure and function. With regard to structure, for example, you will learn terms for the front and back of the body, as well as the top and bottom and inside and outside. *Pathology* can be defined simply as too much or not enough of a body's function. Assessment procedures compare normal structure and function with abnormal structure or function. Abnormal is more easily identified if you know what normal is.

The duality of balance is also expressed by the regulatory functions of the body. Maintaining a healthy balance in the body is part of homeostasis. **Homeostasis** is a condition in which the body's internal environment remains relatively constant within physiological limits. It is maintained by adaptive responses. Specific control and feedback mechanisms are responsible for adjusting body systems to maintain this state.

The duality of wholeness is often how we make sense of our inner and outer worlds. There are many sayings that express this concept. For example, "No rain, no rainbows," or "There cannot be light without darkness." Even your brain compares sensations. Cold is understood as relative to the sensation of hot. Muscles work in groups; one group causes a movement (e.g., kicking a ball), and another group reverses the movement by bringing the leg back. Basic concepts of massage intervention can be as simple as lengthening short tissue and shortening long tissue, to create balance.

The idea of wholeness is presented in many cultures and religions, as well as in science. Because the foundation of massage has evolved from various cultural systems, it is prudent to provide information about overlapping cultural theories. Throughout this textbook, we will explore ways of thinking about body structure and function based on systems that relate to the practice of massage therapy. We will consider systems from China and India that have a deep and enduring history and wisdom. The first concept to consider is the foundation of traditional Chinese medicine (TCM). The cultural terms in this text, such as *yin* and *yang*, represent physiological functions; they are not part of any specific religious system.

Yin and Yang

The duality of wholeness is represented in the yin and yang concept expressed in Asian terminology (Fig. 1.1). For example, the dual aspects of yin and yang combine to form a dynamic unit; many functions of body physiology are complementary, as described by yin/yang principles. Yin corresponds to the Western concept of structure, and yang corresponds to function—opposite but complementary qualities. Yang is said to contain the seed of yin, and yin contains the seed of yang. These seeds are represented by the small black and white spots in the yin/yang symbol (see Fig. 1.1). Nothing can be totally yin or totally yang (Table 1.1). The human body and all its functions can be understood through this concept of the relationship of opposites that creates wholeness. This concept is one of the main themes used throughout this textbook.

Yang (Sympathetic—
using intermittent
function, protective and
supportive function)
Yin (Parasympathetic—
restoring constant
function, vital function)

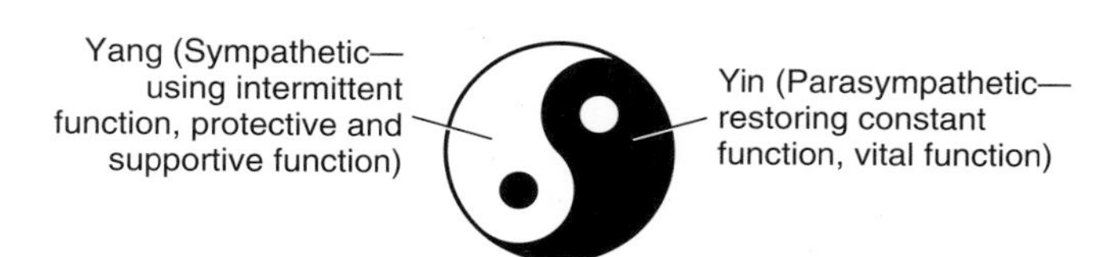

FIG. 1.1 Yin and yang.

Table 1.1 Yang Qualities Versus Yin Qualities

Yang Qualities	Yin Qualities
Day	Night
Immaterial	Material
Produces energy	Produces form
Hot	Cold
Sun	Moon
Expansion	Contraction
Energy	Matter
Above	Below
Fire	Water
Hollow	Solid
Hard	Soft
Superior	Inferior

Practical Application

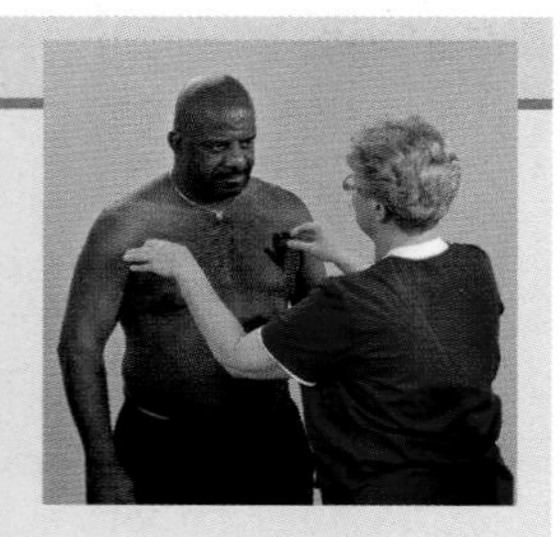

Learners of therapeutic massage must be well versed in gross anatomy. The most effective application of massage methods depends on the practitioner's ability to locate, recognize, and understand the structure the hands are intended to manipulate. Knowing the location of a muscle is not enough—we also must know how muscles function and what effects massage and other soft tissue approaches have on the function of that muscle, as well as the effect of the muscle on the whole body.

Characteristics of Life

What constitutes life? No single criterion defines it. Instead, we speak of the *characteristics* of life, which consist of these factors:

- *Maintenance of boundaries:* Keeping the internal environment distinct from the external environment
- *Movement:* The ability to transport the entire being, as well as internal components, throughout the body
- *Responsiveness:* The ability to sense, monitor, and respond to changes in the external environment
- *Conductivity:* The movement of energy from one point to another
- *Metabolism:* A chemical reaction that occurs in cells to effect the transformation, production, or consumption of energy
- *Growth:* A normal increase in the size and/or number of cells
- *Respiration:* The absorption, transport, use, or exchange of respiratory gases (oxygen and carbon dioxide)
- *Digestion:* The process by which food products are broken down into simple substances to be used by individual cells
- *Absorption:* The transport and use of nutrients
- *Secretion:* The production and delivery of specialized substances for diverse functions
- *Excretion:* The removal of waste products
- *Circulation:* The movement of fluids, nutrients, secretions, and waste products from one area of the body to another
- *Reproduction:* The formation of a new being; also the formation of new cells in the body to permit growth, repair, and replacement

Each characteristic of life is related to the sum of all the physical and chemical reactions that occur in the body. Physiology, or function, characterizes life.

We can study form (structure) without life, such as in cadaver dissection, but we can study physiology only in terms of living dynamics. The concepts in this textbook represent the study of life and the dynamic process of living. Therefore anatomy and physiology are presented together.

Understanding organizational and systemic physiology is important because it helps you to understand how and why methods of bodywork are beneficial. Although we touch the anatomy, physiology produces the benefits of the massage.

We need to understand how stimulating physiological changes can influence structure as part of the dynamic process of change that unfolds constantly in our bodies and in our lives as a whole.

It is also important to know the historical and cultural roots of massage and to understand the basic concepts of the theoretical foundation of these systems. All human beings have similar anatomy and physiology, regardless of their place of birth, cultural influences, and genetic makeup. What differs is language and theory. We need to understand that usually the apparent differences between massage and bodywork systems amount to differences in terminology only. These different words that are used for similar concepts can become confusing unless they are clarified early in the learner's education in massage therapy. Throughout this text, examples of the terminology of various bodywork systems and their concepts are compared with the anatomy and physiology terms and concepts used in this course.

MENTORING TIP

Learning a new language is confusing. The more you use the language, however, the more you will come to understand it. It is helpful to listen to the language of science being spoken. You can do this by finding anatomy and physiology lectures on YouTube. Make sure the content is valid by comparing it to the content in the textbook. YouTube also has some great animations. Start with the search terms *anatomy* and *physiology*.

Review What You Have Learned

- Define *anatomy*—anatomy is the study of body structure.
- Define *physiology*—physiology is the study of body function.
- List five categories of anatomic study:
  1. *Developmental anatomy:* The study of the way anatomy changes over the life cycle.
  2. *Gross anatomy:* The study of body structures large enough to be visible to the naked eye.
  3. *Regional anatomy:* The study of all structures in a particular area.
  4. *Systemic anatomy:* The study of the body systems contributing to similar functions.

5. *Surface anatomy:* The study of organs and structures recognizable from the skin surface.

- Describe two physiological fields of study:
  1. *Systemic physiology:* The study of body systems.
  2. *Pathophysiology:* The study of disease and changes in body function during illness.
- Relate the TCM theory of yin and yang to the Western theory of structure and function—yin is to structure (anatomy) as yang is to function (physiology).
- Define the 13 characteristics of life.

  Characteristics of life are common to all living things. An individual living creature is called an *organism*. Living organisms share many characteristics: (1) maintenance of boundaries, (2) movement, (3) responsiveness, (4) conductivity, (5) metabolism, (6) growth, (7) respiration, (8) digestion, (9) absorption, (10) secretion, (11) excretion, (12) circulation, and (13) reproduction.

ORGANIZATION OF THE BODY'S STRUCTURE

SECTION OBJECTIVES

Chapter objectives covered in this section:

3. List and discuss the levels of organization of the body.
4. Explain the importance of understanding the relationships among the structures and functions of the body as a whole.

Using the information presented in this section, the learner will be able to:

- Describe the sequence of simple to complex structures of the body.
- Define each of these terms: chemical level, organelle level, cellular level, tissue level, organ level, and system level.

From the simplest to the most complex, the structures of the body are able to perform their functions in a logical and well-coordinated manner (Fig. 1.2). This organization is one of the vital characteristics of body structure and function.

Patterns of dysfunction also present a logical order of progression in a well-coordinated manner. Disease processes usually begin at the most basic level and, if left uninterrupted, progress to complex, multisystem involvement. Our bodies work toward balance, which reflects a logical progression of cause and effect. When we understand the patterns of effective function and dysfunction, we can create a map to follow for a return to balance and health.

Both living and nonliving things have certain elements in common that link them and others that distinguish between and differentiate them. For this reason, a study of anatomy and physiology must begin with an investigation of the basic chemical and physical components. It is important for you to understand the basic units of the foundation of life because the massage therapy you provide will influence your client's tissues on both the chemical and cellular levels.

Chemical Level

Every substance has chemical and physical properties that give it a unique identity. Chemical properties demonstrate the way the substance reacts with other substances or the way it responds to a change in the environment.

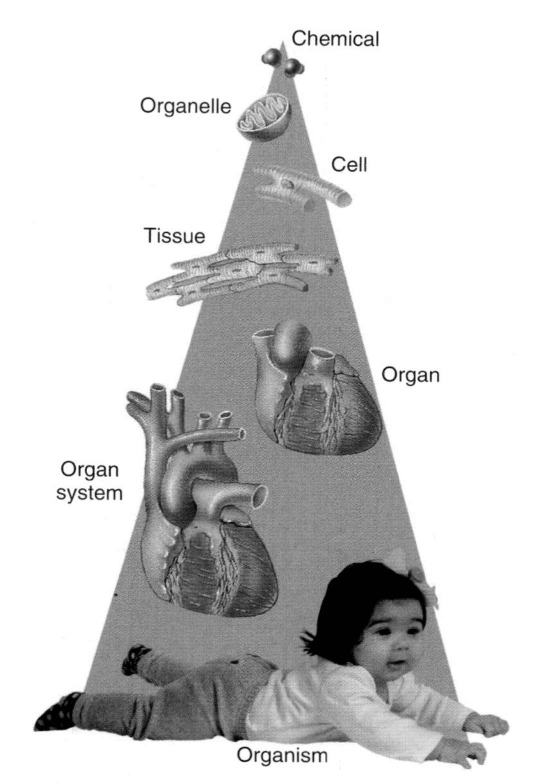

FIG. 1.2 Organizational scheme of the body.

Physical properties are characteristics, such as color, taste, texture, and odor. For example, salt is a chemical. Salt is used to dry food because the chemicals in salt attract water. This is a chemical property. We also can identify salt because of the way it tastes. This is a physical property.

Atoms and Molecules

An **atom** is a small particle of an element. An **element** is a substance composed of a single kind of atom. Atoms are made up of smaller particles called *protons, neutrons*, and *electrons*. Protons, which carry a positive charge, and neutrons, which have a neutral charge, form the nucleus of an atom. They attract electrons, which are negatively charged particles that travel around the nucleus in specific orbital patterns. The atoms most commonly found in living things are hydrogen, carbon, nitrogen, and oxygen.

Electrons are involved in all chemical reactions that bond atoms to make a molecule. A **molecule** is a combination of two or more atoms. It is the smallest part of a substance that can exist independently without losing the physical and chemical properties of that substance. The function of a molecule is related to its structures. The structure of a molecule depends on the patterns of the chemical bonds.

Molecules can form elements or **compounds**, which are substances made up of several types of atoms (Table 1.2). These substances, called *matter*, exist as solids, liquids, or gases, depending on the attraction of the molecules. When the molecules exist close together, the substance is solid; conversely, when the molecules are farthest apart, they form a gas.

Table 1.2 Elements Found in the Body: Their Symbols and Percentage of Body Weight

Element (Atomic Number)	Symbol	Weight in Body (%)
Oxygen (8)	O	65
Carbon (6)	C	18.6
Hydrogen (1)	H	9.7
Nitrogen (7)	N	3.2
Calcium (20)	Ca	1.8
Phosphorus (15)	P	1
Potassium (19)	K	0.4
Sodium (11)	Na	0.2
Chlorine (17)	Cl	0.2
Magnesium (12)	Mg	0.06
Sulfur (16)	S	0.04
Iron (26)	Fe	0.007
Iodine (53)	I	0.0002

Chemical Bonds

The forces that hold atoms together in a molecule are chemical bonds. They occur through chemical reactions. The most important structural feature in a chemical reaction is the stability of the outer shell of the atom, where the electrons are located. *Shells*, or *electron shells*, are envelopes or layers of electron orbit patterns. If the outer shell is full and does not react chemically, the atom is inert.

If the outer shell of an atom is not full, the atom is chemically reactive. An atom can achieve a state of maximal stability by forming one of three types of bonds to fill the outer electron shell: an ionic bond, a covalent bond, and a polar covalent bond.

Ionic Bond

An atom can gain or lose electrons to fill or empty its outer shell. When this happens, the atom is no longer electrically neutral because the ratio of protons to electrons is no longer equal. The atom becomes an electrically charged ion with a negative charge (anion) or a positive charge (cation). Negatively and positively charged ions attract each other to form a stable union. Soluble negatively charged molecules with ions that conduct electrical currents are called *electrolytes*. This type of bond is important in nerve and brain function.

Covalent Bond

When two or more atoms share electrons, a covalent bond is created; this is the most stable kind of association atoms can form with one another. This sharing completes the outer shell. Carbon dioxide (CO_2) is an example of a covalent bond.

Polar Covalent Bond

Molecules with polar covalent bonds, called *polar molecules*, are electrically neutral because they have the same number of protons and electrons. However, the electrons can be arranged in the shells so that one side of the molecule is more negative and the other side more positive. Water is an example of a polar molecule. Polar molecules attract each other, with the positive side of one attracting the negative side of a different molecule. A strong attraction exists between water molecules, and this attraction is called *hydrogen bonding*. Hydrogen bonds help create larger molecules such as **proteins** and **deoxyribonucleic acid (DNA)** (Box 1.2).

Chemical reactions take place when chemical bonds are formed and broken, and new ones are formed. In a chemical reaction, the number of atoms remains the same, but the atoms become linked in a different way, forming a new substance (Fig. 1.3).

Metabolism

Metabolism is the word we use to describe all the physiological processes that take place in our bodies. Metabolism is how we convert the food we eat and the air we breathe into the energy that we need to function.

Energy is the capacity to work. *Work* is defined as a movement or a change in the physical structure of matter. Energy exists in two forms, potential and kinetic. If an elastic band is held in a stretched position, it has the *potential energy* to return to its original shape. *Kinetic energy* occurs when the elastic band actually moves. Energy is constant; it is not lost but is converted from one form to another.

During chemical reactions in the body, most of the energy is converted to heat to maintain the core body temperature. For example, if the body is cold, the muscles contract and relax quickly, increasing the metabolism (chemical reactions) and producing more heat.

The body stores potential energy as high-energy compounds. Chemical reactions form these compounds or break them down. **Metabolites** are molecules synthesized or broken down inside the body by chemical reactions.

The two forms of chemical reactions are as follows:

- **Anabolism**: Chemical reactions that use energy as they join simple molecules to form more complex molecules of carbohydrates, lipids, proteins, and nucleic acids.
- **Catabolism**: Chemical reactions that release energy as they break down complex compounds. Hydrolysis is a catabolic reaction that uses water to break down larger molecules. Dehydration is an anabolic reaction involving the removal of water while small molecules combine to create larger ones.

The energy used in anabolism and catabolism comes from **adenosine triphosphate (ATP)**, which is the primary carrier of chemical energy in the cells. ATP contains many **high-energy bonds** that, when broken, supply energy for the work of the body.

Enzymes are proteins that speed up chemical reactions but are not consumed or altered in the process. Enzyme activity is altered by factors such as temperature, acidity, and alkalinity. Enzyme activity is commonly lower in cold and acidic conditions.

Acidity and Alkalinity

The body has to maintain a balance between acidity and alkalinity to support normal function. The acidity or alkalinity of a solution is measured in terms of pH (Fig. 1.4). pH is actually a measure of hydrogen ion concentration in a solution. Deionized, distilled water is considered to have a pH of 7, which is neutral. Tap water could be a little higher or a little lower. If

Box 1.2 What Are DNA and RNA?

DNA, or deoxyribonucleic acid, is the hereditary material in humans and almost all other organisms. The human genome is composed of all the DNA within a cell. Nearly every cell in a person's body has the same DNA. Most DNA is located in the cell nucleus (where it is called *nuclear DNA*), but a small amount of DNA can also be found in the mitochondria (where it is called *mitochondrial DNA*).

The information in DNA is stored as a code made up of four chemical bases: adenine (A), guanine (G), cytosine (C), and thymine (T). Human DNA consists of about 3 billion bases, and more than 99% of those bases are the same in all people. The order, or sequence, of these bases determines the information available for building and maintaining an organism, similar to the way in which letters of the alphabet appear in a certain order to form words and sentences.

DNA bases pair up with each other, A with T and C with G, to form units called *base pairs*. Each base is also attached to a sugar molecule and a phosphate molecule. Together, a base, sugar, and phosphate are called a *nucleotide*. Nucleotides are arranged in two long strands that form a spiral called a *double helix*. The structure of the double helix is somewhat like a ladder, with the base pairs forming the ladder's rungs and the sugar and phosphate molecules forming the vertical sidepieces of the ladder.

An important property of DNA is its ability to replicate or make copies of itself. Each strand of DNA in the double helix can serve as a pattern for duplicating the sequence of bases. This is critical when cells divide because each new cell needs to have an exact copy of the DNA present in the original cell (see the following figure).

Cytosine and guanine always pair. Adenine and thymine always pair.

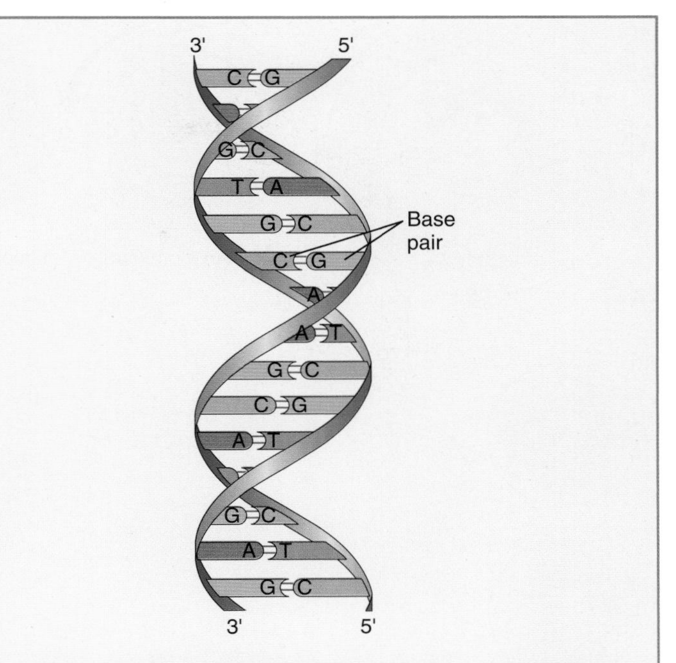

Modified from Copstead-Kirkhorn LE, Banasik JL. *Pathophysiology*. 4th ed. Saunders; 2010.

Ribonucleic acid (RNA) is a molecule that consists of a long chain of nucleotide units similar to DNA. RNA is transcribed (copied) from DNA by enzymes. RNA carries information from DNA to organelles, called *ribosomes*, which can read RNA and translate the information. This enables the cell to make the proteins necessary for the body to function.

From US National Library of Medicine. *What is DNA? Genetics Home Reference.* Sept 3, 2019 <https://ghr.nlm.nih.gov/handbook/basics/>.

the pH is lower than 7, the fluid has more hydrogen ions and is acidic. If a solution has a pH higher than 7, it has fewer hydrogen ions and is alkaline. Each line on the pH scale is a factor of 10. Therefore a pH of 8 is 10 times more alkaline than a pH of 7; a pH of 5 is 100 times more acidic than a pH of 7.

The pH of the body is 7.4, which is slightly alkaline. For the enzymes of the body to be active and for the chemical reactions to proceed normally, the pH has to be maintained at this level.

Buffers are compounds that help maintain the hydrogen ion concentration. Proteins, hemoglobin, and a combination of bicarbonate and carbonic acid compounds are examples of buffers present in body fluids.

Inorganic and Organic Compounds

Inorganic compounds are chemical structures that do not have carbon and hydrogen atoms. **Organic compounds** are chemical structures that have carbon and hydrogen atoms. Much of our body consists of organic compounds. The food we eat is made mostly of organic compounds called **nutrients**. When we digest them, we are catabolizing them. A variety of nutrients in the diet are required by the body for normal function. Organic compounds important in the body are carbohydrates, proteins, fats or lipids, nucleic acids, and vitamins. Inorganic nutrients that the body needs are water and minerals.

Carbohydrates

Carbohydrates make up 2% to 3% of our body weight. Sugars and starches are examples. Carbohydrates may be simple or complex. They supply most of the energy for cells.

Simple sugars, such as glucose and fructose, dissolve easily in water and are transported easily in blood. Complex sugars are formed by the combination of two or more simple sugars and must be broken down by the digestive tract before being absorbed into the body.

Lipids

Lipids are fats. Lipids make up 10% to 12% of our body weight. Lipids are insoluble in water and have to be transported in the blood by special proteins. Lipids are used to form important structures, such as cell membranes and certain hormones, and are an important source of energy. When the lipid supply exceeds the demand, lipids are stored as fat reserves for future use or as important body insulators. Fatty acids, glycerides, steroids, and phospholipids are examples of lipids found in the body.

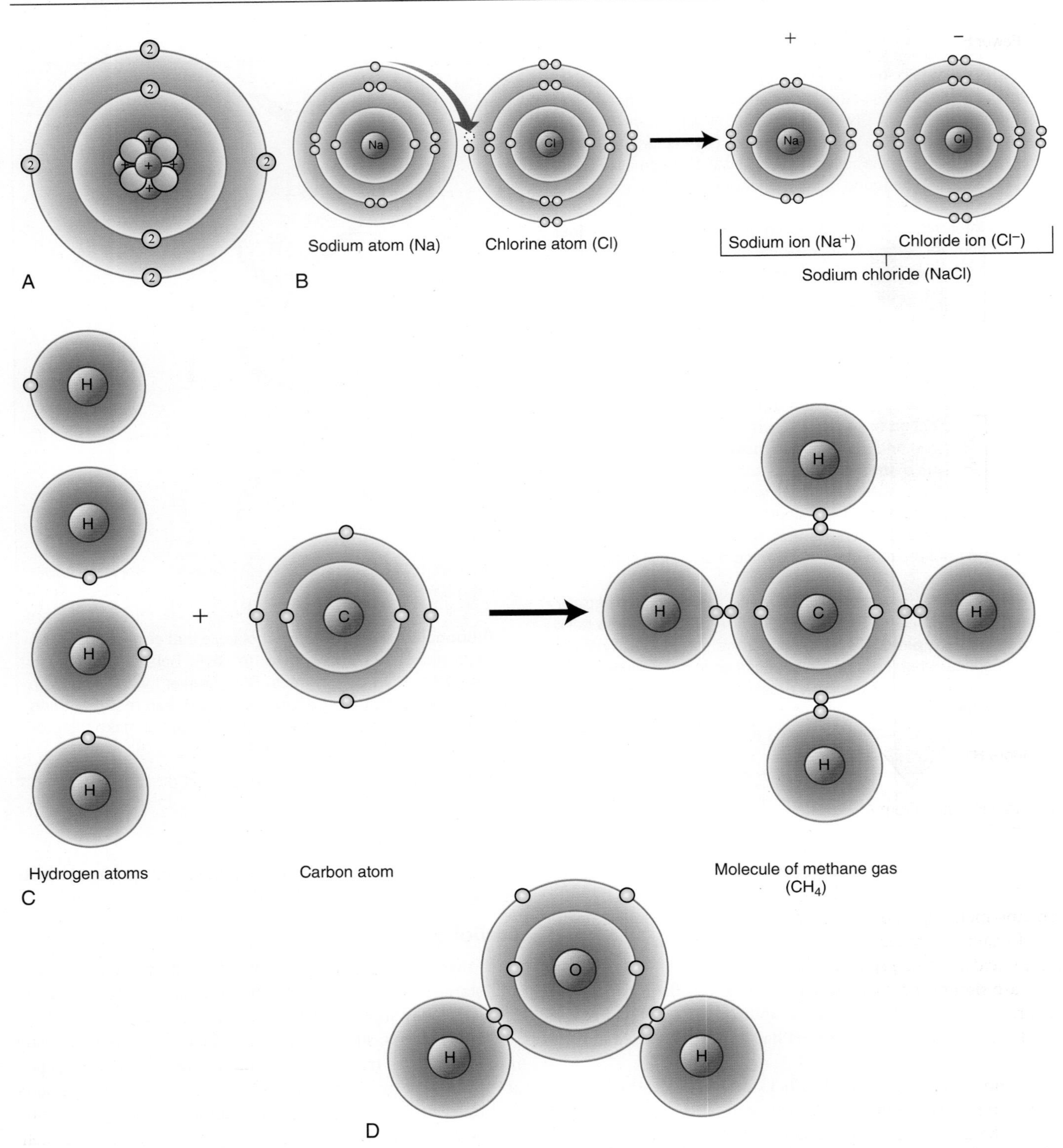

FIG. 1.3 (A) Model of the atom. The nucleus, made up of protons (+) and neutrons, is at the core. Electrons (–) inhabit outer regions called *energy levels*. (B) Ionic bonding. The sodium atom donates the single electron in its outer energy level to a chlorine atom that has seven electrons in its outer level; now each atom has eight electrons in its outer shell. Because the electron-to-proton ratio changes, the sodium atom becomes a positive sodium ion and the chlorine atom becomes a negative chloride ion. The positive-negative attraction between these oppositely charged ions is called an *ionic bond*. (C) Covalent bonding. Two hydrogen atoms move together, resulting in the overlapping of their energy levels. Neither atom gains nor loses an electron; rather, the two atoms share the electrons, forming a covalent bond. (D) Water is a polar molecule, as shown in the diagram. The two hydrogen atoms are nearer one end of the molecule, giving that end a partial positive charge. The opposite end of the molecule has a partial negative charge. ((A to C) From Thibodeau GA, Patton KT. Structure and Function of the Body. 13th ed. Mosby; 2008; (D) From Colville T, Bassert JM. *Clinical Anatomy and Physiology for Veterinary Technicians*. 3rd ed. Elsevier; 2016.)

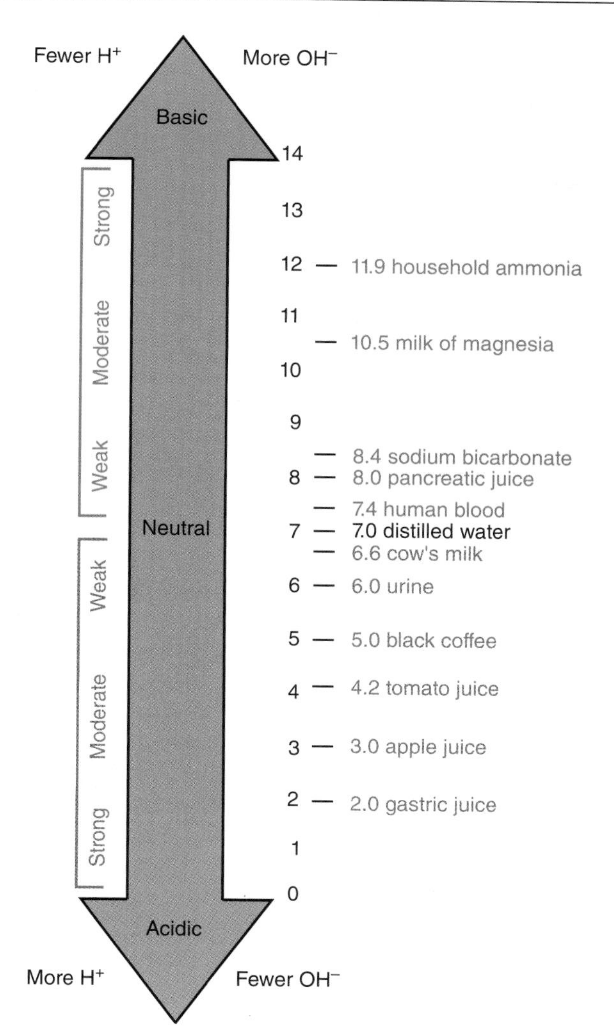

FIG. 1.4 pH scale. (From Applegate E. *The Anatomy and Physiology Learning System*. 4th ed. Saunders; 2011.)

Proteins

Proteins make up about 20% of body weight. Proteins consist of chains of molecules, called *amino acids*, and chains of amino acids, called *peptides*. In our bodies about 20 amino acids are significant. Each amino acid has a different chemical structure that determines its properties. Proteins form the structural framework of the body.

Enzymes that facilitate chemical reactions are proteins. The blood contains proteins in the plasma, and they are used to transport gases (hemoglobin) and hormones (plasma proteins). The antibodies, part of the body's defense system, are proteins, too. Many hormones are proteins.

Nucleic Acids

Nucleic acid is the major component of ova (eggs) and sperm; it conveys information about the genetic cycle. The two types of nucleic acids are deoxyribonucleic acid (DNA) and ribonucleic acid (RNA) (see Box 1.2).

Organelle Level

Molecules combine in specific ways to form **organelles**, the basic structures found in cells (Fig. 1.5). Each type of organelle performs a specific function within the cell. The cell is just a small version of the human as a whole, and an organelle's function is unique, as are the functions of our body systems. Some of these functions include digestion, respiration, and the creation of immunities.

More than two dozen organelles have been identified, but we will discuss only the most common ones.

Practical Application

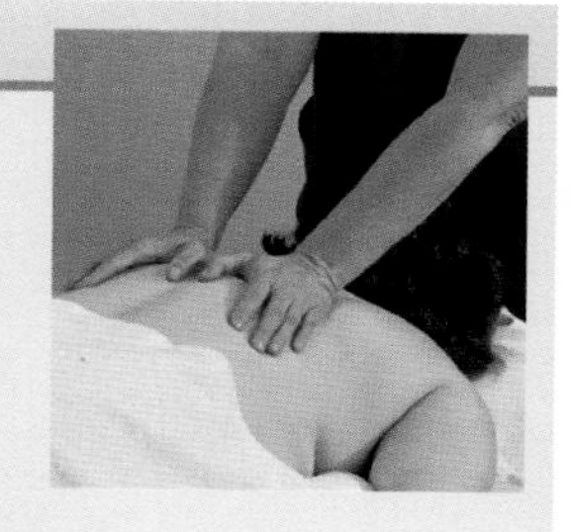

In the study of therapeutic massage, remain mindful of the basic chemical foundations of life and the dynamic processes of change. Change is balanced by stability. We function according to a continual process in which old bonds are being broken and new ones are being formed during every millisecond of our lives, whether in cellular functions or social relationships. Each time we apply massage to a client's body, we become part of the stimuli that activate chemical reactions within that body.

A more detailed study of the electrical and chemical levels of life, beyond this basic overview, would be valuable not only for an appreciation of the elegance in the simple physical basis of life but also for an understanding of the metaphor in terms of the way we relate to our clients, our families and friends, and the people of this world.

Cell Membrane

Also known as the *plasma membrane*, the cell membrane is the outer boundary of a cell. The membrane is composed of lipids, carbohydrates, and proteins and is called the **phospholipid bilayer**. Its molecules are arranged in such a way that they resemble a sandwich. The function of the cell membrane is to contain the inside of the cell and allow the transport of certain substances into and out of the cell by means of various proteins embedded in the cell membrane. Proteins on the surface of the cell function as markers that identify the cell or work as receptors for chemical signals.

The cell membrane is **impermeable** if it does not allow substances to pass through it; the membrane is **semipermeable** if it stops some substances from entering the cell but allows others to pass freely through it; and the membrane is **selectively permeable** if it allows only specifically selected substances to enter the cell. A substance's electrical charge, chemical composition, and size and shape determine whether the cell membrane will allow it to pass through. The transport of substances across the cell membrane without the use of energy is called **passive transport**. Types of passive transport include diffusion, osmosis, filtration, carrier-mediated transport, and vesicular transport.

- **Diffusion** is the movement of ions and molecules from an area of higher concentration to an area of lower concentration.
- **Osmosis** is the diffusion of water from a region of lower solution concentration to a region of higher solution concentration across a semipermeable membrane.

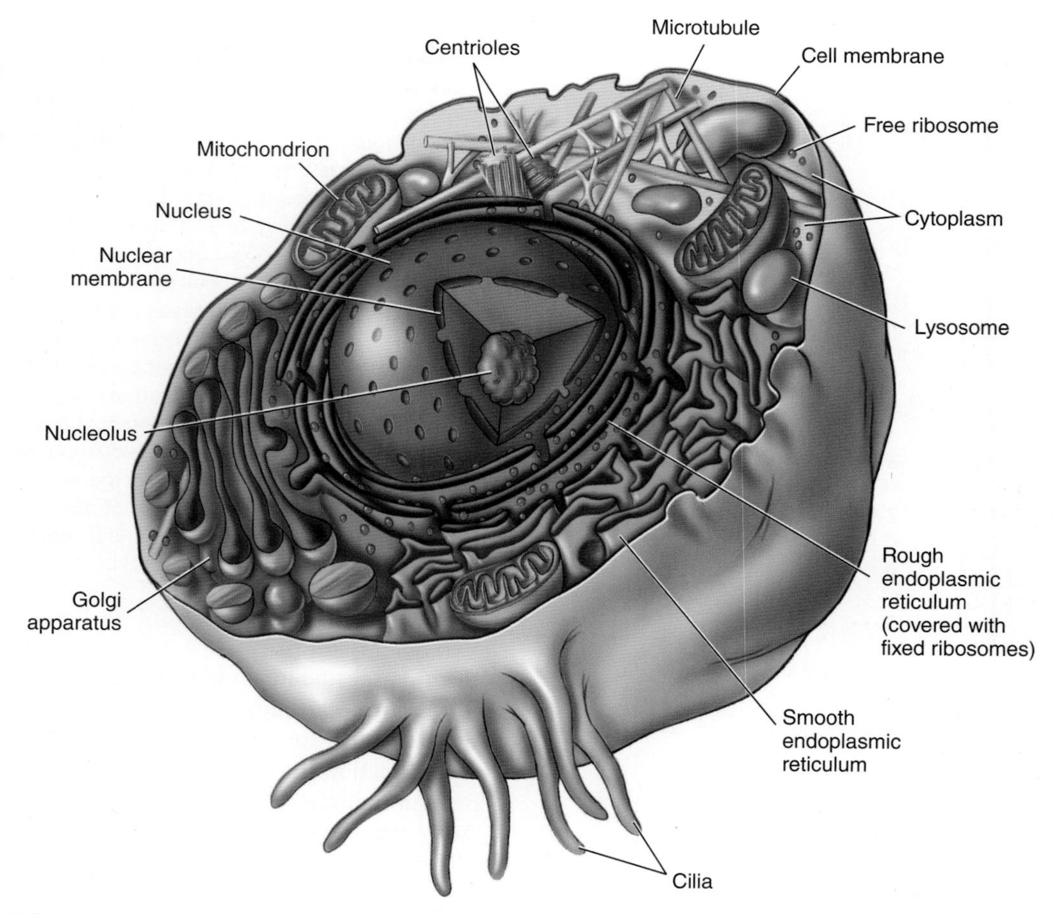

FIG. 1.5 Generalized cell. (From Herlihy B. *The Human Body in Health and Illness*. 4th ed. Saunders; 2011.)

- **Filtration** occurs when hydrostatic pressure forces water across a semipermeable membrane. This occurs in the body when filtration moves fluid out of capillaries and into the renal tubules of the kidney to form urine.
- *Carrier-mediated transport* occurs when integral proteins bind to specific ions or other substances, such as glucose and amino acids, and carry them across the cell membrane into the cell.
- *Vesicular transport* occurs when small, membrane-lined sacs form from the cell membrane, creating vesicles that surround a substance and move it into or out of the cell. Bringing substances into the cell by forming vesicles is called **endocytosis**; transporting substances out of the cell is called **exocytosis**.

Active transport of substances across a cell membrane requires energy in the form of ATP. Active transport uses energy to create **ion pumps**. The most common ion pump is the sodium-potassium pump. Under normal circumstances, the extracellular fluid (fluid outside the cell) contains more sodium than the intracellular fluid (fluid inside the cell); but the extracellular fluid contains less potassium than the intracellular fluid. The sodium-potassium pump pumps sodium out of the cell and potassium into the cell to maintain homeostasis. Cells are negatively charged inside and positively charged outside. This difference in charges, known as the *transmembrane potential*, is maintained by ionic pumps that move substances by means of active transport. Maintenance of the transmembrane potential is important because it is necessary for many functions, such as muscle contraction, secretion by glands, and the transmission of nerve impulses.

Cytoplasm

The material enclosed by a cell membrane is called **cytoplasm**. It contains the nucleus and organelles. The fluid portion of the cytoplasm is called the *intracellular fluid* or **cytosol**. Cytoplasm, which is not classified as an organelle, is the medium that surrounds all the organelles. The fluid portion, or cytosol, contains many protein enzymes that function as catalysts in cell processes. The **cytoskeleton** is the internal scaffolding that anchors the organelles and allows the cells to move or to maintain or change their shape.

Endoplasmic Reticulum

The endoplasmic reticulum is a network of interconnected tubes, flattened sacs, and channels distributed throughout the cytoplasm. Rough endoplasmic reticulum is found in cells in which large amounts of proteins are made. Smooth endoplasmic reticulum is involved in the metabolism of lipids (fats); it also assists in eliminating toxins caused by drugs and in deactivating steroids. The smooth endoplasmic reticulum of muscle cells (sarcoplasmic reticulum) uses large amounts of calcium to trigger muscle contractions.

Golgi Apparatus (or Complex)

The Golgi apparatus processes and packages protein and some carbohydrates for distribution to other parts of the cell or for secretion from the cell.

Lysosomes

Lysosomes contain enzymes that function as the digestive system of the cell. These enzymes are enclosed in membranes to keep them from breaking down the cell itself.

Microvilli

Microvilli are small, fingerlike projections of the cell membrane that serve to increase the surface area. They are found in cells that are involved in absorbing substances from the extracellular fluid.

Mitochondria

The **mitochondria** may be the largest and one of the most numerous of the organelles. They produce ATP, which provides the energy for cell activity.

Peroxisomes

Peroxisomes are similar to lysosomes, except that they help to detoxify the cell of substances, such as alcohol and hydrogen peroxide.

Ribosomes

Often the most numerous of the organelles, ribosomes are the sites where amino acids are combined to create various proteins.

Nucleus

The nucleus controls the daily activities of the cell and all cellular reproduction. Usually the largest of the organelles, the nucleus contains the chromosomes (threads of DNA). DNA is a double-helix strand held together by hydrogen bonds. The nitrogenous bases adenine, thymine, cytosine, and guanine are arranged in different ways to form the genetic code of DNA. The lineup of these bases that provide the code for a specific protein is known as a *gene*. A gene exists for every type of protein manufactured in the body. Inside the nucleus is the nucleolus, which contains RNA structures that form ribosomes. The nucleus has the information needed for the manufacture of more than 100,000 proteins, and it controls which proteins are synthesized and in what amounts during a given time.

Cellular Level

A **cell** is the basic structural and functional unit of an organism. Cellular function is maintained by the organelles. Cell functions reflect the characteristics of life:

- Maintenance of boundaries
- Movement and responsiveness
- Conductivity
- Growth
- Respiration
- Digestion
- Absorption
- Secretion
- Excretion
- Circulation
- Reproduction
- Metabolism

Cells are self-regulating, which allows them to adjust to constant changes and interact with their surroundings. Cells are surrounded by a dilute saltwater solution called *interstitial fluid*. Interstitial fluid is a type of extracellular fluid. Fluid found inside cells is called *intracellular fluid*. Disease is most likely to appear when cellular homeostasis has been lost.

Chemically, a cell is composed of carbon, hydrogen, nitrogen, oxygen, and trace amounts of several other elements. Cells are made up of approximately 15% protein, 3% lipids, 1% carbohydrates, 1% nucleic acids, and 80% water. Although cells are diverse in size and shape, almost all of them have the same parts and general form. Cells are surrounded by cell membranes. All cells contain cytoplasm and organelles.

Cell metabolism, which involves two metabolic processes, catabolism and anabolism, can be identified and measured in terms of our recurring theme, the duality of wholeness. Anabolism uses energy to build molecules the body needs. Catabolism breaks down complex molecules into smaller molecules and releases energy for the organism to use.

The life cycle of a cell involves a series of changes from the time it is formed until it reproduces. The cycle can be divided into two major periods:

- Growth, or **interphase**, during which the cell carries on most of its activities.
- Reproduction (**mitosis**), or cell division, in which the cell reproduces itself by dividing in half. **Meiosis** is a form of mitosis that halves the number of chromosomes in reproductive cells (ova or sperm) before they combine and multiply.

Cell division is regulated by growth factors in the extracellular fluid that bind to receptors in the cell membrane and trigger cell division. Growth factors are hormone-like regulatory chemicals. The main growth factors are growth hormone; nerve growth factor; epidermal growth factor; and erythropoietin, which stimulates the production of red blood cells.

Cell division is suppressed by repressor genes. If the rate of cellular growth exceeds that of repression, tissues enlarge. If cell growth is uncontrolled, a tumor or neoplasm results.

Cells change size in response to hormones, nutrient availability, and changes in their functions. **Atrophy** is a decrease in the size of a cell. **Hypertrophy** is an increase in the size of a cell.

Muscle cells, in particular, can adapt their size to their functions. Hypertrophy most often occurs when a person is continually using muscle cells, such as in weight training; atrophy occurs in underused muscle cells, such as when a muscle is immobilized while a broken bone heals.

Cell Differentiation

No matter what a cell does or where it is located in the body, its basic maintenance functions are the same: nutrition, metabolism, respiration, excretion, organization, and responsiveness. When a cell must adapt to perform specialized duties, the structure of the cell, and in turn some of the specialized functions, are modified. This form of specialization is referred to as *cell differentiation*. For example, fat cells are modified to store energy, but they have lost the functions of contraction and secretion. Muscle cells have well-developed functions of contractility but diminished functions of secretion and reproduction.

Tissue Level

A **tissue** is a group of similar cells specialized to perform a specific function. The cells of a tissue are embedded in or surrounded by material called the **matrix** or **extracellular matrix (ECM)**. The ECM is a complex network of material, such as proteins and polysaccharides, which are secreted locally by cells and remain closely associated with them. The extracellular matrix performs a number of functions. For example, it provides structure and support through adhesiveness so the cells in the tissue stick together. The matrix is also involved with biochemical signaling and communication among cells in the tissue. The composition of the ECM changes based on the tissue type.

In most cases, cells connect directly with one another, which allows for better, more stable intercellular communication. Desmosomes are small contact points; they are filaments that extend between cells and function as welds. Gap junctions are formed when channels of the cell membranes adhere to one another. Tight junctions are the type of configuration implied by the name: whole membranes fused together around the cells to create impermeable structures. The exception is blood plasma, which is a liquid matrix. Plasma maintains tissue structure but does not hold it in a solid mass.

The four principal types of tissue—epithelial, connective, muscle, and nervous—can be identified by their structures and functions.

Epithelial Tissues

Epithelial tissues cover and protect the surface of the body. They also cover and line certain internal structures (Fig. 1.6). They line cavities, form glands, and specialize in moving substances into and out of the blood during secretion, absorption, and excretion. Because they are subjected to a considerable amount of wear and tear, epithelial cells reproduce constantly. If a person is suffering from stress overload or any homeostatic imbalance, the condition is often is seen first in the epithelial tissues because of the fast turnover of cells. For example, a skin wound should heal quickly because the skin is made of epithelial tissue. However, if someone is stressed, a skin wound may heal much more slowly.

Typically, little matrix material is found in epithelial tissues. The matrix tends to form continuous sheets of cells, with the cells held closely together. The surface of most epithelial tissue is not in contact with other tissues but rather is exposed to the external or internal environment. This surface is the **apical surface**. The other surface faces the inside of the body and is known as the **basal surface**.

A permeable, thin **basement membrane** attaches epithelial tissues to the underlying connective tissues. Because epithelial tissues contain no blood vessels, they must obtain oxygen and other nutrients by means of diffusion from capillaries in the connective tissues.

The epithelial tissues make up three types of membranes—cutaneous, serous, and mucous. A **membrane** is a thin, sheet-like layer of tissue that covers a cell, an organ, or a structure; lines tubes or cavities; or divides and separates one part from another. Each membrane has epithelial tissue on the surface and a specialized connective tissue layer underneath.

- *Cutaneous membranes:* Cutaneous membranes cover the surface of the body, which is exposed to the external environment. The largest cutaneous membrane, more commonly known as our skin, accounts for about 16% of our body weight.
- *Serous membranes:* Serous membranes line body cavities that do not open to the external environment and cover many of the organs. These membranes secrete a thin, watery fluid that lubricates organs to reduce friction as they rub against one another and against the walls of the cavities. Serous membranes line the peritoneal, pleural, and pericardial cavities. The peritoneal cavity is around the intestines; the pleural cavity is around the lungs; and the pericardial cavity is around the heart.
- *Mucous membranes:* Mucous membranes are found on the surfaces of tubes that open directly to the exterior, such as those lining the respiratory, digestive, urinary, and reproductive tracts. The film of mucus secreted by these membranes coats and protects the underlying cells.

Connective Tissue

Connective tissue is the most abundant tissue in the body and is the most widely distributed of the four primary types of tissue. Connective tissue is specialized to support and

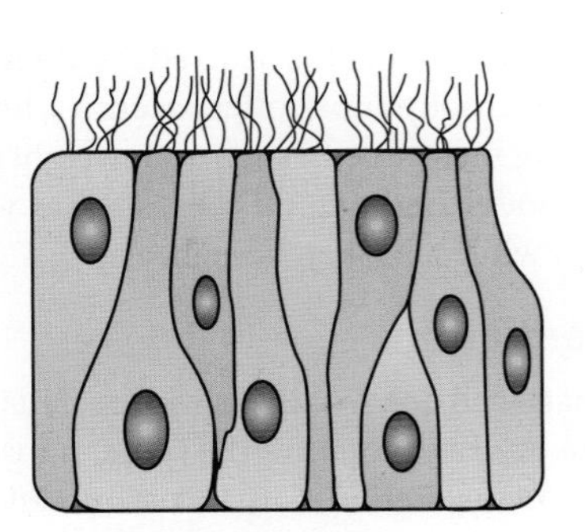

FIG. 1.6 Epithelial tissue.

Practical Application

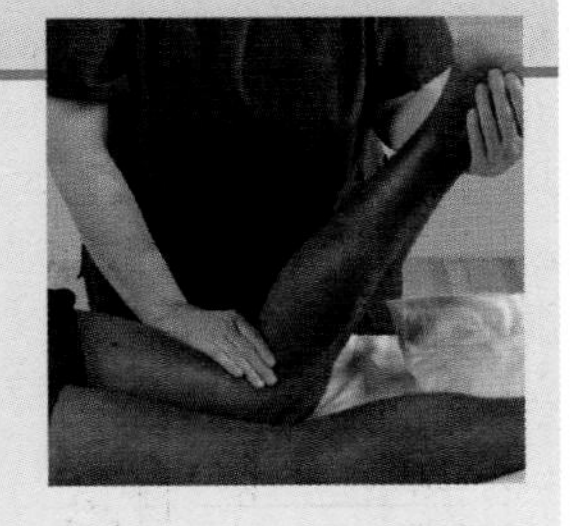

Therapeutic massage focuses on the skin as the primary point of touch. Of particular importance is the sensory function of the touch receptors in the skin. (Skin is discussed more extensively in Chapter 11.) Passive and active methods of joint movement support the normal function of the connective tissue membranes that line all synovial joints and secrete synovial fluid.

hold together the body and its parts, to transport substances through the body, and to protect the body from foreign substances. All forms of connective tissue are made up of matrix, fibers, and cells.

The properties of the connective tissue cells and the composition and arrangement of the matrix elements account for the amazing diversity of connective tissues. Exciting research is underway to help us learn more about the structure and function of connective tissue. This research may eventually explain some of the ways massage provides benefits.

Connective tissue cells are commonly spaced far apart, and the space between cells is filled with substantial amounts of matrix. It consists of protein fibers embedded in an amorphous mixture of huge protein-polysaccharide (proteoglycan) molecules. Within the matrix of connective tissue is a shapeless ground substance containing molecules that expand when combined with electrolytes and water molecules. The matrix of connective tissue may be 90% ground substance. The remainder is made up mainly of one or more types of fibers:

- **Collagenous fibers**: Collagenous fibers are tough and strong and have minimal stretch capability. They have a high degree of tensile strength, meaning they can withstand longitudinal stress. These fibers occur in bundles. Because of their color, they are referred to as *white fibers*. **Collagen** makes up more than one-quarter of the protein in the body. As we age, the molecular structure of collagen changes, which accounts for the appearance of changes in our tissues.
- **Reticular fibers**: Reticular fibers are delicate fibers found in networks that support small structures, such as capillaries, nerve fibers, and the basement membrane. These fibers are made of a form of collagen called *reticulin*.
- **Elastic fibers**: Elastic fibers are extensible and elastic. Found in stretchy tissues, they are made from a protein called *elastin*, which has the ability to return to its original length, much like a rubber band does after being stretched. Because of their color, these fibers are called *yellow fibers*.

Each major type of connective tissue has a fundamental cell type that secretes the matrix and fibers (Table 1.3).

A watery ground substance creates a fluid connective tissue, such as blood. By changing the proportion of collagen and elastic and reticular fibers, the tissue can be made as tough as a tendon or as flexible as the tissue that covers muscles. Adding calcium salts to the ground substance makes the tissue become rigid, like bone.

Connective tissue is *thixotropic*; this means that the substance solidifies when cold or undisturbed but becomes more fluid when warmed or stirred (gelatin is an example). If not stretched and warmed by muscular activity, connective tissue tends to stiffen and become less flexible.

Table 1.3 Connective Tissue Cell Types

Cell Type	Matrix and Fibers
Fibroblast	Connective tissue
Chondroblast	Cartilage
Osteoblast	Bone
Hemocytoblast (hematopoietic stem cell)	Blood

The collagen fibers of connective tissue tend to bind together by means of hydrogen bonding when they are in a state of disuse or chronic pressure. Inflammation is a factor in the bonding process known as *adhesion*, in which tissues are abnormally joined together. The result is also called an *adhesion*. Nerves and blood vessels may get caught in adhesions; the result is a reduced range of motion and pain.

Although connective tissue is found in all areas of the body, some areas contain more than others. The brain has little connective tissue, whereas ligaments, tendons, and skin have high concentrations of it. The number of blood vessels in connective tissue varies. Cartilage has none, but other types of connective tissue have a large number of blood vessels.

Connective tissue contains cells that help with repair, healing, and storage, as well as other cells that help with defense. Fibroblasts, which make fibers, and mesenchymal cells, which make ground substance, repair injured tissue. (Connective tissue disease is discussed in greater detail in Chapter 8.)

Three other types of cells are also commonly found in connective tissue:

- *Macrophages* are large, irregularly shaped cells. They develop in the bone marrow and move throughout the connective tissue, searching for microorganisms, damaged cells, and foreign particles. When these targets are found, the macrophages dispose of them by ingesting and digesting them, a process known as **phagocytosis**.
- *Mast cells* also develop in the bone marrow. Their functions focus on releasing chemicals (e.g., heparin and histamine) as part of the inflammatory response, the allergic response, and pain.
- *Adipose cells* are large cells stored in white or brown fat in the dermis, which is the deep layer of the skin. Adipose cells are also found in other parts of the body. When clustered together, they are known as *adipose tissue*.

Types of Connective Tissue

Dense Regular Connective Tissue

- *Structure:* The matrix consists mainly of collagen fibers produced by fibroblasts, with fibers oriented in parallel. The ligaments and tendons formed by this type of tissue have a small number of cells, and blood flow to the area is limited.
- *Function:* Dense regular connective tissue provides strength and resistance while allowing some degree of stretch.

Dense Irregular Connective Tissue

- *Structure:* Collagen and elastin fibers are interwoven and oriented in an irregular pattern to create the matrix. The tissue has little blood flow and is concentrated in the dermis, in the joint capsules and surrounding muscles, and in some organs.
- *Function:* Dense irregular connective tissue can withstand intense pulling forces and resist impact.

Loose (Areolar) Tissue

- *Structure:* A loose, irregular configuration of fibroblastic cells, macrophages, and lymphocytes is contained within a fine network of mostly collagen and elastin. Fluid-filled spaces separate the cells and fibers from one another.

- *Function:* Areolar tissue is distributed throughout the body and is the substance on which most epithelium rests. Areolar tissue is the packing material between glands, muscles, and nerves; it attaches the skin to the underlying tissues and supplies nourishment because of its high level of vascularity.

Adipose Tissue

- *Structure:* Adipose tissue is composed of fat cells with little matrix between the cells. Support is provided by reticular and collagenous fibers. Most adipose tissue is found in the buttocks, anterior abdominal wall, breasts, arms, and thighs.
- *Function:* The storage and release of fat are regulated by stimulation by hormones and the nervous system. Adipose tissue is a source of fuel; it helps insulate and pad organs and tissues, and it stores fat-soluble vitamins.

Types of Cartilage

Cartilage is a type of connective tissue composed of chondrocytes surrounded by an extensive matrix. Collagen gives cartilage its flexibility, and the strength and water-binding capacity of the ground substance make cartilage rigid, yet able to spring back when compressed. Because cartilage has little blood flow, it heals slowly. The three types of cartilage are hyaline cartilage, fibrocartilage, and elastic cartilage.

Hyaline Cartilage

- *Structure:* Hyaline cartilage is semitransparent. It has a milky bluish color and a strong, solid matrix. It is flexible and insensitive.
- *Function:* Hyaline cartilage is found at the ends of bones in most synovial joints, where it provides additional weight-bearing support or attaches to other bones, as occurs with costal cartilage. Hyaline cartilage provides the support and flexibility found in the trachea, lungs, and nose.

Fibrocartilage

- *Structure:* Fibrocartilage is composed of large amounts of dense fibrous tissue and small amounts of matrix; this arrangement creates a more rigid structure than hyaline cartilage. Fibrocartilage is found mainly in the symphysis pubis (the joint between the left and right pubic bones) and the intervertebral disks, between adjacent vertebrae of the spinal column, and in tendon attachments.
- *Function:* Fibrocartilage can withstand compression and impact forces, diffusing the force so that it is not focused on specific areas of the bone.

Elastic Cartilage

- *Structure:* As its name implies, elastic cartilage is a flexible form of hyaline cartilage with a large concentration of elastic fibers.
- *Function:* Elastic cartilage provides flexibility and support to the external ear and the larynx (voice box).

Other Forms of Connective Tissue

Bone

- *Structure:* Bone is the most rigid of the connective tissues because of its hard, mineralized matrix.
- *Function:* Bone provides the framework for supporting the body, protects the internal organs, serves as storage for minerals, and produces blood cells.

Blood

- *Structure:* Blood cells float within an extremely loose matrix, a fluid known as *plasma*, which contains no fibers.
- *Function:* Blood helps maintain homeostasis by transporting substances, resisting infection, and maintaining heat.

Connective Tissue Membranes

Connective tissue membranes are composed of several types of connective tissue. They are classified as synovial membranes.

Synovial membranes line the joint spaces in the mobile joints. This type of membrane is also found in bursae, which are protective sacs found near joints, between layers of muscle and connective tissue, and wherever the body needs extra protection. Synovial fluid is a thick lubricant secreted by these membranes to keep themselves slippery.

Fig. 1.7 shows all the types of tissue, cartilage, and fiber discussed thus far in this chapter.

Fascia

Simply described, fascia is formed by crimped/wavy collagen fibers and elastic fibers arranged in distinct layers, with the fibers aligned in a different direction in each layer. These fibers are embedded in a gelatin-like structure called *ground substance.*

Superficial fascia is sometimes called *subcutaneous fascia*; that is, it is tissue containing body fat that is located under the skin but on top of muscle. It forms an elastic sliding structure that is essential for thermal regulation, metabolic exchanges, and the protection of vessels and nerves.

Deep fascia is stiffer and thinner than subcutaneous fascia; it resembles duct tape. Deep fascia surrounds and compartmentalizes the muscles and forms the structures that attach soft tissues to bone. This type of fascia also forms a complex latticework of connective tissue (resembling struts, crossbeams, and guide wires) that helps maintain the structural integrity and function of the body. The deep fascia cannot be stretched, but the tautness of the tissue can be reduced by reducing muscle pull into the deep fascia.

The muscle system is part of the fascial continuum and can be considered *myofascia.*

The extracellular matrix in muscle is important to the structural support of tissue and the transmission of mechanical signals between fibers and tendons.

As you continue to learn, you will find that agreement on terminology is lacking in both the sciences and the massage therapy community. The term *fascia* is an example. Because massage methods can target fascial structures, these forms of application have multiple names. Researchers on fascia are attempting to standardize the terminology, but the work is ongoing. Currently, two working definitions are used:

A **fascia** is a sheath, a sheet of connective tissue that forms to attach, enclose, and separate muscles and other internal organs.

The **fascial system** is a network of interacting, interrelated, interdependent tissues that compose a complex whole,

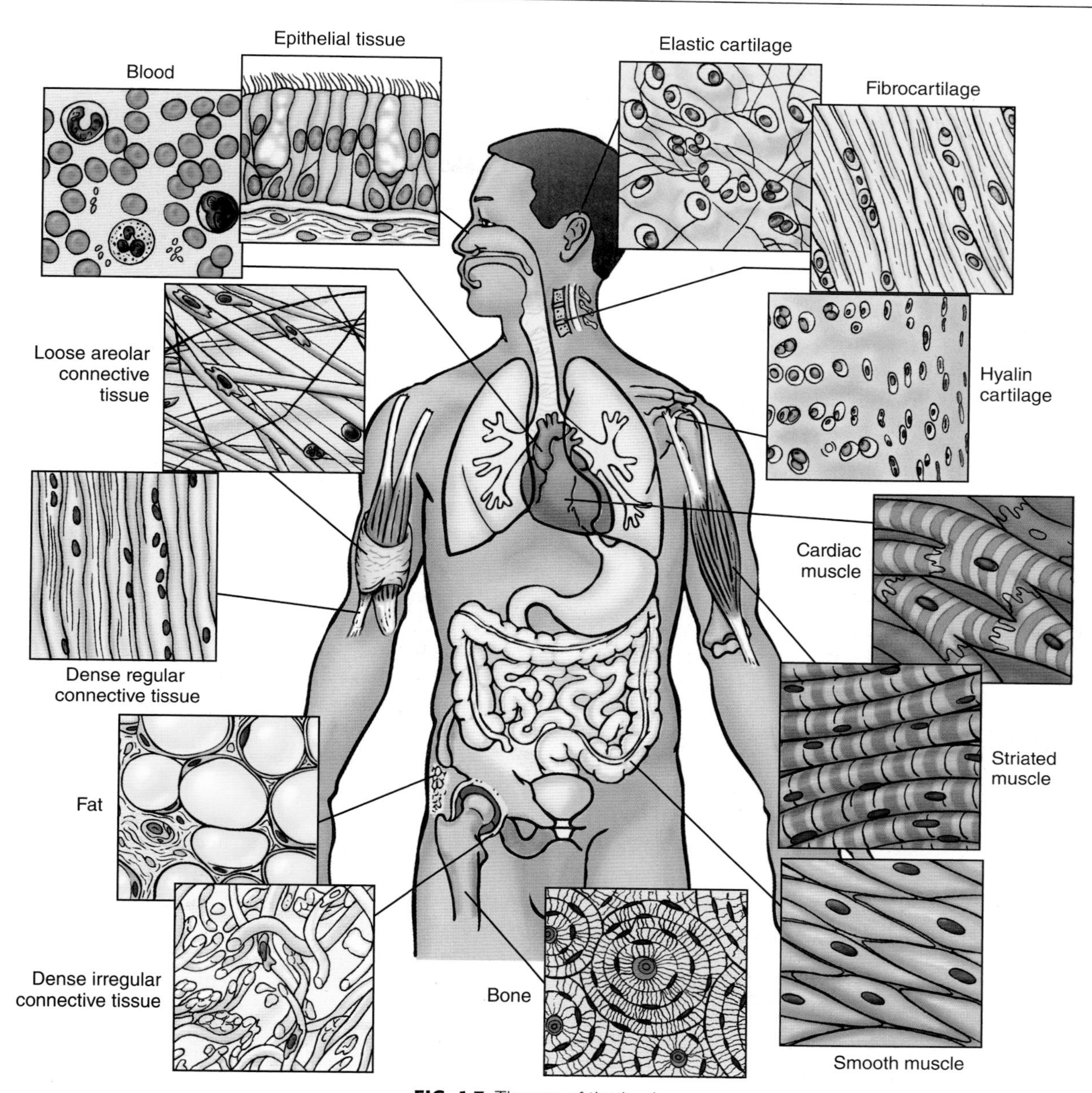

FIG. 1.7 Tissues of the body.

all collaborating to perform a movement. The fascial system consists of the three-dimensional continuum of soft, collagen-containing, loose, and dense fibrous connective tissues that permeate the body (Adstrum et al., 2016).

Because fascia is located almost everywhere in the body, the topic comes up many times in this textbook. The fascial system is part of all organs, muscles, bones, and nerve fibers. These fascial elements interconnect to form a functional structure that enables all body systems to operate in an integrated manner. Some specialized fascial structures include adipose tissue, adventitia (the outermost connective tissue covering of an organ, vessel, or other structure), neurovascular sheaths, aponeuroses, deep and superficial fasciae, epineurium, joint capsules, ligaments, membranes, meninges, myofascial expansions, periosteum, retinacula, septa, tendons, visceral fasciae, and all the intramuscular and intermuscular connective tissues. You will learn more about these structures as you progress through the textbook.

Muscle Tissue

The main characteristic of **muscle tissue** is its ability to provide movement by shortening through contraction. Contraction assists in maintaining posture and produces heat. Contraction results from the action of contractile proteins found inside muscle cells. Muscle cells are longer than they are wide, creating a distinctive pattern that resembles fibers; for this reason, the cells often are referred to as *muscle fibers.*

Muscle tissues can be categorized by their appearance, function, and location:

- **Skeletal muscle fibers** are large, cross-striated cells that make up muscles connected to the skeleton.
- They are controlled by the nervous system, and actions can be considered voluntary, meaning the muscle can be moved deliberately by the organism.
- **Cardiac muscle fibers**, which are found in the heart, are smaller, striated fibers. Their structure is not as organized as that of skeletal muscles.

Practical Application

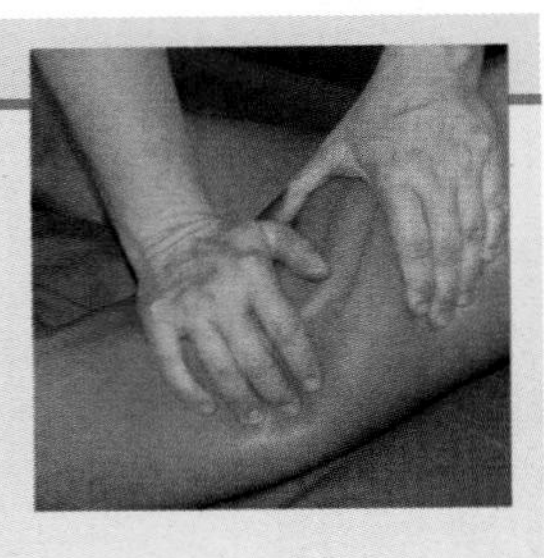

Many of the benefits of massage and bodywork therapies derive from the effects of these treatments on the connective tissue, even if we do not completely understand the mechanisms. It is biologically plausible that connective tissue is responsive to mechanical forces applied during massage. These forces may influence the consistency of the ground substance and the directional pattern of the fiber configuration. The gel of the ground substance is considered thixotropic (remember, that means that it liquefies when agitated and returns to a gel state as it stands). Manipulating connective tissue seems to soften the ground substance and increase the water-binding capacity, which makes the tissue more pliable (i.e., induces a more liquid state). Massage may also help distribute a slippery substance called *hyaluronan* (also called *hyaluronic acid* or *hyaluronate*) between fascial layers, supporting normal sliding. The nerves within connective tissue are likely stimulated. We do not know for sure what is happening to connective tissues during massage application, but research is ongoing.

- **Smooth muscle fibers** are neither striated nor voluntary. Found in the organs and viscera, they help regulate blood flow through the cardiovascular system, move substances (e.g., food and waste) through the intestines, and squeeze secretions from glands.

Muscle tissue is discussed in greater detail in Chapter 9.

Nervous (Neural) Tissue

The functions of **nervous tissue** (Fig. 1.8) are to coordinate and regulate body activity. Nervous tissue is able to do this because it is specialized to develop more excitability and conductivity than other types of tissue. Nerve cells are divided into two types: *neurons*, which are the actual functional units, and *neuroglia*, which connect and support the neurons. Nervous tissue is discussed in depth in Chapters 4 and 5.

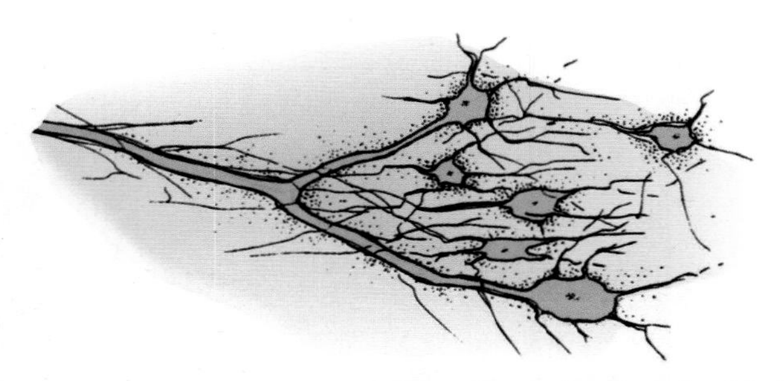

FIG. 1.8 Nervous tissue. (From LaFleur Brooks M. *Exploring Medical Language: a Learner-Directed Approach*. 5th ed. Mosby; 2002.)

Organ Level

Organs are groups of two or more kinds of tissue that combine to perform a special function. Organs in the body include the heart, lungs, brain, eyes, stomach, spleen, bones, pancreas, thyroid, kidneys, liver, intestines, uterus, bladder, and skin (the largest human organ).

According to Asian healing theories, the functions of the organs can be associated with energy patterns. Organs that are hollow and work intermittently are thought of as yang organs. Extensions of the yang organs make contact with the exterior of the body. Examples are the stomach, with the mouth opening to the exterior, and the bladder, which empties through the urethra. Organs that are solid and must work all the time to maintain homeostasis are yin organs. Instead of filling and emptying, they store the various essences of life extracted from the food and air. Examples are the heart and lungs. The relationships of the organs are presented in the five-element (phases) meridian theory, which is explained in Chapter 3.

System Level

Organs that combine to perform more complex body functions are referred to as *systems*. The number and types of organs found in a system are determined by its functions. The human body has 11 systems:

- Integumentary and exocrine
- Skeletal
- Muscular
- Nervous
- Endocrine
- Cardiovascular
- Lymphatic and immune
- Respiratory
- Digestive and excretory
- Urinary/renal
- Reproductive

All organ systems are regulated by the nervous and endocrine systems. In this textbook, Chapters 4, 5, and 6 cover the nervous and endocrine systems, which are collectively called *systems of control*.

A metaphor for this interaction is the gas pedal and brake pedal in a car. The nervous system is the main control system. It is divided into a somatic function (the movement of bones, muscles, and joints) and an autonomic function (the life-sustaining functions of organs). The autonomic nervous system divides again into the sympathetic division (gas pedal) and the parasympathetic division (brake pedal). Massage interacts with the gas and brake functions; that is, the sympathetic and parasympathetic systems, which balance the autonomic nervous system to help the body maintain homeostasis.

All the organ systems affect one another:

- The digestive system provides fuel for energy that all other organ systems use and eliminates waste.
- The cardiovascular system keeps all other organ systems functioning by supplying blood, nutrients, and oxygen to body cells.
- The respiratory system brings in the oxygen that the cardiovascular system delivers to body cells.
- The skeletal system provides physical protection and structural support for other organ systems.
- The urinary system is essential to maintaining fluid and pH balance within all organ systems. This allows them to function optimally.
- The integumentary (skin) and immune systems prevent infections that could affect all other organ systems.

Organism Level: The Body as a Whole

We are more than the sum of our parts. Each part of the body works with the other parts to support the whole. The mutually dependent nature of cells and the organization of complex systems allow us the endless possibilities of diversity that we experience. The cooperation, interdependence, and respect the body displays for itself could be a wise metaphor for the larger organism of the world in which we are the cells—that is, fundamental units of life.

After the overview information has been developed in Chapters 1, 2, and 3, each of the systems is discussed individually.

Review What You Have Learned

- Describe the sequence of simple to complex structures of the body.

  Simple structures create the foundation for complex structures. All structures of the body are interrelated and interdependent so body functions (e.g., respiration, movement, homeostasis) can be efficiently coordinated. Uninterrupted dysfunction in simple structures creates dysfunction in complex structures; for example, as occurs in a viral infection.
- Define chemical level, organelle level, cellular level, tissue level, organ level, system level, and organism level.
  - Chemical level: Composed of atoms that combine to form molecules.
  - Organelle level: Composed of molecules that combine to form the specialized structures (organs) of cells.
  - Cellular level: Composed of organelles that combine to form the basic structural units of an organism.
  - Tissue level: Composed of groups of similar cells specialized to perform a specific function.
  - Organ level: Composed of groups of two or more kinds of tissue that combine to perform a special function.
  - System level: Composed of groups of organs that combine to perform more complex body functions.
  - Organism level: Composed of the unity of all structural levels (simple to complex) that can carry out the various processes of life.

BIOLOGICAL PLAUSIBILITY, CLINICAL PLAUSIBILITY, AND EVIDENCE-INFORMED PRACTICE

SECTION OBJECTIVES

Chapter objectives covered in this section:

5. Use valid criteria to evaluate the plausibility of massage therapy effects and to support evidence-informed professional practice.

Using the information presented in this section, the learner will be able to:

- Define biological plausibility, clinical plausibility, and evidence-informed practice.
- Describe the relationship between correlation and causation.

As massage therapists, we have an ethical responsibility to make clinical decisions and to develop care plans based on the outcomes requested by the client. This is called *critical thinking* and *clinical reasoning*. Your knowledge of anatomy and physiology, first about normal function and subsequently about what occurs in dysfunction, will lay the foundation for your professional massage practice.

Our understanding of how therapeutic massage creates benefits for clients is not yet perfectly clear. Research is ongoing, and some trends are emerging. The relaxing effect of therapeutic massage seems to help normalize functions of the nervous and endocrine systems, reducing physical and emotional stress responses. The nurturing presence of a massage therapist can calm a person. A calmer person generally functions more effectively. Many other claims about massage benefits are not yet supported by research. This textbook considers the concept of **biological plausibility** when considering the benefits of massage. Stated benefits of massage therapy should not conflict with the current scientific understanding of anatomy and physiology. Massage that is applied to mimic normal function, based on our current knowledge of anatomy and physiology, is a logical approach.

Biological plausibility is demonstrated when a therapy, such as therapeutic massage, is scientifically plausible because the biological rationale is logical, even if proof is insufficient. The approach and explanation should, at the very least, make biological sense. Until research into massage becomes more sophisticated and consistent, it is important to avoid unproven claims and to get comfortable with the thought processes of "maybe, might, could, seems logical," and "not sure."

Clinical plausibility considers the results from actual practice settings with real clients. Data from case reports, case series, and small clinical trials may suggest benefits from methods as recorded by actual practitioners. Clinical plausibility is not anecdotal (based on personal stories). Instead, multiple clinical examples are compiled and analyzed to identify trends. Plausibility, both biological and clinical, does not prove or disprove the validity of a method. Instead, plausibility guides informed decision-making. Biological knowledge changes as information evolves, which redefines what is biologically plausible. This means that it is difficult to state absolutes about science. Science is an ongoing investigation. As new information is identified, what is plausible can change.

Evidence-informed practice uses the best available information during the clinical reasoning process to develop and implement therapeutic massage care plans for clients.

The massage therapy community, as well as individual massage practitioners, needs to be cautious before making claims about how massage interacts with the client's body. In the absence of solid research on the effect of massage on the human body, the massage therapist needs to understand normal anatomy and physiology functioning, which is the foundation of wellness and resilience. Then it is possible to understand how dysfunction occurs, producing distress and pathology. We also need to be cautious about claims made for the effects of massage. Just because a client moves better does not necessarily mean massage directly affects a specific joint. The ability to move more freely could occur for many reasons, including lying on the massage table for a time.

Correlation and Causation

An important relationship exists between correlation and causation. **Correlation** is a relationship you observe between two or more events that appear to be related. Correlation often is mistaken for causation, because common sense seems to dictate that one caused the other. For example:

Observation: When I wash my car, it rains.

Correlation: Washing the car and a rainstorm can happen at the same time.

Causation: However, washing the car did not make it rain, nor did a rainy day make me wash the car.

Causation means that one event is the result of the occurrence of another event. This is also referred to as "cause and effect."

Causation is difficult to determine. Scientific research is a way to determine causation. Massage professionals need to be cautious about confusing correlation with causation with regard to massage effects. Unfortunately, this happens far too often, which undermines the credibility of massage therapy.

We can sort out whether an accurate cause-and-effect relationship exists or whether events simply happened at the same time. In 1965 Sir Austin Bradford Hill (1897–1991), an epidemiologist, outlined the minimal conditions needed to establish a causal relationship between two items. This was during the time smoking became linked to lung cancer. Bradford Hill identified nine areas to be addressed to help determine causation; these became known as the Bradford Hill criteria (Fedak et al., 2015):

1. *Strength of the association:* The stronger the association between an event or intervention and the outcome, the more likely the relationship is to be causal.
2. *Consistency of findings:* The same results must occur among different populations and study designs, and at different times.
3. *Specificity of the association:* There must be a one-to-one relationship between cause and outcome.
4. *Temporal sequence of association:* The event or intervention must precede the outcome.
5. *Biological gradient:* Change in effects should follow from corresponding changes in exposure (dose response).
6. *Biological plausibility:* A potential biological mechanism should exist.
7. *Coherence:* The relationship of the intervention to the outcome is based on known biology.
8. *Experimentation:* Stopping the intervention alters the frequency of the outcome.
9. *Analogy:* Similar relationships have been shown to be causal.

The nine points can be simplified into two primary areas that can help massage therapists build an evidence-informed approach to a professional therapeutic massage practice.

- Evidence from multiple studies in which an intervention and an outcome have a causal association. Multiple research studies on a particular topic are combined in *meta-analyses* and *systematic reviews*, which lead to the acceptance of a causal relationship. Learning to read research about massage critically and to use a research database (i.e., PubMed) to find relevant research are crucial skills.
- Current knowledge of anatomy and physiology may logically connect the intervention and the outcome (biological plausibility). Learning and applying the content of this textbook to critical thinking addresses this point. Massage therapists need to understand how the body works to understand how therapeutic massage may provide benefits (Howick et al., 2009).

Review What You Have Learned

- Define biological plausibility, clinical plausibility, and evidence-informed practice.
  - *Biological plausibility:* Exists when a therapy, such as therapeutic massage, is scientifically plausible because the biological rationale is logical, even if proof is insufficient.
  - *Clinical plausibility:* Considers the results from actual practice settings with real clients.
  - *Evidence-informed practice:* Uses the best available information during the clinical reasoning process to develop and implement therapeutic massage care plans for clients.
- Describe the relationship between *correlation* and *causation*.
  - *Correlation:* Two or more events appear to be related; this is easily mistaken for
  - *Causation:* One event is the result of the occurrence of another event (cause and effect)

Throughout this textbook, you will find Practical Application boxes to help make the information applicable to the practice of therapeutic massage. These boxes are based on various forms of evidence, including biological and clinical plausibility. This first chapter has begun the learning journey (Activity 1.1).

SUMMARY

This chapter has laid the foundation for your study of anatomy and physiology. The relationship among structure, function, and homeostasis, in terms of Western and Asian thought, has been presented. The determination of life based on the characteristics of life and the biological organization of life, from the parts of the atom to the systems of the body, have been laid out sequentially, and each level reveals the components that build the next level of body organization. As a massage therapist, if you are to plan and competently organize an effective massage session that meets the outcome goals of your client, you must have knowledge of the structure and function of the human body. We will continue to build levels of knowledge on this foundation as our study of the human body progresses. It is important to be able to use critical thinking to explain and justify the benefits of massage therapy, as well as a client-centered approach to massage application and care.

As research progresses, there will be an increase in the understanding of massage applications related to the benefits realized supporting causation.

Biologically plausible explanations can serve as platforms for this research. It is important to be aware of how easily correlation can be mistaken for causation. A strong foundation in the essential sciences, targeted specifically to massage therapy practice, helps prevent this error in thinking.

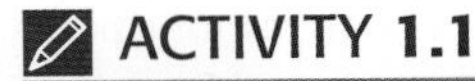

ACTIVITY 1.1

Describe a situation in which you had to determine if related events were a correlation or actually based on causation.

CRITICAL THINKING AND CLINICAL REASONING

Each chapter of this textbook features a critical thinking and clinical reasoning application of the content as it relates to the practice of massage therapy. A client scenario is presented, along with recommendations for additional research, often through the use of the websites MedlinePlus and PubMed. Questions based on the chapter content are provided to guide the discussion. The questions have no specific correct answers. However, your responses should be supported by evidence-informed practices, and if sufficient research is not available, the responses should be based on biological plausibility.

In this first chapter, the author's decision-making process regarding the scenario is included after the scenario and questions. The author's responses for the remainder of the chapters are found on the Evolve website. Compare and contrast your thoughts and discussion with those of the author and determine where you agree or disagree.

Scenario

The massage client is 38 years old. The client has been receiving massages to manage general aches and pains related to work activities. They just completed a yearly medical exam, and some health concerns were noted.

At 200 lb, the client is 30 lb overweight, and a blood test showed they are prediabetic (i.e., blood sugar level of 110 to 125 mg/dL). Prediabetes exists when a person's blood glucose levels are higher than normal, but not high enough for a diagnosis of diabetes. The condition is related to dysfunction in the endocrine system. Treatment consists of losing a modest amount of weight (5% to 10% of total body weight—10 to 20 lb for this client) by following a careful diet and getting moderate exercise, such as walking 30 minutes a day, 5 days a week. The client is especially concerned because people with prediabetes have a 50% greater risk of heart disease or stroke, and diabetes runs in their family. The client has a sinus infection they thought was an allergy, was prescribed an antibiotic and was sent for diabetes management education.

Explore MedlinePlus

Use the search terms *prediabetes* and *diabetes*.

Also search for information about massage therapy. Search terms: massage, therapeutic massage, massage therapy.

Discuss These Points

- How does the vocabulary in this chapter help you to understand the client's physical problems? How do the types of anatomic study contribute to your understanding of the client's situation?
  - Developmental anatomy
  - Gross anatomy
  - Regional anatomy
  - Systemic anatomy
  - Surface anatomy
- How might the information be categorized in each of the main areas of physiological study?
  - Systemic physiology: The study of body systems (e.g., cardiophysiology)
  - Pathophysiology: The study of disease and the functional changes in the body during the course of an illness
- Which of the characteristics of life are most affected by the treatment recommendations for prediabetes?
  - Maintenance of boundaries: Keeping the internal environment distinct from the external environment
  - Movement: The ability to transport the entire being, as well as internal components throughout the body
  - Responsiveness: The ability to sense, monitor, and respond to changes in the external environment
  - Conductivity: The movement of energy from one point to another
  - Metabolism: A chemical reaction that occurs in cells to effect transformation, production, or consumption of energy
  - Growth: A normal increase in the size and/or number of cells
  - Respiration: The absorption, transport, and use or exchange of respiratory gases (oxygen and carbon dioxide)
  - Digestion: The process by which food products are broken down into simple substances to be used by individual cells
  - Absorption: The transport and use of nutrients
  - Secretion: The production and delivery of specialized substances for diverse functions
  - Excretion: The removal of waste products
  - Circulation: The movement of fluids, nutrients, secretions, and waste products from one area of the body to another
  - Reproduction: The formation of a new being; also the formation of new cells in the body to permit growth, repair, and replacement
- How and at what various levels of organization is this client's body being affected?
  - Cellular level
  - Organelle level
  - Tissue level
  - Organ level
  - System level
- Consider the benefits of massage for the clients. Up to now, they have used massage for general muscle discomfort. However, this diagnosis means they will need to exercise more. Will a cause-and-effect relationship be established with regard to their current massage outcomes?
- How might the diagnosis of prediabetes alter the massage application?

Author's Response: Critical Thinking and Clinical Reasoning

NOTE: Author's Response to the Critical Thinking and Clinical Reasoning activity for Chapters 2 to 12 is found on the Evolve website.

When reviewing information in the scenario and when reading information on MedlinePlus, it is helpful to have an expanded vocabulary. Whenever you encounter terms that are unfamiliar, it is important that you look up the definitions of the terms. Medical dictionaries are available online for easy use.

The client's diagnosis of prediabetes primarily involves the systemic anatomy, more so than any other anatomical classification. All areas of physiology study are relevant. The diagnosis of prediabetes is pathophysiology. Blood sugar/glucose regulation is an aspect of organizational physiology, and it is important to know the possible effects of prediabetes on the client's systemic physiology. The recommendation of exercise involves movement, and weight loss involves metabolism and digestion.

Blood sugar/glucose is carried through the body via circulation. Insulin works at a cellular level. The body gets glucose from the food eaten, and it travels through the bloodstream. But without insulin, glucose cannot get into the cells. In diabetes, the pancreas does not make enough insulin or the body cannot respond normally to the insulin that is made. This causes the glucose level in the blood to rise. Normal glucose levels provide fuel for all the cells in the body. However, at elevated levels, glucose becomes a slow-acting poison. High sugar levels interfere with the ability of cells in the pancreas to make insulin. That organ overcompensates, and insulin levels stay too high. Eventually the pancreas is permanently damaged.

Almost any part of your body can be harmed by too much sugar. Elevated levels of blood sugar can cause changes that lead to hardening of the blood vessels, a condition called *atherosclerosis*. Damaged blood vessels cause problems such as:

- Kidney disease
- Stroke
- Heart attack
- Vision loss or blindness
- Nerve damage *(neuropathy)*
- Slow wound healing and poor circulation in the legs and feet

Because the client has a family history of diabetes, they already know they need to get the situation under control. Fortunately, with prediabetes, lifestyle changes can stabilize the condition. Exercise is important. The client is already seeking massage for a general mobility outcome, and massage should help support increased physical activity while minimizing the discomfort sensations. If you use PubMed to look for research related to massage and exercise, you will find a few studies that indicate that massage can reduce the perception of delayed-onset muscle soreness. They are as follows:

Wijianto W, Ega Fahla Agustianti. The effect of active and passive recovery exercise in reducing DOMS (delayed onset muscle soreness): critical review. *Gaster.* 2022;20(1):111–120. Querido SM, Radaelli R, Brito J, Vaz JR, Freitas SR. Analysis of recovery methods' efficacy applied up to 72 hours postmatch in professional football: a systematic review with graded recommendations. *Int J Sports Physiol Perform.* 2022;17(9):1326–1342.

In addition, blood glucose levels are responsive to stress. This mechanism is explained by the American Diabetes Association on its website: https://diabetes.org/. Research supports massage therapy as a means of managing anxiety and stress. An important example of such research is Wang R, Huang X, Wang Y, Akbari M. Non-pharmacologic approaches in preoperative anxiety, a comprehensive review. *Front Public Health.* 2022;10:854673.

Given these facts and studies, it seems reasonable (clinically plausible) to include stress management outcomes in the massage plan for this client.

Reminder: For all other textbook chapters, the author's responses to the Critical Thinking and Clinical Reasoning activity can be found on the Evolve website.

Visit the Evolve website: https://evolve.elsevier.com/Fritz/essential/

The Evolve website provides support for the review of the chapter content and chapter quizzes to help you prepare for the MBLEx or other massage therapy certification or licensing exams. End of chapter questions for discussion and review answer key and rationales and author's response to critical thinking and clinical reasoning scenarios.

AUTHOR'S NOTE

Your Essential Sciences studies will prepare you for critical thinking as a future massage therapist. The content of this Essential Sciences textbook will also prepare you for your massage therapy licensing exams. Most of you will take the Massage & Bodywork Licensing Examination (MBLEx), administered by the Federation of State Massage Therapy Boards.

This edition has been redesigned to better prepare learners for licensing exams. At the end of each chapter, you will find 20 multiple choice questions. Because these questions are used for review and discussion, it is as important to understand why wrong answers are wrong as it is to know why the correct answer is correct. The answers to the questions, with rationales and explanations about why the correct answer is correct and why wrong answers are wrong, can be found on the Evolve site. Guidance is also provided on how questions are developed and how the textbook content can be presented in a multiple choice question format. At the end of the question section here in the textbook, you will find an exercise that asks you to write more questions. Use the various questions in the chapter as examples. This is one of the best study strategies for test taking.

It is important to understand that the actual licensing exam you take may not contain any of the specific questions found in this textbook or in the review material and practice tests on the Evolve site. Therefore just because you can answer any of these questions correctly does not mean you will pass the licensing exam. The questions are content and style examples to help you prepare—this is why understanding why wrong answers are wrong is just as important as identifying the correct answer. Also, make sure you understand all the terminology used in the questions and possible answers in the review and discussion questions. Look up words you do not understand.

MULTIPLE CHOICE QUESTIONS FOR REVIEW AND DISCUSSION

The answers, with rationales, can be found on the Evolve site.

1. The substance between cell tissues that is made up of ground substance and fibers is called _______.
   a. Extracellular matrix
   b. Nucleic acids
   c. Basement membrane
   d. Meiosis
2. Which organelles are involved in the manufacture of proteins?
   a. Nucleus
   b. Mitochondria
   c. Lysosomes
   d. Ribosomes

3. When a cell is able to perform a specialized function, the structure of the cell is modified. This is called _______.
   a. Hypertrophy
   b. Atrophy
   c. Differentiation
   d. Meiosis
4. The basement membrane connects epithelial tissue to _______.
   a. Muscle tissue
   b. Nervous tissue
   c. Neutrophil tissue
   d. Connective tissue
5. Which of these is considered a cutaneous membrane?
   a. Skin
   b. Mucous
   c. Serous
   d. Collagen
6. Which membranes line cavities not open to the external environment, as well as many organs?
   a. Basement membranes
   b. Mucous membranes
   c. Serous membranes
   d. Cutaneous membranes
7. A massage practitioner is charting the location of a bruise. If the bruise is charted as located on the thigh, which term correctly correlates with its location?
   a. Systems anatomy
   b. Regional anatomy
   c. Pathophysiology
   d. Collagenous fibers
8. Which term would represent a direct relationship between a method and an outcome when explaining the benefits of massage?
   a. Causation
   b. Biological plausibility
   c. Correlation
   d. Critical thinking.
9. With regard to the relationship of anatomy and physiology, the phrase "structure and function" means _______.
   a. Gross anatomy translates to regional anatomy.
   b. Anatomy guides physiology and is modified by function.
   c. Systemic physiology involves organizational anatomy.
   d. The duality of wholeness is represented in catabolism and anabolism
10. How do we use physiology in the application of massage?
    a. Location of structures to be manipulated
    b. Specific positioning of the client for assessment
    c. Decision-making related to projected outcomes
    d. Directional communication in charting
11. The process of homeostasis is a logical, well-coordinated pattern of balance. When balance is disrupted, patterns of dysfunction occur. Often disruption of homeostasis begins at what level of body organization?
    a. Chemical
    b. Cellular
    c. Tissue
    d. Organ
12. Massage creates chemical reactions by _______.
    a. Generating a stimulus
    b. Encouraging interphase
    c. Supporting hypertrophy
    d. Disrupting differentiation
13. Why is the study of chemical actions in the body important to the massage professional?
    a. Charting depends on these interactions.
    b. Many massage benefits are derived from chemical reactions.
    c. Validation of subtle energy will be atomic.
    d. Chemical reactions are responsible for all pathologic conditions.
14. The diverse forms of connective tissue are attributed to _______.
    a. Properties of cells and the composition of the matrix
    b. Extensive distribution of blood vessels
    c. Distribution of chondroblasts in the matrix
    d. Collagen formation of ground substance
15. Which type of cartilage is most likely to be damaged by wear and tear on the hip or knee joint?
    a. Hyaline cartilage
    b. Fibrocartilage
    c. Elastic cartilage
    d. Reticular cartilage
16. Massage methods applied to connective tissue may have benefits because of the thixotropic properties of the tissue. This means _______.
    a. Massage stimulates mast cells to release histamine to reduce inflammation
    b. Massage separates the desmosomes and gap junctions to allow flexibility
    c. Massage increases the secretion of synovial fluid to increase joint mobility
    d. Massage may act to alter the water amount in the ground substance and encourages a softer, more pliable tissue texture
17. A massage therapist notices that a client's heart rate has lowered and the client's breathing has become slower and deeper. Which term best describes this massage outcome?
    a. Characteristics of life
    b. Organizational physiology
    c. Change in physiology
    d. Change in anatomy
18. A client reports that he has some hormonal imbalances relating to a diet low in lipids. Which statement is most correct?
    a. The diet is acidic and high in fat.
    b. The diet is low in amino acids.
    c. The diet is excessively low in fat.
    d. The diet has insufficient carbohydrates.
19. Your massage client describes a blog post indicating that massage therapy would remove the toxins in the liver. Which of these tools will you need to best explain why this information is incorrect?
    a. An explanation of the characteristics of life and correlation

b. A biological explanation of the metabolism of the fascia
c. Research evidence shows that this is biologically implausible
d. Clinical plausibility based on your experience as a practitioner

20. You are preparing a presentation about the benefits of massage and its ability to maintain homeostasis through methods that primarily affect the fascia. You have noticed that after a connective tissue–focused massage application, the client is more relaxed; therefore the massage had an effect on homeostasis. Which statement is most correct based on this information?
a. Clinical observations do not necessarily indicate causation.
b. The connective tissues, including the fascia, are not involved in homeostasis.
c. Biological plausibility is necessary to support evidence-informed practice.
d. Correlations are sufficient for evidence-informed practice.

Write Your Own Test Questions

Create at least three more multiple choice questions. Make sure to develop plausible wrong answers and double-check that the correct answer is clearly correct. Then write a rationale for each question. The more questions you write, the better you will understand the material.

Mechanisms of Health and Disease

CHAPTER 2

https://evolve.elsevier.com/Fritz/essential/

CHAPTER OBJECTIVES

After completing this chapter, the learner will be able to:

1. Define homeostasis and adaptive capacity.
2. Compare the concept of homeostasis with traditional Chinese medicine and Ayurveda.
3. Define and relate feedback loops to homeostatic self-regulation mechanisms.
4. List and define biological rhythms and list their influences on health.
5. Define disease terminology.
6. Identify major risk factors for disease development.
7. List sources of disturbances in homeostasis.
8. Describe the body's response to homeostatic disturbances.
9. Define pain and list the types of pain.
10. Describe methods used for pain management.
11. Explain the difference between salutogenesis and pathogenesis.
12. Define stress and list the factors contributing to the stress response.
13. Describe ways to manage stress.
14. Define resilience and list factors that build resilience.
15. List the stages in the cycle of life.
16. Identify relevant health-supporting information and give some examples of ways to use this information to educate others.

CHAPTER OUTLINE

KEY TERMS

acute pain: Pain that is usually temporary, of sudden onset, and easily localized. Acute pain can be a symptom of a disease process or a temporary aspect of medical treatment.

afferent: (AF-er-ent) Toward a center or point of reference.

allodynia: (AL-uh-DIN-ee-uh) Pain, generally on the skin, caused by something that would not normally cause pain.

anaplasia: (an-ah-PLAY-zee-a) Meaning "without shape"; the term describes abnormal or undifferentiated cells that fail to mature into specialized cell types. Anaplasia is a characteristic of malignant cells.

benign: (be-NINE) Usually describes a noncancerous tumor that is contained and does not spread. More broadly, *benign* can also be defined by a term such as "nonthreatening" to cover instances when the word is not associated with cancer.

biological rhythms: The internal, periodic timing of an organism; also known as a biorhythm.

cancer: Malignant, nonencapsulated cells that invade surrounding tissues. They often break away, or metastasize, from the primary tumor and form secondary cancer masses.

chakra: (CHUHK-ra) A wheel-like energy center believed to receive, assimilate, and express life force energy.

chronic pain: Pain that continues or recurs over a prolonged time, usually for longer than 6 months. The onset may be obscure, and the character and quality of the pain may change over time. Also called *persistent pain*.

circadian rhythms: (sur-KAY-dee-uhn) Biological rhythms that work over 24 hours to coordinate internal functions, such as sleep.

dosha: (DOH-sha) Physiological function; described in Ayurveda.

efferent: (EF-er-ent) Away from a center or point of reference.

etiology: (e-tee-OL-o-jee) The study of the factors involved in the development of disease, including the nature of the disease and an individual's susceptibility.

health: A condition of homeostasis that results in a state of physical, emotional, social, and spiritual well-being; the opposite of disease.

hyperalgesia: (HY-per-al-JEE-ze-uh) An abnormally increased sensitivity to pain, resulting in hypersensitivity to stimulus.

hyperplasia: (hye-per-PLAY-zee-a) An uncontrolled increase in the number of cells of a body part.

inflammation: (in-flah-MAY-shun) A protective response of the tissues to irritation or injury; this response may be chronic or acute. The four primary signs are redness, heat, swelling, and pain.

interoception: (in-te-ro-CEP-tion) The body's ability to recognize and interpret its own internal cues.

malignant: Describing an abnormal tissue growth that invades normal tissue; cancerous.

neoplasm: (NEE-o-plazm) The abnormal growth of new tissue. Also called a tumor, a neoplasm may be benign or malignant.

neuropathic pain: (neu-ro-PATH-ik) Pain caused by a lesion or disease of the somatosensory nervous system.

neuroplastic pain: (neu-ro- PLA-stik) Pain symptoms caused by learned neuropathways in the brain and are not due to structural damage or disease in the body.

nociceptive pain: (no-ci-CEP-tive) Pain as a result of the activation of type C and A-delta nociceptive neurons. The receptors of these neurons have high stimulation thresholds, which make them sensitive to stimuli that can damage normal tissues or may become damaging if prolonged.

opportunistic pathogens: (PATH-uh-jen) Organisms that cause disease only when a host's immunity is impaired.

pain: An unpleasant sensation. Pain is a complex, personal, subjective experience with physiological, psychological, and social aspects. Because pain is subjective, it is often difficult to explain or describe.

paresthesia: (par-es-THE-si-a) An abnormal sensation, typically described as pins and needles or crawling insects.

pathogen: (PATH-uh-jen) A disease-causing organism; a type of infectious agent.

pathogenicity: (PATH-o-jen-ISS-i-tee) The ability of an infectious agent to cause disease.

pathology: (pah-THOL-o-jee) The study of disease as observed in the structure and function of the body.

phantom pain: A form of pain or other sensation experienced in a missing extremity after a limb amputation.

resilience: (re-SIL-ience) The capacity to recover quickly from difficulties; toughness.

salutogenesis: (salu-to-JEN-a-sis) The process of healing, recovery, and repair. The term was first used by Aaron Antonovsky to contrast with pathogenesis.

seasonal rhythms: Annual functions, such as feeling more alert in the spring and wanting more sleep in the winter.

sensitization: (sen-si-ti-ZA-tion) An increased responsiveness to stimuli.

somatic pain: (so-MAT-ik) Pain that arises from the body wall. Superficial somatic pain comes from the stimulation of receptors in the skin, whereas deep somatic pain arises from the stimulation of receptors in skeletal muscles, joints, tendons, and fascia.

stress: Any external or internal stimulus that requires a change or response to prevent an imbalance in the internal environment of the body, mind, or emotions. Stress may be any activity that makes demands on mental and emotional resources.

ultradian rhythms: (ul-TRA-di-an) Biological rhythms that repeat at a rate ranging from every 90 minutes to every few hours (e.g., appetite).

virulent: (VIR-u-lent) A quality of organisms that enables them to readily cause disease.

visceral pain: (VIS-er-al) Pain that results from the stimulation of receptors or an abnormal condition in the viscera (internal organs).

LEARNING HOW TO LEARN

To learn new information, you must learn the meanings of unfamiliar terms. When the textbook content seems complicated and overwhelming because of all the unfamiliar terms, your brain needs more frequent breaks. For example, you might want to study for 10 minutes and then break for 10 minutes. Sweep the floor or put on some music and dance—move your body to rest your brain.

When you are learning the meanings of new terms, it is helpful to review the list just before bed, sleep on all the information, and then review the material again first thing in the morning.

This chapter aims to provide a context for understanding why it is important to understand the anatomy, physiology, kinesiology, biomechanics, and pathology of the human body. Some may ask, "Why do I have to know this stuff?" This chapter begins to provide the answers to that question. The start of the answer is "Because you want to be able to intelligently explain the benefits of massage."

Massage therapy clients most often request that massage provide these types of outcomes:

- Relaxation/well-being
- Stress management
- Pain management
- Functional mobility

Commonly a client wants all four of these outcomes, along with the unspoken outcomes of a pleasurable, safe, nurturing, compassionate, and nonjudgmental touch. All these outcomes are necessary for health and well-being and are directly or indirectly related to an understanding of the mechanisms of health and disease.

Massage therapy application typically progresses through these sequences:

General → specific → general
Surface → deep → surface

This textbook is organized in the same way. The first three chapters present a general and surface overview of body organization, health and disease, and the language of science (medical terminology). Chapters 4 through 10 explore the human body in specific and deep detail as it relates to massage therapy. Finally, Chapters 11 and 12 are more general and cover content more broadly, highlighting important information about the body that will help you understand the influences of therapeutic massage and general health maintenance.

Chapter 1 sets the stage, providing an overview and an introduction to the study of the body in structure and function. This chapter provides a wider view of how anatomy and physiology affect each of us in daily life.

You may need to use a medical dictionary to look up unfamiliar terms. The brief overview of anatomy and physiology in Chapter 1 should have provided enough of a basis for you to understand this chapter; however, exploring terminology by looking up definitions is a great learning experience!

Once you understand the importance of anatomy and physiology in relation to how we function, the relevance of the more detailed study in future chapters becomes clear.

HOMEOSTASIS

SECTION OBJECTIVES

Chapter objectives covered in this section:

1. Define *homeostasis* and adaptive *capacity*.
2. Compare the concept of homeostasis with traditional Chinese medicine and Ayurveda.

After completing this section, the learner will be able to:

- Define homeostasis in relation to adaptive capacity.
- Compare Asian yin/yang theory to homeostasis.
- Explain how the Asian five-element theory describes homeostasis.
- Explain how the Ayurvedic theories describe homeostasis.

Our body cells survive and thrive in healthy conditions only when the temperature, pressure, and chemical composition of their fluid environment remain relatively constant. The overall structures of our bodies do not change noticeably from moment to moment. We go to bed at night, and unless major trauma has occurred, our bodies function pretty much the same when we wake up. This consistency is due to the constant balancing activities of our physiology.

Recall from Chapter 1 that homeostasis is the relatively constant internal body state maintained by the physiology of the body. Regulatory mechanisms constantly adjust and adapt to keep our body's temperature and chemical composition in balance within our internal fluid environment. When this balance is interrupted, homeostasis is altered, and the body is more susceptible to a disease process.

Stress can be defined as any stimulus, internal or external, that creates an imbalance in the internal environment. If we are exposed to stress, certain mechanisms attempt to counteract the responses to that stress and bring the conditions back into balance. Thus the body of a person exposed to stress could respond—even before the person has any awareness of the stress—and bring itself back into a balanced state, or homeostasis. This ability is called *adaptation*. If adaptation does not occur, homeostasis is lost, resulting in dysfunction. The ability to adapt is called *adaptive capacity*. **Health** can be described as the effectiveness of the body's ability to maintain homeostasis and a strong adaptive capacity. Dysfunction and disease can happen when the adaptive capacity is diminished.

Two models can help explain health and disease: salutogenesis and pathogenesis. Both describe ways to achieve health, but from different perspectives. **Salutogenesis** begins with a focus on healthy function; **pathogenesis** begins with a focus on disease (Box 2.1).

Adaptive capacity is diminished by the following:

- Too great a demand to adapt (e.g., being involved in a car accident in which a loved one is injured).
- Insufficient ability to adapt because of poor nutrition, sleep disturbances, and other negative factors.
- Dysfunction in the body's organ systems, such as an inability to make the hormone insulin.

Interventions that can support a return to health are the following:

- Reduce the demands (salutogenesis)
- Make healthy lifestyle changes (salutogenesis)
- Use medical treatment (e.g., medication, surgery) to replace substances that are lacking or to correct the dysfunction (pathogenesis)

Box 2.1 Salutogenesis—Moving Toward Health

Salutogenesis is both a theory and a model of how and why people stay healthy. In contrast, the pathogenic model is illness focused. Both models are needed, and each complements the other. Salutogenesis focuses on discovering the elements of health and identifying healthy or salutary factors and behaviors. *Salutary* means favorable to the health of the mind or body. Pathogenesis focuses on understanding the causes of disease and identifying disease risk factors. Both support health and quality of life, but from different perspectives.

Aaron Antonovsky introduced salutogenesis as a model of health creation in his 1979 book *Health, Stress and Coping*. An important aspect of salutogenesis is having a sense of coherence (SOC). SOC is built on optimism with the ability to assess life situations realistically and find and use resources to solve problems and adapt to life circumstances. Developing a sense of coherence is a learning process. A strong SOC can help us find and use resources to cope with stressors and manage tension. We become resilient. SOC and salutogenesis are a process. We are all somewhere between total wellness and total illness.

Modified from Mittelmark MB, Bauer GF. The meanings of salutogenesis. In: Mittelmark MB, Sagy S, Eriksson M, et al., eds. *The Handbook of Salutogenesis*. Springer; 2017. Available at: https://www.ncbi.nlm.nih.gov/books/NBK435854/ https://doi.org/10.1007/978-3-319-04600-6_2.

Adaptive Capacity and Massage Care Planning

The state of a client's adaptive capacity determines the category of care for the massage application. The four general categories of care for massage are *therapeutic change, condition management, restorative care*, and *well-being/palliative care*.

Therapeutic Change

Clients who have a good-quality adaptive capacity are able to respond to the stress of a *therapeutic change* approach to massage. The goal is to reverse a current condition from a pathological state to a healthy state.

Example

A massage therapy client has been ill with an upper respiratory infection and was coughing and experiencing difficulty breathing. As a result, the client's back, chest, shoulders, and neck have become stiff and tender. It has been 2 weeks since the infection subsided. The client is now healthy but still has stiffness in their back, chest, and shoulders. Specific therapeutic massage interventions can be used to reverse the condition, because the client has sufficient adaptive capacity to respond.

Condition Management

If a massage client has a reduced adaptive capacity, then the category of care is *condition management*. The massage application does not attempt to reverse the condition but rather targets more general outcomes that support sleep and stress management. Specific therapeutic massage intervention is minimal and targeted to the client's most aggravating symptoms.

Example

A client who smokes cigarettes is prone to bronchitis and has recurring headaches related to soft tissue changes in the neck and persistent neck and shoulder pain from coughing. The client has a poor to moderate adaptive capacity. The focus of the massage is a general and nonspecific approach. The specific intervention will target the most troubling symptom experienced in that session.

Restorative Care

A **restorative care** approach to massage helps the body to return to a state of calm and allows it to relax and repair. The client is generally healthy and has adaptive capacity. This care approach can be considered preventative and part of health maintenance. A regular appointment schedule is recommended. Regular functional assessment monitors for indications of reduced adaptive capacity and minimal interventions are used to restore function.

Example

A client has a mentally demanding occupation and also jogs and bikes regularly. The client understands the importance of ongoing self-care and health maintenance. Receiving a massage every other week supports a healthy lifestyle.

Well-being/Palliative Care

If the client's adaptive capacity is significantly reduced or nonexistent, the approach to care is *palliative*. The goal of palliative care is to create pleasing sensations to reduce discomfort, but without any expectation of improvement other than symptom management.

Example

A client is recovering from pneumonia. The client has been extremely ill, and just in the past few days has been able to breathe without supportive oxygen. They are stiff and aching from extended immobility adaptive capacity is minimal. The category of care is well-being/palliative. The client enjoys having their feet and shoulders massaged, and this is the plan for the massage.

Homeostasis, Traditional Chinese Medicine, and Ayurveda

Various cultures around the world have used analogy to describe the concept of homeostasis. Briefly exploring these cultural explanations is helpful. For example, in traditional Chinese medicine (TCM), homeostasis is represented as the delicate maintenance of the balance of yin and yang. No matter how complicated, the signs and symptoms of the disease can be explained in terms of yin and yang relationships, which are the foundation of TCM (Box 2.2).

Asian Five-Element Theory

Most healing arts describe the balanced state of homeostasis in their own terminology. Yin and yang represent the organ relationships. The Asian five-element theory is an analogy for the life elements: fire, earth, metal, water, and wood. These elements are found in nature, and their characteristics are reflected in our bodies in a way similar to the characteristics of life described in Chapter 1.

Each element can support or control another to support balance. Fire is hot and consumes, but it needs fuel, which is wood. This analogy describes how our food is used as fuel to provide energy for body function or metabolism. The fire breaks down the wood to release the energy. Think of how your body uses the process of catabolism to break apart large molecules into smaller units that are used by the body.

After the fire burns the wood, ash is left over and feeds the earth. Our body does the same thing by eliminating the leftovers from digestion and metabolism. These organic and

Box 2.2 Characteristics of Yin and Yang

Fire is yang.	Hard is yang.
Water is yin.	Soft is yin.
Hot is yang.	Excitement is yang.
Cold is yin.	Inhibition is yin.
Restlessness is yang.	Rapidity is yang.
Excessive fatigue or sleepiness is yin.	Slowness is yin.
Dry is yang.	Transformation/change is yang.
Wet is yin.	Conservation/storage is yin.

Modified from Maciocia G. *The Foundations of Chinese Medicine.* 2nd ed. Churchill Livingstone; 2005.

inorganic substances return to the earth, where they form organic and inorganic (or metal) materials. Metal can also be thought of as minerals. Our bodies need certain minerals to function properly. For example, zinc and iron are minerals necessary for health. In the Law of Five Elements, metal must be taken from the earth and concentrated.

Fire and water are used to separate the metal from the earth. Think of how water is used to separate gold from the earth, and fire is used to melt iron ore. As the fire concentrates the metal, water is separated and becomes the next element of the five elements. Water in some form is necessary for life as we understand it. You can live quite a long time without food but not very long without water. Water is necessary for our food/fuel (wood) to grow on the earth. Metals become tools strong enough to harvest the wood to maintain the fire.

Although these examples of relationships found in nature are not exactly the same as the physiology of the body, they help describe the way the body functions, using concepts that are already familiar to us.

We can find examples of five-element imbalances in our world today. An excess of mining, for example, is disturbing the stability of the earth. Without tree roots to hold the earth in place, water washes away the soil, which is the food for plants. We are burning (fire) energy (fuel) faster than the earth can renew it, and the waste that results far exceeds what the earth can purify and return to the soil. The waste enters the water, making it unfit to drink. It is not difficult to understand that our planet is becoming unable to maintain homeostasis. Just as we get sick when homeostasis is lost, the world in which we live will get sick if it is unable to maintain balance (Fig. 2.1).

Ayurvedic Theories

Ayurveda is an ancient and indigenous healing system native to India. Ayurveda is thought to have appeared in India nearly 5000 years ago. It emerged from an ancient body of knowledge called the *Vedas*, a Sanskrit word meaning "knowledge."

The word *Ayurveda* means knowledge or science of life. Many of the beliefs and practices of Ayurveda are similar to those of ancient Chinese medicine. One premise of Ayurveda is that the body is a projection of consciousness. Similar underlying principles are fundamental to other ancient healing practices, and more current methods include behavioral medicine and mind/body approaches.

Ayurveda is based on the premise that an individual is made up of five primary elements. The elements differ from the Asian model, but the whole picture of balance is similar. The Ayurvedic elements are ether (space), air, fire, water, and earth. In this ancient healing system, elements can combine to create various physiological functions called **doshas**.

The *Vata dosha* is formed from ether and air. Vata governs the principles of movement and is seen in nerve impulses, circulation, respiration, and elimination.

The *Pitta dosha* is a combination of fire and water and represents the process of transformation. Metabolic transformation begins at a cellular level and moves up through all body functions. One example of Pitta is the transformation of food into usable nutrients.

The *Kapha dosha* blends the water and earth elements. These elements hold our cells together and build our muscles, fat, and bones. They also form some of the protective lining and fluids, such as the mucosal stomach lining and cerebrospinal fluid.

We are created with our unique proportions of Vata, Pitta, and Kapha, which allow for the great diversity of human beings.

Healing systems indigenous to India are also based on chakras (Fig. 2.2). A **chakra** is a wheel-like energy center

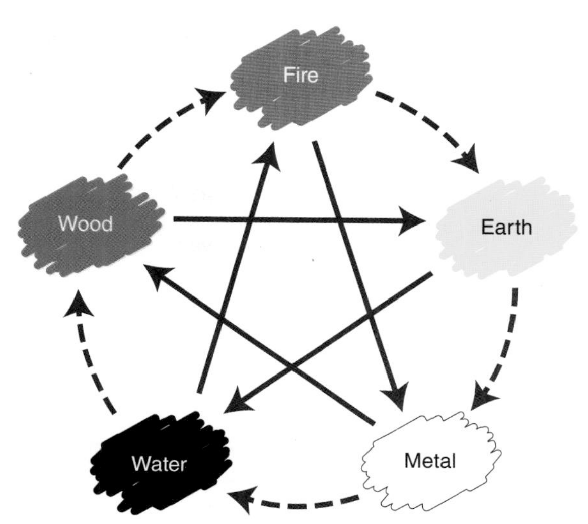

FIG. 2.1 Five-element wheel → supports → controls. (From Anderson SK. *The Practice of Shiatsu.* Mosby; 2008.)

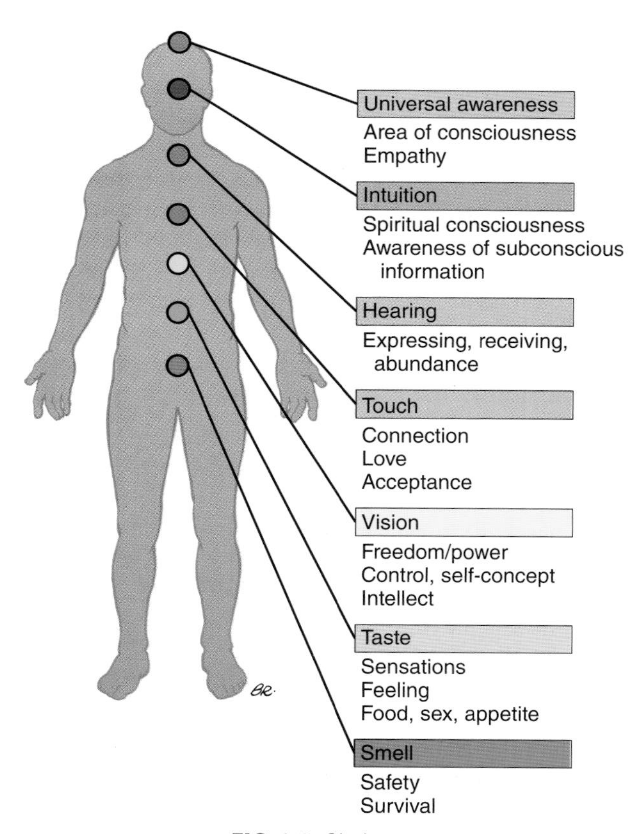

FIG. 2.2 Chakras.

believed to receive, assimilate, and express life force energy. These spinning wheels of bioenergetic activity (life force) are thought to emerge from the major nerve ganglia of the spinal column, beginning on the posterior (back) side of the body and radiating through the body to the front (anterior) side. There are seven major chakras, beginning with the first chakra at the top of the head. The seven major chakras correlate with the endocrine system on a physical level, with basic states of consciousness on a mind level, and with a process of life fulfillment on a spiritual level.

The seven chakras, the three doshas of Ayurveda, and the five elements of TCM must be balanced for us to maintain healthy bodies. A person's character is an expression of the harmonious and smooth interaction among these chakras, doshas, or elements.

The same concept of balance found in Eastern healing systems is the foundation of the body/mind relationship in health and disease that has developed in Western science in recent years. It is important to realize that regardless of the healing system, the physiology and the processes are the same; only the terminology is different.

Practical Application

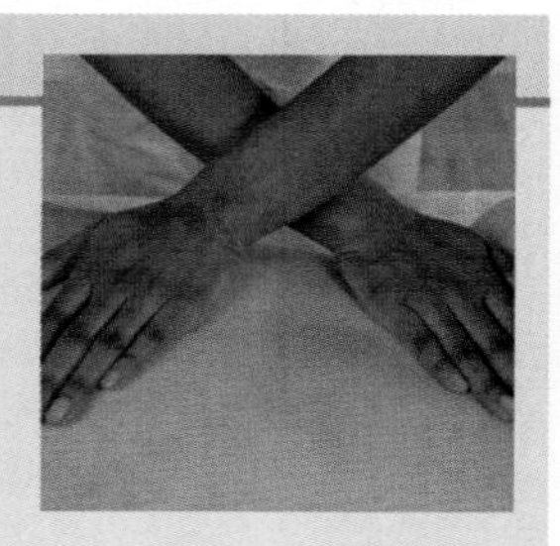

Some of you studying this textbook may wonder about the benefits of learning about TCM, Ayurveda, chakras, or other healing systems based on ancient cultures. You may be asking yourself, "What does this information have to do with anatomy, physiology, and pathology?" On a practical level, the current practice of massage therapy is built on the foundation of these ancient healing traditions. The way anatomical and physiological functions are named and explained can add insight to the study of what can be called *Western science*. Scientists are actively researching the Western scientific basis of the ancient healing traditions. Healthcare systems are now commonly encompassing integrated healthcare practices that blend many healthcare traditions, including the wisdom of the ancient systems.

Review What You Have Learned

- Define homeostasis in relation to adaptive capacity.
  Higher adaptive capacity allows for more efficient maintenance of homeostasis.
- Compare the yin/yang theory of TCM to homeostasis.
  The yin/yang theory concerns the internal balance of elemental, energetic, and spiritual forces, just as homeostasis concerns the internal balance of temperature, pressure, and chemical composition.
- Explain how the Asian five-element theory describes homeostasis.
  The interrelationships of fire, earth, metal, water, and wood, as found in nature, can be used to describe the interrelationships of physiological function.
- Explain how the Ayurvedic theories describe homeostasis.

Elements (ether, air, fire, water, and earth) combine to create three doshas (Vata, Pitta, Kapha), which are associated with form and function. The seven major chakras correlate with the central nervous system and endocrine system on a physical level, as well as with aspects of mental and spiritual balance. The three doshas and seven chakras can be used to describe how the interrelationships of form, function, mind, and spirit affect physiology.

FEEDBACK LOOPS

SECTION OBJECTIVES

Chapter objective covered in this section:

- Define and relate feedback loops to homeostatic self-regulatory mechanisms.

After completing this section, the learner will be able to:

- Explain how stress causes adaptation.
- List the three components of a feedback loop.
- Define the terms *afferent* and *efferent*.
- Describe negative and positive feedback loops.

Self-regulation requires interaction and communication using a well-developed control system. This control system is called a *feedback loop*. Every system in the body contributes to maintaining homeostasis, but the nervous and endocrine systems are the most important. Nerve impulses or chemical messengers transmit the information needed to maintain homeostasis through these feedback loops.

Every feedback loop is made up of three components:

1. A sensor mechanism that responds to the change in homeostasis. This change is referred to as a *stimulus*. The sensor usually creates an electrical or chemical signal.
2. An integration or control center that analyzes and integrates all signals received and, if necessary, initiates a response.
3. An effector mechanism that responds to information from the control center and creates a change to bring back homeostasis.

The terms *afferent* and *efferent* are directional terms. They are used to describe the movement of a signal from a sensor to an integrating or control center or, in reverse, the movement of a signal from the control center to some type of effector mechanism. **Afferent** means that a signal is traveling toward a particular center or point of reference. **Efferent** means that a signal is traveling away from a particular center or point of reference. Effectors are the various organs of the body that can reestablish homeostasis by changing the hormone balance, blood flow, breathing rate, and so forth.

The term *negative feedback* refers to the feedback that reverses the original stimulus, stabilizes physiological function, and helps us maintain our constant internal environment (Fig. 2.3). Most feedback loops are of this type. For example, increasing and maintaining the tension in a muscle helps us to relax the muscle later. During massage we sometimes tell the client to contract a shortened muscle, actually making it shorter. This increase in stimulus is processed in the central nervous system (CNS) (the brain and spinal cord) as *too much*

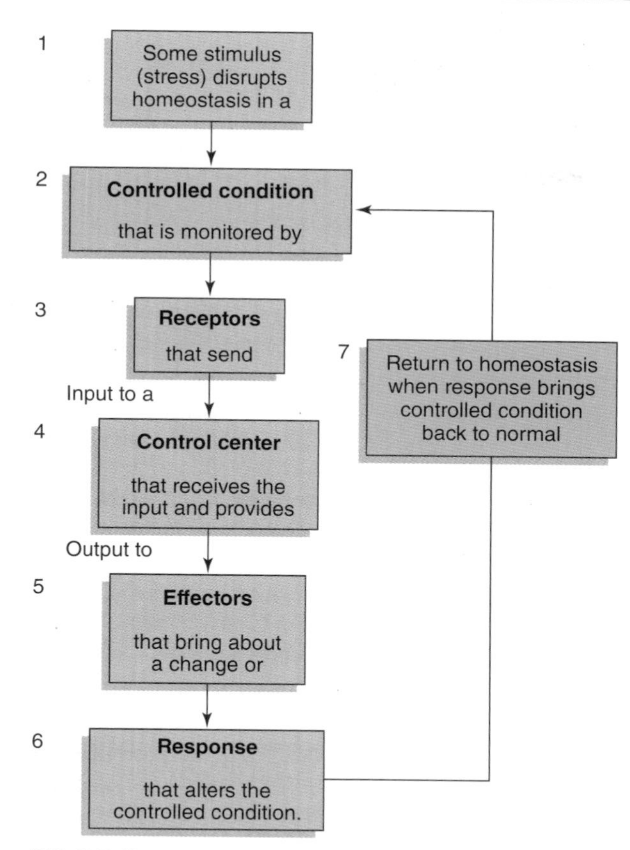

FIG. 2.3 Components of a negative feedback system (loop).

shortening. The CNS sends a signal back out to the effector (the muscle) to stop contracting so much. The shortened muscle can then be lengthened to its normal position, and balance is restored.

Positive feedback enhances the original stimulus and thus maintains or accelerates a disturbed state of homeostasis. Therefore the purpose of positive feedback is not to maintain a stable internal environment but rather to continue the disturbed state of homeostasis until something outside the loop stops it.

The contractions that occur during labor and delivery of a baby are an example of a positive feedback loop. Owing to the release of certain hormones, the contractions become stronger and stronger until the baby is born. The birth of the baby is what eventually stops the feedback loop.

Another example of a positive feedback loop is the way the body responds to invading pathogens. **Pathogens** are disease-causing organisms. The body's immune system has specialized cells, called *lymphocytes*, that respond to these pathogens. As a result of the release of certain hormones and chemicals by body tissues, lymphocytes know to attack pathogens. These lymphocytes stimulate even more lymphocytes to respond and attack the pathogens. This buildup of lymphocytes is a positive feedback loop that continues until the infection is contained. It is the containment of the pathogens that eventually stops the feedback loop.

Some continuing positive feedback loops may become harmful if the loop does not cease when the cycle no longer serves a purpose. An example of this is a muscle spasm that causes pain, which results in increased spasm. This is referred to as the *pain-spasm-pain cycle*. Pain creates a protective spasm, which in turn increases the pain. The cycle continues until some sort of intervention—such as massage therapy—stops it.

The systems of control become the physiological foundation of self-regulation. Self-correcting systems use feedback loops to influence their expression. The body can use this information to coordinate activities (negative feedback), which allows us to remain in a relatively constant state despite being immersed in waves of change.

Review What You Have Learned

- Explain how stress causes adaptation.

  Adaptation is the response of an organism to stress (a demanding change in the environment). Stress creates a stimulus, which engages a response (adaptation). If a body cannot adapt effectively to stress, homeostasis is disturbed.
- List the three components of a feedback loop.
  - A *sensor mechanism* responds to the change (stimulus) in homeostasis.
  - A *control center* analyzes and integrates all signals received.
  - An *effector mechanism* responds to information from the control center and creates a change to return the system to homeostasis.

Practical Application

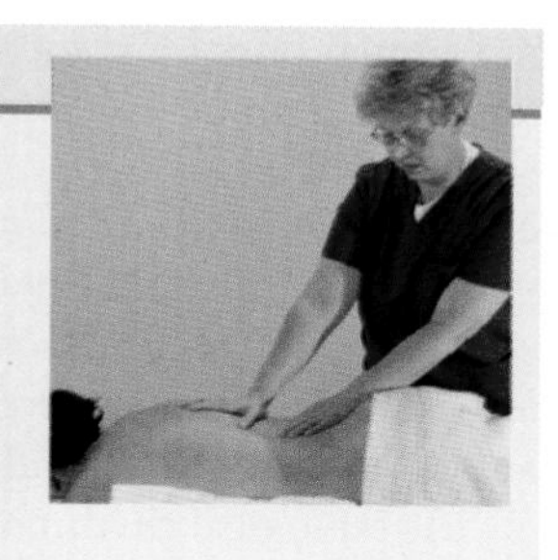

An individual whose body is unable to maintain homeostasis has two main problems: *too much* of something and *not enough* of something else. We can begin to think about how massage can support homeostasis by using these two principles.

Therapeutic massage can support or stimulate homeostatic processes. The stimuli produced by the massage methods are received by the receptors of the nervous or endocrine system. These receptors send signals through *afferent* pathways to the control centers of the central nervous system, where the signals are interpreted. Messages are returned by way of *efferent* pathways to the effector targets, which respond by reestablishing balanced function. For example, the effector targets may trigger a change in muscle length, from too short to a little longer; or they may reduce or increase the arousal responses of the autonomic nervous system (ANS), depending on the need. The goal is always to restore homeostasis.

More simply, if some function is excessive (too much), we want to reduce it. If a function is deficient (not enough), we want to increase it.

Massage approaches are often nonspecific; that is, the stimuli used usually disrupt the general existing pattern of too much or not enough. This disruption requires a response through the feedback mechanism. The objective is to reestablish homeostasis, in much the same way we push a reset button on a machine.

- Define the terms *afferent* and *efferent*.
  Afferent means a signal is traveling *toward* a particular center or point of reference.
  Efferent means a signal is traveling *away* from a particular center or point of reference.
- Describe negative and positive feedback loops.
  Negative feedback reverses the original stimulus, which stabilizes physiological function and helps maintain homeostasis (e.g., sweating, which cools our bodies in response to heat).
  Positive feedback enhances the original stimulus and thus maintains or accelerates disturbed homeostasis (e.g., the pain-spasm-pain response).

BIOLOGICAL RHYTHMS

SECTION OBJECTIVES

Chapter objective covered in this section:

4. List and define biological rhythms and list their influences on health.

After completing this section, the learner will be able to:

- Define three major biological rhythms.
- Explain how biological rhythms relate to health and disease.

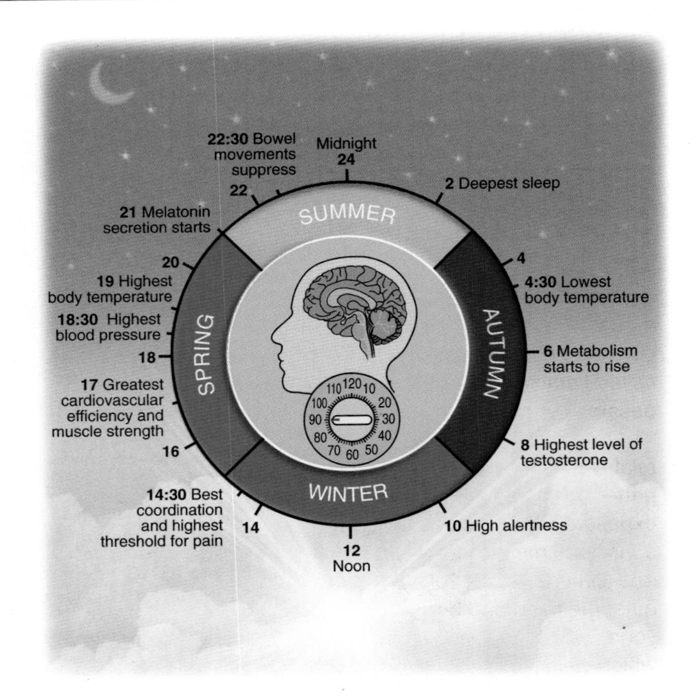

FIG. 2.4 Biological rhythms. Circadian rhythms work in a 24-hour period and involve body functions, such as sleep. Ultradian rhythms repeat themselves every few hours and influence functions, such as appetite. Seasonal rhythms are annual functions, such as feeling more alert in the spring and wanting more sleep in the winter.

Biological rhythms are the internal, periodic timing components of an organism that are generated within the body. **Circadian rhythms** work in a 24-hour period to coordinate internal functions, such as sleep. **Ultradian rhythms** repeat themselves every 90 minutes to every few hours (e.g., endocrine function and temperature regulation). **Seasonal rhythms** are annual functions, such as feeling more alert in the spring and wanting more sleep in the winter. Some forms of depressive disorders—as well as many sleep, neurologic, cardiovascular, and endocrine disorders—recently have been associated with dysfunction of the body's biological rhythms. Many of the conveniences we use, such as laptops, smartphones, and tablets, have put us out of sync with the natural rhythms of light and dark, the seasons, and the cycles of the moon (Fig. 2.4).

The biological rhythms of the body are interconnected and kept balanced by negative feedback loops. Synchronization of the rhythms of the heart, respiration, and digestion promotes this balance, or homeostasis, to support a healthy body. For example, balance among parts of the nervous system influences the heart and vascular systems; these, in turn, modulate the heart rate and blood pressure. The nasal cycle, an ultradian rhythm is characterized by alternating congestion and decongestion of the nostrils due to vasodilatation and vasoconstriction and affecting the ANS. Breathing rhythms through the nose affect the limbic/emotional area of the brain, influencing thinking and behavior (Timmons, 1994; Chaitow et al., 2014; Zelano et al., 2016; Jyothish et al., 2021). Respiration and heartbeat continuously interact at many different levels, representing two of the main oscillatory rhythms of the body and providing major sources of interoceptive information to the brain. **Interoception** is the body's ability to recognize and interpret its own internal cues, such as hunger, thirst, exhaustion, and pain. continuously updating the conscious and unconscious representations of the physiological condition of the body (Zaccaro et al., 2022).

A condition called *circadian misalignment* is caused by changes in light exposure, sleep, or the timing of eating. These changes can adversely affect a person's health by decreasing immune response and promoting a predisposition to type 2 diabetes, obesity, and abnormally elevated levels of fats (lipids) in the blood (hyperlipidemia) (Baron and Reid, 2014; Liu et al., 2021; Parameswaran and Ray, 2022). These disorders are the underlying causes of many chronic health issues. Ongoing research is unraveling the importance of regular sleep-wake cycles and eating patterns. Massage therapy may counteract the negative effects of stress and improve sleep quality by providing tactile-kinesthetic stimulation and increasing parasympathetic activity (Nerbass et al., 2010; Jane et al., 2011; Wang et al., 2013; Chompoopan et al., 2022).

Biological rhythms can be affected by the rhythms of music; by repetitive sounds, such as a bubbling brook and a breeze in the trees; or by visual patterns. Chaotic or abrupt noise can be a disruptive factor, whereas surf and similar nature sounds usually have a calming effect.

Studies have shown that the rhythmic physiological patterns of a dog's or cat's breathing or heart rate can benefit elderly people. The rhythmic patterns of drumming, clapping, singing, chanting, and movement in our religious and social rituals interact with biological patterns, resulting in a calming or exciting organization or disruption of body rhythms.

The rhythmic and ordered approach used in massage and bodywork methods seems to have effects similar to those just described, especially when a calm and focused practitioner

Practical Application

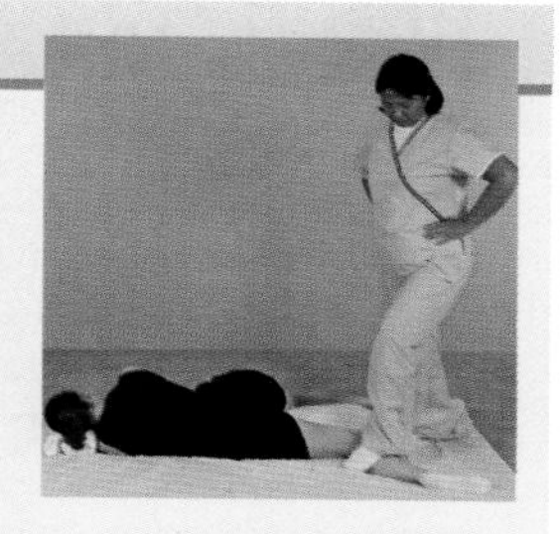

When a person experiences positive emotional states, the tendency is for the biological rhythms to begin to oscillate together; this is called *entrainment*. Entrainment is the physical phenomenon of resonance tendency, in which oscillating bodies move in a synchronized, harmonic manner. Research on entrainment dates to 1665, when Dutch scientist Christian Huygens noticed that when several clocks were placed near each other, their pendulums became synchronized.

One of the most important entrainment functions is the relationship of circadian rhythm to light-dark cycles and sleep patterns. We can enhance entrainment processes by having exposure to natural light and by using techniques that shift the conscious mind to focus on our breathing patterns and heart rate (Jiménez et al., 2022; Pavan et al., 2022). Many disciplines quiet the mind and body during meditation. Examples include yoga, which focuses attention on the breath, and Qigong, which focuses on the point below the navel. These systems center attention on body areas that have known biological oscillators. The Ayurvedic chakra system correlates with biological oscillators.

provides these methods. The length of application seems to be important as well. A session that lasts between 45 and 90 minutes falls within the ultradian rhythm pattern, thus working within the natural balance of the body.

Currently, researchers are examining the possibility that disease processes result from disruptions in body rhythms, as well as from the effects of work environments that directly disturb or alter natural body rhythms.

Review What You Have Learned

- Define three major biological rhythms.
- *Circadian rhythms* (e.g., sleep) work in a 24-hour period to coordinate internal functions.
- *Ultradian rhythms* (e.g., appetite arousal) repeat every 90 minutes to every few hours.
- *Seasonal rhythms* (e.g., feeling more alert in the spring) are annual functions.
- Explain how biological rhythms relate to health and disease.

Biological rhythms have shown to be strong influencers of health and disease. A body that is more in sync with biological rhythms better maintains homeostasis.

A body out of sync with biological rhythms is prone to disturbed homeostasis.

MECHANISMS OF DISEASE: PATHOLOGY

SECTION OBJECTIVES

Chapter objectives covered in this section:

5. Define disease terminology.
6. Identify major risk factors for disease development.
7. List sources of disturbances in homeostasis.
8. Describe the body's response to homeostatic disturbances.

After completing this section, the learner will be able to:

- Define terms that relate to disease.
- Discuss risk factors in disease development.
- List the eight factors most likely to disturb homeostasis.
- List the five types of pathogenic organisms and infectious agents.
- Define two types of tumors.
- Explain the factors known to play a role in the development of cancer.
- Define the inflammatory response.
- List the five primary signs of the inflammatory response.

Massage, other forms of soft tissue bodywork, exercise, and movement therapies focus on maintaining health—a balanced state of physical, emotional, social, and spiritual well-being known as *homeostasis*. As discussed previously, health results from the effective adaptation of an organism to change. When a disease process disturbs homeostasis, a variety of feedback mechanisms usually attempts to return the body to health. Disease occurs when the demand to adapt exceeds the body's ability to do so, and imbalance results. In acute conditions, the body recovers its homeostatic balance within the normal healing cycle. In chronic diseases, the normal state of balance may never be restored.

A number of terms are used when we describe a disease state:

Pathology is the study of disease.

Disease can be described as an abnormality in the function of the body, especially when the abnormality threatens well-being.

Epidemiology is the field of science that studies the frequency, transmission, occurrence, and distribution of disease in human beings.

Etiology is the study of all the factors involved in causing a disease.

Idiopathic refers to diseases with undetermined causes.

Pathogenesis describes the development of a disease. For example, flu begins with a *latent or nonactive stage*, during which the virus becomes established. When a disease is infectious, this is the *incubation stage*. After the disease runs its course, body functions return to normal during the *convalescence stage*.

Diagnosis occurs when a licensed medical professional categorizes a disease by identifying its signs and symptoms.

Signs are objective changes that can be seen or measured by someone other than the client.

Symptoms are subjective changes noticed or felt only by the client.

Acute diseases have a specific beginning and signs and symptoms that develop quickly, last a short time, and then disappear.

Chronic diseases have a vague onset, develop slowly, and last for a long time—sometimes for life. Some chronic disorders are initiated by an acute injury or disease.

Subacute refers to diseases that have characteristics that fall between those described as acute or chronic.

Syndromes are groups of signs and symptoms that identify a pathological condition, especially when they have a common cause.

Communicable diseases can be transmitted from one person to another. Communicable diseases are infectious diseases that spread through contact with infected individuals. They are also called *contagious diseases.* Contact with the bodily secretions of individuals with a communicable disease, or with objects that they have contaminated, can also spread this kind of disease. *Infectious diseases* are airborne and can be caught at any time. Diseases can also be transmitted by bites from insects and other creatures.

Congenital diseases are present at birth, not acquired during life.

Inherited diseases are due to genetics.

Prognosis is the expected outcome in a client who has a disease.

Remission is the reversal of signs and symptoms that may occur in clients who have chronic diseases. Remission can be temporary or permanent.

Pharmacology deals with the preparation and actions of medications and their uses in treating or preventing a disease.

Causes of Disease

Certain predisposing conditions may make a disease more likely to develop. Usually called *risk factors,* these conditions may put a person at risk for a disease, but they do not actually cause a disease (Box 2.3 and Activity 2.1).

Disturbances in homeostasis may arise from many different sources, but eight factors are most common:

1. *Genetic mechanisms:* Altered or mutated genes can cause abnormalities. *Predisposition* is the genetically determined tendency toward disease development. Genetic disease is caused directly by genetic abnormality. A person's body type is also determined by genetics (Fig. 2.5).
2. *Physical and chemical agents:* Toxic or destructive chemicals, extreme heat or cold, mechanical injury, radiation, and metabolic agents (e.g., alcohol, cigarettes, and drugs) can affect the normal homeostasis of the body.
3. *Malnutrition:* An insufficient or imbalanced intake of nutrients can cause a variety of diseases.
4. *Degeneration:* Tissues sometimes break apart, or degenerate. Degeneration is a normal consequence of aging. Degeneration of tissues can also result from disease or wear and tear. Osteoarthritis is an example of wear and tear that occurs in joints. The cartilage on the ends of the bones in the joint degenerates.
5. *Hypersensitivity of the immune system:* Some diseases occur because the immune system attacks the body; this is called *autoimmunity.* Diseases can also occur because of mistakes or overreactions by the immune response. Allergy is the hypersensitivity of the immune system to relatively harmless environmental factors. Steroids are commonly used to treat autoimmune diseases.
6. *Immune suppression* or *immune deficiency:* Some diseases are caused by the failure of the immune system to defend against pathogens. The chief characteristic of immune deficiency is the development of unusual or recurring severe infections or cancer.

Box 2.3 Major Risk Factors for the Development of Disease

1. *Genetic factors:* Several types of genetic risk factors exist. Body type (somatic type) is an example of a genetic trait that can predispose a person to disease. For example, osteoporosis is more prevalent in White females with a slight build. A family history of disease processes and causes of death can usually reveal possible familial genetic traits. Nonetheless, steps can be taken to support the body against the genetic tendency toward a disease process; for example, a person can make changes in their diet and lifestyle.
2. *Age:* Biological and behavioral factors increase the risk that certain diseases will develop at certain times in life. For example, musculoskeletal problems are common between 30 and 50 years of age.
3. *Lifestyle:* The way we live and work can put us at risk for some diseases. Many researchers believe that the high-fat, low-fiber diet common among people in developed nations increases the risk of certain types of cancer. Smoking, excessive use of alcohol, lack of exercise, and poor sleep habits are examples of unhealthy lifestyles.
4. *Stress:* Stress can be defined as any substantial change in a person's routine or any activity that causes the body to adapt. Stress makes demands on your mental and emotional resources. Research has shown that as stressors accumulate, you become increasingly susceptible to physical, mental, and emotional problems and accidental injuries.
5. *Environment:* Some environmental situations put us at greater risk of getting certain diseases. For example, living in a place that has high concentrations of air pollution may increase the risk of respiratory problems.
6. *Preexisting conditions:* A primary (preexisting) condition can put a person at risk for a secondary condition. For example, a viral infection can compromise your immune system and make you more susceptible to a bacterial infection.

7. *Pathogenic organisms and infectious agents:* Pathogenic organisms include viruses, bacteria, fungi, protozoa, and worms. The ability of infectious agents to cause disease is called **pathogenicity**. An organism that lives in or on another organism to obtain nutrients from it is called a *parasite.* Organisms that easily cause disease are **virulent**, and organisms that cause disease only when the immunity is diminished are **opportunistic pathogens**. The presence of microscopic or larger parasites may interfere with the normal body functions of the host and cause disease (Box 2.4).
8. *Tumors and cancer:* Abnormal tissue growths caused by uncontrolled cell division (**hyperplasia**) result in a **neoplasm**, or tumor. Tumors can cause a variety of physiological disruptions. A tumor is named according to its tissue type; a lipoma, for example, is a benign tumor of adipose (fat) tissue.

A **benign** tumor is contained and encapsulated. Benign tumors are relatively harmless, remain localized within the tissue from which they arose, and usually grow slowly. Benign

ACTIVITY 2.1

Using the various factors, including risk factors that disrupt homeostasis, do a personal health assessment.

Example

1. Genetic mechanisms: My family has a history of strokes, heart attacks, and joint problems.
2. Physical and chemical agents: I grew up in an environment with heavy secondary cigarette smoke.
3. Nutrition: I do not eat enough fresh vegetables, and I eat on the run all the time.
4. Degeneration: I have degenerative disk problems.
5. Immune hypersensitivity: I have some allergies to pollens.
6. Immune deficiency: I get upper respiratory problems when my immune system is not functioning well.
7. Viruses: I am susceptible to flu, colds, and herpes simplex when stressed and tired.
8. Fungi: I used to get yeast infections in my teens and 20s.
9. Protozoa: N/A
10. Pathogenic animals: N/A
11. Tumors and cancer: N/A
12. Inflammatory response: I have chronic inflammation in my back.
13. Environment: I work in a clean environment with natural light. I live in an area I like, but my sleep is sometimes interrupted by highway noise.
14. Age: I am in my 40s and am experiencing age-related hormonal changes and weight gain.
15. Lifestyle: My lifestyle is extremely busy, full of demands from many people. I work 60 to 70 hours per week, but I am able to maintain a regular sleep schedule. I exercise moderately, eat too much fat, have never smoked, and do not drink alcohol or use drugs.
16. Stress: I am a single parent of three. I have many people in my life with many different needs. I have many agencies to answer to and feel stressed by the bureaucratic expectations.
17. Preexisting conditions: I have disk dysfunction, an endocrine problem, inner ear balance syndrome, a breathing pattern disorder, and dyslexia.

Considering this information, how would you rate your personal health history on a scale of 1 to 10, with 10 being excellent health? To what types of disease processes do you feel you are most susceptible? What could you do to support your personal homeostasis?

Conclusions

In general, my health is good, an 8 out of 10. The inner ear problem creates physiological confusion and nausea that add to my stress levels. The back and endocrine problems have stabilized but have to be managed. The breathing pattern disorder is under control. I take fairly good care of myself and use some nutritional supplements to balance my diet. If I get enough sleep and exercise, I do better. I feel that I am most susceptible to cardiovascular disease, joint problems, and osteoporosis. Continued attention to diet and exercise, coupled with therapeutic massage to manage my back and my stress level, seems to be working.

Your Turn

1. Genetic mechanisms ____________________
2. Physical and chemical agents ____________________
3. Nutrition ____________________
4. Degeneration ____________________
5. Immune hypersensitivity ____________________
6. Immune deficiency ____________________
7. Viruses ____________________
8. Fungi ____________________
9. Protozoa ____________________
10. Pathogenic animals ____________________
11. Tumors and cancer ____________________
12. Inflammatory response ____________________
13. Environment ____________________
14. Age ____________________
15. Lifestyle ____________________
16. Stress ____________________
17. Preexisting conditions ____________________

Considering this information, how would you rate your personal health history on a scale of 1 to 10, with 10 being excellent health? To what types of disease processes do you feel you are most susceptible? What could you do to support your personal homeostasis?

tumors can become serious if the location and size interfere with body functions by blocking functional tissue or causing pain by pressing on pain-sensitive structures.

A **malignant** tumor **(cancer)** is a nonencapsulated mass that invades surrounding tissue (Fig. 2.6). In addition, malignant cells can break away from the primary tumor and form secondary cancer masses. This ability to break away is called *metastasis*. The cells most commonly migrate by way of the lymphatic system or blood vessels. Cancer cells that do not metastasize can spread another way by growing rapidly and extending the tumor into nearby tissues. Malignant tumors can replace part of a vital organ with abnormal tissues, a life-threatening situation. For example, osteosarcoma is a cancer of the bone.

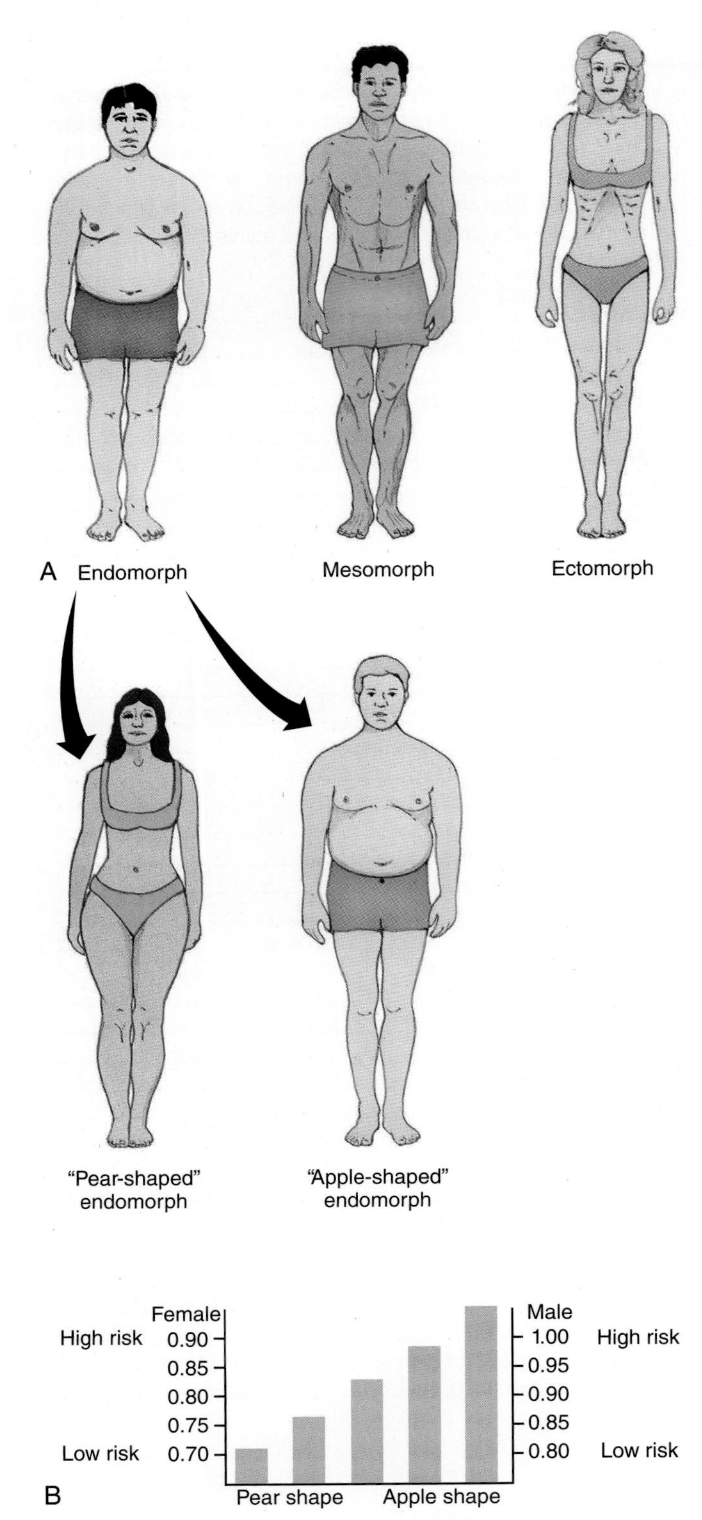

FIG. 2.5 **(A)** The three main body types. **(B)** Health risk for endomorphs. (Modified from Patton KT, Thibodeau GA. *Anatomy and Physiology*. 7th ed. Mosby; 2010.)

Box 2.4 Pathogenic Organisms and Treatment Medications

1. Bacteria, *Rickettsiae* species, and *Chlamydiae* species: Tiny cells without nuclei that secrete toxins, eat body cells, or form colonies.
2. Fungi: Simple plant-like organisms that lack chlorophyll. Fungi are generally molds or yeast.
3. Pathogenic animals: Large, multicellular organisms, such as roundworms, flatworms, flukes, mites, and lice.
4. Protozoa: Large, one-celled organisms with organized nuclei (e.g., an ameba).
5. Viruses: Microscopic, intracellular parasites that consist of a nucleic acid core with a protein coat. Viruses invade a host cell and take over the cell's function to produce more viruses.
6. Medications and herbs used to prevent or treat pathogenic organisms are classified by type:
   - Bacteria: Antibiotics
   - Viruses: Antivirals and vaccines
   - Fungi: Antifungals
   - Worms: Anthelmintics
   - Lice: Pediculicides
   - Scabies: Scabicides

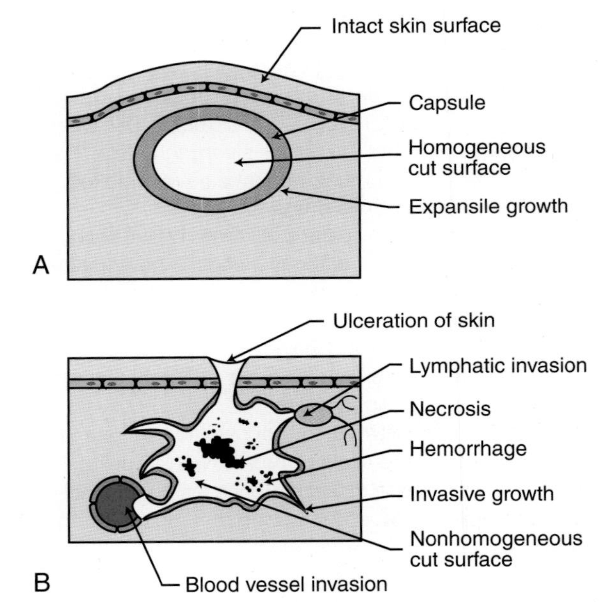

FIG. 2.6 Gross appearance of a benign **(A)** and a malignant **(B)** tumor.

Generally speaking, cells that divide many times display increased mutation (change) rates. Cells in the lymphatic system, epidermis, bone marrow, and gastrointestinal tract are more prone to develop cancer than the cells of organs that do not divide rapidly, such as nerve and muscle tissue. The mechanism of all cancers is a mistake or problem in cell division called *anaplasia*.

Anaplasia is the reproduction of abnormal and undifferentiated cells that fail to mature into specialized cell types. The result is a tissue that is not related to the needs of the body and that does not contribute to the functioning of the body.

Mature specialized cell types display boundary recognition, so they do not invade surrounding tissue. Abnormal undifferentiated cancer cells lack the ability to recognize boundaries and therefore invade and destroy surrounding tissue.

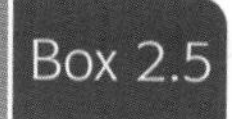

Box 2.5 Factors Known to Play a Role in the Development of Cancer

1. *Age:* Certain cancers are found primarily in young people (e.g., leukemia) and others primarily in older adults (e.g., colon cancer). The age factor may result from changes in the genetic activity of cells over time or from the accumulated effects of cell damage.
2. *Carcinogens:* Carcinogens are chemicals that affect genetic activity in some way, causing abnormal cell reproduction. Many industrial products are carcinogens. A variety of natural vegetable and animal materials are also carcinogenic.
3. *Environment:* Exposure to damaging types of radiation, chronic mechanical injury, viruses, and chronic irritants can cause cancer. For example, sunlight can cause skin cancer, and inhaling asbestos fibers can cause lung cancer.
4. *Genetic factors:* More than a dozen forms of cancer are known to be inherited. Cancers with known genetic risk factors include basal cell carcinoma (a type of skin cancer), breast cancer, and neuroblastoma (a cancer of nerve tissue).

Box 2.6 Warning Signs of Cancer

1. Sores that do not heal
2. Unusual bleeding
3. A change in a wart or mole
4. A lump or thickening in any tissue
5. Persistent hoarseness or cough
6. Chronic indigestion
7. A change in bowel or bladder function
8. Bone pain that awakens a person at night and is located only on one side

From Thibodeau GA, Patton KT. *The Human Body in Health and Disease.* 5th ed. Mosby; 2010.

Box 2.7 Inflammatory Process

Inflammation is a complex process. It requires four main elements:

- Changes in the blood circulation
- Changes in vessel wall permeability
- White blood cell (WBC) response
- Release of inflammatory mediators

Changes in blood flow involve the relaxation of smooth muscle cells in arterial walls so that blood moves into capillaries, creating redness, swelling, and warmth of the tissue. The first response of arterioles (small arteries) to an injury is vasoconstriction. *Vasoconstriction* is the narrowing of the hollow center of a blood vessel. Vasoconstriction lasts only a few seconds and is followed by vasodilation. *Vasodilation* is the enlarging of the hollow center of a blood vessel. This results in the flooding of the capillary network with arterial blood. The influx of blood dilates the capillaries, which cannot actively regulate the blood flow. From the capillaries the pressure is transmitted to venules (small veins). Increased pressure in the capillaries and venules forces plasma through the vessel wall into the surrounding tissue, leading to edema (the buildup of fluid in the tissues).

The permeability of the capillaries and venules changes in response to inflammation because of (1) increased pressure inside the congested blood vessels, (2) slowing of the circulation, which reduces the supply of oxygen and nutrients to cells, (3) adhesion of WBCs and platelets (cells involved in blood clotting) to the vessel walls, and (4) the release of inflammatory mediators. The blood flow in dilated capillaries and venules is slow, which leads to congestion.

The WBCs become sticky and adhere to the lining of the capillaries and venules. Adhesion of WBCs is one of the most common triggers for the release of mediators of inflammation.

The most important and common inflammatory mediators are histamines (increase blood vessel permeability), bradykinin (among other functions, elicits pain), and arachidonic acid and its derivatives, such as prostaglandins. Arachidonic acid plays a significant role in inflammation related to injury and many diseased states, and prostaglandins are responsible for inflammation features such as swelling, pain, stiffness, redness, and warmth. As a group, the inflammatory mediators have numerous effects on blood vessels, inflammatory cells, and other cells in the body. The most important effects are vasodilation or vasoconstriction, altered vascular permeability, activation of inflammatory cells to destroy pathogens, pain, and fever.

The process by which prostaglandins are synthesized can be blocked by aspirin. Corticosteroid hormones have antiinflammatory effects largely because they inhibit the formation of arachidonic acid.

Cancer specialists, or oncologists, have summarized some major signs of early stages of cancer (Box 2.5). Early detection of cancer is important because it is most easily treatable during the development of primary tumors, before the onset of metastasis and the development of secondary tumors. Several warning signs of cancer are listed in Box 2.6.

Surgery, radiation therapy, and medication are usually used in a cancer treatment program. Chemotherapy medications used to treat cancer are called *antineoplastics*. Most of the drugs in this category prevent the growth of rapidly dividing cells. However, as a side effect, antineoplastics affect epithelial cells, which also rapidly divide. Consequently, these drugs interfere with the function of the epithelial tissues and tissue repair.

Inflammatory Response

The body commonly responds to homeostatic disturbances by initiating the inflammatory response, which may occur as a response to any tissue injury. The inflammatory response is a normal mechanism that usually speeds recovery from an infection or injury. However, disease symptoms can occur when the inflammatory response activates at inappropriate times or when it is abnormally prolonged or severe, resulting in damage to normal tissues (Box 2.7).

Inflammation may also accompany specific immune system reactions. It occurs only in living tissue; necrotic or dead tissue cannot generate an inflammatory response. For example, a gangrenous foot cannot become inflamed. Because the body cannot combat infection in necrotic tissue, a foot that is affected by gangrene must be amputated.

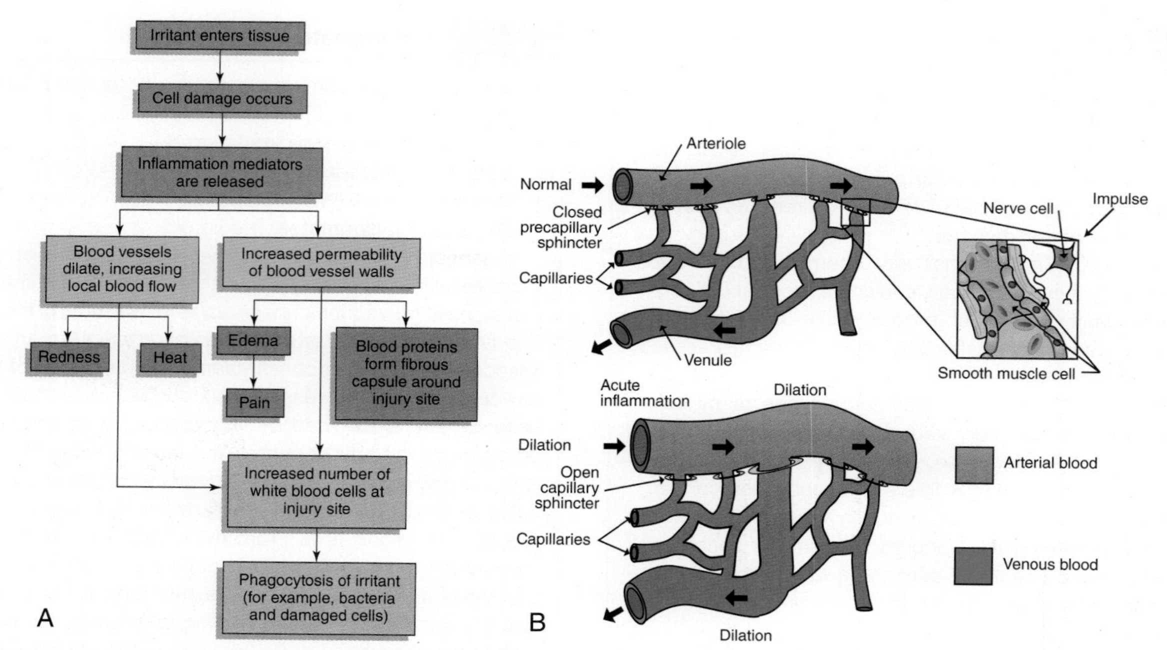

FIG. 2.7 (A) Inflammatory response. **(B)** Circulatory changes in inflammation. Relaxation of the precapillary sphincter in the arterioles results in flooding of the capillary network and dilation of capillaries and postcapillary venules. (**B**, Modified from Damjanov I. *Pathology for the Health Professions.* 3rd ed. Saunders; 2006.)

The inflammatory response has five primary signs (Fig. 2.7):

- *Heat* and *redness:* As tissue cells are damaged, they release inflammatory chemicals (mediators), such as histamine, prostaglandins, and compounds called *kinins.* Some inflammatory mediators (histamine and bradykinin) cause blood vessels to dilate, increasing blood volume in the tissue. Increased blood volume produces the heat and redness of inflammation. This response is important because it allows white blood cells (immune system cells) to travel quickly and easily to the site of injury. These cells attach themselves to the pathogens to be destroyed, especially if they are tagged with antibodies, which are proteins that mark pathogens.
- *Swelling, pain,* and *loss of function:* Some inflammatory mediators increase the permeability of blood vessel walls, allowing water to move through them. As water leaks out of the vessel, tissue swelling, or edema, results. The pressure caused by edema triggers pain receptors. The fluid that accumulates in inflamed tissue is called *inflammatory exudate* and has the beneficial effect of diluting the irritant that is causing the inflammation. Inflammatory exudates are removed slowly by lymphatic vessels (Box 2.8). As a result of the swelling and pain, a loss of function occurs in the area.

Bacteria and damaged cells are held in the lymph nodes and destroyed by white blood cells. This causes the lymph nodes to enlarge when they process a large amount of infectious material.

The normal inflammatory response is the process that heals the body. The goal is to promote regeneration, which is the replacement of dead cells with living, functional cells, and to keep replacement of functional tissue with scar tissue to a minimum (Boxes 2.9 and 2.10 and Figs. 2.8 and 2.9). However, if the inflammation lasts too long or becomes too widespread, the result is an inflammatory disease. (More information on the inflammatory response is presented in Chapter 11.)

Box 2.8 Types of Inflammatory Exudates

An exudate is a fluid with a high content of protein and cellular debris that is found in or on tissues, usually as a result of inflammation. Exudates vary in their composition of proteins, fluid, and cell contents and in their types of cells. Inflammatory exudates contain important proteins, such as fibrin and immunoglobulins (antibodies). If the skin is slightly burned, a blister forms that is filled with a clear exudate; this indicates a low protein content. These are known as *serous exudates*.

Sometimes inflammation results in fibrous exudates that are thick and sticky because a meshwork of proteins is present in the exudate. This type of inflammation can increase adhesion and scar tissue in the area, partly because of the thick, sticky exudate.

Yellow-white fluid in an infected, inflamed area is called *pus* or *purulent exudate*. Purulent exudates may collect in different ways, such as a capsule that surrounds the injury site and thus forms an abscess. If the body's immunity level is low, purulent exudates may spread over a large surface of tissue.

If the fluid that collects is tinged with blood, the blood vessels are injured, or the tissue is crushed, the result is a *hemorrhagic exudate*.

Review What You Have Learned

Define terms that relate to disease.

Review these terms: pathology, disease, epidemiology, etiology, idiopathic, pathogenesis, diagnosis, signs, symptoms, acute diseases, chronic diseases, subacute,

Box 2.9 Tissue Repair

The processes of inflammation eventually eliminate the irritant causing the problem. Tissue repair can then begin. *Tissue repair* is the replacement of dead cells with living cells.

Tissues have two cell types: *parenchymal cells*, which perform the tissue functions, and *stromal cells*, which provide the tissue structure. In a type of tissue repair called *regeneration*, just the parenchymal cells are involved. The new cells are similar to those they replace. Another type of tissue repair is *replacement*, which involves the stromal cells. The new cells are formed from connective tissue. These stromal cells are different from those they replace, and the result is a scar. Collagen is the chief constituent of scar tissue. The factors that promote collagen formation are vitamin C and adequate nutrition, particularly protein, intake. Fibrous connective tissue often replaces the damaged tissue, resulting in a condition called *fibrosis*. Most tissue repairs are a combination of regeneration and replacement.

Cells regenerate to different degrees and at different rates. *Labile cells* regenerate easily and quickly; these include the cells of the lymphatic system, epidermis, bone marrow, and gastrointestinal tract. *Stable cells*, the most common cell type, regenerate at slower rates; these include the cells of the parenchymal, or epithelial, portion of an organ or gland and the connective tissue, or stroma. For example, intestinal cells regenerate in 1 to 2 days, liver cells in 3 to 5 days, and kidney cells in 7 to 14 days. Total tissue repair can take 4 weeks or longer. Permanent cells (e.g., nerve and muscle cells) do not regenerate well, if at all, and if they do regenerate, the process is slow, taking months. Bone regenerates extremely well.

Massage practitioners should wait at least 30 to 45 days before working aggressively on an area of tissue repair so as not to disturb the formation of the repair. Moderate mobilization of the healing tissue supports tissue repair.

Box 2.10 Inflammatory Disease

Local inflammation occurs in a small area. If the irritant spreads throughout the body or causes changes in other areas, the inflammation is said to be *systemic*. When inflammation becomes chronic and stays active for a longer period than benefits the body or is more intense than seems necessary, it may be called an *inflammatory disease*. Systemic inflammations that may become diseases include arthritis, asthma, eczema, and bronchitis.

Chronic Inflammation

Chronic inflammation persists from 6 weeks to years. Medically, inflammation is considered chronic if the area is infiltrated by white blood cells (WBCs), if growth of new capillaries occurs, and if fibroblasts are in the area. Chronic inflammation is implicated in many disease processes, from arthritis to autoimmune disease. Chronic inflammation may cause the development of fibrosis. The fibroblasts produce collagen and fibrous tissue, causing fibrosis and resulting in scar tissue and adhesion formation. Chronic inflammation may also cause a sinus or a fistula. A **sinus** is a tract leading from a cavity to the surface. A **fistula** is a tract that is open at both ends and allows an abnormal connection between two surfaces. For example, fistulae may form between the bladder and the vagina.

Chronic inflammation may lead to ulcer formation if the surface covering of an organ or a tissue is lost because of cell death and is replaced by inflammatory tissue. The most common locations of ulcers are the stomach, intestines, and skin.

Treatments

Antiinflammatory and steroid medications are used to treat inflammation. Antihistamines and aspirin can be used to suppress inflammatory responses. Ice and other forms of cold hydrotherapy may also be beneficial if the inflammation is localized (e.g., shoulder bursitis or ankle sprain).

syndromes, communicable diseases, congenital diseases, inherited diseases, prognosis, remission, pharmacology.

Discuss risk factors for disease development.

Risk factors are predisposing conditions that increase the likelihood a disease will develop.

List the eight factors most likely to disturb homeostasis.

Genetic mechanisms, physical and chemical agents, malnutrition, degeneration, hypersensitivity of the immune system, immune system suppression/deficiency, pathogenic organisms and infectious agents, tumors, and cancer.

List the five types of pathogenic organisms and infectious agents.

Viruses (e.g., colds and flu), bacteria (e.g., *Salmonella* spp., *Mycobacterium tuberculosis*), fungi (e.g., yeasts and *Trichophyton rubrum*, which causes athlete's foot), protozoa (e.g., *Plasmodium falciparum*, which causes malaria), worms (i.e., flatworms, flukes, and tapeworms).

Define two types of tumors.

Benign tumors remain contained and encapsulated and are relatively harmless.

Malignant tumors (cancer) are nonencapsulated and invade surrounding tissues by means of cell migration (called *metastasis*), unregulated growth, and tissue replacement.

Explain the factors known to play a role in the development of cancer.

Anaplasia is the mechanism of all cancers. Anaplasia is the reproduction of abnormal and undifferentiated cells, which fail to mature into specialized cell types. Abnormal undifferentiated cancer cells lack the ability to recognize tissue boundaries and therefore invade and destroy surrounding tissues.

Define the inflammatory response.

The inflammatory response is a normal mechanism that usually speeds recovery from infection or injury.

List the five primary signs of the inflammatory response.

Heat, caused by increased blood volume; redness, caused by increased blood volume; swelling, caused by excess water (inflammatory exudate), which dilutes irritants; pain, caused by pressure from swelling that triggers pain receptors; and loss of function, caused by swelling and pain.

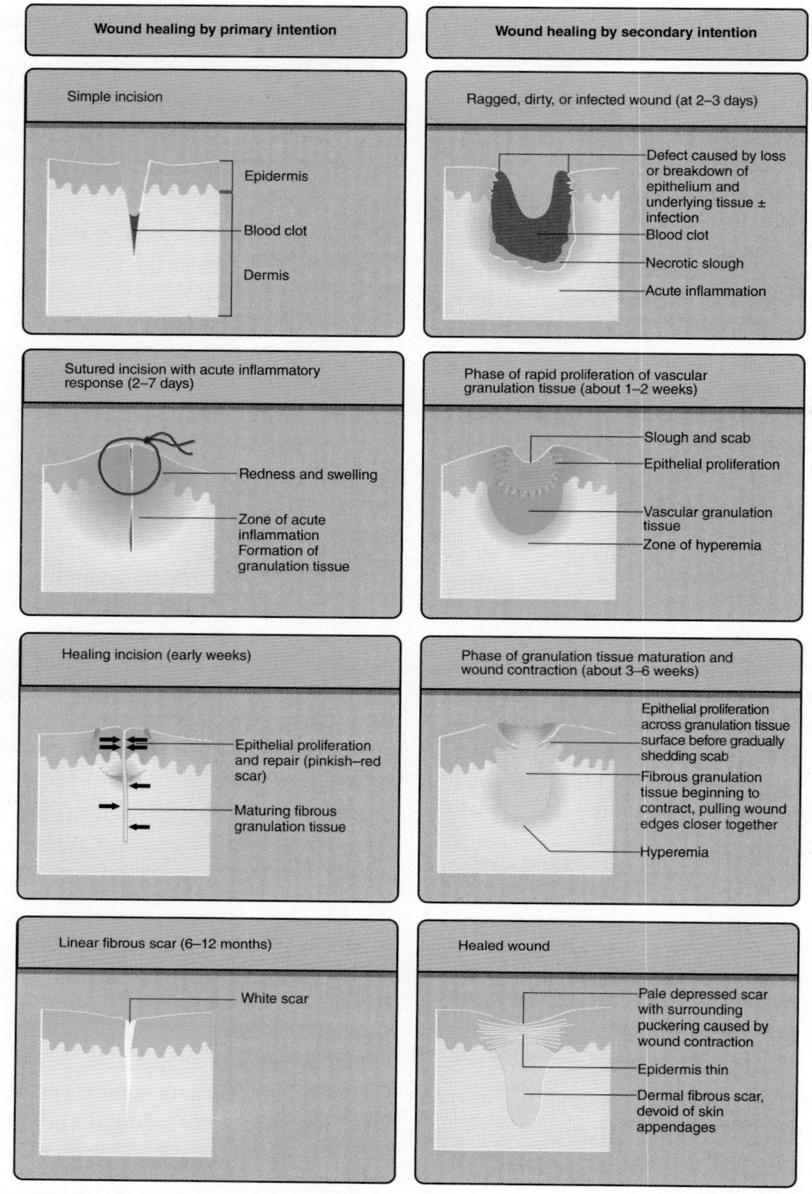

FIG. 2.8 Skin wound healing. The healing of skin wounds reflects mechanisms of healing in general. This figure illustrates the healing of superficial wounds by primary intention and deeper wounds by secondary intention. Wound healing is accelerated by bringing the edges of the wound together through the use of bandaging and sutures. If this were a muscle injury (strain), muscle spasms around the site of the injury would bring the ends closer together to encourage healing. (From Young B, Stewart W, O'Dowd G. *Wheater's Basic Pathology: A Text, Atlas, and Review of Histopathology.* 5th ed. Churchill Livingstone; 2015.)

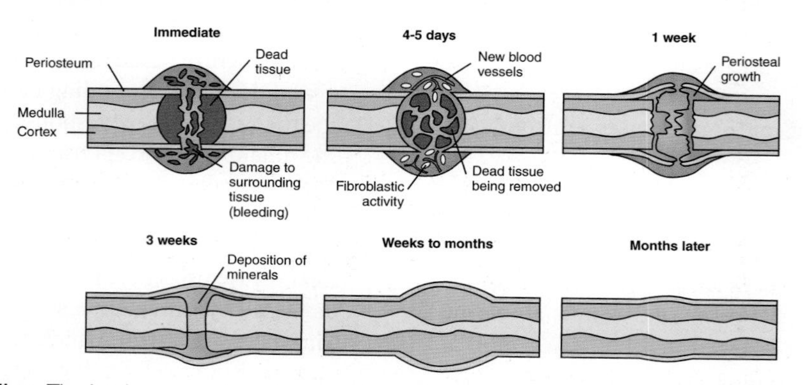

FIG. 2.9 Bone fracture healing. The basic mechanisms involved in the healing of bone fractures are similar to those for the healing of skin or other tissues. An adequate blood supply, nutrition, and rest are necessary for appropriate healing. A deficiency in protein, essential fatty acids, vitamin C, or zinc delays healing. The acute inflammatory process also supports healing; therefore the use of antiinflammatory medications in the first week after injury can slow the healing process.

Practical Application

By understanding the process of tissue healing, the massage therapist is able to support the normal progress of the inflammatory response. This chart provides recommendations for massage interventions during the tissue healing process.

Massage Interventions for Different Stages of Tissue Healing

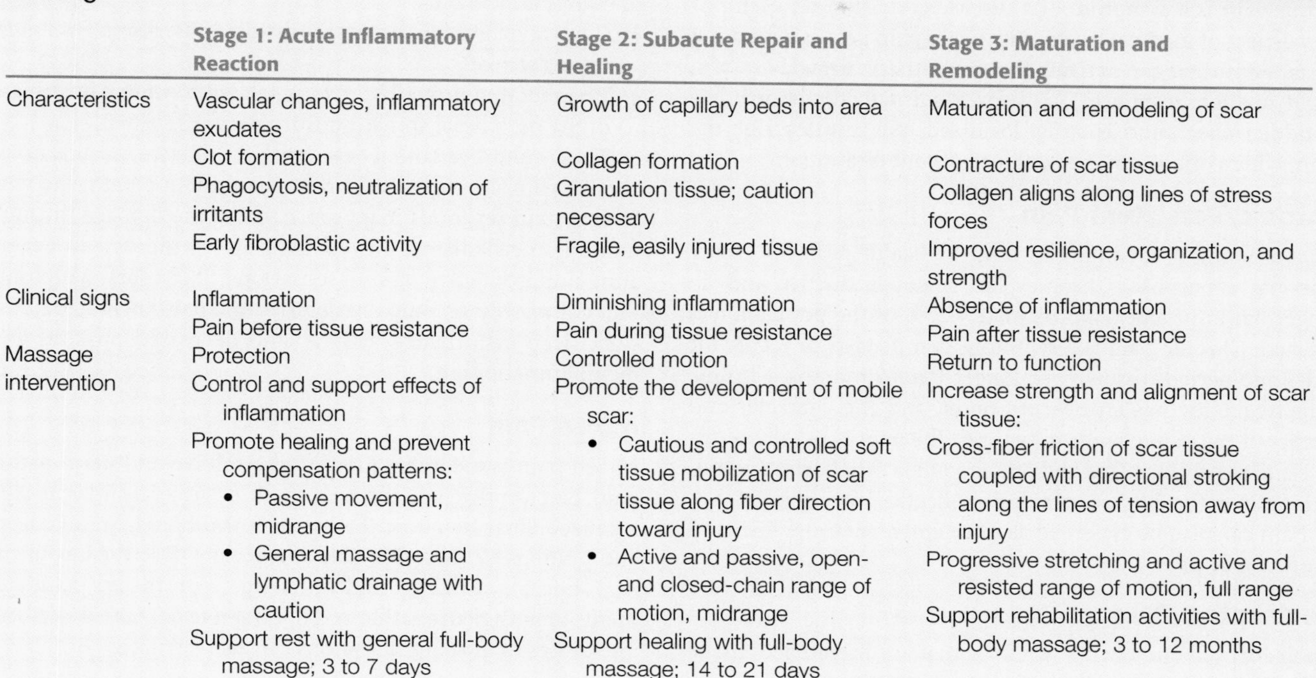

	Stage 1: Acute Inflammatory Reaction	Stage 2: Subacute Repair and Healing	Stage 3: Maturation and Remodeling
Characteristics	Vascular changes, inflammatory exudates Clot formation Phagocytosis, neutralization of irritants Early fibroblastic activity	Growth of capillary beds into area Collagen formation Granulation tissue; caution necessary Fragile, easily injured tissue	Maturation and remodeling of scar Contracture of scar tissue Collagen aligns along lines of stress forces Improved resilience, organization, and strength
Clinical signs	Inflammation Pain before tissue resistance	Diminishing inflammation Pain during tissue resistance	Absence of inflammation Pain after tissue resistance
Massage intervention	Protection Control and support effects of inflammation Promote healing and prevent compensation patterns: • Passive movement, midrange • General massage and lymphatic drainage with caution Support rest with general full-body massage; 3 to 7 days	Controlled motion Promote the development of mobile scar: • Cautious and controlled soft tissue mobilization of scar tissue along fiber direction toward injury • Active and passive, open- and closed-chain range of motion, midrange Support healing with full-body massage; 14 to 21 days	Return to function Increase strength and alignment of scar tissue: Cross-fiber friction of scar tissue coupled with directional stroking along the lines of tension away from injury Progressive stretching and active and resisted range of motion, full range Support rehabilitation activities with full-body massage; 3 to 12 months

PAIN

SECTION OBJECTIVES

Chapter objectives covered in this section:

9. Define *pain* and list the types of pain.
10. Describe methods used for pain management.

After completing this section, the learner will be able to:

- Describe pain sensations.
- Explain the difference between hurt and harm.
- Define *acute* and *chronic/persistent pain.*
- Define and provide examples of nociceptive, neuropathic, neuroplastic, and mixed pain.
- Describe five common pain sensations.
- Discuss the pain-spasm-pain cycle.
- Define *somatic pain* and *visceral pain*.
- Identify viscerally referred pain patterns.
- Define *referred pain*.
- Define *phantom pain*.
- List common types of cancer-related pain.
- List factors that influence the pain threshold and pain tolerance.
- List various pain management strategies.

As a massage therapist, you must have current and accurate information about pain. Pain is a major health issue. The National Center for Complementary and Integrative Health reports that massage therapy is recommended as a pain management strategy. The Centers for Disease Control and Prevention (CDC) 2022 Clinical Practice Guideline for Prescribing Opioids for Pain recommends a variety of nonpharmaceutical subacute and chronic pain treatments, which include massage therapy. The CDC considers acute pain duration of less than 1 month, subacute pain duration of 1 to 3 months, and chronic pain duration of more than 3 months. Medical care staff are encouraged to educate and recommend pain management strategies that do not involve prescription medication including opioids. Evidence suggests therapies that do not involve medications may work better for some conditions and have fewer risks and side effects (Dowell et al., 2022). Learn more about the CDC 2022 Clinical Practice Guideline for Prescribing Opioids for Pain at https://www.cdc.gov/opioids/patients/guideline.html

Massage therapists need to be able to adapt the massage application to pain-based conditions and also to work with other health and medical care professionals in an informed and professional manner.

DEFINING PAIN

Pain is difficult to define and classify. Defining pain in descriptive and measurable terms is not easy, because pain has physiological, psychological, and social aspects. Pain is a complex, private, and abstract experience. It is the No. 1 symptom or complaint that causes people to seek health care. In addition, effective management of pain is a major challenge. The International Association for the Study of Pain (IASP) is the leading professional organization for science, practice, and education in the field of pain. The IASP is the basis for this content.

Acute Pain

Acute pain is a symptom of a disease condition or a temporary aspect of medical treatment. Acute pain acts as a warning signal because it can activate the sympathetic nervous system (fight-or-flight response). Acute pain is usually temporary, has a sudden onset, and is easily localized. We can describe the pain, which often subsides with or without treatment.

Chronic/Persistent Pain

Chronic pain is identified as a major health problem. Acute pain has a purpose. Chronic pain is nonproductive and no longer has any value. Approximately 25% of the population is affected. Chronic pain is a symptom that persists or recurs for indefinite periods, usually for longer than 6 months. Chronic pain frequently has an obscure onset, and the character and quality of the pain change over time. The pain is usually is diffuse and poorly localized and often requires the efforts of a multidisciplinary healthcare team for its effective management.

Pain can also be classified as nociceptive, neuropathic, and neuroplastic pain.

Nociceptive Pain

Nociceptive pain occurs when actual or threatened tissue damage occurs as a result of the activation of nociceptors. Nociceptive pain typically starts as acute pain that lessens with time and tissue healing. This protective and productive response is a normal and appropriate function of the nervous system.

Neuropathic Pain

Neuropathic pain refers to pain that is generated or sustained by the nervous system. It is the result of nerve damage or a malfunctioning nervous system and involves problems with signals from the nerves. Neuropathic pain is commonly associated with a variety of neurodegenerative, metabolic, and autoimmune diseases. By definition, neuropathic pain is chronic and may escalate over time. There are two categories of neuropathic pain:

- Central neuropathic pain results directly from CNS injury (e.g., a stroke).
- Peripheral neuropathic pain is related to injury or disease of the peripheral somatosensory nervous system.

These conditions often begin with productive, normal nociceptive pain. However, in chronic neuropathic pain, the nervous system responds inappropriately to the damage through multiple mechanisms, misreading sensory inputs and generating nonproductive painful sensations. Secondary symptoms that commonly accompany neuropathic pain include depression, sleep disturbance, fatigue, and decreased physical and mental functioning.

Mixed Pain

Mixed pain is a combination of nociceptive and neuropathic pain. Nociceptive pain can be somatic or visceral and is usually localized. It is often described as achy, throbbing, or dull, deep, and pulling. Neuropathic pain is typically described as burning, shooting, tingling, and radiating. With mixed pain, elements of both neuropathic and nociceptive pain are described. The causes of the pain sensations can also be mixed (Box 2.11).

Neuroplastic Pain

Neuroplastic pain is when pain symptoms are caused by learned neuropathways in the brain and are not due to structural damage or disease in the body. Pain can modify the way the CNS

Box 2.11 Pain Classification

- Pain can be categorized according to the anatomical sites where the pain is felt (e.g., headache, neck, and back pain).
- Pain can be classified according to the tissues involved (e.g., musculoskeletal, visceral, neuropathic).
- Pain can be classified by the pathological process involved (e.g., cancer pain, osteoporotic pain, osteoarthritic pain, repetitive strain injury, fibromyalgia, thoracic outlet syndrome, carpal tunnel disorders).

  There are many named pain conditions:
  - Neuropathic pain
  - Peripheral neuropathies
  - Central pain
  - Phantom pain
  - Sciatica
  - Chronic regional pain syndrome
  - Neuropathic cancer pain
  - Irritable bowel syndrome
  - Painful diabetic neuropathy
  - HIV/AIDS pain
  - Postherpetic neuralgia
  - Treatment-induced pain
  - Burn pain
  - Trauma pain
  - Perioperative and postoperative pain
  - Dental and intraoral pain
  - Orofacial pain (neural and muscular)
  - Chronic pelvic pain
  - Vulvodynia
  - Interstitial cystitis
  - Endometriosis
  - Cardiac pain
  - Medication-induced pain
  - Ocular pain
  - Sickle cell pain
  - Fibromyalgia

These conditions are complex and multifaceted. They include biological changes in neuroendocrine function, psychological perceptual concerns, and effects on social interaction and support. A multidisciplinary approach, known as biopsychosocial care, is needed to help individuals in pain achieve quality of life.

Modified from the Interagency Pain Research Coordinating Committee (IPRCC), Department of Health and Human Services. *Federal Pain Research Portfolio Analysis Report.* Federal Research Pain Strategy | IPRCC (nih.gov).

processes sensory signals. Structural and functional changes can occur at every level of the nervous system, including the periphery, the spinal cord, and the higher brain centers, after injury, inflammation, and other damaging events. These changes may increase the magnitude of the perceived pain and may contribute to the development of chronic pain syndromes and increased pain sensitivity. *Neuroplasticity* is the brain and nervous system's ability to form new pathways or synapses and adapt to change. Neuroplastic changes may be responsible for the persistent pain as a nonbeneficial neuroplastic adaptation. Sometimes a person becomes more sensitive to stimuli and experiences more pain with less sensory stimulation. Rather than the nervous system functioning properly to sound the alarm about tissue injury, in neuropathic pain the peripheral or central nervous system malfunctions and becomes the cause of the pain.

Neuroplastic changes commonly occur with neuropathic pain. After a peripheral nerve injury, anatomical and neurochemical changes can occur within the CNS that can persist long after the injury has healed. When the problem begins in the peripheral nerves, it is called *peripheral sensitization*. The increased responsiveness in the CNS is called *central sensitization*. Central sensitization is a factor in chronic pain in which peripheral stimuli are interpreted as more painful than in a normal function. Central sensitization results in the amplification of peripheral signals. It is not an independent pain generator in peripheral neuropathic pain conditions. There are three main dysfunctions:

- **Allodynia** is pain, generally on the skin, caused by something that would not normally cause pain. Allodynia is believed to be a hypersensitive reaction that may result from central sensitization.
- **Hyperalgesia** is an increased pain response—basically, pain that is more painful than it should be.
- **Paresthesia** is the experience of unpleasant or painful feelings even when nothing is touching you, and no stimulus.

Quite often people may experience chronic pain as a result of more than one painful condition. Among the most difficult aspects of treating a person in pain is identifying the type or types and the mechanism (or mechanisms) of pain. Often our clients come for massage with more than one type of chronic pain and more than one mechanism underlying their complaints. Assessing which mechanisms of pain a person is experiencing—in other words, assessing a client's pain and building their pain profile—is not simple, but this step is vital.

The experience of pain is both conscious and subconscious, allowing each individual to decide what the pain means to him or her.

The subconscious part of the brain experiences pain and interprets it as harm—regardless of whether actual damage is occurring. Sometimes we hurt (e.g., after surgery or because of an old injury), but we are not in any danger (harm). If we experience chronic pain (e.g., back pain [hurt]), we must come to grips with the realization that the pain is not productive and does not harm us, even if it does hurt. The problem is that pain often is more about hurt than actual harm. The conscious part of the brain can identify what is causing the pain and coordinate the changes necessary to alleviate the harm or understand the hurt. A conscious understanding of the pain experience allows the individual to get on with living despite the pain perception and find a "new normal."

As massage therapists, we need to understand that any pain experience is complex, and there are no simple solutions. Massage therapy shows strong potential for helping people as part of a multidisciplinary, integrated team. Nonpharmaceutical methods are needed to help people manage conditions involving long-term pain. Chronic/persistent pain is now considered a separate condition from acute pain. This difference is the reason current effective treatments for acute pain do not work for chronic/persistent pain. For example, opiate medications are appropriate for the short-term treatment of acute pain. However, you cannot treat chronic pain using acute pain measures. Attempts to do this are one of the factors that have led to the current opiate addiction crisis (Smith, 2018; Tick et al., 2018; Nielsen et al., 2022).

Practical Application

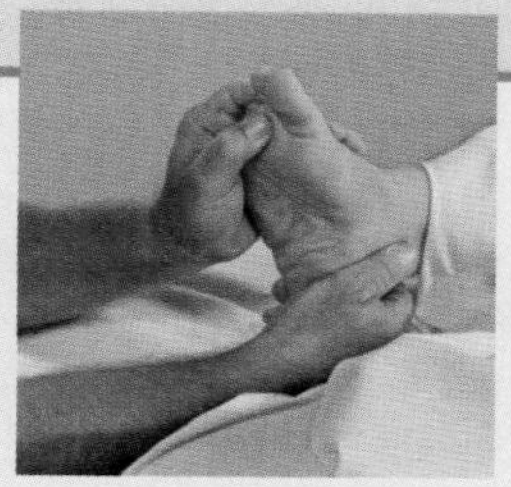

Pain is an unpleasant sensory and emotional experience associated with actual or potential tissue damage. Pain can be acute, persistent (chronic), or both at the same time. Unpleasant acute pain promotes survival and can be considered productive pain. However, acute pain can become complicated by sensitization in the periphery and within the central nervous system, leading to chronic nonproductive pain experiences. Persistent (chronic) pain is pain that lasts after the usual time for healing. It is now known that chronic pain is more complex. Chronic pain is a disease in its own right, one that fundamentally alters the nervous system. This concept is a change in basic assumptions in the pain field.

PAIN SENSATIONS

Nociception is the sensing of danger through stimulation of the nervous system. Pain and itch are both forms of nociception. Pain tells the body that either an injury has occurred, or one is imminent. Itch (pruritus) signals the presence of an irritant or a potential toxin. In both cases, the skin is vital to signaling. The nerve endings transmit the signal through circuits of multiple nerve cells toward the brain.

We need the sensations we experience as pain and itch to keep us safe. These sensations give us enough information about potential tissue damage to help us protect ourselves from greater damage. Pain often initiates a person's search for medical assistance. The subjective description and indication of the location of the pain help pinpoint the underlying cause of the disease.

The receptors for tissue damage, called *nociceptors*, are simply the branching ends of the dendrites of certain sensory neurons. Neurons are nerve cells, and dendrites are branches of the neuron cell body. Injured tissue releases bradykinin, which causes the release of inflammation-producing chemicals such as histamine and prostaglandins. Inflammatory mediators make nociceptors more sensitive to the normal pain response.

Sensory receptors that detect the potential for tissue harm transmit signals to the CNS that may be interpreted as pain. Pain receptors adapt only slightly or not at all. Adaptation is the reduction or disappearance of the perception of a sensation, even though the stimulus is still present. An example is getting used to our clothes soon after dressing. If adaptation to pain occurs, the stimuli cease to be sensed, and tissue damage can result (Box 2.12).

Box 2.12 Cancer Pain Is Different

Cancer pain is different from other forms of acute or chronic pain. Pain is often of a mixed type. The psychosocial aspects of pain may involve worries about an uncertain future and loss of control, with the potential for disfigurement from surgery and even the possibility of death.

When cancer invades a tissue, neuroimmune interactions result in the excretion of cellular and neuroinflammatory substances. These substances promote new nerve growth, and the new nerves increase the individual's sensitivity to pain. Cancer pain syndromes, both from the cancer and the medical treatment, remain a challenge. Neuropathy, inflammation, and ulceration of the mucous membranes, as well as pathologic fractures resulting from reduced bone density, all are sources of pain. For these and other cancer pain syndromes, complementary and integrative health (CIH) approaches, combined with multimodal therapies, are considered best practice. Analgesic medications, including opiates, may be necessary to manage cancer pain. Adding nondrug therapies to the treatment plan is also indicated. Extensive research has shown the benefits of massage therapy as a pain management strategy

Modified from Arnstein P. Adult cancer pain: an evidence-based update. *J Radiol Nurs.* 2018;37:15–20. Available at: https://www.sciencedirect.com/science/article/pii/S1546084317301165#bib35.

Specific Types of Pain

- *Pricking or bright pain:* This type of pain exists when the skin is cut or jabbed with a sharp object. The pain is short-lived but intense and easily localized. It is sometimes called *superficial somatic pain.*
- *Burning pain:* This type of pain is slower to develop, lasts longer, and is localized less accurately (e.g., when the skin is burned). This type of pain often stimulates cardiac and respiratory activity.
- *Aching pain:* Aching pain occurs when the visceral organs are stimulated. The pain is constant, not well localized, and commonly referred to areas of the body distant from the site of the damage. Aching pain is important because it may be a sign of a life-threatening disorder in a vital organ.
- *Deep pain:* The main difference between superficial and deep pain is the nature of the pain evoked by noxious stimuli. Unlike superficial pain, deep pain is poorly localized, nauseating, and commonly associated with sweating and changes in blood pressure. Deep pain initiates the reflex contraction of nearby skeletal muscles, a response similar to the muscle spasm associated with injuries to bones, tendons, and joints. The steadily contracting muscles become ischemic (lacking in oxygen), and ischemia stimulates the pain receptors in the muscles. The pain, in turn, initiates more spasms, setting up a vicious circle. Recall the pain-spasm-pain cycle in the discussion about positive feedback loops (Fig. 2.10).
- *Muscle pain:* If a muscle contracts rhythmically and has an adequate blood supply, pain usually does not result. However, if the blood supply to a muscle is occluded (closed off), the same rhythmic contraction soon causes pain. The pain persists even after the contraction until blood flow is reestablished. If a muscle with a normal blood supply is made to contract continuously without periods of

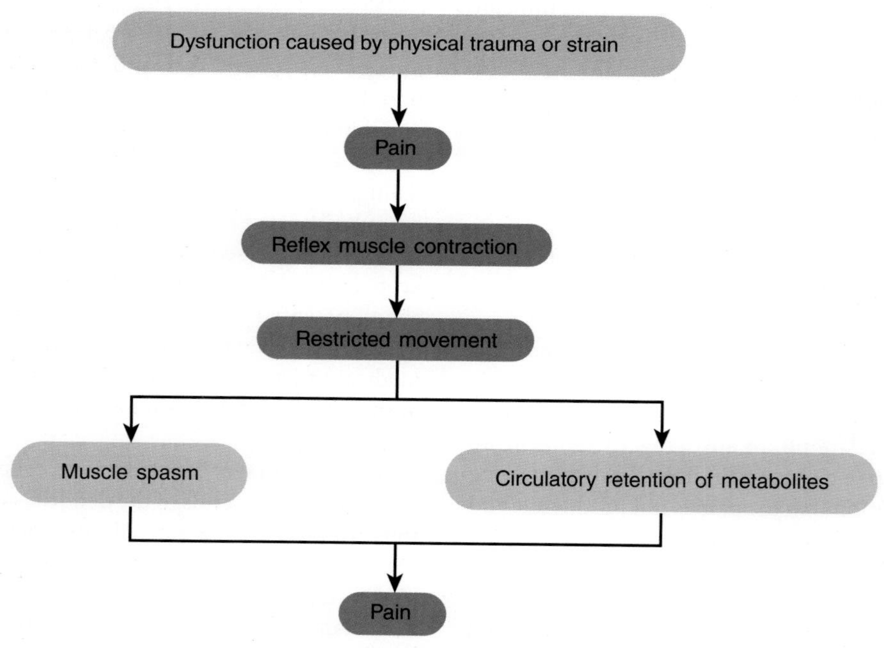

FIG. 2.10 Muscle spasm cycle.

relaxation, it begins to ache because the maintained contraction compresses the blood vessels supplying the muscle, reducing the blood supply.

Somatic and Visceral Pain

We can look at pain in two other ways: somatic and visceral. **Somatic pain** arises from the stimulation of receptors in the skin (superficial somatic pain) or stimulation of receptors in skeletal muscles, joints, tendons, and fasciae (deep somatic pain). **Visceral pain** results from the stimulation of receptors in the viscera, which are internal organs.

Superficial somatic pain is transmitted along finely myelinated (myelin is fatty insulation) A-delta nerve fibers at a fast rate; an analogy for this is a highway or an expressway. Deep somatic pain and most visceral pain are transmitted slowly by unmyelinated (no insulation) C nerve fibers; an analogy for this is a dirt road.

This difference in the transmission of pain signals explains why superficial somatic stimulation transmitted on A-delta fibers can block or mask deep somatic or visceral pain. Stimulation of more A fibers than C fibers blocks the C fiber transmission from entering the spinal cord. If the signal does not enter the spinal cord, it cannot be felt as pain.

Methods of touch and pressure and most methods of movement are transmitted on A fibers; any stimulus of this type increases A fiber transmission, blocking pain signals. Treating pain in this way is called *counterirritation* (Fig. 2.11).

Referred Pain

The ability of the cerebral cortex of the brain (the thinking part of the brain) to locate the origin of pain is related to experience. In most instances of somatic pain and some instances of visceral pain, the brain accurately projects the pain back to the stimulated area.

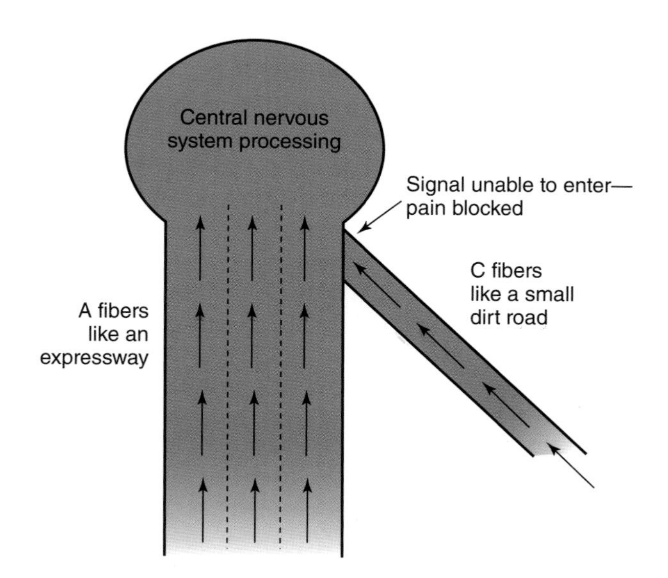

FIG. 2.11 Gate control theory of pain (based on Melzack and Wall's gate control theory).

Visceral pain also may be felt in a surface area far from the stimulated organ. This phenomenon is called *referred pain*. In general, the area to which the pain is referred and the visceral organ that is stimulated receive their nerves from the same section of the spinal cord. Because of this association, the brain may misinterpret the source. For example, the pain of a heart attack is typically felt in the skin over the heart and along the left arm. The same factor is at work in the referred pain in the shoulder caused by gallstones. The schematic in Fig. 2.12 illustrates cutaneous (skin) regions to which visceral pain may be referred. If a client has a recurring pain pattern that resembles the patterns in this figure, they should be referred to a physician for an accurate diagnosis.

Irritation of the viscera frequently produces pain that is felt not in the viscera but in some somatic structures that may be a considerable distance from the viscera. Such pain is said to be *referred* to the somatic structure. Deep somatic pain may also be referred, but superficial pain is not. When visceral pain is local and referred, it sometimes seems to radiate from the local to the distant site.

Visceral pain, like deep somatic pain, initiates reflex contraction of nearby skeletal muscle. Because somatic pain is much more common than visceral pain, the brain has learned to project the pain to the somatic area and initiate the reflex contraction there.

Knowledge about referred pain and the common sites of pain referral from each of the viscera is important to massage practitioners and other healthcare professionals. The most common example of referred pain is that of a heart attack, which is commonly experienced as chest pain. Another example is pain in the tip of the shoulder, which may be due to irritation in the central portion of the diaphragm.

However, remember that sites of reference are not stereotyped, and unusual reference sites occur with considerable frequency. Heart pain, for instance, may be experienced as purely abdominal, may be referred to the right arm, and may even be referred to the neck.

As previously noted, experience plays a key role in identifying referred pain. Although pain originating in an inflamed abdominal organ usually is referred to the midline, in clients who have had previous abdominal surgery, the pain of an inflamed abdominal organ commonly is referred to the surgical scar. Pain originating in the maxillary sinus is usually referred to nearby teeth, but in clients with a history of traumatic dental work, such pain is regularly referred to the previously traumatized teeth. This is true even if the teeth are distant from the sinus.

When pain is referred, the reference usually is to a structure that developed from the same embryonic segment or is located in the same dermatome (nerve map) as the structure in which the pain originates (Fig. 2.13). For example, during embryonic development, the diaphragm moves from the neck to its adult location in the abdomen and takes its nerve supply, the phrenic nerve, with it. One-third of the fibers in the phrenic nerve are afferent, and they enter the spinal cord at the level of the second to fourth cervical segments, the same location where afferent nerves from the tip of the shoulder enter. Similarly, the heart and the arm have the same embryonic segmental origin.

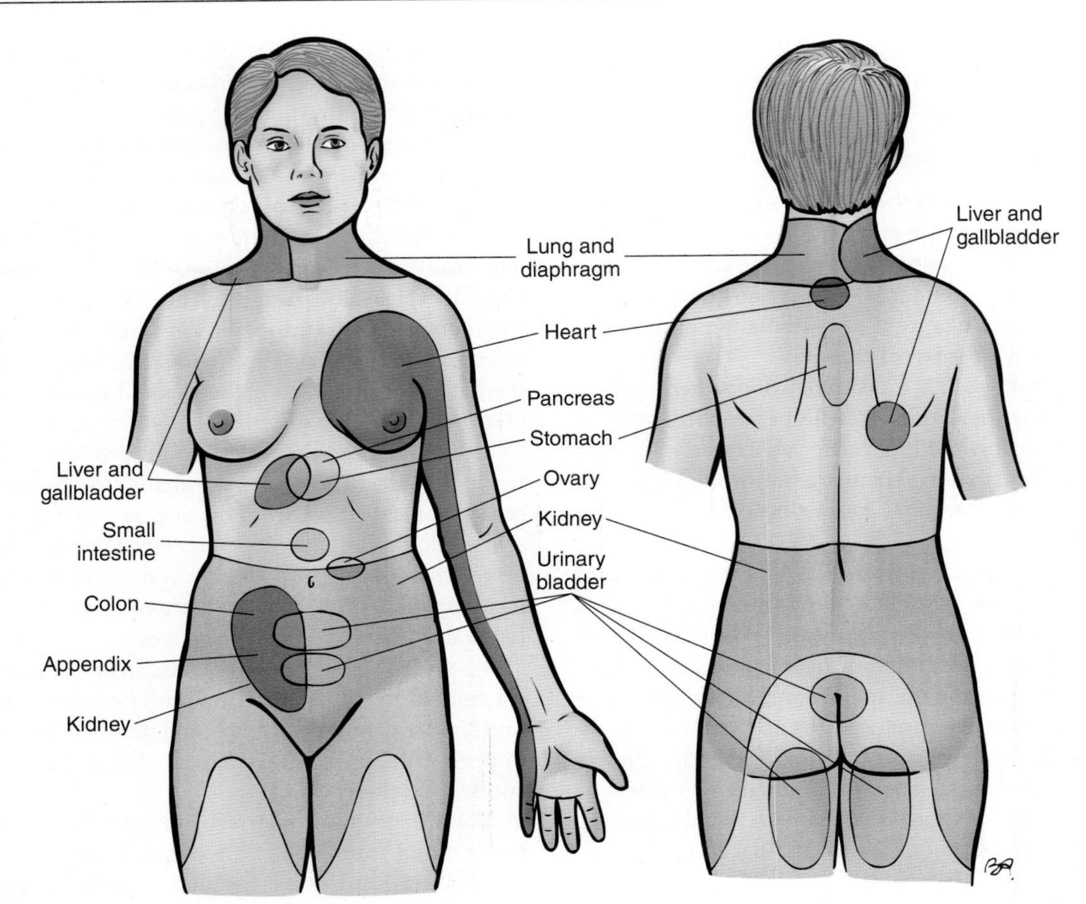

FIG. 2.12 Referred pain. The diagram indicates the cutaneous areas to which visceral pain may be referred. Massage professionals who encounter pain in these areas should refer the client for diagnosis to rule out visceral dysfunction. (From Fritz S. *Mosby's Fundamentals of Therapeutic Massage.* 5th ed., Mosby; 2013.)

Phantom Pain

A kind of pain commonly experienced by people who have undergone limb amputation is called **phantom pain**. The person experiences pain or other sensations in the extremity as though the limb were still there. Phantom pain is believed to occur because the remaining proximal portions of the sensory nerves that previously received impulses from the limb are stimulated by the trauma of the amputation. Stimuli from these nerves are interpreted by the brain as coming from the nonexistent (phantom) limb. New research about phantom pain indicates a connection to established patterns in the brain as a cause.

Cancer-Related Pain

The two most common causes of cancer pain are the cancer itself and the treatments used to treat cancer. The pain related to the cancer itself includes the pressure of a tumor on one of the body's organs, bones, or nerves. Sometimes cancer can cause pain when blood vessels become obstructed by the tumor.

Examples of Treatment-Related Pain

- Chemotherapy: peripheral neuropathy, bone and joint pain
- Surgical treatments and procedures

Most types of cancer pain can be managed with drug and nondrug therapies. How much pain the person experiences depends on where the cancer is located, what kind of damage it is causing, and the various medications and other treatments used to treat the cancer.

Common Types of Cancer-Related Pain

- Acute pain that lasts a short time. The intensity of the pain experienced can range from mild to severe.
- Chronic/persistent pain that will not go away or that comes back often. The intensity of the pain experienced can range from mild to severe.
- Breakthrough pain is an intense pain experience. It may occur as the effects of pain medication begin to diminish. It may also be triggered by a specific activity or may occur for no observable reason.
- Neuropathic pain may occur if the treatment damages the nerves. The pain is often burning, sharp, or shooting (see Box 2.12).

Pain Threshold and Pain Tolerance

Pain may be brought on by mechanical, electrical, thermal, or chemical stimuli. We do not appear to adapt to pain or accommodate it. We all have about the same threshold for pain.

A *pain threshold* occurs when stimulation becomes intense enough to initiate the firing of pain receptors.

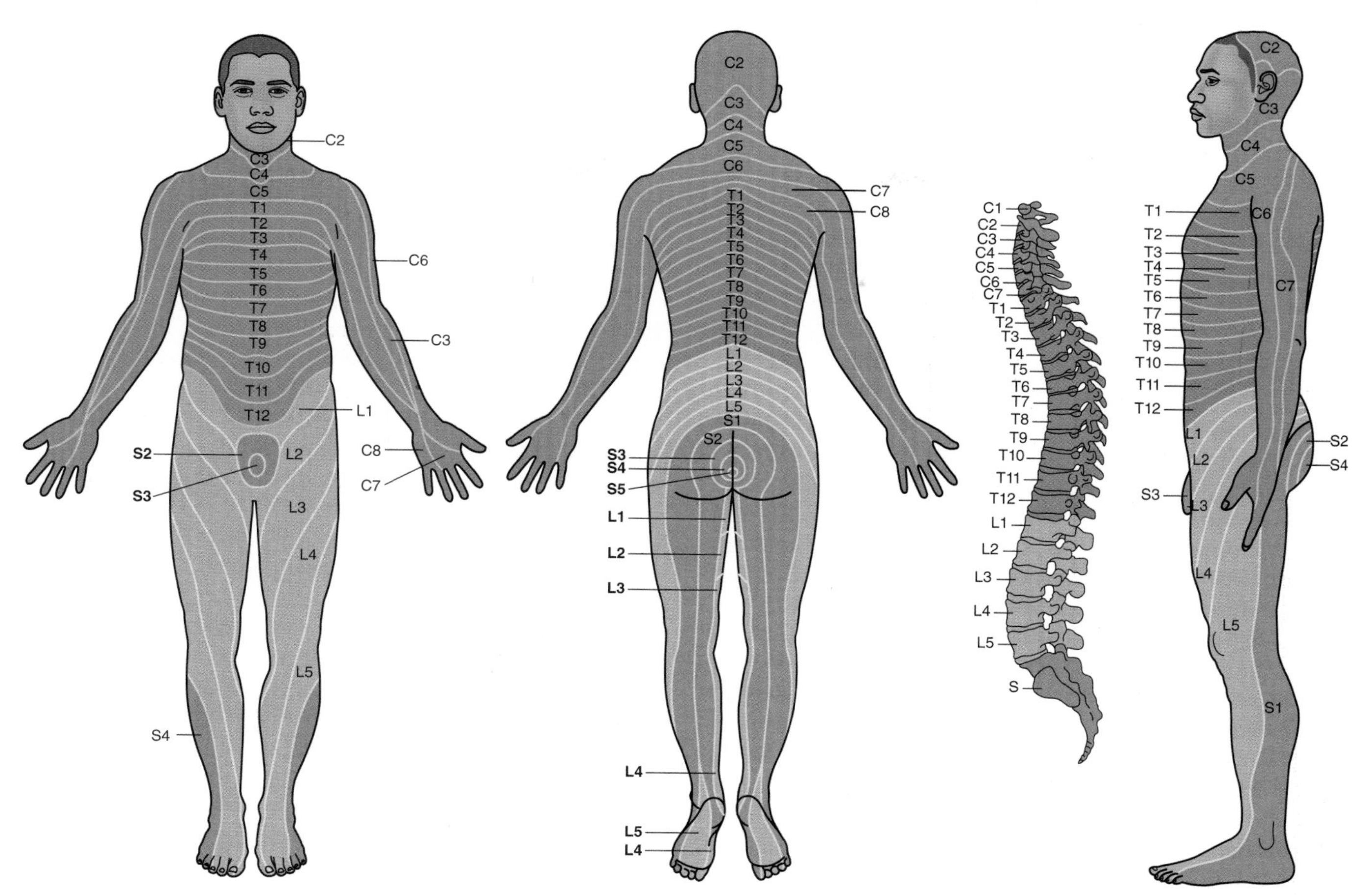

FIG. 2.13 Dermatomal map: posterior, anterior, and lateral views. A *dermatome* is an area of skin in which sensory nerves derive from a single spinal nerve root. In these figures, the boundaries of dermatomes are sharply defined. However, in each person, innervation overlaps with adjacent dermatomes.

Pain tolerance is the response to pain. It varies considerably and is influenced greatly by cultural and psychological factors. Pain tolerance is modified by age and emotional and mental states.

Subjective measurements of the intensity of pain are more reliable than observable measurements. Only the person in pain can determine the severity experienced. Pain is rarely the same at all times. It is perceived differently over time, and it differs with various precipitating and aggravating factors.

The cause, the severity, and the type of pain experienced must be identified if it is to be treated optimally. Assessing the severity and degree of pain is difficult because pain cannot be measured objectively; a thorough history must be obtained and a systematic physical assessment conducted. Some questions that might be asked are:

- Is the pain acute or chronic?
- What is the location of the pain?
- What is the quality of the pain (e.g., sharp, burning, pricking)?
- How intense is the pain?
- When does the pain occur (in other words, what is the timing)?
- What factors affect the intensity of the pain (Activity 2.2)?

ACTIVITY 2.2

List three personal factors that could change your pain tolerance.

Examples

Things that could increase my pain tolerance:

1. Reading an enjoyable book
2. Going for a walk
3. Practicing relaxation techniques

Things that could reduce my pain tolerance:

1. Being tired and upset with the kids
2. Driving in heavy traffic
3. Loud music

Your Turn

Things that could increase my pain tolerance:

1. ____________________
2. ____________________
3. ____________________

Things that could decrease my pain tolerance:

1. ____________________
2. ____________________
3. ____________________

Pain Management

"Pain management" is a catchall phrase used to describe multiple types of healthcare services for pain. Pain management can include these types of services:

- Acute care for injuries and illness
- Postoperative pain care
- End-of-life, or palliative, care
- Burn unit services
- Wound care
- Chronic pain management

These different types of care are usually considered to fall into three broad categories:

- Acute pain management
- Terminal, or palliative, care
- Chronic pain management

Acute pain is usually caused by tissue injury. Inflammation is commonly present (Box 2.13).

The management of chronic pain is more difficult. Some options work for certain individuals but not for others. Many of these strategies come under the heading of neuromodulation or distracting the brain from signals it is getting from the body's periphery.

The following pain management strategies can be used alone or in combination for both acute and chronic pain (Box 2.14).

Evolution of Our Understanding of Pain

Ongoing discussions and research are increasing our understanding of the pain experience (Box 2.15). As this section has described, the pain experience is complex. Pain neuroscience is the biology, psychology, and sociology of what happens during a pain experience for individuals. Evolving information about the science of pain will influence the practice of massage therapy, both in how massage treatment plans are developed and how we educate ourselves and our clients about management strategies.

The *Neuromatrix Theory of Pain* is an explanatory model of how pain is produced and therapeutically managed. The neuromatrix theory of pain provides a framework that may explain why selected nonpharmacological methods of pain relief, such as massage, are effective. The concept of a pain "neuromatrix" suggests that the perception of pain is influenced by multiple factors. The theory was developed by Ronald Melzack and Patrick David Wall and is an expansion of their original gate control theory of pain, proposed in 1965.

Since 1965 ongoing research has broadened our understanding of pain mechanisms, and this understanding has evolved to include the neuromatrix theory of pain. Most pain experts consider the neuromatrix pain theory an accurate understanding of the nature of pain.

The neuromatrix theory of pain addresses the complex nature of pain in these ways:

- Pain is an output of the brain that is produced whenever the brain concludes that the body is in danger and action is required. Each person's brain has developed an individual neural network, referred to as the *body-self neuromatrix*. Pain is a multisystem output that is produced when an individual's pain neuromatrix is activated.

Box 2.13 ICE/RICE/PRICE/POLICE/MEAT MCE/MICE/CRIME

ICE/RICE/PRICE/POLICE/MEAT/MCE/MICE/CRIME are all acronyms for methods to manage acute soft tissue injury, such as a sprain or strain. The process began with ICE and has since evolved altering methods and letters to the acronyms:

I—Ice. Ice or cryotherapy is the application of cold typically with an ice pack applied to the injured area. Ice lowers skin and tissue temperature which decreases nociceptive signally and can lead to a reduction in pain sensation. There is some controversy over the use of ice since it can reduce the productive acute inflammatory response. However, ice is a much better pain management strategy than pain medication. When applying ice to a local area do not apply it directly to the skin to prevent frostbite. Ice application should not exceed 20 minutes.

C—Compression. Compression after an injury helps in the prevention of further swelling and a bit of immobilization. Compression to a local area is usually applied using an elastic bandage wrap. The bandage should not be so tight that it causes discomfort or interferes with blood flow.

E—Elevation. Elevating the injured area results in a decrease in hydrostatic pressure, which in turn, reduces the accumulation of interstitial fluid and manages edema.

Next R and P were added:

R—Rest. The intention of rest is to support the healing process. Not excessive rest but taking it easy for 24 hours may be prudent.

P—Protection. Protection prevents further injury and involves some type of immobilization such as the compression bandage or reduced weight-bearing or demand such as crutches or a sling.

The result is PRICE. However, over time best practices indicated that PRICE needed updating, and POLICE came into being. The R was removed, and an OL was added:

OL—Optimal Loading. Optimal Loading uses movement, weight-bearing, and resistance to stimulate the healing process of bone, tendon, ligament, and muscle. The intensity of the loading increases as the healing progresses. The right amount of activity can help manage swelling.

Then the use of ice/cryotherapy was thought to interfere with the productive inflammatory response in the acute phase of healing so MEAT emerged.

MEAT—The acronym stands for Movement, Exercise, Analgesics, Therapy.

The MEAT protocol has elements of Optimal Loading by recommending movement, exercise, and therapy such as physical therapy. The use of analgesics is to reduce pain enough to support movement, exercise, and therapy. Analgesic medication is usually also antiinflammatory, which will certainly interfere with the normal healing process so maybe ice remains the best form of pain management. And the variations continue:

MCE: Move safely, Compression, Elevation

AND ICE IS AGAIN PART OF THE PROTOCOL … MAYBE.

MICE: Motion, Ice, Compression, Elevation

CRIME: Compression, Rest, Ice, Motion, and Elevation.

Box 2.14 The Opiate/Opioid Crisis

Narcotics fall into two categories:

- Opiates—narcotic analgesics derived from the opium poppy (natural).
- Opioids—narcotic analgesics that are at least partly synthetic and are not found in nature.

The terms are often used interchangeably.

The misuse of and addiction to opiates and opioids—including prescription pain relievers, heroin, and synthetic opioids, such as fentanyl—is a national crisis that affects public health.

Predicting whether an individual tends to become addicted to opiate medications is difficult. Addiction is a disease that affects brain function and behavior. The person feels as if they cannot function without the drug. Addiction causes a person to obsessively seek out the drug, even though using it causes behavior, health, or relationship problems.

Misuse of opioids has been a problem for centuries, but the current situation is different. Opioids are a type of medicine often used to help relieve acute pain from toothaches and dental procedures, injuries, surgeries, and cancer. Opioids are safe when used correctly for a brief time (a few days) for acute pain or appropriately for longer periods for cancer pain or end-of-life pain. People who do not follow the doctor's instructions and those who misuse opioids can become addicted.

In the late 1990s doctors thought people would not become addicted to prescription opioid pain relievers, unlike the case with nonmedical opiate use, such as heroin, for which addiction is common. Based on the pharmaceutical companies' assurances that the new synthetic opiate–type medications were safe, healthcare providers became more comfortable prescribing them, and this led to misuse of these medications before it became clear that they are highly addictive. This issue has become a public health crisis with devastating consequences, including increases in opioid misuse and related overdoses, as well as the rising incidence of *neonatal abstinence syndrome* due to opioid use and misuse during pregnancy. The increase in the use of injection drugs also has contributed to the spread of infectious diseases, including human immunodeficiency virus (HIV) infection and hepatitis C.

Pain severity and pain sensitivity are not huge factors in opioid misuse. However, those who reported less ability to tolerate physical or emotional distress were more likely to misuse opioid analgesics and become dependent. The endogenous (made in the body) opioid system is closely related to the dopamine reward system and to the oxytocin system, which affects bonding and close social interactions, thus leading to feelings of well-being. The opioid medication induces sensations that make the addict feel almost as if they are being supported by caring people, and it also reduces feelings of distress.

Distress refers to the "bad" type of stress (the opposite of good stress, called eustress), and occurs when adaptive demands are excessive and disease-producing stress can occur. Distress can lead to suffering. Although pain is a phenomenon that affects many levels of the nervous system, suffering is highly individual and results from mental and emotional responses to pain. Suffering is both a cause and an effect of distressing emotions associated with chronic pain: anxiety, irritability, anger, fear, depression, frustration, guilt, shame, loneliness, hopelessness, and helplessness. Opiate/opioid abuse and misuse likely may be more related to distress than to pain. Signs and symptoms of distress include:

- Poor self-care and personal hygiene
- Being demanding of others
- Loss of motivation
- Perspiring excessively
- Having breathing difficulties
- Muscular spasms
- Obvious intense pain
- Extreme fatigue
- Complaints of sleep problems
- Anxiety and panic attacks
- Irritability and displaying agitation

Narcotics include:

- Opium
- Codeine
- Fentanyl
- Heroin
- Hydrocodone
- Hydromorphone
- Methadone
- Morphine
- Oxycodone
- Oxymorphone
- Paregoric
- Sufentanil
- Tramadol

MedlinePlus: Opioids and Opioid Use Disorder (OUD): Available at: https://medlineplus.gov/opioidsandopioidusedisorderoud.html.

- An individual's neuromatrix consists of genetic neural programs, individual experience, and behavior. The intensity and location of sensory inputs from the skin, organs, and other somatic receptors influence the perception of a situation as dangerous, triggering the activity of the body's stress-regulation systems.
- Pain becomes chronic as the pain neuromatrix is strengthened by nociceptive and nonnociceptive mechanisms; this means that less input, both nociceptive and nonnociceptive, is required to produce pain. This is called **sensitization**.

Pain research has helped explain that acute pain and chronic pain are different, and actual tissue damage does not always correspond to the intensity of the pain experience. The conscious awareness of pain is a subjective experience that is brain/CNS based. What has emerged is the importance of *pain neuroscience education*. Educating ourselves and our clients reduces fear and stress. Pain management must be person centered, multidimensional, and comprehensive, taking into consideration the biopsychosocial, spiritual, and cultural factors affecting the person. Pain management should be an interprofessional team effort.

Review What You Have Learned

- Describe pain sensations.

  Pain is an unpleasant sensory and emotional experience associated with actual or potential tissue damage. Pain can be acute or persistent (chronic) or both at the same time. Sensory receptors called *nociceptors* detect tissue damage.

Box 2.15 Findings and Recommendations of the National Pain Strategy (NPS) Update

The public at large and people with pain would benefit from a better understanding of pain and its treatment to encourage timely care, improve medical management, and combat stigmatization.

- Increased scientific knowledge regarding the pathophysiology of pain has led to the conclusion that chronic/persistent pain can be a disease in itself that requires adequate treatment and research commitment.
- Chronic/persistent pain is a biopsychosocial condition that often requires integrated, multimodal, and interdisciplinary treatment, all components of which should be evidence based.
- Data are lacking on the prevalence, onset, course, impact, and outcomes of most common chronic pain conditions. The greatest individual and societal benefit would accrue from a focus on chronic/persistent pain.
- Every effort should be made to prevent illnesses and injuries that lead to pain, the progression of acute pain to a chronic condition, and the development of high-impact chronic pain.
- Significant improvements are needed to ensure that pain assessment techniques and practices are high quality and comprehensive.
- Self-management programs can improve the quality of life and are a key component of acute and chronic pain prevention and management.
- People with chronic/persistent pain need treatment approaches that consider individual differences in susceptibility to pain and response to treatment, as well as improved access to treatments that are based on their preferences and are in accord with the best evidence on safety and effectiveness.
- Treatments that are ineffective, that have risks that exceed their benefits, or that may cause harm to certain subgroups need to be identified and their use curtailed or discontinued.
- Much of the responsibility for front-line pain care rests with primary care clinicians, who are not sufficiently trained in pain assessment and comprehensive, evidence-based treatment approaches.
- Greater collaboration is needed between primary care clinicians and pain specialists in different clinical disciplines and settings, including multispecialty pain clinics.
- Significant barriers to pain care exist, especially for populations disproportionately affected by and undertreated for pain, and these barriers need to be overcome.
- People with pain are too often stigmatized in the healthcare system and society, which can lead to delayed diagnosis or misdiagnosis, bias in treatment, and diminished effectiveness of care.

Modified from National Institutes of Health (NIH): National Pain Strategy. https://www.iprcc.nih.gov/national-pain-strategy-overview

Inflammatory mediators are then produced, such as histamine and prostaglandins, which make nociceptors more sensitive. Acute pain typically diminishes as the tissue heals. Chronic/persistent pain may persist for many reasons, including nerve damage and hypersensitivity of the nervous and immune systems.

- Explain the difference between hurt and harm.

  Hurt describes a pain sensation that is not currently causing damage (harm). It can be difficult for a person to consciously distinguish between what hurts and what is harmful.
- Define *acute* and *chronic/persistent pain*.
  - *Acute pain* is usually temporary, has a sudden onset, and is easily localized.
  - *Chronic/persistent pain* is persistent or indefinite, has an obscure onset, and is poorly localized.
- Define and provide examples of nociceptive, neuropathic, neuroplastic, and mixed pain.
  - *Nociceptive pain* results when tissue damage occurs or threatens, and the nociceptors (tissue damage nerve receptors) are activated. Nociceptive pain usually is acute (e.g., a burn).
  - *Neuropathic pain* is the result of nerve damage or a malfunctioning nervous system and involves problems with signals from the nerves. Neuropathic pain is typically chronic. It can be divided into two categories: central neuropathic pain, which results from CNS injury (e.g., a stroke), and peripheral neuropathic pain, which relates to injury or disease of the peripheral somatosensory nervous system (e.g., traumatic brain injury and nerve entrapment).
  - *Neuroplastic pain* occurs when changes in the nervous system result in changes related to pain experiences. These structural and functional changes can occur at every level of the nervous system (e.g., increased somatic representation of a painful area in areas of the brain).
  - *Mixed pain* is a condition in which both nociceptive and neuropathic pain occur (e.g., a burn that is healing).
- Describe five common pain sensations.
  - *Pricking or bright pain:* Exists when the skin is cut or jabbed, is short lived but intense, and is easily localized. Also called *superficial somatic pain*.
  - *Burning pain:* Slower to develop, lasts longer, and is localized less accurately (e.g., when the skin is burned).
  - *Aching pain:* Occurs when the visceral organs are stimulated. The pain is constant, is not well localized, and commonly is felt distant from where the damage is occurring.
  - *Deep pain:* Poorly localized, nauseating, and commonly associated with sweating and changes in blood pressure. Deep pain initiates the reflex contraction of nearby muscles.
  - *Muscle pain:* Occurs if the blood supply to a muscle is occluded (closed off). The pain persists even after the contraction until blood flow is reestablished.
- Discuss the pain-spasm-pain cycle.

  In the context of muscle pain, steadily contracting muscles become ischemic (lacking in oxygen), which stimulates pain receptors in the muscles. The pain, in turn, initiates more spasms.
- Define *somatic pain* and *visceral pain*.

- *Somatic pain* arises from receptors in the skin (superficial somatic pain) or from receptors in skeletal muscles, joints, tendons, and fasciae (deep somatic pain).
- *Visceral pain* results from stimulation of the receptors in the viscera (internal organs).
- Identify viscerally referred pain patterns.
  Irritated or damaged viscera (internal organs) may produce pain in distant somatic structures. Study the patterns shown in Fig. 2.12.
- Define *referred pain.*
  Referred pain is felt in distant somatic structures but originates in viscera or deep somatic structures. Visceral pain and deep somatic pain may refer to pain, but somatic pain does not.
- Define *phantom pain.*
  Phantom pain is commonly experienced by people who have undergone limb amputation.
- List common types of cancer-related pain.
  - *Acute pain:* Lasts a short time.
  - *Chronic pain:* Does not go away or comes back often.
  - *Breakthrough pain*: Intense and may occur as the effects of pain medication wear off.
  - *Neuropathic pain:* May occur if treatment damages the nerves.
- List factors that influence the pain threshold and pain tolerance.
  - *Pain threshold:* The point where stimulation becomes intense enough to activate pain receptors.
  - *Pain tolerance:* The response to pain; it is influenced by culture, psychology, age, emotion, and mental state.

MECHANISMS OF HEALTH AND WELL-BEING

SECTION OBJECTIVES

Chapter objectives covered in this section:

11. Explain the difference between salutogenesis and pathogenesis.
12. Define *stress* and list the factors contributing to the stress response.
13. Describe ways to manage stress.
14. Define *resilience* and list factors that build resilience.

After completing this section, the learner will be able to:

- Define *health*.
- Define *stress*.
- Describe the parts of the autonomic nervous system and the two functions of the ANS.
- List various effects of excessive stress.
- Explain how humans adapt to and manage stress.

A state of good health is supported by a balanced lifestyle. On the continuum of imbalance, disease reflects a state of too much or not enough. Health is a state of being just right, or homeostasis. *Well-being* is a state of being comfortable, happy, and healthy. It is a complex and evolving concept that reflects how we feel about ourselves and our lives.

Health is influenced by many factors, including inherited and constitutional conditions. Lifestyle, activity level, rest, loving relationships, exercise, diet, empowering beliefs and attitudes, self-esteem, authentic personality, and freedom from self-hindering patterns all support health. Individuals need to understand their own bodies, minds, and spiritual selves as they seek balance. It is this awareness that allows the body to maintain a dynamic state of homeostasis (Activity 2.3).

Stress and Stress Management

Maintaining and supporting good health require effective management of stress and stressors. Stress is a state of real or perceived threat to homeostasis. Maintenance of homeostasis requires the activation of a network of responses involving the endocrine, nervous, and immune systems, collectively known as the **stress response**. Activation of the stress response is a primitive survival physiological sequence The stress response is primarily managed by the hypothalamic-pituitary-adrenal (HPA) axis. The HPA axis is made up of the hypothalamus, the pituitary gland, and the adrenal glands that form a neurohormone feedback system (Smith and Vale, 2022). Long-term stress resulting in overactivation of the HPA axis can result in the development of physical and mental health conditions.

The stress response requires energy expenditure, which then results in physiological processes necessary for cellular functioning, energy production, and the elimination of waste substances. Energy is required for the activation of the immune system in response to possible inflammatory processes. Biological energy is stored and released by chemical reactions. If the chemical reaction becomes unbalanced and free radicals build up, oxidative stress occurs. Oxidative stress results in cell damage, which is part of the aging process and many chronic diseases. Stress management and a healthy lifestyle are effective ways to manage oxidative stress (Feelisch et al., 2022).

Hans Selye, MD, PhD, identified "biologic stress" as the neuroendocrine response of the body to exposure to stressors. This information became the foundation for mind-body medicine. Over the years research has expanded and validated Dr. Selye's work. For massage therapy practice, Selye's general adaptation syndrome (GAS) is a functional framework for critical thinking. Selye suggested that the GAS be divided into three stages (Box 2.16 and Fig. 2.14; Selye, 1978):

- The first stage is the alarm reaction, also called the fight-or-flight response, which is the body's initial reaction to the perceived stressor.
- The second stage is known as the resistance reaction; the secretion of regulating hormones (cortisol) allows the body to continue fighting a stressor long after the effects of the alarm reaction have dissipated.
- The third stage is the exhaustion reaction; it happens if the stress response continues without relief.

The ANS (see Chapter 5) is responsible for monitoring, regulating, and coordinating almost all the body's systems—temperature, pH, oxygen levels, volume of blood, blood pressure, intake of food, digestion and absorption of food and water, and excretion of waste products. The response of the ANS to a stressor is the fight-or-flight response. Whenever we perceive that we are physically or psychologically threatened, a reflex alarm system in our brain triggers the release of electrical impulses and a variety of hormones. The alarm reaction is designed for short-term activation to deal with physical

ACTIVITY 2.3

This activity will provide you with an extensive look at your health profile. Give three different responses to each of these statements.

Examples

My lifestyle supports health in these ways:

1. I am involved in work that I love.
2. I am surrounded by information.
3. I am financially stable.

My lifestyle does not support health in these ways:

1. I work too many hours.
2. I am overwhelmed by too much to know and understand.
3. I have a lot of debt.

Your Turn

My lifestyle supports health in these ways:

1. ______
2. ______
3. ______

My lifestyle does not support health in these ways:

1. ______
2. ______
3. ______

My activity level supports health in these ways:

1. ______
2. ______
3. ______

My activity level does not support health in these ways:

1. ______
2. ______
3. ______

My rest pattern supports health in these ways:

1. ______
2. ______
3. ______

My rest pattern does not support health in these ways:

1. ______
2. ______
3. ______

My relationships support health in these ways:

1. ______
2. ______
3. ______

My relationships do not support health in these ways:

1. ______
2. ______
3. ______

My aerobic exercise supports health in these ways:

1. ______
2. ______
3. ______

My aerobic exercise does not support health in these ways:

1. ______
2. ______
3. ______

My diet supports health in these ways:

1. ______
2. ______
3. ______

My diet does not support health in these ways:

1. ______
2. ______
3. ______

My beliefs and attitudes support health in these ways:

1. ______
2. ______
3. ______

My beliefs and attitudes do not support health in these ways:

1. ______
2. ______
3. ______

My self-esteem supports health in these ways:

1. ______
2. ______
3. ______

My self-esteem does not support health in these ways:

1. ______
2. ______
3. ______

My personality supports health in these ways:

1. ______
2. ______
3. ______

My personality does not support health in these ways:

1. ______
2. ______
3. ______

Now, review the information you just wrote down. Pick one area to improve and list three ways you will accomplish that outcome.

1. ______
2. ______
3. ______

threats in which the emergency resolves quickly (in a few seconds or minutes).

Many of the stressors today are psychological in origin, and they are chronic, lasting days, weeks, months, and even years in some cases. Modern stressful events such as job security, financial problems, health worries, difficult neighbors, relationship problems, and so on, cannot be resolved by fighting or running away. Regardless, these psychological stressors still trigger the fight-or-flight response. Exercise can help to counter the stress response by reducing blood clotting, boosting immune function, reducing blood pressure, relaxing muscles, increasing metabolism, and diminishing the sensitivity of the sympathetic nervous system

The fight-or-flight response is controlled by the ANS, which is the part of our nervous system that controls the automatic functions of the body. Put simply, the ANS has two functions and parts:

1. The sympathetic nervous system triggers the biochemical and physiological changes brought about by the fight-or-flight response. Think of it as the accelerator on a car.

Box 2.16 Hans Selye's Stress Research

Hans Selye's groundbreaking research on stress began in 1935 and was formalized in his book *The Stress of Life*, published in 1956. Selye's research (1978) laid the foundation for current concepts about stress.

Many hormones regulated by the hypothalamus come into play during stress. The hypothalamus has connections with the cortex and limbic system and controls the pituitary gland. The pituitary gland regulates the secretion of hormones by the thyroid gland, adrenal cortex, ovaries, and testes. Thus stress easily becomes an event that affects the whole body.

One of the hormones secreted by the adrenal cortex is cortisol. Cortisol maintains blood glucose levels, facilitates fat metabolism, and affects protein and collagen synthesis. Increased cortisol secretion in stressful situations reduces the immune reaction, and the antiinflammatory effect of cortisol can slow healing as well. In generalized stress conditions, the hypothalamus acts on the anterior pituitary gland to cause the release of adrenocorticotropic hormone, which in turn stimulates the adrenal cortex to secrete glucocorticoid. Glucocorticoids are a class of adrenocortical hormones that protect the body against stress and aid in protein and carbohydrate metabolism. Cortisol is an example. Glucocorticoids also provide an antiinflammatory effect, assist in the release of amino acids from muscle, mobilize fatty acids from fat stores, increase the ability of skeletal muscles to maintain contraction and thus prevent fatigue, and increase the production of adenosine triphosphate (ATP). ATP is a complex organic chemical that provides the energy to drive many processes in living cells

In addition to causing the release of glucocorticoids, the adrenal medulla stimulates the release of epinephrine (adrenaline) and norepinephrine to help the body in its response to stress. However, during periods of prolonged stress, continued release of these hormones may have harmful side effects, such as an impaired immune response, diminished blood glucose levels, and altered protein and fat metabolism. These effects, in turn, reduce the body's resistance to stress. Therefore the continued release of epinephrine and norepinephrine increases the possibility of high blood pressure, impaired digestion, diminished tissue repair, and other negative effects.

Modified from Selye H. *The Stress of Life*. 2nd ed. McGraw-Hill; 1978.

2. The parasympathetic nervous system reverses the fight-or-flight response and returns all hormones, organs, and systems to prestress levels. Think of it as the brake on a car.

The fight-or-flight response can also be divided into two categories:

- Short-term fight-or-flight response: sympathetic adrenomedullary (SAM) system

  The short-term response is the primary system triggered within us in response to short-term threats. Electrical impulses from the hypothalamus, a gland located in the brain, travel along nerves that directly connect to the adrenal glands and stimulate the release of the stress hormones adrenaline and noradrenaline. The body cannot sustain this short-term fight-or-flight response for long because it would become exhausted. If the stressor is a more chronic one, then this triggers the secondary, longer-term fight-or-flight response to take over.
- Long-term fight-or-flight response: hypothalamic-pituitary-adrenal (HPA) axis

The longer-term fight-or-flight response is triggered hormonally and involves the hypothalamus, pituitary, and adrenal glands. The adrenal cortex (the outer part of the adrenal glands) releases stress hormones (e.g., cortisol). Chronic activation of this longer-term fight-or-flight response can be a causative factor in several psychological and physiological health problems (Box 2.17).

Selye introduced the terms "eustress" and "distress" to distinguish stress responses that were initiated by positive emotions from those triggered by negative, unpleasant causes. A stressor is not always a negative event. A wedding and a funeral may be equally stressful.

Both exposure to intense or extreme stressors (too much) and deprivation of necessary stimuli (too little) can cause imbalance and thus many problems. Too much heat, cold, noise, activity, exercise, food, or social demands, or not enough food, touch, social interaction, or sleep can be detrimental to health. **Interoception** is the way we sense, interpret, integrate, and regulate signals from within ourselves. Stress perception is both external from the environment and internal from body processes. Detrimental effects of stress occur because of our continuing need to respond or change our bodies to maintain homeostasis (Fig. 2.15 and Activity 2.4).

The active process by which a person predicts, prepares for, and responds to challenges and adapts to changes is called *allostasis* (Katsumi et al., 2022). This involves multiple mediators (autonomic, cortisol, immune/inflammatory, metabolic, neuromodulators within the brain) that interact and promote adaptation in the short run, as long as they are turned on efficiently when needed and turned off promptly when no longer needed. Overuse (too much stress) or dysregulation among the mediators (e.g., too much or too little cortisol; too much or too little production of inflammatory cytokines) results in cumulative change, which is referred to as *allostatic load* and *overload*.

As the key organ of stress and adaptation, the brain directs health-related behaviors (caloric intake, alcohol, smoking, sleep, and exercise) that contribute to or reduce physiological dysregulation, increasing or decreasing the allostatic load/overload (McEwen et al., 2015). Dysfunction of interoception may be a key component of many neurological, psychiatric, and behavioral disorders (Chen et al., 2021; Nord and Garfinkel, 2022). Brain development and healthy or unhealthy neural function determine in part whether the response to challenges, or stressors, is efficient or dysregulated. The development of self-esteem and locus of control, as well as good self-regulatory behaviors, are key factors that determine whether a challenge, such as going to a new place or giving a speech, will result in positive stress, with a satisfying outcome, or have negative consequences (see Box 2.16).

Tolerable stress describes coping successfully with stressful life events. There is minimal allostatic load because an

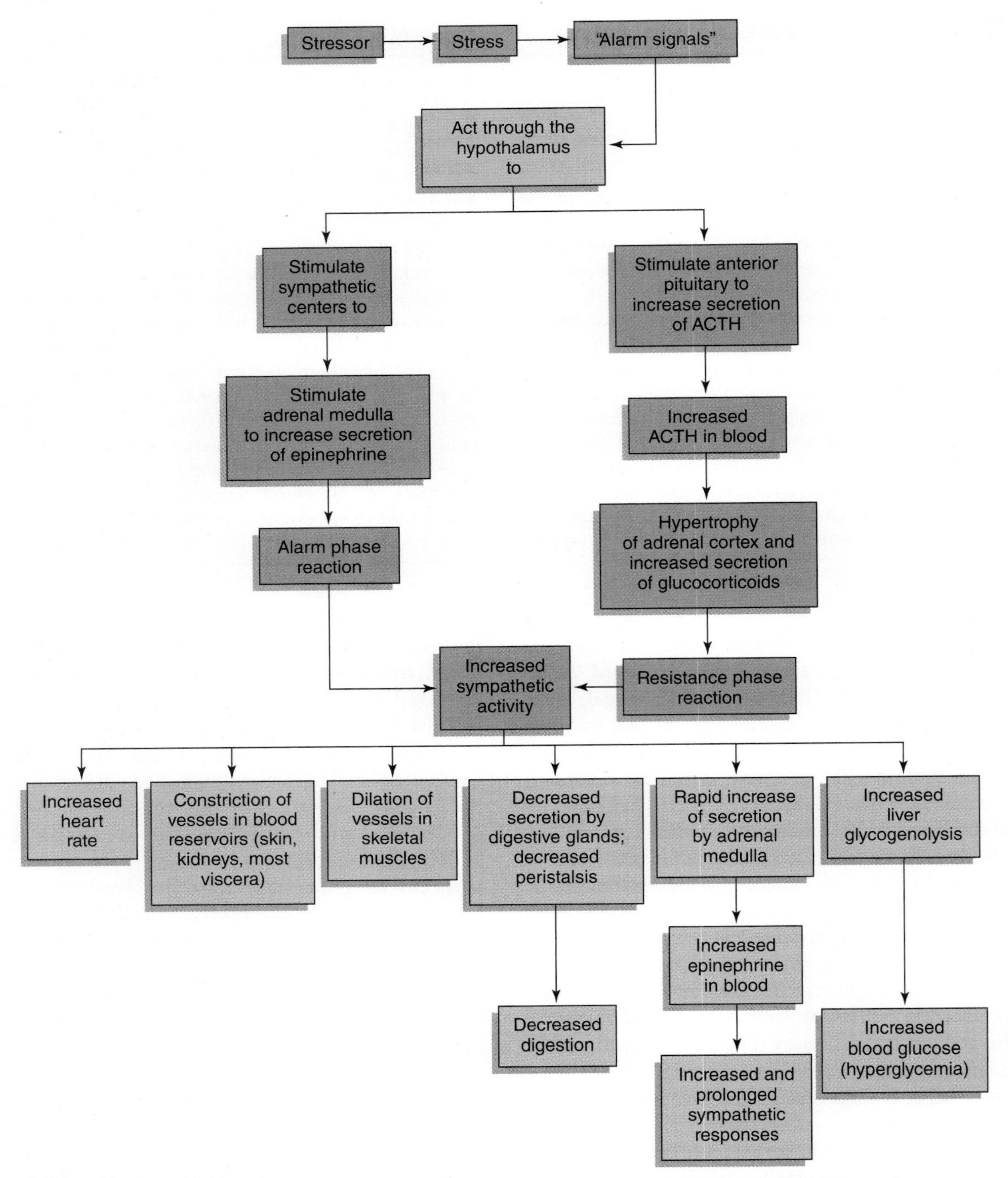

FIG. 2.14 Stress response. The word *stress* is currently used to refer to any stimulus that directly or indirectly stimulates neurons of the hypothalamus to release corticotropin-releasing hormone. Many hormones regulated by the hypothalamus come into play during stress. The main stress response of the autonomic nervous system can be summed up as the fight-or-flight response; this response is activated by an increase in the activity of the sympathetic nervous system. Some of the manifestations of sympathetic arousal are dilation of the pupils, an increased heart rate and blood pressure, an increased respiratory rate, dry mouth, and sweating hands. A manifestation of stress is the tensing of muscles, particularly in the neck, shoulders, and torso. Prolonged tension causes effects such as stiffness of the neck, backache, headache, and clenching of the teeth. *ACTH*, Adrenocorticotropic hormone.

individual has good internal resources and external support (Bobba-Alves et al., 2022). *Toxic stress* refers to a situation of unsuccessful coping because of a lack of internal coping skills and poor external support. *Allostatic overload* applies to toxic stress situations that cause physiological dysregulation and accelerate the development of disease (McEwen et al., 2015; Finlay et al., 2022a,b).

Perception of Stress

An individual's perception of stress is a significant factor related to stress coping. The brain cannot distinguish between a real or a potential threat. It does not matter if you are chasing someone who threatened you or if you are playing a video game in which you are chasing someone who is a threat. The

Box 2.17 Stress-Induced Disease

Stress affects all the body's organ systems, in a variety of ways.

1. *Digestive tract:* Diseases that may be caused or aggravated by stress include gastritis, stomach and duodenal ulcers, ulcerative colitis, and irritable colon.
2. *Reproductive organs:* Stress-related problems include infertility or difficulty conceiving, menstrual disorders or absence of menstrual periods in females, and impotence and premature ejaculation in males.
3. *Bladder:* A common stress response is sensitivity or irritability in the bladder, causing bladder urgency, bed-wetting, or incontinence.
4. *Brain:* Many mental and emotional problems—including anxiety, psychosis, and depression—may be triggered by stress.
5. *Hair:* Some forms of hair loss and baldness have been linked to elevated levels of stress.
6. *Mouth:* Sores, ulcers, and oral lichen planus (thrush) often seem to develop when a person is under stress.
7. *Lungs:* Asthma symptoms often worsen under high levels of mental or emotional stress.
8. *Heart:* Heart rate disturbances and angina attacks often occur during or after periods of stress.
9. *Muscles:* Muscle tension and its associated pain are often the result of stress, as are muscle twitches and nervous tics. The muscular tremor of Parkinson disease is also more marked at such times.

brain can respond to both only by triggering the fight-or-flight response. Stress is not simply a case of cause and effect. A variety of factors influence whether the fight-or-flight response is triggered, how long it remains switched on, and the degree to which it has a negative effect on us. Factors that influence the fight-or-flight response, some of which we can influence to reduce our stress, include:

- Perception of the event
- Social support
- Beliefs
- Diet
- Cumulative stressors
- Degree of control over the stressor
- Unpredictability of the stress
- Duration of the stressor

Some of the manifestations of arousal of the sympathetic nervous system are dilation of the pupils, increased heart rate and blood pressure, increased respiratory rate, dry mouth, and sweating hands. Gastrointestinal tract activity is diminished. Also, stress inhibits the production of thyroid, reproductive, and growth hormones to conserve energy. One of the manifestations of stress is the tensing of muscles, particularly in the neck, shoulders, and torso. Prolonged tension causes responses such as stiffness of the neck, backache, headache, and clenching of the teeth. Therapeutic massage is particularly helpful in managing this aspect of stress. Anything that is perceived as a threat—whether real or imagined—arouses fear or anxiety. How a person responds is influenced by other conditions; some are under conscious control, and some are not. A person's physical and mental health, hereditary predisposition and genetics, past experiences, current coping habits (learned and inborn), diet, environment, and social support all determine which stimuli are interpreted as stressors. Most stress management methods support the functions of the parasympathetic ANS (rest and restore).

People who experience excessive or ongoing stress often say they feel overwhelmed by tension, anger, fear, and frustration and the resulting anxiety. This causes adrenaline levels to rise, blood pressure and heart rate to increase, and breathing to change. Stressed individuals often experience one or more of these effects:

- Overbreathing often results in overoxygenation of the blood, which reduces carbon dioxide levels and leads to breathing pattern disorders. (This is discussed in more detail in Chapter 12.) This response can mark the beginning of panic attacks.
- Sleep disorders and depression commonly accompany long-term stress. A decrease in memory and in the ability to concentrate and solve problems also is common, as are complaints of stomach pain, heart palpitations, fatigue, and muscle aches.
- Blood levels of glucose and fatty acids rise, and the combination eventually causes plaque to be laid down in the arteries. This causes the development of coronary artery disease.
- Immune function becomes less effective, and the body is less capable of dealing with pathogens and cancer cells. Susceptibility to infection increases.
- Water retention caused by certain hormones increases blood volume, which can cause high blood pressure.
- Mood and behavior are affected by stress as well. An ongoing interplay occurs between physiological and psychological stress. This is best described by the chicken and egg question—which came first? Certainly, psychological stress can result in a physiological response, and the physiological stress response alters perception, mood, thought processes, and behavior, thus creating psychological stress. Another consequence of chronic stress is stress-induced disease, although the exact cause-and-effect relationship often is unclear.

Important Factors in Stress Management

Adaptation

One of the remarkable effects of change, internal and external, is the body's ability to adapt (Tian et al., 2022). The body is better able to adapt if changes occur gradually. Sudden changes, along with a diminished physiological reserve, can have dramatically negative effects on the body. Genetic makeup contributes to the effects of stress on the body. It is responsible for how well the organs adapt and respond to stressful situations. With age, the ability to adapt diminishes. Individuals who are fit mentally and physically are able to adapt to stress more easily than others. Those who are strongly motivated to live are well known to be capable of surviving the worst onslaughts made on their minds and bodies. Restorative and optimal amounts of sleep are important for restoring energy, regenerating tissue, and coping with stress. Irregular cycles of sleep and wakefulness can reduce immunity and physical and psychological functioning. Proper nutrition protects us from the detrimental effects of stress. Poor nutrition is itself a stress-causing agent.

A Homeostasis—ability to adapt—but at limit
B High stress load
C Falling apart—too much to carry and manage
D Stress coping. Reduce the load—eliminate some stressors and add social support
ME
SOCIAL SUPPORT
TRASH

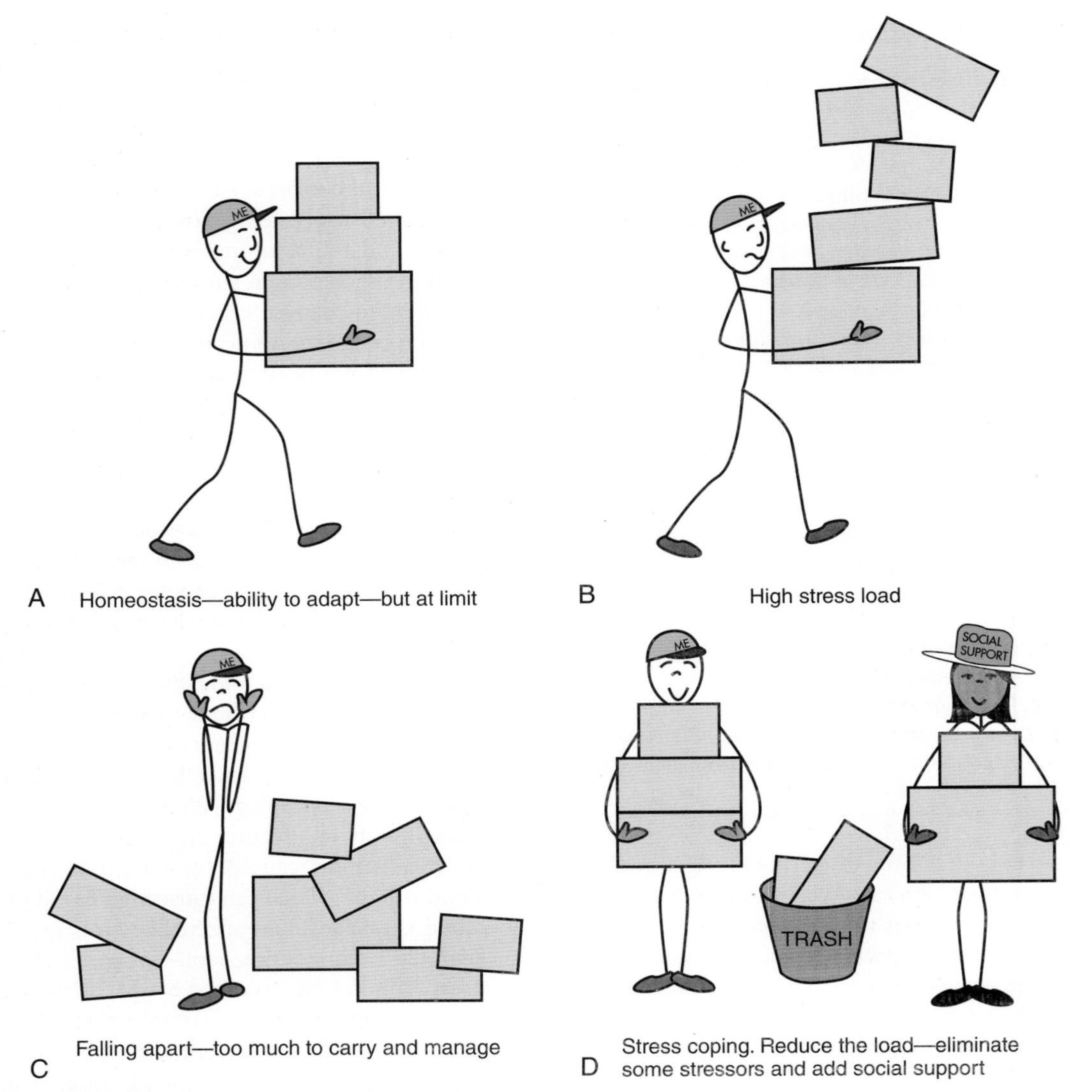

FIG. 2.15 Stress load. (A–D) It is not always the type of stress that causes problems, although some types of stress are more demanding than others. More often, the amount of the stress load and the need to balance many different things cause breakdown. Many stressors cannot be easily altered, and some cannot be altered at all. However, the stress load can be managed through physical mechanisms, such as exercise, diet, and relaxation methods, which allow the body to better cope with those stressors that cannot be changed. The stress load can be lightened by eliminating stressors that are possible to eliminate and by asking for help from social support, such as family, friends, and coworkers.

ACTIVITY 2.4

In Fig. 2.15, A, fill in the boxes with the stressors you can manage. In part B, fill in the stressors from part A, but also put in some additional stressors. In part C, fill in the stressors you listed in part B and add two more that would make the load too heavy. In part D, identify the stressors you can manage yourself. Write those in the boxes carried by the figure representing you. Identify two stressors that can be eliminated by putting them in the trash basket. Then identify two stressors that you can have someone help you with and write them in the boxes carried by the figure representing social support.

Medical Assistance

People are seeking medical assistance to help sort out and identify stress-related symptoms. Because each person responds to stress differently, accurate diagnoses become difficult. This lack of specificity has led to frustration in both clients and healthcare providers. As more research is done in the area of coping and adaptive capacities, the situation is continuing to improve. In contemporary health care, excessive long-term stress now is recognized as an important and widespread cause of disease.

Psychophysiology is the study of the interplay between psychological and physiological stressors and neuroimmunology; it is sometimes referred to as *psychoneuroimmunology*, or the study of the mind-immunity link within the larger field of the mind/body connection.

Additional Stress Management Techniques

A variety of approaches allow for additional ways of managing stress, as well as pain. Such approaches include massage and other forms of bodywork, along with acupuncture, meditation, and relaxation methods that use breathing, biofeedback, music therapy, hypnosis, exercise, and other forms of movement therapy.

The ancient wisdom of Indigenous peoples is now being understood through investigation by Western scientific methods. For example, therapeutic massage has been shown to reduce the levels of hormones associated with stress and to diminish the arousal level of the sympathetic nervous system—this results in the reestablishment of homeostatic balance.

Management of stress may require a multidisciplinary approach to resolve it or to achieve effective long-term management, and massage methods can play a part. A person's perception of stressful events, combined with the amount of stress, not the type of stress, determines the response. Anything that can change the perception of a threat to a perception of safety or that can reduce the intensity of the physical stress response promotes mechanisms of good health. These supportive changes include allowing for effective sleep, reducing pain, and establishing a sense of affiliation that supports effective social contact, as well as enhancement of the restorative and self-regulating processes of the body.

The stress response and stress syndrome are discussed throughout the text as they relate to each system studied.

Resilience

Resilience is the process of adapting well in the face of adversity, trauma, tragedy, threats, or significant sources of stress, such as family and relationship problems, serious health problems, or workplace and financial stressors. It means "bouncing back" from difficult experiences. Resilience involves maintaining flexibility and balance in your life as you deal with stressful circumstances and traumatic events. This happens in several ways, which people can develop in themselves. To develop resilience:

- Identify productive ways to alter demanding situations that enable you to control your reaction to adversity, even if you are unable to alter the situation. Discover ways to grow and learn by dealing with difficult situations.
- Develop realistic plans—along with the steps to carry them out—to deal with your problems and meet the demands of daily living. Also make sure to step back to rest and reenergize. Cultivate a positive view of yourself and confidence in your strengths and abilities, including your skills in communication and problem-solving.
- Allow yourself to experience strong emotions but develop the capacity to manage strong feelings and impulses and realize when you may need to avoid experiencing them at times to continue functioning. Actively seek ways to replace the losses encountered in life.
- Rely on yourself and others. Spend time with loved ones to gain support and encouragement, while also nurturing yourself. Relationships that create love and trust, provide role models, and offer encouragement and reassurance help bolster resilience.
- Realize and nurture your physical, mental, and spiritual health and pursue your sense of purpose and aspirations with persistence and patience while adapting to change.

Review What You Have Learned

- Define *health*.

  Health is the capacity to maintain homeostasis in response to stress.
- Define *stress*.

  Stress is anything that causes the body to respond or change to maintain homeostasis.
- Describe the parts of the ANS and the two functions of the ANS.
  - The sympathetic nervous system triggers the fight-or-flight response (accelerator pedal).
  - The parasympathetic nervous system reverses the fight-or-flight response (brake pedal).
- List various effects of excessive stress.

  Overbreathing, muscle stiffness, anxiety, depression, fatigue, heightened blood pressure, digestive problems, sleep disorders, and inhibited immune system function.
- Explain how humans adapt to and manage stress.

Mental and physical health influence adaptive capacity and resilience. A balanced lifestyle contributes to mental and physical health. Stress management techniques include massage, meditation, mindful breathing, and exercise.

Practical Application

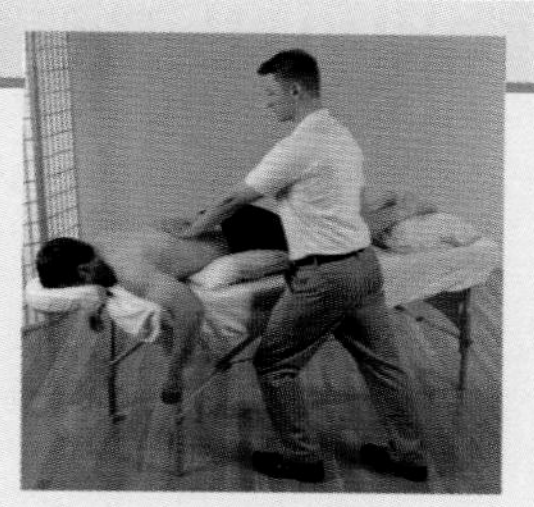

Massage therapy seems to introduce a different sort of stimulus. The body can respond to this stimulus through physiological coping mechanisms. Because unresolved stress increases the intensity of the stress syndrome, the signals introduced by massage help reset the system. Massage methods are usually pleasurable and comforting, and they can provide a soothing rhythmic pattern with which the recipient's body can entrain.

Massage is based on the premise of providing a safe touch that delivers balanced sensory stimulation, thus supporting good health for its recipients. Therefore massage can be an effective stress management tool.

THE LIFE CYCLE

SECTION OBJECTIVES

Chapter objectives covered in this section:

15. List the stages in the cycle of life.
16. Identify relevant health-supporting information and give some examples of ways to use this information to educate others.

After completing this section, the learner will be able to:

- Define *life*.
- Define *life cycle*.
- List six basic phases of the life cycle.
- Define *death*.
- Identify periods during the life cycle when humans are most vulnerable.
- Explain the aging process.
- Identify behaviors that support longevity.

Life can be defined as the expression of the functions (see Chapter 1) that distinguish living organisms from inorganic matter. The term *cycle* can be defined as a complete set of regularly recurring events in the same sequence within a specified period.

The life cycle can be understood as the expression of functions of life that begin and end in an expected and organized pattern:

- A human being is conceived by the joining of two cells, a process that reinforces the yin/yang concept of two opposites blending to make a whole.
- Cells multiply, divide, and differentiate, forming the human being.
- Birth brings forth an independent human, which remains in a dependent functioning state while accelerated growth and development occur.
- The human matures, connects, creates, and contributes.
- The human ages, and function declines.
- The human body dies.

During the beginning and ending of the life cycle—infancy and old age—the body is presented with its greatest challenges to homeostasis. The homeostatic mechanisms in infants and children are less regular than those in adults, because the young are in the process of creating their bodies. From adolescence through middle adulthood, humans have the most efficient bodily functions (Box 2.18).

Box 2.18 The Different Types of Life Cycles

As in every type of cycle (e.g., night and day, the seasons of the year), the life cycle is composed of a repeating pattern of events. All living things move from one life stage to the next, a pattern that is repeated over and over, generation after generation.

The Biological Life Cycle

The human biological life cycle consists of eight stages:

1. Conception
2. Birth
3. Infancy
4. Childhood
5. Adolescence
6. Adulthood
7. Old Age
8. Death
9. *Conception:* Conception is the act in which elements of the male (sperm) and female (ovum) combine to create an embryo. A human begins as a single cell, the tiniest building block of life. The human cells duplicate and specialize and become the fetus.
10. *Birth:* The baby moves out of the womb. The development of the infant, which weighs on average 5 to 10 pounds at birth, takes about 40 weeks from the time the first cell starts growing.
11. *Infancy:* Infancy extends from birth through the first year of life. The infant is dependent on caregivers to remain alive.
12. *Childhood:* From 1 year to about 12 years, a human is a child. For the first 2 years after infancy, the child is called a *toddler*.
13. *Adolescence:* Humans are adolescents roughly from age 12 to 18 years. In this stage, starting with puberty, The adolescent is preparing for adulthood, growing to maximum size, and is physically able to reproduce.
14. *Adulthood:* Humans reach the end of adolescence at 18 to 20 years, and adulthood begins. The life cycle usually starts over again during this stage, when, through reproduction, adults give birth to their own children.
15. *Older Adults:* This is the time of the life cycle when the body begins to break down. By the time humans reach 75 to 80 years of age, they typically are considered elderly.
16. *Death:* Death is the final stage of the life cycle. Humans die when their bodies are no longer able to carry on life functions.

The Psychological Life Cycle

Psychology provides another way to look at the human life cycle. Not only do we grow through stages physically, but we also grow emotionally. We can use Maslow's Hierarchy of Needs as a model for a psychological life cycle.

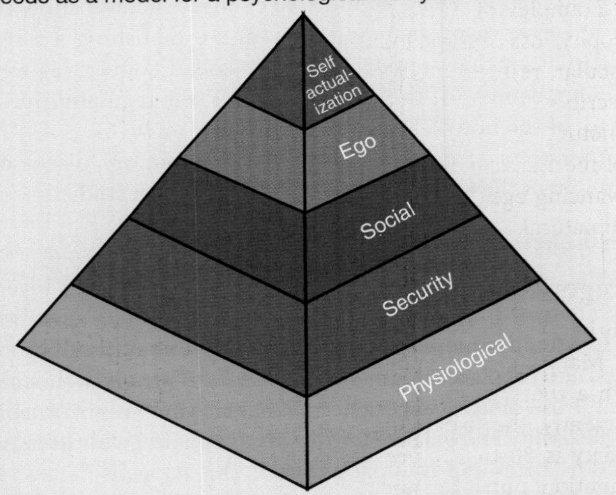

(Redrawn from Maslow AH; revised by Frager RD, et al., eds. *Motivation and Personality*. 3rd ed. Harper & Row; 1987. Reprinted with permission from Ann Kaplan.)

Maslow's Hierarchy of Needs

1. Physiological: At this stage we are most concerned with survival.
2. Security: In this stage of security, we stabilize resources to ensure survival.
3. Social: When we are secure enough to believe we can survive, we are able to develop family and friends.
4. Ego: The ego stage begins as we seek status within the social structure.
5. Self-actualization: This is the stage in which we are confident enough in our status, social support, security, and survival that we can begin the process of achieving our life's purpose.

Chakra System

A third way to view the cycle of life is by considering the symbolic stages of life referred to in the chakra system:

1. Root chakra 1: Conception, survival, preservation
2. Water chakra 2: Gestation, specialization
3. Solar plexus chakra 3: Birth, willpower
4. Heart chakra 4: Living, compassion
5. Throat chakra 5: Dying, communication
6. Brow chakra 6: Death, transformation, self-realization
7. Crown chakra 7: Expansion, purpose

The Aging Process

Normal aging affects the repair and replacement of the structural components of the body. Advancing age creates changes in cell numbers and their ability to function effectively. Changes occur in the production of hormones and in the receptors in target tissues that bind those hormones. Some hormonal levels increase, whereas others remain unchanged or decline.

There are many theories on aging, but the actual mechanics remain elusive to research. Three areas of research look at the physiological mechanics of aging, which seem to be associated with the following:

- Cellular changes produced by genetic and environmental factors
- Changes in cellular regularity and central processing
- Degenerative extracellular and vascular changes
- Oxidative stress

Examples of decreased functional ability include muscle atrophy, loss of the skin's elasticity, and changes in the cardiovascular, respiratory, and skeletal systems. The term *atrophy* describes the wasting effects of advancing age. In addition to structural atrophy, the functioning of many physiological control mechanisms also declines and becomes less precise with advancing age. The aging process is cumulative, progressive, and natural.

Longevity

Any behavior that supports cellular function enhances longevity. Many who live to advanced ages have lived simple lives with a sense of purpose, physical work, and social support. Currently, the usual life span of human beings in Western society is 80 to 100 years, but in societies that offer proper sanitation, nutrition, and health care, living beyond 100 years is becoming more common.

Life expectancy, or the average life span, has increased; females between the ages of 80 and 100 are the fastest growing segment of many populations. In general, females live longer than males because of the influences of genetics, hormones, immunity, and social roles.

Many scientific advances are increasing the potential for a long and physical life. However, the most important components continue to be a balanced lifestyle with a sense of purpose.

Health Education, Resources, and the Massage Therapist's Responsibilities

The health messages we provide to clients are an important part of massage therapy (Boulanger and Campo, 2013; Kennedy et al., 2018). The terms "massage" and "massage therapy" do not mean the same thing. This is an important concept. Researcher Ann Blair Kennedy and others have made important distinctions by explaining *massage* as a patterned and planned soft tissue manipulation and *massage therapy* as a more complex therapeutic interaction that includes elements of health education and messaging, therapeutic relationships, communication, and the therapeutic context (Kennedy et al., 2015). Massage therapy consists of the application of massage, as well as the non-hands-on components of therapeutic interaction, including health promotion and educational messages for self-care and health maintenance (Kennedy et al., 2016).

Massage therapists often work with retention-based clients (i.e., clients seen regularly), which allows for reinforcement of health promotion messages. It is important for therapists to make sure they are giving correct, evidence-informed information and to stay within their scope of practice. Massage therapists can include information about evidence-informed beneficial lifestyle behaviors in the massage session. The information should be general and informative, but not prescriptive (Box 2.19).

Discussing simple and general stress and pain management strategies with clients is appropriate for the massage therapist. Teaching clients about pain neurobiology also is appropriate, especially for those who have chronic/persistent pain. The content in this chapter can be a foundation for this type of information. Massage therapists can discuss moderate, nonprescriptive exercise information related to the benefits

Box 2.19 Public Health

Public health is the science of protecting and improving the health of people and their communities. This work is achieved by promoting healthy lifestyles, researching disease and injury prevention, and detecting, preventing, and responding to infectious diseases. Health should be seen as more than simply a life without illness. The World Health Organization (WHO) acknowledges this in its definition of health. WHO defines health as a state of complete physical, mental, and social well-being, and not merely the absence of disease or infirmity.

Overall, public health is concerned with protecting the health of entire populations. These populations can be as small as a local neighborhood, or as big as an entire country or region of the world.

Public health professionals try to prevent problems from developing or recurring. They implement educational programs, recommend policies, administer services, and conduct research. In contrast, clinical professionals, such as doctors and nurses, focus primarily on treating individuals after they become sick or are injured. Public health also works to limit health disparities. A large part of public health is promoting healthcare equity, quality, and accessibility.

The Centers for Disease Control and Prevention (CDC) is the United States leading public health agency. It is dedicated to saving lives and protecting the health of Americans. The CDC focuses on controlling disease outbreaks, working with other federal agencies to make sure food and water are safe, helping people avoid the leading causes of death (e.g., heart disease, cancer, stroke, and diabetes), and working globally to reduce threats to the nation's health. The CDC works to strengthen local and state public health departments and promote proven health programs.

The CDC's headquarters are in Atlanta, Georgia. The agency has a staff of more than 14,000 employees, in nearly 170 occupations, who work in all 50 states and more than 50 countries. You can learn more about the CDC by visiting its website: https://www.cdc.gov.

of massage therapy and the evidence-informed outcomes for massage: that is, well-being/relaxation, stress management, pain management, and functional mobility.

Review What You Have Learned

- Define *life*.
  Life is the expression of biological functions (movement, reproduction, and so on) that living animals and plants display, which distinguishes them from inorganic matter.
- Define *life cycle*.
  The life cycle is the expression of biological functions that begin and end in an expected and organized pattern.
- List six basic phases of the life cycle.
  Conception, fetal development, birth, physical/functional growth, physical/function decline (aging), death.
- Define *death*.
  Death is the phase in which biological function (yang) separates from inorganic matter (yin).
- Identify periods during the life cycle when humans are most vulnerable.
  Humans are most vulnerable at the beginning and end of the life cycle (infancy and old age).
- Explain the aging process.
  Normal aging concerns the regular repair and replacement of body structures. Advanced aging concerns the eventual decline in cellular capacity for repair and replacement.
- Identify behaviors that support longevity.

Developing a sense of purpose, living a healthy lifestyle, and maintaining social support.

SUMMARY

In this chapter, we looked at homeostasis and factors influencing health and disease. Homeostasis consists of balancing mechanisms that are in constant communication with each other in a feedback loop system. Many factors can disrupt homeostasis, yet in most situations, the body can respond effectively and restore efficient functioning. We are equipped with the ability to deal with many different types of stressors. However, stress coping mechanisms can be overloaded by an accumulated load of unresolved stress, which contributes to the development of disease and pain.

There are many reasons for pain, types of pain, and ways to manage pain. Acute pain can be a friend by alerting us to an emergency. Even chronic/persistent pain can be a gauge by which to monitor the effectiveness of therapy and the return to health (or as near to health as possible). The perception of a threat often makes a significant difference in the body's response to life events. Perception is something that can be altered with diligent work and awareness, coupled with professional assistance when necessary.

We are conceived and born; we live and die. As we travel through life, each event is equally important in the total experience of being. It is the goal of the massage professional to promote health and well-being throughout all the stages of existence.

As massage therapists, we can be educators in wellness and coaches in the ongoing dynamic of homeostasis by becoming competent and able to recognize and support health mechanisms in ourselves and the clients we serve. We must assess for and identify disease, be able to refer clients effectively as necessary, and develop appropriate treatment plans for clients with disease processes. We must also integrate our skills proficiently with those of others in the healthcare community when medical professionals supervise us. Massage can be a valuable tool in the treatment and management of many health concerns, especially those related to stress. The information in this chapter is essential for the massage professional to be able to plan and organize an effective therapeutic massage session.

CRITICAL THINKING/CLINICAL REASONING

Each chapter will feature a critical thinking and clinical reasoning application of the content related to the practice of massage therapy. A client scenario will be presented, with recommendations for additional research, often using MedlinePlus or PubMed. Relevant questions based on the chapter content outline are provided to guide the discussion. There are no specific current answers to the questions. However, responses should be supported by evidence-informed practices and based on biological plausibility (see Chapter 1) if sufficient research is not available. The authors' decision-making process with regard to the scenario and questions is presented on the Evolve site. Compare and contrast your thoughts and discussions to those of the authors and determine where you agree or disagree.

SCENARIO

The client is a 24-year-old student who came to your office for a massage. The client was referred to you by their parents who are regular clients and felt that a massage could help with school stress, especially since finals were coming up.

First session history intake process reveals that the client is under considerable stress from a full load of college classes. In addition, they work approximately 15 hours a week as a server at a local restaurant. Medical history reveals the client experiences seasonal allergies. The client has ongoing neck pain from carrying trays of food at the restaurant.

The client has limited personal time and rarely exercises. The neck pain is described as a dull ache that comes and goes and includes a headache and stiffness, which they said is a level 5 to 6 (on a 0 to 10 Visual Analog scale, with 0 being no pain and 10 being unbearable pain).

Your assessment shows a mildly restricted range of motion in their neck during left lateral flexion, with moderately palpable muscle tenderness in the right trapezius. There is increased muscle tone in the right paracervical muscles.

Discuss the client's health status and plan different ways we might help her.

Explore MedlinePlus

Use the search terms *stress* and *pain*.
https://medlineplus.gov/stress.html
https://medlineplus.gov/pain.html

Also look to see whether current research is available on massage therapy, stress, and pain.

Search PubMed

Use these search terms: massage therapy and stress, massage therapy and neck pain, massage therapy and headache, and massage therapy and pain management.
https://www.ncbi.nlm.nih.gov/pubmed/

Discuss These Points

- How are the client's situations and behaviors challenging adaptive capacity?
- What overlapping themes related to homeostasis are influencing the client?
- How might the current status relate to feedback loops and biological rhythms?
- What sort of disease-based terminology might be used to describe the neck discomfort?
- What are the main risk factors for homeostatic disruption?
- How might the pain the client is experiencing be classified and addressed?
- If the client were to choose the salutogenic model for developing a massage care plan, how would that differ from a pathogenic-based massage care plan?
- The client is stressed by multiple factors. How might massage be a stress management strategy?
- How would you describe the level of resilience, and what education-based information could you provide without violating the massage therapy scope of practice?
- How does age affect the client's current status and ability to respond to the behavioral changes needed to improve the current quality of life?
- Do you agree with this statement: The neck pain and headaches are caused by their job and are not related to being a college student.

The authors' responses to these questions and their decision-making process can be found on the Evolve website.

Visit the Evolve website: https://evolve.elsevier.com/Fritz/essential/

The Evolve website provides support for the review of the chapter content and chapter quizzes to help you prepare for the MBLEx or other massage therapy certification or licensing exams. End-of-chapter questions for discussion and review answer key and rationales and authors' responses to critical thinking and clinical reasoning scenarios.

MULTIPLE CHOICE QUESTIONS FOR REVIEW AND DISCUSSION

The answers, with rationales, can be found on the Evolve site.

These questions are used for review and discussion. It is as important to understand why wrong answers are wrong as it is to know why the correct answer is correct. The answers to the questions, with rationales and explanations about why the correct answer is correct and why wrong answers are wrong, can be found on the Evolve site. At the end of the question section here in the textbook, you will find an exercise that asks you to write more questions. Use the various questions in the chapter as examples. This is one of the best study strategies for test-taking.

It is important to understand that the actual licensing exam you take may not contain any of the specific questions found in this textbook or the review material and practice tests on the Evolve site. Therefore just because you can answer any of these questions correctly does not mean you will pass the licensing exam. The questions are content and style examples to help you prepare—this is why understanding why wrong answers are wrong is just as important as identifying the correct answer. Also, make sure you understand all the terminology used in the questions and possible answers in the review and discussion questions. Look up words you do not understand.

1. The massage outcome is determined to be a reduction in blood pressure. Which of these is most correct?
   a. This is a positive feedback response.
   b. This is a virulent response.
   c. This would be a negative feedback loop.
   d. This would be a reduction of a fistula.
2. When massage stimulates sensory receptors to create a response within the homeostatic mechanism, this is considered ______.
   a. Salutogenesis
   b. A feedback loop
   c. General adaptation syndrome
   d. Threshold and tolerance
3. What do these terms have in common: biofeedback, massage, aromatherapy, medication, and hypnosis?
   a. Strategies for pain management
   b. Methods of massage
   c. Risk factors for resilience
   d. Methods of controlling inflammation
4. A client informs the massage practitioner they are experiencing hair loss, mouth ulcers, and bladder urgency. How are these symptoms related?
   a. They are examples of inflammatory stress.
   b. They are stress/pain modulators.
   c. They are genetic disease risk factors.
   d. They are stress-related disease symptoms.
5. Feedback is an essential aspect of homeostasis because of ______.
   a. Afferent discharge
   b. Effector response
   c. Information exchange
   d. Efferent signaling
6. Massage is part of a feedback loop in the ______.
   a. Controlled condition
   b. Control center
   c. Response
   d. Stimulus
7. Many benefits of massage are a result of ______.
   a. Nonspecific stimulus that encourages a feedback response to a more optimum function
   b. Precise application of selected stimulus-creating positive feedback
   c. Positive feedback response to return function to homeostasis

d. Specific treatment for nociceptive and neuropathic pain

8. People experience relaxed mood states when biological rhythms______.
   a. create sympathetic patterns
   b. are oscillated independently
   c. downregulate resilience
   d. reflect parasympathetic patterns
9. A client was treated successfully for lung cancer and is in remission. However, this client continues to experience pain sensations in the extremities and back. What best explains the client's situation?
   a. The cancer treatment caused ongoing nociceptive pain.
   b. Persistent discomfort is related to neuroplasticity.
   c. Mixed pain was treated inappropriately with an opiate medication.
   d. The sensations stem from neuromatrix dysfunction.
10. Relaxation methods that focus on breathing produce benefit because ______.
    a. Cortisol increases during parasympathetic response.
    b. The respiratory rate is a major biological oscillator.
    c. Sympathetic mechanisms are generated.
    d. Breathing function regulates the nociceptive system.
11. Inflammation that persists beyond beneficial healing is considered an inflammatory disease. This chronic type of local inflammation may be helped by which form of massage?
    a. Extensive application of deep transverse friction
    b. Light surface stroking
    c. Controlled use of friction, stretching, and pulling
    d. Brisk beating and pounding
12. Systemic inflammatory disease is related to ______.
    a. condition resolution
    b. local injury
    c. oxidative stress.
    d. contraindication to massage
13. A client's lower back pain returns within 3 hours of receiving a massage. What organ may be the cause of referred back pain?
    a. Bladder
    b. Kidney
    c. Stomach
    d. Gallbladder
14. Massage used as a pain management strategy is a form of ______.
    a. Stimulus-induced analgesia
    b. Opiate antagonist
    c. Dermatomal inhibition
    d. Prostaglandin stimulation
15. If a pathological condition occurs because of a state of "too much" or "not enough," then health would occur because of ______.
    a. Increased immune activity
    b. Decreased sympathetic arousal response
    c. Effective feedback and adaptive capacity
    d. Tolerance and hardiness
16. When a person perceives an event as a threat, this activates the alarm reaction. What is the first response?
    a. The sympathetic centers activate.
    b. The hypothalamus is stimulated.
    c. The adrenal cortex releases glucocorticoids.
    d. The adrenal medulla releases epinephrine.
17. Many aspects of ancient healing wisdom are being shown as valid stress management strategies because these practices ______.
    a. Support an increase in the heart rate
    b. Reduce sympathetic arousal
    c. Increase the production of glucocorticoids
    d. Increase the blood glucose level
18. A client comes to you complaining of aching pain just under the ribs right of the midline, under the right scapula, and in the right neck and shoulder area. The pain has been occurring more frequently and is now almost constant. The referred pain pattern might indicate problems with what organ?
    a. Bladder
    b. Kidney
    c. Stomach
    d. Gallbladder
19. A massage client does not provide effective feedback about the amount of pressure requested for the massage. The client had asked for very deep pressure. As the massage professional, you keep asking whether the pressure is causing pain, and the client says no. It seems that any deeper pressure may cause bruising and other tissue damage. This client may be exhibiting ______.
    a. Counterirritation
    b. Reduced influence of beta-endorphins
    c. High pain tolerance
    d. Hyperstimulation analgesia
20. A client, who is 69, has had to deal with multiple stressors, including a family death and having their car stolen. The client is not sleeping well and shares with the massage therapist that they are feeling overwhelmed. Which of these most logically explains the client's feelings?
    a. The client has a reduced stress threshold, which is straining the cortisol enhancement of the immune system.
    b. The client's ability to adapt to the multiple stressors is challenged by advanced age.
    c. The client's adaptive capacity is adequate, but the family death is enough to increase mental strain.
    d. The client's stress response is increasing adaptive capacity, which is challenged by age-related immune suppression.

Write Your Own Test Questions

Create at least three more multiple choice questions. Make sure to develop plausible wrong answers and double-check that the correct answer is correct. Then write a rationale for each question. The more questions you write, the better you will understand the material.

Terminology: Scientific, Medical, Social, and Cultural Communication

CHAPTER 3

https://evolve.elsevier.com/Fritz/essential/

CHAPTER OBJECTIVES

After completing this chapter, the learner will be able to:

1. Identify the importance of terminology essential for the practice of therapeutic massage.
2. Use medical terminology to interpret the meanings of anatomical and physiological terms.
3. Define terms used to describe regions of the body and surface anatomy.
4. Define terms used to describe the positions of the body and the parts of the body in relation to other body parts.
5. Define *kinesiology*, body planes, and terms of movement.
6. Describe and use quality of life terminology.
7. Explore terminology used in Indigenous and cultural-based healing systems.
8. Use a charting method that incorporates a clinical reasoning/problem-solving model.

CHAPTER OUTLINE

Key Terms

activities of daily living (ADLs): Normal activities we carry out each day. They include self-care, such as eating, bathing, dressing, grooming, going to work, housekeeping duties, and leisure activities.

acupuncture: The practice of inserting needles at specific points on meridians, or channels. This stimulates or sedates energy flow to regulate or alter body function. A branch of Chinese medicine, acupuncture is the art and science of manipulating the flow of Qi, the basic life force; and of xue, the blood, body fluids, and nourishing essences.

biomechanics: The principles and methods of mechanics applied to the structure and function of the human body.

charting/documentation: The process of keeping a written record of a client or patient. The most effective charting methods follow clinical reasoning, which emphasizes a problem-solving approach. Many systems of charting are used, but they all have similar components based on the problem-oriented medical record (POMR) and SOAP (subjective, objective, analysis/assessment, and plan).

combining vowel: A vowel added between two roots or a root and a suffix to make the pronunciation of the word easier.

kinematics: **(kin-i-MAT-ics)** A branch of mechanics that involves the aspects of time, space, and mass in a moving system.

kinesiology: **(ki-ne-ze-OL-o-je)** The study of movement that combines the fields of anatomy, physiology, physics, and geometry and relates them to human movement.

kinetics: **(ki-NET-ics)** The forces that cause movement in a system.

mechanics: The branch of physics that deals with the study of forces and the motion produced by their actions.

medical terminology: Terms used to describe the human body, medical treatments and conditions, and processes of health care in a science-based manner.

motion: A change in position with respect to some reference frame or starting point.

prefix: A word element added to the start of a root to change the meaning of the word.

quality of life: Individuals' perceptions of their position in life in the context of the culture and value systems in which they live and in relation to their goals, expectations, standards, and concerns.

root: A word element that contains the basic meaning of the word.

suffix: A word element added to the end of a root to change the meaning of the word.
terminology: A vocabulary used by people involved in a specialized activity or field of work. Also, the study of the meaning of words used in a language.
word elements: The parts of a word: the prefix, root, and suffix.

LEARNING HOW TO LEARN

This chapter is about learning a language. As you encounter each new word, translate it into an example that you understand. For example, the definition of **terminology** is a vocabulary used by people involved in a specialized activity or field of work; also, the study of the meaning of words used in a language. How would you explain this definition to yourself? Maybe you would describe terminology as the words used to describe a unique language people use to understand one another at work or when talking to one another about a task. The learning happens as you try to figure out how to say the same thing differently.

Especially when learning the definition of words, you must review the material over and over again. You need to see the material at least four times—ideally at least six times. Each time you review the same information, you need to do it uniquely. Examples are flashcards, singing the terms and definitions, listening to someone else read them to you, writing the terms and definitions, listening to music while reviewing, and reading the terms and definitions aloud. This book offers activities to help you with new types of review methods.

You also need to review the material over several days, and then once every week or so to keep yourself from forgetting it. The adage "Use it or lose it" is especially true when it comes to terminology! Remember to take your "brain breaks"—study for about 30 minutes, then take a short break. Mindless tasks are productive during brain breaks. Water the plants, take out the trash, or do some dishes.

We need to be able to communicate using terms that are meaningful and understandable. Consider these definitions:

- A *word* is a speech sound or series of speech sounds that symbolize and communicate a meaning.
- A *term* is a word or an expression that has a precise meaning peculiar to a science, art, profession, or subject.
- A *vocabulary* is made up of the words used or understood by a particular person or group; it also includes technical terms used in a particular field, subject, science, or art.
- *Communication* is the exchange of information.
- *Terminology* is a vocabulary used by people involved in a specialized activity or field of work; it is also the study of the meaning of words used in a language. *Terminology* is a language of communication, with a system of words used to name things in a particular discipline.

For example, the title of this textbook is *Mosby's Essential Sciences for Therapeutic Massage*. The words in this title have a meaning relevant to your massage therapy studies. The word *essential* means "relevant and necessary." Something is relevant if it is pertinent, connected, and applicable to a given purpose. Our purpose is the study of therapeutic massage. *Science* refers to a system of acquiring knowledge through observation and experimentation to describe and explain natural phenomena. The word *science* comes from the Latin *scientia*, meaning knowledge. Science can be any systematic field of study or the knowledge gained from it. Knowledge is an understanding gained through experience or study by learning facts and information, resulting in the ability to do something. Because the word in the title is *sciences*, it means more than one science (Box 3.1). *Therapeutic* refers to the capability to restore and maintain health.

Box 3.1 Branches of Science

Physics is the science that deals with matter and energy and their interactions. Matter makes up physical objects. It deals with the fundamental particles of which the universe is made and the interactions between those particles, the objects composed of them (e.g., nuclei, atoms, molecules), and energy.

Chemistry is the science that deals with the composition, structure, and properties of substances and with the transformations that they undergo. We learned a little bit about chemistry in Chapter 1.

Biology is the science of living organisms and vital processes. It describes the characteristics, classification, and behaviors of organisms; how species come into existence; and the interactions of species with one another and with the environment. We started learning about biology in Chapter 1, and Chapter 2 was all about biology. Much of the information in this textbook is based on biology.

Earth science or geoscience is the study of the planet Earth. Eventually, we will even cover a little bit about earth sciences in this book.

According to the Model Practice Act developed by the Federation of State Massage Therapy Boards, massage therapy is a healthcare profession:

> *(A) The practice of Massage Therapy means the manual application of a system of structured touch to the soft tissues of the human body, including but not limited to: (1) Assessment, evaluation, or treatment; (2) Pressure, friction, stroking, rocking, gliding, kneading, percussion or vibration; (3) Active or passive stretching of the body within the normal anatomical range of movement; (4) Use of manual methods or mechanical or electrical devices or tools that mimic or enhance the action of human hands; (5) Use of hot or cold applications; (6) Use of hydrotherapy; and (7) Client education (Section 104. Practice of Massage Therapy).*

As defined by the Massage Therapy Body of Knowledge (MTBOK) massage therapy is a healthcare and wellness profession involving the manipulation of soft tissue. In 2013 the Entry Level Analysis Projects (ELAP), which was sponsored by the Coalition of National Massage Therapy Organizations, defined bodywork and massage as follows:

Bodywork—A broad term that refers to many forms, methods, and styles, including massage, that positively influence the body through various methods that may or may not include soft tissue deformation, energy manipulation, movement reeducation, and postural reeducation.

Massage—The ethical and professional application of structured, therapeutic touch to benefit soft tissue health, movement, posture, and neurological patterns. *Healthcare-oriented massage* is a massage performed in medical or healthcare-oriented environments to facilitate therapeutic change, condition management, or symptom management. *Wellness-oriented massage* is a massage performed in wellness or relaxation-oriented environments to facilitate stress reduction, relaxation, or wellness https://elapmassage.org).

In her 2015 doctoral dissertation "A Qualitative Study of the Massage Therapy Foundation's Best Practices Symposium: Clarifying Definitions and Creating a Framework for Practice," researcher Ann Blair Kennedy offered this definition of massage therapy practice:

> *Massage therapy practice is a client-centered framework for providing massage therapy through a process of assessment and evaluation, plan of care, treatment, reassessment and reevaluation, health messages, document, and closure to improve health and/or well-being. Massage therapy practice is influenced by the scope of practice and professional standards and ethics (Kennedy, 2015).*

The purpose of this textbook is to provide you with the knowledge you must have to be able to function professionally in a massage therapy practice. Massage professionals work with their clients' anatomy and physiology; this is an aspect of the science of biology. We need to be able to communicate intelligently with clients, colleagues, and other healthcare professionals. Therefore standard terminology is necessary. Without a common language, healthcare practitioners cannot effectively communicate.

Massage therapists have an ethical responsibility to develop and continually improve these skills:

- Communicate with their clients in a common language
- Understand and communicate across disciplines with other healthcare professionals
- Communicate cross-culturally to appreciate different perspectives on health and healing

This chapter introduces you to the basic concepts necessary to accomplish these goals:

- Enable communication in standardized scientific and medical terms
- Consider a model of cross-cultural terminology
- Use a clinical reasoning approach in client care

Terminology relevant to massage is an ongoing study. Terminology is an area of study that requires memorization, which occurs only with repetition and periodic review. It is like learning a new language. To become proficient, you need to speak and use it often.

LANGUAGE OF SCIENCE AND MEDICINE

SECTION OBJECTIVES

Chapter objectives covered in this section:

1. Identify the importance of terminology essential for the practice of therapeutic massage.
2. Use medical terminology to interpret the meanings of anatomical and physiological terms.

After completing this section, the learner will be able to:

- Identify three word elements used in medical terms.
- Use a medical dictionary.
- Combine word elements into medical terms.
- Identify abbreviations used in health care and their meanings.

Medical terminology uses terms derived from Latin or Greek to describe the human body, medical treatments and conditions, and processes of health care in a science-based manner.

Most scientific and medical terms are derived from fundamental elements of Latin or Greek, the most widely known language bases in the Western world. These elements are combined to form scientific terms, which include medical terms. Once you know the meaning of the fundamental elements, a term can be interpreted easily by separating the word into its elements: prefix, root, and suffix.

Each of the following sections includes a list of some of the more common word elements. These lists are not meant to be all-encompassing; rather, they provide enough examples for you to gain a general understanding of most of the terms encountered by therapeutic massage professionals.

Practical Application

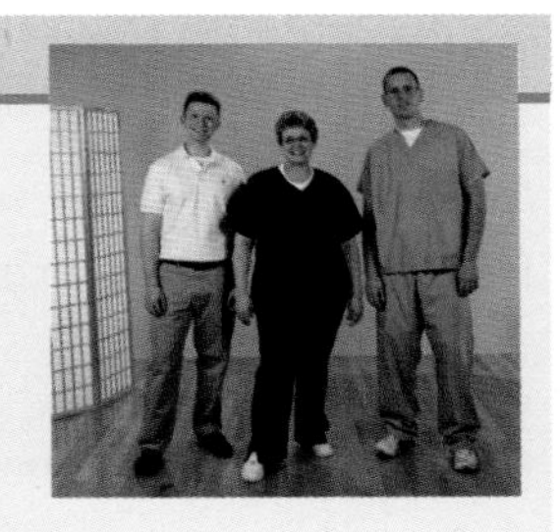

Most learners are required to take tests to measure their competency in therapeutic massage. Sometimes the tests are given in school in the form of quizzes and exams. Mandated licensing tests and voluntary certification tests demonstrate that you have skills that exceed the entry-level requirements of licensing. For all these tests, you must be able to read and understand the questions.

Sometimes test takers become confused because they do not know the meanings of the words in the questions. This is where ongoing study of and practice using medical terminology can help. If you know the meanings of the word elements that make up the terms, you can figure out what the word means. Even if you are not sure of the definition of the word, you may still be able to make a well-educated guess about the meaning of the question. If you spend time becoming confident with scientific terminology and the meaning of common word elements, it will help you be a more confident test taker.

WORD ELEMENTS USED IN MEDICAL TERMS

Prefixes

A **prefix** is an element placed at the beginning of a word to change the meaning of the word. A prefix cannot stand alone; it must be combined with another **word element**. A vowel, called a **combining vowel**, is often used to join word elements. The combining vowel used most often is *o*, but occasionally *i* or another vowel is used. Presents a list of the more common prefixes and some examples of accompanying combining vowels. These prefixes will help you to recognize and understand scientific and medical terminology (Table 3.1).

Roots

The **root** (or stem) word element provides the fundamental meaning of the word. Roots are combined with prefixes and

Table 3.1 Common Prefixes and Their Meanings

Prefix	Meaning	Prefix	Meaning	Prefix	Meaning
A-, an-	Without or not	Febr(i, o)-	Fever, boil	Onc(o)-	Tumor, mass
Ab-	Away from	Fract-	Break, broken	Ortho(o)-	Straight, erect, correct
Acr(o)-	Extremity, tip	Fund-	Base, bottom	Osm(io, o)-	Smell, odor
Ad-	Toward	Gen-	Beginning, origin, produce	Oxy-	Sharp, acute, acid
Alba-	White	Gluc-	Sweet, sugar, glucose	Palp-	Touch, feel
Ambi-	Both, on sides	Gyn(a, e, eco, o)-	Female	Pan-	All
Ana-	Upward, backward, excessive, through	Hemi-	Half	Para-	Abnormal, near
Andr(o)-	Male	Heter-	Other, different	Path(o)-	Disease, suffering
Ankyl(o)-	Crooked, fused, stiff	Hol-	Whole, all	Pept(o)-	Digestion
Ante-	Before, forward	Hom(eo, o)-	Unchanged, alike, same	Per-	By, through
Anti-	Against, opposed	Hyg(ei, ie)-	Health	Peri-	Around
Audi-	Hear	Hyper-	Excessive, too much, high	Phag(o)-	Eat, consume
Auto-	Self	Hypo-	Under, decreased, less than normal	Pharmaco-	Drugs, poison, medication
Bi-	Double, two	Iatr(o)-	Physician	Physio-	Natural, physical agents
Bio-	Life, living matter	Idio-	Distinct, peculiar to the individual	Poly-	Many, much
Brach-	Short	Immuno-	Protection	Post-	After, behind
Brady(o)-	Slow, short, dull	In-	In, into, within, not	Pre-	Before, in front of, prior to
Carcin(o)-	Cancer, malignant	Infra-	Beneath	Pro-	Before, in front of
Cata-	Down, negative, under, against, lower	Inter-	Between	Pseudo-	False
Caud-	Tail, inferior	Intra-	Within	Quadr(a, i)-	Four
Cent(i)-	Hundred	Intro-	Into, within	Re-	Again
Chron(i, o, us)-	Time, long time	Iso-	Equal, like, identical	Retro-	Backward
Circum-	Around	Juxta-	Adjoining, near to	Schist(o)-	Split, divided
Contra-	Against, opposite	Kyph(o)-	Bend, hump	Scler(o)-	Hard
Counter-	Against, opposite	Lact(o)-	Milk	Semi-	Half
Cry(mo, o)-	Cold	Later(al, o)-	Side	Sepsi-	Putrid, rotten
De-	Down, from, away from, not	Leuk-	White	Son(o)-	Sound
Dext-	Right	Levo-	Left	Steno-	Contracted, narrow
Di-	Two, double, twice	Macro-	Large	Strat(i)-	Layer
Dia-	Across, through, apart	Mal-	Bad, illness, disease	Sub-	Under
Dis-	Separation, away from	Mega-	Large	Super-	Above, over, excess
Dys-	Bad, difficult, abnormal	Micro-	Small	Supra-	Above, over
Ecto-	Outer, outside	Mono-	One, single	Therm-	Warm
Endo-	Inner, inside	Multi-	Many	Tract-	Pull down
Epi-	Over, on, upon	Necr(o)-	Death, destruction, corpse	Trans-	Across
Eryth-	Red	Neo-	New	Ultr(a, o)-	Excessive, extreme, beyond
Esthesi-	Sensation	Noct(i, o)-	Night	Uni-	One
Etio-	Cause	Non-	Not	Zyg(o, us)-	Yoke, join, together
Ex-	Out, out of, from, awway from	Olig-	Small, scanty		

suffixes to form medical and scientific terms. In medicine, the root word often refers to a part of the body. As with prefixes, a combining vowel is often added when two roots are combined or when a suffix is added to a root. The combining vowel is usually *o*, but occasionally it is *i*. Table 3.2 presents some of the more common root words and their accompanying combining vowels.

Suffixes

A **suffix** is a word element that is added to the end of a root to change the meaning of the word. Suffixes cannot stand alone. The suffix is the starting point when you want to interpret a scientific term. Roots that end in a consonant require a combining vowel when a suffix is added. If the root ends with a vowel and the suffix begins with a vowel, the vowel at the end of the root is deleted. Table 3.3 presents a list of some of the more common suffixes.

References

A medical dictionary is a necessity. A good dictionary holds an enormous amount of information. It is the place to begin your research to clarify the meanings of words and topics. When selecting a medical dictionary, you should choose one that is encyclopedic and illustrated. Consider using *Mosby's Dictionary of Medicine, Nursing, and Health Professions*. A dictionary's table of contents indicates how expansive it is and whether it contains a special section on medical terminology. Even with all the electronic technology available, it's still a smart idea to have a good old-fashioned paper medical dictionary for the convenience of accessing the reference material.

Electronic reference resources are also helpful. Excellent websites and apps are available that provide electronic medical dictionaries, encyclopedias, and other reference materials.

Activity 3.1 gives you a chance to create some medical terms of your own.

ACTIVITY 3.1

The beauty of medical terminology is that it allows new words to be created as needed. From the lists of prefixes, root words, and suffixes, make up five silly words and define them.

Example

Oligorhinoscoliosis: *oligo*, small; *rhino*, nose; *scoliosis*, curve

Your Turn

- 1.
- 2.
- 3.
- 4.
- 5.

Abbreviations

Abbreviations are shortened forms of words or phrases. They are used primarily in written communications to save time and space. Table 3.4 lists some of these abbreviations. Most medical dictionaries have a more extensive list of accepted abbreviations. If you are unsure whether an abbreviation is acceptable when charting and keeping records, write out the full term to ensure accuracy.

Using too many abbreviations creates confusion. Massage therapists need to use the standard abbreviations accepted in the profession and not make up abbreviations or use texting abbreviations. These can become outdated quickly, and not everyone understands their meaning.

If you use abbreviations when charting, you should provide an abbreviation key with the clinical notes. Abbreviations are not understood universally, and a key ensures accurate interpretation of your notes by the client or a fellow healthcare professional.

Review What You Have Learned

- Identify three word elements used in medical terms.
  - *Prefix*—placed at the beginning of a word to change its meaning.
  - *Root*—the fundamental meaning of the word, placed after the prefix and before the suffix.
  - *Suffix*—placed at the end of a word to change its meaning.
- Combine word elements into medical terms.
  - See Activity 3.1.
- Identify abbreviations used in health care and their meanings.
  - See Table 3.4.

GENERAL STRUCTURAL PLAN OF THE BODY

SECTION OBJECTIVES

Chapter objectives covered in this section:

3. Describe terms used to describe regions of the body and surface anatomy.
4. Define terms used to describe the positions of the body and the parts of the body in relation to other body parts.
5. Define *kinesiology*, body planes, and terms of movements.

After completing this section, the learner will be able to perform the following:

- Explain the structural plan of the human body.
- Identify regions of the body and surface anatomy.
- Locate abdominal quadrants and regions.
- Use proper terms to indicate the positions of the body.
- Use directional terms to describe the relationship of one body area to another.
- Define *kinesiology*.
- Define the body planes and demonstrate the movements that occur in each plane.
- Name and demonstrate movement terms.

THE BODY MAP

The layout of a map is fairly universal. North is usually placed at the top, a legend identifies the number of miles per inch, and symbols indicate types of roads and landmarks. The locations of body areas are also universal. The map of the body begins with the body in the anatomical position (Fig. 3.1).

The following information provides the basic knowledge you need to read the body map and provide accurate descriptions to guide others around the body.

Table 3.2 Common Root Words and Their Meanings

Root (Combining Vowel)	Meaning	Root (Combining Vowel)	Meaning	Root (Combining Vowel)	Meaning
Abdomin(o)-	Abdomen	Hemat(o)-	Blood	Psych(o)-	Mind
Aden(o)-	Gland	Hepat(o)-	Liver	Pulm(o)-	Lung
Adren(o)-	Adrenal gland	Hydr(o)-	Water	Py(o)-	Pus
Angi(o)-	Vessel	Hyster(o)-	Uterus	Rect(o)-	Rectum
Arteri(o)-	Artery	Ile(o)-, ili(o)-	Ileum	Rhin(o)-	Nose
Arthr(o)-	Joint	Laryng(o)-	Larynx	Salping(o)-	Eustachian tube, uterine tube
Bronch(o)-	Bronchus, bronchi	Mamm(o)-	Breast, mammary gland	Splen(o)-	Spleen
Card-, cardi(o)-	Heart	Mast(o)-	Mammary gland, breast	Sten(o)-	Narrow, constriction
Cephal(o)-	Head	Men(o)-	Menstruation	Stern(o)-	Sternum
Chondr(o)-	Cartilage	My(o)-	Muscle	Stomat(o)-	Mouth
Col(o)-	Colon	Myel(o)-	Spinal cord, bone marrow	Therm(o)-	Heat
Cost(o)-	Rib	Nephr(o)-	Kidney	Thorac(o)-	Chest
Crani(o)-	Skull	Neur(o)-	Nerve	Thromb(o)-	Clot, thrombus
Cyan(o)-	Blue	Ocul(o)-	Eye	Thyr(o)-	Thyroid
Cyst(o)-	Bladder, cyst	Ophthalm(o)-	Eye	Tox(o)-	Poison
Cyt(o)-	Cell	Orth(o)-	Straight, normal, correct	Toxic(o)-	Poison, poisonous
Derma-	Skin	Oste(o)-	Bone	Trache(o)-	Trachea
Duoden(o)-	Duodenum	Ot(o)-	Ear	Ur(o)-	Urine, urinary tract, urination
Encephal(o)-	Brain	Ped(o)-	Child, foot	Urethr(o)-	Urethra
Enter(o)-	Intestines	Pharyng(o)-	Pharynx	Urin(o)-	Urine
Fibr(o)-	Fiber, fibrous	Phleb(o)-	Vein	Uter(o)-	Uterus
Gastr(o)-	Stomach	Pnea-	Breathing, respiration	Vas(o)-	Blood vessel, vas deferens
Gloss(o)-	Tongue	Pneum(o)-	Lung, air, gas	Ven(o)-	Vein
Gyn-, gyne-, gynec(o)-	Female	Proct(o)-	Rectum	Vertebr(o)-	Spine, vertebrae
Hem-, hema-, hem(o)-	Blood				

Table 3.3 Common Suffixes and Their Meanings

Suffix	Meaning	Suffix	Meaning	Suffix	Meaning
-able	Capable of, suitable for	-graph	Diagram, recording instrument	-phylaxis	Protection
-ago	Disease	-graphy	Making a recording	-plasty	Surgical repair or reshaping
-algesia	Pain	-hood	State, quality of, condition	-plegia	Paralysis
-algia	Pain	-iasis	Condition of	-pnea	To breathe
-ase	Enzyme	-ician	One skilled in, one who practices	-porosis	Passage
-asis	State or condition of, usually abnormal	-ism	Condition	-ptosis	Falling, sagging
-cele	Hernia, herniation, pouching	-itis	Inflammation	-rrhage, -rrhagia	Excessive flow
-cide	Kill, causing death	-ity	Quality of, state of	-rrhea	Profuse flow, discharge
-cule	Very small	-ive	Having power to, that which performs	-sclerosis	Dryness, hardness
-cyte	Cell	-ize	To treat by a special method	-scoliosis	Curvature, crooked
-dom	State of being	-kinesis	Motion	-scope	Examination instrument

Table 3.3 Common Suffixes and Their Meanings—cont'd

Suffix	Meaning	Suffix	Meaning	Suffix	Meaning
-duct	Tube, channel	-lemma	Sheath, covering	-scopy	Examination
-eal	Pertaining to	-logy	The study of	-sepsis	Putrefaction
-ease	Condition	-lysis	Destruction of, decomposition	-some	Body
-ectasis	Dilation, stretching	-malacia	Softening	-stasis	Maintenance, maintaining a constant level
-ectomy	Excision, removal of	-megaly	Enlargement	-stenosis	Narrow, tighten, short, constrict
-ema	Swelling, distention	-oid	Form, like, resemble	-stomy, -ostomy	Creation of an opening
-emesis[a]	Vomiting	-oma	Tumor	-thymia	Thymus gland, mind, soul, emotions
-emia	Blood condition	-opsy	View of	-tomy, -otomy	Incision, cutting into
-ferent	Bear, carry	-osis	Condition	-tonia	Stretching, putting under tension
-feron	To strike	-otomy	Cutting into	-trophic	Related to growth, development, or nutrition
-form	Shape, structure	-paresis	Paralysis	-ule	Little, small
-genesis	Development, production, creation	-pathy	Disease	-uria	Condition of the urine
-globin	Protein	-penia	Lack, deficiency	-version	To turn
-gram	Record	-phobia	An exaggerated fear	-vert	Turn

[a]One of the few suffixes that can stand alone.

Table 3.4 Common Abbreviations and Their Meanings

Abbreviation	Meaning	Abbreviation	Meaning	Abbreviation	Meaning
ABD	Abdomen	Dx	Diagnosis	OTC	Over the counter
ADL	Activity of daily living	ext	Extract	P	Pulse
ad lib	As desired	ft	Foot (or feet)	PA	Postural analysis
alt dieb	Every other day	fx	Fracture	PM, p.m.	Afternoon
alt hor	Alternate hours	GI	Gastrointestinal	PT	Physical therapy
alt noct	Alternate nights	GU	Genitourinary	Px	Prognosis
AM, a.m.	Morning	h, hr	Hour	R	Respiration; right
a.m.a.	Against medical advice	H_2O	Water	R/O	Rule out
ANS	Autonomic nervous system	Hx	History	ROM	Range of motion
approx	Approximately	IBW	Ideal body weight	Rx	Prescription
as tol	As tolerated	ICT	Inflammation of connective tissue	SOB	Shortness of breath
BM	Bowel movement	id	The same	SP, spir	Spirit
BP	Blood pressure	L	Left, length, lumbar	Sym	Symmetric
Ca	Cancer	lig	Ligament	T	Temperature
CC	Chief complaint	M	Muscle, meter, myopia	TLC	Tender loving care
c/o	Complains of	ML	Midline	Tx	Treatment
CPR	Cardiopulmonary resuscitation	meds	Medications	URI	Upper respiratory infection
CSF	Cerebrospinal fluid	n	Normal	WD	Well developed
CVA	Cerebrovascular accident (stroke)	NA	Not applicable	WN	Well nourished
DJD	Degenerative joint disease	OB	Obstetrics		
DM	Diabetes mellitus				

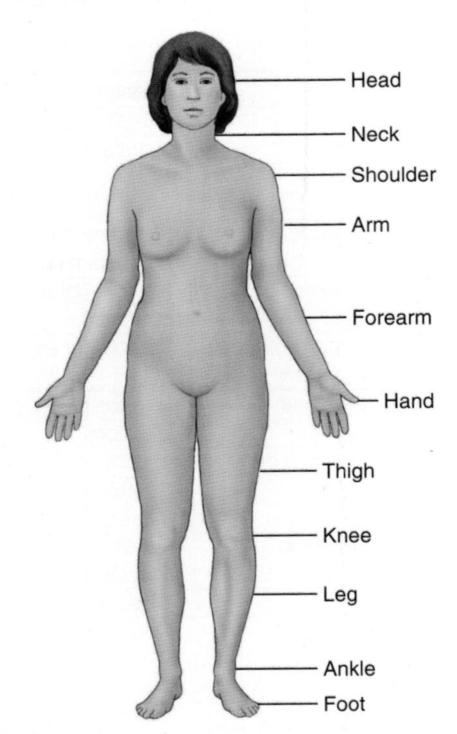

FIG. 3.1 Anatomical position. The individual is standing upright, facing forward, feet slightly separated, and arms at the sides with the palms facing forward. Structures are named, and their positions are described using this standard position. (Modified from Muscolino JE. *Kinesiology: The Skeletal System and Muscle Function*. 2nd ed. Mosby; 2011.)

Regions of the Body and Surface Anatomy

Regional terms are used to designate specific areas of the body. Study Fig. 3.2 carefully.

Structural Plan

The structural organization of the body follows a clear plan. Each human being has a vertebral column that supports the trunk and determines the central axis of the body. The spine also supports two body cavities: the dorsal cavity, which holds the brain inside the skull and the spinal cord in the vertebral column; and the ventral cavities, which are the combined thoracic, abdominal, and pelvic cavities (sometimes referred to as the *abdominopelvic* cavity). Human beings are bilaterally symmetric beings, with left and right mirror images. Also, the body is segmented; this is most obvious in the vertebral column, ribs, and spinal cord. The body is designed as a tube within a tube. The digestive system is a tube that lies within the greater tube of the trunk (Figs. 3.3 and 3.4).

Terms Related to the Structural Plan

These terms are used to describe the structural plan of the body:

- *Soma, somato:* Root words that mean "the body," as distinguished from the mind. Somatic organs and tissues are associated with the skin and skeleton (e.g., bone and skeletal muscles, extremities, and the body wall) and can be commonly controlled voluntarily.
- *Axial:* Areas and organs along the central axis of the body, including the head, neck, trunk, brain, spinal cord, and abdominal organs.

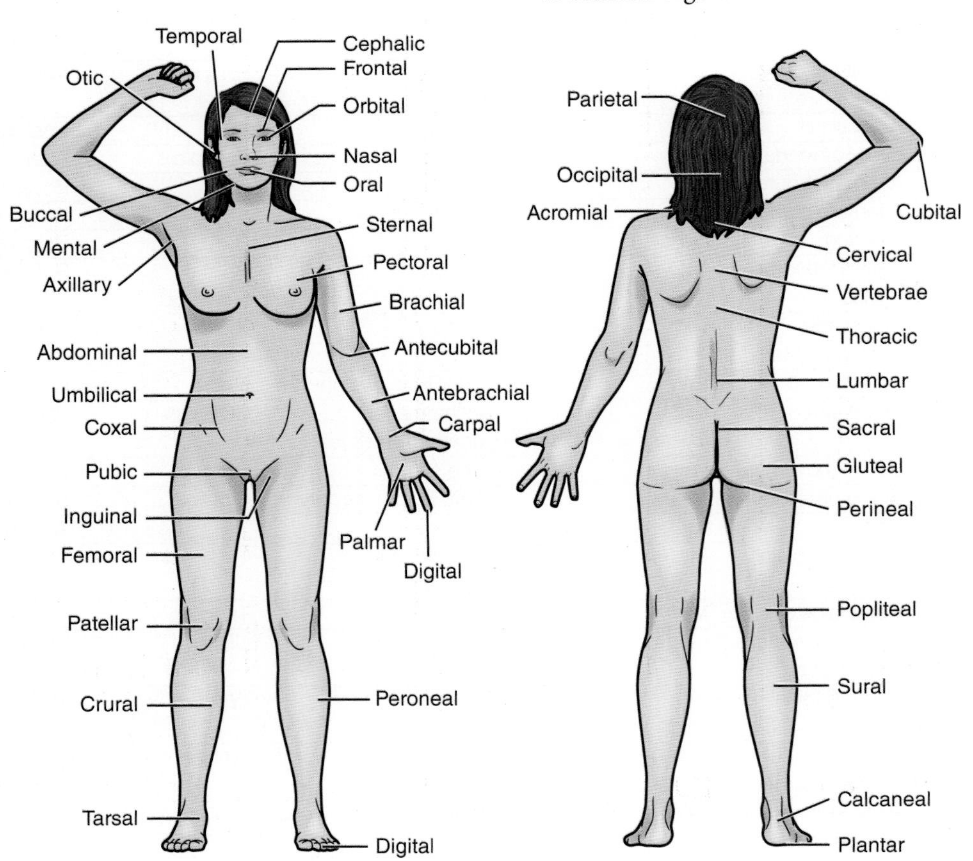

FIG. 3.2 Anatomical regions and surface anatomy.

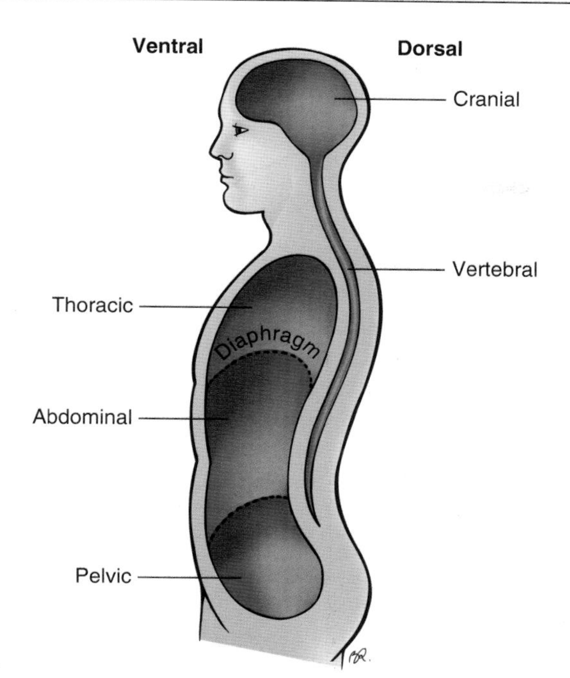

FIG. 3.3 Body cavities. (From Fritz S. *Mosby's Fundamentals of Therapeutic Massage*. 5th ed. Mosby; 2013.)

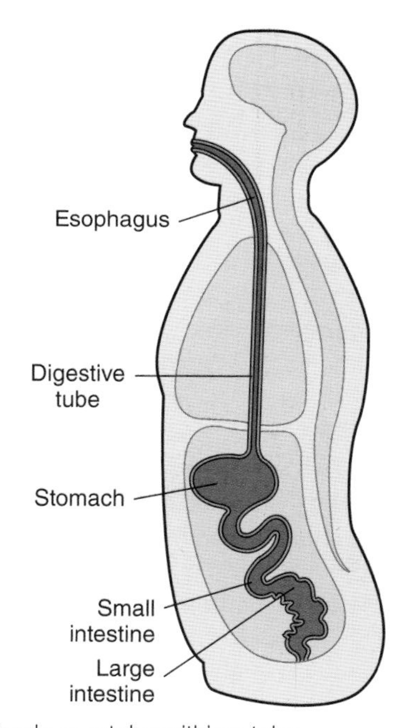

FIG. 3.4 The body as a tube within a tube.

- *Appendicular:* The limbs, joined to the body as lateral appendages.
- *Torso, trunk:* Structures related to the main part of the body, including the chest, abdomen, and vertebral cavity. The head and limbs are attached to the trunk.

Posterior Region of the Trunk

The two dorsal cavities are located toward the back of the body.

- *Cranial cavity:* Found in the skull, containing the brain and related structures.
- *Vertebral cavity:* Extending from the base of the cranial cavity and containing the spinal cord.

The back, or posterior surface, of the trunk is divided into regions named for the corresponding vertebrae in the spinal column.

- *Cervical region:* The neck (7 cervical vertebrae)
- *Thoracic region:* The chest (12 thoracic vertebrae)
- *Lumbar region:* The low back (5 lumbar vertebrae)
- *Sacral region:* The sacrum (5 sacral vertebrae fused into one bone)
- *Coccyx:* The tailbone (4 coccygeal vertebrae fused into one bone)

Anterior Region of the Trunk

The ventral cavities are located in the trunk.

- *Thoracic cavity:* Also known as the *chest*; found between the neck and the diaphragm and surrounded by the ribs. The mediastinum is a part of the thoracic cavity in the middle of the thorax, between the pleural sacs containing the two lungs.
- *Abdominal cavity:* Also known as the *belly*; located below the diaphragm, enclosed within the abdominal muscles. This cavity contains the liver, kidneys, spleen, pancreas, stomach, and intestines.
- *Pelvic cavity:* Inferior to the abdomen, inside the pelvic bones; contains a portion of the large intestine, as well as the bladder and the internal reproductive organs.
- *Viscera:* Internal organs of the thoracic, abdominal, and pelvic cavities that are considered to be under involuntary control.
- *Membranes:* Two types, associated with the regions of the trunk: parietal membranes, lining the body cavities, and visceral membranes, covering the visceral organs.

Abdominal Quadrants and Regions

The abdomen is divided into four quadrants and nine regions, the names of which are used to describe the location of body structures, pain, or discomfort. The four quadrants are the right upper quadrant, left upper quadrant, right lower quadrant, and left lower quadrant (Fig. 3.5A). The nine regions are the right hypochondriac, epigastric, left hypochondriac, right lumbar, umbilical, left lumbar, right iliac, hypogastric, and left iliac regions (Fig. 3.5B).

Positions of the Body

Anatomical position is a term used in Western medicine to describe the position of the body and the location of its regions and parts. The central axis of the body passes through the head and trunk. These terms relate to the position of the body:

- *Anatomical position:* The body standing upright with the feet slightly apart, the arms hanging at the sides, the palms facing forward, and the thumbs outward (see Fig. 3.1)
- *Functional position:* The body standing upright with the feet slightly apart, arms hanging at the sides, palms facing the sides of the body, thumbs forward
- *Erect position:* The body standing
- *Supine position:* The body lying horizontally with the face up (Fig. 3.6A)

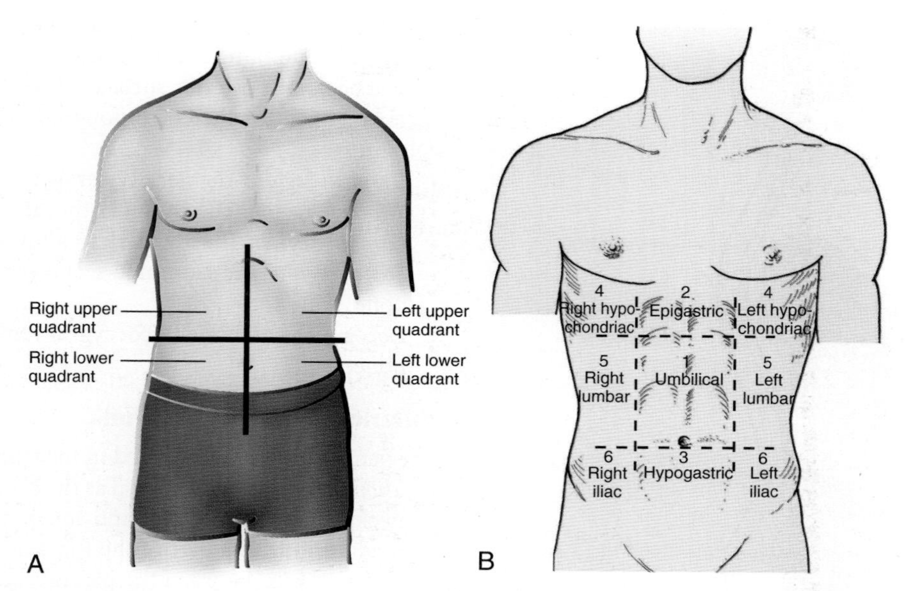

FIG. 3.5 (A) Quadrants of the abdomen. (B) Anatomical regions of the abdomen. (A, From Fritz S. *Mosby's Fundamentals of Therapeutic Massage*. 5th ed. Mosby; 2013; B, From LaFleur-Brooks M. *Exploring Medical Language: a Learner-Directed Approach*. 5th ed. Mosby; 2002.)

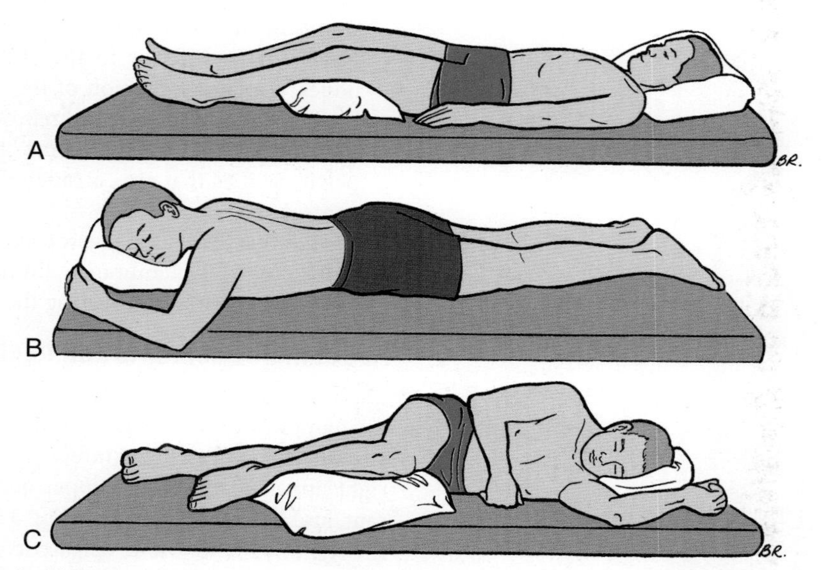

FIG. 3.6 Positions of the body. (A) Supine. (B) Prone. (C) Lateral recumbent. (From Fritz S. *Mosby's Fundamentals of Therapeutic Massage*. 3rd ed. Mosby; 2004.)

- *Prone position:* The body lying horizontally with the face down (Fig. 3.6B)
- *Lateral recumbent position:* The body lying horizontally on the right or left side (Fig. 3.6C)

Directional Terms

Certain terms are used to describe the relationship of one body position to another (Fig. 3.7). These directional terms, which are organized in pairs of opposites, are derived from some of the prefixes listed in this chapter:

- *Anterior (ventral):* In front of, or in or toward the front
- *Posterior (dorsal):* Behind, in the back of, or in or toward the rear
- *Proximal:* Closer to the trunk or the point of origin (usually used on the appendicular body only)
- *Distal:* Situated away from the trunk, or midline, of the body; situated away from the origin (usually used on the appendicular body only)
- *Lateral:* On or to the side, outside, away from the midline
- *Medial:* Relating to the middle, center, or midline
- *Ipsilateral:* The same side
- *Contralateral:* The opposite side
- *Superior:* Higher than or above (usually used on the axial body only)
- *Inferior:* Lower than or below (usually used on the axial body only)

- *Volar (palmar):* The palm side of the hand
- *Plantar:* The sole side of the foot
- *Varus:* Ends bent inward; angulation of a part of the body inward toward the midline
- *Valgus:* Ends bent outward; angulation of a part of the body outward from the midline (e.g., bent toward the wall)
- *Internal:* An inside surface or the inside part of the body
- *External:* The outside surface of the body
- *Deep:* Inside or away from the surface
- *Superficial:* Toward or on the surface
- *Dextral (dextro):* Right
- *Sinistral (sinistro):* Left (*levo* also is used to mean left)

Practical Application

Etymology is the study of the history of words and how their form and meaning have changed over time.

Sometimes terminology is confusing. For example:

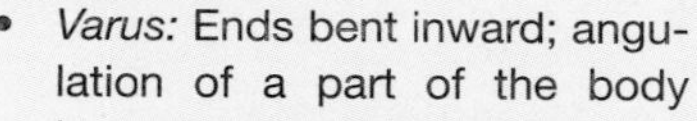

- *Varus:* Ends bent inward; angulation of a part of the body inward toward the midline. Derived from the Latin word *varus*, meaning bowlegged; bent outward; bandy.
- *Valgus:* Ends bent outward; angulation of a part of the body outward from the midline; for example, bent toward the wall. Derived from the Latin word *valgus*, which means knock-kneed, having legs converging at the knee and diverging below.

Varus means bent in. *Valgus* means bent out. Knock-knees look like they are bent in, but it is a valgus deformity. So what is bent out? The tibia is turned outward in relation to the femur (angulation of the distal part of a limb at a joint), resulting in a knock-kneed appearance.

According to the Latin definitions, *varus* and *valgus* both mean bowlegged and knock-kneed. With bowlegs, the knees appear to "bow" out from the body. Knock-knees, on the other hand, occur when the knees appear to bend toward each other.

- *Volar (palmar):* The palm side of the hand
- *Plantar:* The sole side of the foot

The term *volar* is derived from the Latin word *vola*, meaning the hollow of the hand or foot. Now it gets confusing. The dorsum (back) of the hand corresponds to the dorsum (top) of the foot.

KINESIOLOGY

By definition, **kinesiology** is the study of movement. Kinesiology brings together the study of anatomy, physiology, physics, and geometry as a means to understand human movement. Kinesiology uses principles of **mechanics**, musculoskeletal anatomy, and neuromuscular physiology. Mechanical principles that relate directly to the human body are used in the study of **biomechanics**. This may involve looking at the static (nonmoving) or dynamic (moving) systems associated with various activities. Dynamic systems can be divided into **kinetics** and **kinematics**. Kinetics is the study of motion caused by the action of forces. Kinematics is defined as the study of motion without regard to the forces that cause that motion.

Motion is a change in position with respect to some reference frame or starting point. If we are going to observe and describe any type of motion, we have to have an agreed-upon starting point (i.e., reference or baseline position) to:

- Reduce confusion
- Define positional and motion terms
- Identify the position of the segment in space
- Identify whether motion has occurred

Movement has two reference points:

- *Anatomical position:* The body is standing upright with the feet slightly apart, arms hanging at the sides, palms facing forward, and thumbs outward.
- *Functional position:* The body is standing upright with the feet slightly apart, arms hanging at the sides, palms facing the sides of the body, and thumbs forward.

Body Planes and Movements

The body can be divided into sections by imaginary lines and various planes to identify the particular areas (Fig. 3.8). Movements are described as beginning in or returning to the anatomical position (Fig. 3.9). Movement terms define the action as the body part passes through the various planes.

- The *sagittal plane* is a vertical plane that divides the body into left and right. A *midsagittal plane* divides the body into equal left and right parts; a *parasagittal plane* divides it into unequal left and right parts.
- The *frontal (coronal) plane* also runs vertically but divides the body into anterior and posterior (front and back) parts.
- A *transverse plane* divides the body horizontally into two sections, described as *superior* (meaning above) and *inferior* (meaning below). The transverse plane runs perpendicular to the frontal and sagittal planes.

A movement that takes a part of the body forward from the anatomical position within a sagittal plane is called *flexion;* movement backward is called *extension.*

Movements in a frontal plane that take a part of the body toward the midline are called *adduction;* movements away are called *abduction*. Lateral flexion, or side bending, of the head, neck, or trunk also takes place in the frontal plane. A movement in a transverse plane that takes a part of the body away from the midline is called *lateral rotation;* movement inward is called *medial rotation.*

Movement Terms

These terms are commonly used to describe movement in the healthcare profession:

- *Flexion:* A decrease in the angle between two bones as the body part moves out of the anatomical position. Most flexion movements are forward movements. The major exception is knee flexion. Flexion is a sagittal plane movement. Place the fingers of your left hand on your left shoulder. You have just flexed your elbow joint. Make a fist with your right hand. You have just flexed the joints of your fingers.
- *Extension:* An increase in the angle between two bones, usually moving the body part back toward the anatomical

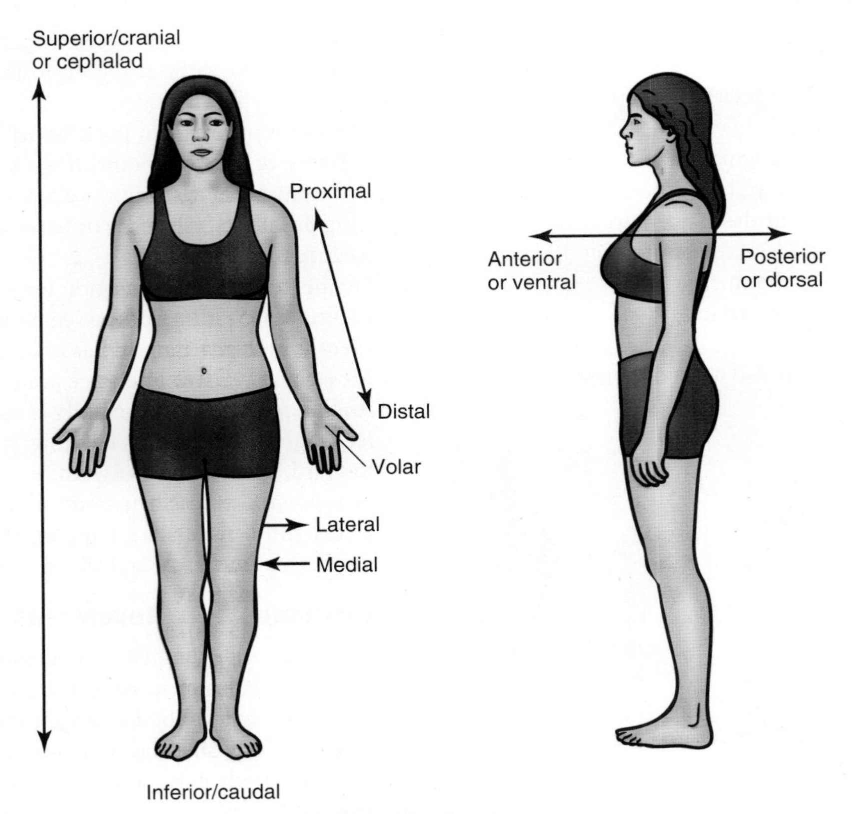

FIG. 3.7 Directional terms.

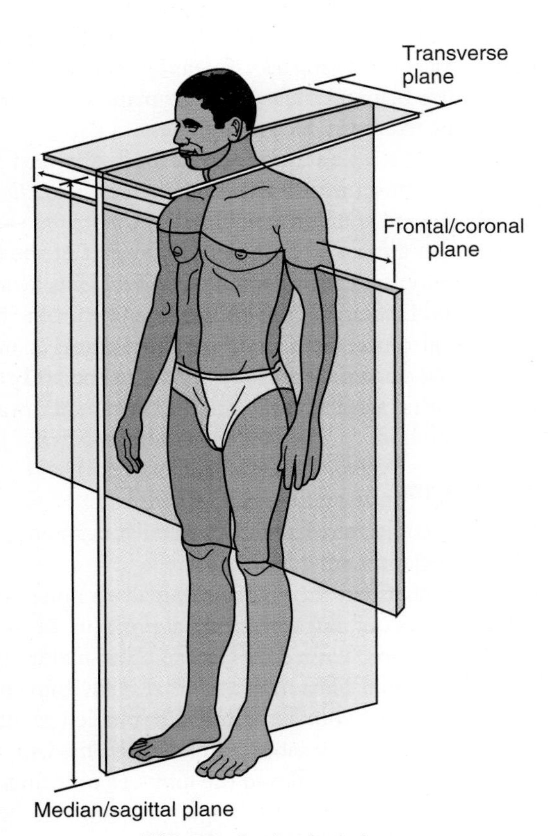

FIG. 3.8 Anatomical planes.

position; most extension movements are backward movements. The exception is knee extension. Extension is a sagittal plane movement.

- Begin with the fingers of your left hand on your shoulder. Now touch the lateral side of your left leg. You have just extended your elbow.
- Begin with your right hand in a fist. Now open your hand so your fingers are straight. You have just extended your finger joints.

- *Hyperextension:* This term has two definitions: (1) any extension beyond normal or healthy extension and (2) any extension that takes the part farther in the direction of the extension, farther out of the anatomical position.
  - Begin by standing in the anatomical position. Now, tip your head back so you are looking at the ceiling. This is hyperextension of the joints of the neck.
  - Begin by standing in the anatomical position. Now, lean back at the waist. This is hyperextension of the trunk.
- *Abduction:* Movement of the appendicular body part away from the midline; abduction is a frontal plane movement.
  - Begin by standing in the anatomical position. Move your arms out to the side away from your body as if you were going to do a jumping jack or were trying to look like the letter Y. Your shoulder joints are now abducted.
  - Begin by standing in the anatomical position. Move your legs out to the side away from your body as if you were going to do a jumping jack or were trying to look like the letter A. Your hip joints are now abducted.

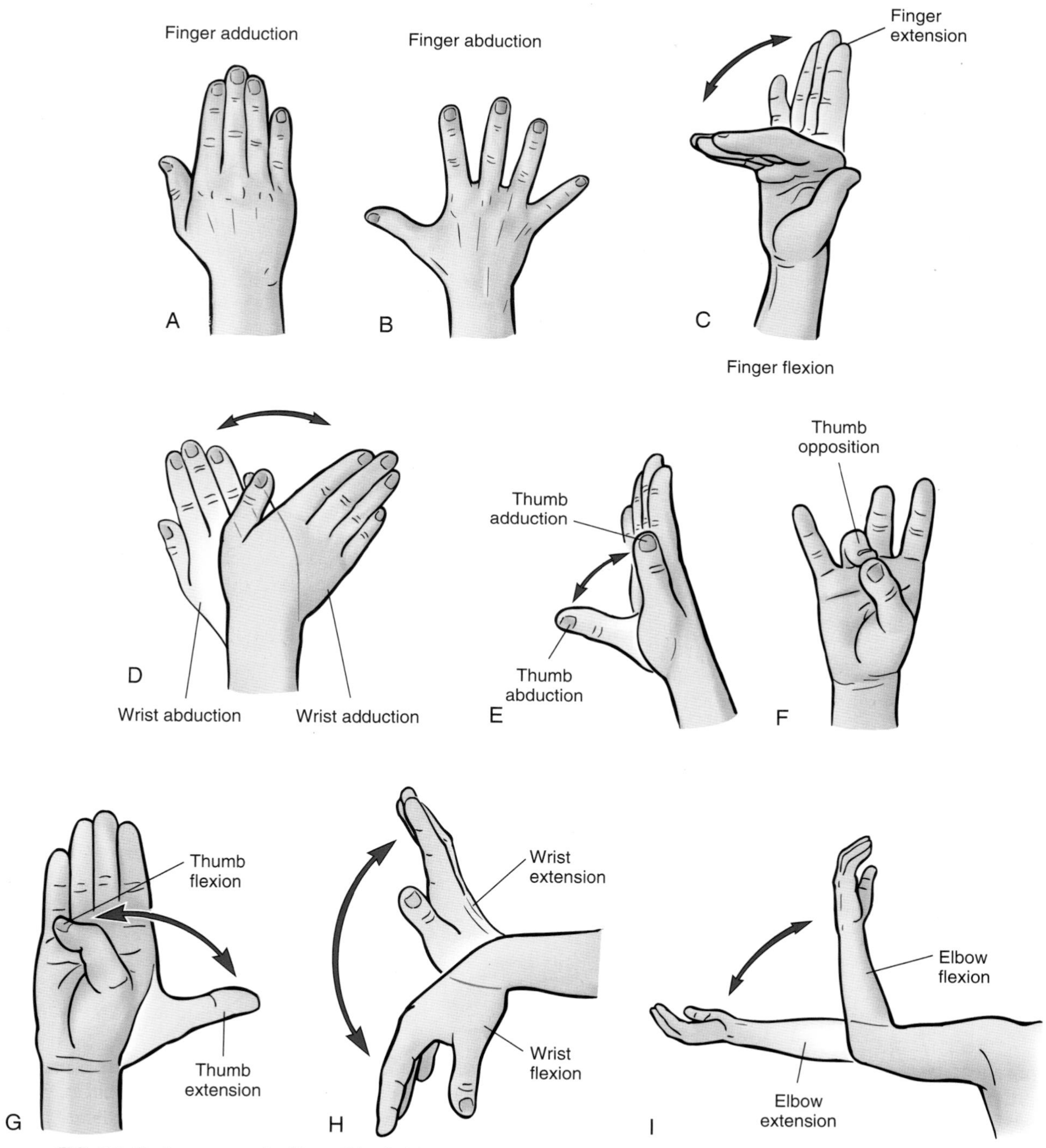

FIG. 3.9 Body movements. (From Fritz S. *Mosby's Fundamentals of Therapeutic Massage*. 4th ed. Mosby; 2009.)

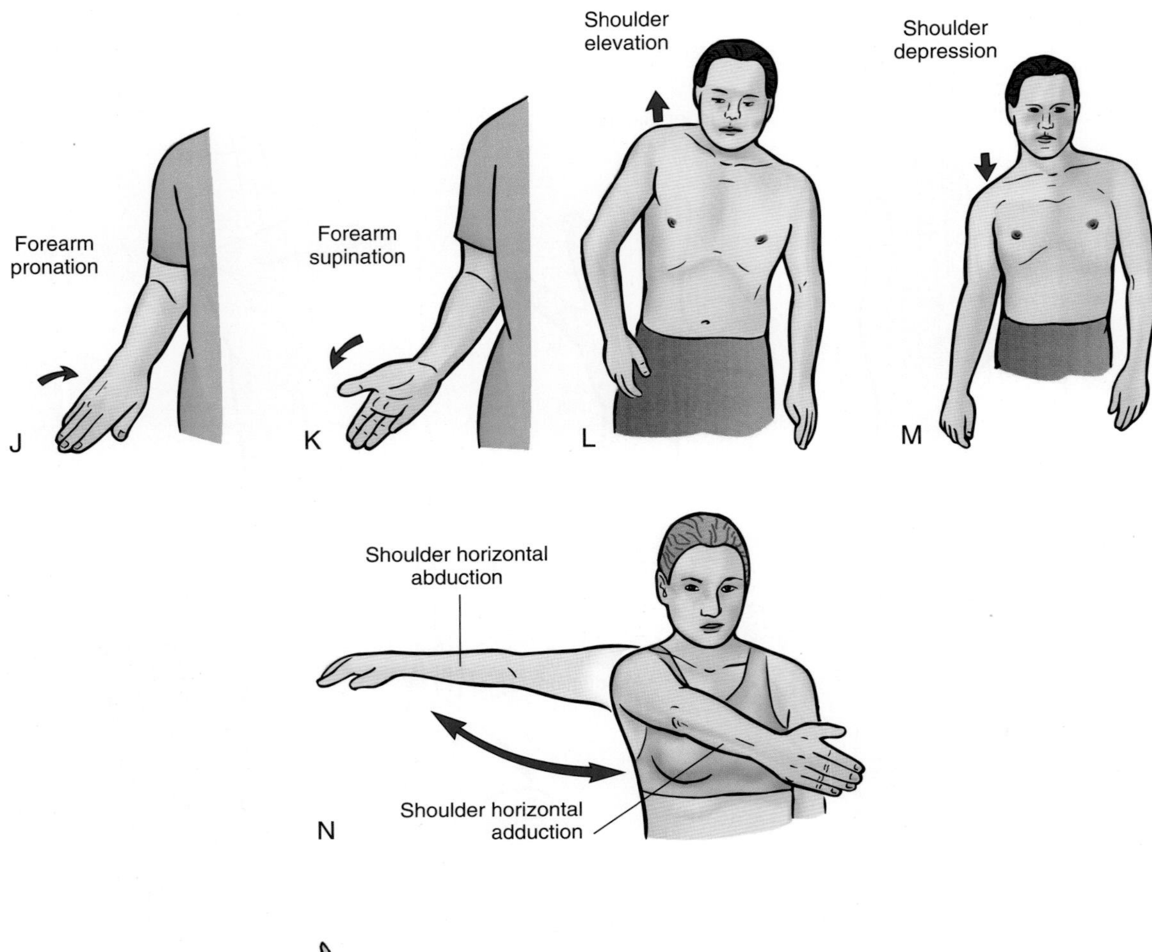

Forearm pronation
J
Forearm supination
K
Shoulder elevation
L
Shoulder depression
M
Shoulder horizontal abduction
Shoulder horizontal adduction
N

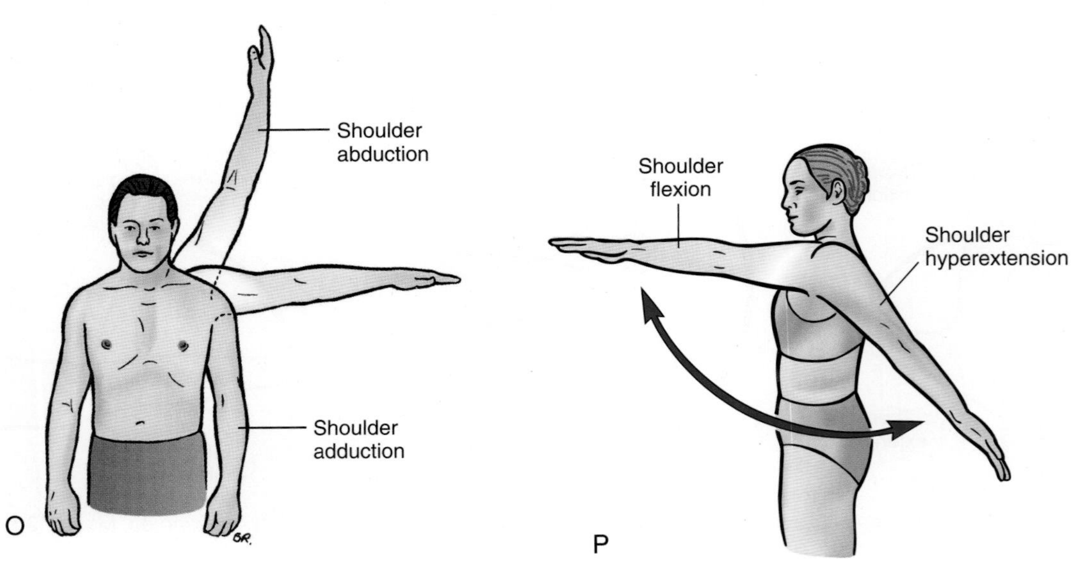

Shoulder abduction
Shoulder adduction
O
Shoulder flexion
Shoulder hyperextension
P

FIG. 3.9, cont'd

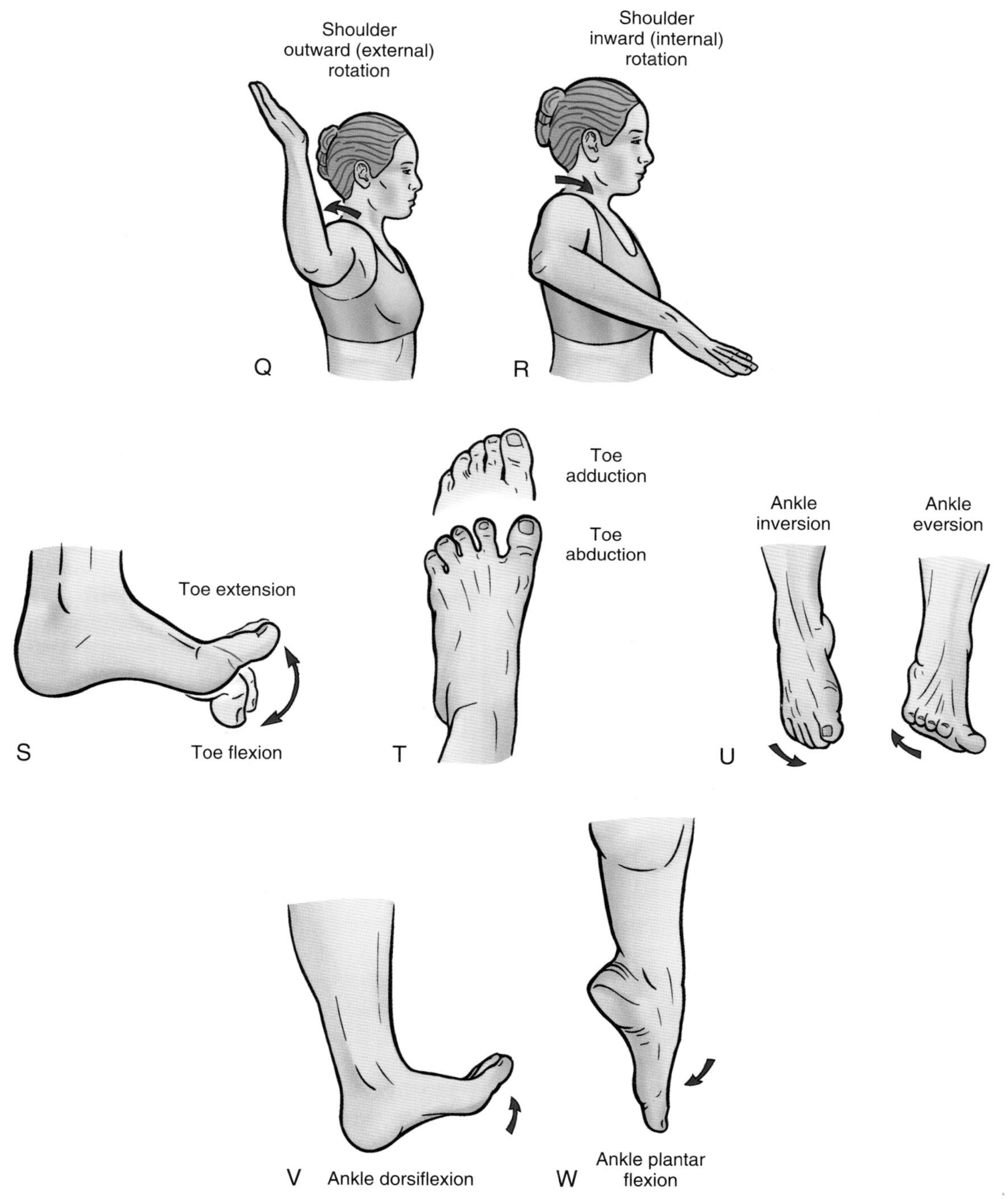
Shoulder
outward (external)
rotation
Shoulder
inward (internal)
rotation
Q
R
Toe extension
Toe flexion
S
Toe
adduction
Toe
abduction
T
Ankle
inversion
Ankle
eversion
U
V
Ankle dorsiflexion
W
Ankle plantar
flexion

FIG. 3.9, cont'd

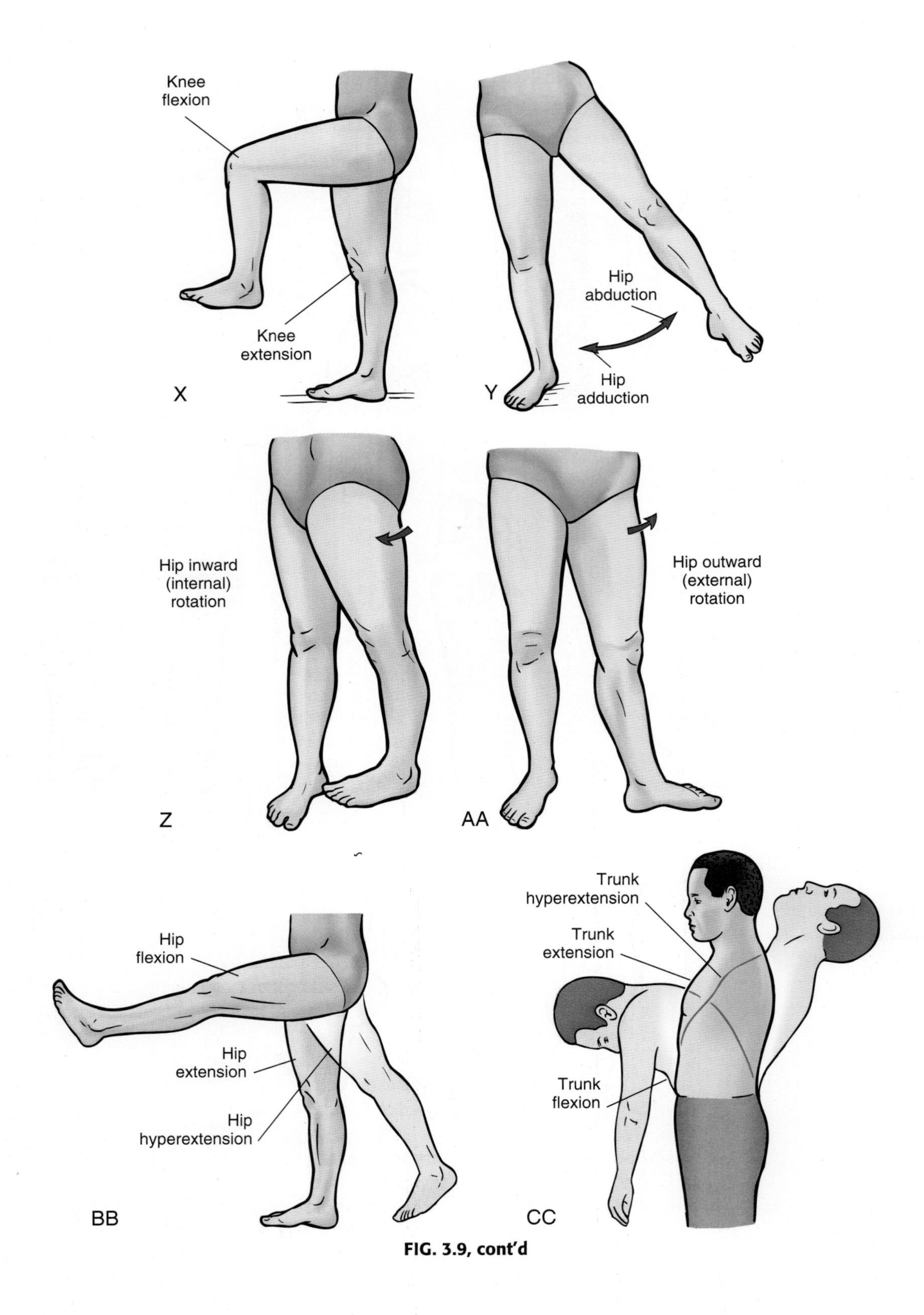
Knee
flexion
Knee
extension
X
Hip
abduction
Hip
adduction
Y
Hip inward
(internal)
rotation
Z
Hip outward
(external)
rotation
AA
Hip
flexion
Hip
extension
Hip
hyperextension
BB
Trunk
hyperextension
Trunk
extension
Trunk
flexion
CC

FIG. 3.9, cont'd

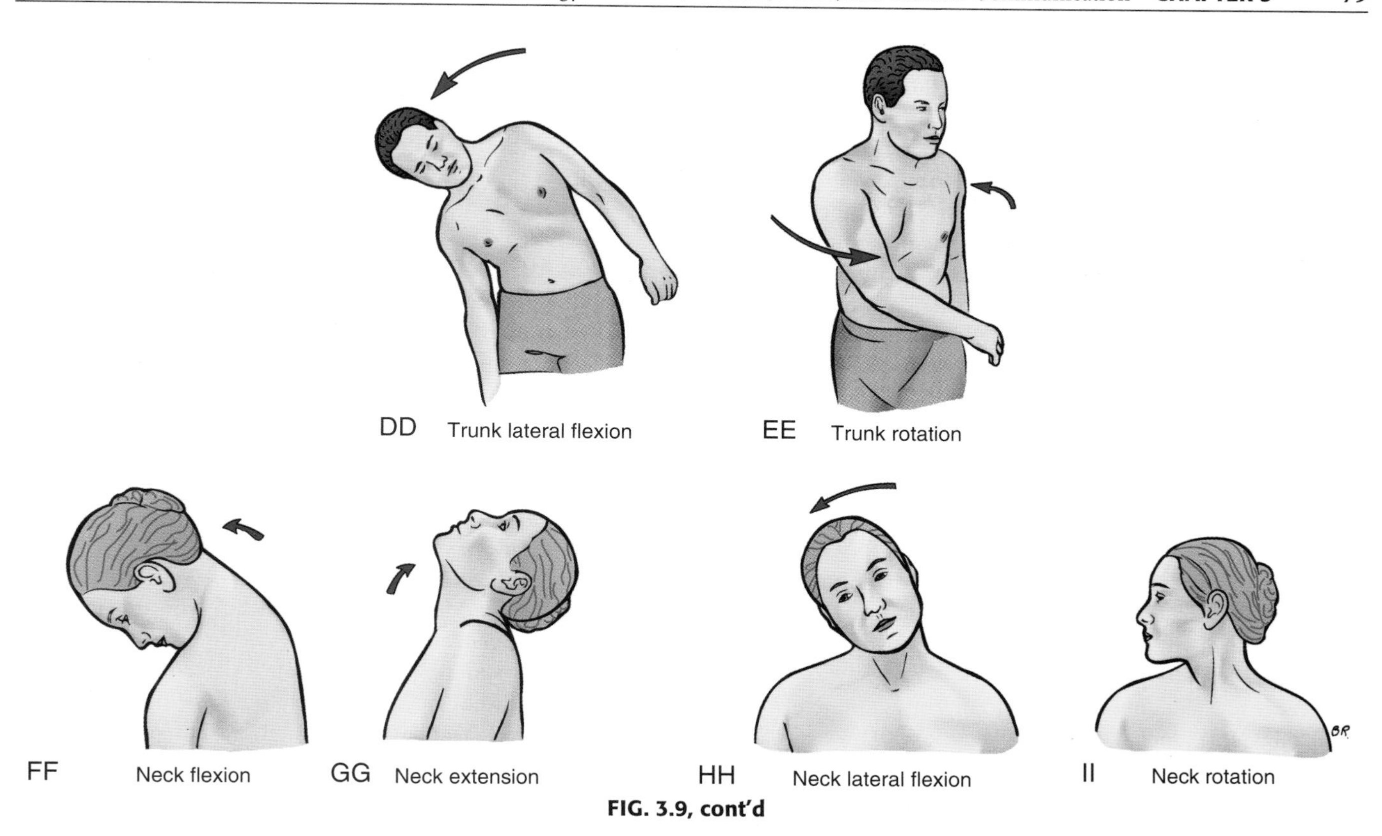

FIG. 3.9, cont'd

- *Adduction:* Movement of the appendicular body part toward the midline; adduction is a frontal plane movement.
  - Begin by standing and positioning yourself to look like the letter Y. Now lower your arms flat to your sides so you look like the letter I. You have just adducted your shoulder joints.
  - Begin by standing and positioning yourself to look like the letter A. Now bring your legs together so that you look like an I. You have just adducted your hip joints.
- *Right lateral flexion:* Movement of the axial body part (head, neck, trunk) to the right; right lateral flexion is a frontal plane movement.
  - NOTE: Lateral flexion terminology is confusing because frontal plane movements are called *abduction* and *adduction*. *Adduction* and *abduction* refer to movement of the limbs, or the appendicular body, not the head, neck, and trunk, which are part of the axial body. Other terms used for lateral flexion are *tilt* and *side bending*. Lateral flexion of the trunk involves moving the shoulders left or right toward the hips; therefore it is exercised in the frontal or coronal plane of motion.
  - Begin by standing in the anatomical position. Now lean (tilt) to the right side at the waist. You have moved your spinal joints into right lateral flexion.
  - Begin by standing in the anatomical position. Now move your right ear toward your right shoulder. You have moved the joints of your neck into right lateral flexion.
- *Left lateral flexion:* Movement of the axial body part to the left; left lateral flexion is a frontal plane movement.
  - Begin by standing in the anatomical position. Now lean (tilt) to the left side at the waist. You have moved into left lateral flexion.
  - Begin by standing in the anatomical position. Now move your left ear toward your left shoulder. You have moved the joints of your neck into left lateral flexion.
- *Right rotation:* Partially turning or pivoting the axial body part in an arc around a central axis to the right; right rotation is a transverse plane movement.
  - Begin by standing in the anatomical position. Twist your head as if you were attempting to look at your right shoulder. Your cervical (neck) joints have just rotated right.
  - Begin by standing in the anatomical position. Twist at the waist as if you were attempting to look behind you and over your right shoulder. Your spinal (back) joints have just rotated right.
- *Left rotation:* Partially turning or pivoting the axial body part in an arc around a central axis to the left; left rotation is a transverse plane movement.
  - Begin by standing in the anatomical position. Twist your head as if you were attempting to look at your left shoulder. Your cervical (neck) joints have just rotated left.
  - Begin by standing in the anatomical position. Twist at the waist as if you were attempting to look behind you and over your left shoulder. Your spinal joints have just rotated left.
- *Medial rotation:* Partially turning or pivoting a body part located in the appendicular body in an arc around a central axis toward the midline of the body; also called *internal rotation*. Medial rotation is a transverse plane movement.
  - Begin by standing in the anatomical position. Now place the palm of your right hand on your lower back. You have just medially rotated your right shoulder.

  - Begin in the seated position. Bring your knees together and move your feet apart. You have just medially rotated your hip joints.
- *Lateral rotation:* Partially turning or pivoting a body part located in the appendicular body in an arc around a central axis away from the midline of the body; also called *external rotation*. Lateral rotation is a transverse plane movement.
  - Begin by standing in the anatomical position. Now place the palm of your right hand on the back of your head. You have just laterally rotated your right shoulder.
  - Begin in the seated position. Place the outside of your left ankle on your right knee. You have just laterally rotated your left hip joint.
- *Circumduction:* Not a movement, but a sequence of movements that turn or pivot the part through an entire arc, making a complete circle. (NOTE: Circumduction involves no rotation and is a multiplanar movement.)
  - Begin by standing in the anatomical position. Raise your arms out to the side (shoulder abduction). Now move your arms in a big circle. You have just circumducted your shoulder joints.
  - Begin by standing in the anatomical position. Now stand on your left foot and make a big circle with the heel of your right foot. You have just circumducted your right hip.
- *Protraction:* Pushing of a part forward in a horizontal plane.
  - Begin by standing in the anatomical position. Flex both shoulder joints, bringing your arms out in front of you. Keep the elbows straight. Now reach forward with both arms. You should feel your scapula bones move apart in the back. You have just protracted your scapula (shoulder blades).
- *Retraction:* Pulling of a part back in a horizontal plane.
  - Begin by standing in the anatomical position. Now move the inside edges (medial border) of your scapula bones together. You have just retracted your shoulder blades.
- *Elevation:* Moving a part upward (superiorly).
  - Shrug your shoulders by bringing the tips of your shoulders up toward your ears. You have just elevated your scapula.
- *Depression:* Moving a part downward (inferiorly).
  - Begin by standing in the anatomical position. Slide your arms down the side of your legs toward your knees. You have just depressed your scapula.
- *Supination:* Movement of the forearm (at the radioulnar joint, not the elbow joint) that turns the palm anteriorly (upward), as in cupping a bowl of soup.
  - Begin in the seated position. Flex your elbows and position your hands as if you were going to type on the computer or play the piano. Now, turn your hands so the palms are facing up and you can look at them. You have just supinated your radioulnar joints.
- *Pronation:* Movement of the forearm (at the radioulnar joint, not the elbow joint) that turns the palm posteriorly (downward).
  - Begin in the seated position. Bring your hands together, palms up as if you are making a bowl to hold water. Now turn your hands as if you were going to type or play the piano. You have just pronated your radioulnar joints.
- *Inversion:* Movement of the sole inward, toward the midline.
  - NOTE: The subtalar joint (talocalcaneal joint) is a joint of the foot and not the true ankle joint. It is located on the rear foot. The subtalar joint is the area between the calcaneus and talus bones. The true ankle joint (talocrural joint) is made up of three bones—two bones from the lower leg (the tibia and fibula) and one bone from the foot (the talus).
  - Begin in the seated position. Now, move your feet so that the bottoms (soles) of your feet touch each other. You have just inverted your feet. This occurs at the subtalar joint.
- *Eversion:* Movement of the sole outward, away from the midline.
  - Begin in the seated position. Now, lift your left leg a little off the floor and attempt to move your little toe toward the outside of your knee. You have just everted your subtalar joint.
- *Plantar flexion:* Movement of the foot downward (may also be called *flexion*).
  - Begin by standing in the anatomical position. Now, raise your body so you are standing on your toes (think ballet dancer). You have just plantar flexed your true ankle joint (talocrural) joint.
- *Dorsiflexion:* Movement of the foot upward (may also be called *extension*).
  - Begin in the seated position. Lift your feet a little off the floor. Now bring the top of your foot up toward your shin. If you were walking, you would be walking on your heels. You have just dorsiflexed your true ankle joint.

Movement is necessary for various **activities of daily living (ADLs)**. ADLs are things we normally do in daily living, including self-care, such as eating, bathing, dressing, grooming, going to work, performing housekeeping duties, and engaging in leisure activities (Activity 3.2). Physical activity involves movement. A common outcome goal for massage is supporting the ability to move without pain and stiffness.

Review What You Have Learned

- Explain the structural plan of the human body.
  - The *axial skeleton* houses the skull, ribs, and spine. The *spine* supports the dorsal and ventral cavities. The *dorsal cavity* houses the brain and spinal cord. The *ventral cavity* includes the thorax, abdomen, and pelvis. The axial skeleton is attached to the *appendicular skeleton* (arms and legs). The *torso/trunk* (spine, ribs, abdomen) is attached to the arms, legs, and head.
- Identify regions of the body and surface anatomy.
  - Review Fig. 3.2.
- Locate abdominal quadrants and regions.
  - Review Fig. 3.5.
- Use proper terms to indicate the positions of the body.
  - Review Figs. 3.1 and 3.6.
- Use directional terms to describe the relationship of one body area to another.
  - Review the directional terms and relate them to your body. Example: Face is *anterior*. Back of skull is *posterior*.

ACTIVITY 3.2

For each of the movements, give an example of a common activity.

- Flexion: Example: I flex my elbow to scratch my nose.
- Extension: __________
- Hyperextension: __________
- Abduction: __________
- Adduction: __________
- Right lateral flexion: __________
- Left lateral flexion: __________
- Right rotation: __________
- Left rotation: __________
- Medial rotation: __________
- Lateral rotation: __________
- Circumduction: __________
- Protraction: __________
- Retraction: __________
- Elevation: __________
- Depression: __________
- Supination: __________
- Pronation: __________
- Inversion: __________
- Eversion: __________
- Plantar flexion: __________
- Dorsiflexion: __________

Shoulder is *proximal* to elbow. Elbow is *distal* to shoulder. Thumb is *lateral* to pinky. Pinky is *medial* to thumb. Right arm is *ipsilateral* to right leg. Right arm is *contralateral* to left leg. Shoulders are *superior* to hips. Hips are *inferior* to shoulders.

- Define *kinesiology*.
  - Kinesiology brings together the study of anatomy, physiology, physics, and geometry as a means to understand human movement.
- Define the body planes and demonstrate the movements that occur in each plane.
  - The *sagittal plane* divides a body into right and left halves. Flexion and extension occur in the sagittal plane. The *frontal plane* divides a body into front and back halves. Abduction and adduction occur in the frontal plane. The *transverse plane* divides a body into top and bottom halves. Lateral and medial rotation occur in the transverse plane.
- Name and demonstrate movement terms.
  - Sitting down requires flexion of hips and knees. Standing up requires extension of the hips and knees. Jumping jacks require shoulder and hip abduction (arms and legs up and out), then adduction (arms and legs down and in).

QUALITY OF LIFE TERMINOLOGY

SECTION OBJECTIVES

Chapter objective covered in this section:

6. Describe and use quality of life terminology.

After completing this section, the learner will be able to:

- Define quality of life.
- Use quality of life terminology in massage practice.

Practical Application

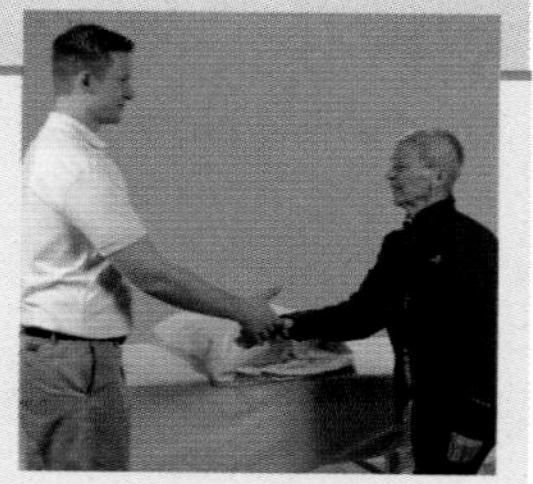

An important aspect of massage is describing clearly the information obtained during the data collection process. The structural plan of the body and the terms used to describe location, position, and movement provide the language we use during the documentation process. We can communicate with peers and other healthcare professionals using this common language. When we use these terms in our charting, others should be able to interpret accurately the content recorded in the charts. In addition, we can understand other information in medical records if it is written using standardized language. When we understand medical terminology, we can explain information to our clients without using terms they may not understand. Standardized language supports effective communication.

In Chapter 2 we discussed mechanisms of health and disease. When we speak of a state of health, we understand that to mean that the individual is experiencing a satisfactory quality of life.

The World Health Organization (WHO, https://www.who.int/) is the directing and coordinating authority for health within the United Nations system. In 1948 WHO undertook the task of identifying, defining, and assessing the spectrum of life quality. WHO defined **quality of life** as "… individuals' perceptions of their position in life in the context of the culture and value systems in which they live and in relation to their goals, expectations, standards and concerns."

The categories of quality of life have been described and presented in a language that can be used to communicate clearly with clients, peers, and others. Interestingly, the common outcome goals for massage therapy are related to the quality-of-life categories, called *domains* by the WHO (Box 3.2).

The World Health Organization Quality of Life (WHOQOL) criteria are divided into six domains:

- Physical
- Psychological
- Level of Independence
- Social Relationships
- Environment
- Spirituality/Religion/Personal Beliefs

Twenty-four areas are spread among the six domains.

The language provided by WHO, as well as other documents concerning quality of life, provide a structure for critical thinking, clinical reasoning, communication, and documentation (described later in the chapter) (Activity 3.3).

ACTIVITY 3.3

Using the language presented in Box 3.2, develop a list of questions relevant to massage on one of the six domains. Even better, find five other classmates and divide up the six domains, and each of you develop relevant massage questions. Combine the work from all six of you to develop a massage-related quality-of-life assessment form.

Box 3.2 WHO Quality of Life Domains

The following information is summarized from the *World Health Organization Quality of Life (WHOQOL) User's Manual*. WHO reports are available at http://www.who.int/mental_health/publications/whoqol/en/.

Domain I: Physical Domain

Pain and Discomfort

Pain is judged to be present if a person reports it to be so, even if there is no medical reason to account for it. The assumption is made that the easier the relief from pain, the less the fear of pain and its resulting effect on quality of life.

Examples

- Unpleasant physical sensations such as stiffness, aches, long-term or short-term pain, and itches
- Constant threat of pain
- Extent to which these sensations are distressing and interfere with life

Energy and Fatigue

Energy is the enthusiasm and endurance that a person has to perform the necessary tasks of daily living, as well as other chosen activities, such as recreation. Lack of energy becomes fatigue.

Examples

- Feeling alive
- Adequate levels of energy
- Fatigued but functioning with effort
- Disabling tiredness due to illness, problems such as depression, and overexertion.

Sleep and Rest

Restorative sleep is necessary for quality of life. Problems with sleep and rest affect the person's quality of life. If sleep is disturbed, reasons can be due either to the person's life and circumstances or to factors in the environment, such as noise or interruption.

Examples

- Difficulty going to sleep
- Waking up during the night
- Waking up early in the morning
- Being unable to go back to sleep
- Lack of refreshment from sleep

Domain II: Psychological

Positive Feelings

A person's view of and feelings about the future are seen as an important part of life. Does the individual experience enjoyment of the good things in life?

Examples

- Contentment
- Balance
- Peace
- Happiness
- Hopefulness
- Joy

Thinking, Learning, Memory, and Concentration

A person's view of their ability to think with clarity of thought and ability to gather and absorb new information and make informed decisions that affect quality of life.

Examples

- Thinking
- Learning
- Memory
- Concentration
- Confidence
- Confusion
- Forgetfulness

Self-Esteem

Self-esteem is how people feel about themselves and their perception of self-worth. This might range from feeling positive about themselves to feeling extremely negative about themselves.

Examples

- Feeling of self-efficacy
- Satisfaction with oneself
- Self-control
- Ability to have a good relationship with other people
- Educational experience and success
- Ability to respond to change
- Sense of dignity
- Self-acceptance

Body Image and Appearance

The focus is on the person's satisfaction with the way they look and the effect it has on self-concept, including the extent to which "perceived" or actual physical impairments, if present, can be corrected (e.g., by makeup, clothing, artificial limbs). How others respond to a person's appearance is likely to affect the person's body image considerably.

Examples

- The person's view of their body
- Is the appearance of the body seen in a positive or negative way?

Negative Feelings

Although negative feelings are normal, how often, how much, and to what extent a person experiences negative feelings reflect quality of life and affect the person's day-to-day functioning.

Examples

- Despondency
- Guilt
- Sadness
- Tearfulness
- Despair
- Nervousness
- Anxiety
- Lack of pleasure in life

Domain III: Level of Independence

Mobility

The focus is on the person's general ability to go wherever they want to go without the help of others, regardless of the means used to do so.

Examples

- Ability to perform mobility tasks (e.g., walking, running, reaching, pushing)
- Ability to get from one place to another
- Ability to move around the home
- Ability to move around the workplace
- Access to transportation services.

Activities of Daily Living

The focus is on a person's ability to carry out activities, which they likely need to perform on a day-to-day basis.

Examples

- Ability to perform usual daily living activities
- Self-care

Box 3.2 WHO Quality of Life Domains—cont'd

- Wellness level exercise
- Family care
- Work activities
- Caring appropriately for property
- Participation in hobbies and other recreational activities

Dependence on Medication or Treatments

When an individual feels dependent on medication or some sort of treatment, quality of life is affected. A person's real or perceived dependence on medication or integrative and complementary medicines and treatments such as acupuncture, massage, and herbal remedies for supporting physical and psychological well-being can either enhance or hinder quality of life.

Examples

- Medications or treatment side effects
- Medication or treatment benefits
- Time expended in obtaining treatments
- Convenience of obtaining medication or treatments
- Medication or treatment costs and ability to pay
- Perception of medication or treatment cost/benefit ratio

Working Capacity

Work is defined as any major activity in which the person is engaged. Quality of life can depend on a person's use of their energy for work, satisfaction with the work, and ability to work.

Examples

- Work for pay
- Desire to work but not employed
- Unpaid work
- Voluntary community work
- Full-time study
- Care of children
- Household duties

Domain IV: Social Relationships

Personal Relationships

The extent to which people feel they can share moments of both happiness and distress with loved ones and a sense of loving and being loved affect quality of life.

Experience Companionship, Love, and Support

- Ability to hug and touch and display other forms of physical affection
- Ability to be hugged and touched and to receive physical affection
- Desire for intimate relationships, both emotionally and physically
- Commitment to caring for and providing for other people
- The ability and opportunity to love, to be loved, and to be intimate

Social Support

Social support occurs when family and friends share in responsibility and work together to solve personal and family problems.

Examples

- Support of family and friends
- Ability to depend on support in a crisis
- Availability of practical assistance from family and friends
- Approval and encouragement from family and friends

Sexual Activity

For many people sexual activity and intimacy are intertwined. How a person is able to express and enjoy their sexuality appropriately and without guilt or value judgment is an aspect of quality of life.

Examples

- Healthy sexual expression is practiced.
- The individual is physically able to participate in sexual behavior.
- Supportive sexual partners are available.
- Sexual activity is expressed in intimate relationships.
- The individual is able to choose to participate in sexual relationships.
- The individual is free to express the creative forces of sexuality in a nonphysical way.

Domain V: Environment

Physical Safety and Security

A threat to safety or security might arise from multiple sources, such as other people, political oppression, and natural disasters, and affect quality of life.

Examples

- Sense of freedom
- Feeling of safety and security
- Lack of safety and security
- Protection from physical harm

Home Environment

Home is the principal place where a person lives; keeps most of their possessions; and, at a minimum, sleeps. The quality of the home is assessed on the basis of being comfortable, as well as affording the person a safe place to reside.

Examples

- Crowdedness
- Amount of space available
- Cleanliness
- Opportunities for privacy
- Availability of facilities such as electricity, toilet, running water
- The quality of the construction of the building
- The quality of the immediate neighborhood

Financial Resources

A person's perspective on financial resources is an influence on quality of life.

Examples

- Resources that meet the need for a healthy and comfortable lifestyle
- What the person can afford or cannot afford
- A sense of satisfaction/dissatisfaction with income
- Income that allows independence
- Financial resources that are inadequate to support independence
- The feeling of having enough

Health and Social Care: Availability and Quality

A person's view of the health and social care in the near vicinity, access to that care, and the quality of the care are aspects of quality-of-life experience.

Examples

- Time it takes to get help
- The availability of health and social services
- The quality and completeness of care
- Access to volunteer and community support organizations
- Access to governmental support organizations
- Access to police, fire, and rescue services

Continued

Box 3.2 WHO Quality of Life Domains—cont'd

Opportunities for Acquiring New Information and Skills
The ability of a person to fulfill a need for information and knowledge, whether this refers to knowledge in an educational sense or to local, national, or international news, is relevant to a person's quality of life.
Examples
- Opportunity to learn new skills, acquire new knowledge
- Access to libraries, schools, and organizations involved in learning
- Access to media (television, radio, Internet) to be in touch with what is going on

Participation in and Opportunities for Recreation and Leisure
Quality of life is found in a person's ability, opportunities, and inclination to participate in leisure, pastimes, and relaxation.
Examples
- Access to parks and recreational faculties
- Ability to see friends and spend time with family
- Time to read, watch television, be entertained, or do nothing

Physical Environment (Pollution/Noise/Traffic/Climate)
A person's view of their environment can improve or adversely affect their quality of life.
Examples
- Noise
- Pollution
- Climate
- General esthetic of the environment

Transport
The availability of transport allows the person to perform the necessary tasks of daily life as well as the freedom to perform chosen activities.
Examples
- Available and easy to find
- Reliable
- Affordable
- Easy to use
- Multiple modes of transport available (e.g., bicycle, car, bus)

Domain VI: Spirituality/Religion/Personal Beliefs
Spirituality/Religion/Personal Beliefs
A person's personal beliefs affect quality of life. Beliefs can enhance or degrade quality of life.
Examples
- Ability to cope with difficulties in life
- Give structure to experience
- Ascribe meaning to spiritual and personal questions
- Provide a sense of well-being
- Ability to be hopeful
- Lack of spiritual, religious, and personal beliefs sometimes leads to despondency
- Rigid, imposed spiritual, religious, and personal beliefs sometimes disempowering

Data from *WHOQOL User Manual.* Geneva, Switzerland; 1998:61–71 [revised 2012]. http://apps.who.int/iris/bitstream/handle/10665/77932/WHO_HIS_HSI_Rev.2012.03_eng.pdf?sequence=1&ua=1

Review What You Have Learned

- Define quality of life.
  - Review the WHO definition: Individuals' perceptions of their position in life in the context of the culture and value systems in which they live and in relation to their goals, expectations, standards, and concerns. Now, put it into your own words.
- Use quality of life terminology in massage practice.
  - Therapeutic massage may help clients achieve outcomes in the quality-of-life domains of physical and psychological health.

Practical Application

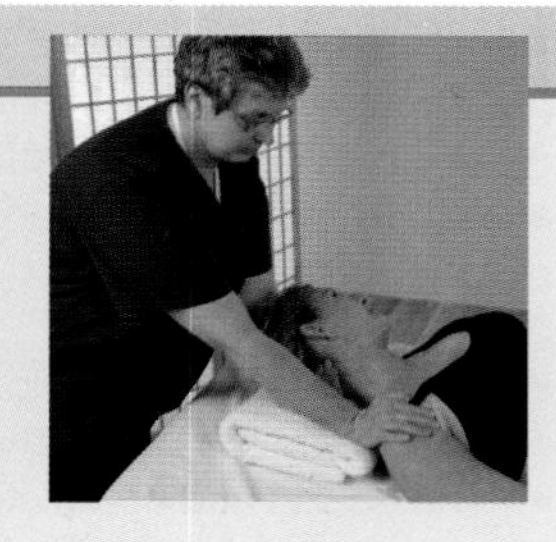

Quality of life terminology can serve as a useful tool for obtaining and documenting a client's history, and for assessment, as you develop the client's initial database. The terminology also helps frame questions during the history-taking process and for developing outcome-based goals for the massage. For example, the energy and fatigue content from domain I can be used as part of the subjective aspect of gathering data from the client (see Box 3.2).

EXAMPLE

Energy and Fatigue

Energy is the enthusiasm and endurance a person needs to perform the necessary tasks of daily living, as well as other chosen activities, such as recreation. Lack of energy becomes fatigue.

Levels

- Feeling alive
- Adequate levels of energy
- Fatigued but functioning with effort
- Disabling tiredness caused by illness, problems such as depression, or overexertion

Questions to Ask

- How would you explain your endurance for performing daily tasks?
- Could you describe your energy level today?

Possible Answers

- Alive and full of energy
- Adequate
- Fatigued but functioning
- Unable to function because of fatigue

Follow-up Questions

- What would you be able to do differently if your fatigue decreased and your energy increased?
- What do you believe is causing you to be fatigued?

- How might massage help you have more energy?
- Would an appropriate outcome goal for massage be to reduce stiffness and improve sleep?

The language in each of the domains in Box 3.2 can be used to form useful questions as you communicate with your clients. The language can also be used to educate clients. For example, consider domain IV, Social Relationships:

- Social support: When family and friends share in responsibility and work together to solve personal and family problems, this provides social support. Examples include:
  - Support of family and friends
  - Ability to depend on support in a crisis
  - Availability of practical assistance from family and friends
  - Approval and encouragement from family and friends

If a client has been diagnosed with a chronic pain condition, you could describe some coping mechanisms in this way:

"Massage therapy can be helpful in managing chronic pain. In addition, the support of family members and friends and their ability to help, especially in a crisis, can be important aspects of coping. I would be happy to teach your family members or friends some basic massage methods they can use to help you between massage sessions."

FOCUS ON PROFESSIONALISM

Massage therapy clients are becoming educated. They no longer consider massage to be just something you do to pamper yourself. Clients expect benefits. They want to relax, feel less stressed, feel less pain, and move more effectively. Clients expect massage to enhance their quality of life. Measures of the benefits of massage are related to aspects of quality of life. If a client finds movement painful, her quality of life is diminished. If a client is stressed and anxious, his quality of life is reduced. Relating massage to outcome goals and describing it as a means to enhance quality of life activities makes sense to clients and helps people understand the value of massage therapy.

CROSS-CULTURAL TERMINOLOGY

SECTION OBJECTIVES

Chapter objective covered in this section:

7. Explore terminology used in Indigenous and cultural-based healing systems.

After completing this section, the learner will be able to:

- Explain the role of intuition in traditional healthcare systems.
- Identify terminology from an ancient Chinese healing model.
- Compare terminology used in various healing traditions.

Terminology is the major source of confusion between Eastern and Western science. Ancient and indigenous healthcare systems each have unique terminology. *Traditional medicine* refers to the knowledge, skills, and practices based on the theories, beliefs, and experiences indigenous to different cultures. Traditional medicine covers a wide variety of therapies and practices and has been used for thousands of years.

The confusion occurs because each system describes the same anatomy or physiology using different words. Western science is a relatively new healing method, one that requires the practitioner to observe, measure, accumulate data, and clinically analyze findings. It has a particular language. Ancient approaches to healing also have a specific language and require observation, measurement, and accumulation and analysis of data; however, they also value and have validated intuition.

Intuition is knowing something without going through a conscious, problem-solving, rational process of thinking. According to researcher and scientist Hans Selye, nothing can be investigated or validated scientifically unless the researcher first has an idea—that is, uses intuition. Without validation, practical application is limited.

Ancient, or Indigenous, healing practices typically do not separate the body, mind, and spirit as Western medicine has done in the past. However, as health becomes better understood, Western medical practices are changing to encompass the whole person. Today technology and advances in research design are revealing the validity of the subtler aspects of ancient healing wisdom. The gap between ancient and new knowledge is narrowing, and with this development comes the need to understand various forms of terminology that describe similar structures and concepts. These other systems do not separate the body from the emotions or the mind. Western mind/body medicine is developing along similar lines.

Watching these older healing theories being discovered, explored, and understood by Western science is exciting. As these systems become more integrated, all will benefit from the blending of human knowledge.

As previously mentioned, the general structural plan of the body can be mapped out using standard descriptions and Western terminology. Other healing systems also map the body, but they use their own standards and terms.

Practical Application

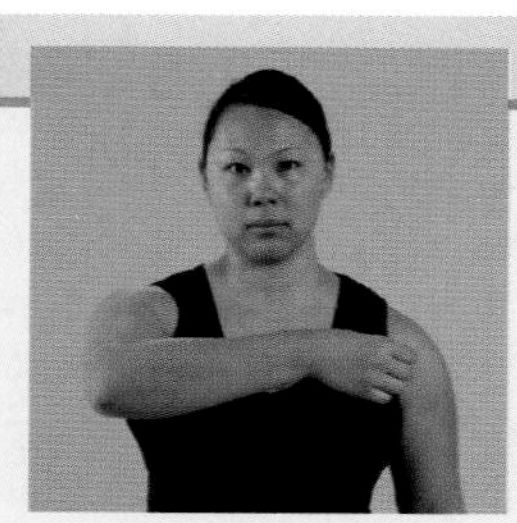

You may be asking yourself why you need to know about these various types of traditional medicine, especially because you are reading a science book. That question has many answers; however, one of the most important reasons is to appreciate the vast diversity of terms used to describe human anatomy and physiological processes. As the concept of integrated health care expands, massage therapists must be able to decipher the language of various cultural systems. The process is akin to becoming bilingual or multilingual. The ability to understand and speak more than one language expands communication possibilities. This textbook provides only a basic introduction to other healthcare traditions. The intent is to create an awareness of the similarities and differences in theory and process for some of the various healing traditions.

It is helpful for the massage therapy learner to understand the Chinese system more fully because historical and current Chinese medicine have an important influence on the practice of massage.

The traditional Chinese health system is among the most ancient. It is based on the continual accumulation of knowledge through centuries of experiential observation. The system is similar to those of other cultural healing systems, which also endeavor to promote health by working toward homeostasis rather than by eliminating symptoms (a Western approach).

The Asian systems (specifically Chinese medicine) are used here as examples of terminology components. The Asian perspective is based on the meridian system. **Acupuncture** points and the five-element relationship system are used to identify and explain anatomical and physiological functions.

In the past, treatments used to help in the survival of and recovery from trauma were mostly a matter of luck. Some believe that before the advent of pain-relieving drugs and treatments, a healer would press, rub, or hit the affected part of the body to alleviate the pain. Sometimes the person who had been burned, bruised, or cut would find that the preexisting pain would dissipate and healing would occur.

The earliest concept of acupuncture involved stimulating a painful point by pressing on it, puncturing it, or burning it. The point was referred to as an *Ah shi point*, which can be loosely translated into, "Ah, yes, that's where it hurts." In Western science, this method of treatment can be explained by the gate control theory, in which one set of sensory signals travels faster to the central nervous system and blocks the transmission of a different set of sensory stimuli that may be distressing.

With the increasing use of acupuncture, the need for a common language to facilitate communication in teaching, research, clinical practice, and exchange of information became apparent. In 1989 the WHO used a group of experts to develop the Standard International Acupuncture Nomenclature, which is now widely used.

Ancient practitioners identified specific points before they recognized any patterns. The mapping of points eventually developed into various healing systems (Box 3.3).

In Western science, acupuncture points have been identified with various anatomical or physiological locations or functions in the body. Many acupuncture points have been associated with the motor points of the nervous system. (A *motor point* is the location where a nerve enters a muscle.) Acupuncture points also correspond to Golgi tendon organs and muscle stretch receptors. These same acupuncture points have been shown to have close correlations with a variety of named tender point phenomena, including trigger points and corresponding pain patterns. A *trigger point* is currently considered a localized area of deep tenderness and increased tissue resistance. The pressure exerted on a trigger point causes referred pain in a predictable area (Fig. 3.10).

Ayurveda, a healing tradition from India, also uses points, called *marmas*. They are clustered around joints where various types of tissue meet, and they also have a high correlation with meridians, acupuncture points, and trigger points.

In the ancient and Western scientific systems, point phenomena have many commonalities, for example:

- They are located in a palpable depression.
- They are associated with a neurovascular formation consisting of free nerve endings, Golgi tendon receptors, spindle cells, pacinian corpuscles, and lymph or blood vessels that pass through the fasciae.

Box 3.3 Acupuncture for Common Conditions

WHO identified symptoms, diseases, and conditions that have been shown through controlled trials to be treated effectively by acupuncture. The findings of this report found acupuncture beneficial for these common conditions:

- Low back pain
- Neck pain
- Sciatica
- Tennis elbow
- Knee pain
- Sprains
- Facial pain
- Headache
- Dental pain
- Temporomandibular joint dysfunction
- Rheumatoid arthritis
- Induction of labor
- Morning sickness
- Nausea and vomiting
- Postoperative pain
- Stroke
- Essential hypertension
- Primary hypotension
- Adverse reactions to radiation or chemotherapy
- Allergic rhinitis, including hay fever
- Depression (including depressive neurosis and depression following stroke)
- Primary dysmenorrhea
- Peptic ulcer
- Acute and chronic gastritis

Data from World Health Organization. *Acupuncture: review and analysis of reports on controlled clinical trials.* Available at http://apps.who.int/iris/bitstream/10665/42414/1/9241545437.pdf; 2003 Accessed 05.05.15.

- They are located on the surface of alpha and delta-fiber afferent, fast-transmitting receptors that are sensitive to sharply pointed stimuli and heat. These points may correlate with the acupuncture points.
- They are deep to the alpha and delta fibers in the same area; they have intramuscularly placed, C-afferent, slow-transmitting fibers, which are more sensitive to chemicals and may correlate with the trigger points.

Particular effects may be demonstrated after acupuncture treatment. Some of these effects involve alterations in the functions of organs or systems. An analgesic effect and also an anesthetic effect occur. The reflexes involved may not yet be fully explained. The mapping of 100 acupuncture points showed them to be located over large nerve trunks and cutaneous neurovascular bundles.

In China, acupuncture was used in combination with herbal medicine, dietetic regimens, and psychological guidance. The use of finger pressure on an acupuncture point has been demonstrated to induce the desired feeling of soreness and fullness that is a forerunner of the anesthetic effect. Electrophysiological studies have shown that firm pressure applied to muscles and tendons has a definite inhibitory effect on the nervous system. Because the body strives toward health, it uses all helpful stimuli to achieve that goal. If, through acupuncture or manual pressure (acupressure), this function can be assisted, health is supported.

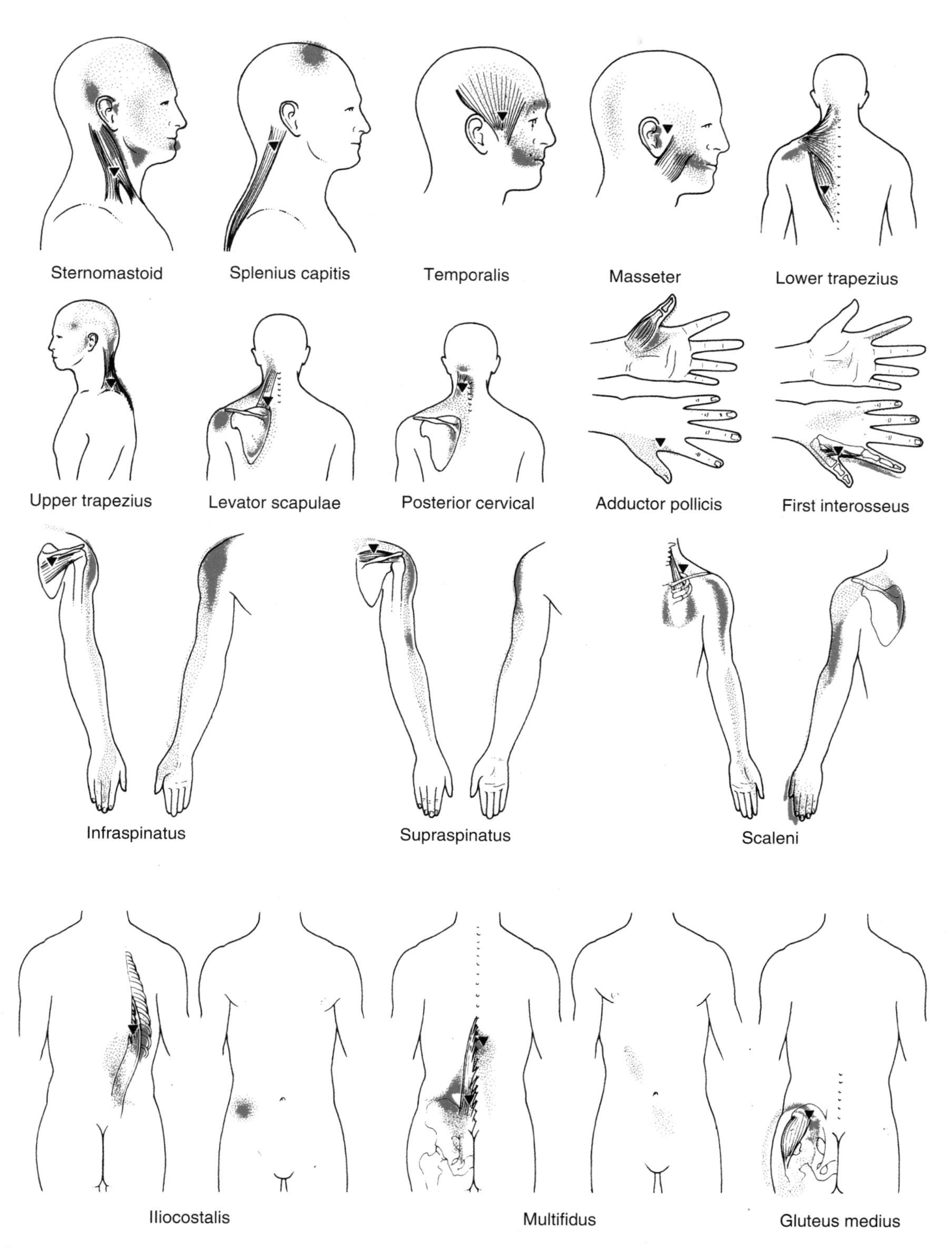

FIG. 3.10 Common trigger point locations in muscles. (From Chaitow L. *Modern Neuromuscular Techniques*. 2nd ed. Churchill Livingstone; 2003.)

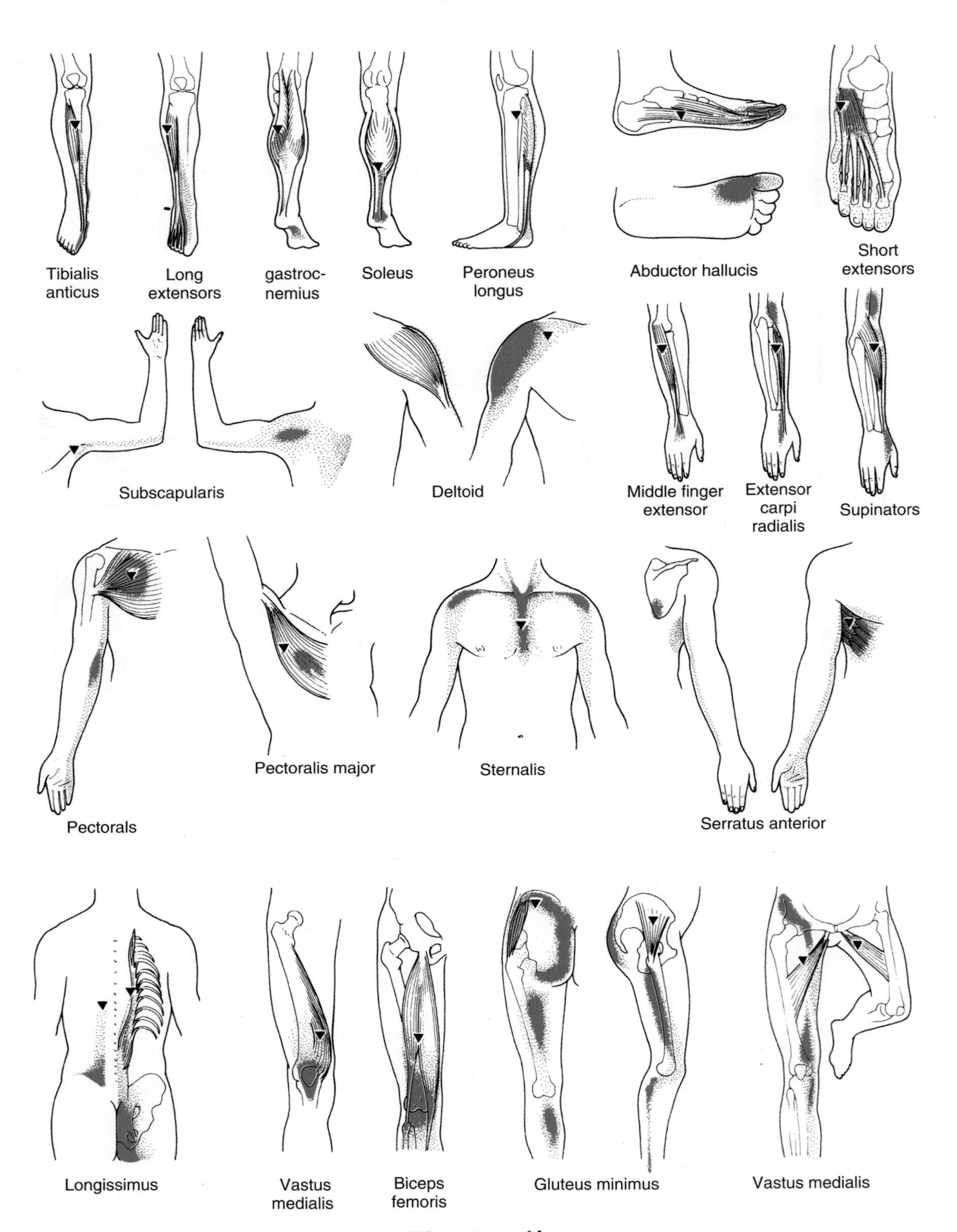

FIG. 3.10, cont'd

Points and Meridians

Acupuncture, acupressure, and cupping are based largely on the theory of the channels and network vessels. In traditional Chinese medicine, this system of points and meridians is known as *jing luo*, which is usually translated into English as either "meridians" or "channels and network vessels." This system of acupuncture points, organized as meridians, is the fundamental infrastructure of Chinese anatomy and physiology. Disturbances in the meridians are reflected in abnormalities along their course (Fig. 3.11).

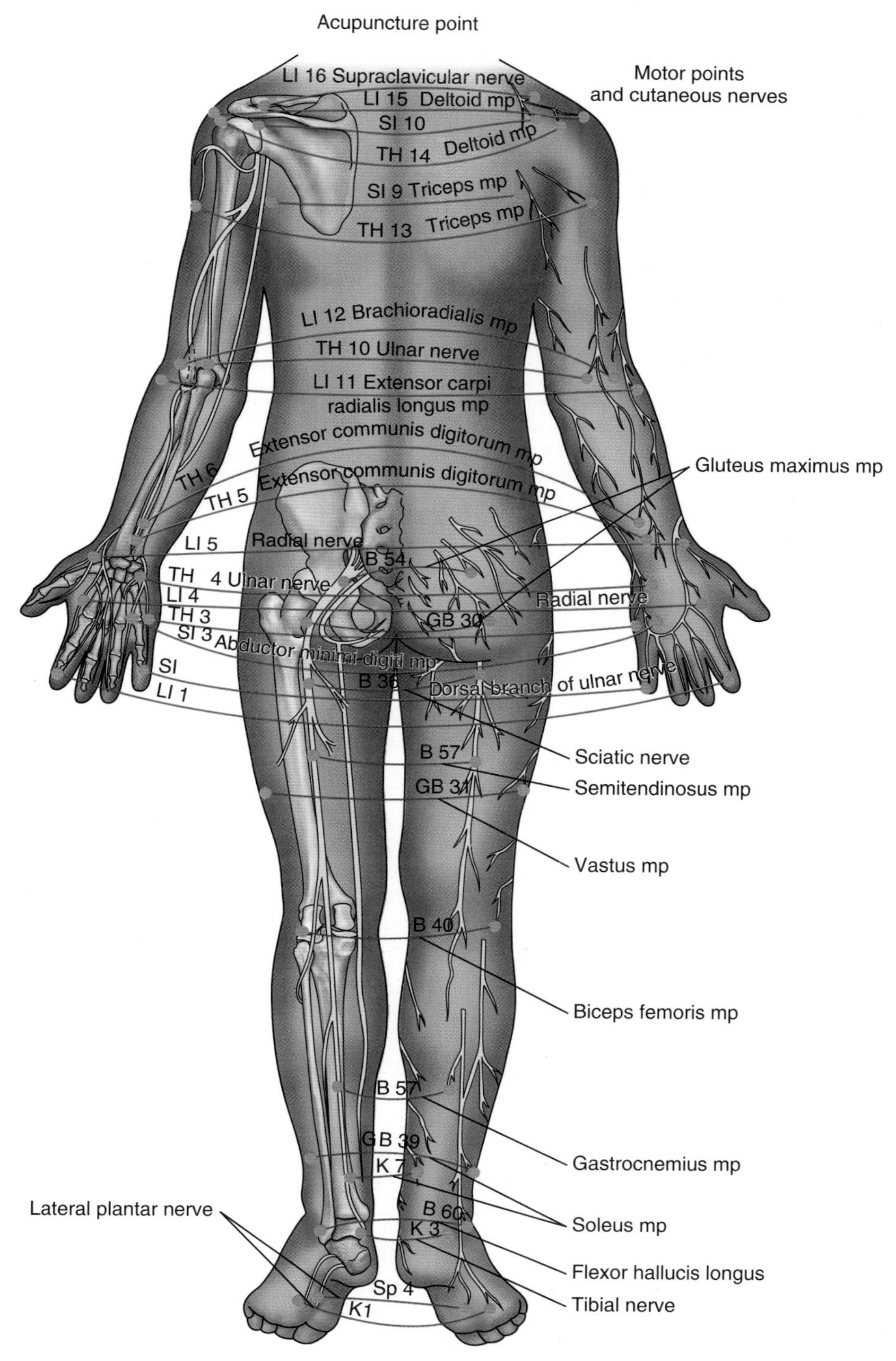

FIG. 3.11 Comparison of traditional acupuncture points, motor points, and cutaneous nerves of the arm and leg. *B*, Bladder; *GB*, gallbladder; *K*, kidney; *LI*, large intestine; *mp*, motor point; *SI*, small intestine; *Sp*, spleen; *TH*, triple heater. (From Fritz S. *Mosby's Fundamentals of Therapeutic Massage*. 5th ed. Mosby; 2013.)

The patterns of acupuncture points on the surface of the body have been charted by practitioners for centuries. They have been grouped in lines (called *channels* or *meridians*). The actual tracts of each meridian were determined by plotting the various sensations that radiated above or below a point when it was pressed. Twelve main meridians have been identified. They are bilateral, symmetrically distributed lines of acupuncture points with an affinity for or effects on the functions or organs for which they are named (Box 3.4 and Fig. 3.12). In addition to the 12 pairs of bilateral meridians, two meridians

Box 3.4 Meridians

Twelve Main Meridians

- The lung meridian (L; yin) begins on the lateral aspect of the chest, in the first intercostal space, and then passes down the anterolateral aspect of the arm to the root of the thumbnail.
- 11 points
- Pathologic symptoms: Fullness in the chest, cough, asthma, sore throat, colds, chills, and aching of the shoulders and back
- The large intestine (LI; yang) meridian starts at the root of the fingernail of the first finger and passes up the posterolateral aspect of the arm over the shoulder to the face, ending at the side of the nostril.
- 20 points
- Pathologic symptoms: Abdominal pain, diarrhea, constipation, nasal discharge, and pain along the course of the meridian
- The stomach (ST; yang) meridian starts below the orbital cavity and runs over the face and up to the forehead, from where it passes down the throat, the thorax, and the abdomen and continues down the anterior thigh and leg to end at the root of the second toenail (lateral side).
- 45 points
- Pathologic symptoms: Bloat, edema, vomiting, sore throat, and pain along the course of the meridian
- The spleen (SP; yin) meridian originates at the medial aspect of the great toe and then travels up the internal aspect of the leg and thigh to the abdomen and thorax, where it finishes on the axillary line in the sixth intercostal space.
- 21 points
- Pathologic symptoms: Gastric discomfort, bloat, vomiting, weakness, heaviness of the body, and pain along the course of the meridian
- The heart (H; yin) meridian begins in the axilla and runs down the anteromedial aspect of the arm to end at the root of the little fingernail (medial aspect).
- 9 points
- Pathologic symptoms: Dry throat, thirst, cardiac-area pain, pain along the course of the meridian
- The small intestine (SI; yang) meridian starts at the root of the small fingernail (lateral aspect) and then travels up the posteromedial aspect of the arm and over the shoulder to the face, where it terminates in front of the ear.
- 19 points
- Pathologic symptoms: Pain in the lower abdomen, deafness, swelling in the face, sore throat, and pain along the course of the meridian
- The bladder (B; yang) meridian starts at the inner canthus and ascends, passing over the head and down the back and the leg to terminate at the root of the nail of the little toe (lateral aspect).
- 67 points
- Pathologic symptoms: Urinary problems, mania, headaches, eye problems, and pain along the course of the meridian
- The kidney (K; yin) meridian starts on the sole, ascends the medial aspect of the leg, and runs up the front of the abdomen to finish on the thorax, just below the clavicle.
- 27 points
- Pathologic symptoms: Dyspnea, dry tongue, sore throat, edema, constipation, diarrhea, motor impairment and atrophy of the lower extremities, and pain along the course of the meridian
- The circulation (C; yin) meridian (also known as *heart constrictor* or *pericardium*) begins on the thorax lateral to the nipple, runs down the anterior surface of the arm, and terminates at the root of the nail of the middle finger.
- 9 points
- Pathologic symptoms: Angina, chest pressure, heart palpitations, irritability, restlessness, pain along the course of the meridian
- The triple heater (TH; yang) meridian begins at the nail root of the ring finger (ulnar side) and runs up the posteromedial aspect of the arm, over the back of the shoulder, and around the ear to finish at the outer aspect of the eyebrow.
- 23 points
- Pathologic symptoms: Abdominal distention, edema, deafness, tinnitus, sweating, sore throat, and pain along the course of the meridian
- The gallbladder (GB; yang) meridian starts at the outer canthus and runs backward and forward over the head, passing over the back of the shoulder and down the lateral aspect of the thorax and abdomen. The meridian passes to the hip area and then down the lateral aspect of the leg to terminate on the fourth toe.
- 44 points
- Pathologic symptoms: Bitter taste in mouth, dizziness, headache, ear problems, and pain along the course of the meridian
- The liver (LIV; yin) meridian begins on the great toe and runs up the medial aspect of the leg and up the abdomen to terminate on the costal margin (vertically below the nipple).
- 14 points
- Pathologic symptoms: Lumbago, digestive problems, retention of urine, pain in the lower abdomen, and pain along the course of the meridian

Midline Meridians

The body has two midline meridians. The conception or central vessel (CV; yin) meridian starts in the center of the perineum and runs up the midline of the anterior aspect of the body to terminate just below the lower lip; it is responsible for all yin meridians (24 points). The governing vessel (GV; yang) meridian starts at the coccyx and runs up the center of the spine and over the midline of the head, to terminate on the front of the upper gum; it is responsible for all yang meridians (28 points).

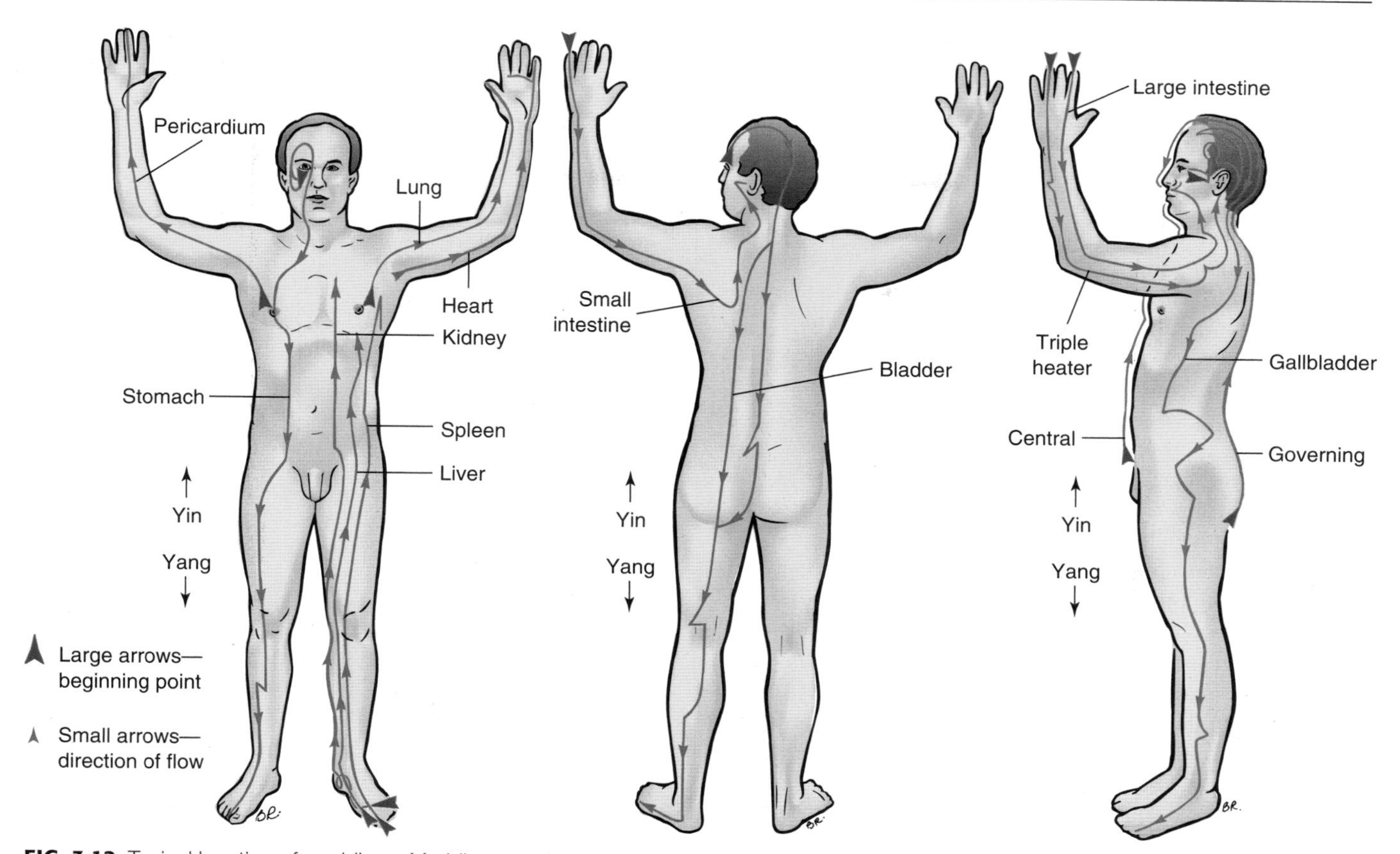

FIG. 3.12 Typical location of meridians. Meridians tend to follow nerves. Yin and yang meridians are paired as follows:

Pericardium	Triple heater
Liver	Gallbladder
Kidney	Bladder
Heart	Small intestine
Spleen	Stomach
Lung	Large intestine

lie on the anterior and posterior midline of the trunk and head. Various extra meridians also exist, and they appear to relate to the organs and functions of the body. Other points on the ear surfaces, the hands, and the face have specific reflex effects.

Unlike the Western concept of individual organs, the Eastern philosophy considers organ systems. Each system includes an organ, essences, and fluids as they interact with the meridians. Ayurveda describes body functions in terms of *doshas*—Vata, Pitta, and Kapha (see Chapter 2). Dr. Randolph Stone, DO, DC, ND (1890–1981) integrated the two systems and added other energetic methods to develop the polarity system. Ancient healing methods have always treated internal functions by means of external stimulation of the body, using methods such as acupuncture and massage. For centuries practitioners have been using these techniques to reestablish homeostasis within the body, so it is reasonable to think that such practices must have some sort of consistent benefit. Current research has validated the cutaneous-visceral connections that are an aspect of these practices.

As discussed in Chapter 2, the nerve reflexes of internal organs manifest on the surface of the body, showing up as referred to pain. These are examples of other manifestations of nerve patterns that connect the internal organs with the surface:

- Pain sensations felt on the skin may be referred to by internal organs (viscerosomatic reflex).
- Muscular splinting may be noted over an area of internal disturbance.
- The autonomic nervous system influences surface areas of the body.
- A stimulus causes shifts in endogenous chemicals (those manufactured inside the body), which can affect organ function (somatovisceral reflex).

Research is helping us to understand some culturally based concepts. For example, a third circulatory system, independent of the blood and lymphatic systems, and a structure of connected nodes and ducts have been identified. This system is called by multiple names, such as the hyaluronic acid–rich node and duct system (NDS) and the primo vascular system. Although it seems to be part of the immune system, little is known about its immunological role. It appears that the NDS has flexible structures, much like lymph nodes, and plays a role in immune cell–mediated local inflammation. The system's structure consists of extremely tiny vessels that integrate features of the cardiovascular, nervous, immune, and hormonal systems. The very tiny vessels, through which a fluid flows, lie next to lymph vessels. Some researchers suspect that these tiny vessels may serve as the pathway for cancer metastasis (Lim et al., 2013; Soh et al., 2013; Stefanov et al., 2013; Rai et al., 2015; Choi et al., 2018).

Other recent findings have given rise to a better understanding of connective tissue, especially a type called the *interstitium*. Traditionally it had been thought that the tiny spaces between cells were filled with a fluid called *interstitial fluid* and that cells were suspended in this fluid. When researchers looked more closely, however, they found a series of fluid-filled sacs in the spaces between cells. Inside these fluid-filled sacs were functional proteins that formed channels connecting all the sacs, creating a flexible structure that interconnects fluid movement throughout the entire body (Benias et al., 2018).

In 2015 the lymphatic system of the central nervous system (CNS) was discovered. Researchers identified functional lymphatic vessels lining the dural sinuses of the CNS. These are venous channels located intracranially between the two layers of the dura mater covering the brain and spinal cord. These structures express all characteristics of lymphatic endothelial cells, can carry both fluid and immune cells from the cerebrospinal fluid, and are connected to the deep cervical lymph nodes. The discovery of this lymphatic system changes how we understand the body's neuroimmunology and helps explain neuroinflammatory and neurodegenerative diseases associated with immune system dysfunction (Louveau et al., 2015). In addition, ongoing studies have identified drainage systems that involve multiple components, including the activity of glial cells and perivascular spaces, which are fluid-filled spaces surrounding certain blood vessels (Englehardt et al., 2016; Abbott et al., 2018).

These discoveries may lead to a better understanding of how various healing systems influence functional processes. Research likely will continue to validate some ancient practices that focus treatment on the wholeness of the person—mind, body, and spirit.

Review What You Have Learned

- Explain the role of intuition in traditional healthcare systems.
  - Intuition is knowing something without going through a conscious, rational process of thinking. Traditional healthcare systems validate intuition as a mechanism to assess health and administer treatment.
- Identify terminology from an ancient Chinese healing model.
  - Ancient Chinese concepts of anatomy and physiology are largely based on the theory of acupuncture points and meridians. Acupuncture points are charted in patterns on the surface of the body and organized along lines called *meridians.*
- Compare terminology used in various healing traditions.
  - Acupuncture points correlate with motor points (where a nerve enters a muscle), trigger points (tender areas that produce referred pain), and marma points (Ayurvedic points clustered around joints where various tissue types meet).

MENTORING TIP

We live in a global society. Many different cultures interact daily. Communication can be a challenge. Many different systems and beliefs about health and illness are found in cultural structures. As health professionals, we need to learn about different cultures and understand the use of massage therapy as part of a variety of healing traditions. We have to learn to communicate with others when English is a second language and we may not speak an individual's first language. Be curious and respectful of cultural diversity. Learn from others and be willing to share your culture as well.

CLINICAL REASONING AND CHARTING

SECTION OBJECTIVE

Chapter objective covered in this section:

8. Use a charting method that incorporates a clinical reasoning/problem-solving model.

After completing this section, the learner will be able to:

- Define critical thinking and clinical reasoning.
- Explain how critical thinking is used in clinical reasoning.
- Describe a problem-oriented medical record (POMR).
- Explain how the SOAP note system supports critical thinking and clinical reasoning.

Effective assessment, analysis, and decision-making are essential to meeting the needs of each client. In attempting to individualize treatment, the practitioner often finds that routines or recipe-type applications of massage and bodywork treatments are of limited value or even ineffective because clients' circumstances vary so widely. Therefore the mark of an experienced professional is thinking in a logical, sensible manner called clinical reasoning.

Clinical reasoning is a learned skill. It enables massage practitioners to gather information effectively, analyze the information, determine the type and appropriateness of a therapeutic intervention, and evaluate and justify the benefits derived from the intervention. Clinical reasoning begins with the broader process of critical thinking. *Critical thinking* is a learned skill for logical and objective thinking.

Individual thought processes can be biased, distorted, partial, uninformed, and emotional and can leave out important information and ideas. Flawed thinking is costly—in time, resources (including money), and quality of life. Unfortunately, flawed thinking is a natural human trait. For this reason, educators, scientists, and other experts have developed processes for effective thinking, for example, the scientific method Therefore productive critical thinking, which is systematically learned, is essential for the massage professional to have career success.

Another example is the documentation process you learn in massage school. It provides a form, such as a SOAP note (discussed later), that serves as a map of the critical thinking process. Many activities in this text are designed to teach and reinforce critical thinking.

We are using clinical reasoning when we use critical thinking skills to make decisions about how we will structure a massage to achieve the client's goals. Clinical reasoning requires a commonly accepted clinical vocabulary. Scientific and medical terminology provides that vocabulary. Because even computers have to speak to each other in a common language, in 2004 the National Library of Medicine created the Unified Medical Language System to facilitate the development of computer systems that work as if they "understand" the meaning of the language of biomedicine and health.

It all begins with critical thinking, which guides clinical reasoning in massage practice and is documented according to a common vocabulary (Boxes 3.5 and 3.6).

Box 3.5 What Is Critical Thinking?

John Dewey was an American psychologist, philosopher, educator, and social activist. In his book, *How We Think*, Dewey (1910) defined critical thinking as "reflective thought": to suspend judgment, maintain a healthy skepticism, and exercise an open mind. Critical thinking in education involves learners doing things such as asking questions, answering questions, examining a problem, and finding a solution while thinking about the things they are doing by reflecting, contemplating feedback, and evaluating.

When you are thinking critically, you examine a problem, find a solution, think about why you were or were not successful, and learn from your successes and failures.

John Dewey said, "One thing more, and that is—you who are learners really have as great an opportunity as any learners of any subject ever had at any time, but it will take a lot of patience, a lot of courage, and, if I may say so, considerable guts!"

From Dewey J. *How We Think.* Health; 1982 (originally published in 1910).

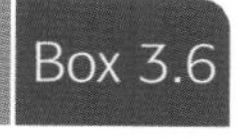

Box 3.6 Characteristics of Critical and Noncritical Thinkers

Critical Thinkers

- Acknowledge what they do not know
- Recognize their limitations
- Are conscious of their errors
- Think before acting
- Keep curiosity alive
- Base judgment on the evidence
- Are interested in others' ideas
- Are willing to listen to ideas even when they may disagree
- Control their feelings
- Are honest with themselves

Noncritical Thinkers

- Believe their views are correct and there is no room for error
- Have no regard for limitations
- See problems and issues as irritations
- Believe their opinions are the only correct ones
- Do not try to understand other views
- Base judgments on first impressions
- Act impulsively
- Are preoccupied with themselves
- Are know-it-alls

Modified from *Master Teacher Development Process Online.* Elsevier; 2005.

Charting/Documentation

Charting/documentation is the process of keeping a record of the clinical reasoning process during professional interactions. Effective charting is more than recording what happened. It is a clinical reasoning methodology that emphasizes a problem-solving approach to client care. Clinical problems are varied and are not necessarily related to dysfunction; rather, the problem involves ways to achieve therapeutic outcomes for the client.

To reason clinically and document effectively, a practitioner must have a comprehensive knowledge of medical terms and abbreviations and a deep familiarity with the anatomy and physiology of clients, both those in balanced states of functioning and those in altered states. Assessment procedures identify deviations from effective and normal functioning, and that information is the basis for formulating the care plan, identifying any contraindications to massage therapy, adapting the massage where appropriate, and evaluating the need for referral.

Electronic health records should be leveraged for what they can do to improve care and documentation, including effectively displaying prior information that shows historical information in a rich context; supporting critical thinking; enabling efficient and effective documentation; and supporting appropriate and secure sharing of useful and usable information with others, including patients, families, and caregivers. Good documentation is a fundamental component of high-quality care. Professional standards for high-quality, computer-based clinical documentation should keep the best elements of paper-based documentation without duplicating its inefficiencies and limitations. The standards should emphasize clarity, brevity, and attention to the needs of other readers, including patients (Akhu-Zaheya et al., 2018). Nevertheless, caution and careful oversight are necessary.

- Never reveal or allow anyone access to your personal identification number or passwords (these are, in fact, electronic signatures).
- Log off when you are not using a system or when you leave a terminal.
- Shred any printouts containing client information.
- Retrieve printouts promptly.

Regardless of whether electronic or paper records are used, no one format is appropriate for all situations. But good documentation always meets five important requirements: (1) factual, (2) accurate, (3) complete, (4) current (timely), and (5) organized.

Types of Charting

A commonly used method of charting is the POMR. Flow sheets and checklists frequently are used to document routine and ongoing assessments and observations. In focus-type charting systems (e.g., SOAP, SOAPIER, PIE, and DAR), the progress notes are used to document the client's progress in meeting established goals, and notes are written to provide documentation related to a specific focus (Kuhn et al., 2015).

A type of POMR commonly used by massage therapists is called *SOAP notes.* The SOAP notes format supports the process of critical thinking applied to clinical reasoning. Because the method is based on an analytical process, after you have learned it, the method can be adapted easily to any other documentation method. The key is to consider a massage session rationally and comprehensively. A charting method provides a structure for and a record of the process.

The SOAP note charting method uses this pattern:

- S—subjective information from the client
- O—objective data based on inspection, palpation, and testing and a record of interventions performed
- A—analysis and assessment of the subjective and objective data, of the effectiveness of the intervention, of the methods used, and of the actions taken during the session
- P—plan, including the methodology to be used in future interventions and the progress of the sessions

The *S* and *O* are the data-collecting (fact-gathering) parts of the SOAP method. The *A* is the most complex of the four parts.

In the DAR form of focus charting, the progress note is written in the DAR format: data, action, and response.

- Data—subjective and/or objective information that supports the stated focus
- Action—what was done
- Response—what happened related to what was done

FDAR is an expansion on DAR charting: Focus (F), data (D), action (A), and response (R). Focus (F) describes the goal.

Database

Any problem-solving charting method must begin with a database. The database is composed of information collected before the process of identifying the client's problems and goals begins. It consists of all the available information that contributes to client care. A database has two parts: (1) the information obtained during a history-taking interview with the client and from other pertinent people, previous records, and healthcare treatment orders (subjective); and (2) the physical assessment (objective).

The first part of the database, the history-taking interview, provides information about the client's health and the reason for the visit, a descriptive profile of the client, a history of the client's current condition, a history of illness and health, and a history of family illnesses. The history also contains an account of the client's current health practices and perception of quality of life.

In the second part, the physical assessment, the extent and depth of the assessment may vary from setting to setting, from practitioner to practitioner, and according to the client's situation. Practitioners of therapeutic massage generally use some sort of visual assessment to look for bilateral symmetry and deviations. Functional assessment reveals restricted, exaggerated, painful, or otherwise altered movement patterns. Palpation is used to identify changes in tissue texture and temperature, locate energy changes, and identify areas of tenderness. Various manual tests may be used to distinguish soft tissue problems from other conditions, such as joint dysfunction.

Analyzing the Data

After collecting all the information, the massage practitioner analyzes it (Box 3.7). Then they identify goals to be achieved based on the examination findings, investigation, and data analysis. This is the *A* part of the SOAP process. The practitioner then decides on a care plan, recording at each session the actions taken and their effectiveness.

Not all therapeutic goals relate to dysfunction. Clients commonly use therapeutic massage to maintain health, manage stress, and fulfill needs for human comfort and well-being. The same analytical process is used to determine the methods that best meet these client goals.

Box 3.7 The Analysis Process

Step 1

- What facts have been gathered from the data provided by the client and from research about the situation presented?
- What is considered normal or balanced function?
- What has happened? (Spell out the events.)
- What caused the imbalance? (Can the cause be identified?)
- What was done or is being done?
- What has worked or not worked?

Step 2

- What are the possibilities? (What could all the information mean?)
- What does my intuition suggest?
- What are the possible patterns of dysfunction?
- What are the possible contributing factors?
- What might work?
- What are other ways to look at the situation?
- What do the data suggest?
- What are possible interventions?

Step 3

- What are the logical progressions of the symptom pattern, the contributing factors, and the current behaviors?
- What are the logical causes and effects of each intervention identified?
- What are the pros and cons of each intervention suggested?
- What are the consequences of not acting?
- What are the consequences of acting?

Step 4

- For each intervention under consideration, what would be the effect on the persons involved—the client, the practitioner, and other professionals working with the client?
- How does each person involved feel about the possible interventions?
- Is the practitioner within the scope of practice to work with such a situation?
- Is the practitioner qualified to work in such a situation?
- Does the practitioner feel confident about working with such a situation?
- Does a feeling of cooperation and agreement exist among all parties involved?

Treatment Planning

The *P*, or *plan*, section of the SOAP method involves the development and implementation of a care plan. The plan is not an exact protocol set in stone, but rather a guideline. After implementing the plan, the practitioner reevaluates and adjusts it as necessary.

SOAP may be summarized as such:

- *S* and *O* are the facts obtained during data collection and what was done during the session.
- *A* is the analysis of the data obtained in *S* and *O* and the research into possibilities, logical causes and effects, consequences, and effects on the people involved.
- *P* is the decision-making and implementation structure.

The practitioner must be able to collect all data from the client history, assessment, and any necessary research. Once all the information has been collected, the massage therapist analyzes it so that they can make decisions about what the data mean and what patterns are represented in the whole person. Because of the amount of information involved and because most human difficulties are multidimensional, involving body, mind, and spirit, all areas must be addressed. In many cases referral is necessary.

Effective practice and ethical behavior require a massage therapist to stay within the competencies of a professionally defined scope of practice and a personal level of training, expertise, and experience. Therefore assessment and analysis may indicate a need to refer the client elsewhere or to use a team approach, working in a multidisciplinary, cooperative effort to provide the best possible care for each client.

Review What You Have Learned

- Define critical thinking and clinical reasoning.
- *Critical thinking* is the learned skill of logical and objective thinking. *Clinical reasoning* is the learned skill of gathering and analyzing information, determining an appropriate intervention, and evaluating the effects of the intervention.
- Explain how critical thinking is used in clinical reasoning.
- *Critical thinking* is necessary for *clinical reasoning*. Logical, objective thinking allows for the gathering of evidence-informed/evidence-based information, the appropriate choice of intervention, and unbiased evaluation.
- Describe a problem-oriented medical record (POMR).
- POMR is a method of charting in which critical thinking and clinical reasoning are used to assess, implement, and evaluate care plans.
- Explain how the SOAP note system supports critical thinking and clinical reasoning.
- *S* (subjective client information) and *O* (objective information assessed by the therapist) provide the gathering of data/evidence. *A* (analysis of information) allows for the appropriate choice of intervention and evaluation. *P* (plan) includes suggested future interventions and the client's progress.

Your ability to apply what you have learned from the study of anatomy and physiology comes from the reasoning and problem-solving processes. With this skill, the information you acquire comes alive and becomes practical. Effective work with clients is a continual learning process of assessing, deciding on interventions, and analyzing effectiveness through evaluation of the client's progress from session to session. Even in the most basic sessions, when the client's goals are pleasure and relaxation, the practitioner must decide on the best ways to encourage the body to respond to meet those goals.

Practical Application

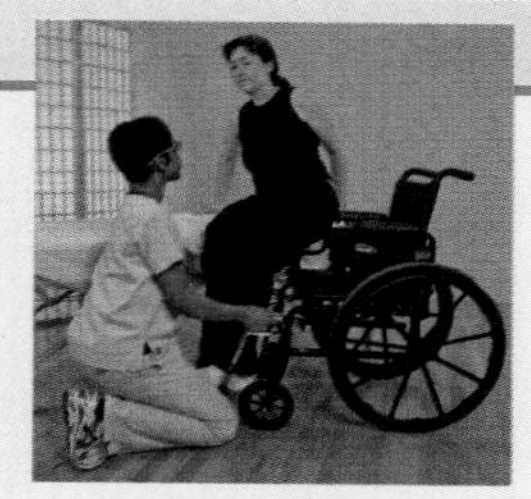

This textbook has been developed on the model of critical thinking and clinical reasoning to ensure that the massage care and treatment plans you develop and implement, as a massage therapist, have the best chance of success. A model is a pattern to imitate. See if you can identify the clinical reasoning model when doing the exercises and activities that encourage analysis and reasoning. Imitating a model is an effective way to begin a learning process. Once you can understand the model and use it effectively, you can vary it as necessary to provide the best response to each set of circumstances. Remember: a model is a tool, not an absolute.

SUMMARY

A competent massage therapist can understand the language of the scientific community, as well as the language and underlying philosophy of other healing practices, such as those of Asia. Even though the main focus of this text is Western science, a tremendous amount of overlap exists between Western and Eastern methods, and therapeutic massage is influenced richly by ancient healing practices.

Cultural healing traditions share similar philosophies but use different terminology. Two additional examples are the chakra system (described in Chapter 6) and the dosha system (described in Chapter 2). Several factors are common to these healing traditions, including the use of soft tissue methods; movement; meditation and inner reflection; exercise; dietary influences, including the use of naturally occurring substances for medicinal purposes; emotional influences; and spiritual connections that make human beings one with their environment and the universe. These ancient systems are often based on metaphors that describe naturally occurring, observable phenomena that are correlated with physical and psychological functions.

Western scientific study is no less colorful, and it weaves a tapestry of its own. It is a young discipline and eventually will reach the harmony of approaches evident in ancient practices. Western methods and ancient healing traditions are not in opposition; rather, they complement each other. Together they blend ancient wisdom and current understanding as we strive for homeostasis. It is impossible to be knowledgeable about every aspect of every healing tradition in the world. Be respectful of cultural traditions.

Professional practices, such as charting and composing reports, require proficiency in the use of language; this is the basis of effective written and verbal communication.

Visit the Evolve website: https://evolve.elsevier.com/Fritz/essential/

The Evolve website provides support for the review of the chapter content and chapter quizzes to help you prepare for the MBLEx or other massage therapy certification or licensing exams. End-of-chapter questions for discussion and review answer key and rationales and authors' response to critical thinking and clinical reasoning scenarios.

CRITICAL THINKING/CLINICAL REASONING

Each chapter will feature a critical thinking and clinical reasoning application of the content related to massage therapy practice. A client scenario will be presented with recommendations for additional research often using MedlinePlus or PubMed. Relevant questions based on the chapter content outline are provided to guide the discussion. There are no specific current answers to the questions. However, responses should be supportive of evidence-informed practices and based on biological plausibility if sufficient research is not available. The author's decision-making process related to the scenario and questions is on the EVOLVE site. Compare and contrast your thoughts and discussion with the author and determine where you agree or disagree.

Scenario

Ethan is an English bulldog rescued from a puppy mill. Inbreeding has resulted in genetic problems for him. A skin condition is most problematic for Ethan. The veterinarian has exhausted traditional treatment methods, and the only medication that has reduced the itching is cortisone injections. The problem appears to be some sort of allergy and autoimmune condition. The name of the condition is *atopic dermatitis*.

The vet recommended acupuncture and referred Ethan to a specially trained vet at an alternative and complementary veterinary clinic. Ethan's vet believes that acupuncture and possibly dietary changes would be beneficial in an integrated medicine treatment plan. After reading the recommended information, Ethan's human companion feels overwhelmed by the large words. You are their massage therapist, and you remember your medical terminology courses from school. The client asks you to help them understand the problems and the possible treatments Ethan would receive. Search MedlinePlus for information on acupuncture and atopic dermatitis.

- Search PubMed for research related to veterinary acupuncture and atopic dermatitis.
- Search Google or similar search engines using the search terms atopic dermatitis dogs.

Discuss These Points

- Why do you think the human companion asked the massage therapist to helpher understand the terminology?
- How did you use medical terminology to interpret the meanings of anatomical and physiological terms when doing the information search?
- What would you explain about Ethan's condition?
- What terms were commonly found in the information?
- How does the atopic dermatitis affect quality of life for both Ethan and the human companion?
- What aspects of culturally based terminology in the chapter helped you understand the content you found during the search process?
- What if a massage client has atopic dermatitis? How would clinical reasoning factor into the massage care plan?

MULTIPLE CHOICE QUESTIONS FOR REVIEW AND DISCUSSION

- The answers, with rationales, can be found on the Evolve site.

Because these questions are used for review and discussion, it is as important to understand why wrong answers are wrong as it is to know why the correct answer is correct. The answers to the questions, with rationales and explanations about why the correct answer is correct and why wrong answers are wrong, can be found on the Evolve site. At the end of the question section here in the textbook, you'll find an exercise that asks you to write more questions. Use the various questions in the chapter as examples. This is one of the best study strategies for test-taking.

It is important to understand that the actual licensing exam you take may not contain any of the specific questions found in this textbook or the review material and practice tests on the Evolve site. Therefore just because you can answer any of these questions correctly does not mean you will pass the licensing exam. The questions are content and style examples to help you prepare—this is why understanding why wrong answers are wrong is just as important as identifying the correct answer. Also, make sure you understand all the terminology used in the questions and possible answers in the review and discussion questions. Look up words you don't understand.

1. The prefix meaning against or opposite is ______.
   a. Circum-
   b. Caud-
   c. Contra-
   d. Brach-
2. The prefix mal- means ______.
   a. Large
   b. One or single
   c. Form or shape
   d. Illness or disease
3. The root word for kidney is ______.
   a. Nephr(o)-
   b. Neur(o)-
   c. Uro-
   d. Phleb(o)-
4. The suffix for pain is ______.
   a. -asis
   b. -ase
   c. -algia
   d. -emia
5. The history-taking interview provides data for which part of the SOAP note charting process?
   a. Subjective data
   b. Objective data
   c. Analysis
   d. Plan
6. For the data collected during the interview process and physical assessment to be focused on a particular outcome for the client, the information must be ______.
   a. Recorded in a SOAP note
   b. Communicated to the client

c. Analyzed using a logical process
d. Written in medical terminology

7. Referral to another healthcare professional is based on which part of the clinical reasoning process?
a. Assessment of data
b. Data collection
c. Plan development
d. History interview

8. The head, neck, trunk, and spinal cord are considered to be ______.
a. Appendicular
b. Thoracic
c. Axial
d. Ventral

9. The bladder is located in which region of the abdomen?
a. Epigastric
b. Umbilical
c. Left iliac
d. Hypogastric

10. The liver is located in which quadrant?
a. Right upper
b. Left upper
c. Right lower
d. Left lower

11. Which movement decreases the angle of a joint?
a. Flexion
b. Extension
c. Retraction
d. Adduction

12. The term meaning on the same side is ______.
a. Lateral
b. Contralateral
c. Ipsilateral
d. Dextral

13. The term meaning closer to the trunk or point of origin is ______.
a. Anterior
b. Posterior
c. Distal
d. Proximal

14. A commonality of the point phenomena is ______.
a. All points are located over motor points
b. All refer pain patterns
c. They are located over A-delta and C-afferent nerve fibers
d. They are located in meridian pathways

15. What do these have in common: circum-, andro-, and steno-?
a. Root words
b. Prefixes
c. Suffixes
d. Abbreviations

16. A massage practitioner identified a tender point in the occipital area. Where is this location?
a. Leg
b. Ankle
c. Neck
d. Arm

17. During the assessment, the client appears twisted. Which of the following would be the most accurate statement?
a. The client has frontal plane distortion.
b. The client is rotated in the transverse plane.
c. The client cannot abduct in the sagittal plane.
d. Flexion and extension are limited in the transverse plane.

18. The use of abbreviations in charting ______.
a. Is universally understood
b. Is more time consuming
c. Requires a deciphering key
d. Clearly communicates information

19. Many ancient healing practices were developed based on ______.
a. Measurement of concrete functions
b. Experiential observation
c. Scientific methods
d. Meridian system

20. A client relies on others to transport them to the massage sessions. They can move about with a walker but cannot navigate stairs. Which of the World Health Organization's Quality of Life Domains is being described?
a. Domain III: Level of Independence
b. Domain II: Psychological
c. Domain V: Environment
d. Domain IV: Social Relationships

Write Your Own Test Questions

Create at least three more multiple choice questions. Make sure to develop plausible wrong answers and double-check that the correct answer is correct. Then write a rationale for each question. The more questions you write, the better you will understand the material.

CHAPTER 4 Nervous System Basics and the Central Nervous System

https://evolve.elsevier.com/Fritz/essential/

CHAPTER OBJECTIVES

After completing this chapter, the learner will be able to:

1. Describe the basic organization of the nervous system.
2. Describe the anatomy of the neuron and neuroglia.
3. Describe the physiology of the neuron and neuralgia.
4. Explain the relationship between neurochemical activity and behavior, including pain behavior.
5. Identify the structures and functions of the brain.
6. Identify the structures and functions of the spinal cord.
7. List drugs that affect the (CNS).
8. Describe common pathological conditions of the CNS and the related indications/contraindications for massage.

CHAPTER OUTLINE

KEY TERMS

amyotrophic lateral sclerosis (ALS): (a-MI-o-TROF-ik) Also called Lou Gehrig disease. A progressive disease that begins in the central nervous system and involves the degeneration of motor neurons and the subsequent atrophy of voluntary muscle.

ascending tracts: Tracts in the spinal cord that carry sensory information to the brain.

axon: (AK-son) A single elongated projection from a nerve cell body that transmits impulses away from the cell body.

brain: The largest and most complex unit of the nervous system; the brain is responsible for perception, sensation, emotion, intellect, and action.

brainstem: The inferior, primitive portion of the brain that contains centers for vital functions and reflex actions, such as vomiting, coughing, sneezing, posture, and basic movement patterns.

catecholamine: (cat-e-CHOL-amine) Any of several compounds occurring naturally in the body that serve as hormones or as neurotransmitters in the sympathetic nervous system.

central nervous system (CNS): The brain and spinal cord and their coverings.

cerebellum: (sair-e-BELL-um) The second largest part of the brain; the cerebellum is involved with balance, posture, coordination, and movement.

cerebrospinal fluid (CSF): (sair-e-bro-SPY-nal) A clear, colorless fluid that flows throughout the brain and around the spinal cord, cushioning and protecting these structures and maintaining proper pH balance.

cerebrum: (se-REE-brum) The largest of the brain divisions; it consists of two hemispheres that occupy the uppermost region of the cranium. The cerebrum receives, interprets, and associates incoming information with past memories and then transmits the appropriate motor response.

dendrites: (DEN-drites) Branching projections from the nerve cell body that carry signals to the cell body.

descending tracts: Tracts in the spinal cord that carry motor information from the brain to the spinal cord.

dorsal root: Also called the posterior root. Posterior attachment of a spinal nerve to the spinal cord. Transmits sensory information into the spinal cord.

enteric nervous system (ENS): (en-TER-rik) A subdivision of the peripheral nervous system (PNS) that controls the digestive system.

essential tremor: A chronic tremor that does not proceed from any other pathological condition.
gray matter: Unmyelinated nervous tissue in the central nervous system.
interoception: (IN·ter·o·sep·shun) The body's ability to identify and process internal actions of the organs and systems inside the body.
monoplegia: (mon-o-PLE-je-a) Paralysis of a single limb or a single group of muscles.
myelin: (MY-e-lin) A white, fatty, insulating substance formed by the Schwann cells that surrounds some axons. Also produced in the central nervous system by oligodendrocytes.
neurolemma: (noo-ri-LEM-mah) Also called the Schwann membrane, sheath of Schwann, and endoneural membrane. The outer cell membrane of a Schwann cell that encloses the myelin sheath found on certain peripheral nerves. Essential in the regeneration of injured axons.
neuroglia: (noo-ro-GLEE-ah) Specialized connective tissue cells that support, protect, and hold neurons together and maintain homeostasis in the nervous system.
neurons: (NOO-ronz) Nerve cells that conduct impulses.
neurotransmitters: (noo-ro-TRANS-mit-erz) Chemical compounds that generate action potentials when released into the synapses from presynaptic cells.
paraplegia: (par-a-PLEE-je-a) Paralysis of the lower portion of the body and of both legs.
peripheral nervous system (PNS): The division of the nervous system that includes the cranial nerves, spinal nerves, and ganglia (bundles of nerves).
quadriplegia: (quad-ra-PLEE-je-a) Paralysis or loss of movement of all four limbs.
Schwann cell: (shwon) A specialized cell that forms myelin.
spinal cord: The portion of the central nervous system that exits the skull and extends into the vertebral column. The two major functions of the spinal cord are to conduct nerve impulses and to serve as a center for spinal reflexes.
status epilepticus: (ep-i-LEP-TIK-us) A medical emergency characterized by a continuous seizure that lasts longer than 30 minutes.
synapse: (SIN-aps) A space between neurons or between a neuron and an effector organ.
ventral root: Also called the anterior root. The anterior attachment of a spinal nerve to the spinal cord; transmits motor information away from the spinal cord. One of two roots that attach a spinal nerve to the spinal cord.
white matter: Myelinated nerve tissue in the central nervous system.

LEARNING HOW TO LEARN

In this chapter we begin to use the terms and concepts described in the first three chapters, which will help you review what you have learned so far. We will also begin to study a body system, including all the parts (anatomy), how it works (physiology), and what can go wrong (pathology). New terms are introduced as well. Learning involves more than memorizing the definitions of words and being able to identify the parts. Each system has a specific job in the body, and all the systems work together. Using analogies, examples, and stories is a fantastic way to help you learn.

An analogy is the comparison of a quality or characteristic to a person or thing. To do this, we use a name, image, adjective, or other word, which is normally used for something else but that is similar, for the purpose of explaining or clarifying. For example: The central nervous system functions as your body's computer.

"This is like that" is an example of a simile. For instance, the nerves are like the electrical wiring in a house.

Stories let you connect the information. For example: Once upon a time, the nervous system and the endocrine system held a meeting because of confusion over who did what. The person who had these body systems was not able to sleep. The nervous system blamed the endocrine system for producing too many hormones; the endocrine system blamed the nervous system for always being on the alert.

It does not matter if the stories are silly. Also check out YouTube, using the search term *nervous system*. Find videos designed for children in grade school. Add the terms *educational videos for kids* to the search. These are especially helpful. Use this strategy for all the body systems.

This is the first chapter in Section II: Systems of Control, which consists of Chapters 4, 5, and 6. Chapter 4 introduces the nervous system in general and then concentrates on the central nervous system (CNS). Chapter 5 covers the peripheral nervous system (PNS), and Chapter 6 covers the endocrine system. Current research indicates that most massage therapy benefits are realized in the nervous system Therefore understanding the nervous and endocrine systems is as important, if not more so, than understanding bones, joints, and muscles.

The essential information related to the systems of control is placed right after Section I: Fundamentals (Chapters 1, 2, and 3) because the nervous system and the endocrine system function as the main regulators of the body. Combined, Chapters 1, 2, and 3 have provided enough of a foundation so that you can understand how the nervous and endocrine systems perform their important monitoring and regulating functions. The nervous and endocrine systems receive information, decide what to do, and then tell the rest of the body how to use the information. Systems of control coordinate the smooth function of the rest of the body's systems to maintain homeostasis.

The nervous and endocrine systems transmit information from one part of the body to another, but they do it in different ways. The nervous system transmits information rapidly, with a short duration of action by nerve impulses conducted from one body area to another. The endocrine system is a network of ductless glands and other structures that secrete chemicals called *hormones* directly into the bloodstream, affecting the function of specific target organs. The action of hormones is slower and longer lasting than that of nerve impulses. Often, the nervous system initiates a response, and the endocrine system sustains it.

Both systems use chemicals. The nervous system uses **neurotransmitters**, which are chemicals that cross a synapse. A **synapse** is a gap between a neuron and another neuron, muscle cell, or gland. Neurotransmitters carry nerve impulses across synapses. As previously discussed, the endocrine system uses hormones. Hormones are often the same chemicals as neurotransmitters. If a chemical is found in the synapses, it is called a *neurotransmitter*. If the same chemical is found in the blood, it is called a *hormone*.

The influence of the nervous system regulates the endocrine system, and the endocrine system influences the nervous system, forming a feedback loop that increases or decreases activity for healthy function. The feedback system and autoregulation, or maintenance of internal homeostasis, are interlinked in all body functions.

As you learn this content, remember that you are learning a new language. Learning all the words, what they mean, and how they are applicable to massage therapy takes effort. Keep in mind that you may have to review the content more than once.

NERVOUS SYSTEM BASICS: OVERVIEW OF THE NERVOUS SYSTEM

SECTION OBJECTIVES

Chapter objective covered in this section:

1. Describe the basic organization of the nervous system.

After completing this section, the learner will be able to:

- List the two main divisions of the nervous system.
- List the two main subdivisions of the peripheral nervous system (PNS).
- List and define the three subdivisions of the autonomic nervous system (ANS).
- List and define three types of nerve cells.

Nervous System Functions

The nervous system is the most complex of the body systems. It has three main functions:

- *Sensing:* Collecting data from the environment, both the external environment and the internal environment
- *Interpreting:* Processing data and formulating a response
- *Acting:* Telling the body to perform the response

Nervous System Divisions

The nervous system is divided into the central nervous system and the peripheral nervous system.

- The **central nervous system (CNS)** is composed of the brain, spinal cord, and their coverings.
- The **peripheral nervous system (PNS)** is made up of the cranial nerves, spinal nerves, and ganglia (bundles of nerves).

The PNS has two main subdivisions. These subdivisions combine and communicate to innervate the somatic and visceral parts of the body:

- *Somatic subdivision:* The somatic subdivision monitors and controls bones, muscles, soft tissues, and skin. The word *somatic* is derived from the Greek *somatikos*, meaning "of the body."
- *Autonomic subdivision:* The visceral, or autonomic, subdivision is associated with the internal glands, organs, blood vessels, and mucous membranes. The word *viscera*, from Latin, is the plural of *viscus*, meaning "internal organ." *Autonomic* is from the Greek word *autonomia*, meaning "independence." When you combine the meanings, you get independence of internal organs. The autonomic nervous system (ANS) was so named because it was originally believed to act independently. However, although it can operate without conscious control, it is actually regulated by parts of the brain. Much of the interaction between body and mind takes place through ANS activity.

The ANS is subdivided even further, into the sympathetic, parasympathetic, and enteric aspects:

- The *sympathetic ANS* activates arousal responses and expends body resources in response to emergencies, excitement, or exercise. The sympathetic ANS is considered the "flight, fight, fear" system, but any highly emotional state of joy, excitement, or elation is also sympathetic in nature.
- The *parasympathetic ANS* reverses the response of the sympathetic ANS by returning the body to a nonalarm state and restoring body resources. The parasympathetic ANS is considered the "rest and digest" system.
- The **enteric nervous system (ENS)** is the third part of the ANS. Enteric means "pertaining to the intestines" and is derived from the Greek word *enterikos*, meaning "intestinal." The ENS has extensive two-way connections with the CNS. It works in concert with the CNS to control the digestive system in the context of local and whole-body physiological demands. The ENS is composed of thousands of small ganglia that lie within the walls of the esophagus, stomach, small and large intestines, pancreas, gallbladder, and biliary tree. The biliary tree is a system of vessels that directs digestive juices from the liver, pancreas, and gallbladder through a common bile duct into the small intestine. The ganglia contain neurons and glial cells. It is believed that the ENS contains as many neurons as the entire spinal cord. It also contains multiple plexuses, which are groups of intertwined nerves that function together. A large nerve, the vagus nerve, is a cranial nerve that comes directly from the brain. It supplies most of the abdominal viscera, among other structures and organs, and plays a key role in ENS functions (Fig. 4.1 and Activity 4.1).

ACTIVITY 4.1

Study the figure and flowchart. Then, on a separate piece of paper, draw the figure and flowchart to see how much you recall.

FOCUS ON PROFESSIONALISM

Massage therapy research is beginning to unravel how massage helps people feel better. In the past, massage therapy science education has been highly focused on musculoskeletal structure and function. Now and into the future, it is becoming apparent that although bones, joints, and muscles are important for an understanding of how massage is performed and related to some of the benefits people experience after massage, the nervous system is much more involved because it is monitoring, controlling, adjusting, and adapting all the time. It is important that we all understand how massage therapy affects the nervous system.

Nervous System Structure

The basic structure of the nervous system is the neuron, or nerve cell. The nervous system is composed of more than 100 billion nerve cells. The nerve cell is an impulse-transmitting fiber connecting the CNS with all parts of the body through the PNS. There are three basic types of neurons:

- *Afferent* (or *sensory*) *neurons*, which carry impulses to the CNS

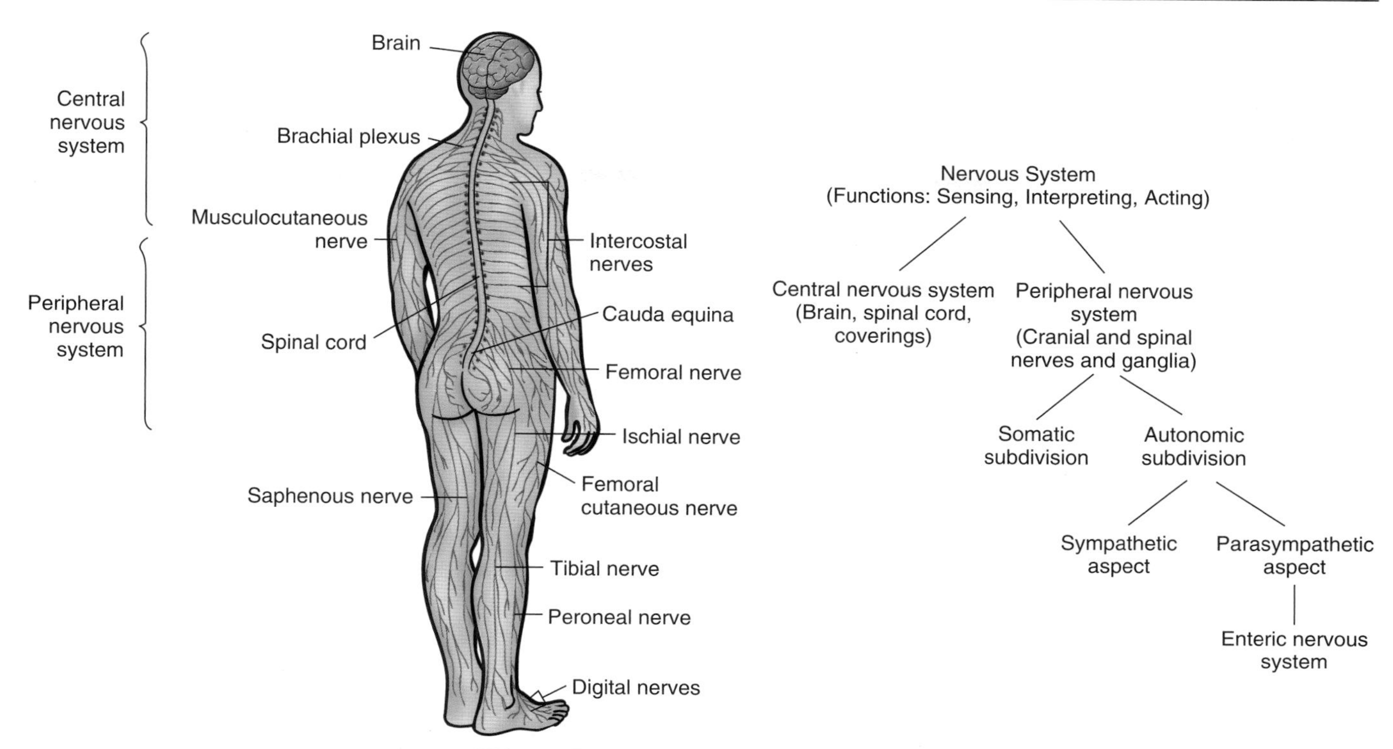

FIG. 4.1 The divisions of the nervous system.

- *Connecting* or *associative neurons* (known as *interneurons*), which transmit nerve impulses between neurons
- *Efferent* (or *motor*) *neurons*, which transmit impulses away from the CNS to muscles, organs, and glands

Review What You Have Learned

- List the two main divisions of the nervous system.
  - The CNS is composed of the brain, the spinal cord, and their coverings. The peripheral nervous system (PNS) includes the cranial nerves, spinal nerves, and ganglia (bundles of nerves).
- List the two main subdivisions of the peripheral nervous system.
  - The somatic nervous system is associated with conscious voluntary function and controls the bones, muscles, soft tissues, and skin. The autonomic nervous system is associated with unconscious involuntary function and controls internal glands, organs, blood vessels, and mucous membranes.
- List and define the three subdivisions of the autonomic nervous system.
  - The sympathetic ANS activates arousal responses and is considered the "flight, fight, fear" system. The parasympathetic ANS reverses the sympathetic ANS arousal responses and is considered the "rest and digest" system. The enteric nervous system (ENS) works in concert with the CNS to control the digestive system.
- List and define three types of nerve cells.
  - Afferent (sensory) neurons transmit impulses to the CNS. Interneurons (connecting or associative neurons) transmit nerve impulses between neurons. Efferent (motor) neurons transmit impulses away from the CNS.

NERVE CELL STRUCTURE

SECTION OBJECTIVES

Chapter objective covered in this section:

2. Describe the anatomy of the neuron and neuroglia.

After completing this section, the learner will be able to:

- Define *neurons*.
- List the parts of the neuron.
- Define *neuroglia*.

Two types of cells are found in the nervous system: neurons and neuroglia.

Practical Application

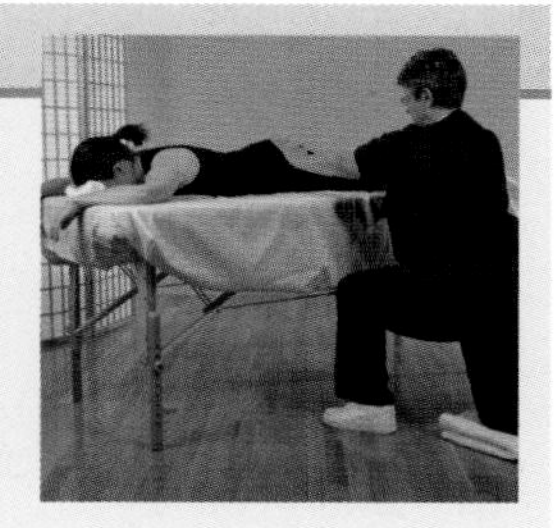

As a massage therapist, when you give a massage, you communicate with the sensory neurons. They are receptors. No matter how quickly, slowly, or deeply the massage is applied; it activates sensory nerves that send information to the spinal cord and brain. There the information is interpreted, and a decision is made about how to respond to the information. That decision is sent back to the rest of the body, where commands are issued, such as "release some chemicals here," "increase circulation there," or "stop contracting and relax." What the body does with the sensory information produced by massage ends up being either a benefit of massage or some sort of adverse (not good) outcome.

Neurons

Neurons are nerve cells. The function of the neurons is to receive and transmit electrical signals from and to other neurons, muscles, or glands (Fig. 4.2). Nerve cells consist of a cell body and its nerve fibers, the axons, and dendrites. The cell body contains a nucleus and its organelles. The **dendrites**, which look like small hairs, are extensions of the cytoplasm of the cell. Their job is to receive signals and carry them to the cell body. The **axon** is an elongated projection that carries signals away from the cell body. An axon may have branches (known as *collaterals*) that allow communication among several neurons.

Neurons are identified by structure or function (Box 4.1; also see Fig. 4.2). The simplest way to classify neurons is based on the function. A sensory neuron detects stimuli from the internal environment (e.g., a decline in the water levels of the blood) and the external environment (e.g., the warmth of the sun on the skin). These neurons send this information to the CNS. Interneurons (the connecting or associative neurons) integrate the sensory information. They analyze it, store some of it, and make a decision for appropriate responses. Motor neurons carry nerve impulses from the CNS out to effectors (muscles and glands) in response to decisions made by the CNS. Stimulation of the effectors causes muscles to contract and glands to secrete.

Unipolar and bipolar neurons are usually sensory neurons. Multipolar neurons are usually motor neurons or interneurons.

Neuroglia

Neuroglia, which are made up of glial cells, are specialized connective tissue cells. The word *neuroglia* means "nerve glue." These cells provide physical support, protection, insulation, and nutrient exchange pathways between the blood and the neurons of the brain and spinal cord. Recent research on neuroglial cells has shown that they have a variety of functions, all of which can be summed up as maintaining homeostasis of the nervous system.

The physiological functions and pathological dysfunction of the neuroglia in the CNS indicate that neuroglial cells play a

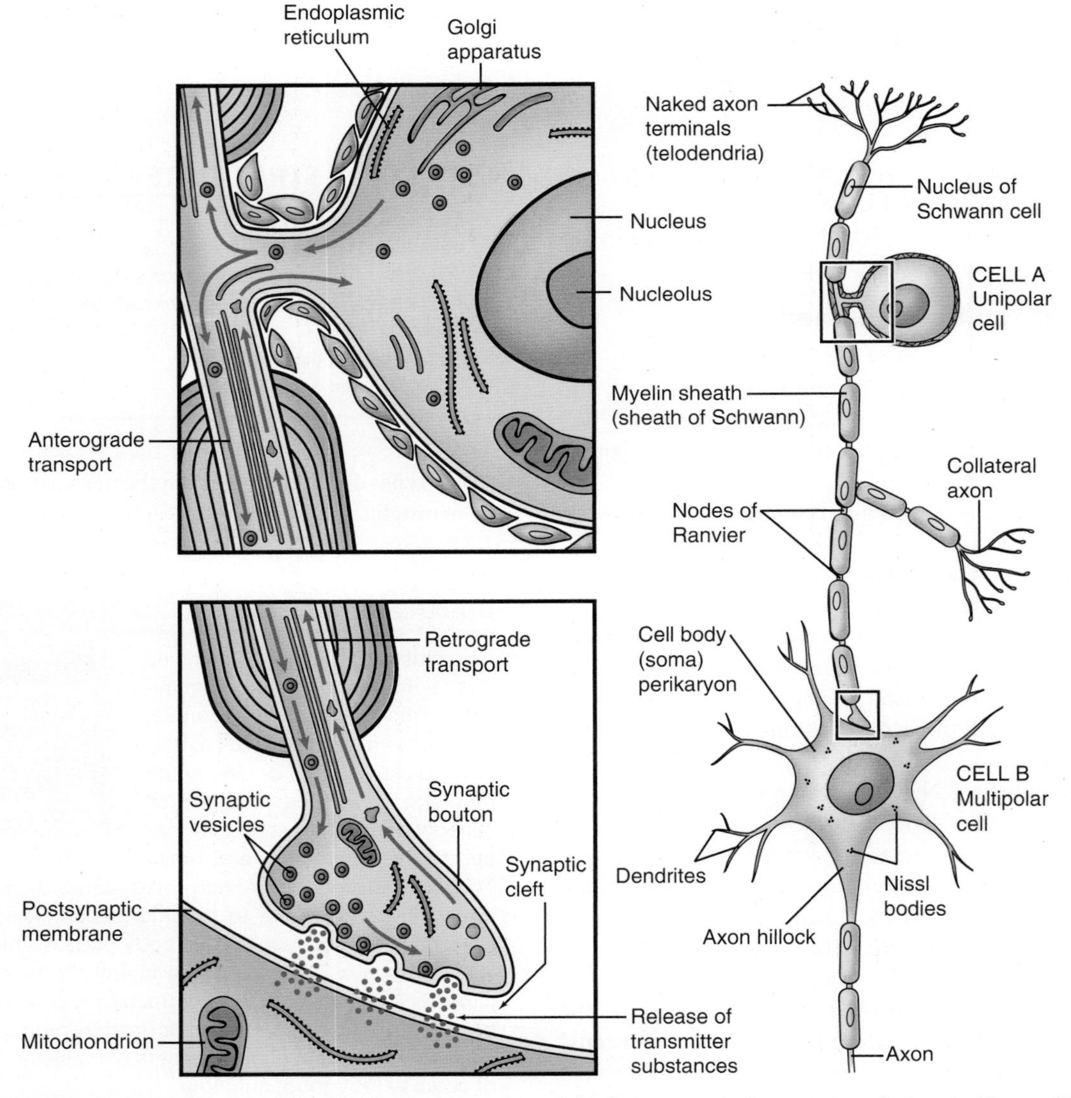

FIG. 4.2 A typical neuron. An electrical impulse travels along the axon of the first neuron to the synapse. A chemical transmitter is secreted into the synaptic cleft to depolarize the membrane (dendrite or cell body) of the next neuron in the pathway.

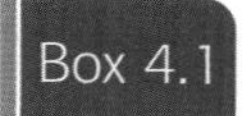

Neurons: Classification by Structure or Function

Three structural classifications of neurons:

1. Neurons that only have one projection to form the cell body, which includes both the dendrite and axon are called *unipolar*.

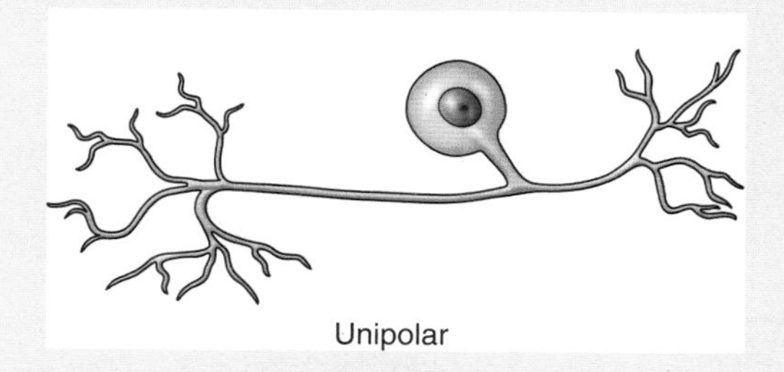

Unipolar

2. Neurons that have only one dendrite and the axon are called *bipolar neurons*.

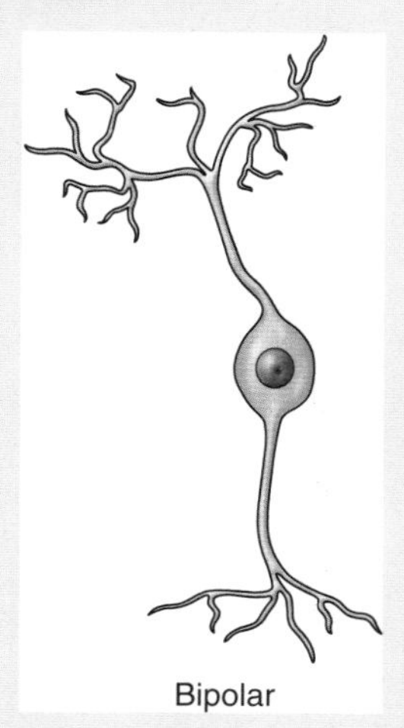

Bipolar

3. Neurons that have multiple dendrites and one axon exiting from the cell body are called *multipolar neurons*.

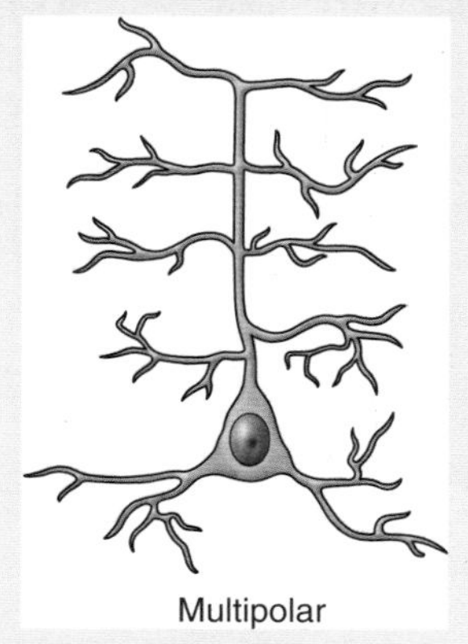

Multipolar

The three functional classifications of neurons are as follows:

1. Sensory or afferent neurons conduct sensory signals to the central nervous system (CNS).
2. Interneurons, or connecting or association neurons, act as bridges in the CNS to conduct signals from one neuron to another.
3. Motor or efferent neurons conduct motor signals away from the CNS to effectors.

role in pathology in the CNS, including neuropsychiatric and developmental disorders and neuroinflammatory responses in the brain. Implications include Alzheimer disease and other forms of dementia, Parkinson disease, some forms of depression, schizophrenia, and autism spectrum disorders. Neuroglial cells are found surrounding the synapses, and they release a wide variety of neuroactive molecules during physiological and pathological conditions. Neuroglial cells modulate the ability of synapses to strengthen or weaken over time in response to increases or decreases in their activity. This ability to change is called *synaptic plasticity*, which is one of the important neurochemical foundations of learning and memory. The four types of neuroglia found in the CNS are the following:

- *Ependymal cells:* Ependymal cells line the walls of the ventricles and form the epithelium, which secretes the **cerebrospinal fluid (CSF)**. Ependymal cells form a permeable barrier between the CSF that fills those cavities and the tissue fluid bathing the cells of the CNS. They also circulate the CSF with their cilia.
- *Astrocytes:* Most, if not all, neural processes involve astrocytes. Astrocytes provide physical and nutritional support for neurons, digest parts of dead neurons, and regulate the content of the extracellular space. Astrocytes secrete neuroactive substances and remove neurotransmitters, thereby influencing the processing of information by the nervous system. Astrocytes regulate synaptic transmission and neurotransmitter function and contribute to memory formation. As mentioned previously, synaptic plasticity underlies higher brain functions, such as learning and memory. Astrocytes are organized as networks and communicate with each other, affecting larger neural circuits. They also provide a link between neurons and the vasculature, potentially changing the cerebral microcirculation.
- *Oligodendrocytes:* Oligodendrocytes provide insulation (myelin) for neurons in the CNS. All white matter tracts contain oligodendrocytes, which form myelin. The most common disease involving oligodendrocytes is multiple sclerosis. It is caused by a loss of myelin in defined areas of the brain and spinal cord, which leads to impairment of axonal conductance.
- *Microglia:* Microglia digests parts of dead neurons and serves as the brain's endogenous defense and immune system. Microglial cells are responsible for protecting the CNS against several types of pathogenic factors.

In the peripheral nervous system, Schwann cells form **myelin**, a fatty, insulating protective sheath around the axons of certain neurons. The outer layer of the **Schwann cell** encloses the myelin sheath and is called the **neurolemma**. The neurolemma plays a role in regenerating an injured axon.

Satellite cells surround the cell bodies of PNS neurons, enclosing them in structures called *ganglia*, which are small bundles of nerve cells (Fig. 4.3).

Ongoing research is finding that the neuroglia is actively involved in most nervous system functions. In the brain, neurons, astrocytes, oligodendrocytes, and microglial cells communicate with each other by direct contact or through

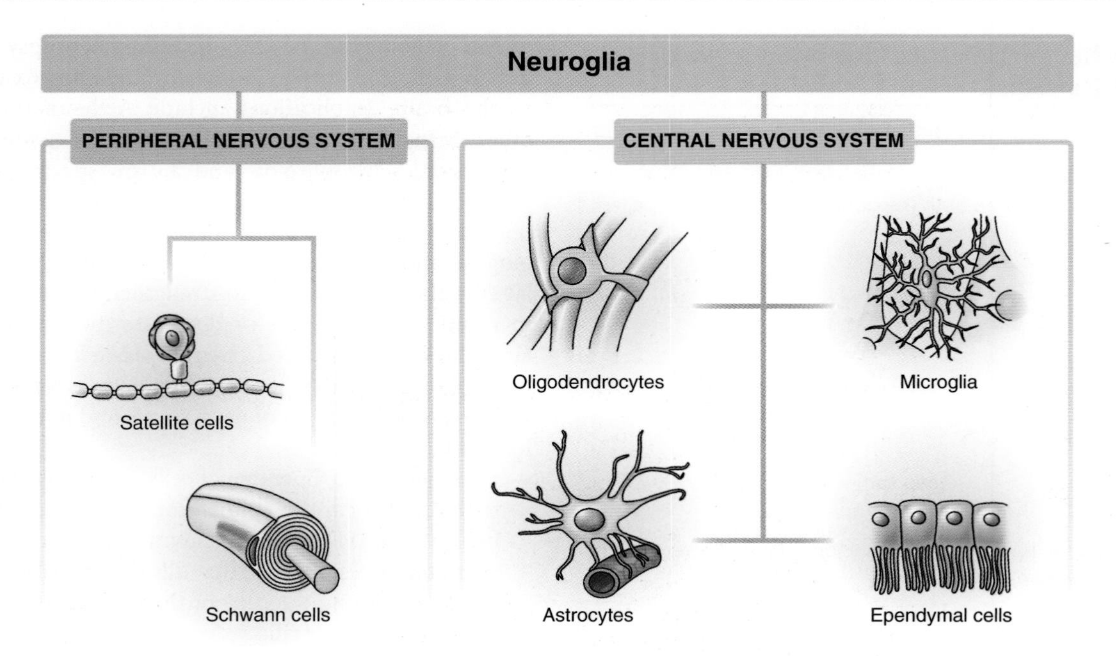

FIG. 4.3 Types of neuroglia found in the central nervous system and peripheral nervous system.

neurotransmitters and various small molecules. Dysfunction of neuroglial communication may cause pathological conditions, including neurodegenerative diseases such as Alzheimer disease, amyotrophic lateral sclerosis (ALS), and Parkinson disease. Psychiatric conditions, such as psychosis, depression, and anxiety, also involve alterations in neuroglial functions. Research is targeting the neuroglia to better understand how these conditions occur and how to improve medical treatment.

Nerve Repair or Regeneration

If a neuron cell body is damaged, the neuron dies. However, in the PNS, if damage occurs only to the axon of a neuron and the neurolemma is not destroyed, the nerve can repair itself. At the point of injury, the myelin sheath and the distal portion of the axon degenerate. The neurolemma then forms a tunnel from the point of injury to the original destination of the axon; that is, another axon, a muscle, or a gland. This tunnel provides a path for the axon to follow as it regenerates. Nerve regeneration can take a long time; just how long is determined by the length of the axon, the location of the injury, the inflammatory response, and the amount of scarring (Fig. 4.4).

In the CNS, oligodendrocytes do not create myelin in the same way the process occurs in the PNS. There is no neurolemma, so no tunnel can form to guide the regrowth of the axon from the injury site. Consequently, regeneration in the CNS is limited. However, extensive and exciting research is being done in the area of CNS regeneration and nerve growth factors. In the near future, scientists may identify nerve growth factors that can be used to assist those with spinal cord and brain injuries.

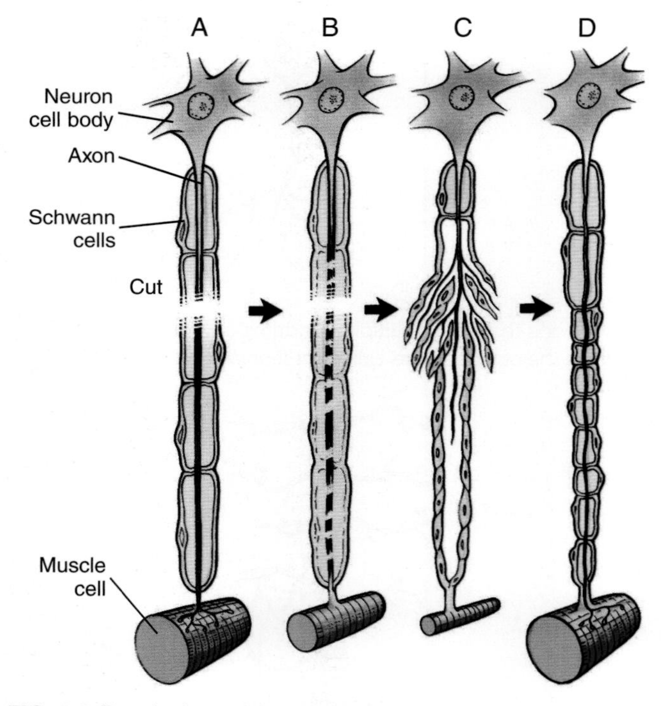

FIG. 4.4 Repair of a peripheral nerve fiber. (A) An injury results in a cut nerve. (B) Immediately after the injury occurs, the distal portion of the axon degenerates, as does its myelin sheath. (C) The remaining neurolemma tunnels from the point of injury to the effector. New Schwann cells grow within this tunnel, maintaining a path for the regrowth of the axon. Meanwhile, several growing axon sprouts appear. When one of these growing fibers reaches the tunnel, it increases its growth rate, growing as much as 3–5 mm/day. (The other sprouts eventually disappear.) (D) The connection of the neuron with the effector is reestablished. (From Patton KT, Thibodeau GA. *Anatomy and Physiology*. 7th ed. Mosby; 2010.)

Review What You Have Learned

- Define *neurons.*
  - Neurons are nerve cells that receive and transmit electrical signals from and to other neurons, muscles, or glands.
- List the parts of the neuron.
  - The cell body contains a nucleus and its organelles. The dendrites are hairlike extensions of the cytoplasm that receive signals and carry them to the cell body. The axon is a cordlike projection that carries signals away from the cell body.
- Define *neuroglia.*
  - Neuroglia are specialized connective tissue cells that maintain nervous system homeostasis by providing support, protection, insulation, and nutrient exchange for neurons. The four types of neuroglial cells are ependymal cells, astrocytes, oligodendrocytes, and microglia.

NERVE CELL FUNCTIONS

SECTION OBJECTIVES

Chapter objectives covered in this section:

3. Describe the physiology of the neuron and neuralgia.
4. Explain the relationship between neurochemical activity and behavior, including pain behavior.

After completing this section, the learner will be able to:

- Define membrane potential.
- Describe a nerve impulse and nerve impulse conduction.
- Describe a synapse.
- Explain neurotransmitters and neurochemicals.
- Explain the relationship between neurochemicals and behavior.

Membrane Potential

Neurons send messages electrochemically. This means that chemicals cause an electrical signal. Chemicals in the body that are electrically charged are called *ions.* Ions can have a positive charge (+) or a negative charge (–).

The term *membrane potential* means that a nerve impulse potentially could be generated. This state is created by the different concentrations of ions in the fluids inside the neuron and around the outside of the neuron. Sodium ions (Na^+) tend to concentrate in the extracellular fluid (outside the cell), and the cell membrane does not allow them to flow into the cell. Potassium ions (K^+) predominate inside the cell membrane. When a neuron is at rest, the outside of its cell membrane is positively charged, whereas the inside of the cell is negatively charged. This difference is called the *membrane potential,* and the cell is said to be polarized, meaning that the ions with the negative pole are outside the cell and the ions with the positive pole are inside the cell.

A neuron that is not stimulated but is polarized has a *resting potential.* This means the neuron is not doing anything; it is resting. However, if it receives a sufficiently strong stimulus, it will generate an impulse.

A stimulus, such as a pressure, light, temperature, or chemical change, results in a brief change in the charge of one segment of the neuron; this is called *depolarization.* During depolarization, protein channels in the cell membrane open and sodium ions flood into the neuron. The outside of that segment of the membrane becomes negatively charged as it depolarizes, and the inside becomes positively charged—and a nerve impulse is created. This flip in charges as the ions flow is called the *action potential,* or *nerve impulse.*

Nerve Impulse

An action potential, or nerve impulse, is a progressive wave of electrical and chemical activity along a nerve fiber. As the electrical signal continues along the nerve fiber, the nerve impulse depolarizes the next section, causing it to reverse its charges, while the previous segment returns to its original polarity, or is *repolarized.* When the nerve segment repolarizes, sodium channels close, potassium channels open, the outside again becomes positively charged, and the inside becomes negatively charged.

The term *excited* is used to describe the segment as the positive and negative charges flip with the action potential, and the term *inhibited* describes the reversal of that action (Fig. 4.5).

A neuron needs a *threshold stimulus* (the minimum level of stimulus needed) to trigger the opening of the first sodium channel. Once that occurs, an "all or none" principle applies, meaning that once an impulse starts, it continues down the entire length of the axon; it does not stop along the way.

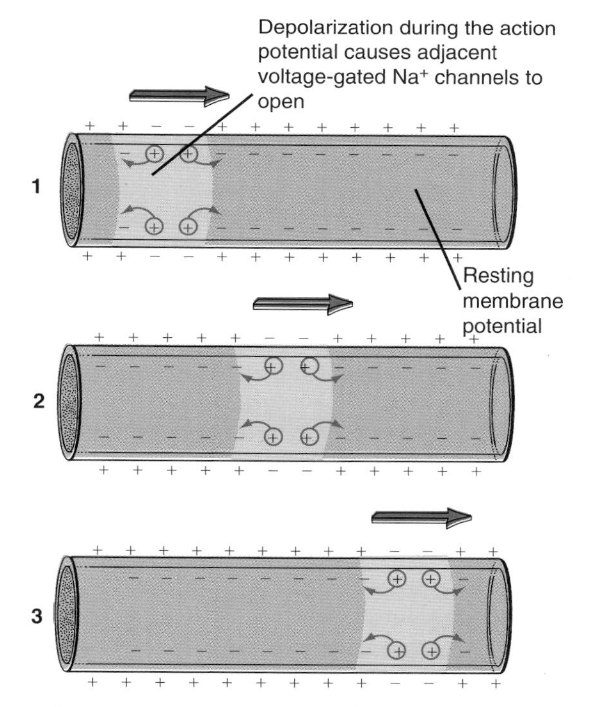

FIG. 4.5 Conduction of the action potential. The reverse polarity characteristic of the peak of the action potential causes local current flow to adjacent regions of the membrane *(small arrows).* This stimulates the voltage-gated sodium ion *(Na^+)* channels to open and thus creates a new action potential. This cycle continues, producing wavelike conduction of the action potential from point to point along a nerve fiber. Adjacent regions of the membrane behind the action potential do not polarize again because they are still in their refractory period. (From Thibodeau GA, Patton KT. *Anatomy and Physiology.* 6th ed. Mosby; 2007.)

After transmitting an impulse, the neuron cannot immediately fire again; it needs time for the sodium and potassium to return to the original location and repolarize the membrane. This time is called the *refractory period*. The refractory period is the brief period after inhibition when the neuron recovers. The absolute refractory period is the time during which a neuron will not respond to any stimuli. This is followed by the relative refractory period when the neuron will respond only to a strong stimulus.

Nerve Impulse Conduction

The path of the nerve impulse is different in myelinated (insulated) and unmyelinated nerve fibers. Conduction is faster in myelinated nerve fibers than in unmyelinated fibers. In the PNS, gaps are present in the myelin insulation where the actual nerve is exposed. These gaps, called *nodes of Ranvier*, occur at regular intervals along the length of the nerve fiber. The electrical impulse jumps from gap to gap, greatly reducing the time it takes to travel down the axon. This is called *saltatory conduction*. The term comes from the Latin word *saltare*, meaning "to dance" (Fig. 4.6).

Synapses and Neurotransmitters

Recall that nerves transmit both electrical and chemical signals. Also recall that a synapse is a space or junction between two neurons or a neuron and an effector organ. An effector organ produces an effect in response to nerve stimulation.

Practical Application

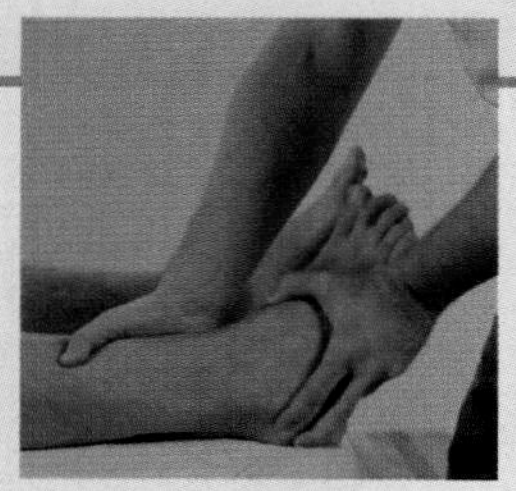

Therapeutic massage methods, such as muscle energy techniques and proprioceptive neuromuscular facilitation, use the refractory period to their advantage. Muscles often resist lengthening by initiating a protective spasm. If the muscle is first contracted and then lengthened, it is less likely to spasm during the refractory period, and the muscle can be restored more easily to a more normal resting length. Because these periods are short, gentle applications of lengthening procedures must be used. Methods that generate any sort of strong stimuli, especially pain, must be avoided. If a stimulus that is too strong is introduced, instead of inhibiting it, the muscle will generate nerve impulses and contract, thus resisting any sort of lengthening or stretching methods.

In a synapse, various chemicals called *neurotransmitters* transfer a nerve impulse across the gap to the next cell. To cross the gap, an electrical signal is transformed into a chemical signal. The neuron sending the signal is referred to as *presynaptic* because it is before the synapse; the neuron or effector organ receiving the signal is *postsynaptic*, or after the synapse. The actual space in the synapse is called the *synaptic cleft* (Fig. 4.7).

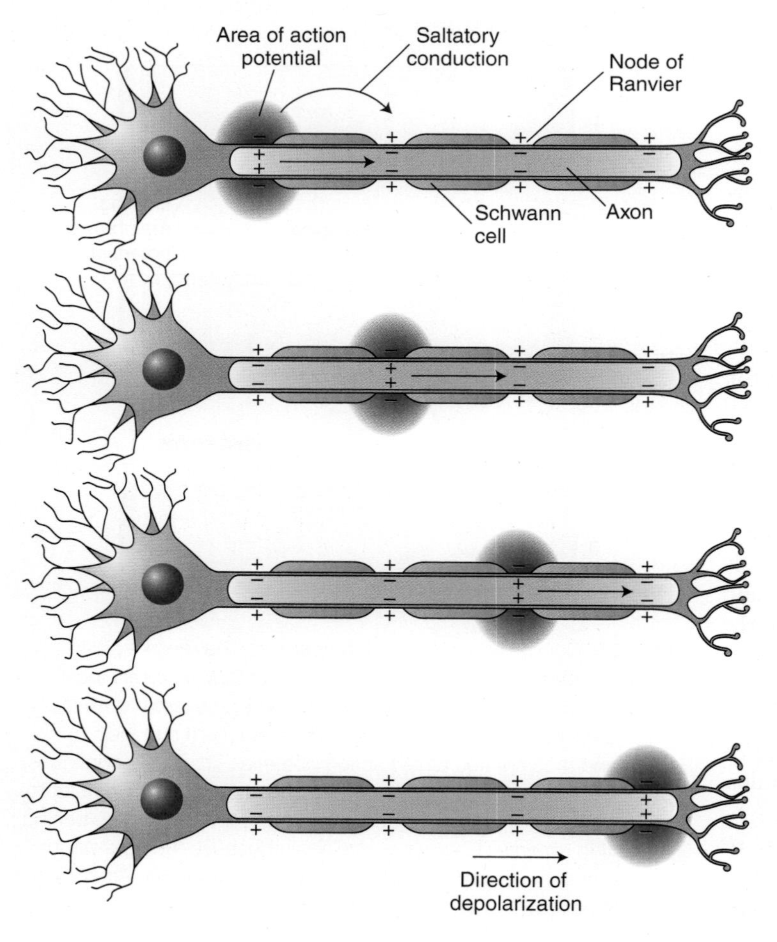

FIG. 4.6 Saltatory conduction. This series of diagrams shows that the insulating nature of the myelin sheath prevents ion movement everywhere but at the nodes of Ranvier. The action potential at one node triggers current flow *(arrows)* across the myelin sheath to the next node, producing an action potential there. The action potential thus seems to leap rapidly from node to node. (From Solomon EP: *Introduction to Human Anatomy and Physiology.* 3rd ed. Saunders; 2009.)

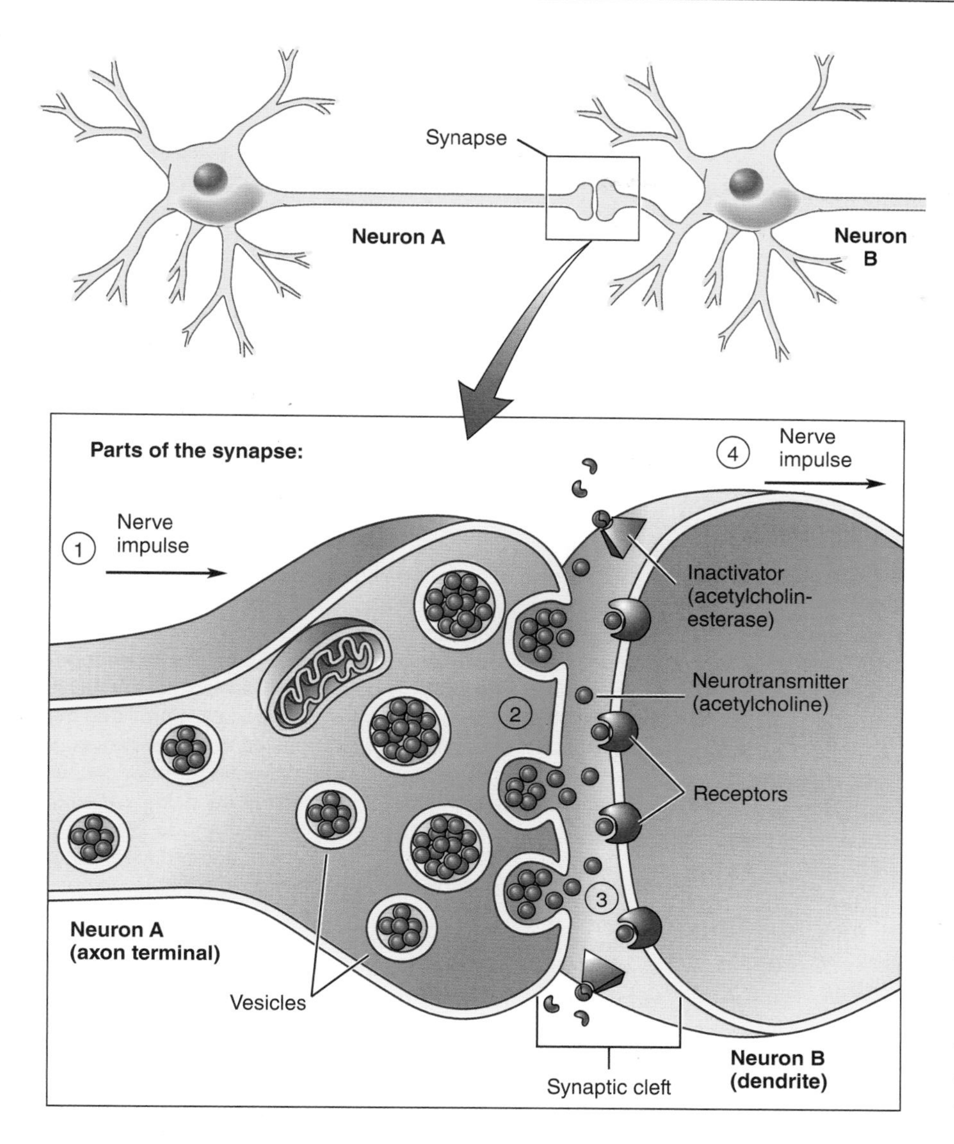

FIG. 4.7 A synapse is the junction between two nerve cells or a nerve and an effector organ, such as an endocrine gland or a muscle. The space in the synapse is called the *synaptic cleft*. (From Herlihy B. *The Human Body in Health and Illness*. 4th ed. Saunders; 2011.)

At the end of the axon of the presynaptic neuron, small sacs, or vesicles, are present. The vesicles contain neurotransmitters. The vesicles release neurotransmitters in response to the nerve impulse. Once released, these chemicals cross the synaptic cleft and bind with specific receptor sites on the postsynaptic neuron or effector organ. This will either generate another action potential, and the nerve impulse continues, or it will prevent another action potential and the nerve impulse stops. As an example, this is the way muscle contraction is controlled. Some muscles are stimulated to contract, whereas others are inhibited from contracting; this process ensures smooth, sequential movements. Another way to think of this is that the two actions, stimulation and inhibition, work the same way as the gas pedal and brakes on a car.

Neurotransmitters that cause the action potential to be transmitted across the synaptic cleft are considered stimulatory neurotransmitters. Those that slow or prevent the transmission of the action potential are inhibitory neurotransmitters.

Vesicles can store thousands of neurotransmitter molecules. After the neurotransmitters bind and their action is completed, they are broken down immediately by enzymes. They diffuse out of the synaptic cleft or are reabsorbed by the axons. This ensures that only one action potential is transmitted by the release of one portion of neurotransmitters.

In certain instances, medication may be used to interrupt the cycle by stopping the metabolism of the neurotransmitter. It does this by preventing binding to the postsynaptic membrane or by slowing the reabsorption of the neurotransmitter into the presynaptic vesicles.

Role of the Neurotransmitters

Neurotransmitters regulate many of the body's activities and senses. Currently more than 50 neurotransmitters have been identified, and many more are suspected to exist. When released into the bloodstream, many of these same chemicals are called *hormones*. Some of the known hormones are thought to work as neurotransmitters, implying a close link between the nervous system and endocrine activity.

Neurotransmitters have three basic chemical categories: amino acids, amines, and peptides. Even a gas such as nitrous oxide can be a neurotransmitter. There are small differences in the actions of these chemicals. For example, peptide chemicals are more complex and can cause a longer effect on the nervous system than a simpler amino acid can.

To be classified as a neurotransmitter, a chemical must have certain characteristics: (1) it must be found in the presynaptic vesicles; (2) it must be able to be removed from the synaptic cleft; and (3) it must be capable of stimulating a nerve impulse. It is important to note here that the receptor dictates the neurotransmitter's effect.

There are neuromodulator chemicals as well. A neuromodulator chemical is a relatively new concept. A neuromodulator is like a neurotransmitter, but it is not reabsorbed by the presynaptic neuron or broken down in the synapse. Instead, neuromodulators spend a significant amount of time influencing, or modulating, a nervous system activity. This can have long-lasting effects on the postsynaptic neuron's metabolic activity and its response to subsequent input. Opioid peptides such as enkephalins, endorphins, and dynorphins are examples of neuromodulators. Although many neurotransmitters function as neuromodulators, not all neuromodulators are neurotransmitters (Boxes 4.2 and 4.3).

Practical Application

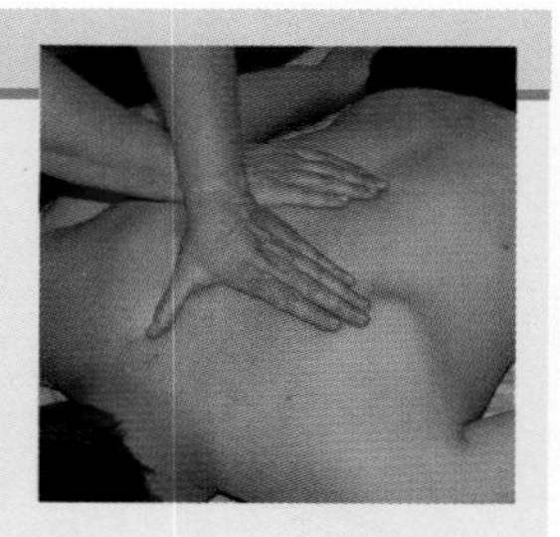

Many words have similar meanings, which can be confusing. Consider this list of terms: neurotransmitters, neuromodulators, neuroactive peptides, peptide transmitters, small-molecule transmitters, chemical messenger, and neurochemical.

Neuropeptides are actually neuromodulators that bind to receptors and activate enzymes, but they are usually listed as neurotransmitters. Endorphins and other endogenous (made in the body) opioids are considered neuromodulators in the CNS but are often found in neurotransmitter lists. Making this all even more complicated, many hormones that are endocrine chemicals are also considered neurotransmitters and neuromodulators.

Neurochemical refers to a chemical having a neural function. *Chemical messenger* is descriptive as well. This overlapping terminology is confusing when it comes to massage-related research. Some massage therapy research indicates that massage influences neurochemicals, and other research says massage does not affect neurochemicals. However, to interpret the research findings, it is necessary to know what neurochemicals are involved. Are they describing true neurotransmitters (e.g., dopamine or gamma-aminobutyric acid [GABA]) or neuromodulators (e.g., endorphins)? When you read research, it is important to know the terminology, even though it can be confusing.

Box 4.2 Cannabis and Endocannabinoids

The body makes cannabis-like substances called endocannabinoids (EC). *Cannabis sativa* plants contain compounds called cannabinoids. Cannabinoids are chemicals that interact with cell receptors throughout the central nervous system. This specialized network of receptors called the endocannabinoid system (ECS) reacts to the presence of cannabinoids to produce a variety of physiologic effects, playing a critical role in maintaining body homeostasis. Endocannabinoids can act as neurotransmitters between neurons in various regions of the brain and are important regulators of neurotransmission. Endocannabinoid signaling is involved in the regulation of the stress response, human memory processes, and inflammation. Neuroinflammatory processes contribute to the progression of normal brain aging, and ECs can control this type of inflammation. Neurodegenerative diseases are suppressed by cannabinoids interacting with microglia that are neuroprotective. On the cellular level, the cannabinoid system regulates the expression of brain-derived neurotrophic factor molecules that enhance the growth and survival of neurons and the development of nervous tissue.

Plant-derived cannabinoids function similarly to endogenous (made in the body) cannabinoids. Cannabidiol or CBD is a nonpsychoactive component of marijuana yet provides the medicinal and therapeutic effects marijuana offers. It occurs in high enough concentrations that extracting it from cannabis plants is relatively easy. For medical cannabis patients, cannabidiol can reduce inflammation, treat mood disorders, manage pain, especially neurogenic pain, and reduce seizure activity. CBD is available in several forms, from edibles to concentrates to topicals.

Exercise will naturally stimulate the endocannabinoid system, and there is some evidence that massage and other forms of manual therapy do as well.

REFERENCES FOR THIS BOX

Alharthi NS. Endocannabinoid system components: a crucial role in regulation of disease. *J Adv Pharm Educ Res*. 2022;12(3):72–81.

Behl T, Makkar R, Sehgal A, et al. Exploration of multiverse activities of endocannabinoids in biological systems. *Int J Mol Sci*. 2022; 23(10):5734.

Ana B-C, Tepavcevic V, Manterola A, et al. Endocannabinoid signaling in brain diseases: emerging relevance of glial cells. *Glia*. 2023; 71(1):103–126.

Buscemi A, Martino S, Scirè Campisi S, Rapisarda A, Coco M. Endocannabinoids release after osteopathic manipulative treatment. A brief review. *J Complement Integr Med*. 2021;18(1):1–7.

Duffy SS, Hayes JP, Fiore NT, Moalem-Taylor G. The cannabinoid system and microglia in health and disease. *Neuropharmacology*. 2021;190:108555.

Desai S, Borg B, Cuttler C, et al. A systematic review and meta-analysis on the effects of exercise on the endocannabinoid system. *Cannabis Cannabinoid Res*. 2022;7(4):388–408.

Body Chemistry of Behavior

Behavior is affected by the type and amount of neurotransmitters released at the synaptic junction. Daily behaviors (e.g., those involved with pleasure, pain, and survival) are determined by the body's chemistry. Too little or too much of any one neurotransmitter or neuromodulator results in a behavior that takes extra effort to manage.

Behavior seems to be the outward manifestation of attempts at homeostasis, and we seek sensations that stimulate our brains. The issue is one of balance. Neurotransmitters and neuromodulators balance one another like the gas pedal and the brake in a car. Those that excite are usually paired with those that inhibit. An ongoing dynamic balance exists in this chemical soup, allowing for behavior that is resourceful

Box 4.3 Important Neurochemicals, Their Primary Actions, and Their Locations

Acetylcholine: Acetylcholine stimulates the skeletal muscles and acts primarily on the parasympathetic nervous system. Acetylcholine can stimulate or inhibit various organs, depending on the receptors to which it is bound. Plentiful in the brain, the chemical is involved in memory. A lack of acetylcholine has been found in many patients diagnosed with Alzheimer disease, although a cause-and-effect relationship has not yet been established. Myasthenia gravis, which is a disease that causes weakening of skeletal muscles, results from a low level of acetylcholine receptors.

Catecholamine: Several compounds occurring naturally in the body that act as neurotransmitters or hormones in the sympathetic nervous system. The catecholamines include epinephrine, norepinephrine, and dopamine. These neurochemicals play a key role in the body's physiologic response to stress and increase the rate and force of muscular contraction of the heart, increasing cardiac output; constrict peripheral blood vessels, increasing blood pressure; elevate blood glucose; and promote an increase in blood lipids by increasing the catabolism of fats.

Epinephrine: Epinephrine can be a stimulant or an inhibitor, depending on the type of receptor bound. Epinephrine is found in several areas of the central nervous system (CNS) and the sympathetic divisions of the autonomic nervous system (ANS). Epinephrine is also involved in fight-or-flight responses, such as dilation of blood vessels to the skeletal muscles, and is classified as a hormone when secreted by the adrenal gland.

Norepinephrine: Like epinephrine, norepinephrine can excite or inhibit and is found in the CNS (especially the hypothalamus and limbic system) and in the sympathetic division of the ANS. Norepinephrine causes constriction of skeletal blood vessels, is considered a feel-good neurotransmitter, and is involved in emotional responses. The release of norepinephrine is enhanced by amphetamines. Cocaine stops the removal of norepinephrine from the synapses, such that stimulation of the synapses continues.

Dopamine: Generally excitatory, dopamine is found in the brain and the ANS. A feel-good neurotransmitter, dopamine is involved in emotions and moods and in the regulation of motor control and the executive functioning of the brain. Release is enhanced by L-dopa and amphetamines. Deficiencies occur in people with Parkinson disease and possibly also in those with schizophrenia. Dopamine is part of the endogenous reward/pleasure, craving/seeking behavior system in the brain. Many addictive drugs stimulate dopamine activity, including cocaine, narcotics, and alcohol.

Histamine: Considered a stimulant, histamine is released by the mast cells as part of the inflammatory process. Histamine causes itching at a cellular level and also works as a vasodilator. Also found in the hypothalamus, the chemical regulates body temperature and water balance and plays a role in emotions. Histamine also stimulates pain receptors to sensitize against further stimulation, as in the case of sunburn.

Serotonin: Serotonin usually works as an inhibitor in the CNS. It is synthesized into melatonin and affects biologic cycles, sleep, and moods. Insufficient levels can result in anxiety or depression. Serotonin is described as one of the feel-good neurotransmitters.

Gamma-aminobutyric acid (GABA): Generally inhibitory and found in the brain, this acid is the most common inhibitory neurotransmitter in the brain.

Glutamate (glutamic acid): Generally excitatory and found in the CNS, glutamate is thought to be responsible for as much as 75% of the excitatory signals in the brain.

Cholecystokinin: Found in the brain, retina, and gastrointestinal tract, the function of cholecystokinin in the nervous system is unclear and may be related to feeding behavior. Cholecystokinin is a gut-brain peptide.

Endorphins, enkephalins, endomorphins, and dynorphins: These endogenous morphines block the brain from feeling pain. Generally inhibitory, they are found in several regions of the CNS, retina, and intestinal tract. They inhibit pain by inhibiting the substance P. Morphine and heroin mimic their effects. Endorphins and enkephalins seem to play a part in mood regulation, pain/pleasure cycles, and the internal reward system of the body.

Somatostatin: Generally inhibitory, somatostatin inhibits the release of growth hormone and is a gut-brain peptide.

Substance P: Substance P is excitatory and is found in the brain, spinal cord, sensory pain pathways, and gastrointestinal tract. Substance P transmits pain information.

Vasoactive intestinal peptide: Found in the brain, some ANS and sensory fibers, retina, and the gastrointestinal tract; the function of this peptide in the nervous system is unclear. It plays a vital role in the regulation of coronary blood flow, cardiac contraction and relaxation, and heart rate.

Oxytocin: Involved in complex emotional and social behaviors, including attachment, social recognition, aggression, and approach and avoidance behavior toward others. It reduces anxiety, increases feelings of trust, helps establish maternal behavior, and is associated with well-being in relationships. Touch causes the body to produce oxytocin, which produces the desire to touch and be touched. It is also involved with uterine contractions and lactation but as a hormone.

Phenylethylamine (PEA): Helps regulate mood, focus, and stress. Exercise seems to increase PEA levels, cause feelings of happiness, and relieve depression. It aids in the transmission of dopamine and norepinephrine and can enhance aggression.

Nitric oxide: A gas that supports the transport of oxygen to the tissues and transmission of nerve impulses. It can function as a neurotransmitter involved in the functions of blood flow to the heart and erectile tissue (e.g., the penis), the sphincters in the gut, and the formation of memory.

Endocannabinoids: Act as neurotransmitters between neurons in various regions of the brain and are important regulators of neurotransmission. Endocannabinoid signaling is involved in the regulation of the stress response, human memory processes, and inflammation. Endocannabinoids can modulate GABA activity.

for each situation encountered. When behavior is effective in achieving some sort of balance, it will be reinforced.

By observing behavior, we can make educated guesses about which neurochemicals are involved. If the behavior is destructive, we may be able to introduce other forms of behavior that are less detrimental but result in similar neurotransmitter activity. It is important to recognize that repeated behavior is accomplishing some form of homeostasis—even destructive behavior, such as drug addiction, excessive exercise, eating disorders, rage, thrill seeking, crisis orientation, and the deliberate creation of pain.

An attempt to eliminate one form of behavior without replacing it with another way to achieve effective homeostasis almost always results in failure and reversion to old behaviors. Consider these examples:

- Substituting movement and aerobic exercise for binge eating may work because the two operate from a similar neurochemical base. Eliminating binge eating without providing a substitute behavior leaves the individual without a way of achieving chemical balance in the brain and body.
- Eating chocolate affects levels of serotonin and phenylethylamine (PEA) (as does eating potato chips, ice cream, and cookies), which are feel-good neurotransmitters. Massage and exercise also stimulate feel-good neurotransmitters. However, eating chocolate is faster and easier. Although chocolate may help a person feel good, if it is the only way the individual can feel good, other problems can arise, such as obesity and heart disease.

Changing a behavior from one that is quick and reliable to one that requires more effort is difficult for some people. The statements "moderation in all things" and "variety is the spice of life" are important and wise advice as far as brain chemistry is concerned. Sprinkled into this mix of expressions are the highs and lows of ecstasy and despair; these feelings are important as well. Having many different ways of feeling good is best.

Understanding what is causing us to feel bad is also important. When we can respond deliberately with our behavior to generate appropriate feelings in response to the situation being faced, instead of reacting and relying on only one type of behavior to meet our needs and cope, our neurochemicals work for us instead of against us.

When medication is used to manage various neurochemicals, mood and behavior are affected. The natural functions of the body allow for a wide range of behaviors through continual adjustment of the balance among neurotransmitters, neuromodulators, and hormones. When neurochemical levels are held in a more static ratio by medication, it means that feelings, moods, and resultant behaviors are held within the expected parameters. However, medication may alter a person's ability to experience the highs and lows of emotional expression appropriate to their daily circumstances. Therefore compliance with taking psychotropic or mood-altering medication is often affected because people sometimes miss the range of emotional experiences and stop taking their medications as prescribed—often with devastating results. Careful monitoring by the medical provider can minimize this situation. But it is important to be able to recognize it (see Box 4.3; also Activity 4.2).

ACTIVITY 4.2

Understanding the neurochemical influences on behavior is important for self-awareness and clinical reasoning when assessing and analyzing a client.

Example

The following is an analysis of an event that resulted in a pattern of behavior:

1. Describe the event in factual terms.
   The hood on the car would not close, and I was late for an appointment.
2. Describe your emotions and feelings concerning the event.
   I became very frustrated and anxious because I could not drive the car with the hood unlatched.
3. Describe the behavior displayed.
   I tried to slam down the hood three or four times and then started to yell at the car.
4. Identify the possible neurotransmitters involved in these feelings and behaviors.
   The catecholamines: epinephrine and norepinephrine.
5. Indicate the mode of action for the neurotransmitters.
   Epinephrine and norepinephrine: mostly excitatory, activating sympathetic arousal.
6. Correlate neurotransmitters with feelings and behaviors.
   I was anxious because I was late. Stress levels that increase sympathetic activity were high before I noticed the problem with the car. The increase in the catecholamines would produce or perpetuate the fight-or-flight behavior, resulting in my hitting the car and yelling.
7. Propose a balancing behavior to reset homeostasis and identify possible neurochemical interactions.
   I could have tightened all my muscles for a few seconds and then relaxed them and repeated this three or four times. This would simulate the activity of fighting or fleeing and use up some of the epinephrine. The goal would be to calm down.

Your Turn

Choose an event from your life in which you were unable to alter an inappropriate behavior pattern. Complete the following exercise on a separate sheet of paper:

1. Describe the event in factual terms.
2. Describe the emotions and feelings concerning the event.
3. Describe the behavior displayed.
4. Identify the possible neurotransmitters involved in the feelings and behavior.
5. Indicate the mode of action for the neurotransmitters.
6. Correlate the neurotransmitters with the feelings and behaviors.
7. Propose a balancing behavior to reset homeostasis and identify possible neurochemical interactions.

Pain Behavior and Behavioral Modification

Pain is a protective sensation for the body and therefore is important to survival. *Pain behavior* refers to the way we act when under the influence of pain perception. It can result from actual tissue damage or, in chronic conditions, it can perpetuate the pain experience (see Chapter 2). Such behavior is caused by brain chemistry, and pain is a complicated neurochemical event. Pain is perceived in the brain. A stimulus that is painful one day may not be painful the next. *Behavioral modification* is a method by which thinking and actions are altered purposefully to support a more satisfying life.

Some drugs interfere with the production of neurochemicals or block the receptor sites for the various chemicals involved in pain sensations. For example, aspirin interferes with the production of prostaglandin such that it cannot sensitize nerve endings to nociceptive stimuli. Anesthetics, including alcohol and barbiturates, depress nociceptive processing so that although the brain identifies pain, the person "does not care" because the pain perception is altered.

The body has a pain-inhibiting system. Receptors for opiates (e.g., morphine) are present on the nerves that transmit pain signals. The body produces endogenous opiates (e.g., endorphins and enkephalins) to block pain impulses in various parts of the pathway, probably as a protective measure.

The neurotransmitter substance P is secreted by pain-transmitting nerve fibers in the spinal cord, but it is blocked by enkephalins. Serotonin modulates the perception of pain. During pregnancy serotonin level gradually increases until it reaches its highest point at the time of delivery, in preparation for birth pain. Some of the food cravings experienced during pregnancy may be caused by the body's need to increase serotonin levels.

Injured tissues release prostaglandins, which make peripheral nociceptors more sensitive to stimuli (hyperalgesia). As a result, less stimulus is needed to begin the signaling of tissue harm. At this point, the pain experience is multifaceted and much more complex than a simple reflex response, such as when we step on a pin or burn a finger. Acute pain occurs with actual tissue damage, and the pain response is productive, leading to protective behavior, reduced movement, and support for tissue healing. However, the important part pain plays in keeping us safe can become dysfunctional, leading to chronic pain.

In chronic pain, sensory nerves can become sensitized and continue to transmit to the CNS even when no tissue damage has occurred. This pain process is nonproductive, but because we are neurologically wired to associate nociceptor signaling with danger and damage, a cascade of pain behaviors follows. Sensory neurons connect peripheral tissues with the CNS. Sensory nerves have the potential to undergo changes. One of the changes, called *sensitization*, occurs in response to a damaging stimulus, and subsequent stimuli are enhanced. In some cases, normally nonnociceptive stimuli elicit pain because the threshold is lower (allodynia); in others, a normally painful stimulus becomes even more painful (hyperalgesia).

Two general mechanisms of sensitization have been identified—one acts at the periphery (peripheral sensitization), and the other acts centrally (central sensitization). Peripheral sensitization results when injury induces the release of several sensitizing agents from damaged cells and immune cells. These sensitizing agents can be considered "inflammatory soup." Central sensitization of nociceptive pathways results from a cyclic feedback system that perpetuates the nociceptor stimuli. Eventually chronic pain conditions result in changes in the CNS, and pain is experienced with little or no peripheral stimuli or nociception. Biochemical changes occur in the brain, resulting in altered perception. Sensation can become misinterpreted and intertwined with past learning, leading to strong emotional overtones to the pain experience.

Recall the gate control theory of pain from Chapter 2. This theory, developed by Ronald Melzack and Patrick Wall, was published in the journal *Science* in 1965. Subsequently, Melzack was challenged to expand the gate control theory primarily because some pain conditions, such as phantom limb pain, did not fit into that model. Melzack built on the gate control theory to describe the neuromatrix theory of pain, which is founded on the concept of the body-self. The body-self is the internal perception of a unified body, like a complex map of the physical body and the experience of being in the body. The understanding of pain is still working from a theory—meaning educated guesses—indicating how abstract and complex the experience of pain is. Ongoing research has resulted in what might be called "pain science." However, a better description is *neuroscience education about pain*. Evidence has shown that neuroscience educational strategies for the client related to neurobiology and neurophysiology can reduce pain perception, increase function, reduce fear and catastrophizing, and improve movement and the way a person thinks about pain experiences (Louw et al., 2011, 2016; Moseley and Butler, 2015; Malfliet et al., 2018; Romm et al., 2021; Sturgeon et al., 2024).

Pain neuroscience education becomes therapeutic when the information helps people change their beliefs about and understanding of pain, reducing their fear and frustration. Recall that in Chapter 2, information was presented about pain. Now the topic appears again—this reinforces how important it is that you, as a future massage therapist, understand the neuroscience of the pain experience. In your profession, you can use this understanding to better help clients realize their pain management outcomes.

Review What You Have Learned

- Define *membrane potential.*
    - The term *membrane potential* means a nerve impulse can potentially be generated. It is created by different concentrations of ions (chemicals with a positive or negative charge) inside and outside the neuron.
- Describe a nerve impulse and nerve impulse conduction.
    - A nerve impulse (action potential) is a progressive wave of electrical and chemical activity along a nerve fiber. Nerve impulse conduction is faster in myelinated nerves than in unmyelinated nerves. In the PNS, the impulse is accelerated by jumping along the nodes of Ranvier (regularly spaced, unmyelinated gaps on nerve fibers). A nerve impulse is followed by a refractory period (a brief period during which the nerve cannot fire).
- Describe a synapse.
    - A synapse is the space or junction between two neurons or a neuron and an effector organ.
- Explain neurotransmitters and neurochemicals.
    - Neurotransmitters are chemicals with certain characteristics: they are found in presynaptic vesicles; they can be removed from the synaptic cleft; and they can stimulate a nerve impulse. A neuromodulator functions much like a neurotransmitter but has longer-lasting effects on

nervous system activity because it is not reabsorbed by the presynaptic neuron or broken down in the synapse. Although many neurotransmitters act as neuromodulators, not all neuromodulators are neurotransmitters.

- Explain the relationship between neurochemicals and behavior.
    - Certain behaviors stimulate certain neurochemicals. This can reinforce both positive and negative behaviors. Massage stimulates the production of various neurochemicals, which may help clients change certain behaviors, including those related to pain.

Practical Application

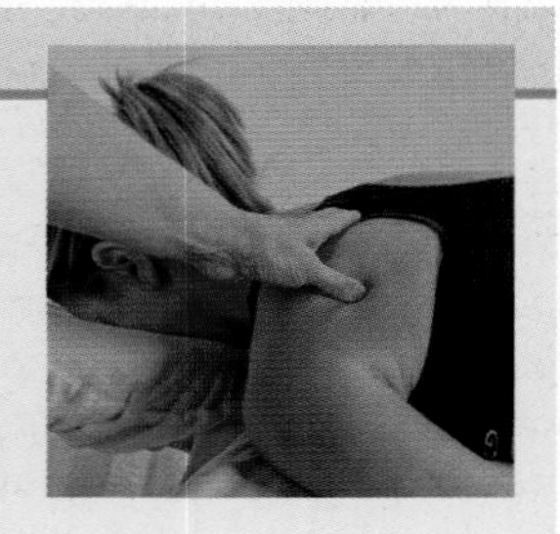

The actions of neurotransmitters are important for many physiological effects. Many drugs of abuse either mimic neurotransmitters or otherwise alter the function of the nervous system. Barbiturates act as depressants, with effects similar to those of anesthetics. They seem to act mainly by enhancing the activity of the neurotransmitter GABA, an inhibitory neurotransmitter. In other words, when barbiturates bind to a GABA receptor, the inhibitory effect of GABA is greater than before. Opiates, such as heroin, bind to a particular type of opiate receptor in the brain, resulting in effects similar to those of naturally occurring endorphins. Amphetamines can displace catecholamines from synaptic vesicles and block the reuptake of catecholamines in the synapse, prolonging the action of catecholamine neurotransmitters.

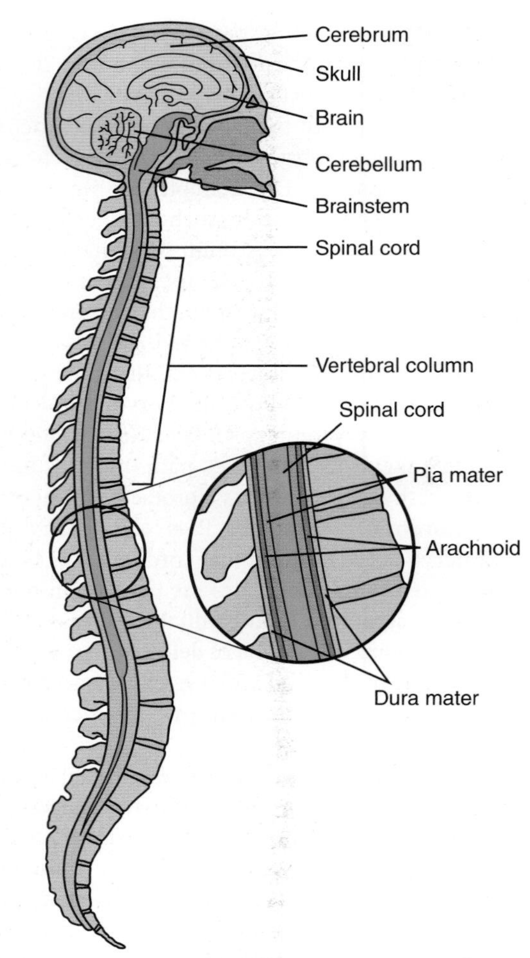

FIG. 4.8 The central nervous system. (From Sorrentino SA, Remmert LN. *Mosby's Textbook for Nursing Assistants.* 8th ed. Mosby; 2012.)

THE CENTRAL NERVOUS SYSTEM

SECTION OBJECTIVES

Chapter objectives covered in this section:

5. Identify the structures and functions of the brain.
6. Identify the structures and functions of the spinal cord.

After completing this section, the learner will be able to:

- List the parts of the CNS.
- Define *meninges*.
- Describe the two main types of extracellular fluid in the CNS.

As mentioned, the CNS has two main components—the brain and the spinal cord (Fig. 4.8).

Brain

The **brain** is the largest and most complex unit of the nervous system. It is composed of approximately 100 billion neurons, which are packed together inside the skull. Besides intellect, emotions, and actions, the brain interprets, regulates, and coordinates physiological activities.

Although the brain weighs an average of only 3 pounds, it makes up more than 97% of the nervous system. The neuroglia accounts for more than half its weight. Composed of more than 85% water, the brain contains a higher percentage of fluid than blood.

The brain is divided into four main areas (Figs. 4.9 and 4.10):

1. Cerebrum
2. Diencephalon (the main structures of the thalamus and hypothalamus)
3. Cerebellum
4. Brainstem (composed of the medulla oblongata, pons, and midbrain)

Cerebrum

The **cerebrum**, also called the *forebrain*, is the largest portion of the brain. It is divided into the right and left hemispheres, which are connected by the corpus callosum.

The right and left hemispheres oversee motor control. Each receives sensory input from the opposite side of the body. The left hemisphere controls the right side of the body, and the right hemisphere controls the left side. The preference for using one brain region more than others for certain functions is called *lateralization*. However, the idea that we can be more left brained (analytical) or right brained (creative) is a myth. It is the connections among all brain regions that enable people to use both creativity and analytical thinking.

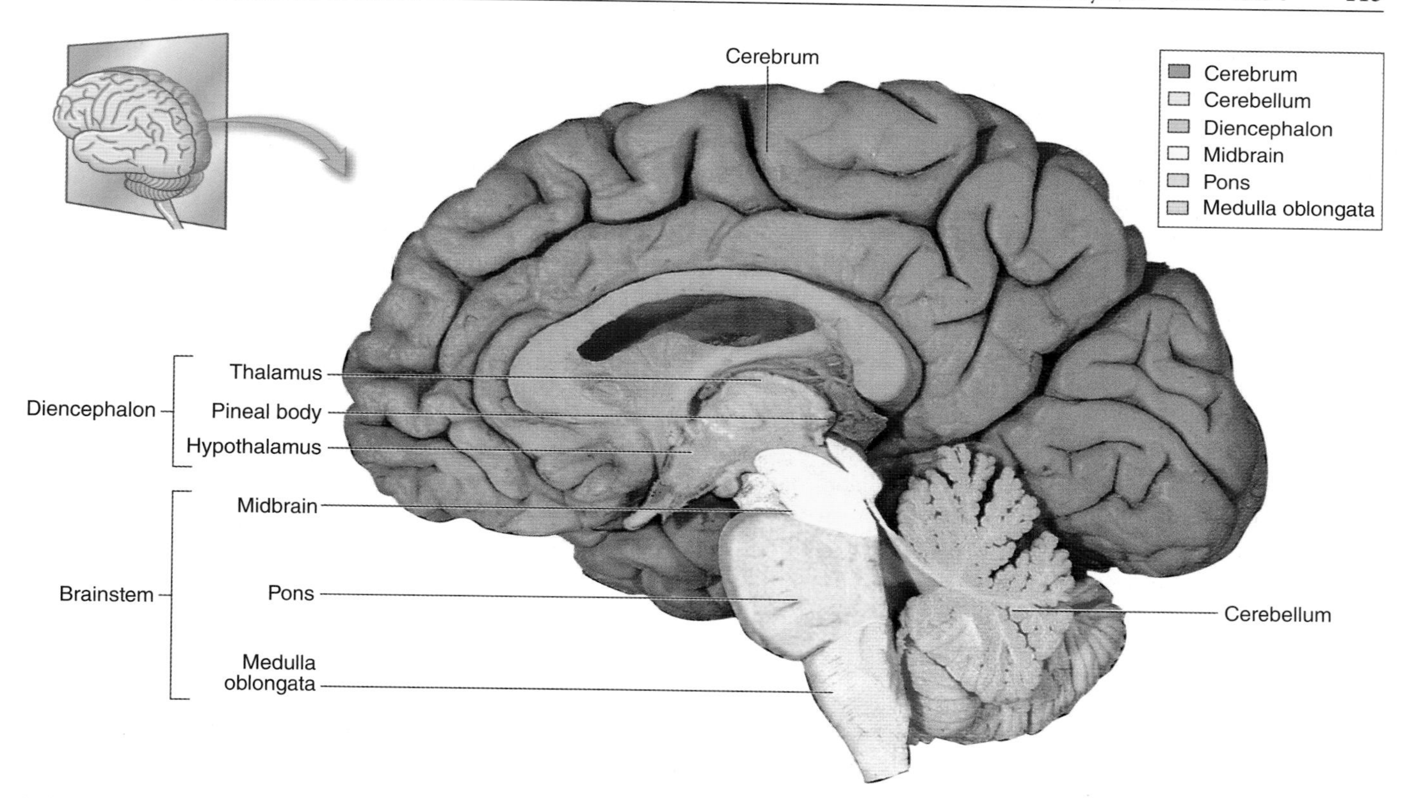

FIG. 4.9 Divisions of the brain. A midsagittal section of the brain reveals features of its major divisions. (From Vidic B, Suarez FR. *Photographic Atlas of the Human Body.* Mosby; 1984.)

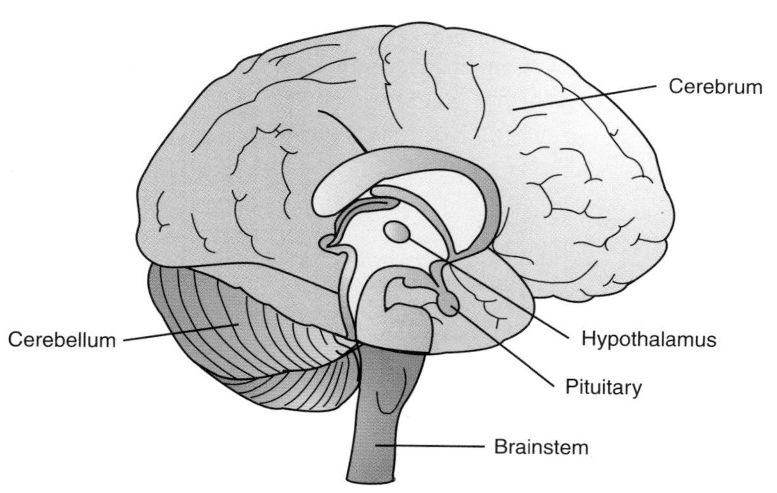

FIG. 4.10 Location of brain structures.

Functions of the Brain's Hemispheres

Each hemisphere of the brain is dominant for some behaviors. However, it seems safe to say that for the most part, we all use both sides of our brains almost all the time.

Most of the cerebrum is composed of white matter. Because the corpus callosum is composed of myelinated axons, it is white. The surface of the cerebrum is covered by the cerebral cortex, a thin layer of matter that is gray because of the presence of dendrites and cell bodies. The basal ganglia are small collections of gray matter in the cerebrum that assist in coordination.

The major functions of the cerebrum are to:

1. Receive sensory information
2. Interpret it
3. Associate it with memories, emotions, and past experiences
4. Transmit the most appropriate motor impulse in response to the input

Each side of the cerebrum is divided into five lobes, four of which are named for the skull bones lying over them.

Frontal Lobe

The anterior portion of the cerebrum, the frontal lobe, is positioned behind the frontal bone and contains the prefrontal cortex (governing personality, intellect, and cognition), the premotor cortex (directing learned motor skills), and the precentral gyrus (managing motor control of muscles). This lobe is responsible primarily for the control of the voluntary skeletal muscles and is active during problem-solving modes and activities that involve concentration and planning. A region known as the *Broca area* is found in the dominant hemisphere and controls the muscle movements involved in speech.

Parietal Lobe

Located next to the parietal bones, the parietal lobe contains the postcentral gyrus, which is the primary sensory area of the brain. This lobe receives and evaluates the sensory information of temperature, pressure, touch, taste, and pain. Its areas of association include speech, thought, and emotions.

Temporal Lobe

Found below the lateral fissure, the temporal lobe is next to the temporal bones. The temporal lobe is responsible for the reception and evaluation of information involved in hearing and smell. The Wernicke area, which is located in the superior portion of the gyrus of the dominant hemisphere, is involved in understanding language. The Wernicke area transmits information to the Broca area in the frontal lobe. The Broca area processes language information comprehended by the Wernicke area and relays it to the precentral gyrus. The areas of association combine complex sensory data (e.g., from music and visual scenes) into comprehensive patterns that form memories.

Occipital Lobe

Located just anterior to the occipital bone of the skull, the occipital lobe is responsible for the mechanical control of eyesight and the integration of visual input with other sensory experiences.

Insula (insular cortex)

The fifth lobe, the insula (also called the *island of Reil*) is located under the lateral fissure and is the part of the limbic system that gives us a feeling or impression of what is real, true, and important. The insula is considered the interoception center of the brain. **Interoception** refers to the processing of visceral-afferent neural signals by the CNS, which results in the conscious perception of bodily processes.

The cerebral cortex contains folds called *convolutions*, or *gyri* (singular, *gyrus*), which increase the area available to the cortex. These folds are separated by *sulci*. The deepest sulci are known as *fissures*. These fissures can be used as landmarks when identifying certain areas of the brain.

- The longitudinal fissure divides the cerebrum into right and left hemispheres.
- The central sulcus, or the *fissure of Rolando*, separates the frontal and parietal lobes.
- The lateral fissure, or the *fissure of Sylvius*, lies above the temporal lobe and below the frontal and parietal lobes.
- The insula lies deep in the lateral fissure.
- The occipital and parietal lobes are separated by the parieto-occipital fissure.

The limbic system is located in the interior of the cerebrum. It is important in emotional responses, including fear, rage, and pleasure. Therefore a built-in reward and avoidance process exists in the brain. The limbic system is connected to the hypothalamus by the fornix, a band of fibers consisting of axons (Fig. 4.11 and Table 4.1).

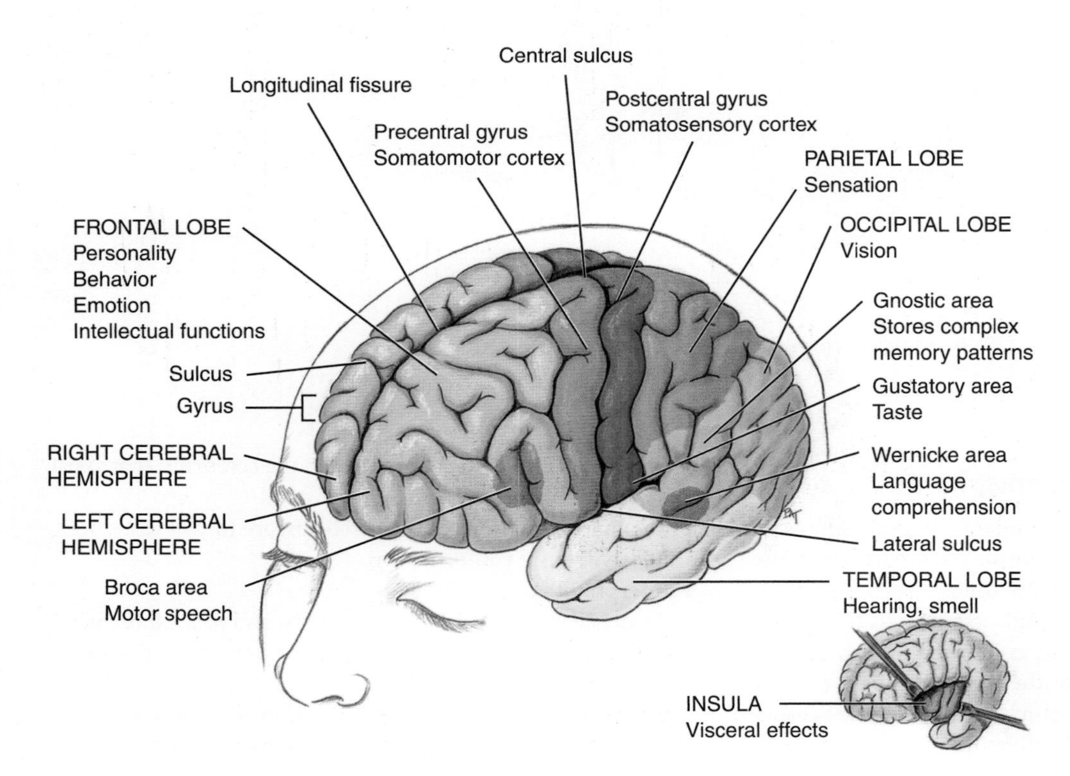

FIG. 4.11 Functional organization of the cerebral cortex. (From Applegate E. *The Anatomy and Physiology Learning System*. 4th ed. Saunders; 2011.)

Table 4.1 Functions of the Cerebral Cortex

Functional Area	Anatomic Area	Functional and Performance Components
Frontal Lobes		
Primary motor area	Precentral gyrus	Execution of movement
Secondary association area	Premotor cortex	Planning and programming of movement Sequencing, timing, and organization of movement Frontal eye field Voluntary eye movements Broca area in the left inferior frontal gyrus Programming of motor speech Supplementary motor area Intention of movement
Tertiary association area	Orbitofrontal and dorsolateral prefrontal cortex	Ideation Concept formation Abstract thought Intellectual functions Sequencing, timing, and organization of action and behavior Initiation and planning of action Judgment Insight Intention Attention Alertness Personality Working memory Emotion
Parietal Lobes		
Primary somesthetic sensory area	Postcentral gyrus	Fine touch sensation Proprioception Kinesthesia
Secondary somesthetic sensory association area	Superior parietal lobule	Coordination, integration, and refinement of sensory input Tactile localization and discrimination Stereognosis
Tertiary association area	Inferior parietal lobule	Gnosis: Recognition of received tactile, visual, and auditory input Praxis: Storage of programs or visual kinesthetic motor engrams necessary for motor sequences Body scheme: Postural model of body, body parts, and their relation to the environment Spatial relations: Processing related to depth, distance, spatial concepts, position in space, and differentiation of foreground from background
Occipital Lobes		
Primary visual sensory area	Calcarine fissure	Visual reception (from the opposite visual field)
Visual association area	Brodmann areas 18 and 19	Synthesis and integration of visual information Perception of visuospatial relationships Formation of visual memory traces Prepositional construction of language comprehension and speech
Temporal Lobes		
Primary auditory sensory area	Superior temporal gyrus	Auditory reception
Secondary association area	Superior and middle temporal gyri (Wernicke area)	Language comprehension Sound modulation Perception of music Auditory memory
Tertiary association area	Temporal pole, parahippocampal gyrus	Long-term memory Learning of higher-order visual tasks and auditory patterns Emotion Motivation Personality
Limbic Lobes		
Tertiary association area	Orbitofrontal cortex in frontal lobe, temporal pole, and parahippocampal gyrus in the temporal lobe Cingulate gyrus in frontal and parietal lobes	Attention Motivation Emotions Long-term memory

Modified from Árnadóttir G. *The Brain and Behavior: Assessing Cortical Dysfunction Through Activities of Daily Living.* Mosby; 1990.

Integrative or Associative Brain Functions

Integrative or associative functions include all the activities that occur in the cerebrum after sensory signals have been received and before motor responses are sent where those signals originated. These responses include consciousness, language, emotions, memory, and learning mechanisms (Fig. 4.12 and Box 4.4).

Consciousness

The term *consciousness* can be defined as the capacity for sensation, thinking, memory, and emotion, thereby creating an awareness of self and the environment. There is a continuum of consciousness, from a high state of consciousness, during which we are alert and hyperaware, to a depressed state of consciousness, such as a coma. Daily life is usually somewhere between those extremes. The level of consciousness is a measurement of a person's responsiveness to stimuli from the environment (Box 4.5). The Glasgow Coma Scale is a neurological assessment tool that provides an objective way to record the conscious state of a person who has experienced trauma or illness (Activity 4.3).

ACTIVITY 4.3

How could you alter your state of consciousness in a health-enhancing way? Write down two methods.

Example
Listen to gentle music for 15 minutes while rocking in a rocking chair.
Your Turn

Practical Application

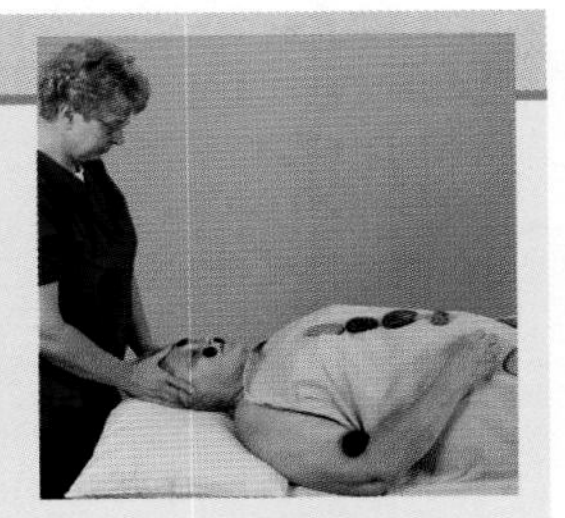

Massage therapy interacts with the cerebral cortex and reticular activating system, the same mechanisms involved in consciousness. Consequently, massage methods often generate the sensations experienced during altered states of consciousness. Most of the major spiritual disciplines have a movement or positional aspect in their practices that contribute to the meditative states experienced by their participants. Some even incorporate touch, which enhances the experience.

Language

Language involves the perception of written and spoken words, in addition to the physical ability to speak and write. For 90% of the population, this takes place in the left hemisphere of the cerebrum in the frontal, parietal, and temporal lobes. The ability to apply labels to processes and subjects inside and outside the body is also tied to sensory systems.

Emotions

We experience and express our feelings and emotions through the limbic system of the brain. Located inside the cerebrum, the limbic system works with other parts of the cerebral cortex. For most of us, the normal expressions of anger, pleasure, fear, and sorrow are under our control. An individual whose limbic system does not interact effectively with the cortex may have episodes of uncontrollable rage or other emotions. Motivation is driven by emotions, especially the pleasure sensations. They cause people to move toward anticipated feelings of pleasure and to move away from feelings or avoid situations remembered from past experiences of distress.

Memory

Memory involves the storage of information in the brain, and it is one of our major mental activities. Two types of memory are short-term (recent) memory and long-term memory. Short-term memory is fragile, unstable, and disappears unless it is reinforced and transferred to long-term memory. The activities in this text are designed to assist in the transference of new data from short-term memory to long-term memory, which can be retrieved days or even years after the initial event.

The temporal lobes are involved with long-term memory. Memory involves repeated impulse conduction over a given neuronal circuit that produces a synaptic change and physical brain alteration. Many research findings indicate that the limbic system—the "emotional brain"—plays a key role in memory as well. Highly emotional events seem to become stored immediately in long-term memory, indicating neurotransmitter involvement in memory structures (Box 4.6).

Learning

Learning can be thought of as the best and simplest way to solve a problem. Anatomically and physiologically, learning involves the use of multiple synaptic pathways to process information. Advanced learning takes place in the association areas of the cerebral cortex, whereas more primitive learning takes place in the brainstem. The ability to read is considered advanced learning, whereas the recognition that something is hot is a more primitive form of learning. Learning involves memory because it is the development of neural structures that remember the way to solve a problem. This process supports survival.

Learning can be thought of as conditioning. Ivan Pavlov's research identified some of the mechanisms of conditioning. In his work, an external stimulus was connected to a natural occurrence in the body. Dogs were conditioned by bells being rung at the same time food was being presented. Soon the dogs learned that the bell and food equaled the same thing, whereupon the sound of the bell alone stimulated digestion and eating behaviors. This is behavioral conditioning that can also be considered a learned habit.

The process of learning is conscious, but after a response has been integrated, it commonly becomes an unconscious habit. Some habits are beneficial, and others no longer serve their original purpose. Breaking a habit is difficult. Learning a new way to do something involves making the thought process take a different path to reach the same result. The body and learned memory tend to resist change, especially because learned behavior is a strong component of primitive survival

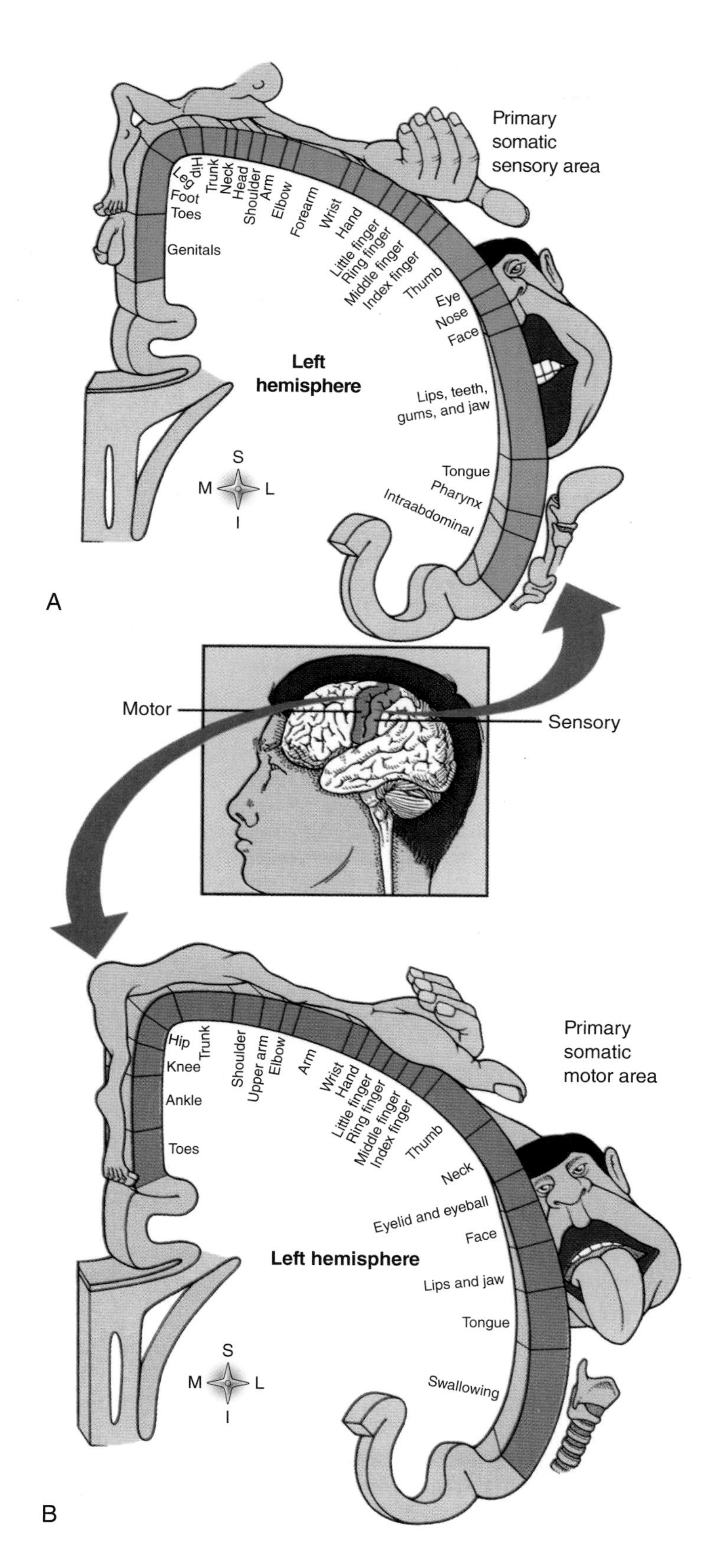

FIG. 4.12 Sensory and motor areas of the brain. The surface area is the largest for sensory interpretation of the face, lips, and fingers. The motor surface area is largest for the hands and face. (From Thibodeau GA, Patton KT. *Anatomy and Physiology*. 6th ed. Mosby; 2007.)

Box 4.4 Body Chemistry–Related Behaviors

We behave in certain ways to increase or decrease levels of neurotransmitters or hormones (e.g., eating or not eating because we are depressed; exercising or not exercising because we are anxious). On the other side, if there is some sort of imbalance in the various neurochemicals, we may find ourselves behaving in ways we do not understand.

Extreme and novel behaviors have the biggest influence.

Soap operas are good examples. Little program content talks about day-to-day life in the midrange of emotional or behavioral expression. Television viewers seldom get caught up in stories about making the bed, changing the oil in the car, or going to the market.

Depression may follow when the release of catecholamines is blocked. Anxiety is aggravated by an increase in catecholamines. Have you ever been depressed or become all worked up about something that was really not that important? The depression lifts, and life goes on.

Researchers are currently investigating the effect of serotonin on migraine headaches.

Too much dopamine in the brain may result in hallucinations and can cause mildly erratic behavior, such as that displayed when a person first falls into romantic love or when an extreme schizophrenic behavior occurs.

Dopamine levels are thought to be involved in attention deficit hyperactivity disorders.

The presence of cholecystokinin and vasoactive intestinal peptides in the eye and the stomach indicates that there is a connection between what we see and what we eat. These same neurochemicals are in the brain. Could this suggest a connection between food, behavior, and emotions? Anyone who has emotional issues around food certainly would not deny that the food we eat changes the way we feel and influences the behavior connected with those emotions.

The following questions are relevant:

- Is the behavior the result of a neurochemical imbalance?
- Is the behavior causing a neurochemical imbalance?
- Is the behavior attempting to regulate a neurochemical imbalance?
- Is the behavior normal but occurring at the wrong time?
- Is the behavior normal for the situation?

Box 4.5 Consciousness and Altered States of Consciousness

Consciousness is awareness of the environment and our relationship to everyone and everything in that environment. Throughout the day changes take place in our level of consciousness, ranging from asleep to wide awake.

Consciousness depends on the excitation of cortical neurons by impulses conducted from the reticular activating system. The reticular activating system consists of centers in the brainstem that receive impulses from the spinal cord and relay them to the thalamus. The thalamus transmits the data to all parts of the cerebral cortex. Substances that stimulate the cerebrum, enhancing alertness, probably act by stimulating the reticular activating system.

We are not always consciously aware of all the functions of our internal body and the external stimuli around us. Subconscious activity occurs beyond the level of consciousness. The ability to not be conscious of all internal and external stimuli and sensations is important. Otherwise, we would be overwhelmed.

Some people have an intensified awareness of ordinary body functions, such as heartbeat, breathing, and stomach noises. This can be very distressing if the person does not know that the sensations are normal. What is abnormal is that the person is aware of these functions. Hypochondriasis is a mental disorder characterized by excessive fear of or preoccupation with a serious illness, despite medical testing and reassurance that no illness exists. Many doctors believe that these individuals may have some sort of abnormal hypersensitivity or inability to filter sensation. Some behaviors associated with autism-type conditions are related to sensation hypersensitivity: smell, touch, sound, and sight.

Altered States of Consciousness

Consciousness may be altered in many ways, including the use of medications, herbs, or foods that change chemical processes; repetitive activities or sounds; and trance. For centuries, many cultures and religions have explored altered states of consciousness and have used them readily in defensive actions, healing, and pain control. Meditation, tai chi, and yoga are examples of ancient methods to achieve altered consciousness. States of higher consciousness refer to the primary activity that actually increases alertness and induces relaxation. Research has confirmed this state to be health enhancing.

We can achieve the same result by gardening, drawing, knitting, or playing a musical instrument. Any rhythmic activity that uses a repetitive motion (e.g., drumming) or natural sounds (e.g., a bubbling brook) can quiet or excite, depending on the speed of the rhythm, the nervous system through entrainment and thereby alter the physiologic processes of the body.

The pleasure derived from the sense of well-being experienced during altered states of consciousness can be addictive. Various plants containing chemicals that alter consciousness have been used over the centuries in awareness rituals. Within the confines of cultural and religious rituals, the limited and judicial use of these plants was controlled. Today most, if not all, of the old discipline and structure are nonexistent, and the risk of drug abuse has made the exploration of altered states of consciousness problematic.

During a massage session, both the therapist and the client can achieve a beneficial altered state of consciousness. When the altered state has been achieved, it should be maintained for at least 15 minutes for optimal therapeutic benefit. The typical time required for the body to respond to the physiologic change is 15 minutes.

Box 4.6 State-Dependent Memory

Sometimes the memory takes the form of state-dependent memory. Memory is thought to occur during a physical alteration in living neural tissue. In state-dependent memory the memory is hard to access unless the state of consciousness is similar to that in effect when the event occurred (Zarrindast et al., 2020). State-dependent memory can take many forms. Sometimes trauma beyond what the conscious centers can integrate is hidden in state-dependent memory. Any form of therapy that can engage the various states of consciousness, such as hypnosis, biofeedback, and various forms of bodywork, may recreate the state of consciousness that holds the key to the memory structure, allowing it to surface. Depending on the person's coping skills, resources, support systems, and professional services available, this awareness of past experience can be a time of conscious understanding and integration of a part of the person's life. However, without the proper resources, this resurfacing of state-dependent memory can be devastating and extremely harmful.

Pleasure states are also encoded in state-dependent memory. Warm feelings (such as being held) or feelings of exhilaration (such as running in the wind on a beautiful spring day) can be remembered and in a sense recreated through various forms of bodywork. These are health-enhancing states that support homeostasis.

behavior. In addition, changing learned behavior takes tremendous energy, and the natural tendency of the body is to conserve energy. Unless the habit is causing us to expend resources in a detrimental way for a sufficiently long time to affect survival, rallying the resources of the body necessary to change the behavior is difficult.

An interesting concept in learning is based on imitation. *Mirror neurons* are a specific type of neuron that discharge both when one executes a motor act and when one observes a similar motor act performed by another individual. These neurons are active during both observation and execution of actions, and researchers think they may play a role in some forms of imitation-based learning. An example of imitation-based learning would be students watching the instructor demonstrate a massage application and then repeating what they saw. Mirror neurons may also play a role in understanding goals and intentions, which is important in learning social skills (Mazurek et al., 2018; Koul et al., 2018; Kemmerer 2021; Koning et al., 2022).

Diencephalon

The diencephalon is located between the cerebrum and the midbrain. It contains the thalamus, hypothalamus, pineal body, and other small structures.

Thalamus

The thalamus is created from the gray matter of nerve cell bodies deep in the white matter of the cortex. It is a relay station to the cerebrum for all sensory input except smell. Signals from the reticular activating system (see the Brainstem section) are sent through the thalamus to the cerebral cortex. The thalamus is also associated with pain, temperature, crude touch, and reflex muscle coordination. Additionally, it associates pleasant and unpleasant feelings with sensory input and then relays information to the limbic system. The thalamus may be involved with internal biorhythm entrainment and supporting internal balance (Jerath et al., 2018; Onder and Green, 2018).

Hypothalamus

The hypothalamus lies below the thalamus and above the pituitary gland. It regulates and coordinates functions such as heart rate, blood pressure, aspects of digestion, appetite and satiety, pleasure, temperature, and general coordination of ANS functions. It also produces releasing hormones that affect pituitary gland hormones, which in turn influence important activities, such as hunger, appetite, sleep cycles, wakefulness, sexual arousal, and water balance in the body. The hypothalamus is associated with the limbic system and is an important link between the nervous and endocrine systems; this allows the mind to affect the body, so it is part of the mind-body connection.

Pineal Body

The pineal body, or gland, is found on the dorsal side of the diencephalon. Approximately 30% of the pineal cells are responsive to external magnetic patterns. The gland functions as an internal biological clock that regulates daily activities (circadian rhythms) and yearly rhythms (circannual rhythms).

Practical Application

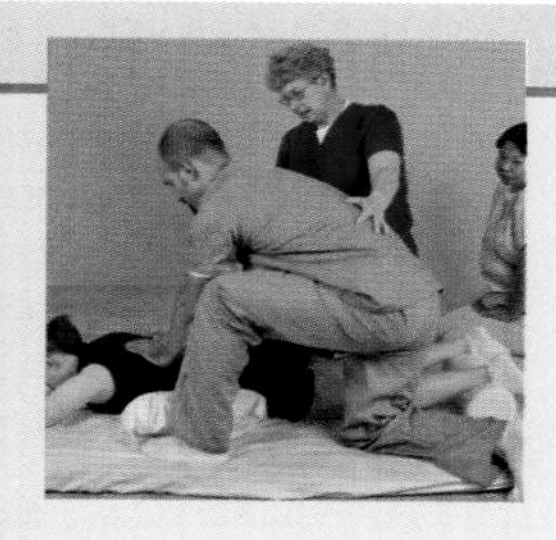

The pleasure center deep inside the hypothalamus involves feel-good neurotransmitters and predisposes a person to addictive behavior to feel good, alter mood, and so forth. Romantic love is a brain bath of norepinephrine and dopamine—feel-good chemicals. The stimulation from therapeutic massage also influences the feel-good neurotransmitters. Abuse of substances—including nicotine, alcohol, and caffeine—and extreme indulgence in eating, sex, gambling, exercise, thrill seeking, pain, violence, and crisis creating—are feel-good chemical substitutes. They have the potential to produce addictive behavior because they interact with feel-good neurotransmitters as well. Many psychotropic or mood-regulating medications act on the feel-good neurotransmitters. The use of chemicals or extreme behaviors to produce pleasure often depletes or inhibits the natural production of the chemicals, resulting in a big downslide after a big high. The extremes of pleasure and discomfort create craving and seeking behaviors that support addictive behavior.

Because therapeutic massage stimulates the release of feel-good neurotransmitters and hormones, the inclusion of these therapies has been shown to support the treatment of addictive behavior by replacing a destructive manner of mood alteration with a constructive, more moderate way to feel good. It is essential that the treatment of complex factors, such as those found in addiction, be monitored and dealt with through a multidisciplinary team approach.

Practical Application

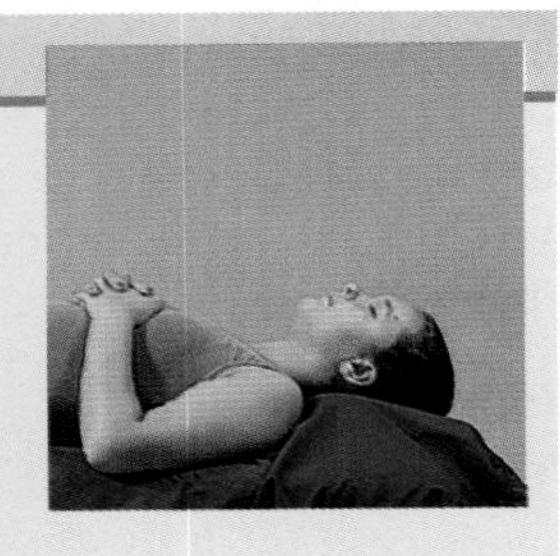

To maintain homeostasis, we need sufficient sleep. During this time of rest, most of the growth and repair of the body take place. Many chronic diseases are associated with disrupted sleep patterns. If sleep can be possibly restored to an effective pattern without the use of medications, often the body can better cope with or even begin to heal a chronic problem over time. Massage is relaxing and conducive to supporting effective sleep patterns, providing benefits to the client and thus reducing the effects of the chronic problem.

Box 4.7 Sleep

Sleep can be divided into two types: slow-wave sleep and rapid eye movement (REM) sleep.

Four stages of sleep have been defined, stage 4 being the deepest sleep.

Slow-wave sleep produces slow-frequency, high-voltage brain waves and is associated with stages 2 and 3. Such sleep is almost entirely a dreamless part of the sleep pattern. At the deeper levels, the activity of the reticular activating system is depressed in the pons and medulla.

REM sleep is associated with dreaming. At intervals of 90 minutes or so, the closed eyes begin to move rapidly. Repeatedly waking a person at the beginning of REM sleep produces anxiety and irritability. If the person is then allowed to sleep, longer than usual periods of REM sleep and dreaming occur for a few nights to allow for catching up. This process is called *REM rebound*.

Many medications, particularly sleeping pills and tranquilizers, suppress REM and stage 4 sleep. Stopping the drug may result in REM rebound, which is sometimes associated with nightmares. Therefore it is important to use medicines with minimal REM rebound when medication is necessary.

Exposure to natural sunlight assists these functions. The pineal body needs darkness to convert serotonin into melatonin, which seems to be involved with sexual activity. Melatonin also triggers the pituitary gland to release luteinizing hormone, which affects sexual maturity and may be involved in puberty and menopause. It is also involved in sleep patterns (Box 4.7).

Brainstem

The **brainstem** is considered the primitive portion of the brain and is divided into three main parts: the midbrain, pons, and the medulla oblongata. A fourth area is the reticular formation and its associated reticular activating system. These areas are control centers for vital survival functions and reflex actions, such as sneezing, coughing, vomiting, and balanced movements. Research shows that the brainstem probably processes much of the sensory data generated by massage modalities.

Midbrain

The midbrain, or mesencephalon, is located in the middle of the brain, below the cerebrum, and between the thalamus and the pons. The midbrain contains reflex centers for visual and auditory stimuli and correlates information about muscle tone and posture. The midbrain contains an important part of the reticular activating system.

Pons

The pons (pons Varolii) is in the middle of the brainstem, between the midbrain and the medulla. The pons assists in the coordinated patterns of breathing, eye movement, and facial expressions and is involved in rapid eye movement (REM) sleep.

Medulla Oblongata

The medulla, or medulla oblongata, connects the pons with the spinal cord and is composed of white matter and the reticular formation, a network of white and gray matter. The fibers handle impulses to lower motor neurons. The fibers on one side of the medulla handle signals to the contralateral side. The medulla regulates the heartbeat, blood pressure, and breathing, as well as such reflex actions as coughing and sneezing. Because the medulla controls vital life functions, injury or disease in the medulla is often fatal.

Reticular Activating System

The reticular activating system is a structural and functional part of the reticular formation in the brainstem. It maintains arousal levels in the cerebral cortex and alerts it to changes in homeostasis, thus keeping us awake and alert. The reticular activating system also helps regulate respiration, blood pressure, heart rate, endocrine secretion, and conditioned reflexes. Epinephrine and amphetamines stimulate reticular activating system conduction, whereas anesthesia and barbiturates depress conduction. Trauma or damage to the reticular activating system can cause a person to become comatose. It is considered the main center of motivation.

Cerebellum

The cerebellum is located in the posterior cranial fossa beneath the posterior portion of the cerebrum. The **cerebellum** is the second largest part of the brain and consists of a cortex composed of gray matter and an inner portion composed of white matter. Like the cerebrum, the cerebellum has sulci and gyri, and it contains two lateral hemispheres that are connected by the vermis. The cerebellum maintains balance and posture and, with proprioceptive input, coordinates everything from normal movements to the complex activities involved in dancing, gymnastics, and giving a massage. The cerebellum, limbic system, and other relay centers of the brain have been shown to work on the same circuit (Box 4.8).

Other Brain Structures

Many structures in the brain support the function of the CNS. Three important structures are the ventricles, meninges, and blood vessels.

Practical Application

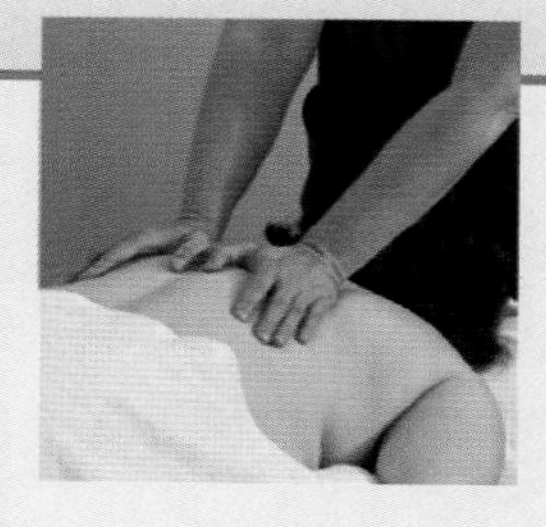

Massage methods that stimulate the cerebellum, such as rhythmic rocking, have a widespread influence. Methods that alter the body's positional sense and initiate specific movement patterns change sensory input from muscles, tendons, joints, and the skin. The output from the cerebellum goes to the motor cortex and brainstem. Stimulation of the cerebellum by alteration of muscle tone, position, and vestibular balance also stimulates the hypothalamus to adjust autonomic nervous system functions and thus restore homeostasis. Rocking produces movement at the neck and head that influences our sense of equilibrium by stimulating the balance mechanisms of the inner ear. Such mechanisms include the vestibular complex and the labyrinthine righting reflexes, which work to keep our heads level. A close relationship exists between the vestibular nerves and the cerebellum.

Rocking also stimulates muscle contraction patterns that pass throughout the body. Pressure on the side of the body may stimulate the righting reflexes.

Box 4.8 Vestibular Apparatus

The vestibular apparatus is a paired organ that is part of the inner ear. Sensations produced in this organ are conveyed to the brain, along with that of hearing, by way of the vestibulocochlear nerve and are related directly to equilibrium, balance, and functions of the cerebellum.

The vestibular apparatus on each side consists of three circular canals that are interconnected and filled with fluid. The canal expands to form fluid-filled structures called *utricles* and *saccules*. The canals, utricles, and saccules have receptors that respond to movement, especially when the head is rotated and when the head moves forward or backward.

Every time the head is moved, the fluid in the semicircular canals is set in motion, generating nerve impulses. The impulses travel to the brainstem and to the cerebellum to provide information about body and head movement, and neurons also provide information to the cranial nerves supplying the eye so that they can adjust eye position according to movement and direction. The motor cortex is stimulated, and the body can increase and decrease tone and maintain balance and equilibrium.

The vestibular apparatuses are important for spatial orientation, our sense of position in gravity, which is aided by vision, proprioceptors, and input from touch and pressure receptors.

Meninges

The meninges are three layers of connective tissue membranes that cover and protect the brain and spinal cord (Fig. 4.13).

The *dura mater*, the outermost layer, is made up of a white, tough, fibrous connective tissue membrane. The dura mater lines the cranial bones and covers the outside of the brain and spinal cord. Portions of the dura mater line the fissures between the left and right hemispheres of the cerebrum and cerebellum and cover the spinal nerve roots. Nerves and blood vessels run through the epidural space next to the dura mater. The middle layer is the *arachnoid mater*, a cobweb-like membrane containing many blood vessels. The third layer, the *pia mater*, is thin and adheres directly to the brain and spinal cord.

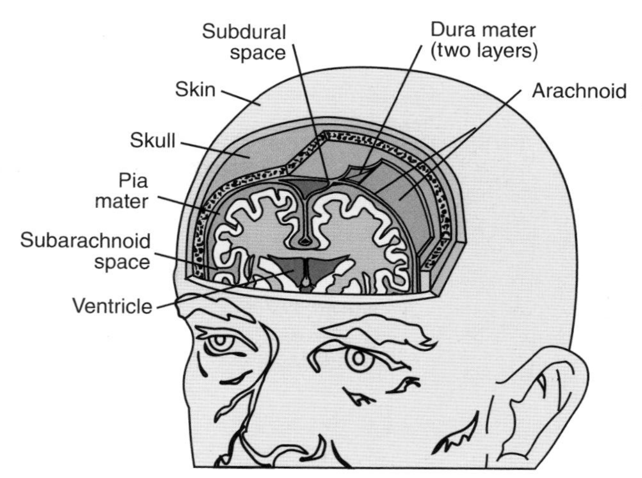

FIG. 4.13 Meninges of the brain.

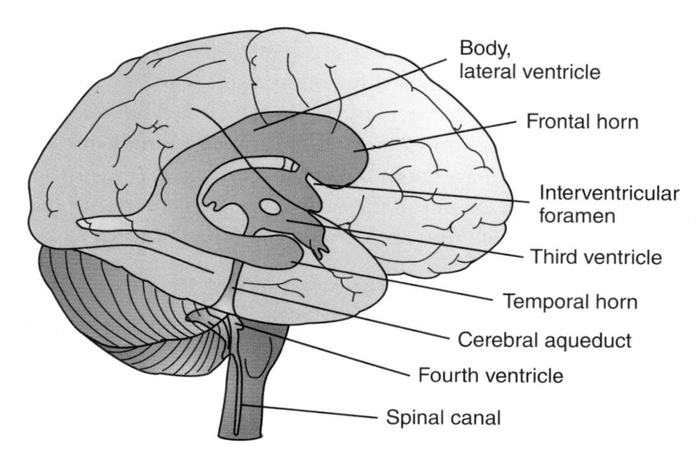

FIG. 4.14 Ventricular system, lateral view.

The meninges form three spaces that add additional cushioning and protection to the CNS:

- *Epidural space:* Found between the skull and dura mater, this space contains connective tissue, including fat.
- *Subdural space:* Found between the dura mater and arachnoid membrane, this space is filled with a cushioning serous fluid.
- *Subarachnoid space:* Found between the arachnoid and pia mater, this space contains the cerebrospinal fluid (CSF).

Ventricles

The ventricles are four fluid-filled chambers found within the brain (Fig. 4.14). There is one in each of the cerebral hemispheres, one positioned just below and between them, and one at the attachment of the cerebrum and the brainstem. CSF fills these ventricles and then passes through several small openings to the subarachnoid space.

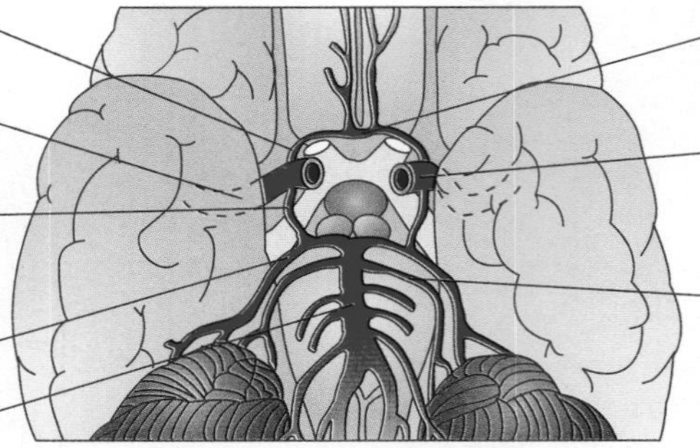

Anterior cerebral artery
Middle cerebral artery
Posterior communicating artery
Posterior cerebral artery
Basilar artery
Anterior communicating artery
Lateral carotid artery
Superior cerebellar artery

FIG. 4.15 Anatomic diagram of the circle of Willis.

Vessels of the Brain

Blood is supplied to the brain through the middle cerebral arteries, which are a continuation of the internal carotid arteries and the basilar artery. These are created from the two vertebrobasilar arteries. These three brain arteries are connected at the midbrain in the circle of Willis, which is a check-and-balance system that provides blood flow to the brain in case of blockage or damage to any of the three arteries (Fig. 4.15). Blood is transported out of the brain by several veins and the dural sinuses, which drain into the internal jugular veins.

Extracellular Fluid and Drainage in the Brain

The fluid around the various cells in the CNS consists of two main types: cerebrospinal fluid (CSF) and interstitial fluid (ISF).

Cerebrospinal fluid is a colorless, watery substance that flows throughout the brain and around the spinal cord, providing cushioning and protection. CSF is classified as one of the circulating fluids of the body. This fluid maintains homeostasis of the brain environment, including the pH balance. CSF is replenished continuously from the fluid filtering out of the choroid plexus, a network of brain capillaries. After circulating through the brain and around the spinal cord, the CSF is returned to the venous system at the dural sinuses.

Interstitial fluid in the brain flows in the spaces among neural cells and capillaries. Collectively these spaces are called the *interstitial system* (ISS). The brain ISS is a dynamic and complex space connecting the vascular system and neural networks, and it plays crucial roles in substance transport and signal transmission among neurons. Because this system is so complex, many of its mechanisms and properties remain unknown (Louveau et al., 2015). However, recent studies have indicated that the brain ISS plays several active roles in brain function, such as communication among neural cells, information processing and integration, and the coordinated response to changes in the external and internal environments of the brain.

The ISF of the brain tissue and the CSF bathing the CNS need to be filtered. Just recently a system for waste clearance from the brain was described (Abbott et al., 2018). Studies have revealed lymphatic vessels in the CNS, where CSF may reach deep cervical lymph nodes (Louveau et al., 2015). A macroscopic waste clearance system has also been identified. Evidence indicates lymphatic drainage of ISF from the brain along perivascular spaces (tiny tubelike structures around blood vessels) (Lei et al., 2017; Wei et al., 2023). A term used to describe this drainage network is the *glymphatic system*. The perivascular tube system also allows for the circulation of several substances in the brain, including glucose, lipids, amino acids, and growth factors. Neurodegenerative diseases, such as Alzheimer disease, have been linked to a failure in the CNS lymphatic system.

Aging and the Brain

Brain aging is inevitable, but age-related changes affect each brain differently. Some cognitive processes do not decline with age. Verbal abilities and implicit memory, a functional form of memory that cannot be consciously recalled, remain stable. As an example, tying shoes is considered an implicit memory. Interestingly, some factors, such as wisdom and procedural knowledge about how to act in certain situations, even improve with age.

Aging is a physiological process that affects all body tissues. In the brain, aging is associated mainly with a decline in attention, memory, and other cognitive functions. Certain parts of the brain shrink, especially those important to learning and other complex mental activities. In certain brain regions, communication between neurons can be reduced. Some general changes are thought to occur during brain aging:

- Shrinkage occurs in the frontal lobe and hippocampus—areas involved in higher cognitive function and encoding new memories. The transferal of new information to memory can take longer but remains possible.
- The outer-ridged surface of the brain thins, resulting in changes in cortical density because of fewer synaptic connections. The decline in synaptic connections may contribute to slower cognitive processing, such as a diminished ability to multitask or do math.
- Myelin is thought to shrink with age, leading to slow processing and reduced cognitive function. White matter consists of myelinated nerve fibers that are bundled into tracts and carry nerve signals between brain cells. Slowed processing can make processing and planning parallel tasks more difficult.

- The aging brain generates smaller amounts of neurotransmitters. The decrease in dopamine, acetylcholine, serotonin, and norepinephrine activity may contribute to declining cognition and memory and increased depression.

A common cause of mental decline in most people is diminished blood flow in small vessels in the brain. These small vessels are easily plugged by cholesterol and fats or ruptured by high blood pressure. These undetected "ministrokes" cause cumulative, progressive damage. Inflammation is another contributor to mental decline. When brain cells die or are damaged for any reason, healthy neuron development is inhibited by inflammatory chemicals that are released by the brain's immune cell system. Brain inflammation can also be caused by infections.

Some behaviors are considered to be protective for brain health:

- Regular physical activity
- Participation in intellectually stimulating activities
- Staying socially active
- Managing stress
- Eating healthfully
- Sleeping well

Practical Application

Therapeutic massage can contribute to a healthy brain by helping to manage stress, supporting restorative sleep, and providing social connection, while also being physically and intellectually stimulating.

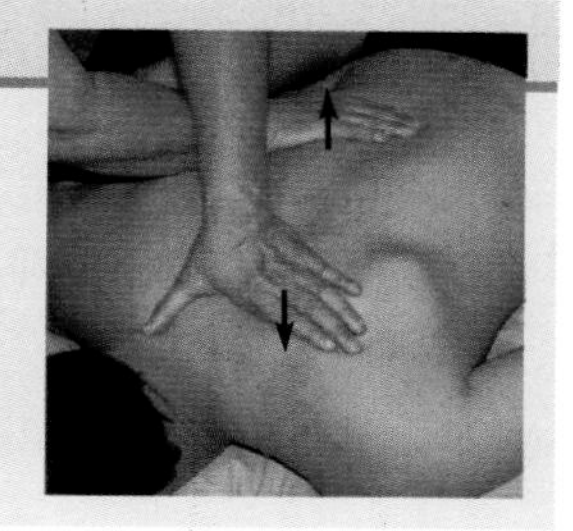

Spinal Cord

The two main functions of the spinal cord are to conduct nerve impulses and to integrate spinal reflexes.

The **spinal cord**, which is made up of white and gray matter, is about 17 to 18 inches long in the average person. The spinal cord is oval and, like the brain, has fissures. The anterior median fissure is deeper and wider than the posterior median sulcus (Fig. 4.16).

The spinal cord begins at the base of the brainstem and exits through an opening in the skull called the *foramen magnum*. The spinal cord continues through the vertebral column to the first and second lumbar vertebrae. At this point, the pia mater continues as the filum terminale and connects to the dura mater at the second sacral vertebra; they both end at the coccyx.

Thirty-one pairs of spinal nerves connect with the spinal cord. When they exit the spinal cord, they are considered part of the PNS.

The section of the spinal cord that corresponds to a single pair of spinal nerves is known as a *segment*. The spinal cord has 31 segments:

- 8 cervical
- 12 thoracic
- 5 lumbar
- 5 sacral
- 1 coccygeal

The spinal nerves are indicated easily in relation to the vertebrae. For example, the nerve between the first and second thoracic vertebrae is T1. Spinal nerves exit the spinal cord through intervertebral foramina. Because the spinal cord is shorter than the vertebral column (ending at the second lumbar vertebra), the spinal nerves from the lower lumbar and sacral regions extend to and exit through sacral foramina. The

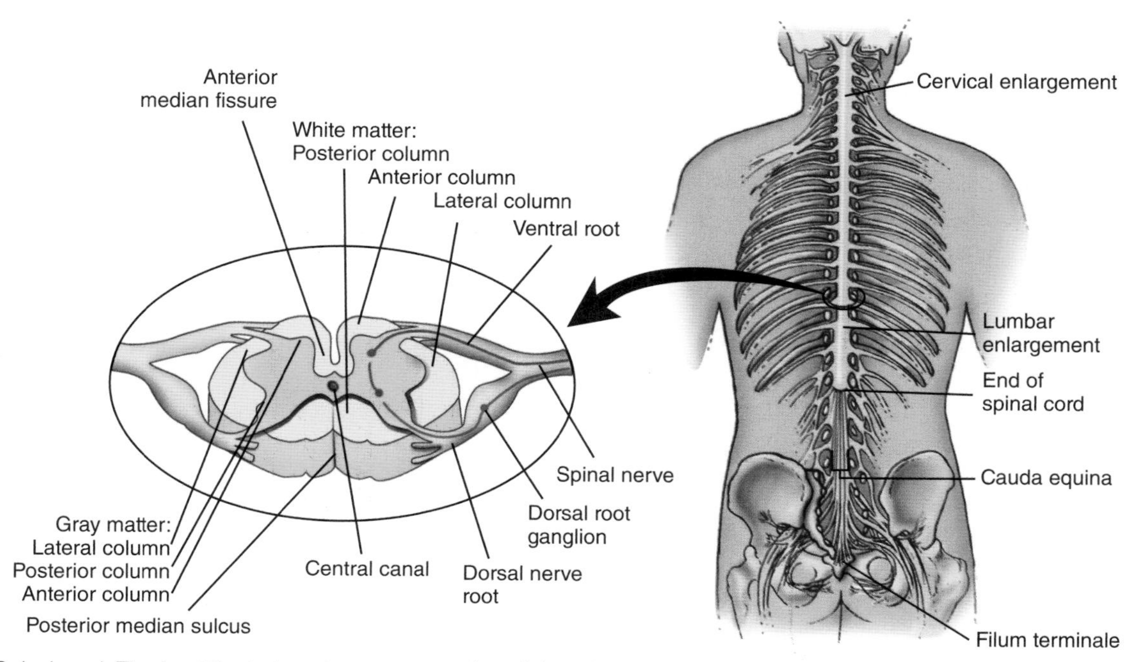

FIG. 4.16 Spinal cord. The *inset* illustrates a transverse section of the spinal cord shown in the broader view. (From Thibodeau GA, Patton KT. *Anatomy and Physiology*. 6th ed. Mosby; 2007.)

spinal and lower lumbar nerves, which are referred to as *cauda equina*, make the lower end of the spinal cord look like the tail of a horse.

Each spinal nerve is attached to the spinal cord by two roots:

- The dorsal (or posterior) root, which carries sensory information
- The ventral (or anterior) root, which carries motor information

The **dorsal root** enlarges to form the dorsal root ganglion. Distal to the dorsal root ganglion, the dorsal root joins with the **ventral root** so that the sensory and motor roots are bound together to form a spinal nerve. Spinal nerves are called *mixed nerves* because they contain both sensory and motor nerve fibers.

Gray matter is located inside the spinal cord and extends the entire length. A cross section shows that the gray matter forms an H pattern.

The dorsal portion of the H forms the dorsal horns and is composed of the associative cell bodies or interneurons. The anterior portion of the H forms the ventral horns, consisting of the cell bodies of motor nerves. In the center of the gray matter is the central canal, which contains CSF.

Surrounding the gray matter are pathways of white matter called *tracts*, created from the myelinated nerve fibers. The axons in each tract are limited to one action, such as transmitting specific touch and pressure sensations. The tracts ascend to and descend from the brain. The **ascending tracts** conduct sensory impulses such as nociception, touch, and temperature up from the spinal nerves through the spinal cord to the brain. The **descending tracts** conduct motor impulses from the brain down the cord to the spinal nerves (Fig. 4.17).

Sensory Ascending Tracts

Sensory receptors are found in the skin, fascia, muscles, and all organs. When stimulated by sensations such as temperature, touch, pressure, joint movement, and muscle action, they respond by generating nerve impulses. These signals travel along the nerve fibers from these receptors to the spinal cord, where they cross to the other side and ascend one of the sensory pathways, or tracts, to the thalamus, medulla, or cerebellum. In the brain, the sensations are integrated into perceptions or filtered as being unimportant. This sensory information is needed to maintain homeostasis.

Some of the most important sensory information supplied to the client's body during massage comes from sensory receptors, specifically from proprioceptors that sense data concerning position and movement. Sensory fibers transmit signals about body position, deep touch or pressure, two-point discrimination (the ability to differentiate between two stimuli applied close to each other), and vibration. The proprioceptors are located in muscles, tendons, ligaments, and joints. Some proprioceptive signals initiate a response in the spinal cord; these are called *deep tendon reflex arcs*.

For a sensory signal to move from a sensory receptor to the brain, it passes through three different neurons.

The first one, referred to as the *primary*, is a relay from the receptor to the brainstem or the spinal cord. This is part of the PNS and is discussed in detail in Chapter 5.

The second neuron extends from the brainstem or spinal cord to the thalamus. The secondary neuron synapses with the tertiary (or third) neuron in the thalamus. The actual crossing of sensory signals from the left to the right side (and vice versa) takes place mostly in the secondary neurons before they enter the thalamus.

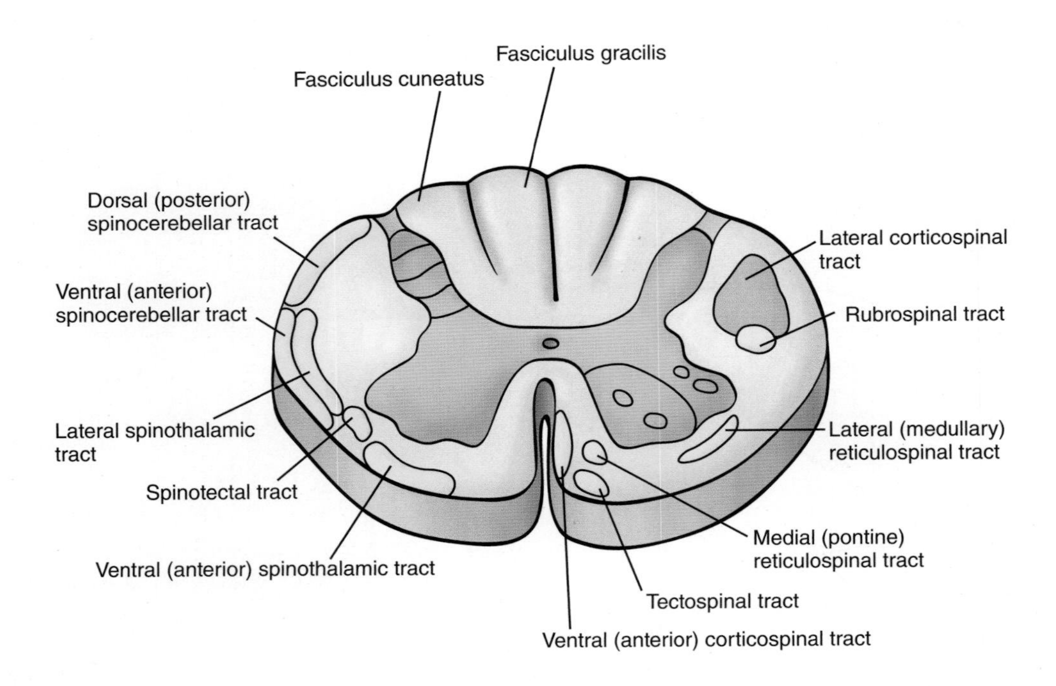

FIG. 4.17 Ascending and descending tracts.

The third neuron ends in the postcentral gyrus of the parietal lobe of the cortex. The axons of these third neurons make up the white matter of the cerebrum, referred to as the *internal capsule;* the dendrites and cell bodies make up the gray matter of the cerebral cortex.

Motor Descending Tracts

Motor tracts transmit information about adaptive responses and sensory experiences concerned with gross movements, posture, and fine motor skills. Signals traveling from the CNS to the muscles use the somatic motor pathways. One of the main motor tracts is the pyramidal, or corticospinal, tract, which ties into the voluntary motor system. The pyramidal fibers handle voluntary and reflex signals to the muscles. The fibers begin in the cortex at the precentral gyrus and descend to the medulla, where they cross to the opposite side of the spinal cord. From that point, they descend through the lateral corticospinal tract to the motor neurons of the skeletal muscles.

One important rule to remember is the *final common path principle.* Each motor unit within a muscle receives impulses that are conducted along a single motor neuron that begins in the anterior gray horn of the spinal cord. This principle is important to healthcare providers who are exploring muscle dysfunction and its relationship to spinal cord injuries. By identifying muscle dysfunction, a common relationship to the spinal nerve can also be determined (Box 4.9 and Activity 4.4).

Box 4.9 Motor Tracts of the Spinal Cord

The spinal cord has five main motor tracts:

1. Lateral corticospinal tracts: These tracts handle voluntary movements, especially the contraction of small groups of muscles such as those in the hands and feet. They affect muscles on the side of the body opposite from the cerebral cortex.
2. Anterior or ventral corticospinal tracts: These tracts handle the same lateral tracts, but the muscles are on the same side of the body as the cortex. The term *pyramidal tracts* refers to the lateral and anterior corticospinal tracts. The neurons from the cerebral cortex cross through the pyramid areas of the medulla.
3. Lateral reticulospinal tracts: These tracts transmit facilitatory impulses from the medulla through the anterior horn motor neurons to skeletal muscles that handle muscle tone and extensor reflexes.
4. Medial reticulospinal tracts: These tracts carry mainly inhibitory impulses from the pons through the anterior horn motor neurons to skeletal muscles that deal with muscle tone and extensor reflexes.
5. Rubrospinal tracts: These tracts transmit impulses that coordinate body movements and maintain posture. The extrapyramidal tracts are composed of the lateral and medial reticulospinal and rubrospinal tracts. They relay motor signals through the cerebrum, thalamus, brainstem, and cerebellum to the gray matter of the spinal cord. At this point most synapse with interneurons, which then synapse with the lower motor neurons. It should be noted that facilitating and inhibiting signals are sent through these motor neurons.

ACTIVITY 4.4

Summarize the ascending and descending functions of the spinal cord.

Example

Ascending	Descending
Sends information to CNS regarding pain	Delivers information to muscles

Your Turn

Upper and Lower Motor Neuron Injury

Injuries to the upper and lower motor neurons result in differing responses in the skeletal muscles. When upper motor neurons are damaged or destroyed by trauma or disease, the result usually is an increase in rigidity and an exaggerated response to reflexes. This is referred to as *spastic paralysis.*

Injuries to the lower motor neurons result in a lack of signal to the muscles, causing the absence of movement. This is known as *flaccid paralysis.*

Review What You Have Learned

- List the parts of the CNS.
  - The CNS is divided into two primary areas, the brain and the spinal cord. The brain is divided into four main areas: (1) the cerebrum (which is covered by the cerebral cortex and divided into right and left hemispheres, connected by the corpus callosum); (2) the diencephalon (the main structures are the thalamus and hypothalamus); (3) the cerebellum (which is divided into five lobes—the frontal lobe, parietal lobe, temporal lobe, occipital lobe, and insula [island of Reil]); and (4) the brainstem (composed of the medulla oblongata, pons, and midbrain). The limbic system, located in the interior of the cerebrum, is connected to the hypothalamus.
  - The spinal cord is contained within the vertebral column, beginning at the brainstem and ending at the first and second lumbar vertebrae. Thirty-one pairs of spinal nerves connect to the spinal cord. The sections of the spinal cord that correspond to pairs of spinal nerves are known as *segments*, making 31 segments: 8 cervical, 12 thoracic, 5 lumbar, 5 sacral, and 1 coccygeal.
  - The ascending tracts conduct sensory impulses such as nociception, touch, and temperature up from the spinal nerves through the spinal cord to the brain. The descending tracts conduct motor impulses from the brain down the cord to the spinal nerves.
- Define *meninges.*
  - The meninges are the three layers of connective tissue membranes that cover and protect the brain and spinal cord: the *dura mater* (outermost layer), the *arachnoid mater* (middle layer), and the *pia mater* (deepest layer).
- Describe the two main types of extracellular fluid in the CNS.
  - The CSF is a colorless, watery substance that flows throughout the brain and around the spinal cord, providing protection and maintaining homeostasis. The ISF in the brain flows in the spaces among neural cells

Practical Application

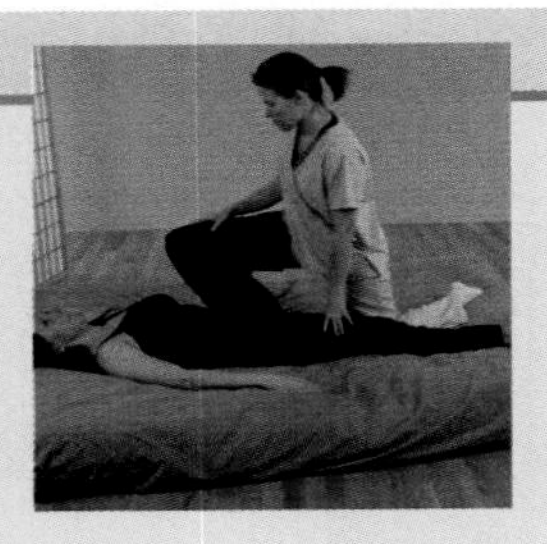

The disability or dysfunction caused by brain and spinal cord injuries is determined by the region and function of the areas affected. The prognosis for trauma to the motor neurons is commonly difficult to identify. Soft tissue methods and other forms of movement therapies seem to be most beneficial as part of the whole healthcare picture. Specific recommendations about massage are difficult to make solely based on the location of damage because the body compensates by rerouting the interrupted signals. This is why clinical reasoning methods are so important. The ability to process a situation and determine the best intervention is an essential skill if you want to succeed as a massage therapy professional.

For example, spastic paralysis results from upper motor neuron injuries. A client with such injuries will have spastic paralysis of the muscles in the affected region. Voluntary control over movement is lost, and limbs may have to be restrained to prevent involuntary movement at inappropriate times. Usually, less muscle atrophy is present, and lymph and blood flow continue because of the working of the muscles. The preferred modalities, when applied to each individual, can moderate some of the random spasms and keep the soft tissues more supple and the joints more mobile, resulting in less rigidity in the muscles.

With lower motor neuron difficulties, the muscles' atrophy and actions and reflexes are slow, limited, or nonexistent. Massage and joint movement may be able to replace the mechanical pumping action of normal muscle contraction and assist in moving the blood and lymph. In addition, keeping the soft tissue pliable may lessen any contractures.

and capillaries. Collectively these spaces are called the *interstitial system* (ISS), which plays crucial roles in substance transport and signal transmission.

PATHOLOGICAL CONDITIONS

SECTION OBJECTIVES

Chapter objectives covered in this section:

7. List drugs that affect the CNS.
8. Describe common pathological conditions of the CNS and the related indications/contraindications for massage.

After completing this section, the learner will be able to:

- Explain the influence of massage methods on CNS pathology.
- Explain how certain drugs affect the CNS.

Pathologies related to the CNS can have profound implications for both physical and mental health. The CNS regulates physiological functions, and it also influences personality and behavior—reflecting, in essence, the concept of self. Damage to the brain and spinal cord can be caused by disease or trauma. Various drugs can be used to treat CNS disorders. However, if used inappropriately, these same chemicals can lead to CNS dysfunction.

Drugs Affecting Central Nervous System Function

Many medications are used to treat dysfunction in the CNS. The main categories are the following:

- Analgesics
- Antianxiety drugs (including tricyclics)
- Anticonvulsants
- Antidepressants
- Antiemetics (nausea, vomiting)
- Antihistamines
- Anti-Parkinson drugs
- Sedative/hypnotics
- Antitussives (relieve coughing)
- Antipsychotics
- Opioids

Most drugs of abuse affect CNS functions. *Physical dependency* (addiction) means that when a drug is withdrawn, severe autonomic excitability occurs. The person thus requires the drug to feel normal. Time and sometimes medical intervention are required before the body reestablishes its ability to self-regulate without the drug.

Tolerance, which occurs with stimulants and depressants, means that larger doses of the drug are required for the same effect because the body has adjusted to the current dose. Amphetamines are dangerous because there is no physical dependency; thus the body gives no physical warnings of abuse. Therefore because of tolerance, a person can approach a lethal dose without being aware of it.

Stimulants that affect the neurotransmitters and receptor sites of the cells in the CNS include caffeine, nicotine, amphetamines, and cocaine. Caffeine is a CNS stimulant that enhances the sense of alertness and diminishes the sense of fatigue and boredom. Nicotine first stimulates and then depresses the nervous system by affecting the release of norepinephrine and mimicking the action of acetylcholine. Amphetamines and cocaine stimulate the release of **catecholamines**, primarily norepinephrine and dopamine, from sympathetic neurons. Their effect on the CNS ranges from a feeling of well-being to euphoria to psychosis.

Depressants (e.g., alcohol, narcotics, minor tranquilizers, and barbiturates) act on the cerebral cortex by blocking norepinephrine and dopamine. The paradoxical effect of alcohol as a stimulant results from its ability to inhibit learned behavior and release primitive biological impulses from inhibitory control. Depressants are also anesthetics. The cortex is depressed first, and then the more primitive centers (brainstem) are depressed as the dosage is increased. Brainstem depression can result in death because respiration and cardiac functions are slowed; if the depression continues, these functions eventually stop.

The hallucinogens include lysergic acid diethylamide (LSD), phencyclidine (PCP), peyote (mescaline), and marijuana (tetrahydrocannabinol). LSD blocks the neurotransmitter serotonin, and PCP blocks acetylcholine. These drugs seem to alter brain function by randomly stimulating and blocking neurotransmitters. A typical action is that smell may be "seen," color may be "heard," and so forth. PCP is considered the most dangerous of the hallucinogens. It uncouples sensory pathways in the brain to produce a sensory deprivation syndrome, creating an increase in body strength accompanied by an acute psychotic reaction. Because of its high fat solubility and the production of long-acting metabolites, PCP may remain in body tissues for months or even years, causing recurring episodes of violence and psychosis.

Adding to the concerns are synthetic designer drugs. These emerging drugs of abuse involve the manipulation of basic chemical structures.

Pathological Conditions

Cerebrovascular Accidents (Strokes)

The most common brain disorder is a cerebrovascular accident (CVA) or stroke. There are two types of strokes: ischemic and hemorrhagic.

- *Ischemic stroke:* Clots can form in the brain's blood vessels, in blood vessels leading to the brain, or even in blood vessels elsewhere in the body and then travel to the brain. These clots block blood flow to the brain's cells. Ischemic stroke can also occur when too much plaque (fatty deposits and cholesterol) clogs the brain's blood vessels. About 80% of all strokes are ischemic.
- *Hemorrhagic stroke:* This type of stroke occurs when a blood vessel in the brain ruptures. As a result, blood seeps into the brain tissue, damaging brain cells. The most common causes of hemorrhagic stroke are high blood pressure and brain aneurysms. An *aneurysm* is a weakness or thinness in the wall of a blood vessel.

When a stroke occurs, blood flow to part of the brain is interrupted. The damage caused by the stroke is determined by (1) the location where the blood flow is cut off and (2) how long the area is deprived of blood flow.

Consequences of a stroke may include these deficits:

- *Hemiparesis:* A partial motor deficit on one side of the body.
- *Quadriplegia:* A total motor deficit in both arms and legs. **Quadriplegia** usually occurs as a result of trauma to the spinal cord, but it can be caused by a stroke.
- *Sensory losses:* The inability to feel pain, temperature, vibration, and so forth.

The limbs initially are flaccid or relaxed. Later they become spastic or contracted. The forearm in flexion and the leg in extension are common sights because of the unequal innervation of extensors and flexors. The cause of the spasticity is thought to be a loss of control of lower motor neurons.

Behavioral changes caused by damage in the associative areas of the cortex are often present. If the left hemisphere is involved, language difficulties such as aphasia (difficulty speaking) occur. A stroke in the right hemisphere produces inattention and lack of concern. Confusion may be present if either hemisphere is affected.

A transient ischemic attack (TIA) is a prestroke condition that mimics a stroke. *Transient* means temporary. TIAs resolve in less than 24 hours. In some cases, when the deficit lasts longer than 24 hours and then clears completely, the condition is called a *reversible neurological deficit* or a *residual ischemic neurological deficit.*

The signs of a TIA are transient blindness in one eye, aphasia, numbness or weakness of the hand or foot, slurred speech, dizziness, ataxia, syncope, and numbness around the lips. The signs may last only a few minutes and then disappear. They are commonly ignored. Because a TIA is often a warning of a major stroke, it is important to know its basic signs.

Cerebrovascular Disease

Cerebrovascular disease is a gradual buildup of arteriosclerotic lesions (thickened, hardened areas of reduced elasticity) in the arteries of the neck and brain. High blood pressure is a strong predisposing factor. Arteries commonly affected are the common carotid, internal carotid, and middle cerebral arteries. Complications of cerebrovascular disease are blood clots and hemorrhage, leading to a stroke.

Aneurysm

An aneurysm is the weakening and bulging of any artery, including those in the brain. If the weakened area bursts, bleeding and complications can be fatal. In the brain, it can lead to a stroke. Sometimes the rupture of a brain artery is preceded by a series of small leaks that produce transient headaches and neck stiffness. These symptoms are common in many other conditions and normal stress, so it is important to have a qualified medical professional rule out more serious conditions before assuming that symptoms are minor or only stress related.

INDICATIONS/CONTRAINDICATIONS for Therapeutic Massage

Therapeutic massage in a supervised setting can be supportive during rehabilitation. The benefits of massage therapy are effective in managing the discomfort caused when the functioning portions of the body must work harder to compensate for nonfunctioning areas. In addition, stress management is an important part of the long-term management of these conditions. Because anticoagulants are commonly used to prevent further CVAs or TIAs, care must be taken when using soft tissue methods so that bruising does not occur during therapy. Careful attention should be paid to any symptom of thrombosis, and the type of massage application chosen should not place heavy pressure over vulnerable vessels to prevent the rare but possible mobilization of an embolism.

Central Nervous System Trauma

A sudden blow to the head or intense shaking of the head may or may not involve a fracture. The fracture itself is usually not important—more significant is the possibility of intracranial bleeding or brain swelling (edema). When bleeding occurs between the dura and arachnoid, it is called a *subdural hematoma*; when the bleeding is located between the skull and the dura, it is referred to as an *epidural hematoma.*

Concussion

A concussion is brain trauma that may be mild, moderate, or severe. Symptoms of mild concussions include a brief loss of consciousness or a state of confusion. A headache and vomiting may follow the episode. In most cases, complete recovery occurs in a matter of a few days to a week, although in rare cases recovery may take longer. Cumulative concussive episodes, even when mild, cause brain trauma.

In cases of moderate to severe concussions, a brain contusion, or bruise, may cause swelling of the brain tissues. This is common in traumas known as *closed head injuries.* Prolonged unconsciousness and problems with vasomotor and respiratory functions may occur. After waking, the person may show behavioral and personality changes, amnesia, and motor and sensory disturbances. The prognosis can range from complete recovery to continued deterioration. Because the amount of internal injury may not be immediately recognizable, any person with a head injury should be referred immediately to a medical professional.

Cerebral Palsy

Cerebral palsy is a general term for brain damage that takes place before, during, or shortly after birth. Damage may involve the whole brain but usually is limited to the pyramidal tracts, which results in motor function disturbance. The most common symptoms include muscle spasticity especially in the feet, legs, and hands; impaired speech, vision, hearing, and tactile sensations; and seizures. Impaired intellectual function may or may not result.

INDICATIONS/CONTRAINDICATIONS for Therapeutic Massage

Therapeutic massage is an effective part of a supervised comprehensive care program. Massage and other forms of bodywork can help manage secondary muscle tension that results from the alteration of posture and the use of equipment, such as wheelchairs, braces, and crutches.

Spinal Cord Injury

Injuries to the spinal cord can result in several neurological problems. Studies of blood flow and metabolism indicate that spinal cord injury involves not only direct neuronal trauma but also direct and delayed vascular trauma. The most commonly injured sites are at the most mobile segments of the spine, such as the cervicothoracic junction (C7 to T1) and the thoracolumbar junction (T12 to L1 through L4). About 40% of spinal cord injuries result in complete interruption of function. The remaining 60% result in impairment or destruction of certain sensory and motor functions.

Injury to or cutting of the spinal cord is followed by a 2- to 3-week period of spinal shock, during which all spinal reflex responses are depressed. The spinal reflexes below the cut or injury become exaggerated and hyperactive. The neurons become hypersensitive to the excitatory neurotransmitters, and the spinal neurons may sprout collaterals that synapse with excitatory input. The stretch reflexes are exaggerated, and the tone of the muscle increases.

If a spinal cord injury occurs above the third cervical spinal nerve, loss of voluntary movement of all the limbs occurs, and respiratory movements are affected if the phrenic nerve is damaged. The phrenic nerve arises from the third, fourth, or fifth cervical nerve and supplies the diaphragm. If the lesion is lower, only the lower limbs are affected, and **paraplegia** results. If the nerves to only one limb are affected, **monoplegia** results.

One of the complications common among people with spinal cord injuries is decubitus ulcers. Because voluntary shifting of weight does not occur, the body's weight compresses the circulation to the skin over bony prominences, causing ulcers to develop. Genitourinary and respiratory complications can also occur.

The function of the autonomic system below the level of the lesion is also affected. Voluntary control of the bladder and rectum is lost if the lesion is above the sacral segments; reflex contractions of the bladder and rectum occur as soon as they become full, resulting in incontinence; and inconsistency of blood pressure can occur. However, paralysis of the muscles of the urinary bladder could also occur, resulting in stagnation of urine and urinary tract infections.

The mass reflex occurs when a slight stimulus to the skin triggers many other reflexes, such as emptying of the bladder and rectum, sweating, and blood pressure changes. People with chronic spinal injuries can be taught to initiate these reflexes by stroking or pinching the thigh, triggering the mass reflex and intentionally giving them some control over urination and defecation.

As a result of the disuse of the bones, calcium from the bones is reabsorbed and excreted in the urine, increasing the incidence of calcium stones in the urinary tract.

INDICATIONS/CONTRAINDICATIONS for Therapeutic Massage

Massage is an effective part of a comprehensive, supervised rehabilitation and long-term care program. Massage and other forms of bodywork can help manage secondary muscle tension resulting from the alteration of posture and the use of wheelchairs, braces, and crutches. Specifically focused massage may help manage bowel paralysis. The circulation enhancement produced by massage may assist in the management of a decubitus ulcer.

Tumors

A brain tumor rarely develops in a neuron because neurons have a significantly diminished ability to divide. Most tumors are formed from the neuroglia, the tissues of the membranes, and the blood vessels found in and around the brain. Most tumors that develop in the brain are benign. However, because there is no space for them to expand, they compress the brain and its supporting tissues, sometimes with fatal results. Malignant brain tumors usually grow from cells of malignant tumors that exist elsewhere in the body, often in the lung or breast.

Signs and symptoms of compression caused by a brain tumor include:

- Loss of sensory or motor function, mainly on one side of the body
- Personality changes, behavioral changes, or both
- Headaches
- Awkward movement or gait (ataxia)

INDICATIONS/CONTRAINDICATIONS for Therapeutic Massage

Massage therapists should be able to recognize the signs and symptoms of a possible brain compression (as previously described) and refer the client to a medical professional for diagnosis and care. During rehabilitation from surgery, massage can be used as supportive care and to improve any compensation patterns that have resulted from brain damage caused by surgery.

Neurodegenerative Disorders

Neurodegenerative disease is an umbrella term for a range of conditions that primarily affect the neurons in the human brain. A variety of degenerative diseases referred to as *dementias* are organic mental disorders caused by a chemical imbalance, endocrine dysfunction, or trauma to the brain, and they can result in the destruction of brain neurons. As the degeneration progresses, symptoms such as memory loss, decreased attention span, diminished intellectual capacity, and loss of control of personality or behavior commonly are observed.

Alzheimer Disease

Alzheimer disease is a type of dementia in which the brain degenerates, resulting in judgment errors, memory difficulties, and a tendency to become confused. Neuronal tangles and plaque found in brain tissue contain amyloid, a pathological, insoluble, starchlike protein. Neurons essential for memory are particularly vulnerable to this degenerative process. The current theory is that Alzheimer disease is determined genetically by amyloid B, which is regulated by a gene located on chromosome 21. Deficiencies in neurotransmitters and dysfunction in neuroglia are also implicated in dementia.

INDICATIONS/CONTRAINDICATIONS for Therapeutic Massage

The degeneration seen in Alzheimer disease may be slowed by therapeutic intervention and medication. Studies indicate that sensory stimulation modalities, such as rhythmic massage and movement, may provide calming and orienting influences.

Amyotrophic Lateral Sclerosis

Also known as *Lou Gehrig disease*, **amyotrophic lateral sclerosis (ALS)** is a progressive disease that begins in the CNS, involves the degeneration of motor neurons, and eventually results in the atrophy of voluntary muscle. Symptoms of ALS include weakness, fatigue, and muscle spasms. The disease is most common in men between 40 and 70 years of age.

INDICATIONS/CONTRAINDICATIONS for Therapeutic Massage

Massage is indicated for ALS, with caution and under a healthcare provider's supervision. The degrees of pressure and intensity must be adjusted as the disease progresses.

Seizures

Seizures, or convulsions, are defined as sudden involuntary muscle contractions. The most common group of seizure disorders is referred to as *epilepsy*, which occurs when the nerve cells of the cerebral cortex send out uncontrolled signals. In many cases, the cause of the neuron stimulation is unknown, but known precipitating factors include hereditary factors, trauma to the head, stroke, brain tumor, and infections.

Minor seizures (absence seizures, formerly known as *petit mal*) may not include actual spasms of the skeletal muscles. Usually seen in children, these seizures are typified by a moment of blankness. Major seizures (tonic-clonic seizures, formerly known as *grand mal*) begin with an aura or sensation, such as a taste, smell, or feeling. The person usually experiences involuntary spasms or continuous tension in the skeletal muscles and loss of consciousness. A sense of confusion and a desire to sleep are common aftereffects.

Most forms of epilepsy can be controlled by antiseizure medication, commonly phenobarbital or phenytoin (Dilantin). The side effects of the medications can include headache, muscle tension, nervousness, joint pain, and sleeping difficulties. A continuous seizure that lasts longer than 30 minutes is called **status epilepticus** and is a medical emergency.

Tremors

Tremors are involuntary muscle twitches. They may be minor and occur in a tired muscle, or they may be exaggerated, such as in St. Vitus dance, Huntington chorea, or Parkinson disease. They are not a form of epilepsy, although they originate in the CNS.

Essential tremor is a chronic tremor that does not result from any pathological condition. The tremor is slowly progressive but usually not debilitating. The onset can occur as early as adolescence but usually occurs in midlife. Essential tremor may be an inherited disorder.

Parkinson Disease

In Parkinson disease, the neurons that release the neurotransmitter dopamine in the brain degenerate, thus slowing or stopping its release. Parkinson disease occurs mainly in the elderly. The symptoms include rigidity of the muscles of the limbs, tremors while the person is at rest, a shuffling gait, and a masklike face. In addition to the movement-related (motor) symptoms, some Parkinson symptoms may not be related to movement (nonmotor). Examples of nonmotor symptoms include apathy, depression, constipation, sleep behavior disorders, loss of the sense of smell, and cognitive impairment.

Pharmacological intervention includes the use of L-dopa (levodopa), the precursor of dopamine; amantadine (Symmetrel), which releases dopamine at the synapse; and benztropine (Cogentin) and trihexyphenidyl (Artane), both of which are anticholinergic drugs. Deep brain stimulation (DBS) is a surgical procedure used to treat several disabling neurological symptoms—most commonly, the debilitating motor symptoms of Parkinson disease, such as tremor, rigidity, stiffness, slowed movement, and walking problems. The procedure is also used to treat essential tremors and dystonia. DBS uses a surgically implanted, battery-operated medical device to deliver electrical stimulation to specific areas in the brain that control movement.

Chorea

Chorea results from the degeneration of neurons in the basal ganglia. The person's normal voluntary movements are replaced by involuntary, dancelike motions. The most common forms are Sydenham chorea and Huntington chorea, a hereditary disease that includes a form of dementia.

INDICATIONS/CONTRAINDICATIONS for Therapeutic Massage

The side effects of medications may be reduced by massage techniques. Massage therapists must remember that clients who show any exaggerated or increased symptoms should be referred to their prescribing physicians. It is important to learn how to respond if a seizure occurs. The National Institute of Neurological Disorders and Stroke recommends these steps:

1. Roll the person over onto their side. This prevents the individual from choking on vomit or saliva.
2. Cushion the person's head.
3. Loosen the person's collar so they can breathe freely.
4. Maintain a clear airway; you may need to grip the lower jaw gently and tilt the head back slightly to open the airway more completely.
5. Do NOT attempt to restrain the person unless failing to do so could result in obvious bodily harm (e.g., a convulsion that occurs at the top of a stairway or on the edge of a pool).
6. Do NOT put anything into the person's mouth—no medicines, no solid objects, no water—nothing. Despite what you may have seen on television, it is a myth that someone with epilepsy can swallow their tongue. However, the person could choke on foreign objects.
7. Remove sharp or solid objects the person might come into contact with.
8. Time the seizure. Note: How long did the seizure last? What were the symptoms? If the person has multiple seizures, how long was it between seizures? Your observations can help medical personnel later.

Additional measures to take include:

- Stay by the person's side throughout the seizure.
- Stay calm. It will probably be over quickly.
- Do NOT shake the person or shout. This will not help.
- Respectfully ask bystanders to stay back. The person may be tired, groggy, embarrassed, or otherwise disoriented after a seizure. Offer to call someone, or obtain further assistance, if the individual needs it.

INDICATIONS/CONTRAINDICATIONS for Therapeutic Massage

Because massage has been shown to increase dopamine activity, its use is indicated in managing Parkinson disease and tremors. In addition, secondary muscle tension can be managed effectively by methods such as massage therapy and other forms of soft tissue manipulation. Make sure to understand the actions and side effects of various treatments.

Headache

Headache is a common symptom with a multitude of causes. Headaches can be caused by stress, muscle tension, chemical imbalance, disordered breathing syndromes, nutritional disruption, side effects from medication, vascular dysfunction, sinus disorders, tumors, and many more internal and external influences. There are two basic headache types:

- *Vascular headaches:* This type of headache is marked by fluid pressure and pain that is felt as a throbbing from the inside of the head out. Vascular headaches are usually classified as migraine, although migraine is only one type of vascular headache. Migraine headache pain is believed to be caused by dilation of the cranial vessels. The pain is knifelike, throbbing, and unilateral. Any visual distortion (e.g., flashing lights) is thought to be caused by vasoconstriction preceding the vasodilation and pain. Cluster headaches occur on one side of the head, with remissions and recurrences lasting for extended periods. They usually occur at night and are associated with other symptoms, such as red eyes and sinus drainage.
- *Tension headaches:* This headache type is due to soft tissue shortening and is typically called a *muscle tension headache*. However, we will learn that headaches are more complicated than short muscles. This headache feels like squeezing on the outside of the head.

Because the brain has no sensory innervations, headaches do not originate in the brain but in the tissues surrounding the brain and in the muscles of the shoulders, neck, and scalp. The pain of a headache is produced by pressure on the sensory nerves, vessels, or meninges or on the muscle-tendon-bone unit. This pressure is caused by two main factors: (1) fluid pressure of various causes, including dilation of blood vessels and (2) soft tissue shortening, including connective tissue changes and muscle shortening.

Headaches are classified as primary and secondary:

- Primary, or benign, headaches (i.e., not due to other underlying problems) have no organic or structural etiology. They include tension headache, vascular (migraine) headache, cluster headache, and medication-overuse headache. Most primary headaches develop slowly over minutes, if not hours.
- Secondary headaches (i.e., due to an underlying cause) are caused by an underlying structural or organic disease. Examples include headaches related to a benign or malignant brain tumor, a brain aneurysm, hematoma, meningitis, brain abscess, cerebral hemorrhage, encephalitis or other infections, or various diseases of the brain, eye, ear, nose, and so on. Fortunately, fewer than 5% of headaches are caused by tumors, and not all people with tumors experience headaches. Symptoms of serious headache that require immediate medical attention are a sudden, sharp, intense, or severe headache; a sudden lack of balance or a fall; confusion; inappropriate behavior; seizures; and difficulty speaking.

Advances in treatment include new drugs and new delivery systems (nasal sprays, needle injections) that may work better and with fewer side effects than older migraine medications.

Neuromodulation devices that use electric stimulation to affect the nervous system also show some promise for treating migraine.

INDICATIONS/CONTRAINDICATIONS for Therapeutic Massage

Massage and other forms of soft tissue therapy are effective in treating muscle tension headache but are much less effective for migraine and cluster headaches. Soft tissue therapy can relieve secondary muscle tension headache caused by the pain of the primary headache. Headache is often stress induced, so stress management in all its forms is usually indicated for chronic headache.

Depression

Depression is associated with a decline in the neurotransmitters norepinephrine, serotonin, and dopamine. Affected individuals can be helped by medications that inhibit the reuptake of norepinephrine (amphetamines) and by monoamine oxidase inhibitors, which reduce the breakdown of norepinephrine. A class of medications known as *selective serotonin reuptake inhibitors* (SSRIs) also helps manage depression. Depression can take several forms:

- *Persistent depressive disorder* (also called *dysthymia*) is a depressed mood that lasts for at least 2 years.
- *Postpartum depression* is much more serious than the "baby blues" that many experience after giving birth. (Baby blues are relatively mild symptoms of depression and anxiety that typically clear within 2 weeks after delivery.) Postpartum depression is accompanied by feelings of extreme sadness, anxiety, and exhaustion.
- *Psychotic depression* occurs when a person has severe depression plus some form of psychosis, such as having disturbed false fixed beliefs (delusions) or hearing or seeing upsetting things that others cannot hear or see (hallucinations).
- *Seasonal affective disorder* (SAD) is characterized by the onset of depression during the winter months, when less natural sunlight is available. Winter depression, typically accompanied by social withdrawal, increased sleep, and weight gain, predictably returns every year in SAD.

Anxiety

Anxiety is a normal reaction to stress. When anxiety becomes an excessive, irrational dread of everyday situations, it becomes a disabling disorder. Anxiety disorders range from feelings of uneasiness to immobilizing bouts of terror. Symptoms include chronic, exaggerated worry, tension, and irritability that appear to have no cause or are more intense than the situation warrants. Physical signs, such as restlessness, trouble falling or staying asleep, headaches, trembling, twitching, muscle tension, and sweating, often accompany these psychological symptoms. Types of anxiety include:

- Panic disorder
- Obsessive-compulsive disorder
- Posttraumatic stress disorder
- Phobias
- Generalized anxiety disorder

Treatment can involve medicines, therapy, or both. Effective treatments include cognitive behavioral therapy, relaxation techniques, and biofeedback to control muscle tension. Medications used to treat anxiety are called *anxiolytics*, or *antianxiety drugs*.

Schizophrenia

Schizophrenia is a common mental disorder. It comprises a large group of psychotic disorders characterized by gross distortions of reality; disturbances in language and communication; withdrawal from social interaction; and disorganization and fragmentation of thought, perception, and emotional reaction. No single cause has been identified, but increased dopamine activity in parts of the brain is strongly indicated. A diagnosis of schizophrenia requires the exclusion of other disorders. Management of chronic schizophrenia requires expert multidisciplinary support, along with psychopharmacological and long-term psychosocial intervention.

Because schizophrenia is associated with increased dopamine levels in the brain, the symptoms are moderated by medications that block or reduce the release of dopamine at the synapses. Large amounts of cocaine and certain amphetamines are associated with increased production of dopamine and may mimic schizophrenic behaviors.

INDICATIONS/CONTRAINDICATIONS for Therapeutic Massage

Therapeutic massage is supportive in a multidisciplinary treatment for depression or anxiety because serotonin, among other neurotransmitters, is influenced by massage. Research has also indicated that massage therapy can reduce the perception of anxiety and the tendency to be anxious. Depression is a serious and, in some cases, potentially life-threatening condition. Know the signs and symptoms of the onset of depression, and of a deepening depression, so that you can refer the client. Some of these signs and symptoms are:

- Persistent sad, anxious, or "empty" mood
- Feelings of hopelessness, or pessimism
- Irritability
- Feelings of guilt, worthlessness, or helplessness
- Loss of interest or pleasure in hobbies and activities
- Decreased energy or fatigue
- Moving or talking more slowly
- Feeling restless or having trouble sitting still
- Difficulty concentrating, remembering, or making decisions
- Difficulty sleeping, early morning awakening, or oversleeping
- Appetite and/or weight changes
- Thoughts of death or suicide, or suicide attempts
- Aches or pains, headaches, cramps, or digestive problems without a clear physical cause and/or that do not ease even with treatment

Infectious Disease

Most CNS infections are bacterial or viral. An infection of the brain is called *encephalitis*. Infection of the meninges is called *meningitis*. The two diseases may appear separately or together. Both have symptoms of fever, nausea, and vomiting. Encephalitis may affect motor function, cause seizures, and produce behavioral and mood changes. Meningitis, which occurs mainly in the subarachnoid fluid, adds stiffness of the neck to the symptom list. As with other infections, the primary treatment of viral infection is support for general immune function. Antibiotics are given for a bacterial infection.

Myelitis is an infection of the spinal cord or brainstem. In the past the poliomyelitis virus was the most common type of infection. It affects motor and sensory functions. Because most forms of myelitis result from viruses, treatment supports the body while the immune functions resolve the infection.

Brain Abscess

A brain abscess is a collection of pus, immune cells, and other material in the brain, usually from a bacterial or fungal infection. As a result, swelling and irritation (inflammation) develop. The germs that cause a brain abscess can reach the brain through the blood, or enter the brain directly, such as during brain surgery or with a skull fracture. In rare cases, a brain abscess develops from an infection in the sinuses. Signs and symptoms include:

- Severe headaches
- Nausea and vomiting
- Changes in personality or behavior
- Changes in speech
- Problems walking
- Increased movement in the arms or legs (spasticity)
- Seizures

INDICATIONS/CONTRAINDICATIONS for Therapeutic Massage

An infectious process is a contraindication to massage intervention unless appropriate medical personnel closely supervise the technique. A person with an unusual or unexplained stiff neck should be referred for diagnosis. A brain abscess can be life-threatening. Early detection is important. If you observe signs and symptoms, refer the client for diagnosis and care.

Review What You Have Learned

- Explain the influence of massage methods on CNS pathology.
  - With nerve damage, massage therapy is effective in managing compensation-related discomfort, as well as in helping to manage secondary muscle tension related to the use of equipment (e.g., wheelchairs and crutches). Massage may help manage bowel paralysis. Circulation enhancement produced by massage may assist in the management of decubitus ulcers. Massage helps manage headaches by addressing secondary muscle tension and by reducing stress. Because massage has been shown to increase neurotransmitter activity (specifically dopamine and serotonin), it is an effective treatment to help manage Parkinson disease, tremors, depression, and anxiety. Massage therapists should always use caution when working with clients using anticoagulants because of the increased potential for bruising. Infectious processes are a contraindication to massage unless medical personnel supervise the technique.
- Explain how certain drugs affect the CNS.
  - Stimulants (caffeine, nicotine, amphetamines, cocaine) promote the release of neurotransmitters such as norepinephrine, causing feelings of alertness and euphoria. Depressants (alcohol, narcotics, minor tranquilizers, barbiturates) act on the cerebral cortex by blocking norepinephrine and dopamine. Hallucinogens (LSD, PCP, mescaline, marijuana, ketamine) alter brain function by randomly stimulating and blocking neurotransmitters.

SUMMARY

Many of the physiological effects of therapeutic massage are caused by interactions with the functions of the CNS. Research has shown that applying massage effectively exerts beneficial influences on the CNS and the associated neurotransmitters and neuromodulators.

You must be competent in interpreting symptoms and behaviors related to the CNS so that you can determine the factors causing distressing symptoms. Clinical reasoning skills and problem-solving techniques allow the therapist to select the methods that will encourage the system's return to effective functioning or create a sense of relaxation and well-being. Knowledge of the CNS also is important because it enables massage professionals to practice safely and to recognize conditions that are contraindications to massage and refer those clients.

This chapter's focus has been on the components and functions of the CNS. Behavior and the nervous system are linked in the feedback loop pattern. Consciousness is a function of the CNS. Soft tissue and movement modalities are supportive, maintaining the health of the CNS. Pathological conditions of the CNS disrupt many types of body functions, and massage methods can provide support by helping the client to cope with many of these dysfunctions.

Visit the Evolve website: https://evolve.elsevier.com/Fritz/essential/

The Evolve website provides support for the review of the chapter content and chapter quizzes to help you prepare for the MBLEx or other massage therapy certification or licensing exams. End-of-chapter questions for discussion and review answer key and rationales and authors' response to critical thinking and clinical reasoning scenarios.

CRITICAL THINKING/CLINICAL REASONING

Each chapter will feature a critical thinking and clinical reasoning application of the content related to massage therapy practice. A client scenario will be presented with recommendations for additional research often using MedlinePlus or PubMed. Relevant questions based on the chapter content outline are provided to guide the discussion. There are no specific current answers to the questions. However, responses should be supportive of evidence-informed practices and based on biological plausibility if sufficient research is not available. The author's decision-making process related to the scenario and questions is on the EVOLVE site. Compare and contrast your thoughts and discussion to the authors' and determine where you agree or disagree.

Scenario

Ms. Ellen Fitch, age 32, was in a serious car accident 16 months ago. She experienced multiple injuries, many of which have affected her CNS functions. She had a skull fracture. She also developed an abscess from a secondary bacterial infection, which has resolved with antibiotic treatment. As a result of the trauma, Ms. Fitch has a closed head injury that affects her linear reasoning. She has difficulty processing any sort of sequence, such as following the steps of a recipe or the instructions for using an appliance. She has a lot of pain, including headache. Concern has arisen that she is developing a dependency on pain medication.

She also suffered a contusion injury of the spinal cord in the lumbar area. She is not fully paralyzed but has weakness in both legs, more so on the left. She can walk using a walker for support, and she is receiving physical therapy, making slow progress.

She is also depressed and experiencing posttraumatic stress symptoms that interfere with her sleep. Ms. Fitch is angry about the accident and obviously stressed. She is unable to work as a retail manager and wonders if she will ever be able to go back to work. Her family and the healthcare team believe that massage can help manage some of the symptoms and aid in her recovery.

You have been asked to analyze her condition and develop a reasonable massage care plan. To help you prepare a justifiable massage care plan, answer these questions:

- Explore
  - Medline Plus, using the search terms *brain abscess, closed head injury, traumatic brain injury, spinal cord injury, posttraumatic stress disorder*
- Discuss
  - To best understand the complexity of Ms. Fitch's current condition, what specific areas of the nervous system were damaged in the car accident?
  - What would be the role of the neuroglia related to the nerve injuries sustained during the car accident?
  - What are the conditions Ms. Fitch is currently dealing with that involve neurotransmitter function? Making an educated guess, which neurotransmitters would be most involved with depression and pain perception?
  - How might the traumatic brain injury complicate the physical therapy rehabilitation for the spinal cord injury and contribute to the posttraumatic stress disorder symptoms?
- Analyze the following suggestions for massage and relate them to the chapter content, as well as to the information in the three preceding chapters.

Massage application that targets pain management incorporates these principles:

1. A general full-body application using a rhythmic, slow approach is provided as often as feasible, at a duration of 45 to 60 minutes.
2. Pressure depth is moderate to deep, with a compressive, broad-based application. No poking, frictioning, or application of pain-causing methods is done.
3. The massage therapist is focused, attentive, and compassionate but maintains appropriate boundaries.

- Create a justifiable and reasonable massage care plan. Include these eight points:

1. Contraindications, cautions, and adaptations needed
2. Primary short-term outcome (4 weeks)
3. Secondary short-term outcome (4 weeks)
4. Primary long-term outcome (12 months)
5. Secondary long-term outcome (12 months)
6. Session frequency (how often) and duration (how long)
7. Massage approach used
8. Massage methods avoided

MULTIPLE CHOICE QUESTIONS FOR REVIEW AND DISCUSSION

The answers, with rationales, can be found on the Evolve site.

These questions are used for review and discussion. It is as important to understand why wrong answers are wrong as it is to know why the correct answer is correct. The answers to the questions, with rationales and explanations about why the correct answer is correct and why wrong answers are wrong, can be found on the Evolve site. Guidance is also provided on how questions are developed and how the textbook content can be presented in a multiple choice question format. At the end of the question section here in the textbook, you will find an Exercise that asks you to write more questions. Use the various questions in the chapter as examples. This is one of the best study strategies for test taking.

It is important to understand that the actual licensing exam you take may not contain any of the specific questions found in this textbook or the review material and practice tests on the Evolve site. Therefore just because you can answer any of these questions correctly does not mean you will pass the licensing exam. The questions are content and style examples to help you prepare—this is why understanding why wrong answers are wrong is just as important as identifying the correct answer. Also, make sure you understand all the terminology used in the questions and possible answers in the review and discussion questions. Look up words you do not understand.

1. The nervous system and the endocrine system coordinate control properties through the ______.
  a. Physiological outcomes
  b. Feedback loops

c. Linear pathways of affect
d. Adrenocortical axis

2. Sensory stimulation of massage causes a chemical change in neurons called ______.
   a. Action potential
   b. Refractory period
   c. Depolarization
   d. Saltatory conduction
3. Which phase of nerve signal conduction is related to methods of massage that use some sort of muscle contraction to prepare the muscle to lengthen?
   a. Action potential
   b. Refractory period
   c. Depolarization
   d. Saltatory conduction
4. A person is clumsy and has a dull or foggy mind in terms of understanding information and making decisions. Which neurotransmitter may be involved?
   a. Norepinephrine
   b. Histamine
   c. Glutamate
   d. Dopamine
5. Neurotransmitters work in excitatory and inhibitory pairs. Which neurotransmitter would provide a balancing action for enkephalin?
   a. Somatostatin
   b. Substance P
   c. Serotonin
   d. GABA
6. A massage client reports that after the massage, they experienced some itchy areas of skin and their clothes felt rough against their skin. Which neurotransmitter may be involved?
   a. Histamine
   b. Acetylcholine
   c. Epinephrine
   d. Cholecystokinin
7. A client reports before the massage that their mind is agitated and wants to scream. The client is talking loudly and pacing. After the massage, the client reports feeling calmer and wants a nap. Which neurotransmitter is largely responsible for the mood change?
   a. Norepinephrine
   b. Dopamine
   c. Serotonin
   d. Substance P
8. The purpose of therapeutic (feel good) pain during massage to manage undesirable pain is to stimulate which neurotransmitters?
   a. Serotonin and endorphin
   b. Epinephrine and histamine
   c. Acetylcholine and dopamine
   d. Histamine and substance P
9. States of higher consciousness are related to ______.
   a. Alertness with relaxation
   b. Decreased health states
   c. Increased sympathetic arousal
   d. Depression with pain
10. Why do the primary motor and the primary somesthetic sensory areas of the brain interfere with the ability to self-massage areas of the back and limbs successfully?
    a. The largest sensory and motor awareness is in these areas.
    b. The distribution of sensory and motor functions to the hands is too small to stimulate sensation.
    c. The distribution of sensory and motor function is larger to the hands than to the back and limbs.
    d. The back and limbs have a predominance of sensory distribution over the motor distribution of the hands.
11. Massage sensations travel on which spinal cord tracts?
    a. Sensory ascending tracts
    b. Motor descending tracts
    c. Corticospinal tracts
    d. Lateral reticulospinal tracts
12. In which pathological process would massage be most beneficial in assisting in the movement of body fluids?
    a. Upper motor neuron injury
    b. Lower motor neuron injury
    c. Aneurysm
    d. Chorea
13. Research indicates that massage increases the availability of the neurotransmitters norepinephrine, serotonin, and dopamine. Which CNS disorder would benefit most from massage?
    a. Stroke
    b. Cerebral palsy
    c. Depression
    d. Schizophrenia
14. A client has essential tremors. Which statement is most correct?
    a. Stress reduction massage would have a significant effect.
    b. Massage will have little effect.
    c. Massage with medication should reverse the condition.
    d. The associated headache is reduced by massage.
15. A client has a spinal cord injury that resulted in paralysis but can walk with difficulty. Which statement is correct?
    a. The client has monoplegia.
    b. The client has paraplegia.
    c. The client has quadriplegia.
    d. The client has ALS.
16. A client fell and hit their head. The client reports they were a bit confused at the time and the next day had a headache. Which term best describes the client's condition?
    a. An aneurysm
    b. A severe contusion
    c. A transient ischemic attack
    d. A mild concussion
17. A medication that would stimulate epinephrine could also result in ______.
    a. Enhanced sleep
    b. Weakening of skeletal muscles
    c. An increase in serotonin
    d. An increase in dopamine

18. Which of the following is most involved in pain mechanisms?
    a. Histamine
    b. Substance P
    c. Acetylcholine
    d. Cholecystokinin
19. A massage session that incorporates rocking affects the vestibular system, including the labyrinthine righting reflexes. Which brain area is also stimulated to coordinate appropriate posture?
    a. Cerebellum
    b. Pons
    c. Motor descending tracts
    d. Sensory ascending tracts
20. The protective membrane that adheres to the brain is the ______.
    a. Dura mater
    b. Arachnoid mater
    c. Epidural mater
    d. Pia mater

CHAPTER

5 Peripheral Nervous System

https://evolve.elsevier.com/Fritz/essential/

CHAPTER OBJECTIVES

After completing this chapter, the learner will be able to:

1. Describe the peripheral nervous system.
2. Relate the reflex mechanisms of the peripheral nervous system to massage application.
3. Explain the structure and function of the autonomic nervous system.
4. Describe the structure and function of the five basic senses: touch, hearing, vision, taste, and smell.
5. Describe pathological conditions of the peripheral nervous system and the related indications for and contraindications to massage.

CHAPTER OUTLINE

KEY TERMS

afferent: (AF-fer-ent) A term for sensory nerves that link sensory receptors to the central nervous system and transmit sensory information.

autonomic (visceral) nervous system (ANS): (aw-toe-NOM-ik) A division of the peripheral nervous system composed of nerves that connect the central nervous system to the glands, heart, and smooth muscles to maintain the internal body environment.

cranial nerves: Twelve pairs of nerves that originate from the olfactory bulbs, thalamus, visual cortex, and brainstem. They transmit information to and from the sensory organs of the face and the muscles of the face, neck, and upper shoulders, as well as organs of the thorax and abdomen.

dermatome: (DER-mah-tohm) A cutaneous (skin) section supplied by a single spinal nerve.

efferent: (EF-fer-ent) A term for motor nerves that transmit motor impulses; they link the central nervous system to the effectors outside it.

enteric nervous system (ENS): A subdivision of the peripheral nervous system that directly controls the gastrointestinal system.

free nerve endings: Sensory receptors that detect itch and tickle sensations.

kinesthesia: (kin-uhs-THEE-zhuh) Sense of movement of body parts.

mechanical receptors: Sensory receptors that detect changes in pressure, movement, temperature, or other mechanical forces.

mixed nerves: Nerves that contain sensory and motor axons.

myasthenia gravis: (my-uhs-THEE-nee-uh) A disease that usually affects muscles in the face, lips, tongue, neck, and throat but can affect any muscle group in the body.

myotome: (MY-o-tohm) A skeletal muscle or a group of skeletal muscles that receives motor axons from a particular spinal nerve.

nerve: A bundle of axons, dendrites, or both.

neurovascular bundle: A spinal nerve, artery, deep vein, and deep lymphatic vessel bound together by connective tissue, traveling the same pathway in the body.

nociceptors: (no-se-SEP-tors) Sensory receptors that detect painful or intense stimuli.

parasympathetic nervous system: The energy conservation and restorative system associated with what is commonly called the ***relaxation response***.

peripheral nervous system (PNS): (pe-RIF-er-al) The system of somatic and autonomic neurons outside the central nervous system. The peripheral nervous system comprises the afferent (sensory) division and the efferent (motor) division.

plexus: (PLEK-sus) A network of intertwining nerves that innervates a particular region of the body.
proprioceptors: (pro-pree-o-SEP-tors) Sensory receptors that provide the body with information about position, movement, muscle tension, joint activity, and equilibrium.
reflex: An automatic, involuntary reaction to a stimulus.
somatic nervous system: (so-MA-tik) A system of nerves that keeps the body in balance with its external environment by transmitting impulses to the central nervous system, skeletal muscles, and skin.
spinal nerves: Thirty-one pairs of mixed nerves that originate in the spinal cord and emerge from the vertebral column; they are part of the peripheral nervous system.
sympathetic nervous system: The part of the autonomic nervous system that provides for most of the active function of the body; when the body is under stress, the sympathetic nervous system predominates with fight-or-flight responses.
thermal receptors (thermoreceptors): Sensory receptors that detect changes in temperature.
vestibular system: (ves-TIB-u-lar) A collection of structures in the inner ear with both sensory and motor functions. The sensory function is responsible for monitoring motion, head position, and spatial orientation. Motor functions relate to balance, posture, normal movement, and equilibrium.

LEARNING HOW TO LEARN

You learn best when you are in a good mood and well rested. We can get into a bad mood when we are stressed, hungry, tired, sad, worried, or even bored. When we are in a good mood, we are calm, have energy, are alert, can focus, and have a sense of well-being. Steps we can take to support a good mood include eating a nutritious diet, getting natural light and moderate exercise each day, and sleeping well at night. Research suggests that sleep plays a key role in memory, both before and after we learn new information. Lack of adequate sleep affects mood, motivation, judgment, and our perception of events. Therefore to learn, sleeping throughout the night (8 hours) is important. Briefly reviewing material before going to sleep is also helpful. The brain takes that information and turns it into a memory.

Remember to study in chunks and give your brain a break. Move your body to rest the brain. Productive mindless activity is beneficial during these brain breaks. Fold laundry, water plants, go outside, or pick up trash while taking a short walk.

This chapter focuses on the anatomy and physiology of the **peripheral nervous system (PNS)**. In Chapter 4, we discussed the basic structural plan of the nervous system before specifically describing the neuron and the central nervous system (CNS). Remember that the nervous system is divided into the CNS, which is composed of the brain, spinal cord, and their coverings, and the PNS, which is made up of the cranial nerves, spinal nerves, and ganglia.

The PNS has two main subdivisions. The *somatic subdivision* monitors and controls bones, muscles, soft tissues, and skin. The *visceral* or *autonomic subdivision* is associated with the internal glands, organs, blood vessels, and mucous membranes.

Also remember that the **autonomic nervous system (ANS)** is divided into two or three subdivisions, depending on the source. This textbook describes the three parts of the ANS:

- The sympathetic aspect of the ANS, which activates arousal responses and expends body resources to respond to emergency situations or any physical activity. The sympathetic ANS is considered the flight-fight-fear system, but any highly emotional state, such as joy, excitement, or elation, is also sympathetic.
- The parasympathetic aspect of the ANS, which reverses the response of the sympathetic ANS by returning the body to a nonalarm state and restoring body resources. You can think of the functions as "rest and digest." The parasympathetic nervous system is associated with the relaxation response.
- The enteric nervous system, which directly controls the gastrointestinal (GI) system and interacts with the vagus nerve.

This chapter explores the PNS in more depth and further explains the importance of the effects of massage on systems of control.

BASICS OF THE PERIPHERAL NERVOUS SYSTEM

SECTION OBJECTIVES

Chapter objective covered in this section:

1. Describe the peripheral nervous system.

After completing this chapter, the learner will be able to:

- Describe the components of the PNS.
- List the cranial nerves and describe the general function of each.
- List the spinal nerves and describe their general function.
- Identify the four nerve plexuses.
- Compare and contrast dermatomes and myotomes.

The PNS is responsible for transmitting messages from the sense organs (e.g., nose, ears, and eyes) and sensory receptors in the soft tissue and bones to the CNS and then relaying messages from the CNS back to the organs, glands, skeletal muscles, and joints to maintain homeostasis and perform functions that help maintain life.

The PNS is composed of the motor nerves, sensory nerves, and ganglia outside the brain and spinal cord. The system consists of 12 pairs of cranial nerves and 31 pairs of spinal nerves, as well as their various branches in the body. Fibers that innervate the body wall are called *somatic fibers*. Those that supply the internal organs are called *visceral fibers*. The ANS consists of the peripheral nerves involved in regulating cardiovascular, respiratory, endocrine, and other unconscious body functions.

Nerves

A **nerve** is a bundle of axons, dendrites, or both. Recall from Chapter 4 that sensory (**afferent**) peripheral nerves transmit information to the CNS; motor (**efferent**) peripheral nerves carry impulses from the brain back to the body. A group of

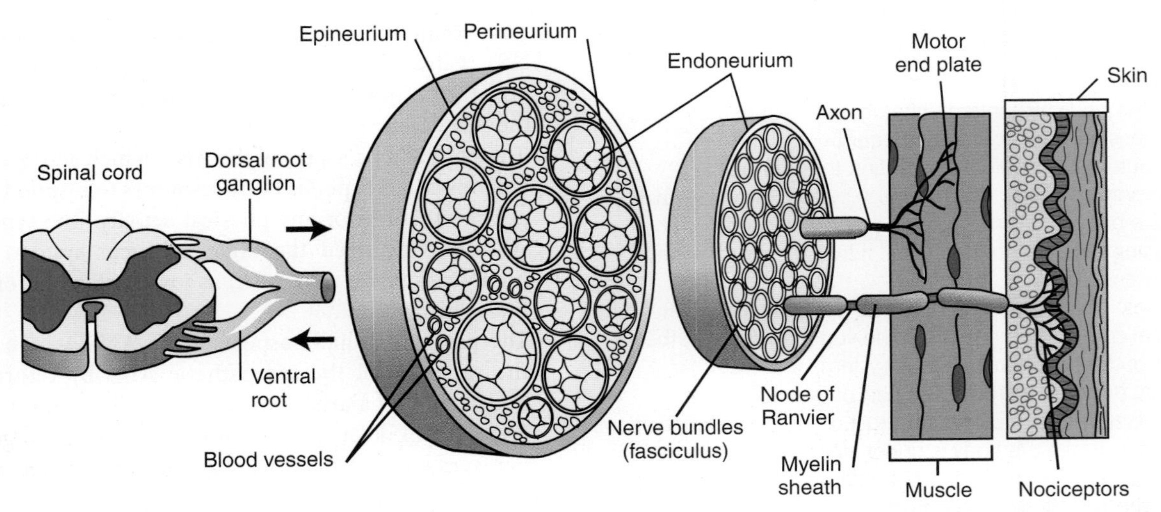

FIG. 5.1 Peripheral nerve trunk and coverings. (Modified from Thompson JM, McFarland GK, Hirsch JE, Tucker SM. *Mosby's Clinical Nursing*. 5th ed. Mosby; 2002.)

nerve fibers in a nerve is called a *fasciculus*. Nerves may be of the motor, sensory, or mixed type:

- Sensory nerves transmit input from sensory receptors that monitor the body's internal and external conditions to the CNS for further processing.
- Motor nerves innervate or provide action-carrying impulses from the brain or spinal cord to a muscle or gland.
- **Mixed nerves** contain sensory and motor fibers.

Connective tissues of the nerve (Fig. 5.1) include the following:

- *Epineurium:* Surrounds the entire nerve
- *Perineurium:* Surrounds each fasciculus
- *Endoneurium:* Surrounds and holds each nerve fiber

Practical Application

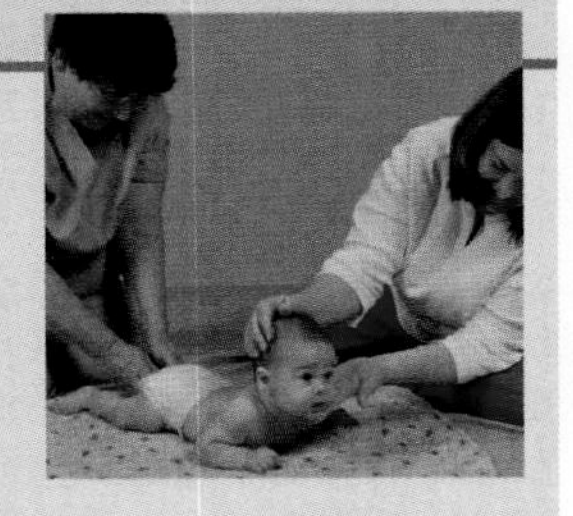

Stimulation of the peripheral nervous system (PNS) and the responses elicited by this stimulation constitute one of the main physiological ways massage and bodywork benefit the client. Therefore it is important that you thoroughly understand the anatomy and physiology of the PNS and the way soft tissue and movement methods interact with the PNS.

Cranial Nerves

Twelve pairs of **cranial nerves** enter (sensory) or leave (motor) the olfactory bulbs, thalamus, visual cortex, and brainstem. These nerves are identified by Roman numerals (according to their order from the anterior to the posterior brain) and by names (which refer to their function or distribution) (Fig. 5.2 and Table 5.1).

Disorders of the cranial nerves can result from a stroke, a tumor, or trauma. A lack of function may indicate damage to a particular nerve. The resulting change in action may help locate the lesion (area of damage). For example, the accessory nerve (cranial nerve XI) affects the trapezius and sternocleidomastoid muscles. Dysfunction in either of these muscles may indicate involvement of these nerves.

The Vagus Nerve

The vagus nerve deserves more discussion, because evidence indicates that massage affects vagal function (Lu et al., 2011; Field, 2018). The connections between the enteric nervous system and the CNS involve the vagus nerve. The vagus nerve is constantly sending updated sensory information about the state of the body's organs to the brain via afferent nerves. Vagus nerve communication between the gut and the brain involves neurotransmitters such as acetylcholine and gamma-aminobutyric acid (GABA). These neurotransmitters lower the heart rate, blood pressure, and other functions related to the parasympathetic division of the ANS.

Vagal tone is an internal biological process that represents the activity of the vagus nerve. Increasing vagal tone activates the parasympathetic nervous system. Other vagus nerve effects include:

- Reducing inflammation
- Regulating stress, anxiety, and fear
- Partly functioning with memory

Vagus nerve stimulation refers to any technique that stimulates the vagus nerve, including manual or electrical stimulation. The relationship between depression, inflammation, metabolic syndrome, and heart disease might be mediated by the vagus nerve (Howland, 2014; Broncel et al., 2020).

Polyvagal Theory

Polyvagal theory suggests that humans have evolved three techniques to survive:

- Freeze or play dead
- Fight or flight
- Social cues from the environment

The polyvagal theory describes the interactive and integrative functions of the nervous system in the evaluation of risk and

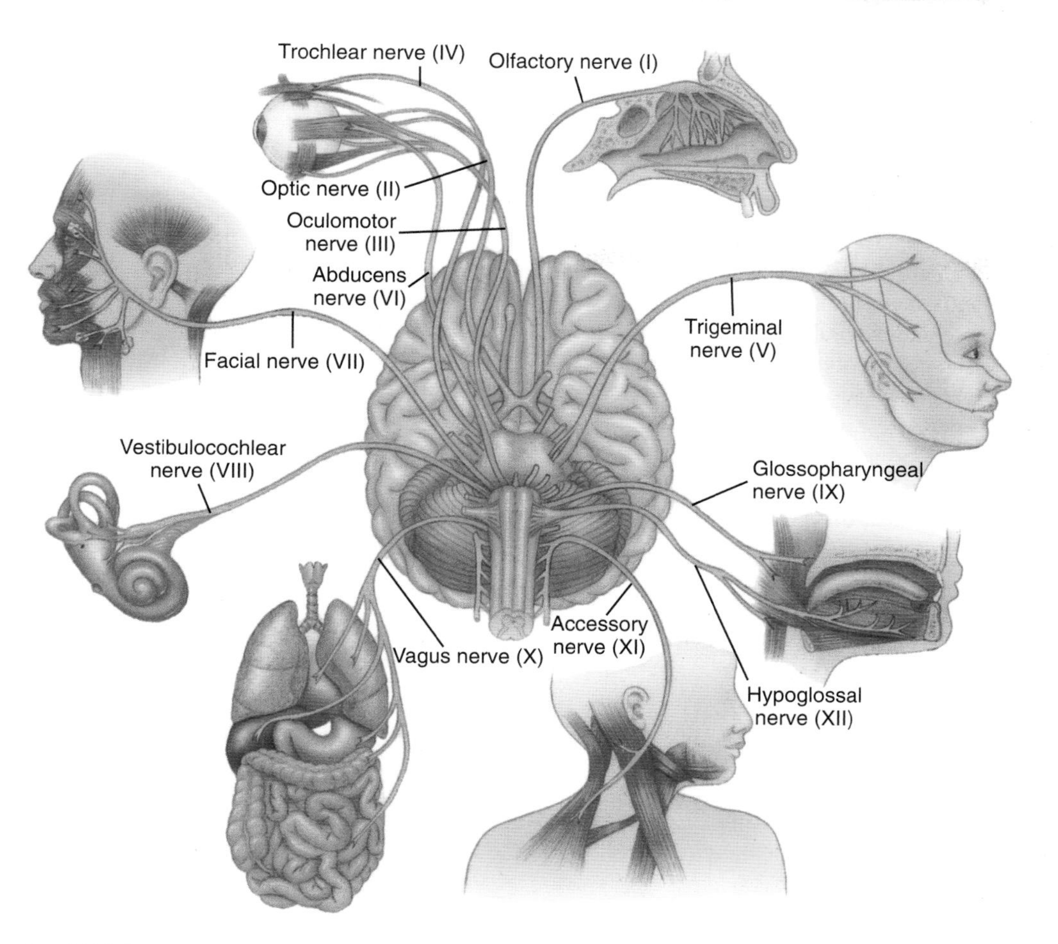

FIG. 5.2 Cranial nerves. The ventral surface of the brain shows the attachments of the cranial nerves. (From Patton KT, Thibodeau GA. *Anatomy and Physiology*. 7th ed. Mosby; 2010.)

Table 5.1 Cranial Nerves

Nerve	Description
I	The olfactory nerves are sensory and transmit information about taste and smell from the nasal cavity to the cerebrum (into the olfactory bulb of the forebrain).
II	The optic nerves are sensory and transmit information about clarity and field of vision from the retina to the midbrain of the cerebrum by way of the thalamus.
III	The oculomotor nerves are sensory and motor. The sensory portion transmits information about eye movement.
	The motor portion originates in the midbrain and controls all external eye muscles (except the superior oblique and lateral rectus muscles) and pupil contraction and relaxation.
IV	The trochlear nerves are composed mainly of motor nerves, which begin in the midbrain. They innervate the superior oblique eye muscles. The few sensory neurons provide proprioceptive information about eye movement.
V	The trigeminal nerves arise in the pons. The motor neurons innervate the muscles involved in chewing. The sensory neurons carry information about sensations and proprioception for the head, face, skin of the face, mucosal linings, eyelids, and tongue. The trigeminal nerves are the largest of the cranial nerves.
VI	The abducens nerves arise in the pons. The motor neurons innervate the lateral rectus eye muscle (an eye abductor). The sensory neurons provide proprioceptive information about eye movement.
VII	The facial nerves have motor fibers that arise in the pons and innervate the muscles that produce facial expression and the glands that release tears and saliva. The sensory fibers carry information about taste to the cerebral cortex. Some of the fibers also relay proprioceptive information about the face and scalp.
VIII	The vestibulocochlear nerves are sensory and are divided into two branches. The vestibular branch begins in the semicircular canals of the ear and carries signals for equilibrium to the pons, medulla, and cerebellum. The cochlear branch arises in the organ of Corti and carries impulses for hearing to the pons and medulla.
IX	The glossopharyngeal nerves contain sensory and motor neurons. The sensory fibers extend to the medulla from the pharynx and the tongue; they are concerned primarily with taste. Another sensory fiber extends from the carotid sinus in the internal carotid artery and aids in the control of respiration and blood pressure. The motor neurons arise in the medulla and affect saliva production, swallowing, and the gag reflex.
X	The vagus nerves contain sensory and motor neurons. The motor fibers originate in the medulla and carry signals that control the muscles involved in swallowing and speaking. Other motor fibers terminate in the muscles of the digestive and respiratory tracts and the heart. The sensory fibers arise from the same structures that the motor fibers innervate and carry information about sensations and proprioception of these organs.
XI	The accessory nerves arise in the medulla and are primarily motor neurons for speaking, turning the head, and moving the shoulders. The few sensory neurons relay proprioceptive information from these muscles.
XII	The hypoglossal nerves originate in the medulla and contain mostly motor neurons, which innervate the tongue and throat. A few sensory neurons carry proprioceptive information from the tongue.

safety (Porges, 2022). Feelings of safety and threat are subjective interpretations of the autonomic nervous system and interoception signaling to higher brain structures (Schwerdtfeger et al., 2022). The polyvagal theory is based on the evolutionary development of two systems: the parasympathetic nervous system connected to the vagus nerve and the sympathetic nervous system. The parasympathetic nervous system's vagus nerve regulation has two divisions affecting heart rate and general arousal, which moderate response to stressors. The vagus nerve consists of the ventral (front) and dorsal (back) aspects.

- The ventral (front) side of the vagus nerve responds to cues of safety and supports feelings of physical and emotional safety in a social environment.
- The dorsal (back) side of the vagus nerve responds to cues of danger. The primitive response is to freeze (Winter and Tyree, 2021).

Polyvagal theory suggests that social connectedness is a core biological function related to survival and the body's responses to stress. This theory considers how the vagus nerve—the longest nerve in the autonomic nervous system running from the brainstem to the colon—functions as a mind and body connection (Neuhuber and Berthoud, 2022). While the vagus nerve plays a role in transmitting emotion-related signals between the brain and the body, more evidence is needed to prove that it has any control over the body's fight, flight, and freeze responses.

Practical Application

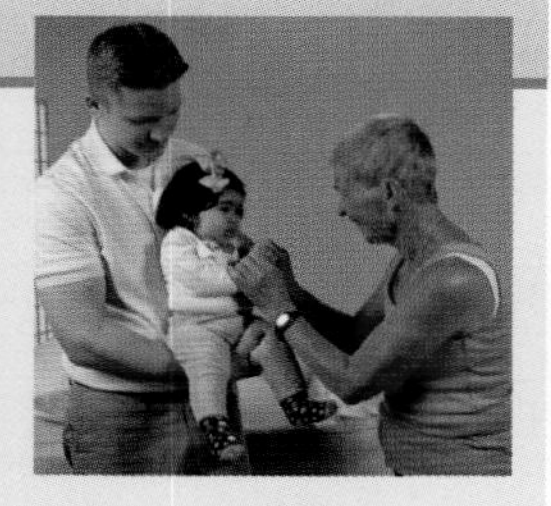

The distribution of the vagus nerve affects many visceral functions. Lower vagal tones are associated with anxiety. High vagal tones indicate that our bodies can quickly return to a calm state after a hyperarousal event. Our heart speeds up as we breathe in and slows down when we breathe out. The greater the difference between the inhalation heart rate and exhalation heart rate the higher your vagal tone. So slow your breathing when you exhale to remain calm. Massage has been shown to support vagus nerve function, especially in premature babies, resulting in better development (particularly in weight gain) and fewer developmental problems. The auricular branch of the vagus nerve supplies sensory innervation to the skin of the ear canal, tragus, and auricle. Massage of the ear may be an effective point of stimulation of the vagus nerve. Foundational to the massage therapy experience is creating an environment of safety as described in the polyvagal theory.

Spinal Nerves

Recall from Chapter 4 that 31 pairs of **spinal nerves** originate in the spinal cord and emerge from the vertebral column. All contain sensory and motor fibers in the same nerve (forming a mixed nerve), making sensation and movement possible. Each nerve attaches to the spinal cord through two short roots on each side, one in the front and one in the back. The anterior, or ventral, root is motor; the fibers originate in the ventral horn cells and innervate skeletal muscles. The posterior, or dorsal, root is sensory; the fibers originate in the sensory receptors and travel to the dorsal roots of the spinal cord. The dorsal root of each spinal nerve is recognized by a swelling, known as the *dorsal root ganglion*, which contains the cell bodies of the sensory neurons.

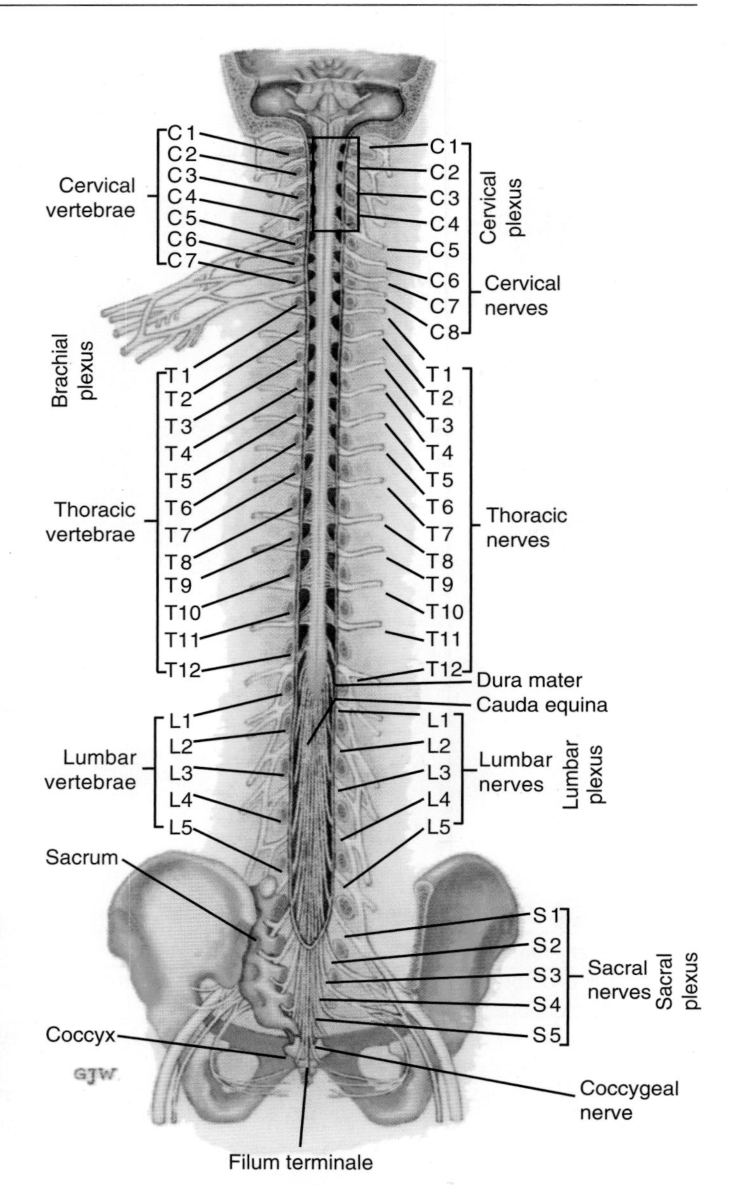

FIG. 5.3 Spinal nerves. Each of the 31 pairs of spinal nerves exits the spinal cavity from the intervertebral foramina. Notice that after leaving the spinal cavity, many of the spinal nerves interconnect to form networks, called *plexuses*. (From Vidic B, Suarez FR. *Photographic Atlas of the Human Body*. Mosby; 1984.)

Table 5.2 Spinal Nerves

Nerve	Location
Cervical (neck)	Eight pairs: C1–C8
Thoracic (chest)	Twelve pairs: T1–T12
Lumbar	Five pairs: L1–L5
Sacral	Five pairs: S1–S5 (These exit through the sacral foramina)
Coccygeal	One pair: Long thoracic nerve

C, Cervical; *L*, lumbar; *S*, sacral; *T*, thoracic.

Spinal nerves are identified by a letter and a number, which refer to their segment of attachment to the spinal cord (Fig. 5.3 and Table 5.2). After the spinal nerves exit the spinal cord, their nerve pathways follow the same pathway as the arteries and deep veins. Deep lymphatic vessels also follow this pathway. Often they are bound by connective tissues that are collectively called a neurovascular bundle.

Nerve Plexuses

Most of the spinal nerves, except those that emerge from the second to twelfth thoracic vertebral spaces, converge in small groups to form an intersecting network known as a *nerve plexus*. Each plexus contains fibers that innervate a specific region of the body. The overlap of nerve function prevents total loss of function if just one nerve in the group is damaged. The four major plexuses are the cervical, brachial, lumbar, and sacral plexuses. Thoracic nerves are the motor nerves to the intercostal muscles and sensory nerves from the skin of the thorax.

Cervical Plexus

The cervical plexus, formed from nerves C1 to C4 and part of C5, consists of sensory distribution from the head, front of the neck, and upper part of the shoulders, of motor impulses to many neck and shoulder muscles, and the diaphragm (Fig. 5.4).

Brachial Plexus

The brachial plexus, formed from nerves C5 to T1, is organized into three divisions: the superior, middle, and inferior trunks. These divisions supply the skin and muscles of the upper limbs (Fig. 5.5).

Thoracic nerves that are not part of the brachial plexus are the motor nerves to the intercostal muscles and sensory nerves from the skin of the thorax.

Lumbar Plexus

The lumbar plexus is composed of nerves L1 to L4. The lumbar and sacral nerves combine to form the lumbosacral plexus (Fig. 5.6).

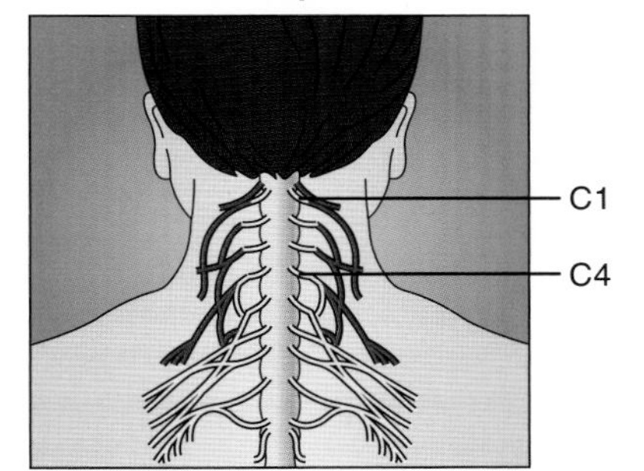

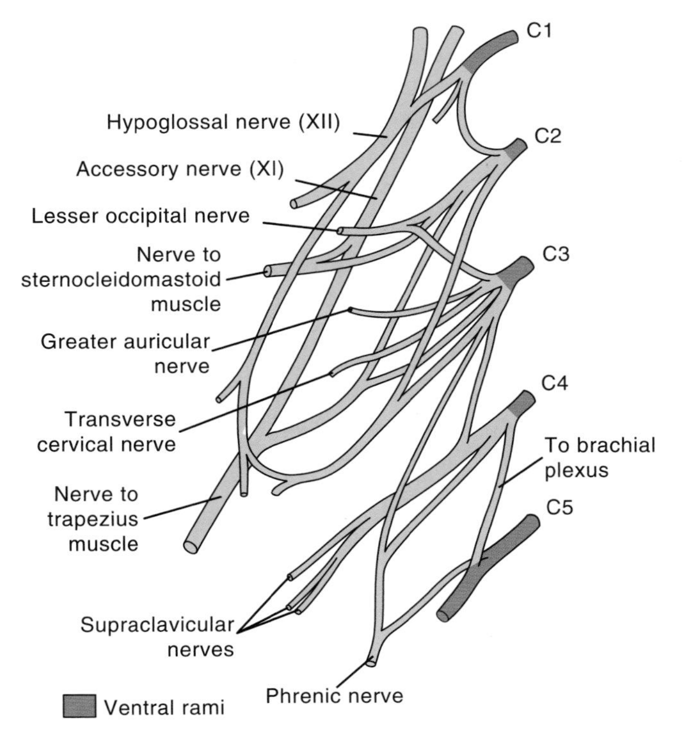

Nerve	Innervation
Ansa cervicalis	Hyoid muscles
Lesser occipital	Skin behind and above the ear
Greater auricular	Skin in front of, below, and over the ear and parotid glands
Transverse cervical	Skin on the anterior portion of the neck
Phrenic	Diaphragm
Supraclavicular	Skin on the shoulders and upper portion of the chest
Segmental branches	Deep neck muscles, midscalenes, and levator scapula muscle

FIG. 5.4 Cervical plexus. Ventral rami of the first four cervical spinal nerves (C1–C4) exchange fibers in this plexus found deep within the neck. Some fibers from C5 also enter this plexus to form a portion of the phrenic nerve. (From Patton KT, Thibodeau GA. *Anatomy and Physiology*. 7th ed. Mosby; 2010.)

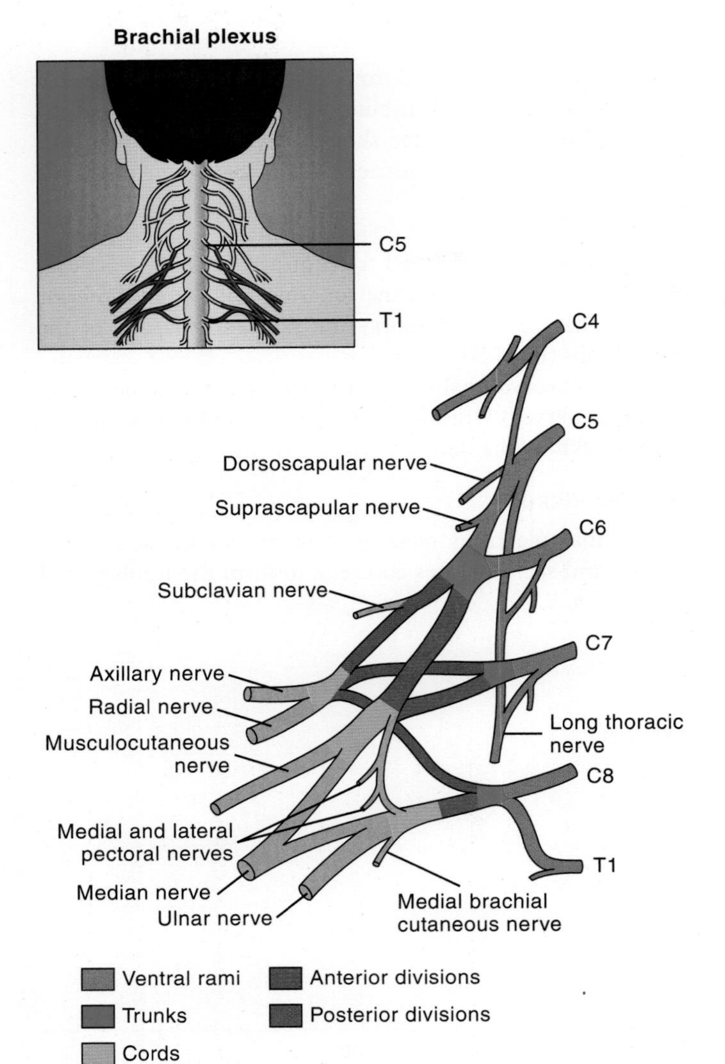

Nerve	Innervation
Dorsoscapular	Superficial muscles of the scapula
Long thoracic	Serratus anterior muscle
Subclavian	Subclavius muscle
Suprascapular	Infraspinatus and supraspinatus muscles
Musculocutaneous	Biceps, brachialis, and coracobrachialis muscles; skin
Subscapular	Subscapularis and teres major muscles
Median	Forearm flexors and palmar surface of the skin of the thumb, index, and middle fingers
Thoracodorsal	Latissimus dorsi muscle
Pectorals	Pectoralis major and minor muscles
Axillary	Deltoid and teres minor muscles and skin
Radial	Triceps and forearm extensors, skin of the forearm and hand, and dorsal surface of the thumb, index, and middle fingers
Medial cutaneous	Skin of the arm
Ulnar	Muscles of the hand and skin of the ring and pinkie fingers

FIG. 5.5 Brachial plexus. From the five rami, C5 to T1, the plexus forms three trunks. Each trunk subdivides into an anterior and a posterior division. The divisional branches reorganize into three cords, and the cords give rise to the individual nerves that exit this plexus. (From Patton KT, Thibodeau GA. *Anatomy and Physiology*. 7th ed. Mosby; 2010.)

Sacral Plexus

The sacral plexus is created from nerves L5 to S3.

Spinal Nerve Injury

Injury to a nerve can stop the transmission of signals to and from the brain, preventing muscles from working and causing loss of feeling in the area supplied by that nerve. Nerves are fragile and can be damaged by pressure, stretching, or cutting. Pressure or stretching injuries can cause the fibers carrying the information to break and can interfere with the nerve function without disrupting the insulating cover. When a nerve is cut, both the nerve and the myelin sheath are damaged.

When nerve fibers are separated during injury, the distal end of the fiber (farthest from the brain) dies. The proximal end (closest to the brain), which contains the cell body of the fiber, does not die, and after some time it may begin to heal. If the myelin sheath is not cut, the nerve fibers may grow down the empty tubes until they reach a muscle or a sensory receptor.

If both the nerve and sheath have been cut, the growing nerve fibers may grow into a ball at the end of the cut, forming a nerve scar called a *neuroma*, which is painful and can cause an electrical feeling when touched.

Injury to the sensory portion of any spinal nerve causes loss of sensation or altered sensation in the innervated area:

- Hyperesthesia (excessive sensation)
- Hypoesthesia (decreased sensation)
- Paresthesia (numbness, tingling, burning sensation)
- Anesthesia (loss of sensation)

Injury to the motor nerves impairs movement or function and results in:

- Impaired movement
- Various forms of paralysis of the muscles due to the damaged nerve
- Gradual weakening and, ultimately, wasting of the muscle
- Uncontrollable twitching (*fasciculations*)

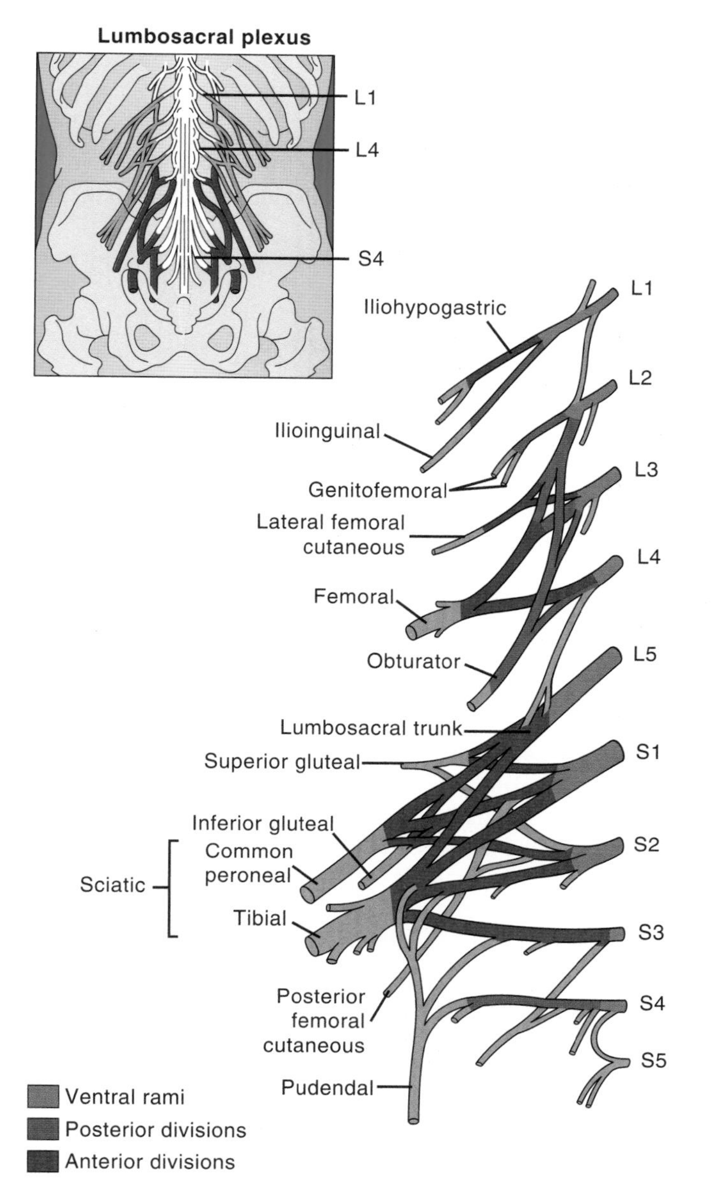

Nerve	Innervation
Iliohypogastric	Abdominal muscles and skin of the abdomen and buttocks
Ilioinguinal	Abdominal muscles and skin of the external genitalia
Genitofemoral	Skin of the external genitalia and inguinal region
Lateral femoral	Skin of the thigh (except the medial cutaneous portion)
Femoral	Hip flexors and extensors and skin of the medial and anterior thigh and medial leg and foot
Obturator	Adductor muscles and skin of the medial thigh
Sacral plexus	Created from nerves L5 to S3
Sciatic	Leg and foot muscles; the skin of the foot, which divides into the tibial and peroneal nerves at the popliteal fossa
Gluteal	Buttocks and tensor fasciae latae muscle
Nerves to hip	Piriformis, quadratus femoris, rotators, obturator internus, and superior and inferior gemellus
Posterior femoral	Skin of the buttocks, perineum, back, cutaneous of the thigh, and leg
Pudendal	Muscles and skin of the perineum (may be considered in the coccygeal plexus)

FIG. 5.6 Lumbosacral plexus. The lumbosacral plexus is formed by the combination of the lumbar and the sacral plexuses, as shown in the *inset*. The ventral rami split into anterior and posterior divisions before reorganizing into the individual nerves that exit this plexus. (From Patton KT, Thibodeau GA. *Anatomy and Physiology*. 7th ed. Mosby; 2010.)

When upper motor neurons are damaged, the results include spasticity or stiffness of limb muscles, overactivity of tendon reflexes (e.g., knee and ankle jerks), and loss of the ability to perform fine movements. When the lower motor neurons are damaged, the result is muscle weakness, twitching, loss of muscle tone, flaccid paralysis, diminished or absent reflexes, and progressive muscle atrophy (Activity 5.1).

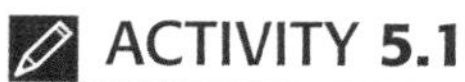

ACTIVITY **5.1**

What could happen if each of the following nerves was damaged?
Phrenic nerve
Thoracodorsal nerve
Radial nerve
Lateral femoral cutaneous nerve
Posterior femoral cutaneous nerve

Myotomes and Dermatomes

Dermatomes

The term *dermatome* indicates the relationship between the spinal nerve and the skin. A **dermatome** is a section of skin supplied by a single spinal nerve. Dermatomes are identified by the number of the nerve. Although Fig. 5.7 shows a clear boundary for each cutaneous segment, the nerve supplies in adjoining dermatomal segments overlap. Knowledge of the dermatome pattern enables a clinician to locate injuries in the spinal cord and spinal nerves.

Myotomes

The term *myotome* indicates the relationship between the spinal nerve and the muscles innervated by it. A skeletal muscle or group of muscles that receives motor axons from a single spinal nerve is known as a **myotome**. As with dermatomes, the

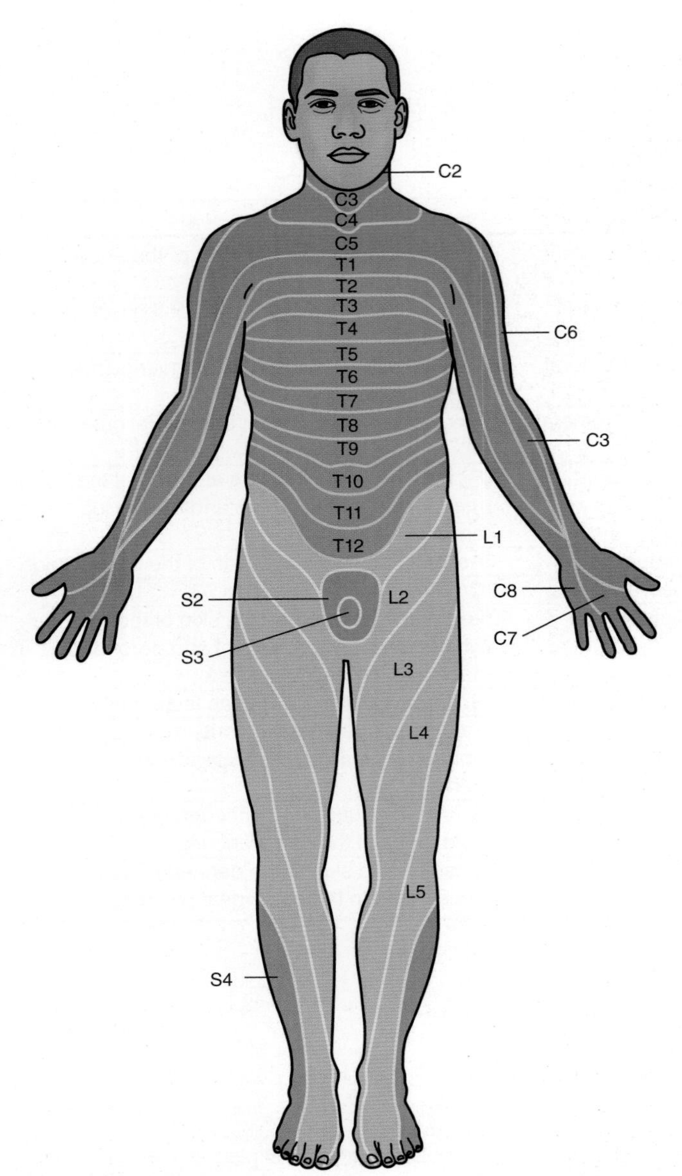

FIG. 5.7 Dermatomal map (*anterior view*) (also see Fig. 2.13). Myotome map.

boundaries of myotomes are not always exact; some muscle groups may be innervated by motor axons from more than one spinal nerve.

Myotomes consist of those of the upper limb nerve roots and those of the lower limb nerve roots. The upper limb nerve roots and their functions are as follows:

- C2—Neck flexion
- C3—Neck side flexion
- C4—Shoulder elevation
- C5—Deltoid muscle (abduction of the arm in the shoulder joint)
- C6—Biceps (flexion of the arm in the elbow joint)
- C7—Triceps (extension of the arm in the elbow joint)
- C8—Small muscles of the hand
- T1—Finger abduction (ulnar nerve)
- T1—Abductor pollicis brevis (median nerve)

The lower limb nerve roots and their functions are as follows:

- L2—Hip flexion
- L3 and L4—Knee extension
- L4—Quadriceps (extension of the leg in the knee joint)
- L5—Tibialis anterior (upward flexion of the foot in the ankle joint)
- S1—Gastrocnemius muscle (downward flexion of the foot in the ankle joint)

Review What You Have Learned

- Describe the components of the PNS.
  - The PNS is composed of motor nerves, sensory nerves, and ganglia outside the CNS. The PNS consists of 12 cranial nerve pairs, 31 spinal nerve pairs, and their branches. Somatic fibers innervate the body wall. Visceral fibers innervate internal organs. The subdivisions of the PNS are the somatic nervous system (function—bones, muscles, soft tissues, skin) and the ANS (function—organs, glands, membranes, blood vessels). Subdivisions of the ANS are the sympathetic nervous system (fight or flight), the parasympathetic nervous system (rest and restore), and the enteric nervous system (digest).
- List the cranial nerves and describe their general function.
  - See Fig. 5.2 and Table 5.1.
- List the spinal nerves and describe their general function.
  - See Fig. 5.3 and Table 5.2.
- Identify the four nerve plexuses.
  - Cervical plexus (C1 to C4/C5), brachial plexus (C5 to T1), lumbar plexus (L1 to L4), and sacral plexus (L5 to S3). Also see Figs. 5.4–5.6.
- Compare and contrast dermatomes and myotomes.
  - A dermatome is a section of skin innervated by a single spinal nerve. A myotome is a skeletal muscle or muscle group innervated by a single spinal nerve (see Fig. 5.7).

REFLEX MECHANISMS

SECTION OBJECTIVES

Chapter objective covered in this section:

2. Relate the reflex mechanisms of the peripheral nervous system to massage application.

After completing this section, the learner will be able to:

- Define a *nerve reflex*.
- List the sensory receptors involved in reflex action.
- Define a *reflex arc*.
- Explain muscle tone.
- Explain fascial tone.

A **reflex** is a biological control system that occurs as a response to a stimulus to return the body to homeostasis. A reflex arc is the mechanism by which the stimulus is linked to the response. A nerve reflex usually is an involuntary action: the message caused by the stimulus is sent, the brain and spinal cord sense the sensory stimulus, and they send a signal (action potential) to an effector organ (muscle) to create an immediate action to counter the stimulus.

Involuntary reflexes involve receptors, neurons, interneurons, and the spinal cord. Conditioned learned reflexes also involve the brain. Almost every reflex is polysynaptic, meaning that internal reflex signals cross many synapses.

Types of Reflexes

The two types of reflexes are a simple (unconditioned or natural) reflex and a complex (conditioned) reflex.

Simple (Unconditioned or Natural) Reflex

With a simple (unconditioned) reflex, the brain is not involved. When the receptor is stimulated, the stimulus is conducted to the spinal cord by the effector. The effector neuron from the spinal cord conducts a response to the muscle or gland. This causes an immediate reaction. It does not involve any thinking or reasoning. It is a natural response that occurs even in newborns (e.g., blinking when bright light falls on the eyes).

Complex (Conditioned) Reflex

A complex reflex involves the brain, but it occurs just as fast as a simple reflex. Salivation on smelling a favorite food is an example of a conditioned reflex. The individual recognizes the smell and based on a previous experience, the response (salivation) occurs. Recognition of the previous experience involves the associative centers of the brain.

Several experiments were conducted by Ivan Pavlov, a Russian biologist, which demonstrated the conditioned reflex. He found that when a bell was rung every time a dog was given food, the dog showed salivation only at the sound of the bell. The ringing of the bell is called the *conditioned stimulus*. The dog had learned to associate the sound of the bell with food, and this made it salivate at the sound of the bell.

Reflexes have a fast response time and allow the body to prevent injury by withdrawing or changing position to compensate for the additional stress. Some of these reflexes persist even when injury or disease affects the spinal cord.

Because of the "wiring" of the body, a simple activity that stimulates a few receptors can involve many neurons going to and from muscles and glands. A brief action, such as bumping the funny bone (the ulnar nerve), requires many neurons. Some conduct signals to and from the spinal cord to prompt withdrawal of the arm; others carry signals to and from the brain, letting us know when to yell "Ow!"

Reflex Patterns

Somatosomatic reflexes involve the stimulation of sensory receptors in the skin, subcutaneous tissue, fascia, striated muscle, tendons, ligaments, or joints, producing a reflex response in segmentally related somatic structures (e.g., from one such site on the body to another segmentally related site on the body, such as the knee jerk that occurs when the patellar tendon is tapped). Massage therapy and hydrotherapy commonly evoke such reflexes.

Somatovisceral reflexes occur where a localized somatic stimulation (from cutaneous, subcutaneous, or musculoskeletal sites) produces a reflex response in a segmentally related visceral structure (internal organ or gland). The vasoconstriction that results from the cooling of the skin is an example. Massage and hydrotherapy commonly affect these reflexes.

Viscerosomatic reflexes occur when a localized visceral (internal organ or gland) stimulus produces a reflex response in a segmentally related somatic structure (cutaneous, subcutaneous, or musculoskeletal). Viscerosomatic reflexes occur when organ dysfunction produces superficial effects involving the skin (including pain and tenderness). Examples include right shoulder pain in gallbladder disease and the typical angina distribution of left arm and thoracic pain produced by cardiac ischemia.

Viscerovisceral reflexes occur when a stimulus in an internal organ or gland produces a reflex response in another segmentally related internal organ or gland, such as the changes in heart rate and blood pressure that relate to baroreceptor stimulation.

Sensory Receptors of the Somatic Nervous System

The **somatic nervous system**, a division of the PNS, primarily affects the skin, muscles, joints, and bones. Our bodies contain many types of receptors located in various areas. Receptors that detect information from outside the body are called *exteroceptors* and are stimulated by actions or changes in our external environment. Two examples are our eyes and ears. Changes in our internal environment stimulate the visceroceptors or interoceptors. These receptors receive signals for monitoring factors such as blood pressure and hunger. Specific to the somatic aspect of the PNS are specialized receptors. In and around the muscles and joints of our body are the proprioceptors, which are affected by changes in position, movement, and tension (Fig. 5.8).

Receptor Adaptation

Most of the time we are not aware of the subtle changes that stimulate sensory receptors or of the adaptations that result from these changes. These natural reflexes, processed in the brainstem or portions of the spinal cord, affect not only our physical response but also the behavior that may result. We can train ourselves to be aware of the stimuli and purposefully adapt our responses; this is another example of a *conditioned reflex*. These learned behaviors are present in our daily actions (e.g., tying our shoes) and are also highlighted in forms of sports training and conditioning. We can learn to shoot a basketball, throw a baseball, or swing a golf club. After the basic skills have been mastered, we do not have to think about most of the actions; these are conditioned reflexive patterns. Personal habits, such as nail biting or eating while watching television, also are conditioned reflexive patterns, and these habits may be hard to break after they become reflexive.

When an appropriate stimulus stimulates a sensory receptor, the receptor sends an impulse to the CNS, where the information is processed. Sensory receptors adapt by becoming less sensitive to a stimulus, and they reduce the number of signals sent, or stop altogether, even if the stimulus is still present. If this did not happen, we would never get used to things (e.g., clothing) because the nervous system constantly

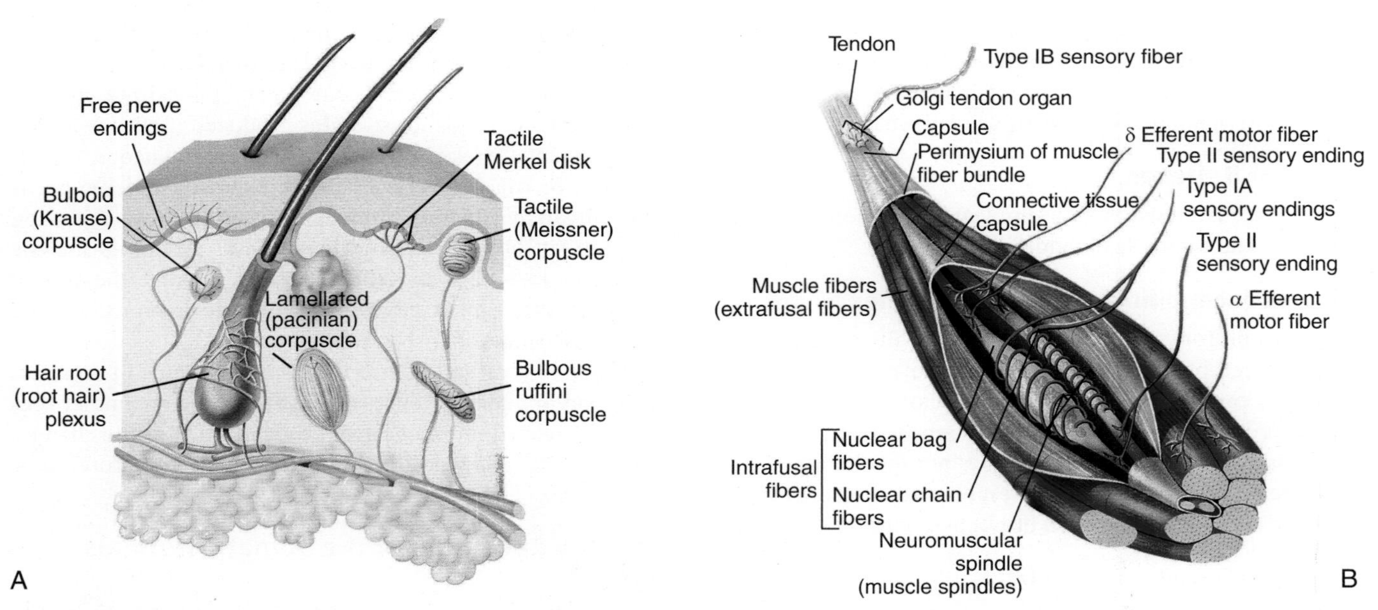

FIG. 5.8 Somatic sensory receptors: (A) exteroceptors and (B) proprioceptors. (Modified from Thibodeau GA, Patton KT. *Anatomy and Physiology*. 6th ed. Mosby; 2007.)

would be aware of the sensations and would be unable to sort through what is important to respond to and what is not. Some forms of minimal brain damage or learning difficulties that involve difficulty focusing or attending to sensory input seem to be perpetuated by a reduced ability for sensory adaptation.

Some of the receptors, especially those associated with pressure and touch, adapt quickly; such receptors play a major role in signaling changes in a particular sensation. Other receptors, such as those that detect tissue harm and body position, adapt slowly and signal information about steady states of the body.

Each sensory receptor is specialized to convert one form of stimulus into action potentials in the sensory nerves. The sensory cortex is activated by the impulse. Changes in the frequency of transmission of action potentials and the number of receptors stimulated determine the intensity of sensation.

Numerous sensory structures are classified as **mechanical receptors**:

- *Mechanoreceptors:* These structures detect changes in pressure, movement, temperature, or other mechanical forces.
- *Lamellar (pacinian) corpuscles:* This type of corpuscle senses brief touch, pressure, and high-frequency vibrations. Located in the submucosal, subcutaneous, and connective tissue of the hands, feet, genitals, joints, and other structures, lamellated corpuscles respond to most forms of rapidly changing mechanical stimulation.
- *Tactile (Meissner) corpuscles:* These corpuscles are touch receptors found in the hairless portions of the skin, mainly on the palms, fingertips, and soles of the feet, and on the eyelids, lips, tongue, and genitals. The corpuscles can identify the exact location and quality of touch (known as *discriminative touch*), the initial onset of touch, and low-frequency vibration. Tactile corpuscles adapt quickly.
- *C-tactile (CT) afferents:* These unmyelinated low-threshold mechanoreceptors are present in the skin of humans and are thought to convey positive and pleasant aspects of touch, due to their optimal firing during gentle, caress-like contact.
- *Hair root (root hair) plexuses:* This type of plexus is a network of dendrites that surrounds hair follicles. Subtle hair movements, such as those caused by light touch or a soft breeze, stimulate hair root plexuses. They respond and adapt quickly.
- *Bulbous (Ruffini) corpuscles:* These structures are touch and pressure receptors located in the deeper areas of hairy portions of our skin and our joints. These spindle-shaped receptors are sensitive to skin stretch. They recognize heavy and continuous touch, pressure, steady position, and direction of movement.
- *Bulboid (Krause) corpuscles*: These mechanoreceptors are located primarily in mucous membranes. They sense texture, low-frequency vibration, and touch.
- *Tactile (Merkel) disks:* These disks are a type of mechanoreceptor that can be found in hairless portions of the skin. They function in discriminative touch.
- *Free nerve endings:* Some free nerve endings detect temperature and are known as **thermal receptors (thermoreceptors)**. One type detects warmth, and another type senses the lack of warmth, or coolness. The brain compares this information to help identify what we would perceive as hot, warm, cool, or cold. The dorsal side of the hand has many thermal receptors, is suited ideally for identifying temperature, and is used commonly by caregivers to check a child for fever. A clinician can use the dorsal side of the hand to assess for warm areas on the body. Other **free nerve endings** detect potential and actual harm, itch, and tickle sensations.
- *Nociceptors:* **Nociceptors** are specific free nerve endings that detect potential and actual harm, and damage-based

stimuli. Often the perception is a pain sensation. Overstimulation of any receptor can signal pain as a protective response.

- *Proprioceptors:* Mechanical receptors that provide us with information about body position and movement are called **proprioceptors**.

Kinesthesia is the sense of movement of body parts, including the ability to feel movements of the limbs and body and the sensation of moving in space.

Proprioception is the sense of the position of body parts. Proprioceptors monitor and provide feedback about the position and movement of the body.

Proprioception and kinesthesia are often used interchangeably, but they are slightly different. Kinesthesia is more about movement and proprioception is more about position.

We maintain posture balance and movement using the input from muscle tension, joint position, and the relative movement of each of our limbs and the movement of the whole body.

Because proprioceptors adapt slowly to sensations, they tend to signal the CNS over longer periods. The motor control centers in the brain receive these signals and coordinate normal muscle actions and patterns of movement.

- Proprioception is our "body sense."
- It enables us to unconsciously monitor the position of our body.
- It depends on receptors in the muscles, tendons, and joints. The proprioceptors are as follows:
- *Muscle spindles* (neuromuscular spindles): Muscle spindles are located primarily in the belly of the muscle. They are stretch receptors that monitor and respond to sudden and excessive lengthening. These same fibers send signals via the spinal cord to inhibit actions in the antagonist muscle (the muscle that creates the opposite movement of an action).
- *Golgi tendon organs*: These fibers, which are found in the tendons and musculotendinous junctions, respond to increases in tension. The signals they send out produce a slight stimulation to the antagonist muscle, which prevents return responses from reaching the signaling muscle, causing it to not shorten.
- *Joint kinesthetic receptors*: The ligaments have receptors that respond to excessive strain or tension applied to a joint. They initiate a signal that results in the inhibition of the adjacent muscle or muscles.

When proprioceptors are stimulated, the somatic reflex arcs process and interpret the signal as a spinal reflex (Activity 5.2). A feedback loop works to protect the muscles and joints from injury. If the demand on either could cause injury, the result often is pain, weakness, or muscle inhibition.

Reflex Arc

As mentioned, a reflex arc describes the pathway of a reflex. The nerve impulse travels from the receptor through sensory neurons to the spinal cord (or brain), then back through motor neurons to an effector. Associative neurons between the sensory and motor neurons help connect the signal pathway for its most efficient routing. The effector is a muscle that contracts or a gland that secretes. A somatic reflex involves skeletal muscle contraction or relaxation, and an autonomic or visceral reflex results in glandular secretion or contraction of a smooth or cardiac muscle.

The somatic reflexes most often stimulated by massage are the *stretch reflex, tendon reflex, flexor reflex*, and *crossed extensor reflex*. These are discussed later in the chapter.

The simplest form of reflex results from a *monosynaptic* (one synapse) and the *ipsilateral* (one-sided) reflex arc. The

Practical Application

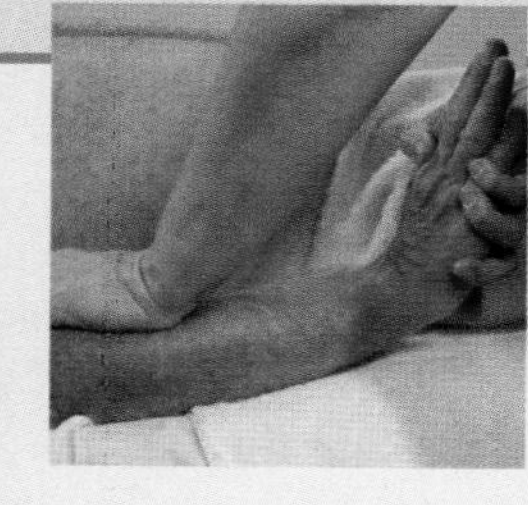

Massage introduces stimulation through touch, pressure, vibration, and movement, causing sensory receptors to respond. Input from the sensory systems plays a role in controlling motor functions by stimulating spinal reflex mechanisms. Sensory receptors code four aspects of a stimulus:

- Modality (or type)
- Intensity
- Location
- Duration

Almost all forms of bodywork use some aspect of touch that stimulates the various touch receptors found in the skin. Methods that use light touch stimulate root hair plexuses, free nerve endings, tactile disks, tactile corpuscles, and bulbous corpuscles. Techniques such as compression; deep, gliding strokes; and joint movement stimulate the pressure receptors, such as the lamellar corpuscles. The rapid, repetitive sensory signals of vibration and percussion techniques directly influence the lamellar corpuscles. Movement affects all the proprioceptors. Remarkably, specialized receptors have evolved to transmit sensory inputs from each of these sensory systems.

ACTIVITY 5.2

Depending on the modality being studied, successful soft tissue and movement treatments in some way stimulate many, if not all, of the various sensory receptors. For each given receptor, identify a technique and explain the way it stimulates the receptor. An example is given to get you started.

Example

Lamellar (pacinian) corpuscles

Answer: Use of a mechanical vibrator to stimulate high-frequency vibrations

Your Turn

Tactile (Meissner) corpuscles

Hair root plexuses

Bulbous (Ruffini) corpuscles

Tactile (Merkel) disks

Thermal receptors

Nociceptors or free nerve endings

Muscle spindles

Golgi tendon organs

Joint kinesthetic receptors

reflex begins with the stimulation of a receptor, which sends out a nerve impulse through an afferent (sensory) neuron. The signal travels to the brain or spinal cord and synapses with an efferent (motor) neuron.

The only true monosynaptic reflex is a deep tendon reflex, which involves just sensory and motor neurons. Deep tendon reflexes are important because they can be used to evaluate the sensory nerve, a portion of the spinal cord, the motor nerve, and the muscle or muscles supplied by the nerve. To evaluate the reflex, a physician or trained medical professional uses a device to tap the tendon, which stimulates the receptor in the tendon. The impulse travels along the sensory nerve to the spinal cord, where it synapses with motor neurons and continues along the motor axon, signaling the muscle to contract. A defect at any point in this arc interferes with the reflex contraction of the muscle.

The important deep tendon reflexes are as follows:

- The biceps and triceps reflexes, which help in the evaluation of spinal cord levels C5 and C6, the brachial plexus, and the biceps and triceps muscles.
- The patellar reflex (the knee-jerk reflex), which helps evaluate spinal cord level L4, the lumbar plexus, the femoral nerve, and the quadriceps muscle.
- The Achilles tendon reflex (the ankle-jerk reflex), which helps evaluate spinal cord level S1, the sacral plexus, and the gastrocnemius and soleus muscles. The result of such an evaluation would be abnormal if, for example, low back pain that radiated to the leg and foot accompanied the stimulus (tendon tapping)—this could indicate a problem at the level of L5 to S1.

Stretch Reflex

The stretch reflex is a protective contraction that results when a muscle is stretched suddenly or intensely. Not to be confused with the action of slow stretching or lengthening, the stretch reflex is a homeostatic mechanism that prevents muscle trauma in response to a stretch. The muscle spindles initiate a nerve impulse that travels to the posterior root of the spinal nerve and into the spinal cord. A nerve impulse then travels back to the same muscle. The impulse reaches the muscle, generating the action potential and causing the muscle to contract. This contraction prevents the muscle spindle from initiating any more nerve impulses. The stretch reflex itself is monosynaptic (one synapse). However, the response becomes a polysynaptic (many synapses) reflex arc. Associative neurons in the spinal cord cause synergist muscles to contract and relay impulses. Other associative neurons interrupt the signal to the antagonist muscles or muscle, allowing it to lengthen.

Reciprocal innervation prevents injury and creates coordinated actions by allowing the signal for contraction of one muscle while inhibiting the signal to its opposing muscle. This is why an antagonist can lengthen when an agonist contracts, and vice versa. Because muscles operate in groups, this stretch reflex coordinates the various contractions and lengthening and the stabilization and balance we need to move effectively.

Tendon Reflex

Also known as the *inverse stretch reflex*, the tendon reflex is a feedback mechanism that controls muscle tension by allowing for muscle lengthening. Golgi tendon organs detect and respond to changes in muscle tension. As the tension increases, often because of an increase in muscle contraction, these sensors initiate a signal that follows the sensory neuron to the spinal cord. Associative neurons inhibit any signal from returning to the same muscle, whereas other neurons continue allowing a signal to reach the antagonist by way of the motor neurons. This causes a slight contraction in the antagonist, which allows the prime mover to lengthen because no impulse is available to generate the action potential.

In some medical texts, the term *tendon reflex* is used to describe a reflex action initiated by tapping a tendon rather than by stretching the muscle belly (which may be called a *muscle reflex* even if the result is the same for both). Keep in mind that such references describe the stimulus and not the resulting reflex action.

The stretch reflex and tendon reflex are simple examples of the way our bodies are programmed to maintain homeostasis. In our normal actions, these reflexes are usually activated for full-body responses instead of isolated muscle groups. The flexor (withdrawal) reflex and the crossed extensor reflex are polysynaptic reflex arcs that work with larger areas and the whole body.

Flexor Reflex

The flexor reflex begins with stimulation of the sensory receptor, often by something painful (e.g., stepping on a pin) or contact with a noxious stimulus (e.g., a hot flame). The signal travels to the spinal cord, crosses associative neurons (as in the tendon reflex), and returns to the muscle involved. This muscle contracts to withdraw; simultaneously, signals have been sent to other muscles on the same limb to do likewise. For example, if you step on a pin with your left foot, your left anterior tibialis muscle, quadriceps (rectus femoris), and psoas contract. The antagonist muscles, including the gastrocnemius, soleus, hamstrings, and gluteus maximus, are inhibited from acting (remember how the associative neurons can block signals), thus allowing the entire leg to remove itself from the stimulus. The withdrawal reflexes are powerful, taking precedence over all other concurrent reflex actions.

Crossed Extensor Reflex

The crossed extensor reflex works in coordination with the flexor reflex. When the initial signal reaches the spinal cord, it not only travels to the flexor muscles on the same side of the body to allow the limb to withdraw but also crosses the spinal cord and travels to the extensor muscles to maintain balance. This action starts the contraction of the right gastrocnemius, soleus, hamstrings, and gluteus maximus while inhibiting the action of the right anterior tibialis, quadriceps, and psoas. The muscles of the torso and arms also can be stimulated or inhibited through this reflex for complete balance if needed.

This reflex action explains why a tension pattern in one part of our body can be seen in other areas. The extensive pathways that the signals follow are called *contralateral reflex arcs*. The initial stimulus given in the previous example was burn-related tissue damage, but the body can respond similarly to other stimuli. If you are standing and begin to walk by lifting your right foot off the floor, the signal of loss of balance begins this process, allowing the right leg and left arm to swing forward (flexing) and the left leg and right arm to keep the body steady (extending). This reflex interaction is known as *gait.*

Proprioception: Gamma Motor Neurons and Muscle Tone

Gamma motor neurons innervate muscle spindles. If a gamma motor neuron is stimulated, contraction occurs at both ends of the spindles, resulting in stretching of the middle region of the spindle where the sensory nerves are located. The sensory nerve endings detect the stretch and produce action potentials that cause the muscle to be more sensitive to stretch. Gamma motor neurons are then responsible for muscle tone. Muscle tone (residual muscle tension or tonus) is the continuous and passive partial contraction of the muscle.

Muscle tone is often assessed by the muscle's resistance to passive stretch during a resting state. A muscle that offers little resistance to stretch is said to be *flaccid.* Flaccidity occurs if the nerve to the muscle is cut. A muscle is *hypotonic* when the gamma motor neuron discharge is low. A muscle that offers great resistance to stretch is said to be *hypertonic* or *spastic.* Spasticity occurs when hyperactive stretch reflexes exist and may be seen in individuals with spinal cord injury or stroke, in whom the inhibitory impulses to the gamma motor neurons from the brain have been removed.

Control of Gamma Motor Neuron Discharge

The gamma motor neurons regulate the sensitivity of the muscle spindles; hence, the stretch reflexes and tone of the muscle can be altered according to the change in posture. Many factors affect the gamma motor neuron discharge. For example, anxiety and stress increase its discharge, resulting in the tensing of muscles and hyperactive tendon reflexes. If the skin of the hand on one side is stimulated by a painful stimulus, the result is increased discharge to the flexors and decreased discharge to the extensors of the same side, facilitating flexion and quick removal. At the same time, the opposite happens on the other side, adjusting posture and weight distribution.

Touch and movement are considered stimuli because they constitute a change in the environment. When the body is called on to restore homeostasis, problematic nerve transmission pathways often can be overridden and a more effective pattern can be established. Learning the receptor language of the body and exploring the reflex patterns initiated by the various forms of stimuli are worthwhile ways to override these nonproductive transmissions. The more this information is incorporated into practical applications, the more effective the therapeutic massage intervention will be.

Fascial Innervations

The extensive nerve supply to the fascia is new to our understanding of somatic nervous system function. Fascia is a form of connective tissue. Some of the functions of fascia are sliding, gliding, and separation of muscle structures; transmission of movement from muscle contraction to bone and joints; suspending organs in place; and providing a supportive and movable covering for nerves and blood vessels as they pass through and between muscles. Anatomists have known for a long time that fascia wraps nerves and nerves pass through fascia. Recent research has found that fascia—once thought to be simply passive connective tissue, like a spider web—is innervated by nerves and functions similar to smooth muscle–like tissue. This means that the brain and the rest of the CNS influence fascia through neural activity to increase or reduce fascial tone, subsequently influencing musculoskeletal function.

Both somatic and autonomic sensory receptors are embedded in the fascia. Typically the receptors monitor stability and movement. The smooth muscle bundles in the fascia function as effectors, and the nervous system can signal increased contraction which would tighten up the fascia. This is an appropriate response if there is instability. Various pain syndromes may be due to an inappropriate response of the fascia to these types of nerve signals. Researchers think that the richly innervated fascia could be maintained in a taut resting state, called *fascial tone,* as a result of the different muscular fibers that pull on it (somewhat like a trampoline). This resting state enables the free nerve endings and receptors in the fascial tissue to sense any variation in the shape of the fascia (and therefore any movement of the body) whenever it occurs. Deep fascia is designed to sense and assist in organizing movements. Whenever a body part moves in any direction, a myofascial tensional rearrangement occurs within the corresponding fascia. Microscopic study has shown that in many places in the fascia, a vein, an artery, and a nerve perforate (poke through) tissue layers. Called *neurovascular bundles,* these points are in the same location as most of the various points used in a variety of massage therapy methods such as trigger points and acupuncture points. It is hypothesized that during injury, these points become sensitized, affecting the muscle nerve receptors and creating dysfunctions in the fascial tone and mechanical strain in the fascial system.

Sensory receptors, embedded in the fascia, report the presence or potential of tissue damage (nociceptors); change in movement (proprioceptors); change in pressure and vibration (mechanoreceptors); change in the chemical milieu (chemoreceptors); and fluctuation in temperature (thermoreceptors). Deep fascia can respond to sensory input by contracting; by relaxing; or by adding, reducing, or changing its composition through the process of fascial remodeling.

The deep fascia is a highly vascular structure with a superficial and a deep layer, each with an independent rich vascular network of capillaries, venules, arterioles, and lymphatic channels. Deep fascia contains myofibroblasts, suggesting contractile ability. Any active contraction would need to be controlled by a nerve supply and myelinated and unmyelinated nerve axons. Schwann cells are found in these deep fascial layers. Electron microscopy and special staining procedures demonstrate that fascia is populated by sensory neural fibers, suggesting that fascia contributes to proprioception and nociception, and may be responsive to manual pressure, temperature, and vibration. Many encapsulated endings found in fascia are mechanoreceptors that respond to mechanical pressure or deformation.

Review What You Have Learned

- Define a *nerve reflex.*
  - Nerve reflexes are usually involuntary actions caused when the CNS receives a message from sensory stimuli and responds by sending a signal (action potential) to an effector organ (muscle) to counter the stimulus.
- List the sensory receptors involved in reflex action.
  - Mechanoreceptors, lamellar (pacinian) corpuscles, tactile (Meissner) corpuscles, hair root (root hair) plexuses, bulbous (Ruffini) corpuscles, bulboid (Krause) corpuscles, tactile (Merkel) disks, C-tactile afferent, free nerve endings (some of which are thermal receptors/thermoreceptors), nociceptors, proprioceptors (muscle spindles, Golgi tendon organs, joint kinesthetic receptors).
- Define a *reflex arc.*
  - A reflex arc is the pathway of a reflex. The nerve impulse travels from the receptor through sensory neurons to the spinal cord (or brain), then back through motor neurons to an effector (a muscle that contracts or a gland that secretes).
- Explain muscle tone.
  - Gamma motor neurons are responsible for muscle tone. Muscle tone is the continuous/passive partial contraction of muscles. Muscle tone can be assessed by muscular resistance to passive stretch. A muscle that offers little resistance to stretch is called *flaccid.* A muscle that offers great resistance to stretch is called *hypertonic* or *spastic.*
- Explain fascial tone.
  - Fascia is innervated by nerves and functions similarly to smooth muscle–like tissue. The CNS influences fascia through neural activity to increase or reduce fascial tone. Subsequently, fascial tone influences musculoskeletal function and vice versa. Fascial layers are perforated by neurovascular bundles (points that commonly correlate with trigger points and acupuncture points). It is hypothesized that tissue injury sensitizes these points, creating mechanical dysfunction.

AUTONOMIC NERVOUS SYSTEM

SECTION OBJECTIVES

Chapter objective covered in this section:

3. Explain the structure and function of the autonomic nervous system.

After completing this section, the learner will be able to:

- Name the two divisions of the ANS and list their functions.
- Describe the Eastern/Western connection as it relates to the functions of the ANS.

Maintenance of the internal environment of the body is the responsibility of the ANS. The ANS controls the actions of the smooth muscles and glands. As in the somatic PNS, ANS information from sensory receptors goes to the brain, which in turn relays the effector response to maintain homeostasis through motor nerves. The sensors are located in areas such as the smooth muscles, blood vessels, lungs, and glands. Motor neurons carry the signals to these same organs to prompt an increase or a decrease in the rate of our heartbeat, breathing, or digestive processes or to initiate glandular secretion. The system is called *involuntary* because its actions normally are outside conscious control. An interesting finding is that fascia is innervated by the ANS and is involved in controlling fascial stiffness.

Divisions of the Autonomic Nervous System

The ANS is divided into the sympathetic and parasympathetic divisions. In general, the **sympathetic nervous system** tends to stimulate and functions primarily when the body is under stress. The **parasympathetic nervous system**, which usually diminishes or inhibits actions, tends to work most often under normal body conditions or to conserve energy (Fig. 5.9). The **enteric nervous system (ENS)** is a third division of the ANS that you do not hear much about. The ENS is a meshwork of nerve fibers that innervate the GI tract, pancreas, and gallbladder. The ENS is sometimes called the *belly brain* (Table 5.3).

Differences Between the Somatic and Autonomic Peripheral Nervous Systems

Our skeletal muscles are innervated by neurons that carry a signal to contract or carry no signal at all, which causes the muscles to relax. The ANS has a different form of control. Most of the organs contain neurons from the sympathetic and parasympathetic divisions; this is called *dual innervation.* By constantly receiving signals from both divisions, the body can maintain or quickly restore homeostasis because the organs can be stimulated or inhibited rapidly.

This form of autonomic antagonism is another example of the duality of wholeness discussed previously in this text. If sympathetic impulses tend to stimulate an effector, parasympathetic impulses tend to inhibit it, and vice versa. This type of antagonistic activity gives precise control, much like the accelerator and brake pedals of a car.

For example, moment-to-moment regulation of blood pressure involves continuously changing sympathetic and parasympathetic signals to the heart. The regulation comes from centers in the brainstem that "turn up" or "turn down" each type of input to keep blood pressure constant as the body changes position or activity.

Another major difference is that in the ANS, two neurons relay the signal from the brainstem or spinal cord to the organ, gland, or smooth muscle innervated. The first neuron synapses with the second, and the second synapses with the receptor.

In the sympathetic nervous system, the synapse, or ganglion, is located near the spinal cord. In the parasympathetic system, the ganglion is near or at the receptor organ, gland, or muscle. The neurotransmitter released at the ganglion synapse near the spinal cord is acetylcholine, just as in the somatic nervous system. The sympathetic postganglionic synapse to the organs releases noradrenaline (norepinephrine), except in the adrenal medulla, which releases adrenaline (epinephrine) and only some noradrenaline. The benefit of adrenaline in the blood is that it reinforces and prolongs the effect of noradrenaline.

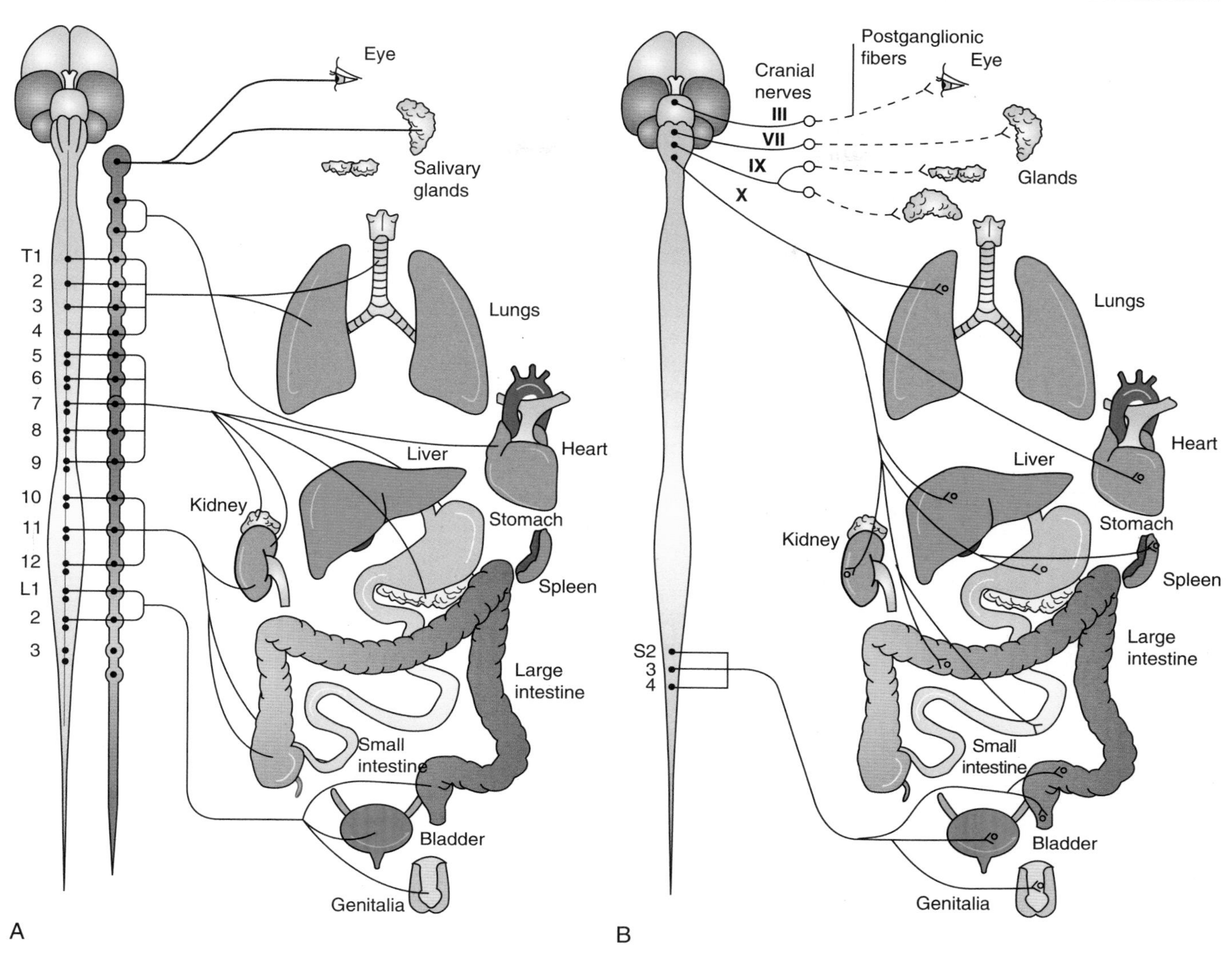

FIG. 5.9 (A) The sympathetic portions of the autonomic nervous system (ANS). (B) The parasympathetic portions of the ANS with the vagus nerve distribution to the enteric devices.

Table 5.3 Enteric Autonomic Nervous System Neurotransmitters

Transmitter	Functions
Nitric oxide	Parasympathetic—important in erection and in gastric emptying
Vasoactive intestinal polypeptide	Parasympathetic—important throughout the body
Serotonin	Important in enteric neurons (peristalsis)
Gamma-aminobutyric acid	Enteric
Substance P	Sympathetic ganglia, enteric neurons

Sympathetic Structure and Function

The sympathetic nervous system begins in the spinal cord, where the neurons exit between the first thoracic vertebra and the second lumbar vertebra. Because of the location, the system often is referred to as the *thoracolumbar division*.

The sympathetic ganglia found near the spinal cord are connected by collateral tissues and form a chain. This interconnected chain allows for many different sources of input of sympathetic activity to each of the effectors, thus producing more sympathetic activity with little input. The preganglionic neurons are short and end in this chain; the postganglionic neurons are much longer and end at the effector organs.

The major function of the sympathetic nervous system involves the emergency response. The signals sent out allow the body to be better prepared for an increase in the intensity of activities that require increased metabolism, higher blood sugar levels, a stronger heartbeat, and dilated bronchi, allowing for more oxygen to the lungs and faster exhalation of carbon dioxide. During this function, the blood is rerouted from the digestive system to the muscles so that they can respond to the increased stress. Sympathetic ANS signaling tends to stiffen fascia.

Whether the stimulus is physical or psychological or whether the threat is real or imagined, all our responses are set into action immediately. Walter B. Cannon described this group of sympathetic responses as a *fight-or-flight* reaction.

These responses are normal and healthy in times of stress. However, chronic exposure to stress or perceived threats to our well-being can affect our health adversely, leading to the dysfunction of sympathetic effectors and perhaps even to the dysfunction of the ANS itself. Excessive sympathetic output causes most of the stress-related diseases. Problems with headaches, GI difficulties, high blood pressure, anxiety, muscle tension and aches, and sexual dysfunction can be related to excessive sympathetic stimulation.

We think of the previously mentioned sympathetic functions as life preserving because they can be used to remove us from dangerous situations and keep us active in self-preservation. However, the sympathetic system is also active during many of our normal daily functions. Dual innervation allows the sympathetic system to oppose the effects of the parasympathetic system, providing balance and maintaining homeostasis. Smooth muscles in the walls of the blood vessels are innervated only by sympathetic fibers. The fibers maintain the tone of the muscles of the arteries, resulting in proper blood pressure whether we are active or at rest. This is another example of general homeostatic balance (Box 5.1).

Freeze Response

A third response to stress has been recognized, called the freeze response. Instead of running away or fighting, the response is to become immobile. It happens when the parasympathetic activation starts to overpower the sympathetic arousal. Freezing is fight-or-flight on hold. It is also called reactive immobility or attentive immobility.

Parasympathetic Structure and Function

The parasympathetic division of the ANS can be thought of as the *rest, digest,* and *restore* system. The parasympathetic nervous system is referred to as the *craniosacral division* because of the location of its nerves. Parasympathetic fibers leave the CNS through cranial nerves, including the oculomotor, facial, glossopharyngeal, and vagus nerves, and at the sacrum and some pelvic nerves. The three long preganglionic neurons that innervate the pupil and the salivary and lacrimal glands end outside the actual organs. The rest of the preganglionic neurons end at the walls of the organs, with the short postganglionic fibers entering the organs. This configuration is the opposite of the sympathetic division, in which the neurons end just before the organ.

The parasympathetic system generally functions as the energy conservation system, which allows the body to rest and restore itself after emergency responses. The result is a relaxation response. To maintain balance with the sympathetic division, the parasympathetic system is dominant under nonstressful conditions; this means that during nonstressful

Box 5.1 Autonomic Nervous System (ANS) Neurotransmitters and Receptors

Acetylcholine is found in the parasympathetic postganglionic synapse. Based on the neurotransmitter secreted, the ANS can be divided into cholinergic (acetylcholine-secreting) and adrenergic (adrenaline-secreting) divisions. All preganglionic and postganglionic fibers of the parasympathetic system belong to the cholinergic division. Postganglionic sympathetic fibers that supply sweat glands and blood vessels of skeletal muscles produce vasodilation and are cholinergic. The postganglionic fibers of the sympathetic system are adrenergic.

Other neurotransmitters, such as dopamine, are secreted by interneurons located in the ganglia. Stimulation of the sympathetic nervous system can excite or inhibit the smooth muscles, depending on the receptors in the organ involved. Receptors are divided into two major groups: alpha receptors, which respond to norepinephrine (noradrenaline) and certain blocking substances, and beta receptors, which respond to epinephrine (adrenaline) and similar blocking substances. Each of these groups can be divided again, into alpha-1 and alpha-2 and beta-1 and beta-2, which better classifies the generalized responses they produce.

When alpha receptors are stimulated, they cause dilation of the pupils and constriction of the smooth muscles and blood vessels. Stimulation of beta-1 receptors, which are found mainly in the heart, increases the force and rate of heart muscle contraction; beta-2 receptors, located in the lungs, cause relaxation of the bronchial muscles, resulting in bronchodilation.

As with sympathetic nerve fibers, the effect of the parasympathetic postganglionic fibers on a target organ depends on the type of receptors present in the cells.

Two types of receptors, nicotinic and muscarinic, have been identified. The nicotinic receptors are present in the parasympathetic and sympathetic ganglions and the neuromuscular junction. The muscarinic receptors are located in target organs supplied by postganglionic parasympathetic fibers. The terms *nicotinic* and *muscarinic* are based on the effects of nicotine, a powerful toxin that can be obtained from a variety of sources including tobacco, and muscarine, a toxin present in poisonous mushrooms. Thus if one ingests a large quantity of nicotine, it produces symptoms according to the presence of nicotinic receptors, such as vomiting, diarrhea, sweating (parasympathetic effects), high blood pressure, rapid heart rate, and sweating. By stimulating skeletal muscles, convulsions may also occur.

The symptoms produced by muscarine poisoning are almost all caused by parasympathetic effects and include vomiting, diarrhea, constriction of bronchi, low blood pressure, and slow heart rate.

Knowledge of the receptors, actions, and distribution of parasympathetic and sympathetic nervous systems is important to all health professionals. Almost all drugs used in conditions (such as asthma, hypertension, the common cold, constipation, diarrhea, and many other conditions) have been developed and are being used based on this knowledge. Side effects of all these drugs can be derived logically if one knows which receptors they affect and whether the drug imitates or opposes the sympathetic and parasympathetic systems.

The effect the neurotransmitter has on a target organ depends on the type of receptor for the neurotransmitter the cells of the organ possess. For example, the effect of postganglionic parasympathetic fibers may be stimulatory or inhibitory depending on the receptor. In general, postganglionic sympathetic fibers are excitatory.

times, more impulses to the effectors are received by parasympathetic fibers than by sympathetic fibers.

The parasympathetic system is active in regulating digestive processes, slowing the heart rate, and constricting eye muscles to focus on near vision. In addition, the parasympathetic system increases glandular secretions, constricts the bronchioles in the lungs, and slows breathing. Parasympathetic stimulation of the nerves to the internal and external genitalia in males and females causes vasodilation in the clitoris and labia minora and erection in the penis.

Reactions to parasympathetic stimulation are highly localized and tend to counteract the adrenergic effects of the sympathetic system (see Activity 5.2, Activity 5.3, Activity 5.4, and Table 5.4). Learning one system is usually simpler because the other is the opposite. Memorizing the fight-or-flight response seems to be the more practical way. These responses make fighting or fleeing possible; for example, pupil dilation improves vision, a faster heart rate increases cardiac output to supply muscles with blood, bronchodilation improves breathing, and slowing of digestive responses reduces interference with fight or flight.

ACTIVITY 5.3

Identify a control process you use to influence the sympathetic and parasympathetic divisions of the autonomic nervous system (ANS) and explain the way it works. An example is provided to get you started.

Example

Sympathetic: Brisk walking for 30 minutes in the morning. The fast pace activates the sympathetic functions and helps wake me up and give me energy for the day.

Parasympathetic: Eating a bowl of cereal before bed. Eating signals digestion and also helps make me sleepy.

ACTIVITY 5.4

After reviewing the effects of sympathetic and parasympathetic stimulation, identify three sensations or body functions related to the autonomic nervous system (ANS) that could be interpreted as some sort of pathological condition. Examples are given to help you.

Examples

Feeling that the heart is pounding
  Sympathetic: Increased rate and strength of contraction
May be constipated
  Sympathetic: Decreased peristalsis (beta receptors)
Frequently finds lighting too dim
  Parasympathetic: Contraction of circular muscle; constricted pupil

Your Turn

1. ______________________________
____
2. ______________________________
____
3. ______________________________
____

Eastern/Western Connection

The ANS is a clear example of the yin and yang concept. The ganglia of the parasympathetic system tend to occupy the same areas traditionally identified as chakras, or energy centers, by traditional Indian medicine. The sympathetic chain ganglia follow one of the paths of the bladder meridian, located on either side of the vertebral column. Specific acupuncture points on this meridian, called *back-shu* points, are considered to be the locations where the Qi of the respective yin or yang organs is assimilated. Practitioners use techniques for stimulating these points to relieve dysfunctions of the corresponding organs. One can see a correlation between sympathetic ANS function and these important organ points in the Asian meridian system.

It is now generally accepted that the traditional meridian system is connected with the fascia. Dr. Helene Langevin and associates have completed multiple studies on the relationship of fascia to acupuncture points and meridians. They have found substantial overlap of acupuncture points and meridians to fascial planes in the body. The needle grasp effect found in acupuncture is also related to the fascia. We now know that the fascia is innervated with both somatic and autonomic sensors and receptors.

Research over the past 20 years has identified the crucial role the ANS plays in stress-related disorders. This research also has validated the effectiveness of many ancient healing, cultural, and spiritual practices that serve to bring the ANS under voluntary control, facilitating conscious control of homeostatic processes.

MENTORING TIP

Whether Western research-based evidence supports the claimed benefits of ancient healing traditions is the subject of debate within the massage therapy community. Evidence-informed practice is an important concept in massage therapy. However, technology may not yet be sophisticated enough to unravel the mysteries of some ancient and cultural forms of healing. Regardless, research continues to reinforce the benefit of including these traditional healing practices in *integrated medicine*. According to Western scientific theory, massage therapy does have enough evidence to be considered evidence-based practice, but the research quantity and quality are improving. The importance of biologically plausible claims was discussed in previous chapters. Division based on "either/or" regarding health care does not serve the growth of the massage profession. Cooperation and ongoing research should close the divide in the future. Massage therapy is rooted in compassion and kindness. It is important to remember this when ambiguity exists.

Review What You Have Learned

- Name the two divisions of the ANS and list their functions.
  - The sympathetic nervous system (also called the *thoracolumbar division*) regulates emergency response/energy expenditure (fight or flight), preparing the body for stressful activities that require increased metabolism, higher blood sugar levels, an increased heart rate, and dilated bronchi (for increased oxygen). The parasympathetic nervous system (or *craniosacral division*)

Table 5.4 Sympathetic and Parasympathetic Effects on Structures and Systems of the Body

Structure/System	Parasympathetic System Response	Sympathetic System Response
Eye		
Radial muscle of the iris	None	Contraction: Results in pupil dilation
Sphincter muscles of the iris	Contraction: results in pupil constriction	None yet identified
Ciliary muscle	Contraction: results in near sight	Reflex action: Farsight
Tear glands	Secretion	None
Skin		
Sweat glands	None	Secretion increased
Arrector pili muscle	None	Contraction, erection of hairs
Cardiovascular System		
Blood vessels to the skin	None	Constriction
Blood vessels to skeletal muscle	None	Dilation
Blood vessels to the heart	None	Dilation
Blood vessels to the intestines	None	Constriction
Heart	Heart rate and contraction force decreased	Heart rate and contraction force increased; vasodilation
Blood coagulation	None yet identified	Coagulation increased in coronary vessels
Digestive System		
Liver	Glycogen synthesis	Glycogen breakdown; glucose synthesis and release
Salivary glands	Mucus secretion	Watery, serous secretion
Intestinal peristalsis	Increased	Decreased
Sphincters	Relaxation	Contraction
Digestive secretions	Stimulation	Possible inhibition
Adipose tissue	None yet identified	Breakdown and release of fatty acid
Skeletal muscles	None	Contraction force increased
Urinary System		
Kidney	Urine production increased	Urine production decreased
Sphincter	Relaxation	Contraction
Respiratory System		
Bronchial muscles	Contraction	Relaxation
Mental activity	Calm	Alertness increased

performs the functions of relaxation response/energy conservation (rest, digest, restore); it reverses sympathetic arousal responses to regulate digestion, slow the heart rate, increase glandular secretions, constrict lung bronchioles, and slow breathing. The freeze response is a form of hyperarousal.

- Describe the Eastern/Western connection as it relates to the functions of the ANS.
  - The parasympathetic nervous system parallels yin. The sympathetic nervous system parallels yang. Parasympathetic ganglia tend to occupy the same areas as chakras. The traditional meridian system correlates with fascial planes.

ACTIVITY 5.5

Using basic massage methods, describe how you would design and implement a 45-minute massage that would result in the following:

A. Sympathetic dominance
B. Parasympathetic dominance

Practical Application

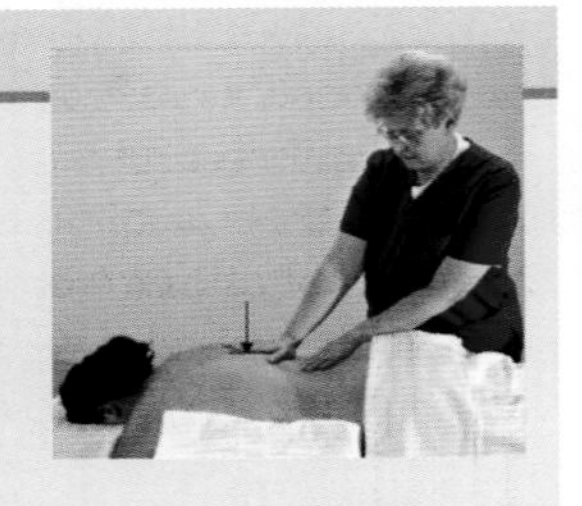

There are four main evidence-informed outcomes related to massage therapy. They are (1) relaxation, (2) stress management, (3) pain management, and (4) functional mobility. Relaxation, stress management, and pain management outcomes are related to how massage interacts with the autonomic nervous system (ANS). The approach to massage that is most apt to achieve these outcomes is a general, full-body nonspecific, nonpainful, pleasurable massage using moderate pressure and moderate drag on the tissue and lasts about 60 minutes. This approach is the single most important skill set that you will deliver as a massage therapist. Typically the interaction is to quiet the sympathetic output and support parasympathetic relaxation, restoration, and rest. Often called relaxation massage, you may find people who indicate that this approach is only basic and does not take much skill. On the contrary, the ability to provide massage to support relaxation outcomes requires great skill and much practice.

FIVE BASIC SENSES

SECTION OBJECTIVES

Chapter objective covered in this section:

4. Describe the structure and function of the five basic senses: touch, hearing, vision, taste, and smell.

After completing this section, the learner will be able to:

- List and describe the five basic senses.
- Describe how the five basic senses contribute to daily function.

With all the possibilities of sensory stimulation, compartmentalizing the types of stimuli and our responses makes studying and understanding the phenomena easier. More than 20 different senses have been identified (Box 5.2). For our purposes, we focus our study on the basic five special senses that we encounter and use daily. The five basic senses are touch, hearing, vision, taste, and smell. Touch is covered in detail in the discussion of the integumentary system in Chapter 11 . Research brings new information about the way senses work, the way they are processed in our brains, and the way they interact to enhance our lives.

Receptors for the general senses are scattered throughout the body and are relatively simple in structure. These receptors are classified according to the nature of the stimulus that excites them. Important sensor classes include:

- Tissue damage/noxious stimuli (nociceptors)
- Temperature (thermoreceptors)
- Chemical stimuli (chemoreceptors)
- Touch/pressure/position (mechanoreceptors)

Box 5.2 Our Many Senses

Balance or vestibular sense allows us to sense body movement, direction, and acceleration and to attain and maintain postural equilibrium and balance. The vestibular labyrinthine system found in both of the inner ears is responsible for the senses of angular momentum, linear acceleration, and gravity.

Thermal sense is the sense of heat and the absence of heat which is the sensation of cold. There are specialized receptors for cold (declining temperature) and heat. The thermoreceptors in the skin are quite different from the homeostatic thermoreceptors in the brain (hypothalamus), which provide feedback on internal body temperature.

Kinesthetic sense provides the brain with information on the relative positions of the parts of the body during movement. Doctors evaluate this sense by telling patients to close their eyes and touch the tip of a finger to their nose.

Pain sense (nociception) signals near-damage or damage to tissue. The three types of pain receptors are cutaneous (skin), somatic (joints and bones), and visceral (body organs). Pain is a distinct phenomenon that intertwines with all the other senses, including touch.

Directional sense, or magnetoreception, is the ability to detect the direction one is facing based on the Earth's magnetic field. Directional awareness is most commonly observed in birds, although it is also present to a limited extent in humans.

Internal sense, or interoception, is the sense from within the body, such as a full bladder or gastrointestinal sensation.

The processes involved in sensations work this way: sensory receptors receive mechanical, chemical, and thermal stimuli and transform them into electrical signals; they then send that information to the brain to be processed and associated with previous experiences (Activity 5.6).

ACTIVITY 5.6

Describe how you could stimulate some of the senses during a massage session.
Your Turn

Touch

Touch, or mechanoreception, results from activation of neural receptors, generally in the skin, including hair follicles, but also in the tongue, throat, and mucous membranes. The sense of touch occurs when some sort of mechanical deformation of the skin and soft tissues of the body occurs, causing a change in the shape of the capsule surrounding the nerve ending. The nerve ending, called *mechanoreceptor*, detects this change in shape and produces an action potential, sending nerve impulses. For a person actually to feel the sensation, the nerve impulses must make their way up to the brain.

Sensory nerve endings monitor what the body touches. The sense of touch is protective. Touch mechanoreceptors are also called *tactile receptors* and provide the sensations of touch, pressure, and vibration. A variety of sensory receptors are found in the skin, but there are seven main ones:

1. Free nerve endings are sensitive to touch and pressure.
2. The root hair plexus is made up of free nerve endings that detect hair movement.
3. C-tactile (CT) afferents are low-threshold mechanoreceptors present in the skin of humans and are thought to convey positive and pleasant aspects of touch,
4. Tactile (Merkel) disks are fine touch and pressure neurons located in the lower epidermal layer of the skin.
5. Tactile (Meissner) corpuscles are fine touch and pressure receptors located in the eyelids, lips, fingertips, nipples, and external genitalia.
6. Lamellar (pacinian) corpuscles are large receptors sensitive to deep pressure and pulsing or high-frequency vibrations.
7. Bulbous (Ruffini) corpuscles are located in the dermis of the skin and are sensitive to pressure and distortions of the skin.

When the tactile receptors are stimulated, the action potential codes for the touch's location on the skin, the amount of force, and its velocity so that the CNS can interpret where the sensation is occurring and whether it is safe or dangerous. Compared to the other senses, touch is hard to isolate because tactile sensory information enters the nervous system from every single part of the body.

A study of the tactile sense has identified a low-threshold mechanoreceptor called C-tactile (CT) afferent. Touch targeted to stimulate this receptor produces nervous system changes that may reduce stress and facilitate social processes. CT fibers respond to gentle stroking. Stimulation during touch supports feelings of safety, connection, and well-being and may be involved in the modulation of pain (Croy et al., 2022).

The physical characteristics of something you are touching can influence your feelings; this interpretation of touch has made its way into our language. Weight is metaphorically associated with concepts of seriousness and importance; for example, a "weighty matter" or "light reading." Roughness and smoothness are associated with difficulty and harshness; think of "a rough day" or "smooth sailing." Hardness and softness are associated with stability, rigidity, and strictness, as in being "hard-hearted" or "soft on someone" (Wein, 2010).

Affectionate touch lowers an individual's stress and anxiety levels. Physical contact affects oxytocin levels.

Hearing

Sounds are vibrations created by mechanical methods that are turned into recognizable patterns of electrical energy in our nervous system. These vibrations can travel through air, water, or solid substances.

The brain can recognize immense variations in pitch, volume, and tone. When several sounds reach the ear, they are transferred to the hair cells in the ear. The lower frequency signals are given priority when transmitted as electrical signals to the brain; thus a slow, deep, even voice is the best one to use when we want to be heard.

Our sense of hearing is well developed even at birth. Newborns can identify the direction of a voice and turn in response. Only in the past decade has investigation been conducted into the ability of the fetus to hear or sense sound carried through the amniotic fluid. Research indicates that the fetus does respond to sound. Music is often used as an adjunct to massage therapy. Hearing soothing sounds supports the relaxation response.

The center of our hearing is the cochlea, named for its shape as a spiral shell (*cochlea* comes from the Greek word for snail). The true organ of hearing is the organ of Corti. This spiral structure within the cochlea contains hair cells that are stimulated by sound vibrations. The hair cells convert the vibrations into nerve impulses, which are transmitted by the cochlear portion of the eighth cranial nerve to the brain.

Practical Application

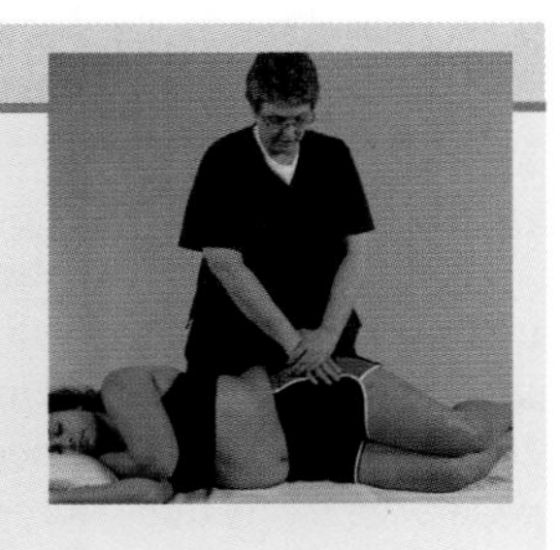

Any movement activity, especially one that causes head movements that affect the inner ear, shifts the perception of balance in the somatic system, thus altering muscle tension patterns. Many of the benefits of massage therapy are derived indirectly through the effect on the inner ear balance system.

Rhythmic rocking is used universally to calm infants, children, and adults because it interacts with balance mechanisms that influence the ANS to initiate parasympathetic functions. The rocking chair can be a lifelong calming companion in our hectic world.

Structures of the Ear

The ear is divided into three main parts: the external ear, the middle ear, and the inner ear (Fig. 5.10).

External Ear

The external ear is funnel shaped to help guide sound waves into the ear. This part of the ear consists of the auricle, sometimes referred to as the *pinna*, and the external acoustic meatus. The auricle is the part of the ear that is visible. The external acoustic meatus is the tubular structure that links the auricle to the tympanic membrane, commonly referred to as the *eardrum*.

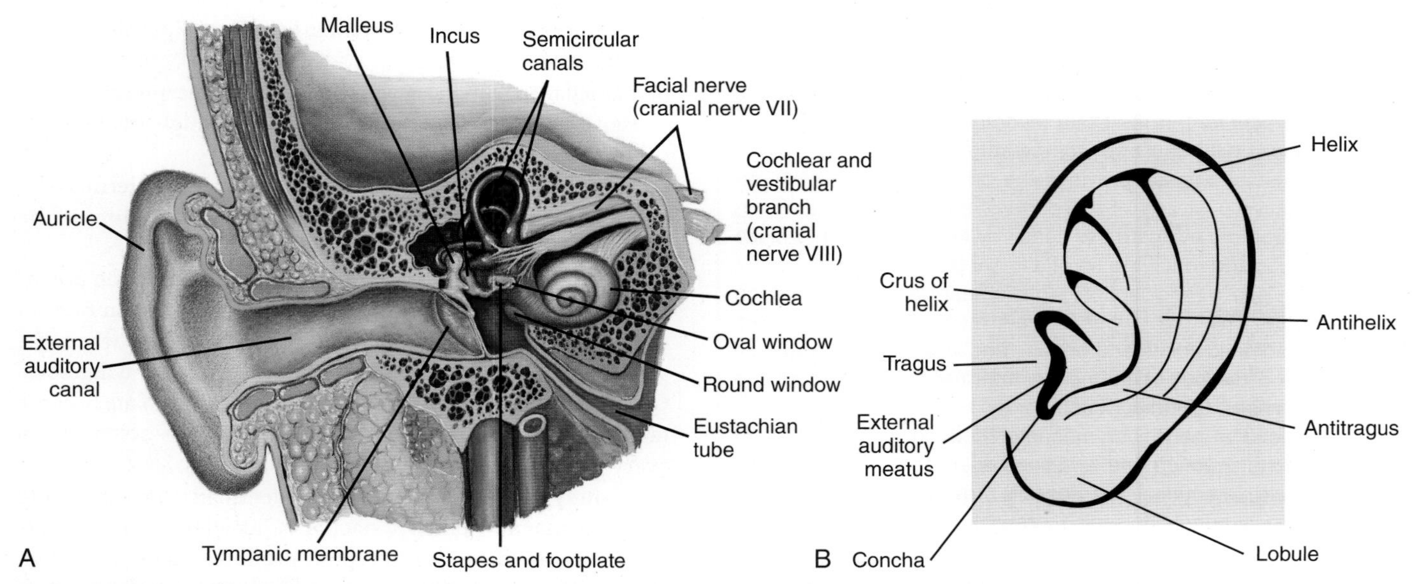

FIG. 5.10 (A) External auditory canal, middle ear, and inner ear. (B) Structures of the external ear (pinna). (A, From Barkauskas VH, Baumann LC, Darling-Fisher CS. *Health and Physical Assessment*. 3rd ed. Mosby; 2002.)

Middle Ear

The middle ear is a cavity linked to the eustachian tube. The eustachian (auditory) tube connects the middle ear with the throat and equalizes pressure between the middle ear and the outside air. Any imbalance in pressure can cause pain and distort or muffle sounds. Activities that open this tube (e.g., yawning, swallowing, chewing) often can relieve the pressure.

The middle ear has a layer of temporal bone that has two openings, commonly known as the oval window and the round window. Three tiny bones known collectively as the *auditory ossicles* extend along the middle ear from the tympanic membrane to the oval window. They are known individually as the malleus, the incus, and the stapes.

Inner Ear

The inner ear is filled with fluid and is responsible for changing sound waves into nerve signals inside the cochlea.

This labyrinthine cavity is made up of the bony labyrinth and the membranous labyrinth. The bony labyrinth consists of a vestibule, a cochlea, and three semicircular canals. The vestibule expands into the middle ear and contains the round and oval windows. The vestibule contains two organs—the utricle and saccule—that are the organs of balance. The vestibular nerve carries signals from the balance organs into the brain.

The membranous labyrinth is separated from the bony labyrinth by a fluid known as *perilymph*. It is the vibrations of the perilymph that stimulate the nerve impulses that deliver sound.

The Sequence of Hearing

1. Vibrations in the air are taken in by the external ear, called the *auricle* or *pinna*.
2. The vibrations are funneled into the external auditory meatus, which leads to the middle ear.
3. Inside the middle ear, the sounds reach the tympanic membrane or eardrum.
4. As the eardrum vibrates in response to the sound vibration, it pulls on the tiny bones called *ossicles* to amplify the sounds.
5. These three bones of the middle ear work together. The motion transfers to the hammer (malleus), which hits the anvil (incus), which pulls on the stirrup (stapes).
6. The stapes rests on the oval window, a membrane at the beginning of the inner ear.
7. Sound waves leave the middle ear and travel to the inner ear, to the cochlea.
8. The sound waves travel through a thin membrane to the middle canal and the organ of Corti. When sound is transmitted to the inner ear, the organ of Corti begins to vibrate up and down, which triggers the generation of nerve signals that are sent to the brain.

Balance and Equilibrium

The **vestibular system** is involved with maintaining body balance and equilibrium. Only the inner ear functions in the vestibular system. The inner ear consists of a group of fluid-filled tubes that run through the temporal bone of the skull. In this region of the inner ear, fluid-filled circular ducts are positioned at right angles to each other, and each duct contains hair cells embedded in a gelatinous substance. These specialized receptor cells respond to vibrations and motion. The semicircular canals are three loops of fluid-filled tubes that are attached to the cochlea in the inner ear.

The semicircular canals and vestibule function to sense movement and position. They help us maintain our sense of balance.

The three semicircular canals lie perpendicular to each other, one to sense movement, such as tilting, twisting, and bending. At the base of the canals are movement hair cells (crista ampullaris). Depending on the movement, the fluid (endolymph) flowing within the semicircular canals stimulates the appropriate movement of hair cells. A static head position is sensed by the vestibule—specifically its utricle and saccule—which contain the position hair cells. Different head positions produce different gravity effects on these hair cells. Small calcium carbonate particles (otoliths) are the ultimate stimulants for the position of hair cells.

The maculae and the cristae are the sensory epithelium of the vestibular system (balance). There are two maculae (the saccule and the utricle), three cristae, and one organ of Corti on each side of the head.

The hair cells (stereocilia) of each macula are linked to an overlying structure; the movement of this structure causes the hair cells to bend. The stereocilia in the cristae are bent in response to the movement of the fluid in a semicircular canal caused by changes in head position.

As we move, the directional hair cells transfer information about our head position and speed of movement. All this sensory information is transformed into electrical signals, which the auditory nerve conducts to the brain. Your brain interprets the incoming information and tells the muscles of the body what to do without your awareness. For example:

- Tilting your head or slamming on your car's brakes causes the overlying mass in the maculae to move relative to the hair cells, bending the stereocilia bundle, and activating the afferent nerve fibers connected to the hair cells.
- When watching a tennis match, you rotate your head to follow the ball. This causes the fluid in the "horizontal canal" to move relative to the crista, and the nerve fibers are stimulated. The end result is that the muscles of your eyes move (again, without your conscious attention) to stabilize the visual field.

If this vestibular balance mechanism is disrupted, the result often is vertigo, or balance problems. If the disruption goes undetected or untreated, the erroneous sensory information can contribute to anxiety and panic disorders.

Vision

The eyeball is a fluid-filled sphere composed of three layers of tissue (Fig. 5.11). The outer layer comprises the sclera and the cornea. The sclera is a white, fibrous structure that maintains the shape of the eye and protects the inner structures. The cornea is the clear portion in the front that allows light to enter the eye.

In the middle layer of the eyeball are the ciliary body, choroid, and iris. The ciliary body, on the anterior portion,

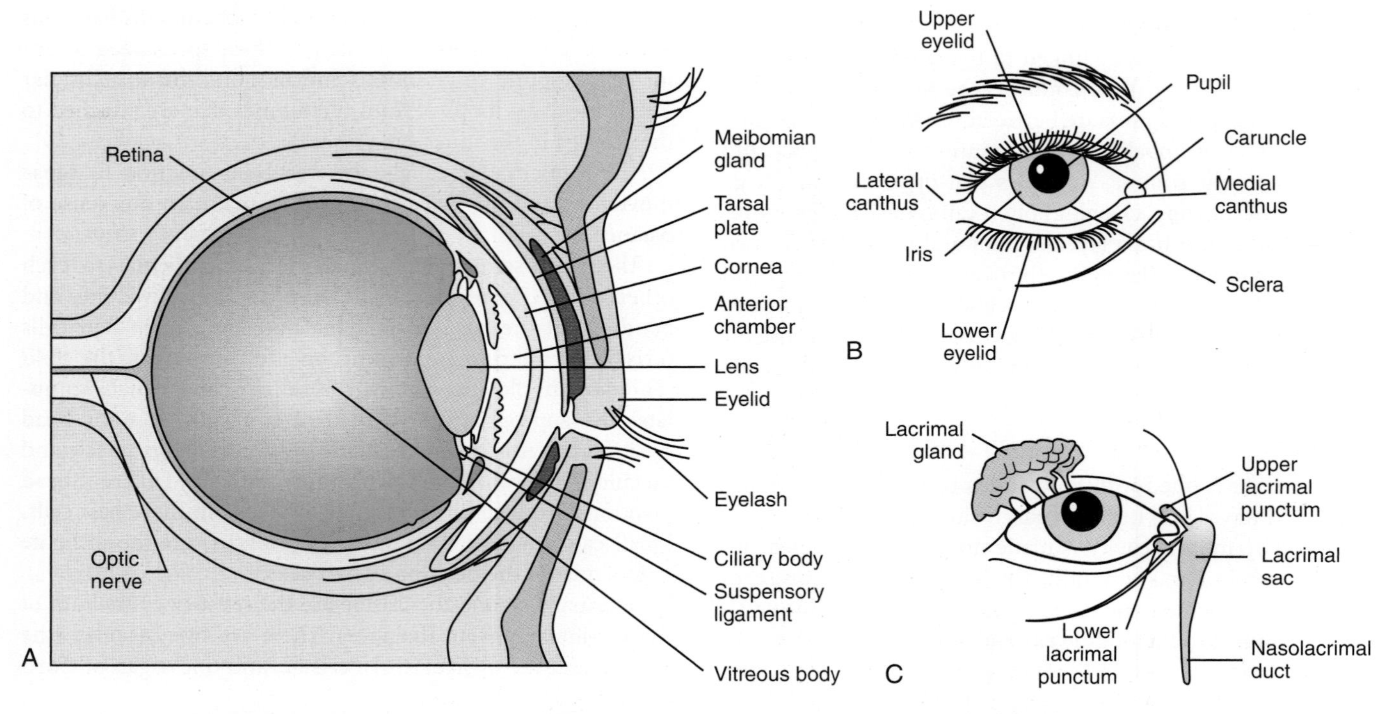

FIG. 5.11 (A) Structures of the eyelid and globe of the eye. (B) Anterior view of the eye. (C) Lacrimal system.

contains smooth muscles attached to the lens by ligaments. The choroid, which covers the posterior of the sclera, is filled with capillaries that nourish the eye. The cells of the choroid contain melanin and absorb light as it enters the eye. The iris, the colored portion of the eye, contains smooth muscles and controls the size of the pupil, which increases or decreases the amount of light allowed to enter the eye. Vision occurs when light rays enter through the lens and are focused on the retina.

The inner layer of the eyeball is the retina, which contains photoreceptor cells and neurons. The rods, which are concentrated on the outer edges of the retina, take in information about the levels of lightness and darkness. The rods are responsible for recognizing shapes and patterns and providing contrast. Cones, which are concentrated at the fovea, or center of the retina, help us identify color and brightness. We can see colors that range from red to purple. Rods and cones receive the mechanical signals, transform them into chemical substances, and create an electrical signal that is sent to the brain by way of the optic nerve. The optic nerve is created from association neurons in the retina. The point where the nerves exit the eye is called the *optic disk*, or *blind spot*, because it has no photoreceptors.

Vision signals are organized and processed in our cerebral cortex. Information received from the left and right eyes stays separate until it converges in the visual cortex. Signals received when we are not paying attention to any specific item are sent to the posterior parietal cortex for processing. Anything we focus on is sent to the visual cortex. Items that reflect a change in the environment cause a signal to be sent to the frontal lobe. These three areas of the brain (cerebral cortex, visual cortex, and parietal cortex) work to process and coordinate visual information.

The eyeball is protected by the skull within cavities known as *orbits*. Six muscles control the movement of the eyeball. These muscles are highly sensitive and coordinate to control the position of the eye. Eyelids and eyelashes close over the eyes for protection and to block light and maintain the distribution of fluid. The lacrimal glands produce tears, which keep our eyes moist, fight infections, and remove foreign particles. These glands, which are located supralaterally, release their product into the eye, where it evaporates or drains into the nasolacrimal duct alongside the nose, thus explaining why the nose becomes stuffed up and runs when we cry.

Taste

Taste is one of the more complex senses. Separating taste from smell is difficult. Specific areas on the tongue correspond to four distinct tastes: sweet, sour, salty, and bitter (Fig. 5.12). Molecules of food bind to receptor sites on the tongue, cheeks, and floor of the mouth. The rest of our tasting is done through our nose and combines with the sense of smell. (You can confirm this by holding your nose and tasting something.)

On average, an adult has more than 10,000 taste buds; however, as we age, our taste buds, which usually last about 10 days, are not replaced as frequently, which may explain why older adults are much less sensitive to taste than younger persons. Most of the nerve fibers that carry taste information to the brain can carry information about more than one taste, although they are mainly sensitive to just one and usually are classified as such.

Practical Application

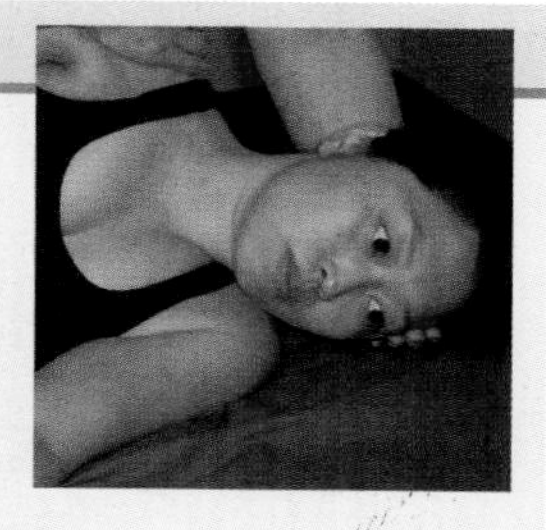

Visual orientation and eye movement are important in posture mechanisms. Visual orientation aids in posture by confirming sensations coming from proprioceptive senses in the muscles and joints. The body shifts positions as necessary to keep the eyes level with the horizontal plane. The position of the eyes is involved in righting reflexes that orient the body in gravity. The combination of proprioceptive, visual, and inner ear (vestibular) information activates various posture or righting reflexes that activate muscular responses to regain balance. Disturbance of the vestibular, visual, or proprioceptive impulses that initiate these reflexes may cause equilibrium disturbances, nausea, vomiting, muscle tension, and other symptoms.

Some forms of movement methods use various eye positions as part of the intervention protocol. The effectiveness of these methods depends partly on the visual orientation aspects of posture. Because of the number of sensory receptors involved with the muscles of the eyes, coupled with the various posture reflexes, subtle movement activates muscle facilitation and inhibition of skeletal muscles, especially in the neck and shoulder area. A simple way to use this response therapeutically during massage is to have the client roll their eyes in slow circles as various massage methods are applied. Muscle groups that would turn the body in the direction of the eye position tense in preparation for movement as antagonist muscles begin to inhibit. A variation is to have the client look at the targeted symptom area, and then look in the opposite direction.

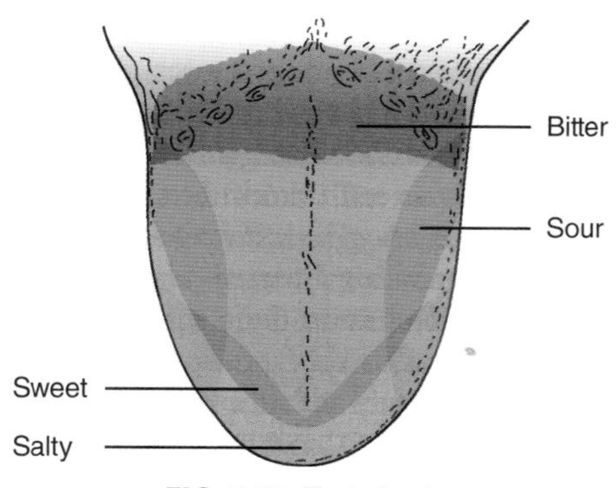

FIG. 5.12 Taste buds.

Our individual preferences for certain tastes may be because of cultural differences or genetics. We can be much more or much less sensitive to certain tastes, making them something we love or something unpleasant. For most of us, bitter tastes are the most easily identified, which may be because most of the poisonous substances around us are bitter.

Smell

The sense of smell is a primitive sense that does not translate well to methods of human communication. For our ancestors, smell was the main lifesaving sense. Today smell still alerts us to dangers. The sense of smell is considered primitive because it deals with our unconscious, animal-like behaviors and experiences and elicits gut-level emotions. The nerves from the nose end in the olfactory bulb in the limbic area of the brain, the portion of the brain that also controls much of our autonomic, involuntary actions. The smell centers in the brain are connected with the limbic system and thus have an emotional and behavioral effect.

Unlike with our other senses, smells are hard to imagine. We can picture a scene, remember a soothing voice, and conjure up a taste that makes our mouth water, but most of us have difficulty imagining a smell. The smell also is the hardest sense to describe to another person.

The more civilized we become, the more we attempt to cover up our body smells and what they mean. Each of us has a unique body odor that changes in response to our emotions. It is true that we can smell fear, danger, anger, and sexual arousal and that we can smell a friend. Memories, associated with déjà vu, are elicited most with our sense of smell. Much of the information we receive from smells helps integrate other information from the senses processed at the same time.

The actual activity of olfaction, or smell, involves chemical receptors found in the roof of the nasal cavity. Blocked nasal passages affect the senses of smell and taste. Fig. 5.13 shows the structures of the nose. As an odor contacts the receptors, they transform chemical signals into electrical signals and transmit them to the temporal lobes of the brain.

The sense of smell is provided by paired olfactory organs located on either side of the nasal septum. Each is comprised of olfactory epithelium, which consists of olfactory receptors, supporting cells, and basal cells (stem cells). There is potential for the basal stem cells to be harvested and used to help treat various diseases and injuries.

Review What You Have Learned

- List and describe the five basic senses.
  1. *Touch* (mechanoreception). Receptors: Mechanoreceptors (tactile receptors). Function: Provide sensations of touch, pressure, and vibration. Process: Mechanical deformation of the skin/soft tissues stimulates mechanoreceptors to send nerve impulses to the brain.
  2. *Hearing*. Receptors: The cochlea contains the true organ of hearing, the organ of Corti. It contains hair cells that are stimulated by sound vibrations. Function/Process: Sound vibrations are converted into nerve impulses, which are transmitted by the cochlear portion of the eighth cranial nerve to the brain.
  3. *Vision*. Receptors: Photoreceptors and neurons in the retina. Function/Process: Rods and cones of the retina (inner layer of the eyeball) receive mechanical signals, transform them into chemical substances, and create electrical signals that are sent to the brain via the optic nerve. Rods process lightness and darkness. Cones help identify color and brightness.

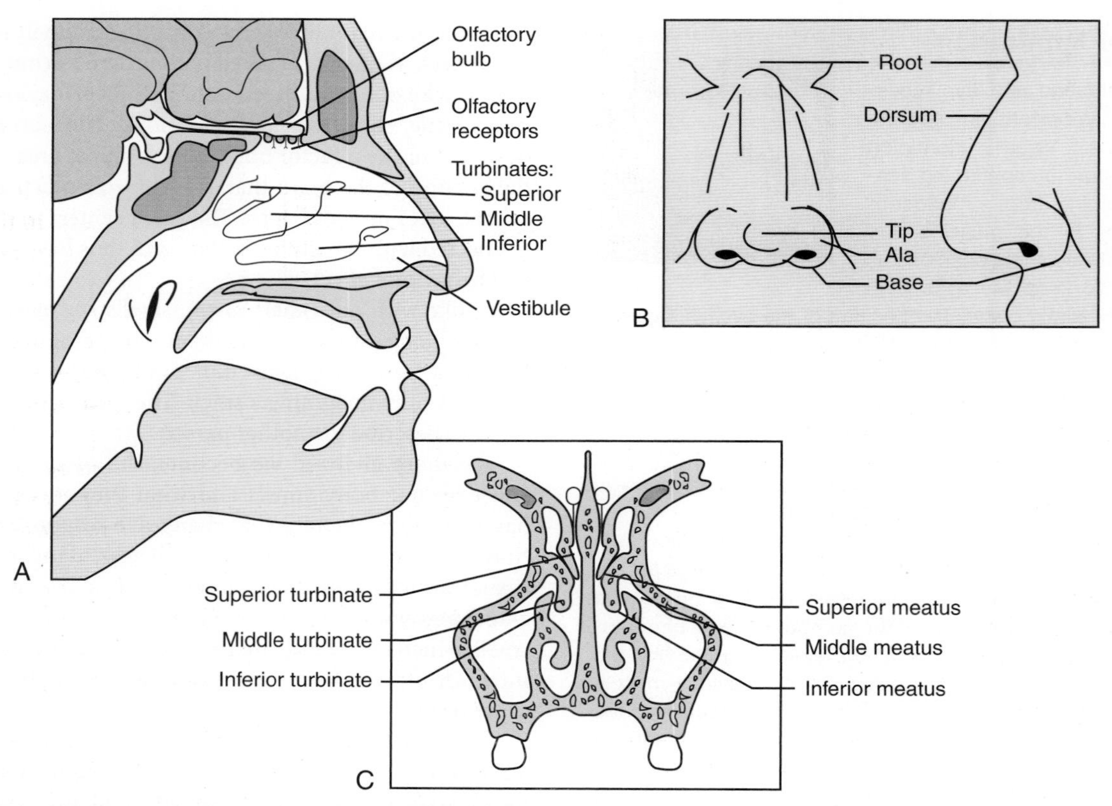

FIG. 5.13 (A) Lateral view of the right nasal cavity. (B) External structure of the nose. (C) Internal structure of the nose.

4. *Taste:* Receptors: Taste buds contain receptor sites on the tongue corresponding to four distinct tastes: sweet, sour, salty, and bitter. Function/Process: Molecules of food bind to receptor sites on the tongue, cheeks, and floor of the mouth and are translated through nerve fibers to the brain. Taste sense is strongly connected to smell.
5. *Smell:* Receptors: Olfactory receptors housed within paired olfactory organs located on either side of the nasal septum. Function/Process: Chemical receptors in the nasal cavity detect odors and transmit electrical signals to the temporal lobes of the brain.

- Describe how the five basic senses contribute to daily function.
  1. *Touch:* Touch sense is protective, sending signals relating sensation location on the skin, force amount, and velocity to the CNS so it can interpret the sensations' cause and any threat to safety.
  2. *Hearing:* Sound recognition and location. The inner ear also functions with the vestibular system, allowing for a sense of movement and position.
  3. *Vision:* Perception of color, shape, and distance of objects in our environment. Aids in posture and navigation of movement. (The combination of proprioceptive, visual, and inner ear [vestibular] information is essential for postural righting reflexes and balance.)
  4. *Taste:* Perception of edible, inedible, and poisonous substances.
  5. *Smell:* Unconscious perception of emotions such as fear, danger, anger, happiness, and security. Influences behavior. Strongly associated with the sense of taste.

Practical Application

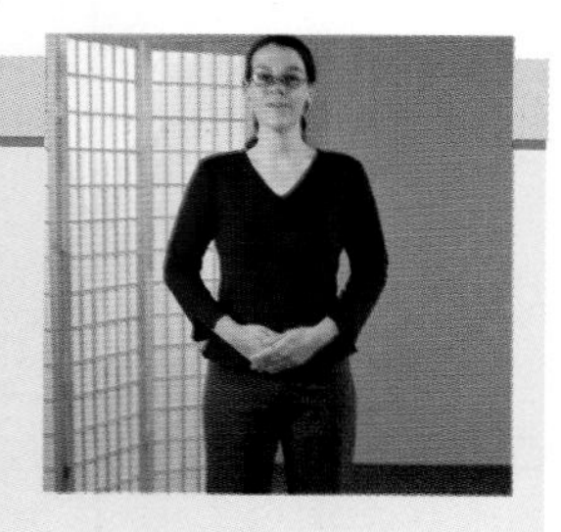

We can use smell therapies, such as aromatherapy, to deliberately influence our physiology and moods. Scents used as the trigger for conditioned learning can help establish a method of reaching a more desirable state of homeostatic balance. The application involves connecting a smell to a particular state of consciousness, be it a calm state or a state of focused arousal. While the person is in the conscious state, they smell the chosen scent. If this is done consistently, the two become connected in the body. Eventually, the smell alone elicits the state of consciousness. This type of conditioned behavior is beneficial for managing pain and anxiety. The scent of lavender is calming. A person can carry drops of lavender or other pleasant aromas on a cotton ball and smell them as needed to support a calming effect.

FOCUS ON PROFESSIONALISM

Therapeutic massage is a full sensory experience involving touch, temperature, sound, vision, and smell. Taste is a sense that is not routinely incorporated into massage but it could be with a selection of herbal teas. The massage environment stimulates the senses. Not only the touch from massage but also soft, warm draping materials; the feel of lubricants; or any adjunct hydrotherapy stimulates the thermoreceptors and touch receptors. Because one of the most important outcome goals of massage is relaxation (parasympathetic dominance), it is necessary to consider the type of sound in the massage environment. For example, external traffic sounds, especially emergency sirens, can interfere with the ability to relax. Music or white noise (e.g., a fan or sounds of nature) can be relaxing if the client enjoys the sounds. Lighting, colors, shapes, and art (e.g., pictures on the wall) are visual stimulation. A client's comfort or discomfort with the visual elements of the massage environment will also influence the response to the massage. The sense of smell is important in evaluating the safety of an environment. A person must enjoy the scent to be able to relax. Each of us, in our role as massage therapists, also stimulates the five senses. Of course, we touch the client, but we also affect the client by the tone of our voice, appearance, and our smell. As massage therapy professionals, ongoing evaluation of how our massage environment and personal interactions influence a client's senses is as important as the massage methods we use.

PATHOLOGICAL CONDITIONS OF THE PERIPHERAL NERVOUS SYSTEM

SECTION OBJECTIVES

Chapter objective covered in this section:

5. Describe pathological conditions of the peripheral nervous system and the related indications for and contraindications to massage.

After completing this section, the learner will be able to:

- Describe the action of medications prescribed for pathologies of the PNS.
- List the common pathologies of the PNS.
- Discuss indications and contraindications, including cautions and adaptations, of massage therapy for pathological conditions of the PNS.

Medications That Affect the Autonomic Nervous System

Certain groups of medications bind to or join with alpha and beta receptors, thereby enhancing or blocking the receptor sites for the binding of norepinephrine (noradrenaline), acetylcholine, or other neurotransmitters and hormones. The effects determine the medication used to modify ANS function. The major problem with many of these medications is the side effects, which range from tachycardia to constipation.

Alpha-Adrenergic Blockers

Alpha-adrenergic blockers (alpha blockers) bind to receptors and thus prevent norepinephrine from binding, causing a decrease in blood vessel tone; this lowers blood pressure and increases circulation. Ergotamine diminishes the intensity of blood vessel contraction in the cranial arteries and can relieve migraine headaches. Hydralazine dilates blood vessels, which reduces blood pressure. Nitroglycerin, one of the most widely known alpha blockers, rapidly dilates arteries and veins, reduces blood pressure, and increases blood flow to the heart muscles. Nitroglycerin is used primarily for patients with angina and coronary artery disease. Alpha blockers are used to treat hypertension.

Beta-Adrenergic Medications

Medications that include epinephrine (adrenaline, which is a beta-1 or beta-2 agonist) or that affect beta-2 receptors by enhancing the uptake of epinephrine (adrenaline) are used most commonly to treat respiratory disorders, such as asthma, chronic bronchitis, and emphysema. Epinephrine-adrenaline inhalers dilate bronchial tubes while causing the walls of the blood vessels to contract, increasing blood flow to the lungs. Other forms of this medication are used as eye drops for glaucoma to reduce internal eye pressure.

Beta-Adrenergic Blockers

Beta-adrenergic blockers (beta blockers) diminish the force and rate of heart muscle contractions and are used to treat hypertension, irregular heart rhythms, and angina.

Chemical substances that mimic the effect of or increase the uptake of norepinephrine (noradrenaline) are called *sympathomimetics*, because they imitate sympathetic stimulation. Besides the bronchodilators used to treat asthma, bronchitis, and emphysema, these drugs include medications used during surgery to counteract the parasympathetic effects of anesthetics and maintain normal blood pressure. Ephedrine is used in many over-the-counter preparations for colds and sinus congestion.

Monoamine oxidase inhibitors are medications that reduce or stop the breakdown of norepinephrine and serotonin; they commonly are used to treat phobias, depression, migraines, and hypertension. The monoamine oxidase inhibitors interact with many other drugs, foods, and herbs, especially those containing the amino acid tyrosine.

Other drugs considered opiates also affect norepinephrine use by mimicking the sympathetic effect. A side effect is constipation.

Parasympathetic Blockers

Many of the alkaloid medications are anticholinergic and block the uptake of acetylcholine. Because of its bronchodilator effect, the atropine-like drug, ipratropium, is used to treat chronic bronchitis and emphysema, as well as some forms of asthma.

Withdrawal from medications or other substances that affect the ANS produces a variety of sympathetic effects (e.g., tachycardia, pupil dilation) and parasympathetic effects (e.g., increased tearing, diarrhea). The distress of withdrawal symptoms continues until the body can restore homeostatic balance without the substance.

Pathological Conditions

Compression Syndromes

Compression syndromes, entrapment neuropathies, and nerve impingement (pinched nerve) are disorders of the peripheral nerves characterized by pain or loss of function of the nerves (motor, sensory, or both) as a result of chronic compression. Tissues that can bind and impinge on nerves are the skin, fasciae, muscles, ligaments, and bones.

The most common type of injury to a nerve is an impingement or "pinching" of the nerve. Nerve impingement often occurs at the spine and can be caused when the nerve becomes sandwiched between two spinal bones, pressed on by a bulging disk, or encroached on by bony overgrowth. In addition to impingement, nerves can become "stuck" to surrounding soft tissues (muscles, ligaments, fascia), usually as a result of repetitive motion injuries. This is commonly referred to as a "trapped" nerve, or *nerve entrapment.*

Regardless of the cause, the symptoms are similar—however, the therapeutic intervention is different. Soft tissue approaches are beneficial in entrapment but less so with bony types of impingement.

Shortened muscles and connective tissue (fasciae) often impinge on major and minor nerves, causing discomfort. Because of the structural arrangement of the body, these impingements often occur at major nerve plexuses. The specific nerve root, trunk, or division affected determines the condition, producing disorders such as thoracic outlet syndrome, sciatica, and carpal tunnel syndrome.

If the cervical plexus is impinged, the person most likely will have headaches, neck pain, and breathing difficulties. The muscles most responsible for pressure on the cervical plexus are the suboccipital and sternocleidomastoid muscles. Shortened connective tissue at the cranial base also presses on these nerves. The cervical plexus is formed by the ventral rami of the upper four cervical nerves. The phrenic nerve is part of this plexus and innervates the diaphragm. Any disruption to this nerve affects breathing. Many cutaneous (skin) branches of the cervical plexus transmit sensory impulses from the skin of the neck, ear area, and shoulder. The motor branches innervate muscles of the anterior neck. Impingement causes pain in these areas.

The brachial plexus is situated partly in the neck and partly in the axilla and consists of virtually all the nerves that innervate the upper limb. Any imbalance that increases pressure on this complex of nerves can result in pain in the shoulder, chest, arm, wrist, and hand. The muscles most often responsible for impingement on the brachial plexus are the scalene, pectoralis minor, and subclavius muscles. The muscles of the arm also occasionally impinge on branches of the brachial plexus. Brachial plexus impingement is responsible for thoracic outlet symptoms, which are often are misdiagnosed as carpal tunnel syndrome. Whiplash injury often causes impingement on the brachial plexus.

Carpal tunnel syndrome is caused by compression of the median nerve as it passes under the transverse carpal ligament at the palmar aspect of the wrist. The condition often occurs in postmenopausal females but also occurs in conditions in which fluid retention causes swelling of the hand and wrist. The syndrome is common in workers who use their hands in repetitive movements, usually because of inflammation that results in compression of the nerve. The symptoms are palmar pain and numbness in the first three digits. Surgically opening the transverse carpal ligament sometimes helps relieve the pain.

Impingement on the lumbar plexus gives rise to low back discomfort, which is marked by a belt-like distribution of pain and pain in the lower abdomen, genitals, thigh, and medial lower leg. The main muscles that impinge on the lumbar plexus are the quadratus lumborum and the psoas muscles. Shortening of the lumbar dorsal fascia exaggerates lordosis and can cause vertebral impingement on the lumbar plexus.

The sacral plexus has about a dozen named branches. About half of these serve the buttock and lower limb; the others innervate pelvic structures. The main branch is the sciatic nerve. Impingement on this nerve by the piriformis muscle gives rise to sciatica. Shortened ligaments that stabilize the sacroiliac joint can affect the sacral plexus. Pressure on the sacral plexus can cause pain in the gluteal muscles, leg, genitals, and foot.

INDICATIONS/CONTRAINDICATIONS for Therapeutic Massage

Various forms of massage reduce muscle spasms, lengthen shortened muscles, and support normal sliding of connective tissue, restoring a more normal space around a nerve and alleviating impingement and entrapment. When massage is combined with other appropriate methods, surgery is seldom necessary. If surgery is performed, the practitioner must consider the potential for scar tissue adhesion to prevent reentrapment of the nerve. The outcome targets maintaining soft tissue suppleness around the healing surgical area and, as healing progresses, using therapeutic massage to deal more directly with the forming scar. In general, work close to the surgical area can begin after the stitches have been removed and all inflammation has abated. Direct work on a new scar is usually safe after 8 weeks into healing. Nerve compression conditions generally resolve, and although the client may be fearful of pain at first, it is important to remember to avoid increasing the fear of movement by overly focusing on the pain experience.

Nerve Root Compression

Many different conditions can result in compression of the nerve root, including tumors, vertebrae changes, and muscle spasms (entrapment) and tissue shortening. Disk degeneration is a common cause. As the degeneration progresses and the fluid content of the disk decreases, the disk becomes narrower. As a result, the amount of space between vertebrae declines. Because spinal nerves exit and enter the spaces between the vertebrae, this situation increases the likelihood of nerve root compression. The condition most commonly occurs in the areas where the spine moves the most: C6 to C7, T12 to L1, L3 to L4, and L5 to S1. The result is radiating nerve pain (radicular), often associated with protective and stabilizing muscle spasms, weakness, or both. It is unclear why some people experience nerve pain with vertebral and disk changes and others do not.

Disk Herniation

Disk herniation occurs when the fibrocartilage surrounding the intervertebral disk ruptures, releasing the nucleus pulposus, which cushions the vertebrae above and below. The resultant pressure on spinal nerve roots may cause pain and damage the surrounding nerves. This condition most often occurs in the lumbar region and involves the L4 or L5 disk and L5 or S1 nerve roots. This particular back pain radiates from the gluteal area down the lateral side or back of the thigh to the leg or foot. Back strain or injury may result in disk herniation and coughing and sneezing occasionally precipitate the condition.

The symptoms of herniation are similar to those produced by a compressed disk but are often more severe. In extreme cases, surgical intervention may be necessary; however, more conservative measures usually are attempted first. Conservative treatment consists of rest, exercise, and other methods, including massage to reduce spasms. Traction can be beneficial.

Spondylolisthesis

Spondylolisthesis occurs when a bone (vertebra) in the spine moves forward out of the proper position onto the bone below it. This movement can cause nerve compression. The condition mostly affects people aged above 50.

Bone disease and fractures can also cause spondylolisthesis. Any activity that hyperextends the spine can lead to a stress fracture on one or both sides of the vertebra. A stress fracture can cause a spinal bone to become weak and shift out of place. The result is a compression of a nerve and radicular pain. Symptoms of spondylolisthesis may range from mild to severe. A person with spondylolisthesis may have no symptoms. The symptoms of spondylolisthesis vary widely depending on the location and severity of the displaced vertebra. Common symptoms include pain or numbness in the region that worsens when the person twists or bends over.

INDICATIONS/CONTRAINDICATIONS for Therapeutic Massage

Various forms of massage are important for managing the muscle spasms and pain associated with nerve root compression and disk herniation. Remember that the muscle spasms serve a stabilizing and protective function called *guarding*. Without some protective spasm, the nerve could be damaged further, but too much muscle spasm increases the discomfort. Therapeutic intervention seeks to reduce pain and excessive tension and restore moderate mobility while allowing for the resourceful compensation produced by the muscle tension pattern. Because low back pain is a common disorder, the massage practitioner must be familiar with its causes and treatment protocols. Limit or avoid the prone position during massage. Lying on the stomach causes hyperextension of the spine. If the prone position is necessary, bolster under the abdomen to maintain a neutral spine.

Viral Infections

Bell Palsy

Bell palsy causes partial or total paralysis of the facial muscles on one side as the result of inflammation or injury to the seventh cranial nerve. The exact cause of the inflammation is unknown, but current research suggests a reactivation of the herpes simplex virus as one of the probable causes. Mechanical causes include bone spurs, tumors, or temporomandibular joint disorders. Bell palsy also occurs in persons affected by diabetes and Lyme disease. The facial nerve swells and is compressed in its narrow course through the temporal bone. The primary method of treatment is oral administration of steroids. The condition usually resolves and normal functioning returns within 6 weeks.

Guillain-Barré Syndrome

Guillain-Barré syndrome, or infectious polyneuritis, may occur 1 or 2 months after a viral infection. Lymphocytes and macrophages invade the myelin sheath, causing partial demyelination. The person develops tingling in the hands or feet, motor weakness, and a decrease in deep tendon reflexes; mild sensory loss ensues. Paralysis usually begins in the legs and moves upward. Facial weakness is common and may appear as Bell palsy. Sometimes respiratory support must be given. Most individuals recover in a few weeks.

Herpes

Herpes zoster, or shingles, is a self-limiting viral disease in which groups of vesicles (fluid-filled blisters) appear along a cutaneous nerve distribution, usually on one side of the trunk. Pain occurs before the rash is visible. The varicella-zoster virus, a member of the Herpesviridae family, is the same virus that causes chickenpox. Some researchers believe that after infection, the virus remains in the body in an inactive state in the dorsal root ganglia. In a healthy person, the immune system keeps the virus in check when it tries to flare up. If the immune system becomes compromised for any reason, it may not be able to contain the virus, and the result is shingles. Primary treatment consists of administration of an analgesic and the antiviral medication acyclovir.

The herpes simplex virus, which is categorized as type 1 or type 2, causes contagious, chronic viral infections that produce painful, fluid-filled blisters on the skin and mucous membranes. Outbreaks seem to be related to stress. Acyclovir can control the symptoms and accelerate healing but does not destroy the virus or cure the infection. Herpes virus lies dormant in the nerve between outbreaks.

Polio

Polio is a viral infection, first of the intestines and then (for about 1% of exposed persons) the anterior horn cells of the spinal cord. The destruction of CNS motor neurons leads to degeneration, atrophy, and finally paralysis of skeletal muscles. Effective vaccines prevent polio, but the virus remains active; however, infection is rare. There is concern about a rise in the number of cases if childhood vaccinations for the virus decline. Post-polio syndrome may occur in individuals who contracted the virus. Symptoms include tiredness, muscle weakness, and muscle and joint pain.

Multiple or Unknown Causes

Multiple Sclerosis

Multiple sclerosis is a disease of autoimmune or viral cause (or both) in which myelin degenerates in random areas of the CNS. Hard, plaque-like lesions replace the destroyed myelin,

INDICATIONS/CONTRAINDICATIONS for Therapeutic Massage

Massage approaches for infectious diseases can be supportive and can reduce stress. Massage can help control the number of recurrent outbreaks by managing stress, especially in recurring viral conditions. The practitioner must follow Standard Precautions with any contagious disease. The person's total stress load is a key factor. When a person is immunocompromised to the extent that they are susceptible to viral and bacterial disease, the stress load is greater. The practitioner should keep in mind that many forms of massage produce stress in a therapeutic sense. One must gauge the intensity and duration of any therapeutic intervention so that the demand on the body to adapt does not overtax an already stressed system, aggravating the condition. The "less-is-more" philosophy of intervention, which calls for shorter, more frequent interventions, often is indicated. Massage is beneficial for post-polio syndrome as part of an integrated healthcare approach.

and inflammatory cells invade affected areas. The myelin around the axons is lost, impairing nerve conduction, and weakness, diminished coordination, gait difficulties, incontinence, vision problems, and speech disturbances occur. Multiple sclerosis is a chronic condition with periodic remissions because the axon is preserved even though the myelin degenerates. Relapse shows some indication of the condition being responsive to stress. Multiple sclerosis should not be confused with amyotrophic lateral sclerosis, which involves the degeneration of motor neurons.

Myasthenia Gravis

Myasthenia gravis is a disorder of neuromuscular transmission that usually affects muscles in the face, lips, tongue, neck, and throat, which are innervated by the cranial nerves; however, the condition can affect any muscle group. Eventually, muscle fibers may degenerate, and weakness, especially of the head, neck, trunk, and limb muscles, may become irreversible. When the disease involves the respiratory system, it may be life threatening.

The disease follows an unpredictable course, with periodic exacerbations and remissions. Spontaneous remissions occur in about 25% of patients. No cure exists, but thanks to drug therapy, patients may lead relatively normal lives except during exacerbations.

The cause of myasthenia gravis is unknown. The condition commonly accompanies autoimmune and thyroid disorders.

INDICATIONS/CONTRAINDICATIONS for Therapeutic Massage

Massage can be an effective part of a comprehensive, long-term care program. Stress management is a key component of an overall care program for any chronic disease. Massage and other forms of bodywork can help manage secondary muscle tension caused by the alteration of posture and the use of equipment such as wheelchairs, braces, and crutches. As previously mentioned, because therapeutic massage produces some stress, the practitioner must gauge the intensity and duration of any therapeutic intervention so as not to aggravate the condition.

Neurotransmitter-Based Disorders

Depression

Depression is one of the more common causes of physical complaints that are a manifestation of underlying psychiatric illness. Many forms of depression respond to medications that increase norepinephrine, dopamine, or serotonin in certain synapses in particular areas of the brain. Although primarily considered a CNS disease, dysfunction can be linked to synaptic transmission as the PNS delivers information to the CNS.

INDICATIONS/CONTRAINDICATIONS for Therapeutic Massage

Massage has the effect of increasing the availability of the neurotransmitters related to depression and may play an important part in the care program for depression. Aerobic exercise is another vital component in depression management. These methods use the PNS as the point of access.

Anxiety States

Anxiety states are classified into two basic types, endogenous anxiety and exogenous (reactive) anxiety. Endogenous anxiety is a biochemical phenomenon that is usually unrelated to environmental stimuli. An example of this type is panic disorder, which involves hyperventilation syndrome and other breathing difficulties, heart palpitations, chest pain, dizziness, sweating, and feelings of impending doom. An increase in the activity of the neurotransmitters GABA, epinephrine, and norepinephrine is implicated. Antianxiety medication often is prescribed.

Breathing pattern disorder may be an underlying factor in anxiety, resulting in a change in body chemistry that alters the feedback loop mechanisms. Restrictions in the soft tissue or the bony structures of the thorax may interfere with appropriate breathing, predisposing a person to breathing in excess of physical need. Massage to the full body, as well as a specific focus on the thorax, can be effective in restoring more balanced function and supporting appropriate breathing. Breathing retraining may be a principal factor in managing anxiety.

Exogenous (reactive) anxiety is prompted by anxiety-provoking stimuli, such as specific events, situations, relationships, and conflicts. Management of this type of anxiety requires dealing with the precipitating difficulties directly or improving mechanisms and skills for coping with environmental or social problems. Making changes in stressful situations, resolving smoldering conflicts, using relaxation methods, and cognitive restructuring of the client's views of the situation are helpful. Professional counseling often is beneficial. Other helpful measures include avoiding caffeine, exercising regularly, eating a healthy diet, and generally gaining control over those things we can control ourselves.

Both types of anxiety can be thought of as activation of the sympathetic ANS. With endogenous anxiety, a faulty internal feedback system results in panic. With exogenous anxiety, the tendency to respond with fight-or-flight behavior is present, but some sort of inhibition of those feelings is in place. What occurs is a fight-or-flight response without the appropriate expression; it therefore is internalized as anxiety.

INDICATIONS/CONTRAINDICATIONS for Therapeutic Massage

Massage and exercise often are effective as part of a comprehensive management strategy for dealing with anxiety symptoms.

Trauma. Trauma results from an event, series of events, or set of circumstances that is experienced by an individual as physically or emotionally harmful or threatening and that has lasting adverse effects on the individual's functioning and physical, social, emotional, or spiritual well-being. A traumatic experience can be a single event or a series of events. It generally overwhelms an individual's ability to cope, and it often ignites the "fight, flight, or freeze" reaction. It frequently produces a sense of fear, vulnerability, and helplessness. A traumatized person can feel a range of emotions both immediately after the event and in the long term. They may feel overwhelmed, helpless, shocked, or have difficulty processing their experiences. Trauma can also cause physical symptoms. It is important to know that the experience of trauma is subjective, individually based on the person's perception.

Trauma can have long-term effects on the person's well-being. If symptoms persist and do not decrease in severity, it can indicate that the trauma has developed into a mental health disorder called post-traumatic stress disorder (PTSD). Symptoms include severe anxiety, flashbacks and persistent memories of the event, and avoidance behaviors. Biological alterations associated with PTSD include changes in limbic system functioning, hypothalamic-pituitary-adrenal axis activity changes with variable cortisol levels, and neurotransmitter-related dysregulation of arousal and endogenous opioid systems. Stress responses of the autonomic nervous system are altered.

INDICATIONS/CONTRAINDICATIONS

A trauma-informed perspective views trauma-related symptoms and behaviors as an individual's best and most resilient attempt to manage, cope with, and rise above experiences of trauma. Trauma-informed care (TIC) involves a broad understanding of traumatic stress reactions and common responses to trauma. Massage therapy can calm the nervous system. However, the manifestations of trauma are complex and the massage therapist needs to expand skills related to TIC and work in an interdisciplinary manner.

Trauma-Informed Care in Behavioral Health Services—NCBI Bookshelf (https://www.nih.gov)

Neuropathy

Neuropathy is the inflammation or degeneration of the peripheral nerves. *Neuralgia* is severe nerve pain caused by a variety of noninflammatory disorders of the nervous system. *Neuritis* is the inflammation of a nerve.

Side effects of various cancer treatments involve neuropathy. Complex regional pain syndrome (reflex sympathetic dystrophy) is also called *causalgia syndrome.* With this syndrome, pain is caused by a soft tissue or bone injury that does not follow a normal healing course. Instead, the pain continues, for no known reason, after the healing process is complete. Ketoacidosis and a hypoglycemic reaction of diabetes cause diabetic neuropathy because they affect the myelin covering of the neuron. The condition is a painful and severe complication of diabetes for which effective control measures are limited. One such pain control measure is hyperstimulation analgesia, which interrupts the pain for a brief period.

Trigeminal neuralgia (tic douloureux) causes sudden, severe pain in the jaw area on one side of the face. Often the pain is caused by chewing or simply by touching the face. Usually, the problem is contact between a normal blood vessel and the trigeminal nerve. This contact puts pressure on the nerve and causes it to malfunction. Extreme caution should be exercised if any form of therapy is to be performed in this area.

INDICATIONS/CONTRAINDICATIONS for Therapeutic Massage

Nerve pain is difficult to manage, does not respond well to analgesics, and often is intractable. Because of its interface with the nervous system, massage may provide short-term, symptomatic pain relief through shifts in neurotransmitters and stimulation of alternate nerve pathways, resulting in hyperstimulation analgesia and counterirritation. Any therapy that increases mood-elevating and pain-modulating mechanisms makes coping with nerve pain somewhat easier for short periods.

Headache

Headache is a common symptom with a multitude of causes. Because the brain has no sensory innervation, headaches do not originate in the brain. The pain of a headache is produced by pressure on the sensory nerves, vessels, meninges, or the muscle-tendon-bone unit.

A tension, or muscle contraction, headache is the most common type. Tension headaches are believed to be caused by a muscle-tendon strain at the origin of the trapezius and deep neck muscles at the occipital bone or the origin of the frontalis muscle on the frontal bone (occipital or frontal headaches). Tension headaches can also originate in the temporomandibular joint muscle complex. Connective tissue structures that support the head may be implicated in headaches if they are shortened and pull the head into nerves, creating pain. Conversely, if connective tissue support structures are lax and fail to support the neck and head, nerve structures may be compressed as well.

The treatment for most headaches is nonsteroidal antiinflammatory drugs, such as aspirin and ibuprofen.

INDICATIONS/CONTRAINDICATIONS for Therapeutic Massage

Massage and other forms of soft tissue therapy are effective in treating muscle tension headaches. Because stress often induces headaches, stress management in all forms is usually indicated in chronic headache conditions.

Vertigo

Vertigo is the sensation that the body or environment is spinning or swaying. It can occur when disturbances occur in the inner ear balance mechanism or between the visual-vestibular balance mechanisms. The most common type of vertigo is benign paroxysmal positional vertigo. This condition occurs when otolith particles in the inner ear stimulate movement sensations that do not exist. Muscle tension, nausea, and mood disturbances, particularly anxiety, can result.

Enteric-Based Pathology

The ENS is now well recognized by gastroenterologists as the "brain in the gut." This is because it controls gut function, including motility, secretion, absorption, blood flow, and aspects of the immune system. Many GI disorders, such as colitis and irritable bowel syndrome (IBS), originate from problems within the gut's ENS. Also, pathophysiological mechanisms underlying CNS disorders often involve the ENS. Many neurotransmitters are common to the CNS and ENS, and similar mechanisms govern the development of both systems. Inflammatory neuropathy of the ENS is emerging as a cause of pathology. The ENS may trigger big emotional shifts experienced by people coping with IBS or with functional bowel problems, such as constipation, diarrhea, bloating, pain, and stomach upset. Enteric neuropathy is a degenerative neuromuscular condition of the digestive system in which the gut stops functioning. The main symptom of enteric neuropathy is severe and constant pain. Other symptoms include nausea, vomiting, diarrhea, constipation, bloating, and abdominal abnormalities.

Dysautonomia

Dysautonomia is a nervous system disorder that disrupts autonomic body processes. Symptoms include the following: Orthostic Intolerance: Dizziness, lightheadedness, or fainting upon standing. Gastrointestinal Issues: Nausea, bloating, constipation, or diarrhea. Temperature Regulation Problems: Excessive sweating or difficulty maintaining body temperature. Heart Rate Abnormalities: Rapid heart rate (tachycardia) or slow heart rate (bradycardia). Urinary Dysfunction: Difficulty emptying the bladder or frequent urination. Management focuses on symptom relief, lifestyle changes, medications, physical therapy, and stress management.

INDICATIONS/CONTRAINDICATIONS for Therapeutic Massage

Movement therapies can help or aggravate vertigo; therefore the practitioner must take care to design an individual therapeutic program based on the client's history. Massage methods can deal effectively with muscle tension and diminish anxiety and nausea, but the benefit is temporary because the symptoms return with a recurrence of vertigo.

Massage therapy that produces a calm state interacts with the brain-gut axis. When a person becomes stressed enough to trigger the fight-or-flight response, digestion slows or even stops. In response to less severe stress, the digestive process may slow or may be temporarily disrupted, causing abdominal pain and other symptoms of functional GI disorders. Persistent GI problems can heighten anxiety and stress. Massage therapy, with the targeted outcome of stress management, could be beneficial in a comprehensive treatment plan for managing dysautonomia.

Review What You Have Learned

- Describe the action of medications prescribed for pathologies of the PNS.
  - Alpha-adrenergic blockers (alpha blockers) lower blood pressure and increase circulation. Beta-adrenergic medications, which include epinephrine (adrenaline, a beta-1 or beta-2 agonist), are commonly used in respiratory disorders, such as in inhalers to dilate bronchial tubes, thereby increasing the blood flow to the lungs. Beta-adrenergic blockers (beta blockers) reduce the force and/or rate of heart muscle contractions. Parasympathetic blockers block the uptake of acetylcholine to reduce parasympathetic activity in the PNS.
- List the common pathologies of the PNS.
  - Compression syndromes (entrapment neuropathies, nerve impingement, nerve entrapment). Potential causes: disk herniation, disk degeneration, spondylolisthesis. Viral infections (Bell palsy, Guillain-Barré syndrome/infectious polyneuritis, herpes/shingles, polio). Multiple/unknown causes: multiple sclerosis, myasthenia gravis. Neurotransmitter-based disorders: depression, anxiety. Neuropathy; headache; vertigo. Enteric-based pathology: colitis, irritable bowel syndrome. ANS dysregulation: dysautonomia.
- Discuss indications and contraindications, including cautions and adaptations, of massage therapy for pathological conditions of the PNS.
  - *Contraindications:* Acute injuries or infections; regional and systemic conditions—applications that may aggravate the condition. *Indications:* Stress and pain management outcomes support the emotional and physical demands related to chronic conditions. Massage is an effective adjunct for three categories of care: palliative, condition management, and therapeutic change. *Adaptations:* The massage therapist should use a less-is-more approach with regard to intensity and duration to make sure not to overtax an already stressed system. The client should be repositioned to limit physical stressors on condition sites (e.g., limiting or adapting the prone position in cases of lumbar nerve root compression). *Caution:* Always follow proper sanitary guidelines, including added precautions if a client has a contagious disease.

SUMMARY

Understanding how the PNS works specifically influences the massage practitioner's ability to plan and arrange an effective massage session. Massage applications and outcomes the client experiences from the massage session depend on the practitioner's knowledge of the physiological effects of massage manipulations and techniques. Understanding the normal function and pathological conditions of the PNS helps the massage professional make good decisions about indications for and contraindications to massage.

In this chapter we studied the PNS, its components, and the names of its many parts. We presented valuable information about reflexes and sensory receptors because these portions of the PNS function directly with massage.

CRITICAL THINKING/CLINICAL REASONING

Each chapter features a critical thinking and clinical reasoning application of the content related to massage therapy practice. A client scenario is presented, with recommendations for additional research, often using MedlinePlus or PubMed. Relevant questions based on the chapter content are provided to guide discussion. There are no specific correct answers to the questions. However, responses should support evidence-informed practices and should be based on biological plausibility if sufficient research is not available. The authors' decision-making process related to the scenario and questions is on the Evolve site. Compare and contrast your thoughts and discussion with the authors and determine where you agree or disagree.

Scenario

A client has been receiving massage therapy on and off for years and was recently referred to you for therapeutic massage. The client experiences a cluster of symptoms that primarily involve the peripheral nervous system, particularly sympathetic ANS function. The client is 54 years old and in relatively good health but complains of a racing heart, stomach upset, and neck and shoulder pain. They also tend to experience left brachial plexus entrapment. Concerning is that the symptom pattern is extremely similar to heart attack symptoms. The client has been thoroughly examined for cardiac pathology, and none currently exists. Their physician attributes most of their problems to stress.

The client has an arthritic knee that was injured during military service and has used various complementary therapies, with varying success. The best pain control is with acupuncture. The client occasionally experiences some inner ear balance issues and seasonal sinusitis. The referring massage therapist indicates that the client gets a little dizzy as soon as they sit up after the massage, but it goes away quickly. The client prefers a general full-body massage with firm pressure.

- Explore: MedlinePlus using the search terms *brachial plexus impingement, heart attack symptoms, stress response*, and *knee arthritis*
- Search PubMed for any research validating the benefits of acupuncture for knee pain.

Discuss These Points

- Which conditions are most related to the somatic nervous system and which to the autonomic nervous system?
- Which reflex pattern would be an indication that a heart attack could be occurring?
- How are the brachial plexus entrapment, stress response, and cardiac symptoms related?
- Which aspect of the somatic nervous system would the massage most influence?
- What symptoms are related to the vestibular system?
- How might massage therapy help reduce stress-related symptoms?
- Do you think the client has any symptoms indicating enteric nervous system involvement?
- Of the five basic senses, which one is most closely related to the vestibular symptoms?
- What do you think the client would have as target areas for the massage application? How would a general nonspecific massage target those areas?

We reinforced the role of the ANS, the body-mind connection. We discussed the five basic senses briefly and related massage to specific functions of the PNS for four of the five. We will discuss touch to a much greater extent in Chapter 11. A student of massage would do well to learn this particular material thoroughly because massage therapy works closely with the PNS. Such an understanding can only further the benefits to the clients we serve.

Visit the Evolve website: https://evolve.elsevier.com/Fritz/essential/

The Evolve website provides support for the review of the chapter content and chapter quizzes to help you prepare for the MBLEx or other massage therapy certification or licensing exams. End-of-chapter questions for discussion and review answer key and rationales and authors' response to critical thinking and clinical reasoning scenarios.

MULTIPLE CHOICE QUESTIONS FOR REVIEW AND DISCUSSION

The answers, with rationales, can be found on the Evolve site.

These questions are used for review and discussion. It is as important to understand why wrong answers are wrong as it is to know why the correct answer is correct. The answers to the questions, with rationales and explanations about why the correct answer is correct and why wrong answers are wrong, can be found on the Evolve site. Guidance is also provided on how questions are developed and how the textbook content can be presented in a multiple choice question format. At the end of the question section here in the textbook, you will find an Exercise that asks you to write more questions. Use the various questions in the chapter as examples. This is one of the best study strategies for test taking.

It is important to understand that the actual licensing exam you take may not contain any of the specific questions found in this textbook or the review material and practice tests on the Evolve site. Therefore just because you can answer any of these questions correctly does not mean you will pass the licensing exam. The questions are content and style examples to help you prepare—this is why understanding why wrong answers are wrong is just as important as identifying the correct answer. Also, make sure you understand all the terminology used in the questions and possible answers in the review and discussion questions. Look up words you do not understand.

1. A client is experiencing radiating pain in the abdomen and buttocks. Which statement is most accurate?
   a. The femoral nerve in the sacral plexus is impinged.
   b. The client has compression of the thoracodorsal nerve.
   c. The client's symptoms involve the lumbar plexus.
   d. The client's symptoms involve the brachial plexus.
2. During the assessment, the massage therapist notices that the client has dilated pupils. What would be the most logical cause of this condition?
   a. The client is experiencing sympathetic dominance.
   b. The client is experiencing parasympathetic dominance.

c. The client has a somatic dysfunction.
d. The accessory nerve is damaged.

3. A client is extremely sensitive to scent and can get anxious if the smell of something is not pleasing. Which statement explains this reaction?
a. Smell is controlled by the vagus nerve.
b. Smell is an aspect of the limbic system.
c. Smell directly affects endocrine function.
d. Smell is a vestibular process.

4. Pain, tingling, and numbness in the arm and hand may result from nerve damage in which plexus?
a. Cervical
b. Brachial
c. Lumbar
d. Sacral

5. During massage, pain that is not related to specific symptoms radiates around the ear. This indicates excessive pressure on which nerve?
a. Greater auricular
b. Thoracodorsal
c. Medial cutaneous
d. Pudendal

6. During the history interview, a client reported that they almost fell downstairs but caught themselves and was able to regain balance. What type of reflex action was required to accomplish this?
a. Monosynaptic
b. Polysynaptic
c. Patellar
d. Pacinian

7. A client is having difficulty being comfortable with the touch of draping material during the massage and cannot get used to the scratchy feeling. The client may be displaying a reduced ability of sensory receptors to ______.
a. Send impulses
b. Adapt to sensation
c. Remain monosynaptic
d. Initiate reciprocal inhibition

8. The sensory receptors most affected by deep compression and slow gliding strokes are ______.
a. Pacinian corpuscles
b. Root hair plexuses
c. Merkel disks
d. Ruffini's end organs

9. Which receptors are most likely to adapt and stop responding to sustained compression during massage on one specific area of the body?
a. Meissner corpuscles
b. Thermal receptors
c. Intrafusal fibers
d. Nociceptors

10. A compressive massage method is applied to the belly of a muscle with the intent of reducing a muscle spasm brought on by a cramp. The receptors most affected are the ______.
a. Joint kinesthetic
b. Golgi tendon organ
c. Muscle spindles
d. Meissner corpuscles

11. As a slow, deep gliding stroke is applied to a client's left upper thigh, the massage practitioner notices and the client describes a twitching of the muscles in the back of the opposite leg. What type of reflex has been stimulated?
a. Stretch reflex
b. Tendon reflex
c. Ipsilateral reflex
d. Contralateral reflex

12. A client requests an outcome from the massage session that includes a good night's sleep and less fidgeting. The massage session then would need to be designed to accomplish what?
a. Cranial sacral plexus inhibition
b. Parasympathetic inhibition
c. Sympathetic inhibition
d. Sympathetic dominance

13. Massage and acupuncture share which physiologic effect related to pain sensation reduction?
a. Increased sympathetic arousal
b. Decreased levels of endorphins
c. Influence of substance P release
d. Decreased parasympathetic arousal

14. The massage method that most affects the inner ear balance mechanisms is ______.
a. Percussion
b. Compression
c. Friction
d. Rocking

15. A client complains of difficulty hitting a golf ball and describes a sense of timing being off. This could be a result of a disruption in what type of reflex?
a. Conditioned reflex
b. Tendon reflex
c. Stretch reflex
d. Mono reflex

16. A client reports being prone to headaches from bright light. This has been a problem only in the past few weeks. The client also reports an increase in their workload. What autonomic nervous system function might be responsible for the sensitivity to light?
a. Parasympathetic dilation of the pupil
b. Sympathetic dilation of the pupil
c. Parasympathetic contraction of the pupil
d. Sympathetic contraction of the pupil

17. A client complains of pain radiating down their arm into the elbow and fingers. The client has not been evaluated by a physician, so a referral is indicated. Which diagnosis by the physician would be most helped by massage?
a. Guillain-Barré syndrome
b. Brachial plexus entrapment
c. Cervical plexus compression
d. Osteoporosis

18. A client reports having herpes zoster and is experiencing pain. Which of these would be the best massage approach?
a. A full-body, 1-hour massage, with attention to Standard Precautions, which uses tapotement, active joint movement, and friction methods

b. A full-body, 90-minute massage that avoids the area of the rash and actively engages the client in muscle energy lengthening and stretching
c. A seated massage over clothing that lasts for 15 minutes
d. A full-body, 1-hour massage, with attention to Standard Precautions, which avoids the area of the rash and focuses on relaxation

19. A client seeks massage after a diagnosis of neuralgia in the left leg. Which would be a realistic therapeutic massage outcome?
a. Reduction of pain and regeneration
b. Long-term symptom diminishment
c. Short-term pain management
d. Short-term regeneration

20. A client complains of a recent inability to sleep and a feeling of agitation. The client reports concern over a change in management systems at work. The physician's diagnosis was exogenous anxiety. Which treatment plan is most appropriate?
a. A mild exercise program, therapeutic massage, and a medication such as imipramine to control symptoms
b. A hypoventilation syndrome management program, including massage and chiropractic manipulation
c. A mild exercise program, cognitive-behavioral therapy, short-term use of diazepam, and relaxation massage
d. Therapeutic massage, meditation, increased caffeine consumption, and bed rest

CHAPTER

6 Endocrine System

https://evolve.elsevier.com/Fritz/essential/

CHAPTER OBJECTIVES

After completing this chapter, the learner will be able to:

1. Describe the physiological processes of the endocrine system.
2. List the traditional endocrine glands.
3. Connect the endocrine system to the nervous system through the hypothalamus.
4. Define endocrine tissues and give examples.
5. Describe the hypothalamic-pituitary-adrenal (HPA) axis and its link to the general adaptation syndrome.
6. List and describe the three main hormone types and their functions.
7. Identify the hormones produced by each endocrine gland and their associated functions.
8. Explain why the gut can be considered an endocrine organ.
9. Describe the hypersecretion and hyposecretion pathological conditions of the endocrine system, and list the associated indications and contraindications for massage.

CHAPTER OUTLINE

KEY TERMS

axis: A series of glands that signal each other in a sequence.

endocrine-disrupting chemicals (EDCs): Environmental substances that alter the function of the endocrine system.

endocrine glands: (EN-doe-krin) Ductless glands that secrete hormones directly into the bloodstream.

endorphins: (en-DOR-finz) Peptide hormones that mainly work in the same way as morphine to suppress pain. They influence mood, producing a mild euphoric feeling (e.g., "runner's high").

exocrine glands: (EK-so-krin) Glands that secrete hormones through ducts directly into specific areas. Exocrine glands are part of the endocrine system.

half-life: The time required for half of a hormone to be eliminated from the bloodstream.

hypersecretion: Excessive release of a hormone.

hyposecretion: Insufficient release of a hormone.

hypothalamic-pituitary-adrenal (HPA) axis: A complex set of direct influences and feedback interactions involving the hypothalamus, the pituitary gland, and the adrenal glands.

microbial endocrinology: (mi-CRO-bi-al en-do-crin-OL-o-gy) The study of the ability of microorganisms both to produce and recognize neurochemicals that originate either within the microorganisms themselves or within the host they inhabit.

microbiome: (mi-cro-BI-ome) Entire collection of microorganisms in a specific area of the body, such as the human gut.

negative feedback system: A control mechanism that provides a stimulus to reduce or diminish a function. For example, a fire alarm causes a series of reactions intended to put out the fire.

neuroendocrine system: Interactions that occur between the nervous system and the endocrine system.

tropic (or trophic) hormones: Hormones produced by the endocrine glands that affect other endocrine glands.

LEARNING HOW TO LEARN

Repetition, repetition, and then more repetition. The key is to make each repetition a little different, so your brain remains interested. In the chapters of this textbook, novel repetition is built right in. The key terms are listed at the beginning of the chapter. Section summaries restate information, and the end-of-chapter multiple questions provide terminology repetition as does the critical thinking activity.

As you have learned, the endocrine system and the nervous system control and regulate the body's response to events and return the body to homeostasis. The endocrine system works in partnership with other systems of the body, especially the nervous system, to maintain homeostasis in the body. In this capacity, the endocrine system is involved primarily with physiological functions using chemicals called hormones. Not only are hormones of the endocrine system involved with maintaining homeostasis, but they also direct the creation of our very form, such as our size, shape, and sexual characteristics. Three major physical form processes are controlled and integrated by hormones:

- Reproduction
- Growth
- Development

Therefore hormonal pathological conditions affect functions, as does the nervous system, and can also affect form. The endocrine system uses negative feedback to regulate physiological functions. A **negative feedback system** provides a stimulus to decrease a function. Negative feedback regulates the secretion of almost every hormone.

The key functions of the endocrine system are as follows:

- Regulation of metabolic functions
- Regulation of chemical reactions
- Regulation of the transport of substances through cell membranes

In Chapter 4, we learned that a chemical found in the synapse is called a *neurotransmitter*. When the same chemical is found in the bloodstream or tissue, it is a hormone. Neurotransmitters act on adjacent cells, whereas hormones may travel long distances in the body before they reach their target cells. The main differences between endocrine system and nervous system control are speed and duration of effect:

- The nervous system is fast acting, with a short duration of effect.
- The endocrine system is slow acting, with a long duration of effect.

This offers a balance of control, with the nervous system responding quickly and the endocrine system taking over to sustain a response (Activity 6.1).

ACTIVITY 6.1

Before we go any further in this chapter, do the following. In 1 minute, list as many physiologic processes influenced by hormones as you can. Come back at the end of the chapter and compare your before and after knowledge.

Example
Pregnancy

OVERVIEW OF ENDOCRINE GLANDS AND TISSUES

SECTION OBJECTIVES

Chapter objectives covered in this section:

1. Describe the physiological processes of the endocrine system.
2. List the traditional endocrine glands.
3. Connect the endocrine system to the nervous system through the hypothalamus.
4. Define endocrine tissues and give examples.
5. Describe the hypothalamic-pituitary-adrenal (HPA) axis and its link to the general adaptation syndrome.

After completing this section, the student will be able to:

- Explain the difference between endocrine and exocrine glands.
- List the endocrine glands of the body.
- List the functions of the hypothalamus.
- Describe the HPA axis and its relationship to stress.

MENTORING TIP

In Chapter 2 we discussed feedback loops as a process to maintain homeostasis. Now we learn that negative feedback loops regulate the secretion of almost every hormone. The term *negative feedback* refers to the feedback that reverses the original stimulus, stabilizes physiological functions, and helps us maintain our constant internal environment.

The systems of control become the physiological foundation for self-regulation. Self-correcting systems use feedback loops to influence their expression. Feedback is a necessary aspect of communication. When we give clients a massage, we need feedback to be able to respond, regulate, and adapt the massage application. If the pressure is too light and the client gives us feedback, then we increase the pressure. If the client tells us that the method is painful, then we alter the approach to remain effective but not painful.

We also need to learn to pay attention to nonverbal feedback. A client may tighten up or flinch if the massage application is uncomfortable. The client may begin to breathe more deeply when the massage pressure is satisfying.

Feedback is good most of the time. Sometimes the process gets mixed, and then the result is not what was anticipated. For example, massage therapy should support productive self-regulation. However, if the massage therapist or the sensations produced by the massage send undesirable signals (e.g., being cranky and grumpy during the massage) or physically nonproductive pain (e.g., poking or pinching someone during massage application), the nervous system and the endocrine system can respond in a defensive way.

Endocrine and Exocrine Glands

The **endocrine glands** are ductless glands that secrete hormones directly into the bloodstream or diffuse into nearby tissues (Fig. 6.1). In contrast, **exocrine glands**, or glands with ducts, such as the salivary and sweat glands, secrete their products directly into ducts that open to specific areas.

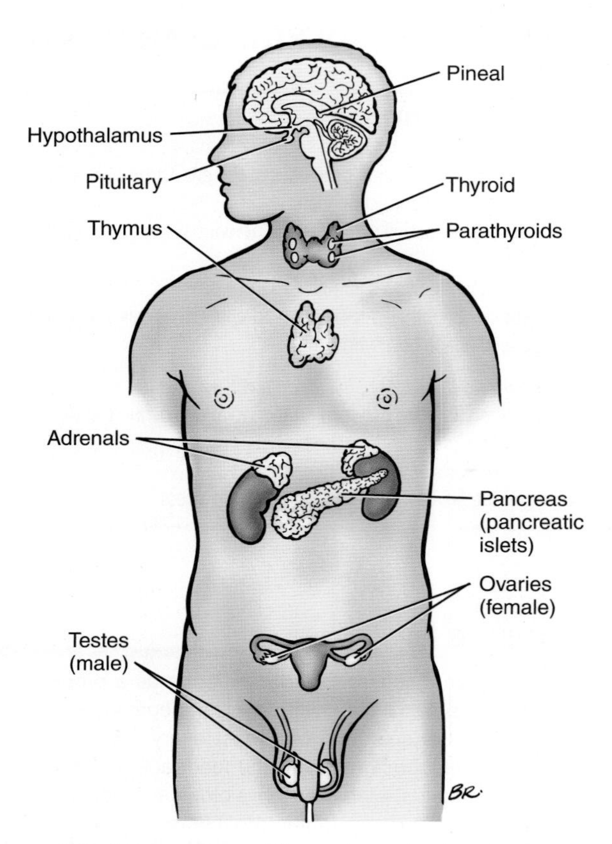

FIG. 6.1 Locations of the major endocrine glands.

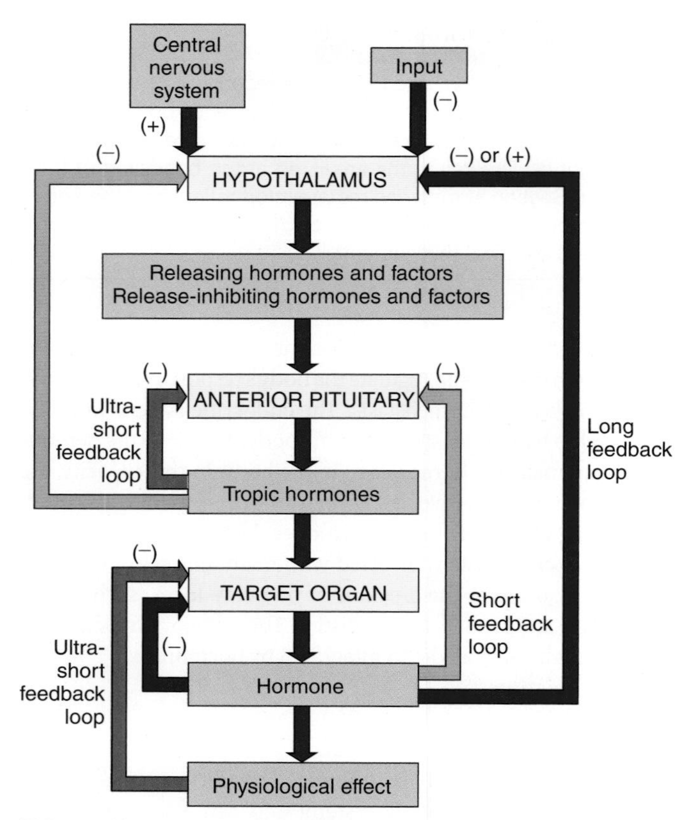

FIG. 6.2 Feedback loops. A general model for control and negative feedback to hypothalamic-pituitary target organ systems. Negative feedback regulation is possible at three levels: target organ (ultrashort feedback), anterior pituitary gland (short feedback), and hypothalamus (long feedback). (From McCance KL, Huether SE. *Pathophysiology: The Biologic Basis for Disease in Adults and Children*. 6th ed. Mosby; 2010.)

The traditional endocrine glands of the body include:

- Pituitary gland
- Hypothalamus
- Thymus
- Pineal gland
- Testes
- Ovaries
- Thyroid
- Adrenal glands
- Parathyroid glands
- Pancreas

Hypothalamus

The hypothalamus is considered part of the nervous system, but it also produces and releases hormones, and thus can be considered a neuroendocrine organ. Pathological conditions are found mainly with hyposecretion (not enough) and hypersecretion (too much). This pattern now should seem familiar as the elegance of the body shows itself in the repetition of basic patterns (Fig. 6.2).

The hypothalamus is the link between the body/mind and nerve/endocrine function. The main purpose of the hypothalamus is homeostasis; for example, its effects on blood pressure, body temperature, and fluid and electrolyte balance. The hypothalamus has the following functions:

- To control blood pressure and electrolyte balance through thirst and salt craving
- To regulate body temperature through the influence of both the autonomic nervous system (ANS) and the behavior that seeks a warmer or cooler environment
- To regulate energy metabolism through influence on feeding behavior, digestion efficiency, and metabolic rate
- To regulate reproduction through hormonal control of sexual and mating behavior, pregnancy, and lactation
- To direct responses to stress by altering blood flow to specific tissues and stimulating the adrenal glands to secrete stress hormones

During stress, the hypothalamus translates nerve impulses into hormone secretions by endocrine glands. The hypothalamus plays a role in:

- Awareness of pleasure and pain
- Expression of emotions, such as fear and rage
- Sexual behaviors

The hypothalamus exerts its primary influence over the pituitary gland, which in turn controls other endocrine glands with tropic hormones. **Tropic** (or **trophic**) **hormones** cause the secretion of other hormones. The hypothalamus secretes releasing or inhibiting hormones that affect the secretion of pituitary hormones.

Psychosocial short stature, failure to thrive syndrome, and delayed tissue healing, which result from stress, emotional disorders, and deprivation are the consequences of suppression of the hypothalamic release of growth hormone–releasing hormone. This hormone signals the secretion of growth hormone from the pituitary gland (Table 6.1).

Table 6.1 Hypothalamic Hormones (Hypophysiotropic Hormones)

Hormone	Target Tissue	Action
Thyrotropin-releasing hormone	Anterior pituitary	Stimulates release of thyroid-stimulating hormone (TSH) Modulates prolactin secretion
Gonadotropin-releasing hormone	Anterior pituitary	Stimulates release of follicle-stimulating hormone (FSH) and luteinizing hormone (LH)
Somatostatin	Anterior pituitary	Inhibits release of growth hormone (GH) and TSH
Growth hormone–releasing factor	Anterior pituitary	Stimulates release of GH
Corticotropin-releasing hormone	Anterior pituitary	Stimulates release of adrenocorticotropic hormone (ACTH) and beta-endorphin
Substance P	Anterior pituitary	Inhibits synthesis and release of ACTH Stimulates secretion of GH, FSH, LH, and prolactin
Dopamine	Anterior pituitary	Inhibits synthesis and secretion of prolactin
Prolactin-releasing factor	Anterior pituitary	Stimulates secretion of prolactin

From McCance KL, Huether SE. *Pathophysiology: The Biologic Basis for Disease in Adults and Children.* 6th ed. Mosby; 2010.

Hypothalamic-Pituitary-Adrenal Axis

When a series of glands signal each other in a sequence, this is called an **axis**. For example, the hypothalamic-pituitary-adrenal axis is a complex set of direct influences and feedback interactions involving the hypothalamus, the pituitary gland, and the adrenal glands. This communication network between the nervous system and the endocrine system is now considered the **neuroendocrine system**. The axis controls the general adaptation syndrome (GAS) described by Dr. Hans Selye, a noted researcher on stress and its effects (Box 6.1).

The **hypothalamic-pituitary-adrenal (HPA) axis** is our central stress response system. The HPA axis's function is kicked off by some sort of stressor. The hypothalamus secretes the corticotropin-releasing hormone, which sends a message to the pituitary. This stimulates the pituitary's ACTH production, and the adrenal glands secrete cortisol and adrenaline. Cortisol raises the blood sugar, and adrenaline raises the heart rate and blood pressure, preparing for the fight-or-flight response of the ANS. These interactions continue until the hormone levels needed for an appropriate response to the stressor are reached. Then a negative feedback loop series of chemical reactions reverses the process to restore homeostasis.

Review What You Have Learned

- Explain the difference between endocrine and exocrine glands.
  - Endocrine glands are ductless glands that secrete hormones into the bloodstream or nearby tissues. Exocrine glands are glands with ducts that secrete hormones into specific areas.
- List the endocrine glands of the body.
  - Pituitary gland, hypothalamus, thymus, pineal gland, testes, ovaries, thyroid, adrenal glands, parathyroid glands, and pancreas.
- Describe the hypothalamus and its functions.
  - The hypothalamus is a neuroendocrine organ—that is, it is part of the nervous system, but it also produces and releases hormones. Its functions are to provide a link between mind/body and nerve/endocrine function; to help maintain homeostasis in many ways (e.g., blood pressure and

Box 6.1 Adipose Tissue Is an Endocrine Tissue

Adipose tissue serves important endocrine functions. It secretes numerous hormone substances, including leptin, resistin, adiponectin, adipsin, acylation-stimulating protein, angiotensinogen, and estradiol. Most of these hormones are involved in several metabolic processes, such as glucose regulation and the metabolism of fat for energy production.

Leptin has received attention because it is involved in appetite and obesity. Leptin acts on receptors in the hypothalamus to inhibit appetite. This system is more sensitive to starvation than to overfeeding. Leptin circulates at levels proportional to body fat.

A condition called *leptin resistance* may be a factor in some types of obesity. This hormone signals the brain that our appetites are satisfied and we can stop eating. Leptin resistance is similar to insulin resistance in diabetics. Leptin resistance occurs when the body fails to transport leptin past the blood-brain barrier to the hypothalamus. For leptin to control body weight and metabolism, it must do so from the hypothalamic centers in the brain. When levels of leptin in the hypothalamus are low as a result of leptin resistance, food cravings and weight gain occur because the body believes that it is hungry and goes into a state of continued fat storage. Recent work from Harvard researchers has tied leptin to a crucial pathway in fat metabolism in muscle. This pathway suggests a role for leptin in clearing fat out of cells and sheds light on the connection between diabetes and obesity.

- Geer EB, Islam J, Buettner C. Mechanisms of glucocorticoid-induced insulin resistance: focus on adipose tissue function and lipid metabolism. *Endocrinol Metab Clin North Am.* 2014;43(1):75–102;
- Birerdinc A, Younossi ZM. Adipose tissue as an endocrine organ. *Clin Liver Dis.* 2014;18(1):41–58;
- Park HK, Ahima RS. Physiology of leptin: energy homeostasis, neuroendocrine function and metabolism. *Metabolism.* 2015;64(1):24–34.
- Kumar SS, Mishra AK, Ghosh AR. Endocrine role of adipose tissue in obesity and related disorders. In: Tappia PS, Ramjiawan B, Dhalla NS, eds. *Cellular and Biochemical Mechanisms of Obesity*. Advances in Biochemistry in Health and Disease. Springer; 2021:23–42.

electrolyte balance, and temperature and metabolic regulation); and to play a role in the expression of emotions, in pain and pleasure awareness, and in sexual behavior.

- Describe the HPA axis and its relationship to stress.
    - The HPA axis is a complex set of relationships and signals involving the hypothalamus, the pituitary gland, and the adrenal glands. The HPA axis acts as our central stress response system. Stressors stimulate the hypothalamus, which sends signals to the pituitary, which stimulates the adrenal glands to secrete cortisol and adrenaline. This continues until negative feedback loops reverse the process to restore homeostasis.

Practical Application

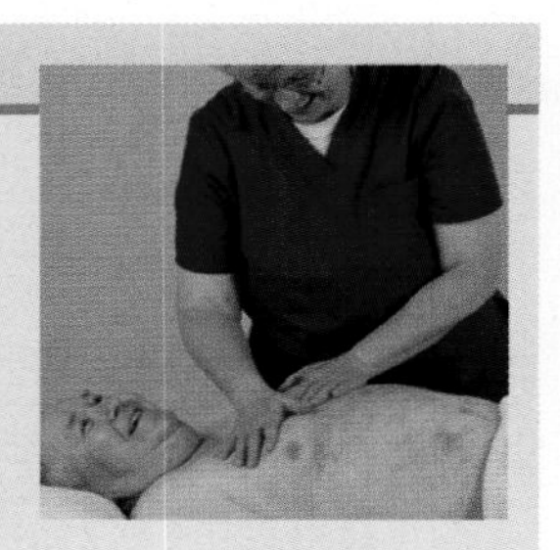

According to the National Institutes of Health, many people use complementary and integrative health care. Complementary healthcare methods, such as massage therapy, are used in conjunction with conventional medicine. Mind/body practices focus on the interactions among the brain, mind, body, and behavior, with the intent to use the mind to affect physical functioning and promote health. At one time these methods were considered alternative or used in place of conventional medicine in pursuit of health and well-being. Now many of these approaches have been integrated into a total health plan. People use massage for a variety of health-related purposes, including relieving pain, rehabilitating sports injuries, reducing stress, increasing relaxation, addressing anxiety and depression, and aiding general well-being. If a non-mainstream practice is used together with conventional medicine, it's considered "complementary."

If a non-mainstream practice is used in place of conventional medicine, it is considered "alternative." True alternative medicine is uncommon. Most people who use non-mainstream approaches use them along with conventional treatments.

The term "integrative health care" has many definitions, but all involve bringing conventional and complementary approaches together in a coordinated way. The US National Center for Complementary and Integrative Health generally uses the term "complementary health approaches" for practices and products of non-mainstream origin and "integrative health" when describing incorporating complementary approaches into mainstream health care.

Other Endocrine Tissues

Endocrine glands are not the only tissues that secrete hormones. Numerous cells and tissues throughout the brain, gut, and cardiovascular system produce hormones as well. New research in **microbial endocrinology** continues to discover endocrine tissues that are separate from the traditional endocrine glands. These local tissue hormones are called *eicosanoids*. The concept of tissue hormones or hormonelike substances (e.g., prostaglandins) has altered and expanded the idea of hormones being carried throughout the blood to distant sites in the body. Prostaglandins not only have a local effect on surrounding tissue, but because they are carried by the blood, they also affect distant sites in the body.

Research now indicates that gut bacteria (microbes) can produce and secrete hormones. The collective bacteria are called **microbiota**. The crosstalk between microbes and hormones can affect host metabolism, immunity, and behavior, and it also exerts control over the HPA axis. The microbiota produces and secretes hormones, responds to host hormones, and regulates the levels of expression of host hormones. The biochemical complexity of the gut microbiota and many of the hormones produced by the microbiota are also neurotransmitters in the central nervous system (CNS). This has broad implications for health maintenance and physical and mental disease.

Examples of endocrine tissues are as follows:

- Placenta
- Heart
- Kidney
- Brain
- Gut
- Adipose tissue (Box 6.2)

Box 6.2 General Adaptation Syndrome

Dr. Hans Selye's research into the effects of stress describes a universal response of the human body to stressors, which he termed the *general adaptation syndrome (GAS)*. There are three stages: alarm, resistance, and exhaustion.

1. **Alarm:** When the stressor is identified, the body's stress response is a state of alarm. The hypothalamic-pituitary-adrenal (HPA) axis is activated. Adrenaline is produced, setting off the fight-or-flight response.
2. **Resistance:** If the stressor persists, attempting some means of coping with the stress becomes necessary. The adrenal glands begin producing cortisol. The resistance stage can be thought of as enduring. Although the body tries to adapt to demands, it cannot keep this up indefinitely, and functioning reserves become depleted. The ability to maintain homeostasis is strained.
3. **Exhaustion:** The body's resources are depleted, and the body is unable to sustain normal function. The ability to maintain homeostasis is lost. Long-term damage may result as the capacity of glands, especially the adrenal gland, and the immune system is exhausted and function is impaired, resulting in illness.

Endocrine Glands and Ancient Healing Traditions

As identified in previous chapters, various ancient healing traditions have described physiological functions using analogies or examples to explain what was observable based on behavior or signs and symptoms of disease. The endocrine glands have important implications in the Eastern chakra system. The chakra system is a mapping of energy centers with interesting anatomical correlations to the ANS plexus and functional aspects interrelated with the endocrine gland functions. Many Eastern healing traditions (e.g., Ayurvedic, Tibetan) work from this knowledge base, just as many Asian healing philosophies were developed around the meridian system.

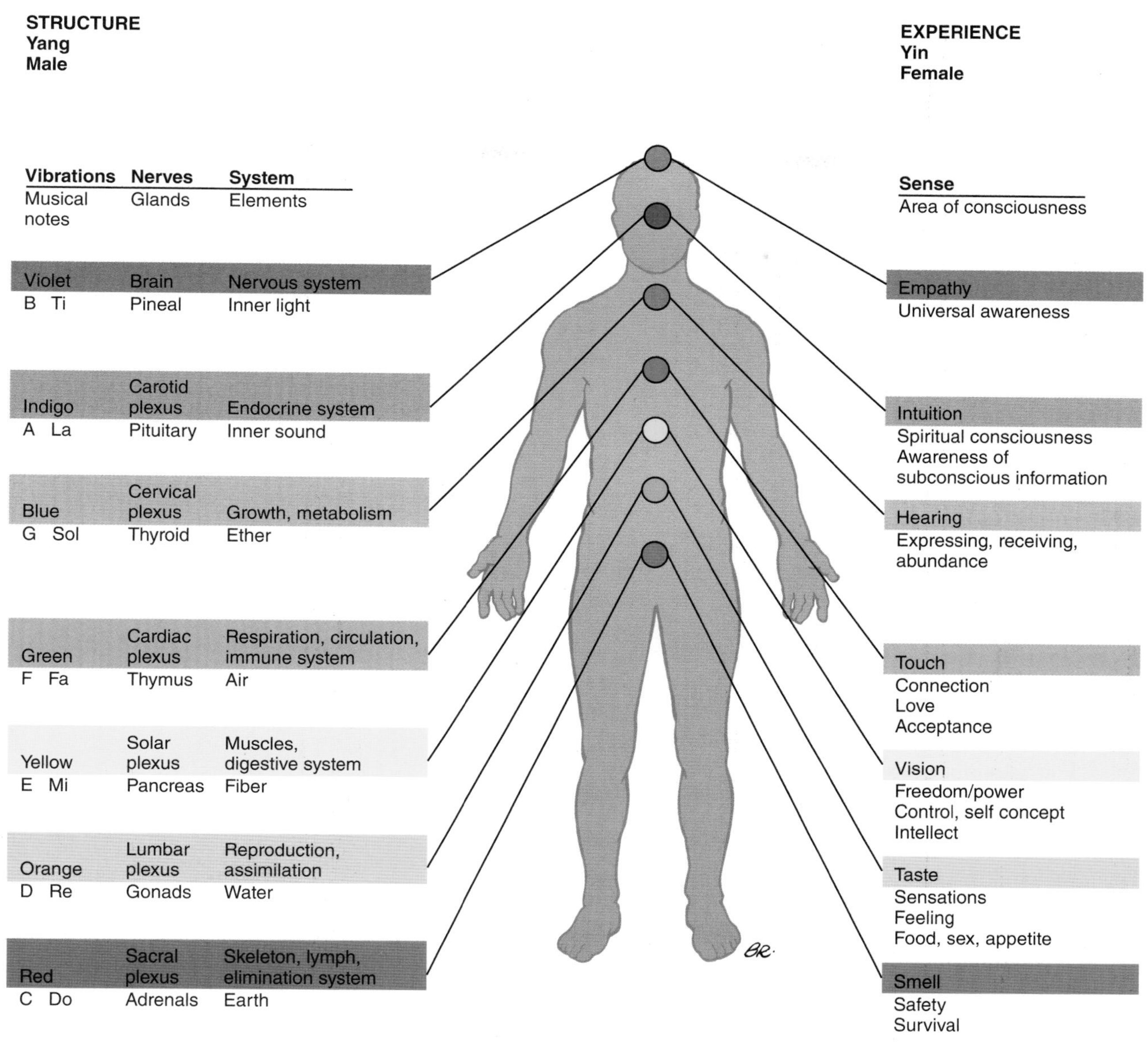

FIG. 6.3 Name and location of major chakras. There is a correlation between each of the major chakras and the endocrine glands.

The body of knowledge of the chakra system is expansive and consistent with Western scientific thought once the language and concepts are understood. Just as the meridian system sees anatomy and physiology as an interrelated system encompassing emotional energy conjoined with the major organs, the chakra system represents similar patterns in relationship to the endocrine functions (Fig. 6.3).

ENDOCRINE GLANDS, TISSUES, AND THEIR HORMONES

SECTION OBJECTIVES

Chapter objectives covered in this section:

6. List and describe the three main hormone types and their functions.
7. Identify the hormones produced by each endocrine gland and their associated functions.
8. Explain why the gut can be considered an endocrine organ.

After completing this section, the learner will be able to:

- List three main hormone types.
- List endocrine glands and describe the functions of their secreted hormones.
- Describe the hormone function of the gut microbiome.

Hormones

Hormones are secreted from endocrine glands and tissues. Each hormone causes a response in a specific target organ or group of cells, rather than on the body as a whole (Fig. 6.4). Exocrine hormones are secreted through a duct into the blood and usually affect a distant organ or tissue. Endocrine hormones are secreted within the tissue and enter the bloodstream through capillaries.

There are three main types of hormones:

- *Amines* are simple molecules.
- *Proteins* and *peptides* are chains of amino acids.
- *Steroids* are derived from cholesterol (Table 6.2).

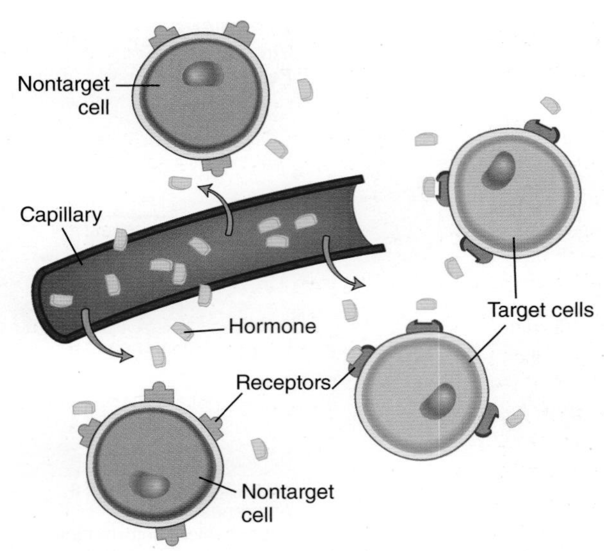

FIG. 6.4 The target cell concept. A hormone acts only on cells that have receptors specific to that hormone because the shape of the receptor determines which hormones can react with it. This is an example of the lock-and-key model of biochemical reactions. (From Lewis SL, Dirksen SR, Heitkemper MM, Bucher L.*Medical Surgical Nursing: Assessment and Management of Clinical Problems*. 9th ed. Mosby; 2014.)

The hormones of the endocrine system maintain homeostasis as we respond to life events and our real or perceived emotions and resulting moods. Functional aspects of hormone molecules include the mobilization of body defenses against stressors; maintenance of electrolyte, water, and nutrient balance of the blood; and regulation of cellular metabolism and energy balance.

Hormones exert their effect on target organs and cells at low blood concentrations. The concentration of a hormone in the blood is determined by the rate of release and the speed of inactivation and removal from the body. The influence of a hormone in the blood can range from seconds to 30 minutes.

The term **half-life** describes the time required for half of the hormone to be eliminated from the bloodstream. After this occurs, the effect is slowed. Hormones require various lengths of time to generate noticeable influences in the body or on behavior. Some hormones promote target organ responses almost immediately, such as the effect of epinephrine on the heart. In contrast, steroid hormones (e.g., testosterone and estrogen) may require hours or days for their effects to be seen.

Endocrine glands release hormones in response to three types of stimuli:

- Hormones are released when a shift occurs in the concentration of a specific substance in the body fluids, such as when the parathyroid gland responds to a rise and fall in calcium levels in the blood.
- Hormones are released when the larger endocrine gland receives instructions from another endocrine organ. For example, the ovaries secrete estrogen under the influence of tropic hormones from the pituitary gland.
- Hormones are secreted when the nerves stimulate the gland, as when the adrenal gland releases adrenaline when stimulated by sympathetic nerves.

Table 6.2 Categories of Hormones

Structural Category	Examples
Water Soluble	
Peptides	Growth hormone
	Insulin
	Leptin
	Parathyroid hormone
	Prolactin
Glycoproteins	Follicle-stimulating hormone
	Luteinizing hormone
	Thyroid-stimulating hormone
Polypeptides	Adrenocorticotropic hormone
	Antidiuretic hormone
	Calcitonin
	Endorphins
	Glucagon
	Hypothalamic hormones
	Lipotropins
	Melanocyte-stimulating hormone
	Oxytocin
	Somatostatin
	Thymosin
	Thyrotropin-releasing hormone
Amines	Epinephrine
	Norepinephrine
Lipid Soluble	
Thyroxine (an amine but lipid soluble)	Thyroxine (both thyroxine and triiodothyronine)
Steroids (cholesterol is a precursor for all steroids)	Estrogens
	Glucocorticoids (cortisol)
	Mineralocorticoids (aldosterone)
	Progestins (progesterone)
	Testosterone
Derivatives of arachidonic acid (autocrine or paracrine action)	Leukotrienes
	Prostacyclins
	Prostaglandins
	Thromboxanes

From McCance KL, Huether SE. *Pathophysiology: The Biologic Basis for Disease in Adults and Children.* 6th ed. Mosby; 2010.

Endocrine glands and other specialized cells secrete hormones into the bloodstream to bind to specific receptors on or in their target cells. Any cell with one or more receptors for a particular hormone is said to be a *target* of that hormone. Cells usually have many different receptors, so they can be target cells for many different hormones.

Each hormone-receptor interaction produces different regulatory changes within the target cell. Hormones bring about their characteristic effects on the normal cellular processes of target cells by increasing or decreasing the rate of those cell processes. Even though the diffusion of a hormone usually occurs system wide through the blood, the effects are more specific because of the specificity of the target cells in organs and tissues.

Pituitary Gland

The pituitary gland, or hypophysis, is located in the head at about eye level. The gland hangs down from the hypothalamus and sits in the sella turcica, a recessed area in the sphenoid bone. About the size of a peanut, the pituitary gland has an anterior lobe and a posterior lobe. The posterior lobe is not a true endocrine gland, because it only stores and releases hormones but does not synthesize them. According to ancient chakra-based tradition, the pituitary gland and its regulating counterpart, the hypothalamus, are related to the crown or brow chakra, with primary functions of integration of emotional patterns and realization of the total self.

The pituitary gland secretes hormones that regulate growth, fluid balance, lactation, and childbirth. The gland is the main source of tropic hormones, hormones that have a stimulating effect on other endocrine glands. The hypothalamus regulates the pituitary gland by *releasing* and *inhibiting* hormones. The negative feedback mechanism affects the pituitary gland by acting on the hypothalamus. The terms *primary* and *secondary* refer to target organ problems as opposed to problems in other organs that affect the target gland. For example, *primary hyperthyroidism* means that the cause is in the thyroid gland. *Secondary hyperthyroidism* refers to the pituitary gland and its influence on the thyroid gland.

The large anterior lobe secretes seven major hormones, and the posterior lobe secretes two major hormones.

Practical Application

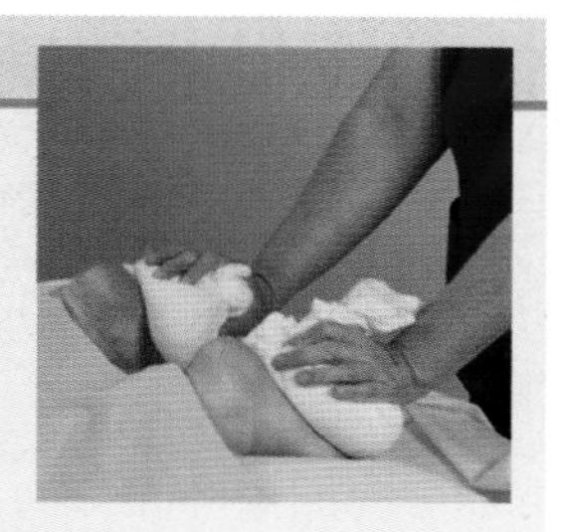

It is important for the body to be able to deal with its stress-load systems. That is why stress management systems are so important. If we analyze ancient and traditional healing practices, we can easily see similarities to the current recommendations for stress management programs.

Because isolation is a recognized problem for many, even within social groups (lonely in a crowd), many types of professionals are concerned about the quality of physical, emotional, and spiritual health for those without touch interactions. The Quality of Life domains (WHOQOL) established by the WHO reflect the importance of the health of the body, mind, and spirit. Psychosocial influences on hypothalamic function reflect the importance of resourceful contact with fellow human beings or loving pets. Even caring for plants has been shown to increase the sense of well-being for some people. We seem to be preconditioned to need others to be healthy. On a professional level, practitioners using a primary modality of touch can offer important health-restoring interventions and act in a preventive role for those at risk from touch deprivation.

Anterior Pituitary Hormones

Growth Hormone (Somatotropin)

Growth hormone, or somatotropin, stimulates most body cells to increase in size and divide. The major target organs are bones and muscles. In the adult, the response of growth hormone is the repair and rebuilding of tissues. Growth hormone follows a circadian cycle, with the highest levels occurring during evening sleep, primarily delta wave sleep. Growth hormone releases stored fat and raises blood glucose concentrations to provide us with energy. Growth hormone is also triggered for release during exercise and periods of hurt, tension, and stress. As we age, the total amount of growth hormone secreted declines.

Growth hormone release can be inhibited by emotional deprivation, excessive blood sugar, and high blood fat levels. Disruption in the sleep pattern interferes with growth hormone functions as well.

Thyroid-Stimulating Hormone

Thyroid-stimulating hormone (TSH) is a tropic hormone that promotes and maintains the growth and development of the thyroid gland and controls the release of thyroid hormones in a negative feedback system. Production of TSH often increases in response to cold temperatures.

Adrenocorticotropic Hormone

Adrenocorticotropic hormone (ACTH) is a tropic hormone that promotes and maintains normal growth and development of the adrenal cortex by stimulating the release of glucocorticoids and androgens. Androgens are hormones, such as testosterone, which produce secondary male characteristics. Stress, mild to moderate fevers, and hypoglycemia can increase the amount of ACTH secreted.

Practical Application

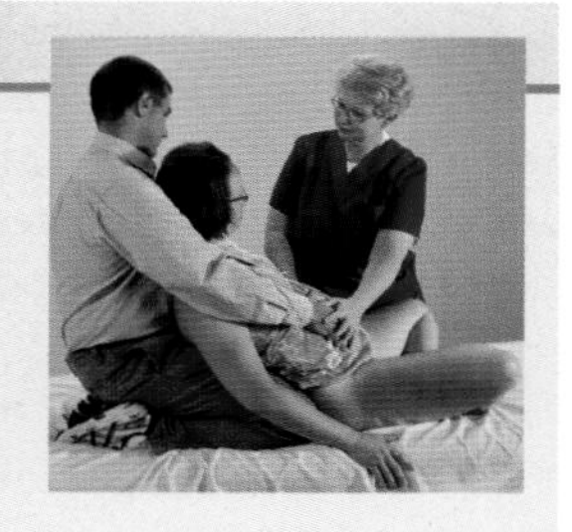

Stress experienced for an extended period causes abnormal glucocorticoid effects on the body that are responsible for some diseases. Glucocorticoids are known to suppress the immune system. Any modality that reduces the effects of stress, including therapeutic massage, promotes appropriate levels of adrenocorticotropic hormone (ACTH) and thus brings the immune system back into balance.

Research has shown that giving and receiving massage reduces sympathetic arousal. This enhances the effects of oxytocin, supporting lactation and bonding between infants and parents. Research has also shown that pleasurable rhythmic skin stimulation increases levels of oxytocin. This could explain some of the feelings of connectedness that occur between the client and the massage practitioner when these types of methods are used.

Follicle-Stimulating Hormone

Follicle-stimulating hormone (FSH) is a tropic hormone in females that stimulates the growth and maturation of ovarian follicles, which contain eggs. FSH also stimulates the secretion of estrogen; in males, it stimulates sperm production.

Luteinizing Hormone

In females, luteinizing hormone is a tropic hormone that causes ovulation (the release of the mature egg) and stimulates progesterone production in the ovaries. In men, luteinizing hormone stimulates the production and secretion of testosterone in the testes.

Prolactin

Although found in males and females, prolactin primarily works in two areas of the female body. First, in combination with other hormones, prolactin plays a part in breast development. Second, prolactin initiates milk production when stimulated by the CNS. Receptors for prolactin in lymphocytes suggest that prolactin is involved in immune function.

Melanocyte-Stimulating Hormone

Melanocyte-stimulating hormone acts on the pigment cells in the skin and the adrenal glands. The exact function is uncertain. One theory suggests that melanocyte-stimulating hormone, ACTH, and other hormones that darken the skin control pigmentation of normal skin.

Posterior Pituitary Hormones

Posterior pituitary hormones are made by hypothalamic neurons and stored in the posterior pituitary gland.

Oxytocin

Oxytocin stimulates smooth muscle contraction, especially in the uterus. Oxytocin is released in large quantities just before a person gives birth. This is part of a positive feedback cycle that ends when the child is born. Pitocin is synthetic oxytocin used mainly to induce labor. Oxytocin stimulates the milk letdown response, which causes the breast ducts to contract and release milk. Oxytocin also may be implicated in bonding behavior or feelings of belonging to another, as occurs between a parent and child. When increased sympathetic activity releases epinephrine, which inhibits oxytocin, problems in lactation and bonding may occur. Oxytocin is found in males and nonpregnant females. The role of this hormone in males has been suggested to be to support pair bonding in couples and enhance parental behavior. Oxytocin appears to work with several other neurotransmitters to foster interpersonal relationships and an individual's ability to withstand stress, empathy, and enduring loneliness (Patin et al., 2017). Massage increases oxytocin and reduces ACTH. Trust and touch are essential parts of sustaining social ties. Oxytocin reduces the stress response and supports the immune system, and it may be the mechanism through which social relationships protect health (Morhenn et al., 2012; Takayanagi and Onaka, 2021; Kageyama and Nemoto, 2022).

Antidiuretic Hormone

Also known as *vasopressin*, antidiuretic hormone (ADH) stimulates the kidneys to remove water from urine and release it into the bloodstream. The release of ADH is stimulated by pain, anxiety, nicotine, tranquilizers, and low blood pressure. The release of ADH is inhibited by alcohol, so the amount of urine produced increases. Because ADH can cause arterioles to contract, it increases blood pressure, which is beneficial during hemorrhaging because of the rerouting of blood to the internal organs. ADH can reduce the rate of perspiration, thus helping a dehydrated person (Fig. 6.5).

Thyroid Gland

The thyroid gland lies on the trachea below the thyroid cartilage and consists of a right and left lobe connected by a bridge (isthmus), resulting in a butterfly shape. The thyroid and parathyroid glands are related to the Eastern energy chakra of the throat, the function of which is communication and creativity in a balanced function.

The thyroid gland regulates metabolism in the body by maintaining an adequate amount of oxygen consumption at the cellular level. The two principal hormones are thyroxine

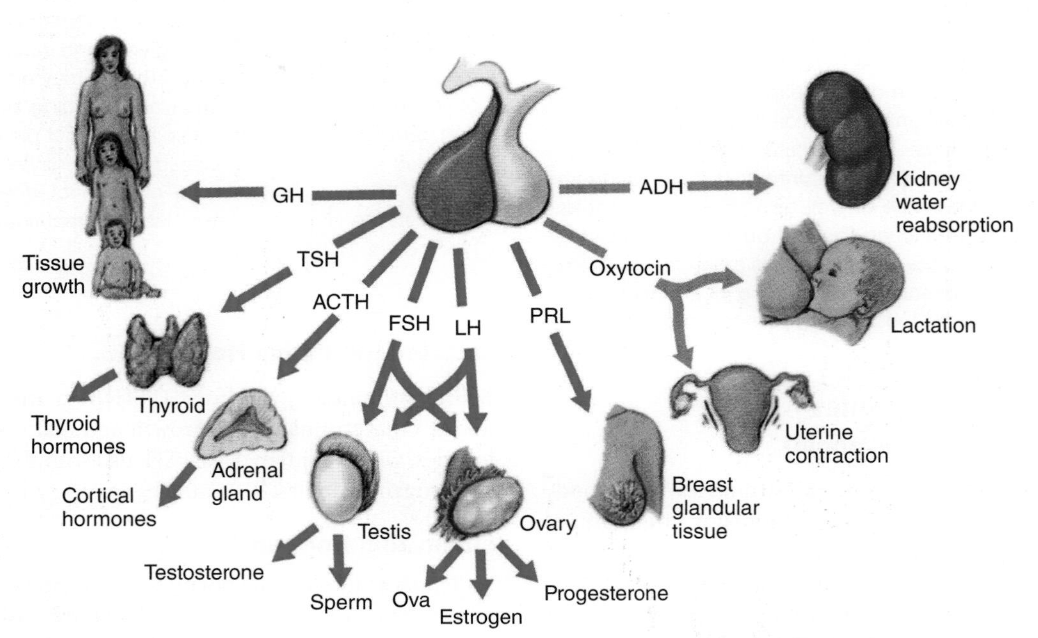

FIG. 6.5 The effect of pituitary hormones on target tissues. *ACTH*, Adrenocorticotropic hormone; *ADH*, antidiuretic hormone; *FSH*, follicle-stimulating hormone; *GH*, growth hormone; *LH*, luteinizing hormone; *PRL*, prolactin; *TSH*, thyroid-stimulating hormone. (From Applegate E. *The Anatomy and Physiology Learning System*. 4th ed. Saunders; 2011.)

and triiodothyronine. TSH from the pituitary gland stimulates these hormones, and iodine is necessary for their synthesis. A third hormone, calcitonin, inhibits bone reabsorption by limiting the rate at which bone tissue releases calcium to plasma. This in turn reduces the blood calcium level and counters the effect of the parathyroid hormones.

Parathyroid Glands

The parathyroid glands are made up of four round, pea-sized bodies located on the posterior surface of the thyroid lobes. Their hormone, parathormone, when combined with vitamin D, reduces the amount of calcium excreted, causes the release of calcium from bone, and absorbs more calcium from the gastrointestinal (GI) tract, increasing blood levels of calcium and phosphorus.

Pancreas

The pancreas is a long, slender gland located behind the stomach. The pancreas is an exocrine and endocrine gland. Although the enzymes of the pancreas aid in digestion, our focus is on its hormone production. Islands of cells called the *islets of Langerhans* are interspersed within the exocrine gland tissues. These islets produce the hormones insulin and glucagon. The pancreas secretes two other hormones in small amounts: somatostatin, which inhibits the release of all islet hormones, and amylin, which acts as an antagonist to insulin.

The beta cells of the islets of Langerhans secrete the hormone insulin, which lowers blood glucose levels by transporting glucose into cells to be used for energy. Insulin binds to the cells and allows glucose and potassium to be transported across the cell membrane. Although insulin receptors are present on most cell membranes, only our muscles, connective tissue, and white blood cells need it for glucose transport. However, glucose is readily available to the liver, brain, and kidneys, no matter what our blood insulin levels are. Insulin removes glucose from the blood, making it available for cellular activity.

Insulin

The pancreas releases insulin when levels of blood sugar, amino acids, and fatty acids rise. Other hormones, including ACTH, growth hormone, epinephrine, thyroxine, and glucocorticoids, also affect insulin secretion. Because these hormones necessitate a response from muscles, the demand for energy increases; thus insulin secretion supplies energy. Fluctuations in blood sugar during experiences of stress put additional strain on the body because the body often actually does not need increased amounts of energy.

Glucagon

Alpha cells of the islets of Langerhans secrete the hormone glucagon, which increases blood glucose, the opposite of the insulin response. Growth hormone stimulates these cells, which are a part of the feedback loop in hypoglycemia. A high protein intake and exercise raise the amount of amino acids in the blood, which also increases glucagon secretion. This happens by requiring the liver to speed up the conversion of glycogen to glucose, as well as by creating glucose from fatty acids, lactic acid, and amino acids. Blood levels of glucose increase but do not enter the cells, so cellular levels of glucose decrease.

Adrenal Glands

We have two adrenal glands, one on top of each of our kidneys. Each gland consists of an inner portion, called the *medulla*, and an outer layer, called the *cortex*.

Adrenal Medulla

The tissue structure of the adrenal medulla is similar to nerve tissue and functions as part of the sympathetic nervous system. The adrenal medulla secretes two catecholamines, epinephrine (sometimes called *adrenaline*) and norepinephrine (or *noradrenaline*). These hormones are active in the sympathetic fight-or-flight, alarm, or response to stress. Epinephrine has its primary influence on the heart, causing an increase in the heart rate, whereas norepinephrine has a greater effect on peripheral vasoconstriction, which raises blood pressure. The hormones produced by the adrenal medulla prolong and intensify the activity begun by the sympathetic nervous system neurons. The hypothalamus, the adrenal medulla, and the adrenal cortex are linked and interdependent in the management of the stress response. When stress-producing events are unresolved within about 15 minutes (Selye's alarm phase), these symptoms activate a more prolonged stress-coping pattern of the adrenocortical responses (Selye's resistance phase). If epinephrine and norepinephrine remain elevated over the long term, they perpetuate predisposing factors for stress-related disease.

Adrenal Cortex

The adrenal cortex secretes three major glucocorticoid hormones (glucose-producing steroid hormones) that are derived from cholesterol. ACTH from the pituitary gland, which receives its messages from the hypothalamus, stimulates the release of these hormones: cortisol, aldosterone, and the gonadocorticoids. The adrenal cortex hormones are involved with the metabolism of most body cells. Without a functioning adrenal cortex, a person could die from excessive stress and its effects.

Cortisol

Cortisol is secreted in minute amounts. If the body does not have sufficient supplies of fat or glycogen stored to use for energy, cortisol synthesizes certain amino acids into glucose (gluconeogenesis), causing a rise in blood sugar. Cortisol also converts starches into glycogen in the liver if the body does not acquire enough carbohydrates to use.

Eating and activity stimulate cortisol secretion, which seems to follow daily biological rhythms. Peak cortisol levels occur shortly after waking, whereas the lowest levels are reached just as the sleep cycle begins. Elevated levels of cortisol in the blood may disrupt the sleep cycle. Any situation that produces acute stress increases blood levels of cortisol, and the sympathetic nervous system overrides any inhibitory effects in feedback loop regulation. This results in a rise in blood levels of glucose, fatty acids, and amino acids—all because of cortisol. Levels of stress are often measured by cortisol levels, and

Practical Application

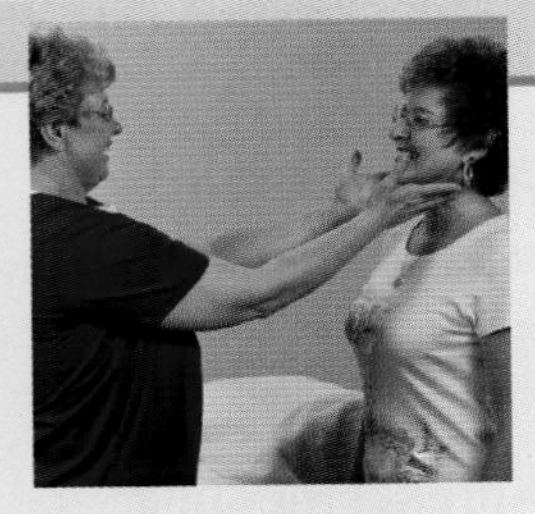

Therapeutic massage methods have been shown to influence the concentration of adrenal medulla hormones, reducing their detrimental effects on the body. Because the effects of catecholamines dissipate within a short time, the usual goal for therapeutic massage is to support the body in a return to homeostasis and prevent a recurrence of the excessive alarm response so that the body can remain in a state of homeostasis.

Because the major repair and energy-restoring mechanisms of the body are supported most effectively in the parasympathetic pattern and because most energy is expended and tissue damage is created during fight-or-flight activity, we can begin to see the wisdom in supporting parasympathetic function to allow sufficient time for restoration and repair of the body. Generally for every 15 minutes of catecholamine-generated sympathetic activity, the body requires about 45 minutes of parasympathetic balancing time. In a healthy, well-balanced person, sympathetic activities account for 25% of daily actions, with parasympathetic restorative actions making up another 25%. The other 50% of the time is taken up with activities that use sympathetic and parasympathetic functions together. However, this seldom happens, and the ratio is often reversed. Dysfunction occurs when sympathetic activity dominates, often because of lifestyle demands. Over time, the body cannot provide enough restorative action, and homeostatic balance is disrupted. Regular therapeutic massage supports homeostasis. Various forms of relaxation, including moderate aerobic exercise and slow, gentle flexibility methods (e.g., yoga) show similar results. The most effective interventions seem to be rhythmic, with a duration of 15 to 60 minutes producing the best results. Because the effects wear off within 24 hours, some sort of relaxation method needs to be done every day to best support well-being.

research in stress management methods often uses cortisol as a measurement criterion, with a drop indicating a reduction in the stress response.

Cortisol contains antiinflammatory agents that limit the amount of substances released during the inflammatory response. Cortisol slows wound healing because of a decreased rate of connective tissue regeneration. Excessively high levels of cortisol, especially over a prolonged period, can cause symptoms such as a decrease in cartilage and bone formation; inhibition of the inflammatory response, which reduces normal signals for tissue repair; depression of the activity of the immune system; increase in fat storage in adipose tissue; depression of brain activity; and promotion of detrimental changes in cardiovascular, neural, and GI function.

Aldosterone

Aldosterone is a mineralocorticoid, a sodium- and potassium-regulating steroid. Aldosterone causes the kidneys to reabsorb more sodium and water and excrete more potassium and hydrogen. Although aldosterone is necessary for our survival, excessive amounts of the hormone lead to sodium and water retention, accompanied by elevation of potassium ions and, in some instances, alteration of the acid-base balance of the blood. Under excessive stress, the hypothalamus secretes corticotropin-releasing hormone. ACTH blood levels rise and trigger an increase in aldosterone secretion. The resulting increase in blood volume and blood pressure helps ensure adequate delivery of nutrients and respiratory gases during the stressful period.

Practical Application

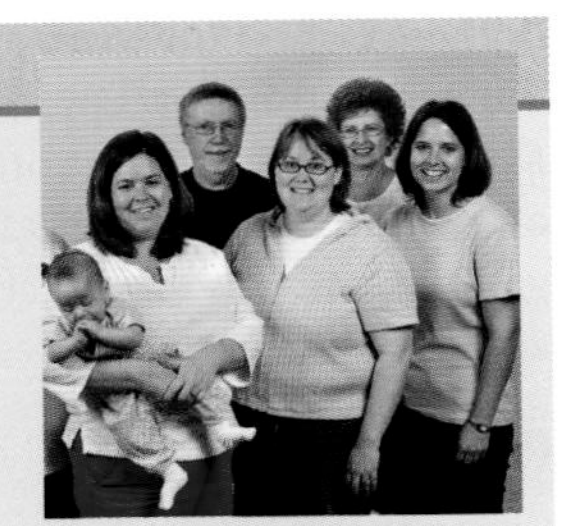

The release of aldosterone is effective when the body is expending physical energy (such as that required in actual fighting). However, it also increases the likelihood of stress-induced disease (e.g., high blood pressure) when the energy expenditure is less than the physiological response. This happens often as people try to deal with increased emotional and mental stress without physical activity. Aerobic activity and moderate weight-resistance exercises help manage this situation, balancing emotional and mental activity.

Gonadocorticoids

Although the ovaries and testes produce most of the sex hormones, the adrenal glands also produce similar male and female sex steroids, called *gonadocorticoids*. Both sexes secrete estrogen, progesterone, and the male androgens, with androgens predominating. This hormone secretion is significant in the fetus and during early puberty. The effect of the adrenal sex hormones increases as we age, and hormone production in the gonads decreases. For this reason postmenopausal females may use adrenal estrogen when ovarian function decreases.

Testes and Ovaries

The male and female gonads are located in the pelvic cavity and produce sex hormones identical to those of the adrenal cortex. Because this is the primary function of the gonads, they secrete larger amounts than the adrenal cortex and, in females, secrete them in a cyclic manner to regulate the menstrual cycle, support pregnancy, and prepare for lactation.

The two primary female sex hormones are estrogen and progesterone. Male sex hormones are called *androgens*. The main male sex hormone is testosterone. These hormones help develop and maintain primary sexual characteristics. Sexual behavior, male and female brain development, and gender behavior have been linked directly to concentrations of these hormones. Testosterone affects the sex drive (libido). Sex hormones influence biological function and behavior throughout life. Males and females are most similar in the beginning and end of life, with the greatest differences from puberty to midlife (the reproductive years) when these hormones are more active.

These sex hormones have other effects on the body. Estrogen, progesterone, and androgens affect epithelial and connective tissue and circulation. Continuing research concerning the sex hormones secreted by the adrenal glands indicates functions of these hormones other than reproduction. Testosterone, along with other androgens, is known to influence hair growth and the distribution of hair in males and females. Androgens also affect the skin and are a factor in acne development.

Androgens and estrogens exert their major influence during puberty. Androgens in particular stimulate the growth and maturation of bone, cartilage, and muscle. Low levels of estrogens promote growth, whereas high levels inhibit growth. Beyond puberty, androgens increase hemoglobin levels, whereas estrogen protects against bone loss and epidermal tissue atrophy. Estrogen can also be synthesized by adipose tissue, which converts naturally occurring androgens.

Besides the primary sex hormones, the ovaries produce relaxin, a hormone that relaxes and dilates the cervix near the end of pregnancy and relaxes pelvic and pubic ligaments to prepare for delivery. The ovaries also produce inhibin, the hormone that inhibits FSH and luteinizing hormone after ovulation and during pregnancy. The testes produce inhibin, which controls sperm production.

FOCUS ON PROFESSIONALISM

Transgender health care is an interdisciplinary field. The terms transgender and gender diverse (TGD) describe members of the many varied communities of people with gender identities or expressions that differ from the gender socially attributed to the sex assigned to them at birth. Gender transition refers to any combination of social, medical, and legal changes a person makes to support their gender identity. Usually, this involves transitioning from one gender role to another or moving away from the gender assigned at birth.

Gender affirmation is an umbrella term for the range of actions supporting living, surviving, and thriving as authentic gendered individuals. TGD health care involves gender-affirming interventions including endocrinology, surgery, voice and communication, primary care, reproductive health, sexual health, and mental health disciplines. Gender-affirming interventions include puberty suppression, hormone therapy, and gender-affirming surgeries, among others.

Gender-affirming hormone therapy is an essential part of gender affirmation for many TGD individuals. Transmen (female sex assigned at birth, male gender identity) typically receive testosterone, whereas transwomen (male sex assigned at birth, female gender identity) often receive estrogens frequently combined with antiandrogens.

Feminizing hormone therapy using estrogens causes changes, including breast growth, softening of the skin, reduction in body hair, and a change in body shape and composition. In the majority of cases, antiandrogen therapy is needed. In some cases, progesterone is also used for its effects on breast development. Transgender women on estradiol therapy may have a higher risk of stroke and venous thromboembolism.

Masculinizing hormone therapy using testosterone causes increased body and facial hair, deepening of the voice, menstrual suppression, and increased muscle development. Testosterone treatment may affect triglycerides and cause moderate to severe acne (T'Sjoen et al., 2019; Bhargava et al., 2021; Green et al., 2022; Coleman et al., 2022).

Pineal Gland

The pineal gland is a tiny gland inside the brain within the diencephalon and surrounded by the pia mater. All the functions of this gland have not been identified. Serotonin, norepinephrine, dopamine, histamine, and other neurotransmitters and hormones have been identified from this gland, but its major function seems to be to secrete melatonin. The gland is light-sensitive and is involved with regulating the rhythmic patterns of the body. The pineal gland also produces a hormone that stimulates the secretion of aldosterone by the adrenal cortex.

Many body rhythms have long been known to move in step with one another or to be entrained. The body temperature, pulse, hormone concentrations, and sleep-wake cycles seem to follow the same beat over 24 hours. The influences of light on the biological clock of the hypothalamus activate many of these rhythms. Melatonin secretion is inhibited when light reaches the eyes and is enhanced during darkness. Light produces melatonin-mediated effects on reproductive, eating, and sleeping patterns. Light intensity, spectrum (color mixture), and timing (day/night or seasonal changes) influence individuals.

Many ancient healing rituals were timed with the rising or setting of the sun. We now understand how sunlight affects body rhythm. Vitamin D, produced by our body when skin is exposed to sunlight, can be classified as a hormone. It is important in the regulation of calcium levels, bone health, immune function, and much more.

The cycles of the moon also are important in the regulation of biological rhythms. Some native traditions refer to the menstrual cycle as the "moon time" because females usually menstruate during the full moon. The word *lunatic* is derived from *lunar* (i.e., of or relating to the moon) because the moon is traditionally associated with increased emotional behavior.

Not only are we deficient in natural light, but we are also starved of the dark. Exposure to artificial light well beyond the natural cycle has influenced the drastic increase in insomnia and disruptive sleep patterns. Our bodies are out of touch with the natural rhythms that they were designed to follow, which puts more stress on our systems. Artificial lights do not provide the full spectrum of sunlight. The incandescent bulbs commonly used in homes primarily provide red wavelengths, whereas the fluorescent bulbs used in many businesses and schools provide yellow-green wavelengths. Animals exposed for extended periods to artificial lighting exhibit reproductive abnormalities and an enhanced susceptibility to cancer. Could it be that some of us are unknowingly experiencing the same effects?

Scientists are just now beginning to understand the reasons for these effects, and as they do, they increasingly are concerned about windowless offices, restricted and artificial illumination of work areas, and the growing number of institutionalized and isolated individuals who rarely feel the energy of the sun, the natural rhythm of the moon, or the quieting enveloping of the dark

Thymus

The thymus is a gland located deep in the sternum and mediastinum of the thorax and between the lungs at the level of the fourth and fifth thoracic vertebrae. Often considered part of the lymphatic system and identified as the master gland of the immune system, the thymus does have endocrine secretions. Thymus hormones are thymopoietin, thymic humoral factor, thymic factor, and thymosin. These hormones function in the growth and development of T-cell lymphocytes in the immune system. The thymus is large in children, providing some evidence that its production of hormones may slow down with aging.

Other Hormones

Endorphins

Endorphins belong to a family of peptide hormones that have many different effects, most notably suppressing pain like that of morphine. Endorphins are synthesized in the brain, primarily in the anterior lobe of the pituitary gland, and bind to receptors in the brain that increase pain thresholds. Endorphins appear to enhance the release of thyroid-releasing hormone from the hypothalamus and also influence the neurosecretion of vasopressin, ACTH, and growth hormone. Endorphins influence mood, producing a mild euphoric feeling. They also help control body temperature; assist with memory and learning; and help regulate the sex hormones that control the onset of puberty, sex drive, and reproduction.

Atrial Natriuretic Factor

Besides pumping blood, the heart secretes an important hormone. Specific cells located in the right atrium produce atrial natriuretic hormone when blood entering the heart stretches cardiac muscle fibers. The atrial natriuretic hormone works like a calcium channel blocker, inhibiting aldosterone secretion and thereby lowering blood pressure by increasing the amount of water excreted. It also inhibits the release of ADH, resulting in the same effect.

Erythropoietin

When oxygen levels in the body decline, the kidneys produce erythropoietin to stimulate the production of red blood cells in the bone marrow.

Insulin-like Growth Factor

Insulin-like growth factor is produced primarily in the liver and looks like the insulin molecule. The factor is released in response to growth hormone and stimulates the growth in the target cells of insulin, matrix production in cartilage, and the growth of fibroblasts in connective tissue. Insulin-like growth factor also synthesizes lipids and glycogen in adipose tissue.

The Gut and Gastrointestinal Hormones

Our human **microbiome** is made up of communities of symbiotic, commensal, and pathogenic bacteria, along with fungi and viruses. Symbiotic and commensal microbes function together and benefit from other microbes and the human host. Pathogenic microbes disrupt homeostasis. The microbiome comprises all the genetic material of all the microorganisms that live on or in specific parts of the body. The idea that the microbiome, particularly the gut microbiome, serves as an endocrine organ has been suggested by several researchers (Evans et al., 2013; Clarke et al., 2014; Gomes et al., 2018). The microbiome of the human gut (the digestive tract; see Chapter 12) produces and responds to hormones. Unlike other endocrine systems or organs that secrete a single or at most a small number of hormones, gut microbes have the potential to produce hundreds of endocrinologically active substances. Not only do bacteria in the gut produce hormonelike substances and regulate hormonal output, but potentially they also respond to the hormonal secretions of the host.

The mucosa of the GI tract produces specific GI hormones and releases them when food is present to help regulate digestion. Three of the most prominent are gastrin, secretin, and cholecystokinin.

Gastrin is produced in the mucosal cells of the stomach and duodenum. It stimulates the release of hydrochloric acid and pepsin from the stomach. These are needed to digest proteins. *Secretin*, produced by the small intestine, stimulates the release of pancreatic enzymes that digest proteins, lipids, and carbohydrates. *Cholecystokinin* is produced in the mucosa of the intestine and secreted into the bloodstream. Cholecystokinin causes the release of bile from the gallbladder (bile is needed for efficient lipid digestion), stimulates the pancreas to release its digestive enzymes, and inhibits the secretion of stomach enzymes.

Tissue Hormones/Eicosanoids

Unlike most hormones that travel to distant target cells, most of the tissue hormones work in the vicinity of or on the exact organs where they are found. These local hormones, called *eicosanoids*, are a group of about 14 unsaturated fatty acid hormones. The primary ones are *prostaglandins, thromboxanes*, and *leukotrienes*. Prostaglandins are important and powerful substances found in a variety of tissues. They play a key role in communication and control of many body functions but do not meet the definition of a typical hormone. Prostaglandins are specific, highly concentrated, and the shortest acting of the naturally occurring biologic compounds. Prostaglandins are important in overall endocrine regulation and vascular, metabolic, GI, reproductive, respiratory, and inflammatory functions.

Inflammation causes the release of prostaglandins and histamines, resulting in vasodilation and pain. Thromboxane is a vasoconstrictor and facilitates blood clotting. Leukotrienes are proinflammatory, and overproduction is a major cause of inflammation in asthma and allergic rhinitis. Aspirin and other antiinflammatory agents act as analgesics by inhibiting the synthesis of prostaglandins. Aspirin also acts as an anticoagulant.

Review What You Have Learned

- List three main hormone types.
    - *Amines* (simple molecules), *proteins/peptides* (chains of amino acids), and *steroids* (derived from cholesterol) (see Table 6.2).
- List endocrine glands and describe their secreted hormone functions.
    - Pituitary gland: Secretes hormones that regulate growth, fluid balance, lactation, and childbirth. Primary

synthesizer of endorphins (hormones with many effects including pain suppression).
  - Thyroid gland: Secretes hormones that regulate metabolism by maintaining adequate amounts of cellular oxygen consumption.
  - Parathyroid glands: Secrete a hormone that, when combined with vitamin D, reduces calcium excretion, causing the release of bone calcium and absorption of calcium from the gastrointestinal tract.
  - Pancreas: Secretes hormones that lower blood glucose levels (insulin) and increase blood glucose levels (glucagon).
  - Adrenal glands: Secrete hormones that are mostly active in sympathetic arousal/stress (e.g., epinephrine [adrenaline], norepinephrine [noradrenaline], and cortisol).
  - Testes/ovaries: Secrete sex-related hormones. Testes secrete testosterone, and the ovaries secrete progesterone and estrogens.
  - Pineal gland: Secretes various hormones, predominantly melatonin, which regulate the body rhythms.
  - Thymus: Secretes hormones associated with the growth and development of T-cell lymphocytes of the immune system.
- Describe the hormone function of the gut microbiome.
  - The gut microbiome has the potential to produce hundreds of endocrinologically active hormonelike substances, regulating digestion, modulating hormonal output, and responding to hormonal secretions of the host.

PATHOLOGICAL CONDITIONS

SECTION OBJECTIVES

Chapter objective covered in this section:

9. Describe the hypersecretion and hyposecretion pathological conditions of the endocrine system and list the associated indications and contraindications for massage.

After completing this section, the learner will be able to:

- Explain endocrine hypersecretion and hyposecretion.
- Describe the causes of nonglandular disorders of the endocrine system.
- Determine the indications and contraindications for massage in specific pathological conditions of the endocrine system.

Primary Mechanisms of Endocrine Disease

Diseases of the endocrine system are numerous. They generally take the form of tumors or other abnormalities and are frequently caused when the glands secrete too much or too little of their hormones. The production of too much hormone by a diseased gland is called **hypersecretion**. If too little hormone is produced, the condition is called **hyposecretion**.

Hypersecretion

Any of several different mechanisms may be responsible for a given case of hypersecretion. Tumors are often responsible for an abnormal proliferation of endocrine cells and the resulting increase in hormone secretion. Another cause of hypersecretion is autoimmunity resulting from abnormal functioning of the immune system. Another possible cause of hypersecretion of a hormone is a failure of the feedback mechanisms that regulate the secretion of a particular hormone.

Hyposecretion

Various mechanisms have been shown to cause the hyposecretion of hormones. Although most tumors cause oversecretion of a hormone, they can also cause a gland to undersecrete its hormone or hormones. Tissue death, caused by a blockage or failure of the blood supply, can cause a gland to reduce its hormonal output. Still, another way in which a gland may reduce its secretion below normal levels is through the abnormal operation of regulatory feedback loops. An example of this is hyposecretion of testosterone and gonadotropic hormones in men who abuse anabolic steroids. Men who take testosterone steroids increase their blood concentration of this hormone above set-point levels. The body responds to this high concentration by reducing its own output of testosterone and gonadotropins, which may lead to sterility and other complications.

Abnormalities of immune function may also cause hyposecretion. An autoimmune attack on glandular tissue sometimes has the effect of reducing hormone output. Some endocrinologists theorize that autoimmune destruction of pancreatic islet cells, perhaps in combination with viral and genetic mechanisms, is a culprit in many cases of diabetes mellitus (type 1, insulin dependent).

Recent research has shown many types of hyposecretion disorders to be caused by insensitivity of the target cells to pituitary tropic hormones rather than by actual hyposecretion. Tropic hormones target other endocrine glands, stimulate their growth, and promote their function (Activity 6.2).

ACTIVITY 6.2

List three causes of hypersecretion.

1. ______
2. ______
3. ______

List three causes of hyposecretion.

1. ______
2. ______
3. ______

Nonglandular Disorders of the Endocrine System

Some endocrine disorders are not caused by the glands themselves. Other potential causes of endocrine disorders include these factors:

- Some cancers can produce hormonelike substances that cause endocrine syndromes.
- An abnormal decrease in the number of hormone receptors on target cells can occur, thus blocking hormonal action.
- Target cells may have abnormal metabolic responses to the hormone-receptor complex.

Endocrine Disruptors

Endocrine-disrupting chemicals (EDCs) are environmental substances that alter the function of the endocrine system, producing adverse health effects. Harmful effects of these contaminants were first reported in the late 1950s in wildlife and later in humans. EDCs mimic the actions of endogenous hormones. They are now prevalent in the environment, and human exposure is linked to chronic diseases, such as obesity and diabetes and a variety of inflammatory and autoimmune conditions. EDCs including diazinon, parathion, malathion, bisphenol A, and polychlorinated biphenyls (Bateman et al., 2017; Jacobs et al., 2017; Nunes et al., 2018; Dalamaga et al., 2024; Hassan et al., 2024).

Pharmacological Use of Synthetic Adrenocorticosteroids

Synthetic steroids (corticosteroids and steroids) are used primarily to reduce the effects of inflammation by reducing capillary dilation and permeability. Steroids also prevent the release of vasoactive substances, such as histamine and kinins. Allergic disorders (e.g., asthma, reactions to bee stings, contact dermatitis, drug reactions, hay fever, and hives) are treated with steroids. Steroids are also used to treat arthritis, bursitis, and autoimmune disorders, such as lupus erythematosus and rheumatoid arthritis. Steroids are useful in treating leukemia, multiple myeloma, Crohn disease, ulcerative colitis, kidney failure, infections, and skin disorders.

Common side effects of synthetic steroid use include symptoms as diverse as mood changes, insomnia, high blood pressure, increased susceptibility to infection, glaucoma, headache, reduced wound healing, sweating, fragile skin, vertigo, stunted growth in children, osteoporosis, and an increased risk of bone breakage.

Using steroids for extended periods without reevaluation is dangerous. Periodic reductions in the dosage often are necessary, but dosages must never be altered or stopped except by licensed medical practitioners. Weaning gradually from large doses of steroids is necessary because they suppress the pituitary gland and ACTH by negative feedback. When ACTH is suppressed, the adrenal glands do not function. When steroid treatment stops, sometimes the adrenal glands do not rebound to a functioning mode, and the person may lapse into Addison disease. A side effect of oral steroid therapy is GI bleeding. Protection of the stomach lining with cimetidine (Tagamet) is often necessary when one uses oral steroids.

INDICATIONS/CONTRAINDICATIONS for Therapeutic Massage

Some forms of massage may be used to manage some of the side effects of synthetic steroids. However, the practitioner should avoid massage methods (e.g., friction) that may cause inflammation when a person is taking synthetic adrenocorticosteroids. Massage is also contraindicated directly over areas where steroids were injected to treat localized inflammation (e.g., bursitis) because it is important for the steroid to remain localized in the tissues.

Pituitary Pathological Conditions

Gigantism

In gigantism and acromegaly, the pituitary gland produces excessive growth hormone. The term *gigantism* refers to the condition that begins in infancy or early childhood. The condition results in excessive growth of the entire body. Acromegaly is an abnormality that occurs in adults in whom the excessive hormone thickens bones and enlarges organs. In secondary Cushing disease, the pituitary gland produces excessive ACTH, resulting in increased production of steroids by the adrenal gland. The symptoms include increased fat on the face and between the shoulder blades, thinning of bones and skin, and bruising. Treatment of gigantism, acromegaly, and secondary Cushing disease may include surgery or radiation therapy. If a pituitary tumor is present, drug therapy with somatostatin is usually the treatment of choice.

Dwarfism

Decreased production of growth hormones and insufficient tropic hormones may cause height deficiencies. In pituitary deficiency, all pituitary hormones are diminished, which leads to the loss of target organ hormones, specifically adrenal steroids, thyroxine, and gonadotropins. Proportionate dwarfism may result. Proportionate dwarfism in children is treated by administration of synthetic growth hormone and, if necessary, replacement of thyroid, adrenal, and sex steroid hormones.

Diabetes Insipidus

In diabetes insipidus (not to be confused with diabetes mellitus), the pituitary gland releases less vasopressin than it should. Scarring or damage from head injuries often causes the condition. The ability of the water in urine to be reabsorbed declines, and urine output increases, sometimes by as much as 20 L per day. Maintaining an adequate fluid intake may control mild cases, but in others, treatment with a synthetic form of vasopressin has proved effective. If the inability of the kidney to respond to vasopressin causes diabetes insipidus, the normal treatment is reducing salt intake and taking medications focused on kidney function. Radiation therapy, surgery, or both are indicated in rare cases in which a tumor causes diabetes insipidus.

Thyroid Pathological Conditions

Hyperthyroidism

Hyperthyroidism, or thyrotoxicosis, is the second most common endocrine disorder after diabetes mellitus and mostly affects females. The most common cause is autoimmune dysfunction. Symptoms include an increased metabolic rate; excessive sweating; weight loss, even with an increased food intake; fatigue; nervousness; loose stools; tachycardia; warm, moist skin; hand tremor; and hyperactivity. Hyperthyroidism behavior can mimic psychosis and is almost always accompanied by a goiter. (A goiter, or an enlarged thyroid gland, may be found in hyperfunction, hypofunction, or normal thyroid function.) Toxic nodular goiter is another form of hyperthyroidism.

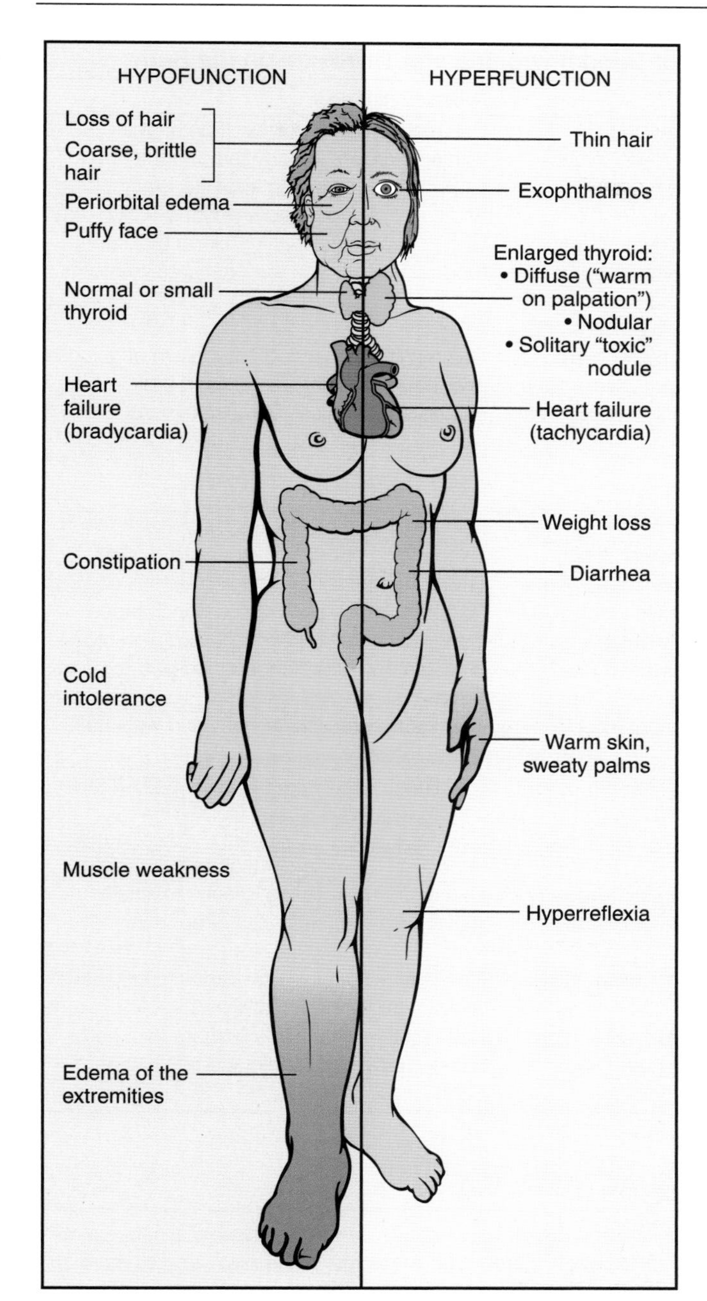

FIG. 6.6 Comparison of hyperthyroidism and hypothyroidism. (From Damjanov I. *Pathology for the Health Professions*. 4th ed. Saunders; 2012.)

The symptoms of Graves disease, also a form of hyperthyroidism, include an enlarged thyroid gland and abnormal eyeball protrusion, called *exophthalmos*. This results from excess fluid behind the eye and may not diminish even after treatment. Graves disease runs in families, is associated with autoimmune problems, and is most common in females between the ages of 20 and 40. Treatments include thyroidectomy; the use of antithyroid medications, such as propylthiouracil (which blocks iodine from being incorporated into thyroxine), or the use of radioactive iodine, which shrinks (destroys) the thyroid gland without affecting other tissues (Fig. 6.6).

Hypothyroidism

Hypothyroidism can result from treatment for hyperthyroidism by radioactive iodine, overdose of antithyroid medication, or partial or complete thyroidectomy. The next most common causes are autoimmune dysfunction and a decrease in thyroid-releasing hormone from the hypothalamus. Symptoms include general aching, weakness, fatigue, a lower metabolic rate, constipation, hoarseness, bradycardia, skin dryness, weight gain (often resulting in obesity), sluggishness, and slowed mental function (sometimes with psychotic behavior). Again, a goiter is often present. Mild hypothyroidism is common in perimenopausal females between the ages of 35 and 45. Because of this, thyroid function should be checked as part of the routine health care of females. Hypothyroidism responds well to oral medication.

If thyroid hormones are absent in the fetus or during infancy, the result can be cretinism, a condition that results in severely stunted physical and mental growth. Hashimoto disease is an autoimmune hypothyroid disorder that is hereditary, is found mainly in females between 30 and 50 years of age, and causes tissue changes in the thyroid gland itself. Myxedema is the most severe form of hypothyroidism, causing many of the previously mentioned symptoms and swelling of the face, hands, and feet (see Fig. 6.6). Table 6.3 presents a summary of the major effects on the body at normal levels and of disturbances in triiodothyronine and thyroxine secretion (Activity 6.3).

ACTIVITY 6.3

Design a personal 15-minute sympathetic activity sequence. Then design a personal 45-minute parasympathetic relaxation sequence. Remember that the idea of balance is important. The body needs glucocorticoids for normal function to achieve homeostasis. Excessive stress and use of steroids, such as pharmacologic agents, may lead to the disruption of this homeostasis.

Example

15-minute sympathetic activity sequence: I will go to the recreation center and spend 5 minutes on the track and 10 minutes on the stair-climbing machine.

45-minute parasympathetic relaxation sequence: I will spend 15 minutes doing slow stretching combined with coordinated breathing. I will take a 15-minute hot bath, and I will read inspirational and heart-warming stories for 15 minutes.

Your Turn

15-minute sympathetic activity sequence

45-minute sympathetic activity sequence

INDICATIONS/CONTRAINDICATIONS for Therapeutic Massage

Therapeutic massage may be beneficial in managing symptoms of hyperthyroidism and hypothyroidism. Thyroid conditions can go undiagnosed because the symptoms are common in many stress-related conditions. Referring clients for medical assessment to rule out thyroid dysfunction is important when they have any hyperthyroid or hypothyroid symptom patterns.

Table 6.3 Normal Versus Major Effects and Disturbances of Triiodothyronine and Thyroxine on the Body

Normal Function	Hyposecretion	Hypersecretion
Maintains basal metabolic rate (BMR) and temperature regulation to promote appropriate oxygen consumption and production of heat and energy; enhances effects of catecholamines and sympathetic nervous system activity.	Can result in BMR less than normal with a decreased body temperature, cold intolerance, decreased appetite, weight gain, muscle and joint pain, decreased sensitivity to catecholamines, and a general slowed state; low thyroid function mimics many disease symptoms and should be checked when any of the aforementioned symptoms are present.	Can result in BMR greater than normal with an increase in body temperature; heat intolerance; decreased appetite; weight loss; and sensitivity to catecholamines, which may lead to hypertension (high blood pressure); mood changes; and anxiety-type symptoms.
Thyroid hormones also promote appropriate carbohydrate/lipid/protein metabolism and glucose catabolism and mobilize fats. Thyroid hormones are also essential for protein synthesis and enhance liver secretion of cholesterol.	Can result in decreased glucose metabolism, elevated cholesterol and triglyceride levels in the blood, decreased protein synthesis, and edema.	Can result in enhanced catabolism of glucose and fats, weight loss, increased protein catabolism, and loss of muscle mass.
Promotes the development of the nervous system in the fetus and infant, as well as normal adult nervous system function.	Can result in slowed brain development in the infant with retardation and mental dulling, depression, paresthesias, memory impairment, listlessness, and hypoactive reflexes in the adult.	Can result in irritability, restlessness, insomnia, overresponsiveness to environmental stimuli, bulging eyes (exophthalmos), and personality changes.
Promotes the functioning of the heart.	Can result in decreased efficiency of the pumping action of the heart, slow heart rate, and lower blood pressure.	Can result in rapid heart rate and high blood pressure and, if prolonged, can lead to heart failure.
Promotes normal muscular development, tone, and function.	Can result in sluggish muscle action, muscle cramps, and myalgia.	Can result in muscle atrophy and weakness.
Promotes growth and maturation of the skeleton.	Can result in growth retardation, skeletal malabsorption, retention of a child's body proportions in adults, and joint pain in the adult.	Can result in excessive skeletal growth initially, followed by early epiphyseal closure and short stature in children; adults experience demineralization of the skeleton.
Promotes gastrointestinal motility and tone and increases secretion of digestive juices.	Can result in depressed gastrointestinal motility and tone and increased secretion of digestive juices.	Can result in excessive gastrointestinal motility, diarrhea, and loss of appetite.
Promotes female reproductive ability and normal lactation.	Can result in depressed ovarian function, sterility, and depressed lactation.	Can result in depressed ovarian function in females and impotence in males.
Promotes secretory activity of the skin.	Can result in skin that is pale, thick, and dry; facial edema; coarse and thin hair; and hard, thick nails.	Can result in skin that is flushed, thin, and moist; may produce thin and soft hair and nails.

Parathyroid Pathological Conditions

An excess of parathormone causes too much calcium to be removed from bone, resulting in weak bones. A deficiency of parathormone can cause hypocalcemic tetany, the symptoms of which include loss of sensation, muscle twitches, uncontrolled spasms, and convulsions.

In hypoparathyroidism, the levels of calcium in blood and urine are less than normal, frequently resulting in spasms of skeletal muscles. Moderate to mild deficiency can result in neuromuscular excitability that could be misdiagnosed as simple muscle tension. Anxiety may result as well. Ruling out hypoparathyroidism in cases of unresolved anxiety and muscle tension is important. Emergency treatment of tetany caused by hypoparathyroidism is an injection of calcium chloride. Calcium and vitamin D supplements are used for maintenance therapy (Activity 6.4).

ACTIVITY 6.4

List three thyroid dysfunction symptoms that may cause a client to seek therapeutic massage. Examples are provided to get you started.

Examples
Nervousness, fatigue, constipation

Your Turn
1. ______
2. ______
3. ______

Pancreatic Pathological Conditions

Hyperfunction

A benign tumor occasionally causes high insulin levels. More commonly, high insulin levels occur in clients with diabetes who take insulin without eating properly. The result is what is known as an *insulin reaction*, which means the body is flooded with insulin. Glucose enters the cells at an increased rate, and the blood glucose level falls, causing hypoglycemia (low blood sugar). When the brain is deprived of glucose, confusion and weakness result. A deficient production of glucagon may cause hypoglycemia.

INDICATIONS/CONTRAINDICATIONS for Therapeutic Massage

The symptoms of hyperparathyroidism include mild to severe skeletal pain and possibly osteoporosis. The client may seek therapeutic massage for these conditions, and the massage therapist must take care to provide the appropriate referral to determine the underlying cause of the problem.

In primary hyperparathyroidism, which usually results from a benign tumor, levels of calcium increase in the blood and urine. In secondary hyperparathyroidism, which mostly results from kidney disease, blood calcium decreases and urine calcium increases. Hyperparathyroidism is much more common than hypoparathyroidism, and it is increasing in frequency.

True hypoglycemia is rare. More common is reactive hypoglycemia, a diet-induced condition that can be corrected by eating a balanced diet on a regular schedule.

Hypofunction

The disorder known as *diabetes mellitus* results from the pancreas not producing enough insulin or stopping insulin production. Because cells do not absorb glucose, the amount in the bloodstream increases (hyperglycemia). Glucose is a powerful diuretic, so glucose entering the urine is accompanied by water. As glucose flows through the kidneys, some of the excess is released in the urine (glycosuria). This causes many of the first symptoms of diabetes, such as dehydration, increased thirst (polydipsia), increased urination (polyuria), and an increased appetite (polyphagia).

When the body is unable to use glucose, it uses fats for energy. The breakdown of fats results in the formation of ketones (ketoacids) as byproducts, increasing body acidity and causing ketoacidosis. In severe cases, the combination of dehydration, high blood sugar, and acidosis may depress the cerebral cortex to the point of coma. This metabolic acidosis stimulates the respiratory center to increase the breathing rate.

There are three types of diabetes mellitus: type 1, type 2, and gestational diabetes.

Type 1, or insulin-dependent, diabetes is usually severe and occurs at a young age. Symptoms develop quickly, and ketoacidosis is often the first manifestation. Ketoacidosis is treatable with saline, bicarbonate, potassium, and insulin. A controlled diet and daily use of insulin are the most common long-term treatments.

Type 2, or non-insulin-dependent, diabetes is usually milder and in most cases begins in adults. However, type 2 diabetes is occurring in younger people. Heredity and obesity are important contributing factors. Symptoms include dehydration, increased thirst and appetite, frequent urination, reduced resistance to infection, blurred vision, and fatigue. These symptoms usually develop over a period of years. Treatment generally begins with dietary changes, such as those recommended by the American Diabetes Association. An exercise program is implemented to control weight and increase general fitness. Weight loss is an important first step because fewer insulin receptors are present and they become less sensitive to insulin in an overweight person. Oral medications can reduce blood sugar levels. Insulin may be used if blood sugar levels remain high, but it is not necessarily a permanent form of treatment.

Gestational diabetes is hyperglycemia (high blood glucose levels) during pregnancy. Gestational diabetes usually develops in the third trimester (between 24 and 28 weeks) and typically disappears after the baby is born.

Complications of diabetes sometimes include vascular disease because diabetes increases the development of arteriosclerosis. High glucose levels also raise the chances of infection because they provide a good medium for bacterial growth. Other complications include kidney disease, heart attacks (people with diabetes have twice the average rate), eye problems (diabetic retinopathy), impotence in males, and loss of menstrual cycles in females. Gangrene of the feet accounts for more amputations of the feet than any other condition, including trauma. Treatment for the complications of diabetes includes meticulous attention to hygiene of the feet and an exercise program for weight loss and fitness. Diabetic neuropathy, a painful and difficult to manage condition resulting from peripheral nerve damage, is more severe with type 1 diabetes because nerve damage results from ketoacidosis (ketoacidosis is not seen as often in those with type 2 diabetes) (Fig. 6.7).

Prediabetes, also commonly referred to as borderline diabetes, is a metabolic condition and a growing global problem that is closely tied to obesity. Prediabetes means that the blood glucose (or blood sugar) levels are higher than normal but not high enough to be called diabetes. Most people at the prediabetes stage should focus first on lifestyle changes, including diet, physical activity, and maintaining a healthy weight. Medications may be prescribed to manage related conditions, and prescriptions will likely be needed if prediabetes progresses to type 2 diabetes.

INDICATIONS/CONTRAINDICATIONS for Therapeutic Massage

A general stress management program supports the management of prediabetes and diabetes. Therapeutic massage can be an integral part of such a program. When we work with clients with diabetes, the bodywork must be part of an overall treatment program with medical supervision. Careful observation of the feet during massage supports a hygiene program. The practitioner should refer the client for immediate medical care if any tissue changes are noted.

In pain management for diabetic neuropathy, massage approaches used as part of a supervised program have proved beneficial for the short-term reduction of pain symptoms (Activity 6.5).

Adrenal Pathological Conditions

In *Cushing syndrome*, corticosteroid levels in the blood and urine are elevated, specifically cortisol and urinary 17-hydroxycorticosteroid—both of which are excretory products of cortisol. The usual cause of Cushing syndrome is taking large doses of corticosteroid drugs for long periods. ACTH is low in primary Cushing disease. ACTH is high in secondary Cushing disease. Usually caused by a pituitary tumor, the secondary condition is referred to as *Cushing disease* instead of *Cushing syndrome*. In both cases, symptoms include fat accumulation, edema, hyperglycemia, muscle weakness,

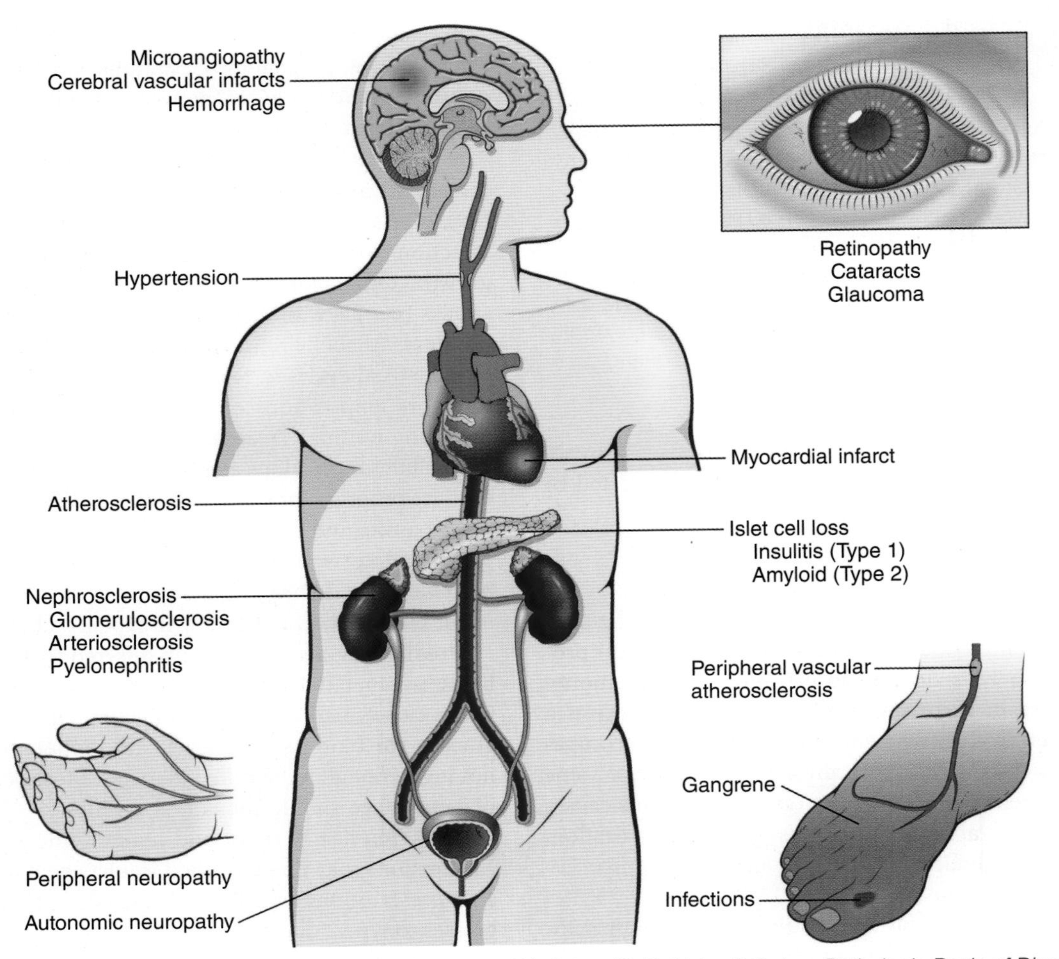

FIG. 6.7 Complications of diabetes mellitus. (From Kumar V, Abbas AK, Aster JC. *Robbins & Cotran Pathologic Basis of Disease*. 9th ed. Saunders; 2015.)

ACTIVITY 6.5

Identify a reason therapeutic massage can be beneficial as part of a total diabetes management program. Justify your position using the clinical reasoning model.

Example

Statement: Therapeutic massage supports weight management programs.

1. What are the facts?
   Weight loss and changes in diet result in chemical changes in the body. Mood-elevating chemicals that are generated from high-sugar, high-fat foods are reduced substantially in a diabetic diet.
   Therapeutic massage increases the feel-good chemicals in the body.
2. What are the possibilities?
   Therapeutic massage can act as a substitute for food to provide stimulation for mood elevation.
3. What are the pros and cons? What are the consequences of not acting (not doing bodywork)? What are the consequences of acting (doing bodywork)?
   Positive consequences include pleasure sensations that do not contribute to the diabetic problem. Negative consequences include the cost and inconvenience that may prevent easy implementation of these methods into a person's lifestyle.
4. What would be the effect on the persons involved: client, practitioner, and other professionals working with the client?
   The person would feel cared for and supported as part of the weight management program by receiving personal attention from a professional during a time in which they may feel deprived.

Your Turn

Statement:

1. What are the facts?
2. What are the possibilities?
3. What are the pros and cons? What are the consequences of not acting? What are the consequences of acting?
4. What would be the effect on the persons involved: client, practitioner, and other professionals working with the client?

suppressed immunity, osteoporosis, acne, and increased facial hair. Diabetes mellitus can be brought on during Cushing disease and can develop into a chronic condition.

Primary hyperaldosteronism (*Conn syndrome* or *aldosterone-producing adrenal tumor*) is caused by an adrenal tumor.

In rare cases, if caused by a nonspecific enlargement of the adrenal glands, the syndrome is referred to as *aldosteronism*. Levels of aldosterone and sodium are elevated in the plasma and urine, and potassium is decreased. Symptoms include headache, tingling and weakness in the limbs, increased thirst, fatigue, hypertension, and an increase in urine volume, especially at night.

Adrenal insufficiency is an endocrine, or a hormonal, disorder that occurs when the adrenal glands do not produce enough of certain hormones. Adrenal insufficiency can be primary or secondary. *Addison disease*, the common term for primary adrenal insufficiency, occurs when the adrenal glands are damaged and cannot produce enough of the adrenal hormone cortisol. The adrenal hormone aldosterone may also be lacking.

Secondary adrenal insufficiency occurs when the pituitary gland fails to produce enough ACTH, a hormone that stimulates the adrenal glands to produce the hormone cortisol. If ACTH output is too low, cortisol production drops. Eventually, the adrenal glands can shrink as a result of a lack of ACTH stimulation. Secondary adrenal insufficiency is much more common than Addison disease.

Symptoms of adrenal insufficiency include weakness, decreased endurance, increased pigmentation of the skin and mucous membranes, anorexia, dehydration, weight loss, intestinal disturbances, anxiety, depression (or similar emotional distress), and a diminished tolerance to cold. The onset is usually gradual and may be mistaken as general stress symptoms.

INDICATIONS/CONTRAINDICATIONS for Therapeutic Massage

Adrenal insufficiency can become serious, and proper diagnosis is essential for appropriate treatment. Because the symptoms occur gradually and mimic generalized stress and fatigue, the condition can go undiagnosed. Refer clients to their provider if symptoms suggest the possibility of adrenal insufficiency. After these conditions have been diagnosed, stress management can be an important part of ongoing therapeutic care.

Pineal Pathology

Conditions such as illness, drug use, jet travel, alterations in eating patterns, weather changes, changes in the work schedule to the night shift, or other disruptions in the sleep-wake cycle can throw biological rhythms out of synchronization. Disruptions in normal biological rhythms (Chapter 2) cause mood changes, affect immune function, alter digestion, and unsettle the entire homeostatic balance. Researchers have identified a common emotional disorder, called *seasonal affective disorder* (SAD), in which mood swings are grossly exaggerated. As the days grow shorter each fall, people with SAD become irritable, anxious, sleepy, and socially withdrawn. Their appetite becomes insatiable; they crave carbohydrates and gain weight readily. Research has shown that phototherapy (the use of bright lights for up to 2 hours daily) reversed these symptoms in nearly 90% of those studied and was more effective than the use of antidepressant drugs. When the subjects stopped receiving phototherapy or were given melatonin, their symptoms returned as quickly as they had lifted, indicating that melatonin may be a key to seasonal mood changes as well.

The symptoms of SAD are virtually identical to those seen in individuals with carbohydrate-craving obesity and premenstrual syndrome, except that carbohydrate-craving obesity affects sufferers daily and premenstrual syndrome affects sufferers monthly. Phototherapy relieves premenstrual syndrome symptoms in some females, according to some research.

Night shift workers show reversed melatonin secretion patterns. When the pineal gland is exposed to light during the night, it releases no hormone; during daytime sleeping hours, the gland releases high levels of melatonin. If these individuals are awakened from sleep and exposed to bright light, their melatonin levels drop. The same sort of melatonin inversion occurs in those who fly from coast to coast. The reversal disrupts sleep patterns. Anything that disrupts sleep eventually causes widespread stress in the body (Activity 6.6).

ACTIVITY 6.6

Develop a daily schedule that supports biologic rhythms, particularly those mediated by the pineal gland. Carry this schedule from awakening to bedtime.

Example
5:30 AM: Wake up
5:45 AM: Quiet meditation
6:00 AM: Exercise outside in the rising sun
7:30 AM: Breakfast
Your Turn

INDICATIONS/CONTRAINDICATIONS for Therapeutic Massage

Relaxation methods, including therapeutic massage, can support effective sleep patterns. Adhering to a bedtime and waketime schedule can reestablish sleep patterns. Sleeping in the dark and experiencing adequate natural light during the day seem to be important. Engaging in moderate exercise during the day and a gentle stretching program before retiring is beneficial. Eating on a regular schedule also reinforces the rhythm.

Review What You Have Learned

- Explain endocrine hypersecretion and hyposecretion.
  - Hypersecretion is the production of too much hormone. Hyposecretion is the production of too little hormone. Causes include tumors, autoimmune disorders, tissue damage or death, and failure to regulate feedback loops.
- Describe the causes of nonglandular endocrine disorders.
  - Causes include some cancers; a reduction in or dysfunction of target cell hormone receptors; EDCs, which mimic endogenous hormones and alter endocrine

function; and steroid use for extended periods without reevaluation, which suppresses pituitary gland function.

- Determine the indications and contraindications for massage in specific pathological conditions of the endocrine system.
  - *Indications:* Massage helps manage the emotional and physical stress and discomfort associated with pathological conditions. *Contraindications:* Inflammation-causing techniques (frictioning) during synthetic adrenocorticosteroid use. Regional contraindication for recent steroid injection sites. Consider referral for potentially undiagnosed conditions and/or condition reevaluation.

SUMMARY

The ability to integrate knowledge into practical applications, including effective clinical reasoning and decision-making, is the foundation of competent practice. The foundation of therapeutic massage is taking a history, doing a physical assessment, determining outcome goals for the client, charting, maintaining an appropriate scope of practice, supporting interdisciplinary teams, and understanding anatomy and physiology. The endocrine system may seem removed from the therapeutic application of massage, but it is not. Massage powerfully interacts with the endocrine system, a major system of control.

Endocrine functions coordinate most body functions with the nervous system. These two systems of control (the nervous system and the endocrine system) provide a correlation to the organic basis for most healing mysteries. As our understanding grows, more of the knowledge found in Eastern and Western healing traditions concerning the body/mind/spirit interconnection will continue to reinforce the importance of integrated health practices and the maintenance of wellness.

Visit the Evolve website: https://evolve.elsevier.com/Fritz/essential/

The Evolve website provides support for the review of the chapter content and chapter quizzes to help you prepare for the MBLEx or other massage therapy certification or licensing exams. End-of-chapter questions for discussion and review answer key and rationales and authors' response to critical thinking and clinical reasoning scenarios.

CRITICAL THINKING/CLINICAL REASONING

Each chapter features a critical thinking and clinical reasoning application of the content related to massage therapy practice. A client scenario is presented, with recommendations for additional research, often using MedlinePlus or PubMed. Relevant questions based on the chapter content are provided to guide discussion. There are no specific correct answers to the questions. However, responses should support evidence-informed practices and should be based on biological plausibility if sufficient research is not available. The authors' decision-making process related to the scenario and questions is on the Evolve site. Compare and contrast your thoughts and discussion with the authors' and determine where you agree or disagree.

Scenario

Darlene Hayes is a new massage client. She has been referred for massage therapy to manage generalized stress as part of a comprehensive, integrated treatment plan for infertility. The underlying problem is polycystic ovary syndrome.

In polycystic ovary syndrome, the pituitary gland may secrete high levels of LH and the ovaries may make excess androgens. This disrupts the normal menstrual cycle and may lead to infertility, excess body hair, and acne. Ms. Hayes and her spouse have been attempting to get pregnant for 2 years. The health screening to determine the problem with conception identified the syndrome, along with prediabetes. Ms. Hayes is 31 years old and a medical assistant. There is a family history of type 2 diabetes.

Ms. Hayes has gained 30 pounds over the past 3 years. She is now on a weight management program that considers the beginning stages of diabetes. The program includes dietary changes, moderate aerobic exercise, and stress management, including meditation and massage. The healthcare team hopes that with weight loss and reduced stress, Ms. Hayes's endocrine system will normalize and she will ovulate on her own, without the use of medication.

- Explore MedlinePlus using the search terms *polycystic ovary syndrome*, and *prediabetes*.
- Search PubMed for the terms *massage therapy and infertility, massage therapy and diabetes, massage therapy and endocrine function, polycystic* ovary syndrome and endocrine-disruptor chemicals, and *hypothalamic-pituitary-adrenal axis and infertility*.

Discuss These Points

- What is the evidence for claims that massage therapy can help infertility?
- Is it possible to correlate in a biologically plausible way massage therapy's ability to reduce the stress response with an improved chance of conceiving?
- What is the indicated outcome for the massage sessions? How does the outcome relate to normal endocrine function?
- What hormones are related to polycystic ovary syndrome and what endocrine functions are disrupted, causing the condition?
- Does any evidence indicate that EDCs are a causal factor in the development of polycystic ovary disease and prediabetes?

The authors' responses can be found on the Evolve website. Chapter 6

MULTIPLE CHOICE QUESTIONS FOR REVIEW AND DISCUSSION

The answers, with rationales, can be found on the Evolve site.

These questions are used for review and discussion. It is as important to understand why wrong answers are wrong as it is to know why the correct answer is correct. The answers to the questions, with rationales and explanations about why the correct answer is correct and why wrong answers are wrong, can be found on the Evolve site. Guidance is also provided on how questions are developed and how the textbook content can be presented in a multiple choice question format. At the end of the question section here in the textbook, you will find an Exercise that asks you to write more questions. Use the various questions in the chapter as examples. This is one of the best study strategies for test taking.

It is important to understand that the actual licensing exam you take may not contain any of the specific questions found in this textbook or the review material and practice tests on the Evolve site. Therefore just because you can answer any of these questions correctly does not mean you will pass the licensing exam. The questions are content and style examples to help you prepare—this is why understanding why wrong answers are wrong is just as important as identifying the correct answer. Also, make sure you understand all the terminology used in the questions and possible answers in the review and discussion questions. Look up words you do not understand.

1. Which action best explains the influence of massage on the endocrine system?
   a. Stimulation of mechanoreceptors
   b. Decrease in lymphatic stagnation
   c. Influence on the autonomic nervous system
   d. Direct release of hormones
2. An elderly client has been more alert and has gained a bit of weight since they have been receiving massage. Which statement is the most logical explanation?
   a. Massage stimulates the hypothalamus.
   b. Excessive pituitary function is inhibited.
   c. The pancreas increases insulin output.
   d. Thyroid function increases melatonin production.
3. A client complains of dry skin, joint pain, and edema. Which endocrine function should the client have checked by a provider?
   a. Glucagon
   b. Androgen
   c. Thymosin
   d. Thyroid
4. A client has a chronic inflammatory condition that is helped somewhat by aspirin. Which statement is most correct in this case?
   a. Prostaglandins, which are tissue hormones, are involved.
   b. Progesterone, which is an androgen, needs to be inhibited.
   c. Pituitary hormones are overactive.
   d. The pancreas and gonads are hyperactive.
5. The hypothalamic-pituitary-adrenal (HPA) axis acts as
   a. a positive feedback loop.
   b. the central stress response system.
   c. the regulator of the microbiome.
   d. an immune system dysregulation factor.
6. A client is experiencing lingering anxiety from a minor car accident 4 hours ago. What difference between the nervous system and the endocrine system would explain this condition?
   a. The nervous system is short acting, and the endocrine system is long acting.
   b. The endocrine system is short acting, and the nervous system is long acting.
   c. The nervous system transports hormones more consistently through blood and tissues.
   d. Neurotransmitters have a long duration of effect, and hormones are short acting.
7. Which of the following supports the function of growth hormone in the adult?
   a. High blood sugar
   b. Loving relationships
   c. Disrupted sleep
   d. Lack of exercise
8. Which anterior pituitary hormone can be influenced positively by cold hydrotherapy applications?
   a. Melanocyte-stimulating hormone
   b. Follicle-stimulating hormone
   c. Thyroid-stimulating hormone
   d. Luteinizing hormone
9. A patient with type 2 diabetes wishes to become a client for therapeutic massage. The nurse practitioner is supportive. Which statement is most accurate as a basic understanding of type 2 diabetes?
   a. A disruption of insulin production occurs in the islet cells of the pituitary gland.
   b. Insulin is a powerful diuretic, so increased edema is a warning sign of diabetic coma.
   c. Insulin is released when blood sugar, amino acids, and fatty acids rise.
   d. Glucagon facilitates the ability of insulin to transport glucose across the cell membrane.
10. The resistance phase of Selye's general adaptation syndrome is most supported by which hormone?
    a. Progesterone
    b. Cortisol
    c. Noradrenaline
    d. Melatonin
11. Prolonged effects of lingering, unresolved stress can predispose a person to type 2 diabetes because
    a. cortisol supports a rise in the blood levels of glucose, fatty acids, and amino acids.
    b. glucocorticoids reduce the activity of aldosterone, predisposing one to ketoacidosis.
    c. catecholamines inhibit the sympathetic dominance pattern, resulting in excessive parasympathetic control over digestive processes.

d. stress shuts down the production of adrenal cortex hormones, putting additional strain on the pancreas for glucose production.

12. A client undergoing gender-affirming hormone treatment is experiencing an increase in facial hair and acne. Which hormones may be involved?
a. Androgen
b. Estrogen
c. Progesterone
d. Endorphin

13. An older adult client with a history of slow tissue healing and gradual weight loss begins to show stabilization of their weight and an increased ability to heal skin abrasions after receiving a weekly massage for 3 months. Which statement offers the most concrete explanation for this outcome?
a. Massage influences positive feedback mechanisms to reduce adrenal output.
b. Massage supports the hypothalamic release of growth hormone–releasing hormone.
c. Massage changes sleep patterns to increase the influence of dopamine.
d. Massage beneficially influences tissue transport systems of neurotransmitters from endocrine tissues.

14. A 38-year-old client describes symptoms of constipation, increased edema, sensitivity to cold, muscle and joint pain, and hair loss. The client indicates that there is an increase in stress in their life; is tired and seems unable to cope as effectively as before. The client had a general physical examination within the past 6 months, but no specific tests were done. Based on these symptoms, which condition might suggest a need for referral?
a. Exophthalmos
b. Hypothyroidism
c. Hyperthyroidism
d. Hypocalcemic tetany

15. A client who is a marathon runner developed an inflammatory condition of the knee. As part of the treatment process, they received an injection of corticosteroid into the area of the knee. The client requests to have a deep massage of the area to reduce the pain. Why is this not appropriate?
a. The massage could reduce the inflammatory response and concentrate the medication at the injection site.
b. Deep massage increases the potential for localized inflammation and would disturb the action of the corticosteroid injection.
c. Deep massage would increase the tension of the muscles, causing instability, and inflammation would decrease.
d. Corticosteroids reduce inflammation and increase tissue repair; because massage increases the tendency for tissue repair, excessive scarring could result.

16. A client has just experienced a job shift change from days to nights and is having difficulty adjusting to the sleep pattern, and feels disconnected and out of sorts. Which endocrine gland initially might be affected, and which massage approach would be most beneficial?
a. Pituitary gland—a massage that focuses on sympathetic stimulations with active participation by the client
b. Adrenal glands—a massage that generates localized inflammatory areas, such as is found with direct pressure and friction on trigger points
c. Thymus gland—a massage that uses sufficient pressure but pain-free compression and rhythmic gliding methods to support parasympathetic dominance
d. Pineal gland—a massage that uses sufficient pressure but pain-free compression and rhythmic gliding methods to support parasympathetic dominance

17. By supporting restorative sleep, on which of the following does massage have the most direct effect?
a. Antidiuretic hormone
b. Cortisol
c. Luteinizing hormone
d. Oxytocin

18. The microbiome influences the endocrine system because
a. microbes can produce and secrete hormones.
b. gut-based microbes affect the thalamus.
c. the microbiome suppresses tissue hormones.
d. antibiotic medication supports gut flora.

19. What two endocrine glands secrete androgens?
a. Adrenal glands and pituitary
b. Ovaries and thyroid
c. Pineal and adrenal glands
d. Testes and adrenal glands

20. Which of the following is the most common tissue hormone?
a. Prostaglandin
b. Cholecystokinin
c. Atrial natriuretic factor
d. Insulin-like growth factor

CHAPTER

7

Skeletal System

https://evolve.elsevier.com/Fritz/essential/

CHAPTER OBJECTIVES

After completing this chapter, the learner will be able to:

1. List the components and seven main functions of the skeletal system.
2. Describe the structure, classification, and development of bone.
3. Identify bony landmarks.
4. Describe the two divisions of the skeleton.
5. List and describe the individual bones of the axial skeleton.
6. Describe the pathology of the skeletal system and the related indications/contraindications for massage.

CHAPTER OUTLINE

KEY TERMS

appendicular skeleton: (ap-en-DIK-u-lar) The part of the skeleton composed of the limbs and their attachments.

articulation: (ar-tik-u-LAY-shun) Another word for joint, the structure created when bones connect to each other.

axial skeleton: (AK-see-al) The axis of the body; the axial skeleton consists of the head, vertebral column, ribs, and sternum.

biomechanics: The application of mechanical principles and engineering to human movement.

cartilage: (car-TI-lage) A tough, flexible connective tissue with a high water content that makes it softer than bone.

compact (dense) bone: The hard portion of bone that surrounds spongy bone and helps provide the firm framework of the body.

endoskeleton: The bony support structure found inside the human body; it accommodates growth.

endosteum: (en-DOSS-tee-um) A thin membrane of connective tissue that lines the marrow cavity of a bone.

kinesiology: (ki-ne-si-OL-o-gy) The study of movement that combines the fields of anatomy, physiology, physics, and geometry and relates them to human movement.

periosteum: (PAIR-ee-OSS-tee-um) The thin membrane of connective tissue that covers bones, except at articulations.

piezoelectric: (PEE-eh-zoh-ee-LEK-trik) The ability to produce electrical current when deformed or compressed, especially in a crystalline substance, such as bone matrix. When electric currents pass through them, these substances deform slightly and vibrate.

sesamoid bones: (SES-ah-moyd) Round bones that are often embedded in tendons and joint capsules. The largest of these is the patella.

spongy (cancellous) bone: The lighter-weight portion of bone, which is made up of trabeculae.

trabeculae: (tra-BEK-u-lay) An irregular meshing of small, bony plates that makes up spongy bone; its spaces are filled with red marrow.

LEARNING HOW TO LEARN

Learning the names of structures (e.g., bones) requires persistent and ongoing review, or else you will forget. Visualize all the people in your massage class or at your workplace. How do you remember their names? Association is one way. Association is when you compare two things. For example, one of the names you will learn is *scapula*, which is your shoulder blade. The association could be this: The word *scapula* reminds you of scraping, and you scrape with a blade. Singing the words enhances remembering.

A mnemonic is another memory tool. For example, the first letter of each word you are trying to remember might become the first letter in the word of a sentence. This is a memory strategy described in this chapter. Labeling, drawing, and coloring activities are also excellent for learning this type of content.

Box 7.1 Kinesiology and Biomechanics

Kinesiology is the study of human movement. There are two aspects of studying kinesiology: (1) the anatomy and (2) the process of movement.

Biomechanics is the study of mechanical principles of function and structure of the human body.

Although the terms are sometimes used interchangeably, this text follows the most current trend in which the term *kinesiology* is used for a broader meaning: the study of human movement with the study of anatomic kinesiology and how the anatomy works to produce movement. The term *biomechanics* refers to the mechanical principles of function, which include information about how the body uses concepts of simple machines, center of gravity, force production, coordination of movement, and so forth.

Often, the words *kinesiology* and *biomechanics* are used interchangeably, which can be confusing. These have similarities and differences, including that they can be defined in several ways. The definitions are as follows:

- **Kinesiology**
  - The study of movement that blends anatomy, physiology, physics, and geometry and relates them to human movement.
  - The science of dealing with the interrelationship of anatomy and the physiology of the body with respect to movement.
  - The study of human movement.
- **Biomechanics**
  - Application of the mechanical principles in the study of living organisms.
  - The science of movement of a living body, including how muscles, bones, tendons, and ligaments work together to produce movement.
  - The study of mechanical principles and actions applied to living bodies. This may involve looking at the static (nonmoving) or dynamic (moving) systems associated with various activities.
  - The application of mechanical principles, such as engineering, to human movement.

From these definitions, you can see how the topics are similar but not identical. Consider how these descriptions support the content of this unit:

- Kinesiology is the study of body movement. It involves anatomy and physiology.
- Developing a treatment plan requires an understanding of kinesiology.
- Biomechanics is the study of the effects of movement on the body. It involves math and measurement.
- Understanding the effects of the mechanical forces applied to the body during massage requires an understanding of biomechanics.

Chapters 7 to 9 target the anatomy and physiology of body parts involved in movement. Chapter 10 is about kinesiology and biomechanics. You must know the parts—bones, joints, and muscles—to understand how we move and the effect of movement on our bodies. These four chapters combined will help you understand why, how, and what happens when we move (Box 7.1).

SKELETAL SYSTEM BASICS

SECTION OBJECTIVES

Chapter objective covered in this section:

1. List the components and seven main functions of the skeletal system.

After completing this section, the learner will be able to:

- Define endoskeleton and exoskeleton.
- List the components of the skeletal system.
- Describe the eight functions of the skeletal system.

What would we look like if we did not have bones? Picture yourself as a mass of soft tissue with little form. Managing the forces of gravity would be almost impossible without the structure supplied by our skeletons. Getting from one place to another would be difficult. We would also be more susceptible to injury. As we explore the most concrete aspect of our anatomy—the skeletal system—the knowledge gives us an understanding of its functions.

Human beings have an **endoskeleton**, which means that our support structure is inside us and we grow around it. Some animals, such as lobsters, have an *exoskeleton*, a support structure that is on the outside of the body. Although an exoskeleton is appropriate for a lobster, it is not appropriate for a human being. Because an exoskeleton does not grow at the same rate as the rest of the body, it can become too small; also, it needs to be shed as a new one is grown. With an endoskeleton, growth is accommodated easily.

The skeletal system comprises the bones, joints, and related connective tissues. The connective tissue component is important for the functioning of the system. Bones connect at a joint, which is also known as an **articulation**. Bones are held together at joints by ligaments and other connective tissues, or both. Muscle contractions produce the forces that move the joints. The actions of skeletal muscles are voluntary and are coordinated by the nervous system. When the structures of the muscles and bones are combined, they form the functional unit known as the *musculoskeletal system*.

Because the bones do not have enough room for all the muscles to attach, the membranes between the bones and the ligaments at the joints function to expand the skeletal structure, allowing adequate space for muscle attachments.

Because muscles attach to bones, learning the names, functions, and various landmarks of the bones first helps in locating the muscles studied later in this section. Other chapters focus on the joints, biomechanics, and kinesiology. Carefully studying each illustration in this chapter will be helpful as you learn about the skeleton. The labeling of the illustrations is often more specific than the major features of the bones discussed in the text.

Main Functions of the Skeletal System

Besides the obvious functions of support and motion, bones have other important roles. The eight major roles of bones are to:

1. Support soft tissues and serve as a framework for the entire body
2. Provide attachment points for muscles and ligaments
3. Protect delicate internal organs, such as the brain, spinal cord, heart, and lungs
4. Serve as levers to provide movement created by the attached muscles
5. Store calcium, phosphorus, and other minerals for release to the body as needed
6. Store lipids in bone marrow for use as energy
7. Produce blood cells in the red marrow
8. Promote endocrine activity

Research in bone biology has found that bone acts as a regulator of several metabolic processes. Based on these functions, the skeleton can be considered an endocrine organ. The osteoblast-derived hormone osteocalcin is involved in several physiological processes. Osteocalcin has been shown to enhance several aspects of energy metabolism, brain development, cognition, reproductive functions, and male fertility (Guntur and Rosen, 2012; Karsenty, 2017; Han et al., 2018).

Section Summary

- Define endoskeleton and exoskeleton.
  - Endoskeleton—a support structure inside a living body with tissue growing around it.
  - Exoskeleton—a support structure outside a living body with tissue growing inside it.
- List the components of the skeletal system.
  - Bones, joints (i.e., articulations), and related connective tissues (e.g., ligaments, which attach bones at joints).
- Describe the eight functions of the skeletal system.
  - Review the list in the preceding section, "Main Functions of the Skeletal System."

BONES

SECTION OBJECTIVES

Chapter objective covered in this section:

2. Describe the structure, classification, and development of bone.

After completing this section, the learner will be able to:

- List the four shared structural features of bone.
- Define *compact* and *spongy bone*.
- Describe two kinds of marrow and their functions.
- Describe the five classifications of bone.

Bones are hard, dense, and slightly elastic organs of the skeleton. Bones have their own system of blood vessels, lymphatic vessels, and nerves. No matter their size, shape, or location, all bones are made of the same fundamental cells and matrix and are covered with the same sheets of connective tissue.

Bones develop into different shapes that serve specific functions. The location and shape of a bone determine its function. The protective bones of the skull differ in shape from the supportive long bones of the limbs. Disease, injury, and aging can all affect the structure and function of bones. The function of a bone can change its structure through a remodeling process, supporting once again the theme of form following function and function determining form.

During infancy, humans have 270 to 300 bones. By the time adulthood is reached, some of the bones have fused. The adult body has 206 bones, with some individual variations; for example, some individuals have more or fewer **sesamoid bones** (a type of bone that develops within a tendon or joint capsule), and others may have an extra rib.

Although all bones support the body, store calcium and other minerals, and house marrow for the production of red blood cells, some bones also play other, more specific roles. For example, the skull and the vertebral column protect the brain and spinal cord.

Bones are composed chiefly of bone tissue, called *osseous tissue*. Bones are not lifeless, but rather are ever-changing. The spaces between the cells of bone tissue are permeated with deposits of inorganic mineral salts of calcium and phosphorus, along with small amounts of magnesium, potassium, sodium, and carbonate ions. Two-thirds of bone tissue is made up of these inorganic minerals, which provide rigidity, and one-third of bone tissue is composed of organic material, which provides elasticity. Without this elasticity, the bone would break readily.

Bones are subject to considerable mechanical strain. They must support the weight of the body; disperse the impact shock of activities such as walking, running, and jumping; and withstand the force of muscle contractions.

Bones have a piezoelectric quality. **Piezoelectric** substances, such as the collagen in bones, deform slightly and vibrate when electrical currents pass through them. In reverse, when stretched, twisted, or compressed, bones produce minute electrical currents; the strength and direction of these currents change with the direction of the stress load. Bone formation patterns follow lines of stress load directed by these piezoelectric currents (Barbosa et al., 2022).

Bone Structure

All bones share four features that allow them to work together as parts of the skeleton.

- A rigid matrix gives bones strength and shape to sustain weight and movement.
- Bones usually articulate with other bones, thereby transferring forces and movement through the skeleton.

- A connective tissue structure, called the *periosteum*, covers every bone and provides vessels for nutrition, bone cells for growth, and attachments for tendons and ligaments.
- Growth of new bone matrix and remodeling of existing bone matrix are responsible for shaping bones.

The structure and function of bones are intrinsically connected. Bones remodel themselves constantly, depending on the functional demand. Although it may seem static, the skeletal system is one of the more dynamic systems of the body.

Bone Tissue

The different areas of a bone contain one of two types of tissue, compact bone or spongy bone (Fig. 7.1).

Compact Bone

Compact (dense) bone has a compact arrangement of hard inorganic matrix. This hard portion of the bone makes up the main shaft of the long bones and the outer layer of all bones. Compact bone protects spongy bone and provides the firm framework of the bone and the body.

The osteocytes in this type of bone are located in concentric rings called *lamellae* around a central canal, called the *haversian canal*, and form cylinder-shaped units that are called *osteons*. Blood vessels are located within the haversian canals. Within the hard layers of lamellae, osteocytes are located within spaces called *lacunae*.

Spongy Bone

Spongy (cancellous) bone has larger spaces within the bony matrix than does compact bone, which makes the bones lighter in weight. Cancellous bone is made of an irregular meshing of small, bony plates called **trabeculae** and is found at the ends of the long bones or the center of all bones except the shafts of long bones. In some bones, the trabecular spaces are filled with red marrow, which produces blood cells.

Spongy bone tissue forms a supporting grid that can be altered mechanically by the construction, destruction, or reorganization of the trabecular network. The piezoelectric current seems to be responsible for guiding these changes, which occur in response to postural change, muscle tension, and the stresses of weight.

Bone Marrow

Bones contain two kinds of marrow, red and yellow.

- Red marrow, which manufactures blood cells, is found at the ends of long bones and the center of other bones of the thorax and pelvis.
- Yellow marrow is largely fat and found mainly in the central cavities of the long bones.

Periosteum and Endosteum

Except for the ends that form joints, bones are covered with **periosteum**. On the inside of this membrane are osteoblasts, which are essential to bone formation during periods of growth and in the repair of bones. In addition to blood and lymph vessels, the periosteum has nerve fibers that alert the person to trauma, such as a blow to the shin or a fractured arm.

A thinner membrane of connective tissue called the **endosteum** lines the marrow cavity of a bone; it too contains cells that aid in the growth and repair of bone tissue.

Bone Development

In the embryo bone, development begins near the end of the second month. The process that creates our skeleton is called *ossification*. Ossification is the process of building bone by depositing calcium salts into tissues. *Calcification* is another term to describe the bone-making process. Ossification is a two-part process:

- Chondroblasts, or cartilage-forming cells, create the cartilage model of bones.
- Osteoblasts, or bone-building cells, develop the bone tissue from the cartilage model.

This process does not create the hard bones with which we are familiar. Instead, these cells remain soft and pliable, allowing the fetus to remain flexible so that it can exit the body more easily during birth.

Shortly after birth, hardening of the cartilage into bones, or *osteogenesis*, occurs as calcium salts are deposited in the gel-like matrix of the forming bones. *Osteocytes* are mature bone cells that maintain the bone throughout our lifetime.

Articular Cartilage

Cartilage is a tough, flexible connective tissue with a high water content, so it is softer than bone. Recall that cartilage forms the skeletal framework in the fetus. In the adult, the only remaining cartilage in bone is called *articular* (or hyaline) cartilage. This cartilage is smooth, slippery, porous, and malleable. It contains no nerves or blood vessels and is found wherever bones come together at synovial or freely movable joints. It allows the bones to move against each other easily.

Synovial fluid is secreted by synovial joints and provides lubrication, oxygen, and nutrition to the joint. Articular cartilage is "massaged" by synovial fluid during joint movement. The degenerative process of arthritis involves the breakdown of articular cartilage.

Because cartilage is an integral component of the synovial joint, it is discussed in more detail in Chapter 8.

Ligaments

Ligaments are dense bundles of parallel connective tissue fibers, primarily collagen. Ligaments connect bones and stabilize the joints and can also serve as muscle attachment sites. They are not typically elastic, nor do they have much stretch. Some joint positions place ligaments under tension, whereas other positions slacken them. Because ligaments are specific to joint function, they are also discussed in more detail in Chapter 8. An important feature of ligaments is that they are poorly vascularized and take longer to heal than muscles.

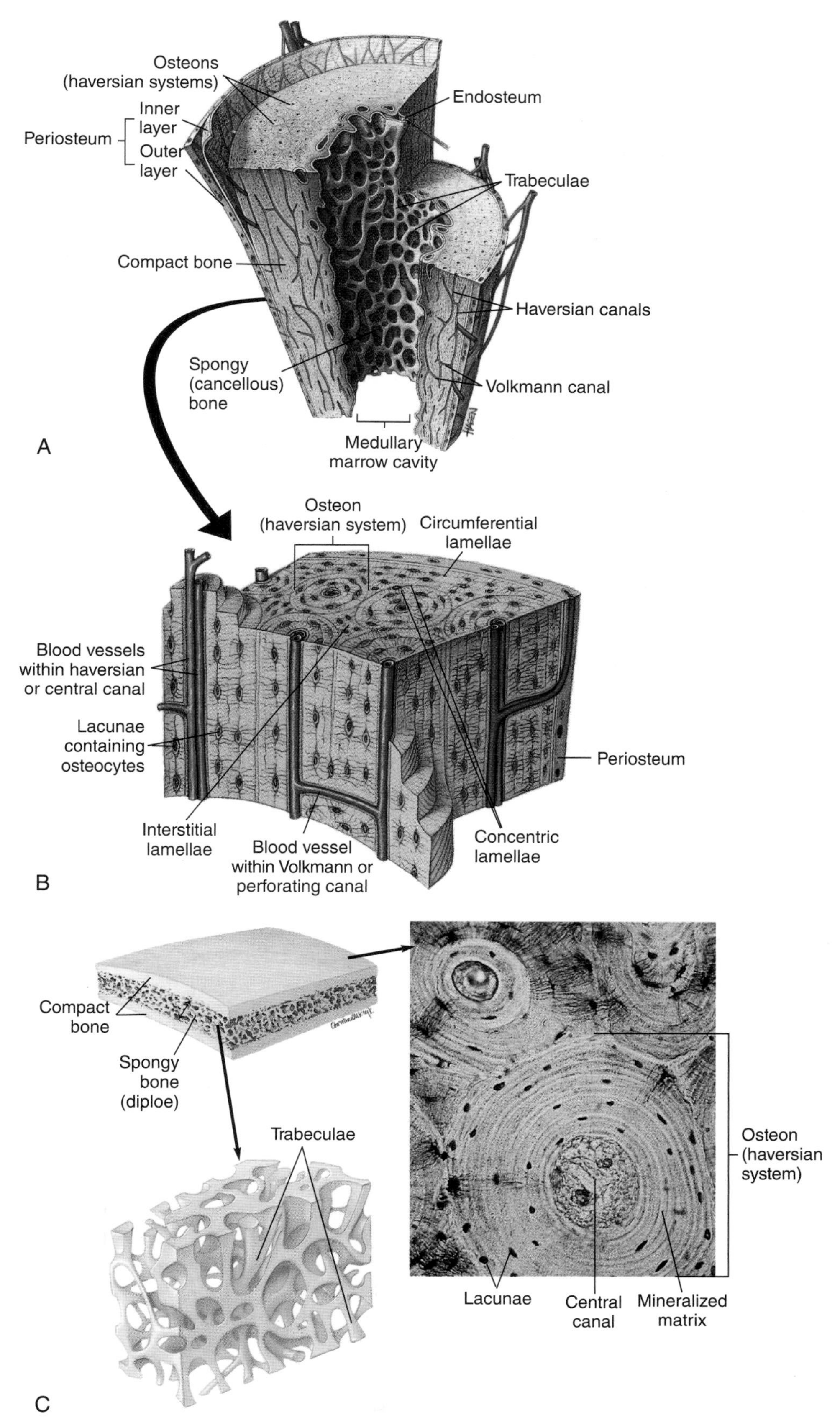

FIG. 7.1 Structure of compact and cancellous bone. (A) Longitudinal section of a long bone showing spongy (cancellous) and compact bone. (B) Magnified view of compact bone. (C) Section of a flat bone. Outer layers of compact bone surround the cancellous bone. The fine structure of compact bone and cancellous bone is shown to the *right*. (From Patton KT, Thibodeau GA. *Anatomy and Physiology.* 6th ed. Mosby; 2007.)

Classification of Bones

The bones of the skeleton are identified by their different shapes. The common classifications are as follows:

- *Long bones:* These are longer on one axis than another. Bones of this type are characterized by a medullary cavity; a hollow diaphysis, or shaft, of compact bone; and at least two epiphyses, or ends, which are active in the growth of long bones. The hollow structure of the diaphysis gives strength with light weight. Most of the bones of the arms and legs are long bones. Examples: femur and ulna.
- *Short bones* (sometimes classified as *cube-shaped bones*): These are predominantly cancellous bones with a thin cortex of compact bone and no cavity. Examples: wrist bones (carpals) and ankle bones (tarsals).
- *Flat bones:* These are generally more flat than round. Examples: ribs and skull bones.
- *Irregular bones:* These have complex shapes that occur as two or more forms within the same bone structure. Examples: vertebrae and scapulae.
- *Sesamoid bones:* These are round bones often embedded in tendons and joint capsules. Sesamoid bones are often considered to be a subdivision of irregular bones. Example: patella.

Bone Growth and Repair

Shortly after birth, we begin the process of changing the pliable cartilage skeleton into the calcified hard bone. In a long bone, the transformation of cartilage into bone begins at the center of the shaft. Later, secondary bone-forming centers develop at the epiphyses. The long bones continue to grow in length at these centers through childhood and into the late teens.

A growth spurt is often seen during puberty because of the influence of the sex hormones estrogen and testosterone. Both hormones promote the growth of long bones; testosterone also increases bone density. At higher levels of estrogen, long bone growth stops. This is the reason females generally are shorter and have bones that are less dense than those of men (Activity 7.1).

ACTIVITY 7.1

Refer to Chapter 6 and explain the influence of sex hormones on bone. Include the page number where you found the information.

An example is provided to get you started.

Example
High estrogen levels slow the growth of females, including their bones, at puberty.

Your Turn
Provide two more explanatory statements.
1. ______________________________
2. ______________________________

Identify two other hormones that affect bone formation. (Hint: See the sections in Chapter 6 on the thyroid and parathyroid glands.)
1. ______________________________
2. ______________________________

By the late teens or early 20s, again through the influence of sex hormones, the growth plate or epiphyseal disk of the long bones closes and the bones stop growing in length. The remnant of the growth plates hardens and can be seen in radiographic films (x-rays) as a thin line across the end of the bone. Physicians can judge the future growth of the bone by the appearance of these lines on the radiographic film. As we grow, our bones widen and lengthen, and the central cavity follows this change in size. This all takes place because bone tissue is added in some areas of bone and reabsorbed in others.

As mentioned previously, children are more flexible because their bodies contain more cartilage, and complete calcification has not yet taken place. In older adults this is reversed; bone cells outnumber cartilage cells, and bone is more brittle because it contains more minerals and fewer blood vessels. This makes bones prone to fracture and slower to heal.

Skeletal Changes Caused by Aging

As we age, various changes occur in the skeleton, such as the loss of calcium and protein. These changes can lead to brittle bones. Loss of calcium begins earlier in females than in males. Also, bone fractures heal more slowly in older persons. Beginning at approximately age 40, the vertebrae begin to thin, and the average person loses about an inch of height every 20 years. The cartilage on the ribs calcifies, leading to a decrease in the diameter of the rib cage and loss of flexibility.

Section Summary

- List the four shared structural features of bone.
  (1) A rigid matrix for strength and shape. (2) Predominantly, articulation with other bones (creating joints for movement). (3) Periosteum, the connective tissue covering of bone (which provides vessels for nutrition, bone cells, and tendon/ligament attachments). (4) Growth and remodeling of bone matrix.
- Define compact and spongy bone.
  - *Compact bone:* Hard outer layer of bone that protects spongy bone and provides a stable framework for the body. *Spongy bone* (i.e., *cancellous bone*): Lighter inner layer of bone made of trabeculae (an irregular meshing of small, bony plates) located at the ends of long bones/the center of other bones. In some bones, trabecular spaces are filled with red marrow.
- Describe two kinds of marrow and their functions.
  - *Red marrow*: Manufactures blood cells, found at the end of long bones/center of other bones. *Yellow marrow*: Mostly fat, found mainly in the center of long bones.
- Describe the five classifications of bone.
  - *Long bones:* Characterized by a medullary cavity; a hollow diaphysis (shaft) of compact bone; and at least two epiphyses or ends. Examples: The femur and ulna. *Short bones (sometimes classified as cube-shaped bones):* Predominantly cancellous bone with a thin cortex of compact bone and no cavity. Examples: Wrist bones (carpals) and ankle bones (tarsals). *Flat bones:* Generally more flat than round. Example: Ribs and skull bones. *Irregular bones:* Have complex shapes with multiple forms. Examples: The vertebrae and scapulae. *Sesamoid bones:* Round bones are often embedded in tendons and joint capsules. Example: The patella.

Practical Application

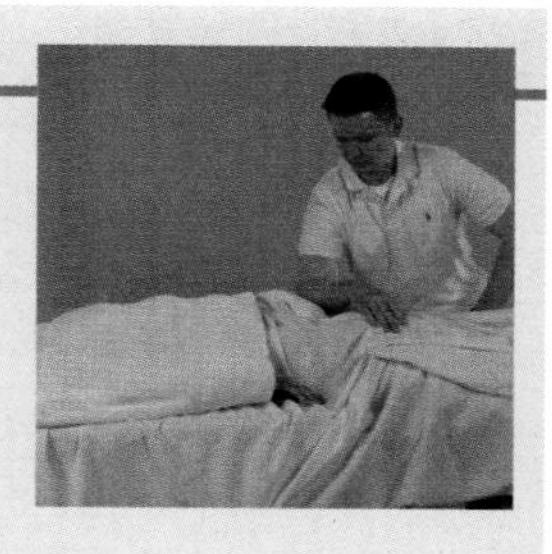

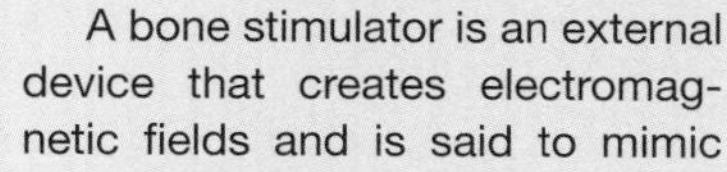

In the 1950s and 1960s it was first recognized that bending bone creates a strain that results in electrical streaming potentials within the bone. This is a piezoelectric effect.

A bone stimulator is an external device that creates electromagnetic fields and is said to mimic the same electrical streaming potentials that the body produces; it therefore stimulates bone healing. Another method of stimulating bone healing is by causing the bone to vibrate slightly a distance away from the fracture site. The vibration occurs at a certain frequency. Our bones heal best at a frequency between 20 and 50 Hz. Researchers have investigated the osteogenic effect (increasing bone cell production) of low-magnitude, high-frequency vibration (LMHFV; 35 Hz, 0.3 g) on the enhancement of fracture healing in rats, and it works. Some believe that the frequency of a cat's purring has a healing influence. The frequency of the cat's purr falls within the range of 27 and 44 Hz.

A tuning fork is a two-pronged fork with tines in the shape of a U. It is an acoustic resonator. When the tines vibrate, they create a sound. When tapped lightly, a tuning fork begins to vibrate at a specific frequency. There are tuning forks made for music, as well as for engineering, physics, and medicine. When a vibrating tuning fork is placed near a break in a bone, a person's pain increases. If the vibrations do not increase the person's pain, it is a lot less likely that the person has suffered a bone fracture.

FOCUS ON PROFESSIONALISM

Because of changes in the skeletal system due to aging, people over the age of 50 often experience stiffness and aching. Massage can help manage these sensations but not necessarily reverse them. Adaptive capacity reduces as we age. The most important activities to support the skeletal system as we age are moderate exercise and weight-bearing exercise. As we work with clients who are older than 50, it is important to remember age-related normal changes in the skeletal system. Realistic expectations related to joint range of motion and bone strength need to be considered when creating care plans for more mature clients.

BONY LANDMARKS

SECTION OBJECTIVES

Chapter objective covered in this section:

3. Identify bony landmarks.

After completing this section, the learner will be able to:

- Define bony landmarks.

The contour of bones varies and includes configurations such as flat areas, knobs, projections, spikes, dents, holes, and ridges. These landmarks often serve as regions for muscle or ligament attachment or provide passage or space for nerves and vessels. It is extremely important that you can identify and palpate the bony landmarks because this knowledge will assist you in learning muscle attachments later in this study.

The landmarks are categorized by shape and function (Activities 7.2 and 7.3).

ACTIVITY 7.2

For each of the landmarks listed, identify an analogy that will help you remember what each represents. A few examples are provided to get you started.

Examples

Foramen: Hula hoop
Groove: Ditch
Sinus: Cave

Your Turn

Canal:
Fissure:
Foramen:
Fossa:
Groove:
Meatus:
Notch:
Sinus:
Sulcus:
Condyle:
Head:
Facet:
Process:
Trochlea:
Crest:
Epicondyle:
Spinous process, or spine:
Trochanter:
Tubercle:
Tuberosity:

ACTIVITY 7.3

Palpating the Landmarks

Using the skeleton in your classroom, practice palpating the bony landmarks by feeling the bones with your eyes closed. When you find a dent, hole, point, knob, ridge, and so forth, identify it as a type of bony landmark (e.g., meatus, tuberosity).

Depressions and Openings

- *Canal:* A tunnel or tube in bone. Example: the carotid canal in the temporal bone.
- *Fissure:* A groove or slit between two bones. Example: the orbital fissure of the sphenoid bone.
- *Foramen:* An opening, or hole, in a bone. Example: the vertebral foramen of a vertebra through which the spinal cord passes.
- *Fossa:* A shallow depression in the surface or at the end of a bone. Example: the infraspinous and supraspinous fossae of the scapula.
- *Groove:* A depression in the bone that holds a blood vessel, nerve, or tendon. Example: the radial groove of the humerus.

- *Meatus:* A tunnel or canal found in a bone. Example: the canal in the skull that extends from the external ear to the eardrum.
- *Notch:* An indentation or large groove. Example: the greater and lesser sciatic notches of the ilium.
- *Sinus:* An air cavity within a bone. Example: the frontal sinuses.

Processes That Form Joints

- *Condyle:* A rounded projection at the end of a bone that articulates with other bones to form a joint. Example: the medial and lateral condyles of the femur.
- *Head:* A rounded projection atop the neck of a bone. Example: the head of the femur.
- *Facet:* A smooth, flat surface. Example: the facet of a rib or vertebra.
- *Process:* Any prominent, bony growth that projects. Example: the olecranon process of the ulna.
- *Trochlea:* A pulley-shaped structure. Example: the trochlea of the humerus.

Processes to Which Tendons and Ligaments Attach

- *Crest:* A ridge on a bone. Example: the iliac crest.
- *Epicondyle:* A projection on a condyle. Example: the medial epicondyle of the femur.
- *Line:* A ridge that is smaller than a crest. Example: the linea aspera of the femur.
- *Spinous process, spine, or spina:* A sharp, bony, or slender projection. Example: the spinous process of the vertebral column or spine of the scapula.
- *Trochanter:* One of two large, bony processes found only on the femur. Example: the greater or lesser trochanter.
- *Tubercle:* A small, rounded process. Example: the adductor tubercle of the femur.
- *Tuberosity:* A large, rounded protuberance. Example: the tibial tuberosity.

Section Summary

- Define bony landmarks.
  - Bony landmarks are areas of bone categorized by their shape and function. They can commonly be palpated through the skin and are used to locate and identify soft tissue structures because they serve as attachment sites for tendons and ligaments.

DIVISIONS OF THE SKELETON

SECTION OBJECTIVES

Chapter objective covered in this section:

4. Describe the two divisions of the skeleton.

After completing this section, the learner will be able to:

- Define axial skeleton and appendicular skeleton.
- Compare the bones of the upper and lower limbs.

The skeleton is divided into two groups of bones: the axial skeleton and the appendicular skeleton.

The **axial skeleton**, which forms the center, or axis, of the body, consists of the head, vertebral column, ribs, and sternum. The axial skeleton provides the body with form and protection.

The **appendicular skeleton is** composed of the limbs (appendages) of the body and their attachments (Activity 7.4). The shoulder and hip girdles, which have similar structures, connect the appendicular skeleton to the axial skeleton.

The bones of our body, in combination with the muscles, provide our fine and gross motor movements. The long bones of the limbs allow for large movements. In the same manner, the short carpals and phalanges of the wrist and fingers and the tarsals and phalanges of the ankle and toes allow for the flexibility needed in the wrist, hands, ankles, and feet.

The more we study the basic construction of the skeletal system, the more we notice its elegant and simple pattern. Simplicity and repetition of form reflect this effective biomechanical design (Fig. 7.2).

ACTIVITY 7.4

Match six similar sets of bones of the upper and lower appendicular skeleton. An example is provided.

Example

Femur/humerus

Your Turn

1. __________
2. __________
3. __________
4. __________
5. __________
6. __________

Section Summary

- Define axial skeleton and appendicular skeleton.
  - The axial skeleton includes the skull, vertebrae, and ribs. It forms the center/axis of the body, protecting the central nervous system and organs. The appendicular skeleton includes the clavicle, scapulae, humerus, ulna, radius, carpals, metacarpals, pelvis, femur, tibia, fibula, tarsals, metatarsals, and phalanges. It forms the limbs (appendages), providing mobility.
- Compare the bones of the upper and lower limbs.
  - Both consist of one large, long bone, two smaller long bones, several small bones (carpals/tarsals), and five digits (phalanges). Compared with upper limb bones, lower limb bones are larger and less mobile.

MENTORING TIP

If you learn the bony landmarks, it will help you learn the muscle attachments in Chapter 9. The relationship of bones, joints, and muscles and the intermingling connective tissue, including tendons, ligaments, and fascia, creates an elegant and dynamic design. Understanding the parts helps you appreciate the whole.

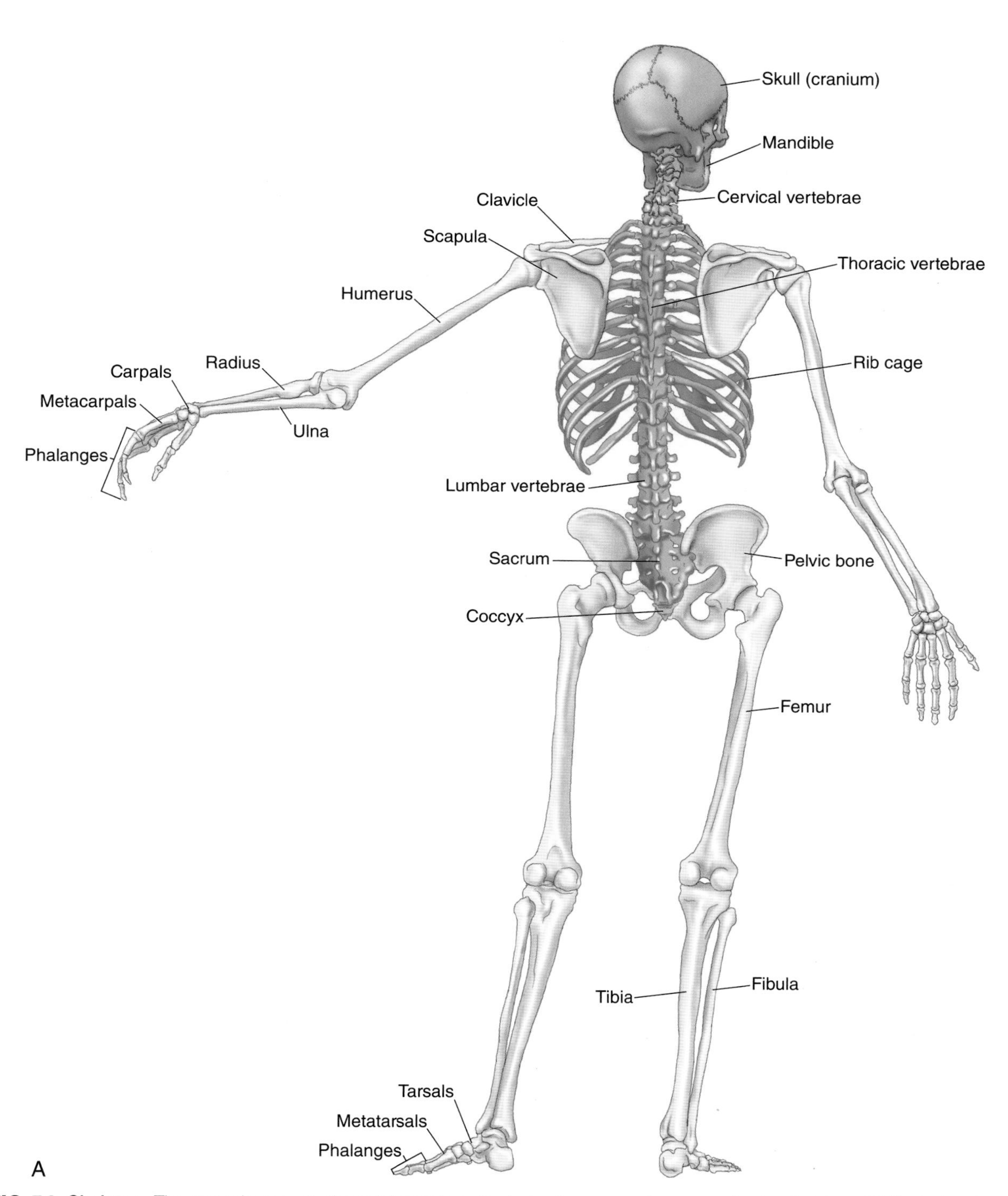

FIG. 7.2 Skeleton. The *green* bones are the axial skeleton; the *beige* bones are the appendicular skeleton. (A) Posterior view.

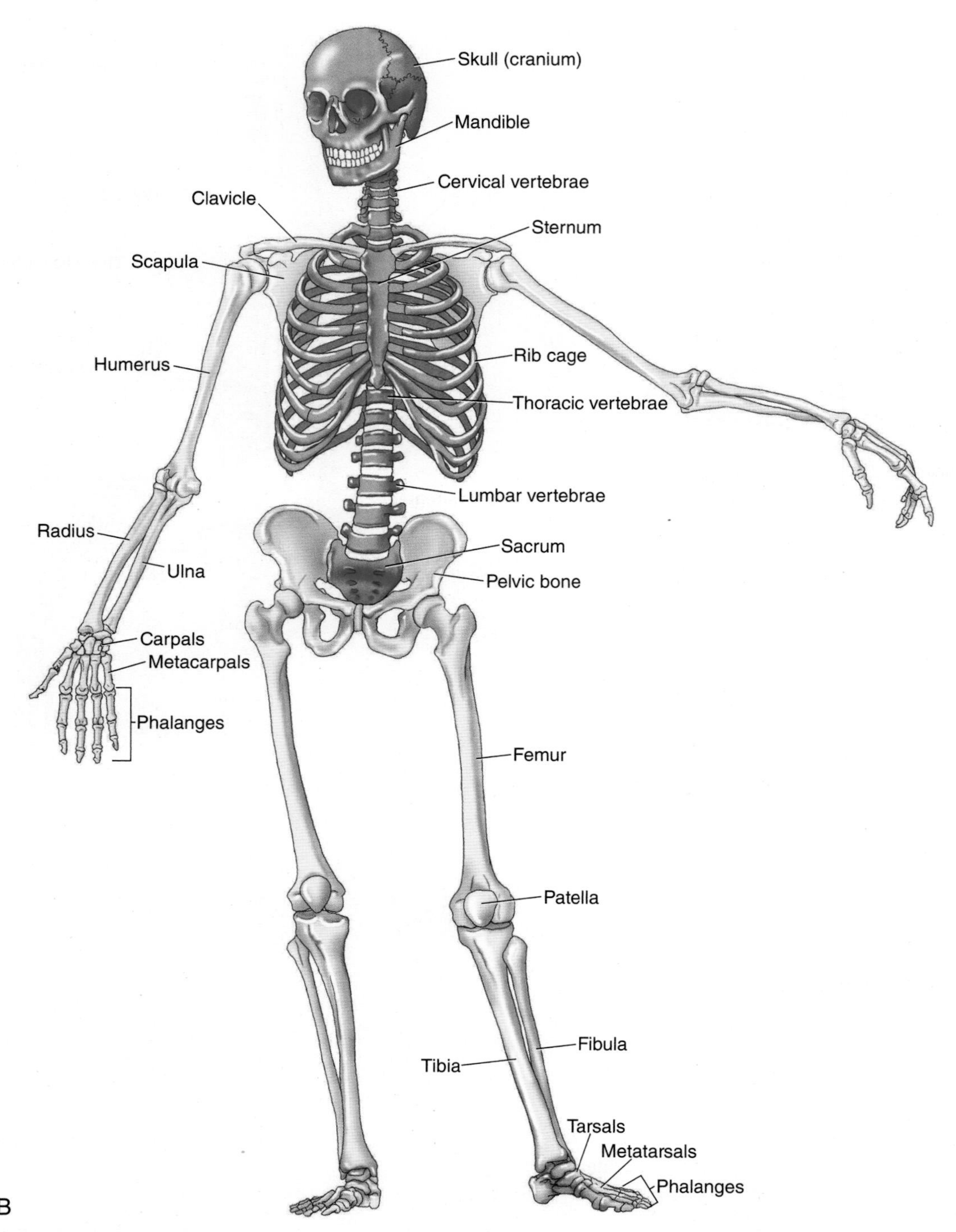

FIG. 7.2, cont'd (B) Anterior view. (From Muscolino JE. *Kinesiology: The Skeletal System and Muscle Function.* 2nd ed. Mosby; 2011.)

INDIVIDUAL BONY FRAMEWORK BY REGION

SECTION OBJECTIVES

Chapter objective covered in this section:

5. List and describe the individual bones of the axial skeleton.

After completing this section, the learner will be able to:

- List the bones of the head, spine, and thorax.
- List the number of cervical, thoracic, and lumbar vertebrae.
- List the bones of the upper and lower limbs.

Bones of the Axial Skeleton

The axial skeleton makes up the central and essential structures of the body. The structures contain vital organs and provide protection. For example, the skull contains the brain, the vertebral column houses and protects the spinal cord, and the ribs contain and protect the heart and lungs. As you study each figure in this section, find the bony landmarks.

Framework of the Head

The bony framework of the head, or skull, is made up of the cranial bones and the facial bones. Fig. 7.3 labels the structure of the head in detail, and the text describes the most prominent areas. Be sure to study the diagram carefully (Box 7.2; Activity 7.5).

The bones of the face provide the framework for the appearance of the face. Facial bones protect the eyeball, structure for the nose, and anchor for the teeth (Box 7.3).

In addition to the cranial and facial bones, other bones of the axial skeleton are found in the neck and head. The six auditory bones, called *ossicles* (three in each middle ear) are discussed in Chapter 5. The hyoid bone is a U-shaped bone attached to the tongue. Although it is attached to other bones by muscles and ligaments, it does not form an articulation with any other bones.

The structure of the skull is important to the function of other systems. Nerves and blood vessels enter and exit the skull through holes, or foramina, in the base. Muscles attach to the various projections and prominences on the outside of the skull. The sinuses are air spaces that resonate with the voice and remove some of the weight of the bones, making the head lighter (Fig. 7.4).

Between the bones of the skull are specialized joints called *sutures*. The four most prominent sutures are as follows:

- Sagittal suture, between the parietal bones
- Lambdoid suture, between the parietal bones and the occipital bone
- Coronal suture, between the parietal bones and the frontal bones
- Squamous suture, between the temporal and parietal bones

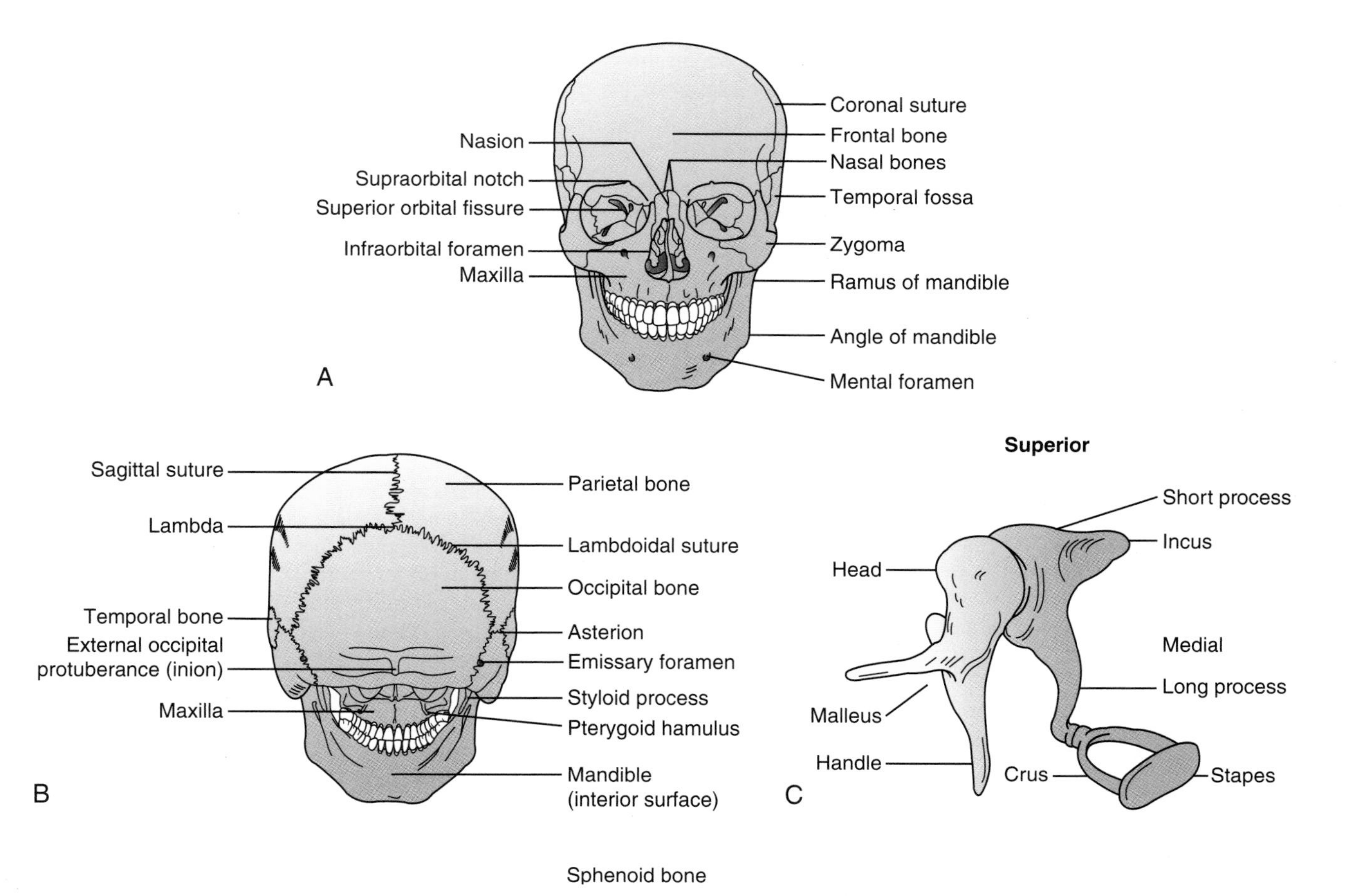

FIG. 7.3 (A) Anterior (frontal) view of the skull. (B) Posterior view of the skull. (C) The three auditory ossicles. The malleus attaches to the inner surface of the tympanic membrane (eardrum). The incus links the malleus to the stapes. The stapes is attached to the wall of the inner ear.

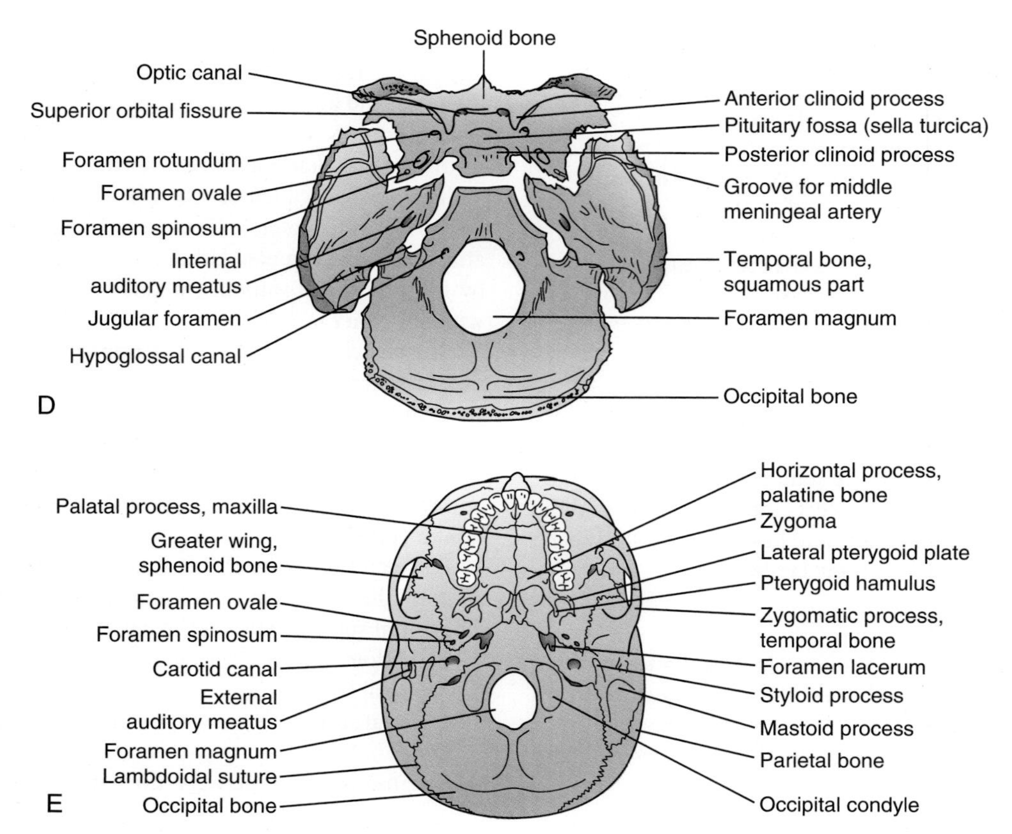

FIG. 7.3, cont'd (D) Detailed view of the internal surface of the base of the skull. The sphenoid, occipital, and temporal bones are presented as slightly separated to show that many of the important apertures traversing the floor of the skull are found within one of these bones or along their mutual borders. (E) Basal view of the skull, showing several of the important foramina that convey nerves and vessels in and out of the cranial cavity.

Box 7.2 Cranial Bones

Eight cranial bones enclose and protect the brain (see Fig. 7.3 and Activity 7.6):

- The **frontal bone** forms the forehead, the anterior portion of the roof of the skull, the top of the eye sockets, and part of the floor of the cranium. The frontal sinuses (air spaces) are within the frontal bone and open into the nasal cavities.
- Two **parietal bones** form most of the sides and top of the cranium.
- Two **temporal bones** form part of the side and part of the floor of the skull. Each temporal bone contains mastoid sinuses, an ear canal, an eardrum, and the middle and inner ears.
- The **ethmoid bone**, which is part of the anterior portion of the cranial floor, is a very light, spongy bone located between the eyes. The ethmoid bone forms part of the medial wall of the eye sockets and most of the nasal roof and contains the ethmoid sinuses. An extension of the ethmoid bone forms most of the superior portion of the nasal septum. If this bone is fractured, its proximity to the brain means that cerebrospinal fluid could leak into the nasal cavity. A runny nose that develops after a head injury could be the result of trauma to the sinuses or an indication of a serious condition.
- The **sphenoid bone** is in the middle of the base of the skull in front of the temporal bones. When viewed from above, the sphenoid bone looks like a bat with its wings extended. The sphenoid sinuses are located within this bone. The sella turcica, or "Turkish saddle," is a cavity on the superior surface of the body of the sphenoid that supports the pituitary gland.
- The **occipital bone** forms the posterior portion and a large part of the base of the cranium. This large, curved bone provides attachments for the muscles of the neck and trunk.

The Infant Skull

In the skull of an infant, bone formation is incomplete in some areas; these soft spots are called *fontanelles*. Found between the cranial bones, fontanelles are formed from very dense connective tissue, which is replaced with bone as the infant grows. The fontanelles allow for compression of the skull as the infant travels through the birth canal and for expansion of the skull as the brain grows. The fontanelles close when the child is 18 to 24 months old. The largest of the fontanelles is the anterior fontanelle, found near the front of the head at the junction between the two parietal bones and the frontal bone (Fig. 7.5).

Framework of the Trunk and Neck

The skeletal structure of the trunk and neck is made up of the vertebral column and the bones of the chest. A child's vertebral column has 33 (or sometimes 34) irregularly shaped bones, which fuse in the lower portion to become 26 bones in the

ACTIVITY 7.5

The names of the cranial bones start with various letters. To help you remember them, make up a sentence that uses the first letter of each name. Get creative!

Example

The cranial bones are the following:
*P*arietal
*S*phenoid
*T*emporal
*F*rontal
*O*ccipital
*E*thmoid
*P*lease *S*top *T*he *F*lying *O*strich *E*gg.

Your Turn

The facial bones are the following:
Nasal
Vomer
Lacrimal
Zygomatic
Palatine
Maxilla
Mandible
Inferior nasal concha

Make up a creative sentence that uses the first letter of each name in whatever order works for you.

Box 7.3 Facial Bones

Fourteen facial bones form the front of the skull (see Fig. 7.3; see Activity 7.6):

- The **mandible**, or lower jawbone, is the only voluntarily movable bone of the skull. The largest of the facial bones, the mandible forms the chin, which is classified as a mental prominence.
- Two **maxillary bones** unite to form the upper jawbone, part of the floor of the eye sockets, part of the roof of the mouth, including the anterior portion of the hard palate, and the outer walls and floor of the nasal cavity. Each maxilla contains the maxillary sinus, a large air space that empties into the nasal cavity.
- Two **zygomatic bones**, or cheekbones, form the prominences of the cheeks and a portion of the floor and outer wall of the eye sockets.
- Two small, oblong **nasal bones**, in the superior middle of the face, form the bridge of the nose.
- Two **lacrimal bones**, each about the size and shape of a fingernail, are posterior and lateral to the nasal bone. These bones form part of the medial wall of the eye sockets.
- The **vomer** is a triangular bone that forms the inferior and posterior nasal septum.
- Two L-shaped **palatine bones** form the posterior portion of the hard palate and part of the floor of the nasal cavity.
- Two inferior **nasal conchae bones** form a portion of the lateral wall of the nasal cavities. The inferior conchae work with the superior and middle conchae of the ethmoid bone to circulate and filter air that enters the nose.

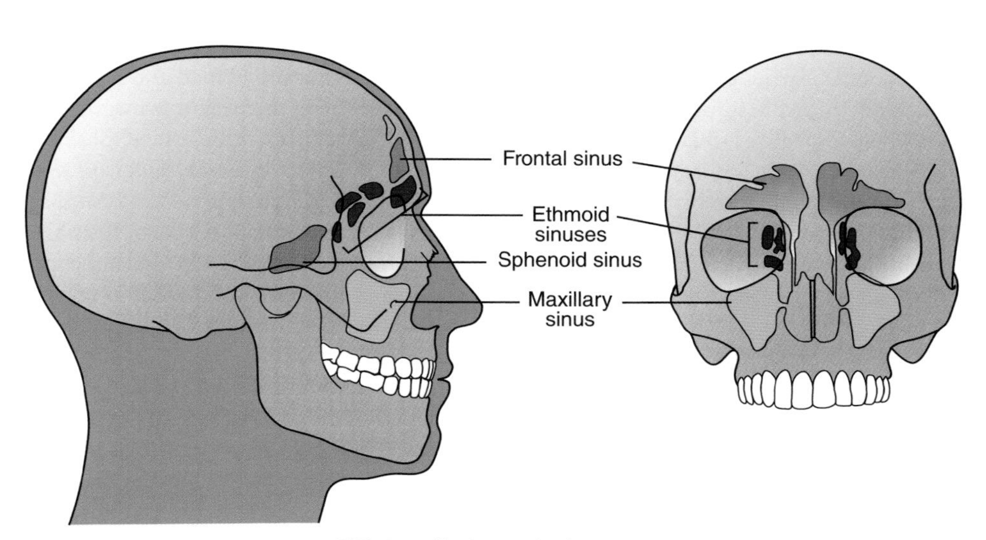

FIG. 7.4 Air sinuses in the nose.

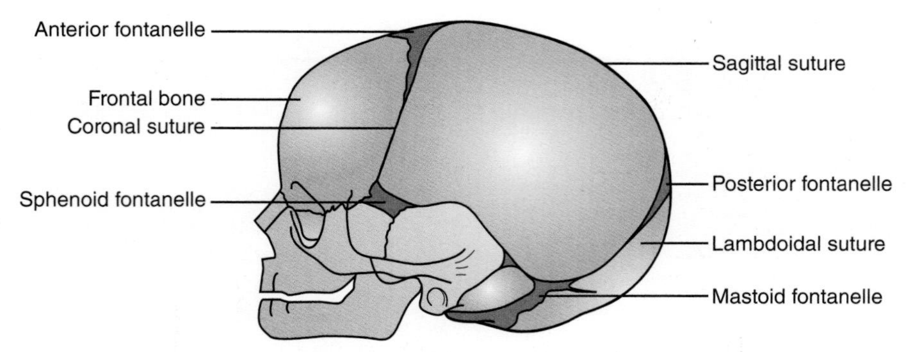

FIG. 7.5 Infant skull.

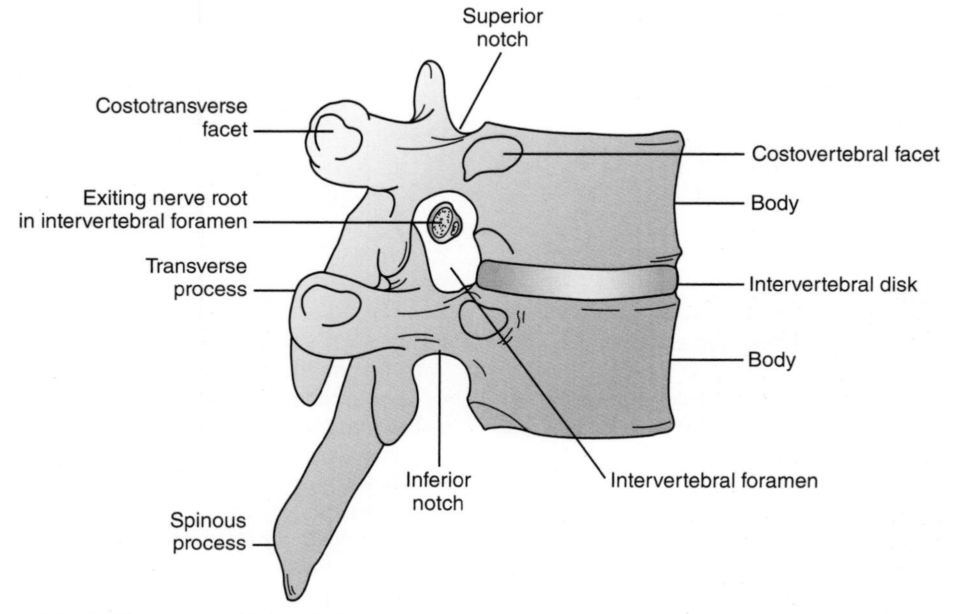

FIG. 7.6 Lateral view of the intervertebral foramen. Vertebrae T5 and T6 have been articulated, and the resultant intervertebral foramen is shown with a segmental nerve in place. Blood vessels (not shown) also enter and leave the interior of the vertebral canal through the intervertebral foramen.

adult. Each of the vertebrae has two main sections: the anterior body and the posterior arch. All vertebrae, except the atlas and the axis, have these characteristic features:

1. A drum-shaped body, or centrum, located toward the anterior, serves as the weight-bearing portion of the bone.
2. A vertebral arch, which encircles the spinal cord, is connected to the body by two pedicles (feet). Two laminae (part of a vertebra) unite posteriorly to form the spinous process. The spinous process usually can be felt just under the skin of the back. The thickened junctions between the pedicles and the laminae have superior and inferior cartilaginous articular facets and a laterally projecting transverse process.
3. A large hole, or foramen, is in the center of each vertebra. All the vertebrae are linked in a series by strong ligaments, and these spaces form the spinal canal, a bony cylinder that protects the spinal cord. As the vertebral bodies stack on one another, a space is created between the upper and lower pedicles, forming the intervertebral foramina, which allows passage of the spinal nerves.
4. Vertebrae that are stacked one on the other. Each vertebra has three joint surfaces, two articular facets that provide the articulating surface for this stacking arrangement, and one intervertebral disk joint.
5. The vertebrae are named and numbered according to their location from the neck downward:
   - 7 cervical vertebrae, called *C1 through C7*
   - 12 thoracic vertebrae, called *T1 through T12*
   - 5 lumbar vertebrae, called *L1 through L5*

The sacrum and coccyx form the base of the vertebral column. During childhood, the sacrum consists of five individual bones, and the coccyx is made up of three to five bones. The individual bones of the sacrum and coccyx fuse in the adult, becoming two solid bones.

Although not technically a part of the vertebrae, the intervertebral disks (or discs; both spellings are correct) between the vertebral bodies act as shock absorbers and spacers and provide flexibility (Fig. 7.6). The disk consists of two components. The outer portion, or annulus fibrosus, is composed of concentric rings of fibrocartilage arranged like the layers of an

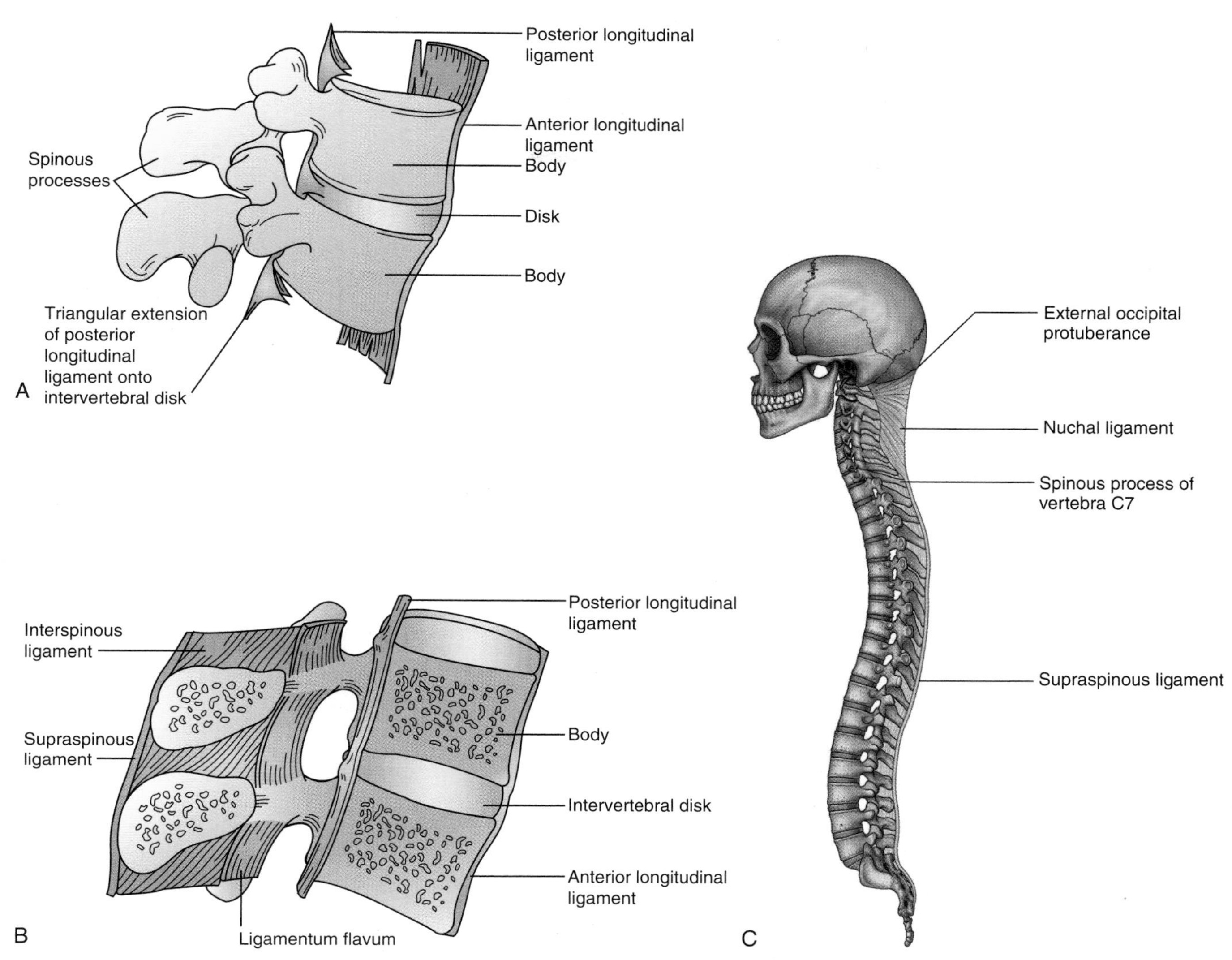

FIG. 7.7 (A) and (B) Vertebral ligaments. (C) Supraspinous ligament and nuchal ligament. (C, From Drake RL, Wayne Vogl A, Mitchell AWM. *Gray's Anatomy for Students.* 2nd ed. Elsevier; 2010.)

onion. Internally, the center, or nucleus pulposus, is made of a gelatinous substance. If a disk ruptures, the fibrocartilage splits and the nucleus pulposus leaks. The disk becomes smaller and is less able to disperse pressure and maintain space between the vertebrae. In severe cases, the ruptured disk vertebra can impinge on nerves.

The vertebral arteries heading toward the brainstem pass through the foramina of the transverse processes of the cervical vertebrae. These vessels are subject to stretching injuries with extreme cervical rotation of the extended neck.

Again, study all illustrations carefully, because the labeling detail is more complete than what is provided in the discussion and major features of bones in the text.

Ligaments

Three ligaments extend the length of the vertebral column:

- The anterior longitudinal ligament attaches to the front of the vertebral bodies and acts to restrain extension.
- The posterior longitudinal ligament attaches to the back of the vertebral bodies and acts to restrain flexion.
- The supraspinous ligament runs along the tips of the spinous processes and restrains flexion.

A strong, fibrous band called the *nuchal ligament* (a thickening of the supraspinous ligament) runs along the notched spinous processes of C2 to C6 and helps support the weight of the head. Other vertebral ligaments are placed between individual vertebrae.

- The ligamenta flava connects the laminae of each adjacent vertebra.
- The interspinous ligaments connect the spinous processes.
- The intertransverse ligaments connect the transverse processes (Figs. 7.7 and 7.8).

Right-side lateral flexion stretches the left intertransverse ligaments, and left-side lateral flexion stretches the right intertransverse ligaments. Vertebral movement patterns are discussed in detail in Chapter 8 (Box 7.4; Fig. 7.9).

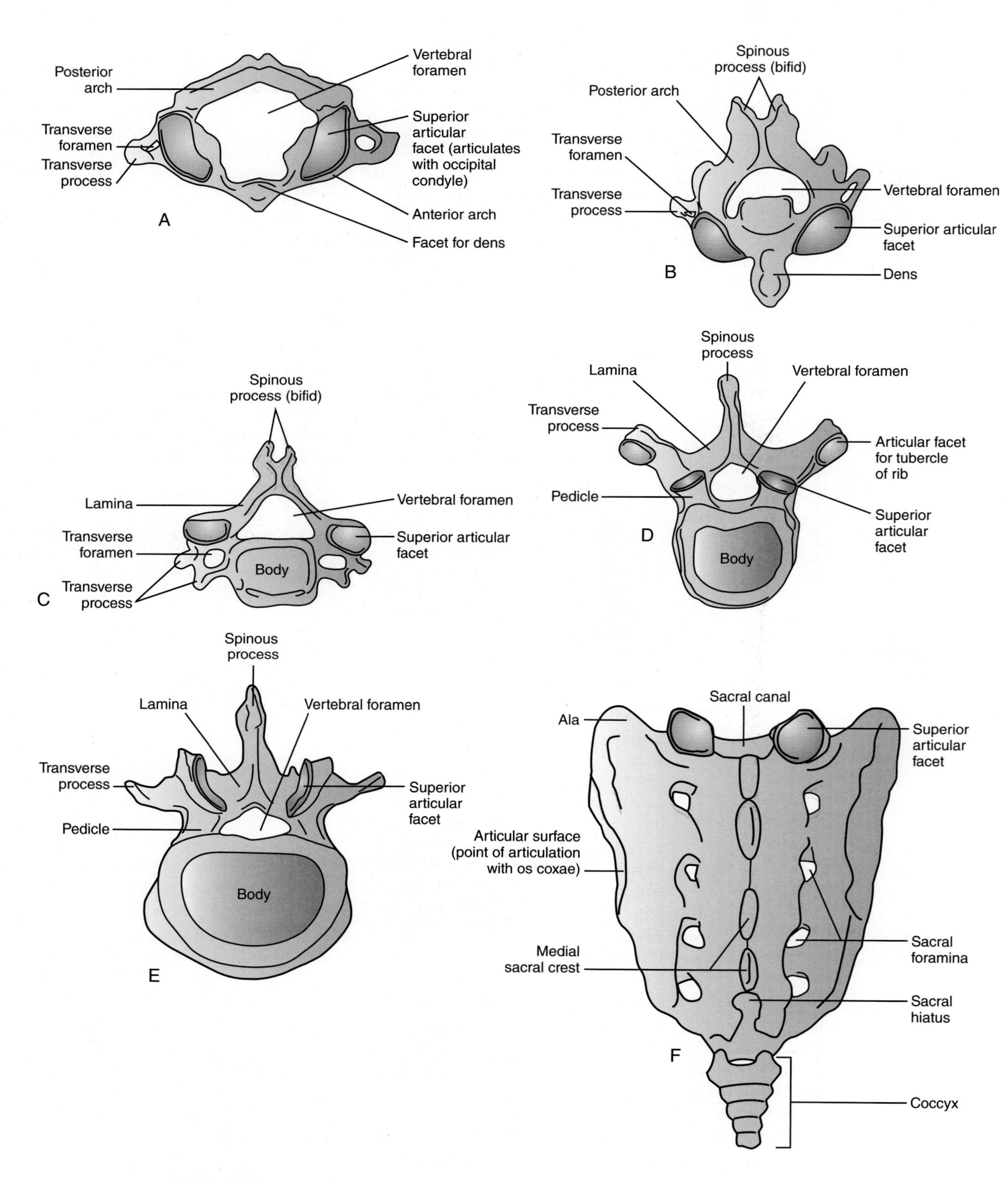

FIG. 7.8 Six types of vertebrae: (A) atlas, (B) axis, (C) cervical, (D) thoracic, (E) lumbar, and (F) sacrum.

Box 7.4 Bones and Structures of the Vertebral Column (see Figs. 7.6–7.9)

Cervical Vertebrae

The seven cervical vertebrae (C1 to C7) are located in the neck.

The first vertebra (C1), called the *atlas*, supports the head. When you nod your head "yes," the occipital bone of the skull rocks on the atlas. The atlas is greatly modified for articulation within the occipital region of the skull. The atlas does not have a body or spinous process; rather, it is essentially a bony ring consisting of anterior and posterior arches and two lateral masses.

The second cervical vertebra (C2), called the *axis*, serves as a pivot when the head is turned from side to side (as in the gesture "no"). The axis has a peglike den, or odontoid process, projecting superiorly from its anterior side.

The pivot joint of C1 to C2 consists of a ringlike structure (the atlas) that rotates around the dens. Considerable movement, especially as seen in rotation, is possible because of the design of this joint.

Thoracic Vertebrae

The 12 thoracic vertebrae (T1 to T12) are located in the thorax of the trunk (the body area between the neck and diaphragm). The main functions of the thoracic vertebrae are to provide spaces on which to build the rib cage, which protects the heart and lungs, and to house the spinal cord.

The posterior ends of the 12 pairs of ribs are attached to these vertebrae at posterior facets and hemifacets (thought of as one-half of a facet).

T1 has a whole facet joint space for the first rib articulation and an inferior hemifacet, which works with the corresponding superior hemifacet of T2 for articulation with the second rib.

T2 to T8 each has superior and inferior hemifacets, which together form the vertebral portion of the articulation with the ribs. T9 has one superior hemifacet, and T10 to T12 each has a whole facet to articulate with the ribs.

The arrangement of the vertebrae in the thorax allows for a certain amount of flexion, extension, side bending, and rotation; but movements generally are limited, with most movement occurring at the thoracic-lumbar junction at T11, T12, and L1.

Lumbar Vertebrae

The five lumbar vertebrae (L1 to L5) are located in the abdomen of the trunk. They are larger and heavier than the other vertebrae, which allows them to support more weight.

The interlocking shape of the lumbar vertebrae makes rotation difficult but facilitates flexion, extension, and side bending. L4 and L5 allow the most motion.

Most disk injuries occur at L4 to L5 and L5 to S1 (the area of the lumbar-sacral junction).

Sacral Vertebrae

The sacral vertebrae are five separate bones in a child; however, they eventually fuse to form a single bone, the sacrum, in an adult.

Wedged between the two pelvic bones, the sacrum completes the posterior part of the bony pelvis. Four transverse ridges are the remnants of intervertebral disks. At the ends of each ridge are paired sacral foramina, through which the sacral nerves pass.

Coccyx

The coccyx, or tailbone, consists of four or five tiny bones in a child. As a person develops, these bones fuse to form a single bone in an adult.

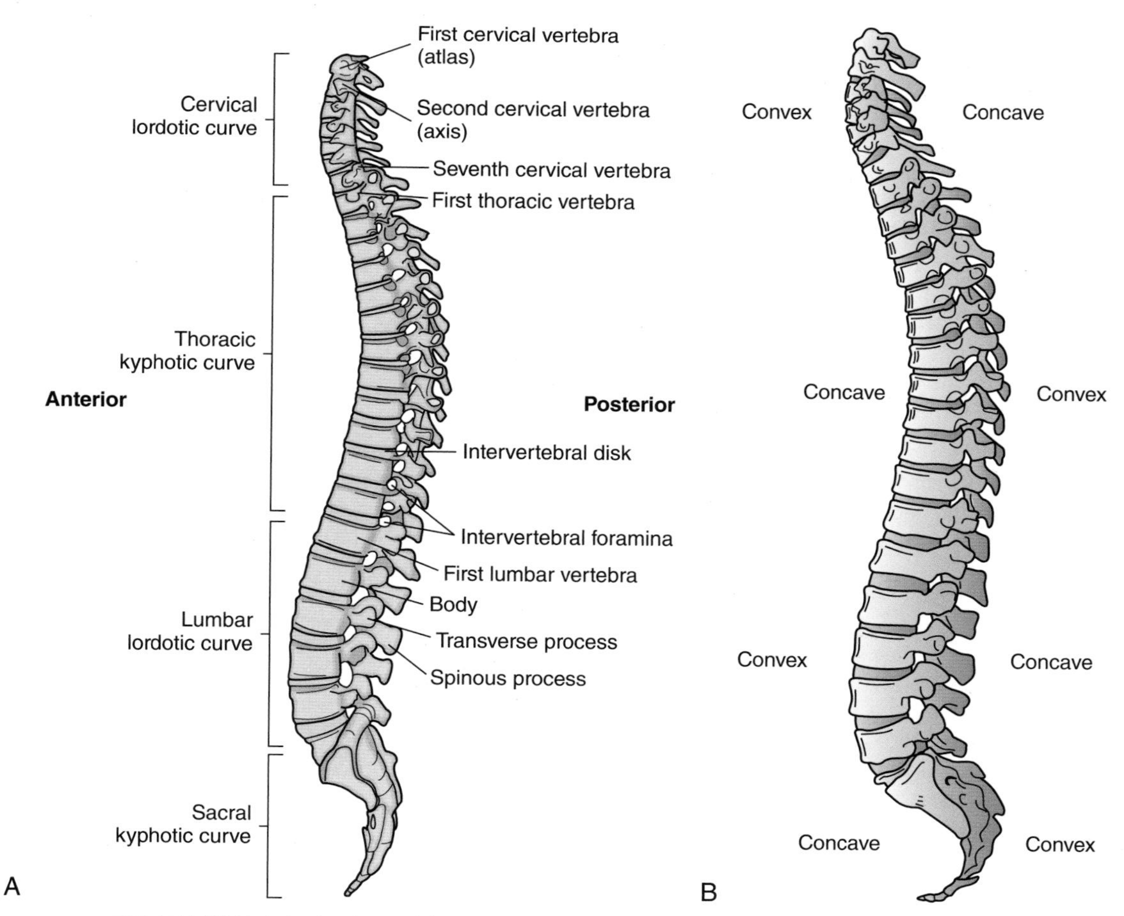

FIG. 7.9 (A) Vertebral column. (B) The convex and concave curves of the vertebral column.

Vertebral Curves

When viewed from the side, the vertebral column has curves that correspond to the groups of vertebrae. In a newborn, the entire column is a concave-forward shape; this is the primary kyphotic curve. When the infant begins to assume an erect posture, secondary lordotic curves are convex forward in shape. For example, the cervical lordotic curve appears when the infant begins to hold up the head at about 3 months of age; the lumbar lordotic curve appears when the child begins to walk. The curves of the vertebral column provide some of the resilience and spring that are so essential to walking and running.

- The cervical region is convex forward or has a *lordosis*.
- The thoracic region is concave forward, called a *kyphosis*.
- The lumbar region is also lordotic.
- The sacrum is also kyphotic.

Vertebral curvatures develop dysfunction generally from exaggerated posture, activity, obesity, pregnancy, trauma, and disease. These conditions have the same name as the normal curves but are considered abnormal if they are exaggerated enough to cause problems. For example:

- Osteoporosis can lead to the development of a hump in the thoracic vertebrae, called *hyperkyphosis* or *dowager's hump*.
- A swayback of the lower back is a hyperlordosis.
- A different type of abnormal curvature is called *scoliosis*. It is a lateral curvature of the spine.

Any exaggerated curve puts a strain on the musculoskeletal posture mechanisms and may predispose a person to pain and impaired movement (see Fig. 7.9).

Bones of the Thorax

The thorax is the region of the trunk between the base of the neck and the top of the abdomen (where the diaphragm muscle is located). The bones of the thorax form a cone-shaped cage that protects the heart, the lungs, and other thoracic cavity structures. Twelve pairs of ribs form the rib cage. The rib cage attaches posteriorly to the spinal column and anteriorly to the sternum or breastbone. The xiphoid process is the inferior portion of the sternum and is used as a landmark in cardiopulmonary resuscitation for chest compressions. Chest compressions are performed above the xiphoid process to avoid breaking it off (Box 7.5; Fig. 7.10).

Bones of the Appendicular Skeleton

The appendicular skeleton may be considered as having two divisions: the upper extremity and the lower extremity.

The upper extremity includes the shoulders or pectoral girdles; the arms between the shoulders and the elbows; the forearms between the elbows and the wrists; and the wrists and hands, including the fingers. In everyday conversation, we refer to the arm as the whole appendage from the shoulder joint to the wrist joint. In anatomical terms, the arm is the portion from the shoulder joint to the elbow joint. The only bony attachment of the upper extremity to the axial skeleton occurs at the sternoclavicular joint, the articulation of the clavicle, and the manubrium of the sternum.

The lower extremity includes the hips or pelvic girdles; the thighs between the hips and knees; the legs between the knees and ankles; and the ankles and feet, including the toes. Note that in anatomical terms, the leg is only the portion from the knee joint to the ankle joint.

Bones of the Upper Extremity

The bones of the upper extremity can be divided into two groups. One group consists of the bones of the pectoral girdle, which include the clavicle, and the scapula (some references include the manubrium, upper thoracic vertebrae, and first two ribs as functional units of the pectoral girdle). The other group includes the bones of the arm, forearm, and hand (Box 7.6; Figs. 7.11 and 7.12).

Box 7.5 Bones of the Thorax (see Fig. 7.10)

The sternum is fairly flat.
The sternum consists of three parts:

- The manubrium at the top
- The body in the middle
- The xiphoid process at the lower end

The ribs are elongated, flattened, and twisted bones.
Most ribs articulate with two thoracic vertebrae at three points:

- The two facets on the head of the rib contact the hemifacets of the vertebral bodies.
- The tubercle contacts the transverse process.

At the posterior end of each rib is a head, which has two facets for articulation with the body (or bodies) of the thoracic vertebra.
The neck of the rib is a constricted portion next to the head.
The tubercle has an articular part, which is connected to the transverse process of a thoracic vertebra, and a nonarticular part for ligament attachment.
The body, or shaft, is long and curved.
The shaft also has a sharp bend, called the *costal angle*.
The anterior end is joined to the costal cartilage.
Each of our ribs attaches to the posterior vertebrae. The intercostal spaces, between the ribs, contain muscles, blood vessels, and nerves.
The 12 pairs of ribs are classified by their anterior attachments:

- The first seven pairs are the true ribs; they attach directly to the sternum by way of their costal cartilages.
- The next five pairs of ribs are known as the *false ribs*. The first three (or the eighth, ninth, and 10th ribs) attach to the cartilage of the above rib.
- The 11th and 12th false rib pairs are referred to as *floating ribs* because they have no anterior attachment.

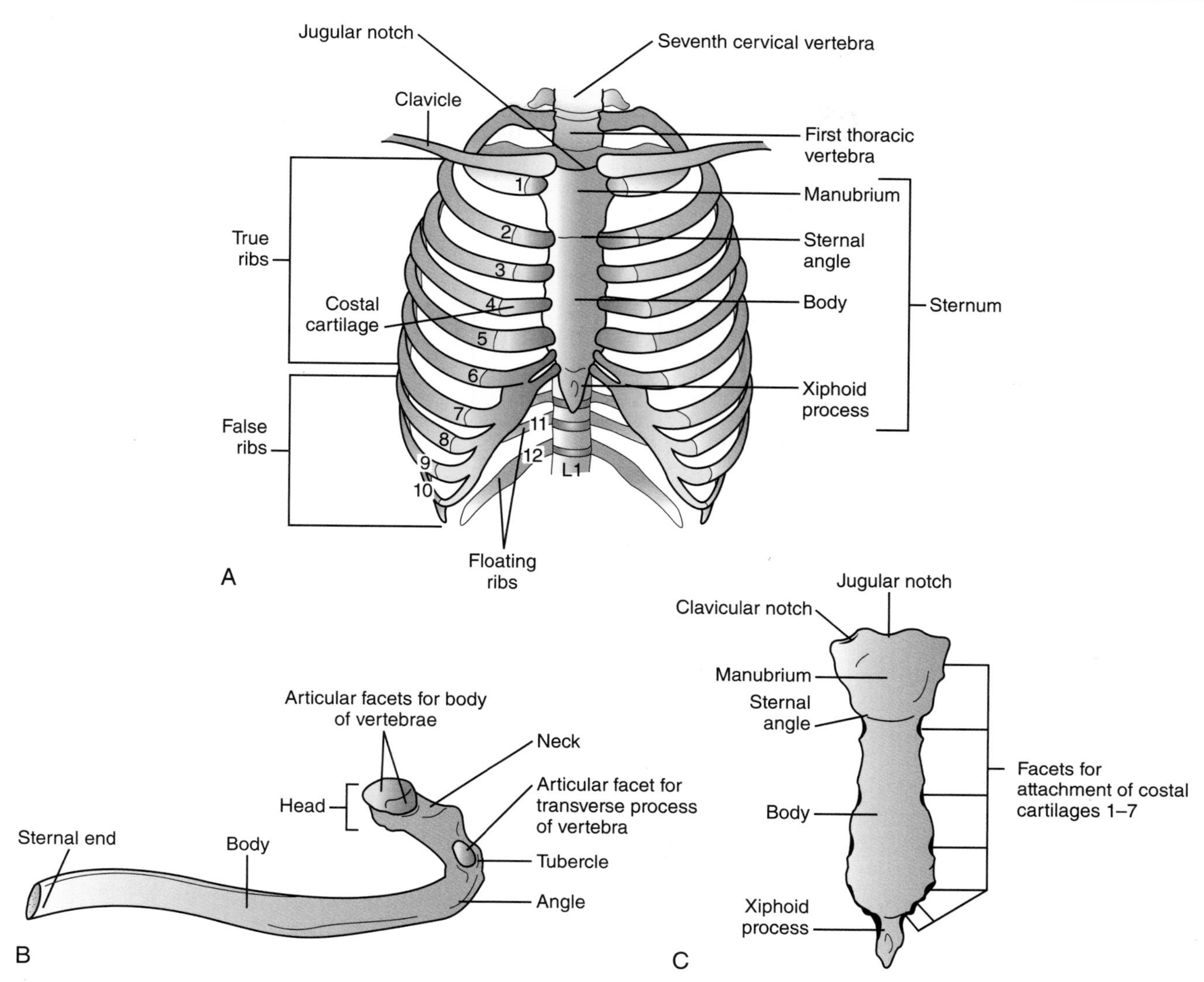

FIG. 7.10 (A) Rib cage. (B) Typical rib. (C) Sternum.

Box 7.6 Bones of the Pectoral Girdle

Clavicle (see Fig. 7.11)

The clavicle, or collar bone, is long and flat and has two bends, which gives it an S shape. This fragile bone transmits force from the arms to the thorax. For this reason, when a person falls with arms outstretched, this bone often breaks or the joint separates when the clavicle hits the acromion.

The lateral clavicle articulates with the acromion of the scapula, and together they form the upper portion of the shoulder.

This structure functions as a strut by keeping the scapula posterior, which maintains the position of the glenoid fossa (the point of articulation of the humerus on the scapula).

The clavicle articulates medially with the manubrium to form the sternoclavicular joint.

Scapula (see Fig. 7.12)

The scapula, or shoulder blade, is an irregular, triangular bone with a flat anterior surface. The edges of the bone are also landmarks and attachment points for muscles; these are the medial, superior, and lateral borders.

The posterior surface has a large spine and two major processes, which are all easy to palpate:

- At the lateral end of the scapular spine is the acromion process, the highest point of the bony portion of the shoulder.
- The coracoid process is a fingerlike projection from the anterior portion of the superior border.

The three corners of this triangular-shaped bone are referred to as the *inferior, superior*, and *lateral angles*.

The scapula has three borders, referred to as the *medial, superior*, and *lateral*.

- The medial border is also known as the *vertebral border*.
- The superior border is the hardest to palpate because it lies under the shoulder muscles.
- The lateral (or axillary) border is the thickest of the three. The lateral border contains the glenoid cavity, a shallow depression that articulates with the head of the humerus to form the shoulder joint.

The scapula has three fossae that are attachment points for muscles that connect the scapula to the humerus:

- Supraspinous fossa, which is on the posterior and upper portion of the scapula
- Infraspinous fossa, which is on the posterior and upper portion of the scapula
- Subscapular fossa, which is on the anterior portion of the scapula

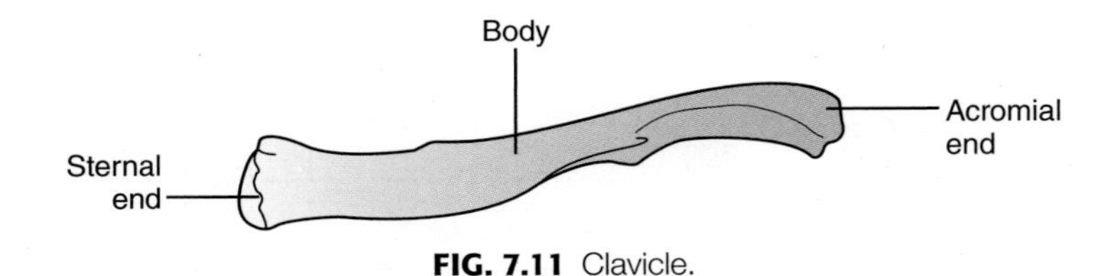

FIG. 7.11 Clavicle.

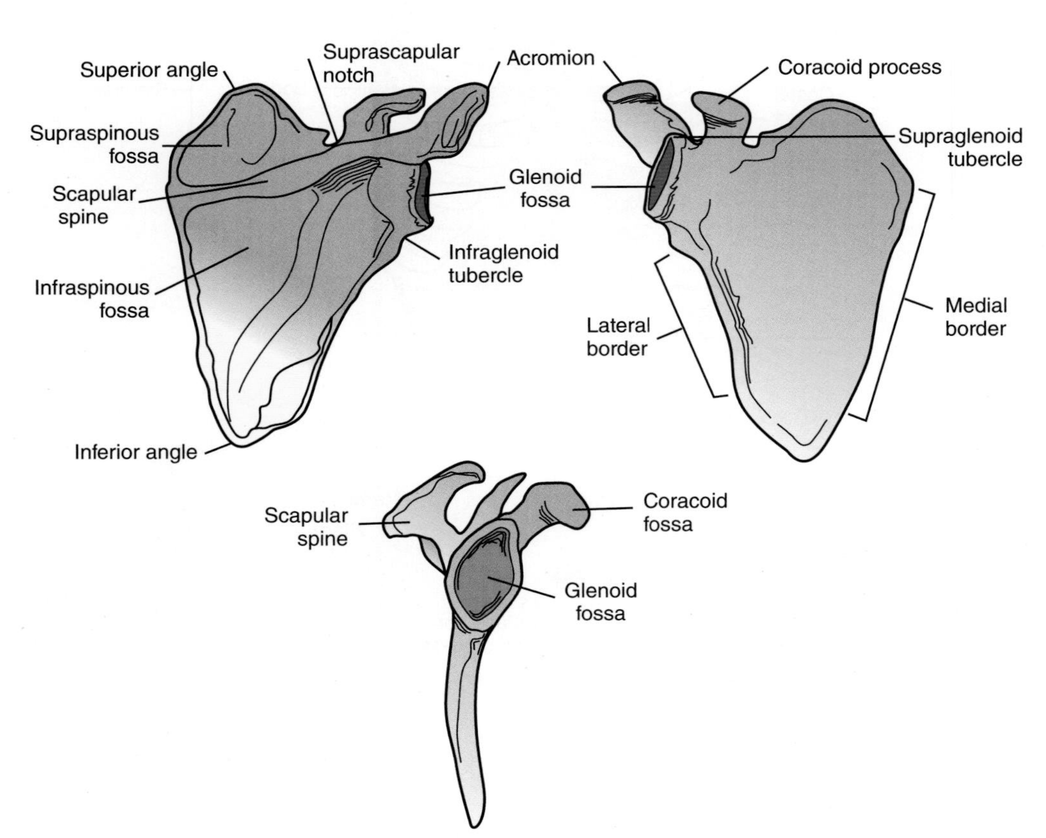

FIG. 7.12 Scapula (three views).

The Humerus, Radius, Ulna, and Bones of the Wrist and Hand

The second group of bones of the upper division consists of the bones of the upper extremity, which are the humerus, radius, ulna, and bones of the wrist and hand. The medial and lateral epicondyles of the humerus are attachment points for muscles and are prone to problems from repetitive use (Fig. 7.13).

The head of the radius, at the proximal end, articulates with the capitulum of the humerus during flexion and extension. During flexion and extension, the radial head slides on the capitulum, and the trochlear notch of the ulna slides over the trochlea of the humerus.

In full flexion, the radial head and the ulnar coronoid process fit into the radial and coronoid fossae of the humerus. At full extension, the olecranon process of the ulna moves into the olecranon fossa of the humerus, which prevents extension beyond 180 degrees. During full flexion, the radius slides into the radial fossa of the humerus. At the distal end of the radius, the articular surface combines with the proximal carpals to form the wrist joint.

The styloid process of the radius is a bony projection at the distal end, just proximal to the thumb. The radius and ulna articulate with each other in three places: proximally near the elbow, in the middle between the shafts, and distally near the wrist. Motion between the radius and ulna is important for orienting the placement of the hand. It is important to remember that all anatomical references are made when the forearm and hand are in anatomical position.

The actions of the joints of the shoulder girdle, arm, and forearm are discussed in more detail in Chapter 8 (Box 7.7; Fig. 7.14).

The two bones of the lower arm—the radius and the ulna—meet at the hand to form the wrist. Technically, the wrist is part of the hand and is considered a joint that consists of eight bones forming the proximal skeletal segment of the hand. The hand is made up of the wrist, palm, and fingers. The bones of the hand are the carpals (wrist bones), metacarpals (in the palm), and phalanges (finger bones). Many skeletal injuries occur with falls on the hand, especially when it is forced into extreme hyperextension. Fractures of the scaphoid and radius

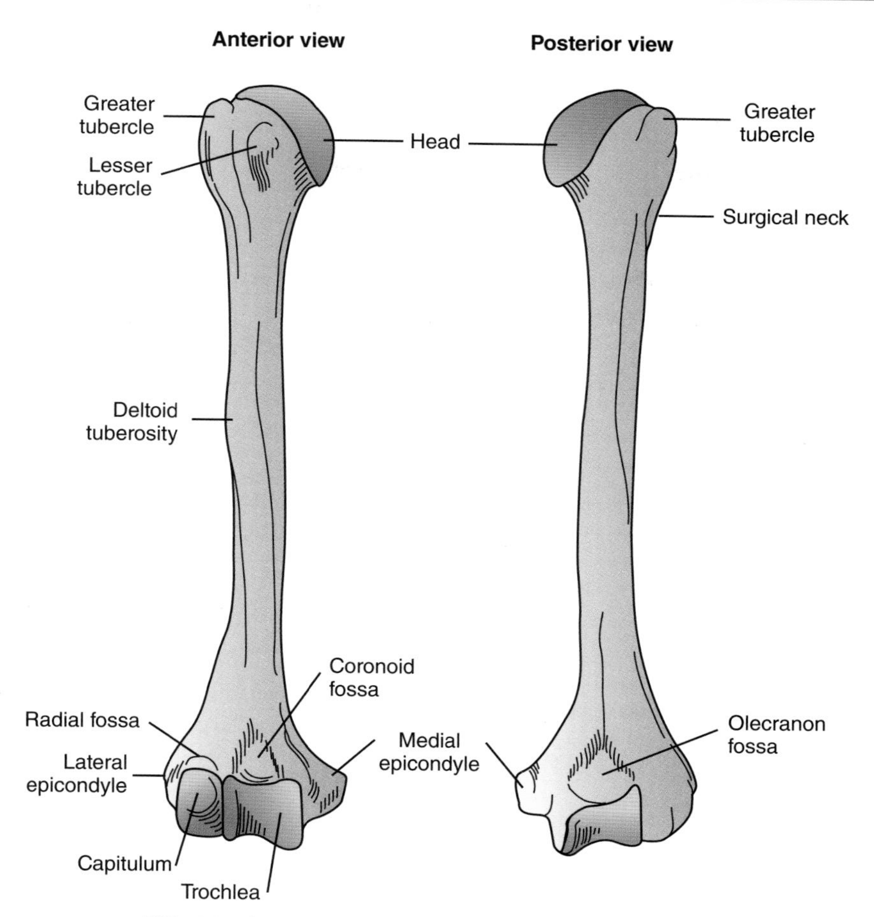

FIG. 7.13 Anterior and posterior views of the right humerus.

Box 7.7 Features of the Humerus, Radius, and Ulna

Humerus (see Fig. 7.13)

The humerus, or arm bone, is a long bone. The head of the humerus, at the proximal end, articulates with the glenoid fossa of the scapula, forming the glenohumeral (shoulder) joint.

The distal end of the humerus articulates with the radius and ulna to form the elbow joint.

On the lateral edge of the distal end of the humerus is a rounded surface called the *capitulum*.

The medial edge of the distal end of the humerus forms a pulley-shaped surface, the *trochlea*.

Just above these projections on the anterior surface are the radial and coronoid (ulnar) fossae.

The *olecranon fossa* is on the posterior surface.

Radius and Ulna (see Fig. 7.14)

The lower part of the upper limb is called the *forearm*. It is composed of two bones: the **radius** and the **ulna**. The radius and ulna lie parallel to each other when the forearm is supinated.

Radius

The radius is bigger and longer than the ulna.

The radius is the bone on the lateral (thumb) side of the arm.

The *radius* is narrow at the elbow and widens just above the wrist.

During pronation, the radius crosses the ulna.

The radius takes most of the strain when weight is placed on the wrist.

The radius is a common site of fractures.

Ulna

The ulna provides most of the stability of the forearm.

Opposite in shape to the radius, the ulna is wider at the elbow and narrower at the wrist.

At the proximal end of the ulna is the trochlear notch, which articulates with the trochlea of the humerus.

The olecranon process is the large projection on the posterior side that is easily palpable. Most individuals refer to it as their *elbow*. This process slides into the olecranon fossa of the humerus during extension.

The coronoid process is located on the ulna, which moves into the coronoid fossa of the humerus during full flexion.

At the distal end of the ulna is the head. The head of a bone is usually found at the proximal end.

The styloid process of the ulna is a bony landmark found proximal to the wrist.

Just beyond the proximal end is an articular disk, which articulates with the carpals to provide some of the movements of the wrist.

are common because forces produced by a fall on the hand are transmitted through the scaphoid and lunate and are absorbed by the radius (Box 7.8; Figs. 7.15 and 7.16; see Activity 7.6).

Bones of the Lower Extremity

The bones of the lower extremity are grouped like those of the upper extremity. The two primary groups of the lower extremity are the bones of the pelvic girdle and the bones of the thigh, leg, and foot. The pelvis supports the trunk and the organs in the pelvic cavity. The pelvis also absorbs stress from the lower limbs when we are moving, whether walking or jumping. The female pelvis is adapted for pregnancy and childbirth and is wider and lighter than the male pelvis. The second group of bones of the lower extremity is structured for weight-bearing during walking and standing; therefore these bones are larger than the bones of the upper limb.

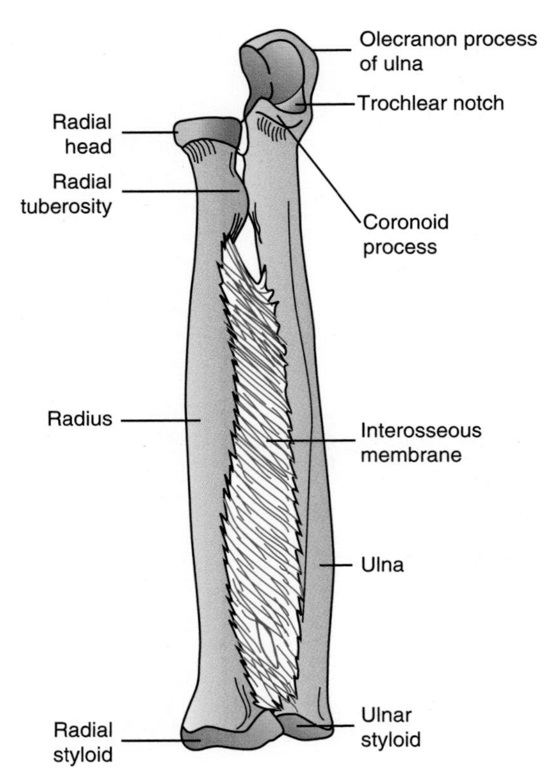

FIG. 7.14 Anterior view of the forearm bones.

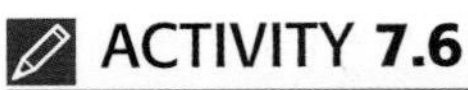

ACTIVITY 7.6

Draw the posterior view of the scapula, and label the following:
Acromion process
Scapular spine
Inferior angle
Superior angle
Lateral border
Medial border
Superior border
Glenoid fossa
Supraspinous fossa
Infraspinous fossa

Bones of the Thigh, Leg, Ankle, and Foot

The second group of bones of the lower division consists of the bones of the lower extremity, which are the femur of the thigh, patella or kneecap, tibia, fibula of the leg, and bones of the ankle and foot. The bones of the ankle and foot pair with the bones of the wrist and hand. Whereas the hand is adapted for mobility and dexterity with the opposable thumb, the foot is much less mobile and provides a platform for us to walk on.

Box 7.8 The Bones of the Wrist and Hand (see Figs. 7.15 and 7.16)

Wrist

The wrist is the joint between the hand and the forearm. The structure of the wrist allows movement of the hand. The hand is an elegant and versatile structure that allows the digits (fingers and thumb) to move independently and form an effective grip.

The wrist contains the carpals—eight small, cube-shaped bones arranged in two rows of four.

In the proximal row are the scaphoid, lunate, and triquetrum, which articulate with the radius to form the wrist joint.

The pisiform is also in the proximal row but does not articulate with the radius.

The distal row contains the trapezium, trapezoid, capitate, and hamate.

The transverse arch of the wrist, formed by the carpals, is anteriorly concave.

A wide, thick ligament, the flexor retinaculum, connects the pisiform and hamate to the scaphoid and trapezium or the anterior side.

The posterior (dorsal) side of the wrist has six tunnels for the extensor tendons.

The palmar side of the wrist has two tunnels to carry nerves, arteries, and flexor tendons.

The carpal tunnel, the largest of the two palmar tunnels, is the most commonly traumatized. The carpal tunnel contains the median nerve, which can become compressed, especially when repetitive movements of the hand and fingers cause friction and inflammation.

Hand

The human hand has 27 bones: carpus or wrist accounts for 8; metacarpals or palm contains 5; the remaining 14 are digital bones, fingers, and thumb. In the palm are five metacarpal bones, long bones that form the framework of each hand.

Knuckles are the rounded distal ends of the metacarpals.

Fourteen phalanges, or finger bones, are found in each hand, two for the thumb and three for each finger.

Each of these long bones is called a *phalanx*.

The first, or proximal phalanx, articulates with a metacarpal.

The second and third are referred to as the *middle* and *distal phalanges*.

The thumb has only a proximal phalanx and a distal phalanx (see Activity 7.8).

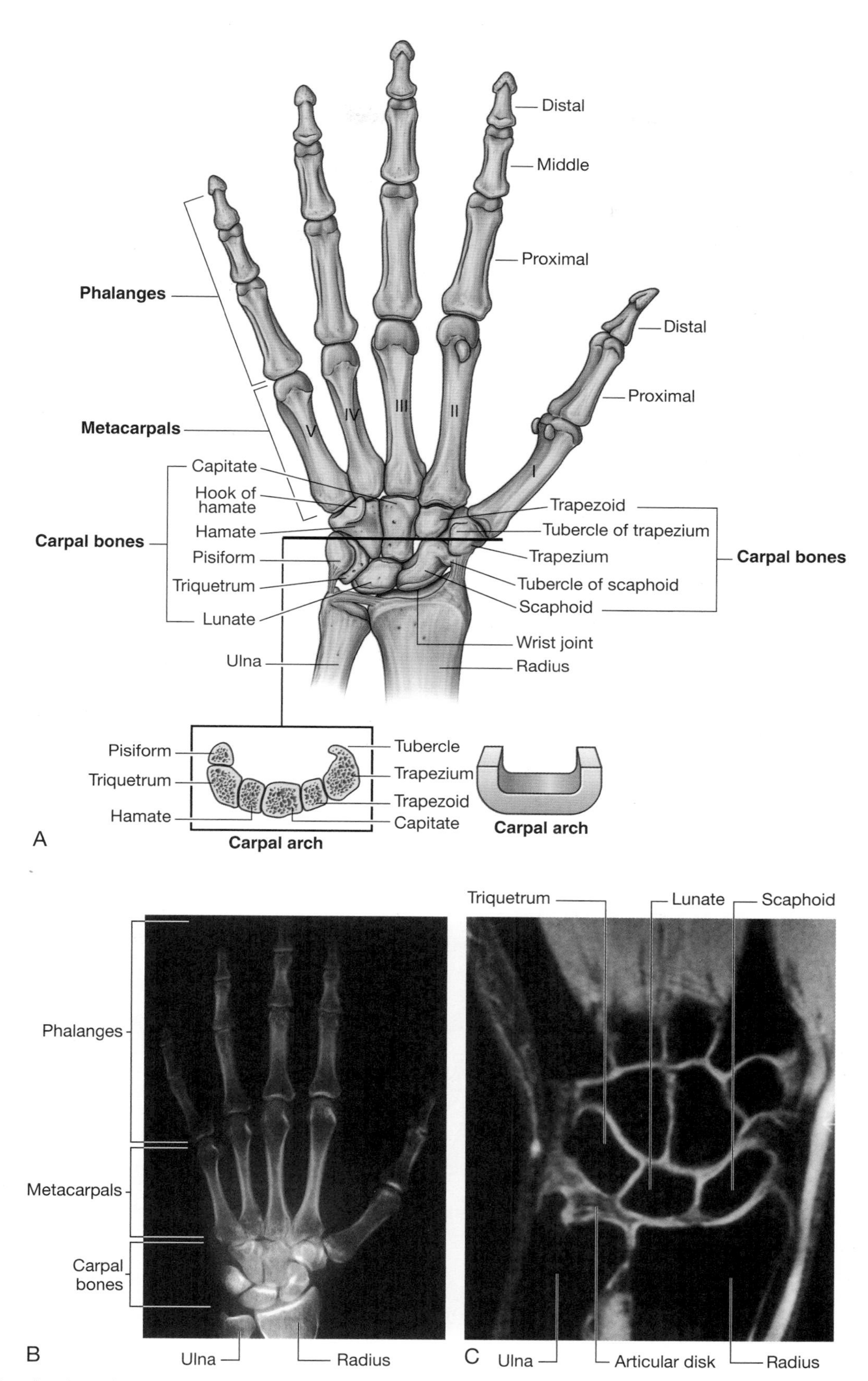

FIG. 7.15 (A) Anterior view of the bones of the hand. (B) and (C) Radiographs of the bones of the hand. (From Drake RL, Wayne Vogl A, Mitchell AWM. *Gray's Anatomy for Students.* 2nd ed. Churchill Livingstone; 2010.)

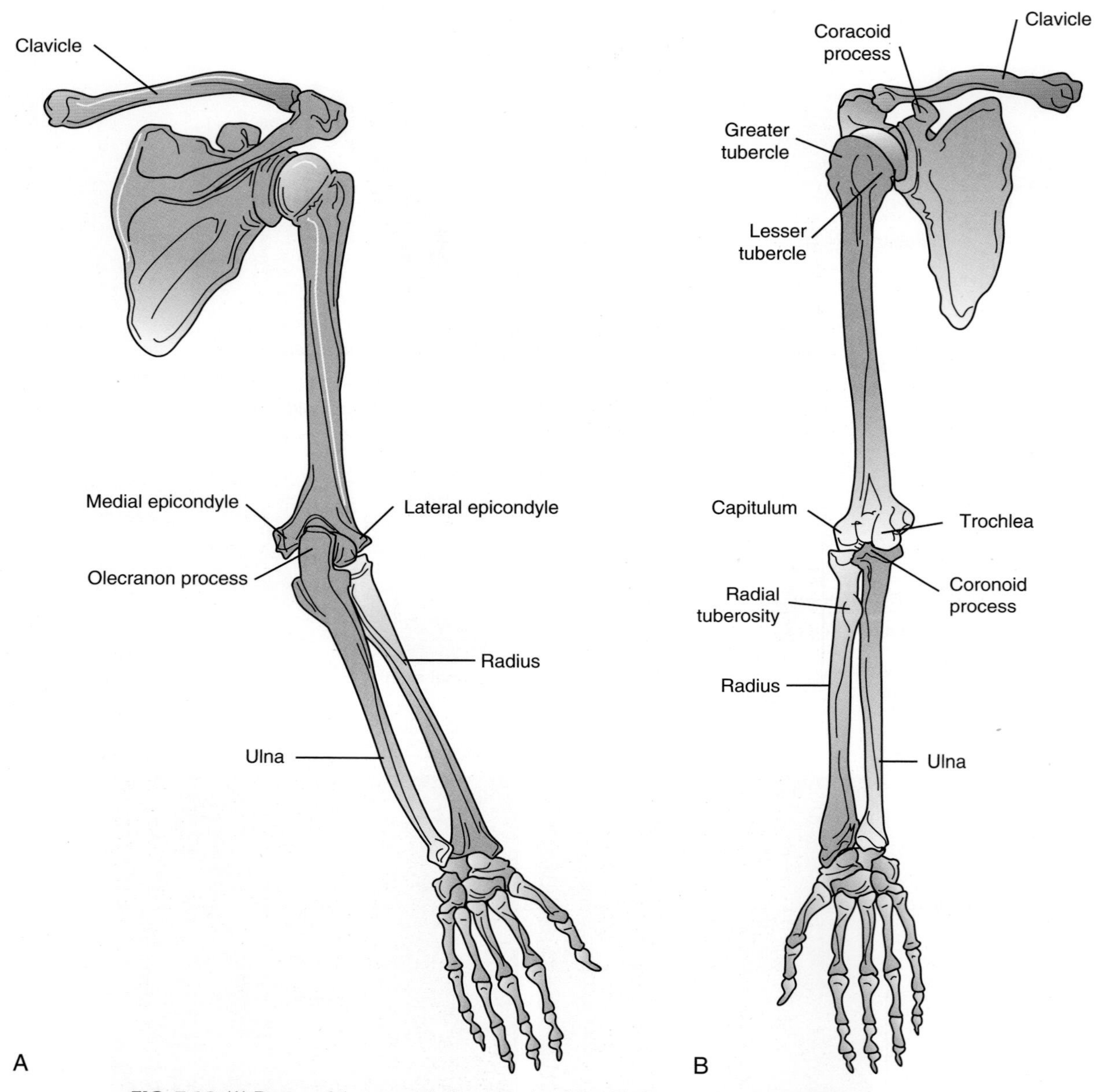

FIG. 7.16 (A) Bones of the upper limb, posterior view. (B) Bones of the upper limb, anterior view.

The bones and joints of the foot form the arches of the foot. The *transverse arch* of the foot is also known as the *instep*. The transverse arch is concave from the medial to lateral aspects of the foot. The *medial longitudinal arch* is the longest and highest arch. This arch is made up of the calcaneus and talus and the navicular, cuneiform, and first metatarsal bones. The *lateral longitudinal arch* is made up of the calcaneus and cuboid and fifth metatarsal bones.

The *plantar aponeurosis* is a large band of connective tissue that begins at the inferior calcaneus and runs along the plantar surface of the foot, attaching to the toes. The plantar aponeurosis adds stability to the arches of the foot but can shorten if the person often wears improperly fitting shoes. Plantar fasciitis is a painful condition caused by this shortening. Inflammation from repetitive use is common in track athletes, dancers, airport workers, and members of many other professions (Boxes 7.9 through 7.11; Figs. 7.17 through 7.23; Activity 7.7). For a complete review of the bones, try Activity 7.8.

ACTIVITY **7.7**

The following list names the bones of the upper extremity:
Clavicle
Scapula
Humerus
Radius
Ulna
Carpals
Metacarpals
Phalanges

Your Turn

Make up a silly sentence to help you remember these bones by using the first letter of each name in whatever order works for you.

ACTIVITY **7.8**

The following list names the bones of the lower limb:
Pelvic bone: Ilium, ischium, and pubis
Femur
Patella
Tibia
Fibula
Tarsals
Metatarsals
Phalanges

Your Turn

Make up a silly sentence to help you remember these bones by using the first letter of each name in whatever order works for you.

Section Summary

- List the bones of the head, spine, and thorax.
  - The head/skull is made up of cranial bones and facial bones (see Figs. 7.3 and 7.4). The spine is made up of the cervical, thoracic, and lumbar vertebrae, the sacrum, and the coccyx. The thorax is made up of 12 sets of ribs (24 total) and the sternum.
- List the number of cervical, thoracic, and lumbar vertebrae.
  - 7 cervical (C1 is atlas, C2 is axis), 12 thoracic, 5 lumbar. Study tip: Visualize a triangle on a clock face—breakfast at 7, lunch at 12, dinner at 5.
- List the bones of the upper and lower limbs.
  - Upper limb (proximal to distal)—clavicle, scapula, humerus, ulna, radius, carpals, metacarpals, and phalanges. Lower limb (proximal to distal)—pelvis (divided into ilium, pubis, ischium), femur, patella, tibia, fibula, tarsals, metatarsals, and phalanges.

Box 7.9 Bones of the Pelvic Girdle (see Fig. 7.17)

The pelvic girdle is a strong, bony ring composed of the pelvic (coxal) bones and the sacrum. Unlike the shoulder girdle, the pelvis is attached anteriorly at the symphysis pubis and posteriorly at the sacroiliac joints.

Three bones fuse as we grow to create the pelvic bones, which form the front and sides of the pelvic girdle. These three bones are as follows:

- The ilium, which forms the superior flared portion
- The ischium, which is the inferior portion and the strongest
- The pubis, which forms the anterior portion of the pelvic bone

In the middle of the pubis is the symphysis pubis, which is the anterior connection of the pelvis. The fibrocartilaginous disk at the symphysis pubis allows this joint to function as a shock absorber.

The posterior portion of the pelvic girdle is created from the sacrum, which is discussed along with the spine.

The lateral portion of the pelvis, where the ilium, ischium, and pubis fuse, creates a deep socket called the *acetabulum*. The acetabulum articulates with the head of the femur to form the hip joint.

At the superior portion is the iliac crest. On the anterior end of the crest is the anterior superior iliac spine (ASIS), which is often used as a bony landmark, especially in assessment and treatment.

The posterior superior iliac spine (PSIS) is a bony prominence at the posterior end of the iliac crest.

Just below the PSIS on each side is the posterior joint of the pelvis, the sacroiliac joint.

On the surface of the body is a small dimple or depression over the sacroiliac joint; the PSIS lies just above it.

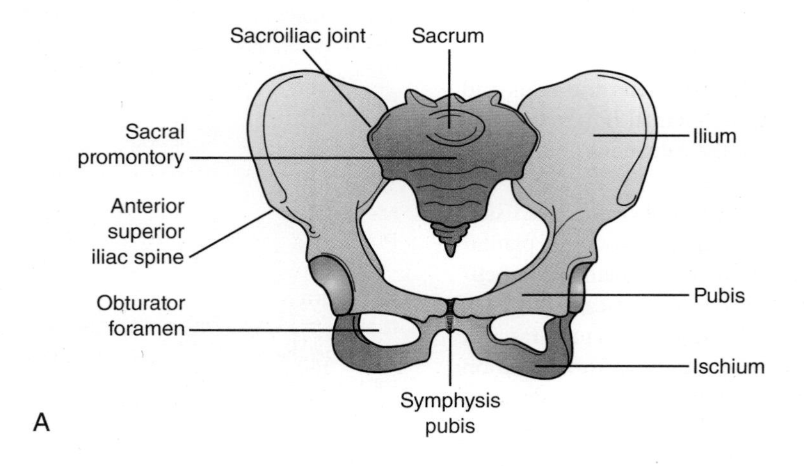

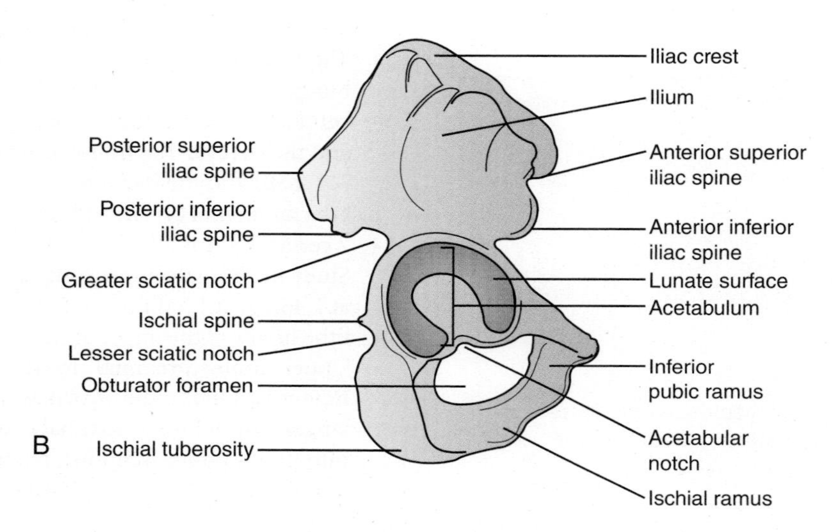

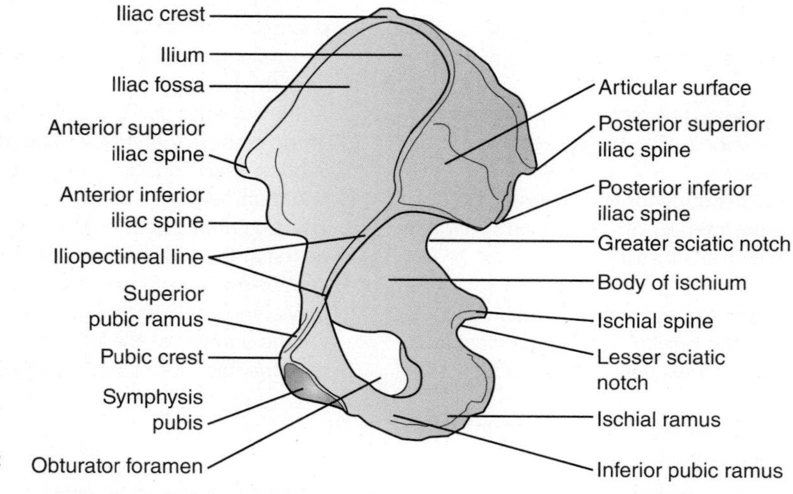

FIG. 7.17 Pelvis. (A) Anterior view. (B) Lateral view. (C) Medial view.

Box 7.10 Features of the Femur and Patella, Tibia, and Fibula

Femur (see Fig. 7.18)

The femur, or thigh bone, is the longest, strongest, and heaviest bone in the body.

At the proximal end is the head, which has a smooth, spherical surface that fits into the acetabulum to form the hip joint.

A depression in the center of the head, called the *fovea capitis*, serves as an attachment for the ligamentum teres.

All areas of the head except the fovea are covered with articular cartilage.

The neck of the femur, distal to the head, is a common site of fracture in the elderly.

The greater and lesser trochanters are projections that serve as muscle attachments.

The shaft of the femur, as in most long bones, is triangular in cross-section.

On the posterior shaft is a prominent ridge, called the *linea aspera*, to which the adductor and vastus muscles attach.

The lateral and medial condyles are smooth surfaces that articulate with the proximal tibia.

Between the condyles on the anterior side is the trochlear (patellar) groove.

The lateral and medial epicondyles, which are on the condyles, are points of muscle attachment.

The intercondylar fossa is a depression on the posterior surface between the condyles that articulates with the intercondylar eminence of the tibia.

The menisci are cartilaginous cushions (lateral and medial) that lie between the femur and tibia.

Patella (see Fig. 7.19)

The patella, or kneecap, is a sesamoid bone encased within the tendons of the quadriceps femoris group, where it crosses the knee joint.

The patella is triangular; the broad superior edge is called the *base*, and the more pointed inferior edge is called the *apex*.

The patella sits in the trochlear groove of the femur.

The two articular facets on its posterior surface fit against the medial and lateral condyles of the femur.

Bones of the Leg (see Fig. 7.20)

The leg comprises two bones, the tibia and the fibula.

Tibia

The tibia, or shin bone, is on the medial, big-toe side of the leg.

The tibia is the longer and stronger of the two bones and is a weight-bearing bone.

At the proximal end are the *lateral* and *medial condyles*, which fit against the identically named surfaces of the femur.

The medial condyle is larger than the lateral condyle.

The *intercondylar eminence*, a ridge that separates the two condyles, moves into the intercondylar fossa of the femur during knee extension.

The *tibial tuberosity*, at the proximal anterior tibia, is the attachment point for the patellar ligament.

The distal end forms the *medial malleolus*, a prominent bony landmark of the ankle.

The tibia articulates with the fibula at the proximal end (the proximal tibiofibular joint) and at the distal end (the distal tibiofibular joint). The tibia also articulates the tarsal (ankle) bone, called the *talus*.

Fibula

The fibula is on the lateral little toe side of the leg. This slender bone does not reach the knee joint and so does not bear weight. The main function of the fibula is to serve as an attachment for muscles and fascia.

The head of the fibula articulates with the tibia.

The distal end of the fibula, which forms the *lateral malleolus* (another prominent bony landmark of the ankle), articulates with the talus.

Despite its small size, the fibula can withstand more tensile pull and strain than any other bone in the body.

As with the forearm, an interosseous membrane connects the tibia and fibula.

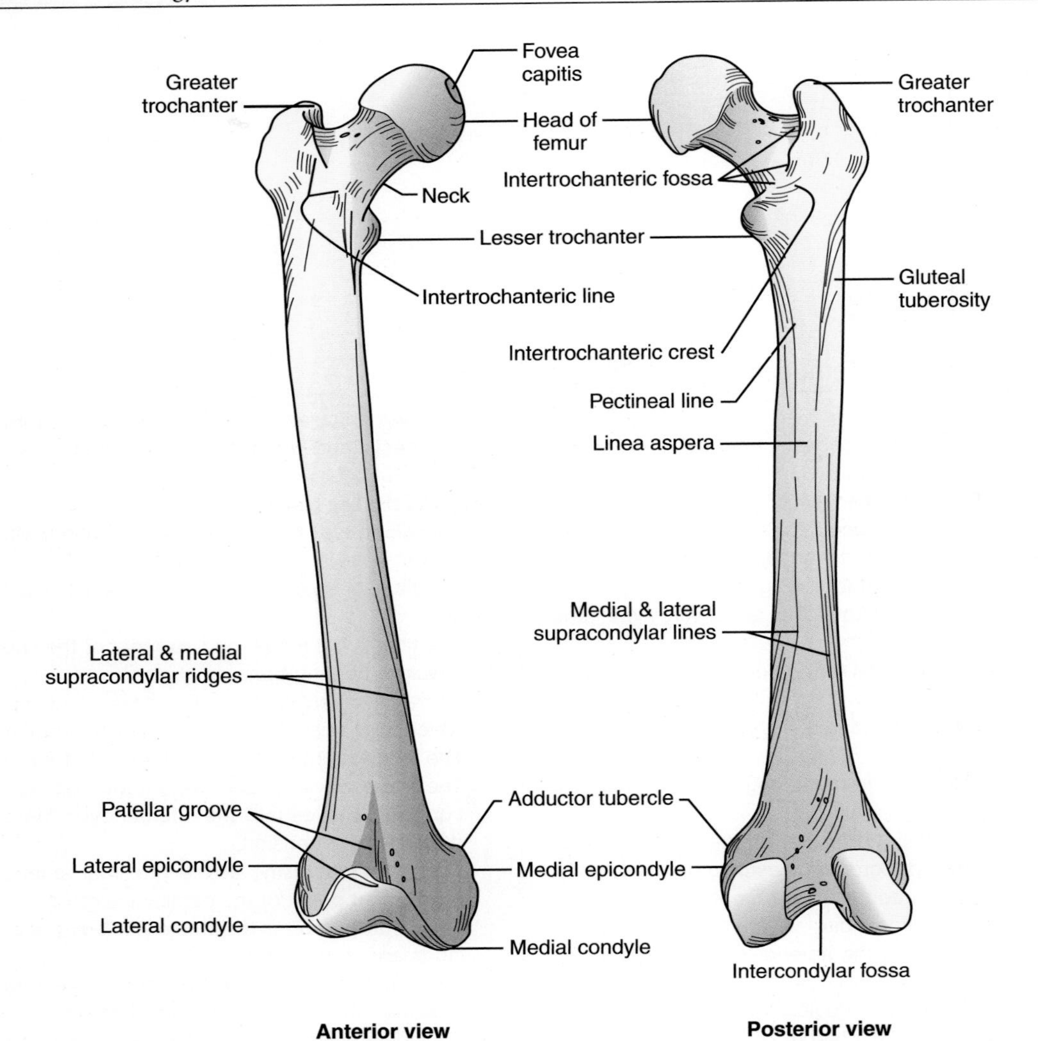

FIG. 7.18 Anterior and posterior views of the right femur.

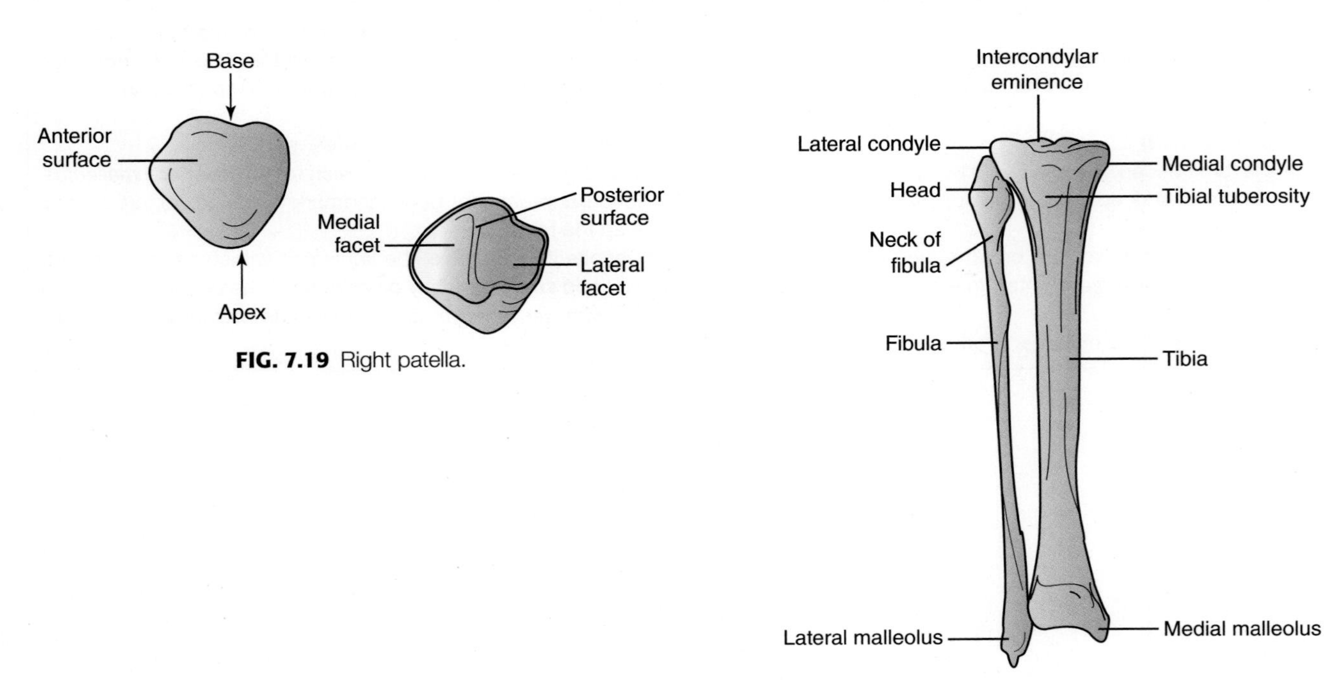

FIG. 7.19 Right patella.

FIG. 7.20 Right tibia and fibula.

Box 7.11 Bones of the Ankle and Foot (see Figs. 7.21–7.23)

Ankle

Ankle structure is similar to the wrist structure. Seven *tarsal (ankle) bones* connect the foot to the leg.

The largest is the *calcaneus*, or heel bone.

The *talus* is the major weight-bearing bone of the foot during upright motions; it is next in size to the calcaneus.

The talus and calcaneus are the most posterior of the tarsal bones; they articulate anteriorly with the other tarsals.

The talus articulates with the tibia and fibula on its superior side and with the calcaneus inferiorly.

Because no muscles are inserted in the talus, motion occurs through the movement of the bone and soft tissue structures around it.

The other tarsals are cube shaped and lie between the talus, calcaneus, and metatarsals; they are the anterior tarsals.

The navicular bone articulates with the talus, cuneiform bones, and cuboid bone.

The cuboid bone articulates with the calcaneus, navicular, third cuneiform, and metatarsals.

Foot

The structure of the foot is similar to that of the hand. The difference lies in the fact that because the foot supports the weight of the body, it must be stronger and does not have to be as mobile as the hand. The foot has 26 bones.

Five short metatarsal bones form the instep.

The heads of these bones form the ball of the foot.

These bones articulate proximally with the three cuneiforms and the cuboid and distally with the phalanges.

The phalanges are organized in the same way as in the hand.

Each toe has three phalanges.

The great toe has two phalanges.

The phalanges are identified in the same manner as in the hand: the *proximal, middle*, and *distal.*

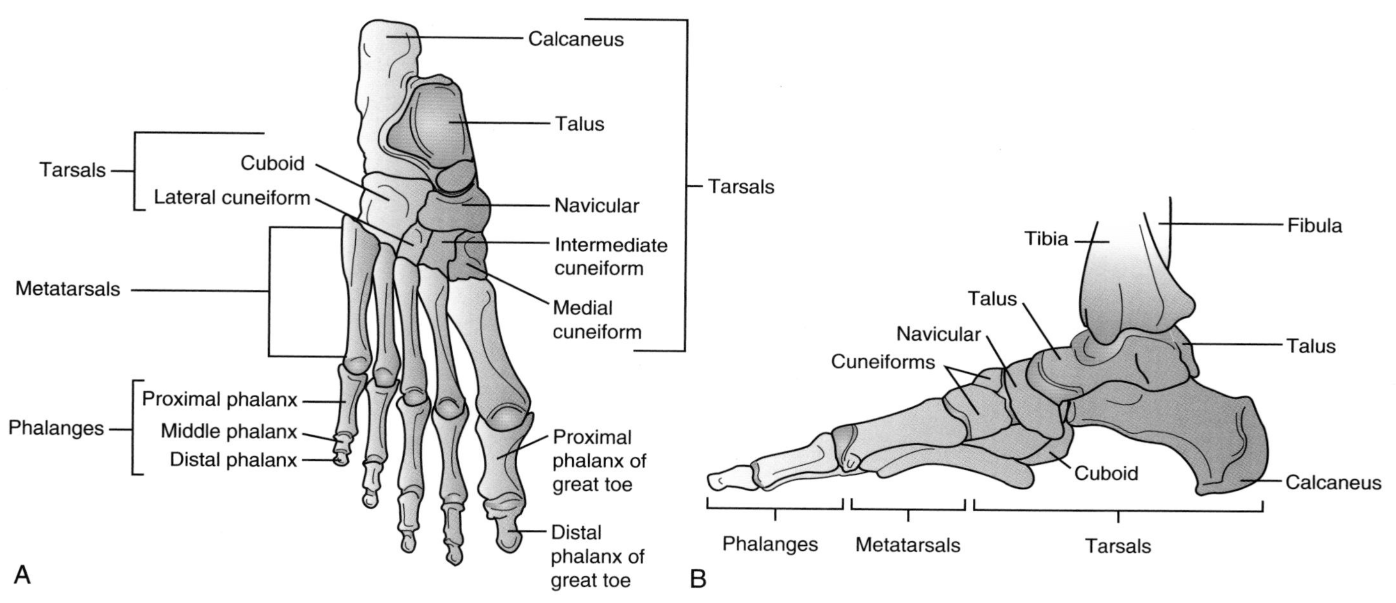

FIG. 7.21 (A) Dorsal view of the bones of the foot. (B) Medial view of the bones of the foot and ankle.

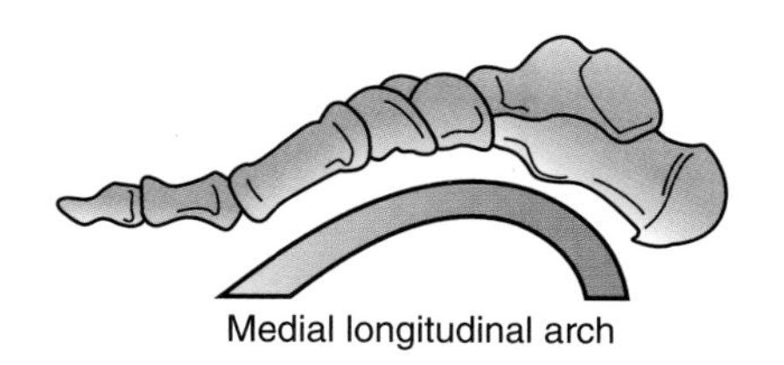

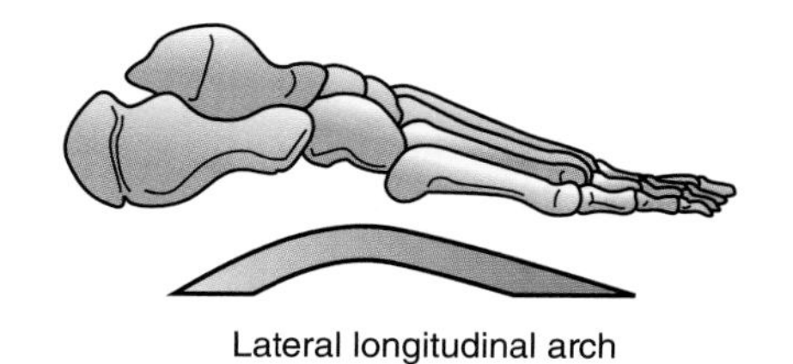

FIG. 7.22 Arches of the foot.

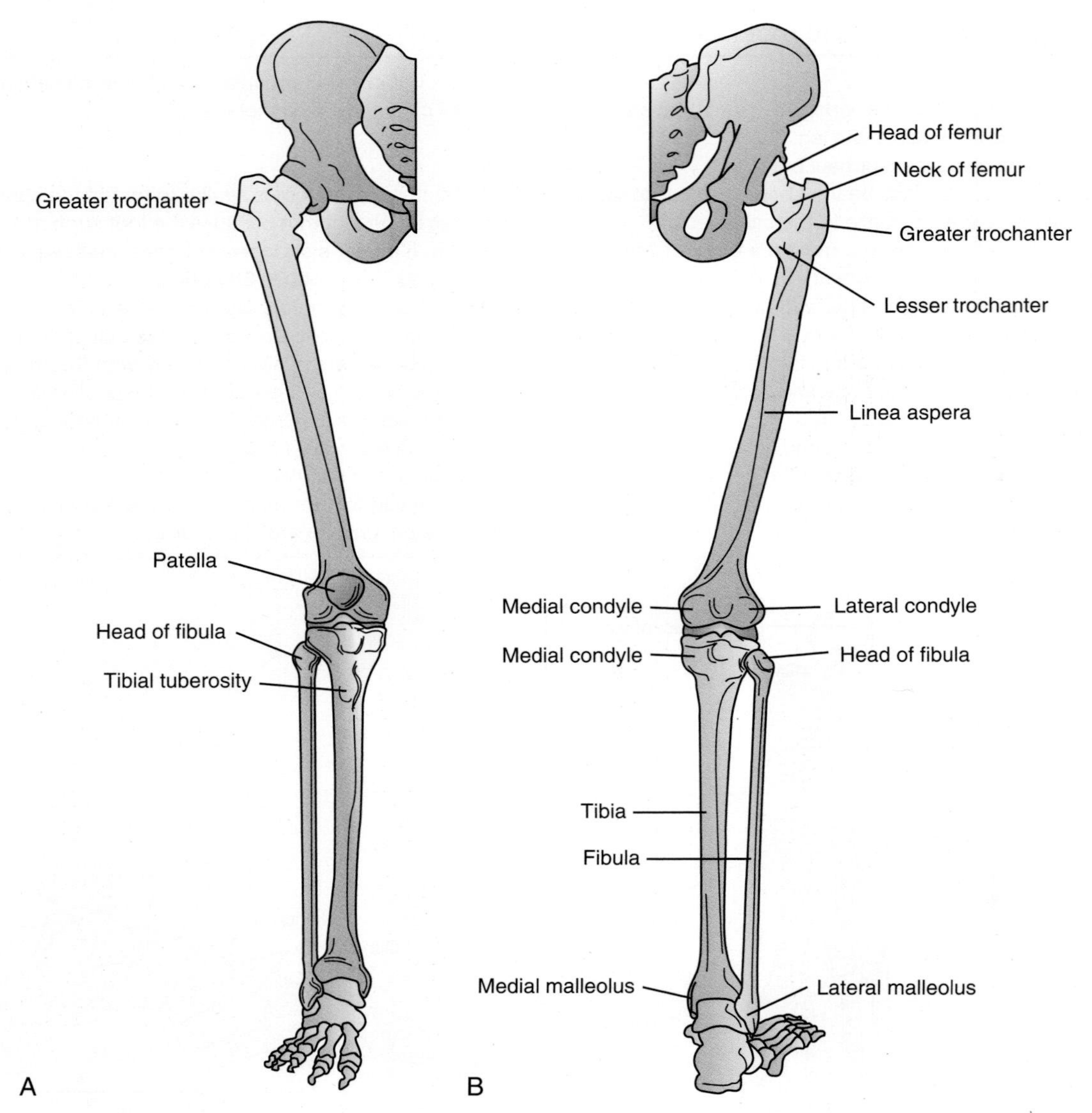

FIG. 7.23 (A) Bones of the lower limb, anterior view. (B) Bones of the lower limb, posterior view.

PATHOLOGICAL CONDITIONS

SECTION OBJECTIVES

Chapter objective covered in this section:

6. Describe the pathology of the skeletal system and the related indications/contraindications for massage.

After completing this section, the learner will be able to:

- Describe the three main stages of bone fracture healing.
- List three common spinal curve abnormalities.
- Determine indications and contraindications for massage based on skeletal pathology.

The most common pathological conditions of the skeletal system are the result of trauma. Other pathologies include developmental conditions and spinal curve abnormalities. Bone demineralization disorders are common, especially in the elderly. Disorders caused by necrosis (tissue death), infectious diseases, tumors, and nutritional deficiencies are less common.

Disorders Caused by Trauma

Fractures

Severe force can fracture almost any bone. The term *fracture* means a break or rupture in a bone (Fig. 7.24). Fractures may be classified as:

- *Avulsion fracture:* A fragment of bone tears away from the main mass of a bone.
- *Compound (open) fracture:* The skin and other soft tissues are torn, and the bone protrudes through the skin.
- *Simple (closed) fracture:* The break in the bone does not break the skin or injure soft tissue.
- *Greenstick fracture:* The break in the bone is incomplete, producing a split, such as might occur in a green piece of wood. This type is most common in children.
- *Impacted fracture:* The broken ends of the bones are jammed into each other.
- *Comminuted fracture:* The break involves more than one fracture line, with several fragments resulting, often with much soft tissue damage.

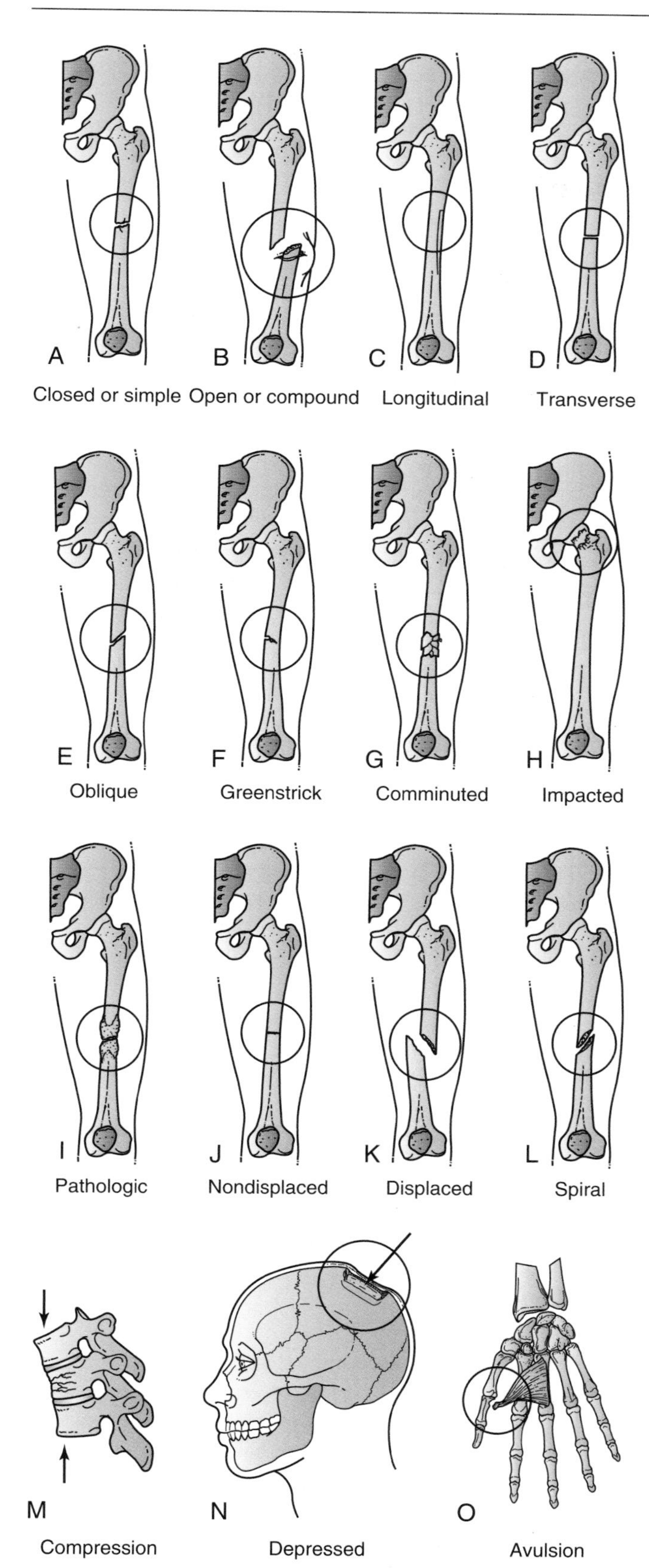

FIG. 7.24 Fracture types. (Adapted from Frazier MS, Drzymkowski J. *Essentials of Human Disease and Conditions.* 4th ed. Saunders; 2008.)

- *Complete fracture:* The break goes across the entire bone.
- *Incomplete fracture:* The break does not go across the entire bone.
- *Compression fracture:* The bone is squeezed or crushed (this type most often occurs in the spinal column).
- *Depressed fracture:* Bone in the skull is driven inward.
- *Stress fracture:* This type of fracture is a crack in the bone, often caused by repeated mechanical stress and strain. Stress fractures may not be readily detected. Referral is indicated if the history points toward a mechanical stress condition, such as participation in a recent athletic event.
- *Spiral fracture:* A break in which the bone is twisted apart. These fractures are common in skiing accidents.

The signs and symptoms of fractures include local swelling, pain, loss of function or abnormal movement of the affected part, and deformities, such as angulation, shortening, or rotation. *Crepitation*, a grating sound produced when bone fragments rub together, also may be heard. Pain may not occur immediately because of the temporary loss of nerve function and shock.

The most important step in first aid for a fracture is to prevent movement of the affected parts. Expert help should be summoned immediately, and the area should be protected to prevent movement, leaving the area "as is" if possible.

A fracture is treated by *reduction*, which means that the broken ends are pulled into alignment and the continuity of the bone is reestablished so that healing can take place. Closed reduction is performed by manual manipulation of the fractured bone so that the fragments are brought into proper alignment; no surgical incision is made. Open fractures occur when the end of a broken bone pushes through the skin. Open fractures are highly contaminated and must be débrided (scraped and cleaned) and irrigated in the operating room to flush out debris.

A fracture may also require internal fixation with pins, nails, metal plates, or screws to stabilize the alignment. Once reduction is accomplished, the bone is immobilized by the application of a cast or an apparatus that exerts traction on the distal end of the bone.

The healing of acute fractures follows the same phases that soft tissue healing does, but it is more complex. Fracture healing involves cell and tissue proliferation and differentiation, bone breakdown by osteoclasts, and bone building by osteoblasts. In general, acute fracture healing has three main stages: fracture hematoma formation, reparative phase, and remodeling phase.

Fracture Hematoma Formation

When a bone fractures, there is trauma to the periosteum and surrounding soft tissue. Acute inflammation usually lasts approximately 4 days.

A hematoma accumulates in the medullary canal and surrounding soft tissue in the first 48 to 72 hours. The exposed ends of vascular channels become blocked with clotted blood, disrupting the blood supply.

The hematoma surrounding the fracture site provides a loose fibrin mesh in which fibroblasts and capillaries form granulation tissue that replaces the blood clot. Osteoblasts and chondroblasts become active in forming new bone and cartilage.

Reparative Phase

Within approximately 7 days the hematoma becomes a soft tissue callus. This temporary bony union is called a *procallus*. Eventually, the procallus is replaced by bone, and a rigid, bony callus is formed.

With adequate immobilization and compression, the bone ends become crossed with new haversian systems that eventually lead to the laying down of primary bone.

Remodeling Phase

In this phase bone has been completely laid down. The fracture has been bridged and firmly united. Excess callus has been resorbed by osteoclasts.

Remodeling or reshaping of the new bone occurs after the callus has been resorbed and trabecular bone is laid down along the lines of stress. Complete remodeling sometimes takes many years.

Often the site of a break is stronger than the surrounding bone because of the increased activity of the osteoblasts and remodeling process, which essentially creates bone-scar tissue.

The healing process for a fractured bone usually takes 6 weeks, and this process must not be interrupted. This is why immobilization and casting often are required. Extensive soft tissue damage, including nerve damage and infection, can result from the fracture. These conditions can continue to cause difficulties long after the bone itself has healed.

INDICATIONS/CONTRAINDICATIONS for Therapeutic Massage

Massage and bodywork are contraindicated locally over a trauma area until healing is complete. Very light, subtle methods of touch therapies (e.g., a gentle laying on of hands) may be beneficial for reducing pain. The process usually is calming and soothing, which encourages healing through stress management. Bodywork methods are beneficial in supporting the rest of the body during the healing process, especially in managing compensation patterns caused by immobilization of an area and in helping the client learn the use of crutches and canes.

Shin Splints

Shin splints involve muscle strain and possibly hairline fractures of the tibia.

Plantar Fasciitis

Plantar fasciitis develops from a strain or injury to the plantar fascia of the foot. The signs and symptoms include acute pain when resuming activity after a period of rest. The pain lessens as the tissue warms and then begins to hurt again with continued use. A deep, sharp, bruised sensation is felt at the arch and the attachment at the heel.

INDICATIONS/CONTRAINDICATIONS for Therapeutic Massage

Massage is beneficial for plantar fasciitis and shin splints as long as it does not cause an increase in pain and inflammation. Tibial fractures are contraindicated and need to be ruled out before massage is applied.

Developmental Conditions

Spina Bifida

If the vertebral arches in a growing fetus do not fuse into the spinous processes, the result is spina bifida. Instead of being protected by bone, the nerves of the dorsal spinal cord may be covered by a thin membrane, skin, muscle, or spinal meninges. This condition may range from a mild case, with the child showing no symptoms, to severe spinal cord damage and paraplegia. The most common site of the defect is the lumbosacral region.

Cleft Palate

A cleft palate is a congenital deformity involving a gap in the roof of the mouth from behind the teeth to the back of the mouth. Newborns with this defect may have difficulty nursing or swallowing because their mouths are open to the nasal cavities above. Newborns suck in air rather than milk, or the milk may enter the nose instead of the throat. The condition is corrected surgically.

Osteogenesis Imperfecta

Osteogenesis imperfecta comprises a group of hereditary disorders that appear in newborns or young children. The bones are deformed and fragile as a result of demineralization and defective formation of connective tissue.

Clubfoot (Talipes)

Clubfoot is the most common of the lower extremity congenital deformities. In most cases one or both feet are bent downward and inverted; in other cases the feet are pointed upward and everted. Mild cases respond to splinting and stretching, but severe cases require surgical correction. Clubfoot is more prominent in boys and may be the result of genetic predisposition or the position of the fetus in the uterus.

Spinal Curve Abnormalities

Abnormal curvatures of the spine (Fig. 7.25) may be congenital, may result from paralysis, weakness, or tension in spinal muscles, or may be the result of asymmetry in the length of the lower extremities. Bad posture habits, especially during periods of accelerated growth, can contribute to the problem. As discussed previously, exaggeration of the thoracic curve is known as *hyperkyphosis* (or hunchback), and excessive lumbar curvature is referred to as *hyperlordosis*. Lateral curvature of the spine is called *scoliosis* and is most often found in young girls, especially during or just after puberty. When discovered and treated early, good results are often seen. One of the major problems caused by any extreme spinal curve is compression of the internal organs.

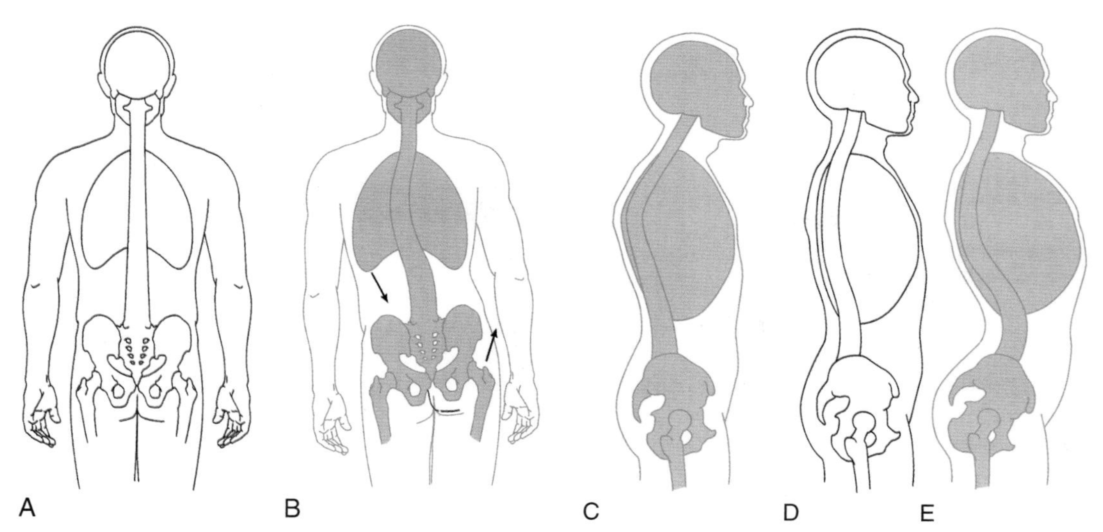

FIG. 7.25 Deformity of the spine. (A) Normal spine. (B) Spinal deformity, scoliosis is a lateral deviation of the spine. (C) Hyperkyphosis, a flexion deformity of the spine. (D) Normal spine (posterior view). (E) Hyperlordosis (side view), an extension deformity of the spine. (Modified from Barkauskas VH, Baumann LC, Darling-Fisher CS. *Health and Physical Assessment.* 3rd ed. Mosby; 2002.)

INDICATIONS/CONTRAINDICATIONS for Therapeutic Massage

If skeletal problems create or are part of a permanent condition, supportive care is required. Any type of aggressive compressive force or joint movement methods are contraindicated for a fragile skeletal structure, regardless of the cause. Light, superficial methods, such as the gentle laying on of hands used in some forms of touch methods, might be indicated. Always consult with the client's physician when conditions indicate extreme caution. Back pain is one of the most common complaints. Most back pain is caused by soft tissue problems and not skeletal changes, and massage can be indicated and beneficial to the client. Massage methods help manage compensatory muscle spasms and connective tissue changes when actual vertebral pathology is present.

Osgood-Schlatter Disease/Apophysitis of the Tibial Tubercle

Osgood-Schlatter disease, which affects the tibial tuberosity, most often occurs in boys between 10 and 15 years of age. The tuberosity becomes inflamed or separated from the tibia because of irritation caused when the patellar tendon pulls on the tuberosity during periods of rapid growth or overuse of the quadriceps femoris group.

General Growing Pains

One of the many causes of growing pains occurs during growth spurts in children and adolescents when the bone grows faster than the attached muscles and other soft tissues. The pain results when the soft tissues pull on the pain-sensitive periosteum.

INDICATIONS/CONTRAINDICATIONS for Therapeutic Massage

Treatment of local areas may be contraindicated if inflammation is present. General growing pains are often soothed by methods that do not introduce any sort of therapeutic inflammation, such as intense stretching and frictioning methods, which should be avoided. Methods that relax and lengthen the muscle and soften the connective tissue are appropriate.

Bone Demineralization Disorders

Osteoporosis

Osteoporosis is a disorder of the bone in which calcium and other minerals are lacking and bone protein is diminished. Osteopenia is a decrease in bone mineral density below normal but not low enough to meet the diagnostic criteria for osteoporosis. Under normal conditions, osteoblasts replace bone. In osteoporosis, this happens much more slowly, leaving the bones soft, fragile, and more likely to break. Osteoporosis primarily affects the spine and pelvis. The condition is seen most often in postmenopausal females as a result of the decrease in estrogen levels. Other causes include deficiencies in the nutritional intake, absorption, or assimilation of protein and minerals; cigarette smoking; and inactivity. Treatments include implementing hormone therapy (primarily estrogen, progesterone, and calcitonin); increasing exercise; and including more sources of calcium, magnesium, boron, and vitamin D in the daily diet.

Paget Disease/Osteitis Deformans

Paget disease, or osteitis deformans, occurs when the bones undergo normal periods of calcium loss followed by periods of excessive new cell growth. Bone cells are replaced with fibrous tissue and blood vessels. As a result, the bones harden, deform, and become susceptible to fracture. Currently, neither the cause nor the cure is known. The condition is most commonly found in men older than 40 years of age.

Osteitis Fibrosa Cystica

In osteitis fibrosa cystica, bone tissue is replaced by fibrous tissue and cysts, making the bones weak and prone to fracture. This disorder is seen in long-standing hyperparathyroidism.

Disorders Caused by Radiation Therapy

When radiation is used to treat a bone disorder or is given as part of the treatment of a malignancy, the bone may become brittle and fragile because of the changes in its structure. This happens if the bone is treated directly or if the treatment site involves bony structures.

INDICATIONS/CONTRAINDICATIONS for Therapeutic Massage

Caution is necessary before any massage and bodywork requiring any amount of compressive force are used on a client with a condition that causes demineralization of bone or that results in brittle, fragile bones. A fragile is carefully supervised by the appropriate medical professionals. Light, superficial methods, such as the gentle laying on of hands used in some forms of touch methods, might be indicated with supervision. Bone involvement may be localized, such as with radiation treatment. In these cases, massage methods can be used on the unaffected areas and avoided over the involved area.

Necrosis (Tissue Death)

Osteonecrosis (Ischemic Necrosis)

Various pathological changes occur in the bone when its blood supply is diminished or cut off, or when infection, malignancy, or trauma occurs, leading to tissue death or necrosis. These conditions are among the common causes of hip pain and disability. The changes usually occur after a primary disease, such as lupus, especially when the disease is treated with glucocorticoids. Symptoms include pain during active motion and at night. Because of the slow, progressive deterioration, necrosis may go undiagnosed.

More commonly known as *Perthes disease*, Legg-Calvé-Perthes disease (also called *idiopathic avascular osteonecrosis of the capital femoral epiphysis of the femoral head*) involves degeneration and necrosis at the head of the femur, followed by recalcification. The disorder, most often seen in young boys, occurs when the vascular supply to the head of the femur is compromised, resulting in developmental deformity. The condition lasts about 3 years and may predispose the child to arthritis in the area as an adult. Symptoms include hip pain and gait abnormalities.

Scheuermann Disease/Idiopathic Juvenile Kyphosis of the Spine

Idiopathic juvenile kyphosis of the spine (Scheuermann disease) is most commonly caused by necrosis or inflammation in bone or a thoracic disk. The disease begins during puberty, is the result of genetic predisposition or trauma (or both), and leads to back pain and hyperkyphosis. The excessive curvature is caused by changes in the structure of the vertebrae, from columnar to wedge shaped.

Osteochondritis Dissecans

In osteochondritis dissecans the cartilage and adjacent bone separate from the bone itself. This disorder is most common in adults and is caused by inflammation and necrosis of the particular area. At the affected joint, portions of dead tissue may break away and lodge in the joint capsule, restricting movement and causing pain. The condition is most often seen in the knee joint.

INDICATIONS/CONTRAINDICATIONS for Therapeutic Massage

Necrosis is usually a localized condition that requires regional avoidance of the involved bone area. Because massage provides the generalized effect of enhanced local circulation, indirect benefits might occur with careful use of these methods. However, because these disorders are pathological conditions, massage must be done with the permission and supervision of the primary healthcare provider.

Infectious Diseases

Osteomyelitis

Osteomyelitis is an inflammation in the bone, bone marrow, or periosteum usually caused by pyogenic (pus-producing) bacteria. The bacteria reach the bone through the bloodstream or by way of an injury in which the skin is broken. Osteomyelitis is most often seen in children, near the joints in the upper or lower extremities. When osteomyelitis is promptly treated medically, the chance of a full recovery is excellent.

Tuberculosis

Tuberculosis is a systemic disease caused by the tubercular bacillus. Involvement in the skeletal system destroys the bone tissue and necrosis. Tuberculosis of the spine, known as *Pott disease*, affects mostly children. The onset of skeletal tuberculosis is insidious, usually marked by vague complaints of pain.

INDICATIONS/CONTRAINDICATIONS for Therapeutic Massage

Massage is contraindicated in infectious diseases unless the massage therapist is carefully supervised by medical personnel. The therapist must always refer clients with vague pain symptoms for proper diagnosis.

Tumors

Tumors in the skeletal system can be primary or secondary. Primary tumors, such as cysts or osteomas (bony knobs in or on a bone), are rare and usually benign. Some tumors are malignant, such as *osteosarcomas*, which often arise in the femur or tibia of a young person. Some of the signs of malignancy are pain, unexplained swelling over a bone, a feeling of warmth on the skin, and prominent veins over the area.

Secondary tumors develop from primary sites, most often in the breast, lungs, or prostate. In older individuals, metastases from epithelial tumors or carcinomas of various organs can spread to the bones.

Tumors also can be found in cartilage. Osteochondroma is a benign tumor of the cartilage and bone tissue of long bones. *Chondrosarcomas* are malignant tumors of the cartilage.

INDICATIONS/CONTRAINDICATIONS for Therapeutic Massage

Prompt referral for diagnosis is necessary for any sign that may indicate the growth of a tumor. Benign tumors are a local contraindication for massage. These therapies are contraindicated for individuals with malignant tumors unless the therapist is supervised directly and carefully by the medical team. General massage to provide system management related to cancer treatment is indicated if additional training is acquired.

Nutritional Disorders

Rickets

Rickets is a childhood disease that is rare in the Western world but still occurs with conditions of extreme nutritional deficiency. Rickets is characterized by numerous bone deformities. Deficiency of the active form of vitamin D prevents the absorption of calcium and phosphorus through the intestine; these minerals are then not available for deposit in the bones, which remain soft and become distorted. The deformity patterns may be noticeable in older clients who had rickets as children.

Scurvy

Scurvy is a vitamin C deficiency. Vitamin C is necessary for the production of collagen in the fibrous tissue and bone matrix. With scurvy, bone density is lost. Treatment involves increasing the vitamin intake, but some damage may be permanent. As with rickets, this disease is rare in the Western world, but it can occur under conditions of inadequate nutrition, such as with eating disorders.

INDICATIONS/CONTRAINDICATIONS for Therapeutic Massage

Regardless of the cause, a fragile skeletal structure is a contraindication for any type of compressive force or joint movement methods, unless these methods are carefully supervised by the appropriate medical professionals. Light, superficial methods, such as the gentle laying on of hands used in some forms of touch methods, might be indicated, with supervision (Activity 7.9).

Section Summary

- Describe the three main stages of bone fracture healing.
  - Stage 1—Fracture hematoma formation (i.e., reaction phase/inflammatory phase). Begins: Onset of injury. Duration: hours to days. Blood cells accumulate near the injury site, clotting to form a hematoma, which acts as a template for callus formation. Stage 2—Reparative phase. Begins: Commonly after 1 week. Duration: days to weeks. A soft tissue callus of fibrous tissue and cartilage forms around the bone ends and then ossifies into a rigid bony callus. Stage 3—Remodeling phase. Begins: Commonly after 6 weeks. Duration: weeks to years. Calcification occurs. Osteoclasts break down old bone/bony callus. Osteoblasts build new bone.
- List three common spinal curve abnormalities.
  - Hyperkyphosis: Exaggeration of the thoracic curve (i.e., hunchback). Hyperlordosis: Excessive lumbar curvature (i.e., swayback). Scoliosis: lateral curvature of the spine.

ACTIVITY 7.9

Locate each of the following bony landmarks on yourself. You may need to refer to the illustrations in this chapter.

Zygomatic bone (cheekbone)
Seventh cervical vertebra (the most pronounced of the cervical vertebrae, especially with the neck flexed)
Mastoid process of the temporal bone
Clavicle (collar bone)
Coracoid process of the scapula
Sternum (breastbone) between the ribs
Jugular notch of the manubrium
Xiphoid process (at the inferior end of the sternum; it has a pointed tip)
Scapula
Acromion of the scapula (the highest point of the shoulder)
Spine of the scapula
Medial or vertebral border
Lateral or axillary border
Inferior angle
Superior angle
Humerus
Greater and lesser tubercles
Bicipital or intertubercular groove (runs between the two tubercles)
Anatomic neck (just below the head of the humerus)
Deltoid tuberosity (the distal attachment point for the deltoid muscle)
Lateral epicondyle (a bump at the distal end)
Medial epicondyle (a bump at the distal end)
Olecranon process (the point of the elbow)
Head of the radius (the bony knob just distal to the lateral epicondyle; you can feel it rolling during supination and pronation)
Pisiform bone (the medial carpal bone on the anterior wrist)
Iliac crest (near the level of the waist)
Anterior superior iliac spine (ASIS)
Posterior superior iliac spine (PSIS)
Sacrum (the curved, triangular bone beneath the lumbar spine)
Coccyx (the caudal tip of the vertebral column, deep between the gluteal muscle masses)
Ischial tuberosity (the "sit bones" in the middle of the lower gluteal muscles)
Pubic symphysis (the anterior midline joint of the pelvic girdle)
Femur
Greater trochanter (large protuberance on the lateral side)
Lesser trochanter (small elevation; on the medial side near the top of the inner thigh)
Medial condyle
Lateral condyle
Patella
Head of the fibula (the bump at the lateral proximal leg)
Tibial tuberosity (the large bump just distal to the patella)
Lateral malleolus
Medial malleolus
Calcaneus

- Determine indications for and contraindications to massage based on skeletal pathology (Activity 7.10).
  - Massage is regionally contraindicated in conditions related to trauma and infection until healing is complete. Conditions affecting bone that result in brittleness and fragility require caution and adaptation of pressure. For example, osteoporosis is a demineralization disorder of the bone in which calcium and other minerals are lacking and bone protein is diminished, resulting in brittle, fragile bones. Supervision and consultation by appropriate medical professionals are necessary. Compressive force and joint movement methods may be contraindicated. Light, superficial methods usually are indicated.

SUMMARY

This chapter focused on the general structure of the skeletal system and the specific anatomy of the bones of the body. The various activities have reviewed and integrated the data so that the names, shapes, and functions of bones are familiar. Information about the skeleton is important to our study of the way the body moves, which continues in Chapters 8–10.

ACTIVITY 7.10

List three benefits of massage in dealing with pathologic conditions of the skeletal system.

Example
Stress management promotes healing.

Your Turn
1. ______
2. ______
3. ______

List three contraindications for the use of massage in dealing with pathologic conditions of the skeletal system.

Example
Necrosis is locally contraindicated.

Your Turn
1. ______
2. ______
3. ______

CRITICAL THINKING/CLINICAL REASONING

Each chapter will feature a critical thinking and clinical reasoning application of the content related to massage therapy practice. A client scenario will be presented with recommendations for additional research often using MedlinePlus or PubMed. Relevant questions based on the chapter content outline are provided to guide the discussion. There are no specific current answers to the questions. However, responses should be supportive of evidence-informed practices and based on biological plausibility if sufficient research is not available. The author's decision-making process related to the scenario and questions is on the Evolve site. Compare and contrast your thoughts and discussion with the author and determine where you agree or disagree.

Scenario
Doris has osteoporosis. She fits the profile: White; slight build; and a smoker, although she quit smoking 10 years ago. She has not had any broken bones, nor has she begun to experience the trademark kyphosis that so often occurs.

Doris is taking medication to treat her condition and has begun exercising and lifting light weights. She has been getting massages on and off for many years. She just relocated to Florida from Minnesota because she has friends there and is frankly nervous about falling on the ice during winter. She is getting ready to have her first massage with a new massage therapist.

Explore These Sites
- MedlinePlus: Search terms—*geriatrics, osteoporosis*
- https://www.womenshealth.gov/a-z-topics/osteoporosis
- National Institute on Aging support
- PubMed: massage and balance; geriatrics and massage therapy

Discuss These Points
- What functions of the skeletal system are affected related to aging, especially after age 65?
- What parts of the bone are affected by osteoporosis?
- What bones in the axial skeleton are most likely to fracture because of osteoporosis?
- What bones in the appendicular skeleton are most likely to fracture because of osteoporosis?
- What medications might Doris be taking, and are there any cautions for massage application? What cautions might these medications create for the massage application?
- Since falls are a leading cause of serious injury in older people, what precautions need to be taken in the massage therapy setting?
- Is there any evidence to support massage therapy for improving balance that would reduce falls?

Visit the Evolve website: https://evolve.elsevier.com/Fritz/essential/
The Evolve website provides support for the review of the chapter content and chapter quizzes to help you prepare for the MBLEx or other massage therapy certification or licensing exams. End-of-chapter questions for discussion and review answer key and rationales and author's response to critical thinking and clinical reasoning scenarios.

MULTIPLE CHOICE QUESTIONS FOR REVIEW AND DISCUSSION

The answers, with rationales, can be found on the Evolve site.

These questions are used for review and discussion. It is as important to understand why wrong answers are wrong as it is to know why the correct answer is correct. The answers to the questions, with rationales and explanations about why the correct answer is correct and why the wrong answers are wrong, can be found on the Evolve site. Guidance is also provided on how questions are developed and how the textbook content can be presented in a multiple choice question format. At the end of the question section here in the textbook, you will find an Exercise that asks you to write more questions. Use the various questions in the chapter as examples. This is one of the best study strategies for test taking.

It is important to understand that the actual licensing exam you take may not contain any of the specific questions found in this textbook or the review material and practice tests on the Evolve site. Therefore just because you can answer any of these questions correctly does not mean you will pass the licensing exam. The questions are content and style examples to help you prepare—this is why understanding why wrong answers are wrong is just as important as identifying the correct answer. Also, make sure you understand all the terminology used in the questions and possible answers in the review and discussion questions. Look up words you do not understand.

1. The continual changing of bone in response to functional demands is called _______.
   a. Remodeling
   b. Oppositional growth
   c. Haversian
   d. Articulation
2. Which of the following is a depression on a bone?
   a. Condyle
   b. Fossa
   c. Line
   d. Tubercle
3. Which of the following bones is located in the appendicular portion of the skeleton?
   a. Ethmoid
   b. Clavicle
   c. Sternum
   d. Coccyx
4. Which suture joins the parietal bones and occipital bone?
   a. Squamous
   b. Coronal
   c. Lambdoidal
   d. Sagittal
5. Which of the following landmarks is located on the humerus?
   a. Glenoid fossa
   b. Xiphoid process
   c. Radial styloid
   d. Olecranon fossa
6. The coracoid process is located on which bone?
   a. Scapula
   b. Sternum
   c. Femur
   d. Talus
7. When one is palpating the posterior cervical area, the fibrous structure felt is the _______.
   a. Kyphosis ligament
   b. Odontoid process
   c. Nuchal ligament
   d. Demifacets
8. The costal angle is located on which bone?
   a. Sternum
   b. Clavicle
   c. Atlas
   d. Rib
9. The foot typically contains how many bones?
   a. 31
   b. 26
   c. 12
   d. 22
10. Which sequence of terms would all be bony landmarks?
    a. Trabeculae, lacunae, crest
    b. Epicondyle, sulcus, fissure
    c. Periosteum, osteon, trochanter
    d. Sesamoid, axial, meatus
11. Which sequence of terms are all axial skeleton bones?
    a. Coccyx, occipital, sternum
    b. Rib, sacrum, tibia
    c. Femur, clavicle, ulna
    d. Vertebrae, mandible, ilium
12. Which of the following are bony landmarks of the humerus?
    a. Radial tuberosity and styloid process
    b. Iliac fossa and coracoid process
    c. Olecranon fossa and lesser tubercle
    d. Intercondylar fossa and intertrochanteric line
13. Which of the following is located in the vertebral column?
    a. Manubrium
    b. Lamina
    c. Vertebral border
    d. Scaphoid
14. Which spinal deformity has the concavity in the lumbar and the convexity in the thorax?
    a. Scoliosis
    b. Scurvy
    c. Whiplash
    d. Lordosis

15. A client experienced an accident in which the trunk was thrust into an extension. Which of the following structures might have been injured?
    a. Deltoid ligament
    b. Anterior longitudinal ligament
    c. Anterior superior iliac spine
    d. Linea aspera
16. A young client is experiencing a growth spurt and complains that the bones in their legs ache. What is responsible for this phenomenon?
    a. Increased testosterone promotes long bone growth.
    b. Increased estrogen promotes long bone growth.
    c. Decreased estrogen supports long bone growth.
    d. Decreased testosterone promotes long bone growth.
17. If an intervertebral disk rupture actually occurs, what is the possible outcome?
    a. Narrowed disk space because of leakage of the nucleus pulposus
    b. Narrowed intervertebral space because of rupture of the fontanelle
    c. Impingement of the nerve from pressure exerted by the sella turcica
    d. Increased space in the foramen impinging on the spinal cord
18. A client complains of pain in the lower back. Observation indicates an excessive lumbar curve. This is called ______.
    a. Scoliosis
    b. Kyphosis
    c. Lordosis
    d. Talipes
19. A female client, age 67, has a history of smoking. This could indicate caution for compressive force used during massage for which reason?
    a. Osteonecrosis
    b. Osteomyelitis
    c. Osteochondritis dissecans
    d. Osteoporosis
20. A client complains of pain in the tibia. The client completed a marathon 24 hours before the massage session. What contraindication to massage may account for the pain?
    a. Stress fracture
    b. Compound fracture
    c. Dislocation
    d. Whiplash

Joints

CHAPTER 8

https://evolve.elsevier.com/Fritz/essential/

CHAPTER OBJECTIVES

After completing this chapter, the learner will be able to:

1. Describe the basic principles of joint design.
2. List the mechanical forces that act on the body.
3. Identify and describe three categories of joints.
4. Demonstrate the principles of joint motion.
5. Identify and palpate individual joints of the skull, shoulder, elbow, wrist, and hand.
6. Identify and palpate individual joints of the pelvis and hip, knee, ankle and foot, spine, and thorax.
7. Design a joint movement sequence for the body.
8. Identify pathological conditions of joints and describe general treatment protocols used for intervention.

CHAPTER OUTLINE

KEY TERMS

amphiarthrosis: A nonsynovial cartilaginous joint that is slightly movable.

anatomic range of motion: The amount of motion available to a joint based on the structure of the joint and determined by the shape of the joint surfaces, joint capsule, ligaments, muscle bulk, and surrounding musculotendinous and bony structures. The anatomical ROM is the limit of passive ROM.

arthrokinematics: (AR-thro-ki-ne-MA-tiks) The movement of bone surface in the joint capsule, including roll, spin, and slide.

articulation: (ar-tik-u-LA-shun) A place where two or more bones meet to connect parts and allow for movement in the body.

ball-and-socket joint: A joint that allows movement in three planes around a central point. Ball-and-socket joints are ball-shaped convex surfaces fitted into concave sockets. This type of joint gives the greatest freedom of movement but also is the most easily dislocated.

bursa: (BER-sah) A flat sac of synovial membrane in which the inner sides of the sac are separated by a fluid film. Bursae are located where moving structures rub over each other and are considered high-friction areas.

closed kinematic chain: The positioning of joints in such a way that motion at one of the joints is accompanied by motion at an adjacent joint.

close-packed position: The position of a synovial joint in which the surfaces fit precisely together and maximal contact occurs between the opposing surfaces. The compression of joint surfaces permits no movement, and the joint has its greatest stability.

condyloid (condylar) joint: A joint that allows movement in two planes, but one motion predominates. The joint resembles a condyle, which is a rounded protuberance at the end of a bone forming an articulation.

diarthrosis: (dye-ar-THRO-sis) A freely movable synovial joint.

edema: (eh-DEE-ma) Fluid accumulation in the tissues.

effusion: (ef-FU-sion) Fluid accumulation in a body cavity, such as the joint space enclosed by the joint capsule.

fibrocartilage: (fye-bro-KAR-ti-lij) A connective tissue that permits little motion in joints and structures. It is found in places such as the intervertebral disks and the menisci of the knees.

gliding joint: A joint that allows only a gliding motion in various planes; is also called a *synovial plane joint*.

hinge joint: A joint that allows flexion and extension in one plane, changing the angle of the bones at the joint, like a door hinge.

hyaline cartilage: (HYE-ah-lin) The thin covering of articular connective tissue on the ends of the bones in freely movable joints in the adult skeleton. Hyaline cartilage forms a smooth, resilient, low-friction surface for the articulation of one bone with another; distributes forces; and helps absorb some of the pressure imposed on the joint surfaces.

hypermobility: A range of motion (ROM) of a joint greater than would be permitted normally by the structure. Hypermobility may result in instability. Some hypermobility may be present without instability if sufficient dynamic stabilization is present.

hypomobility: A range of motion (ROM) of a joint less than what would be permitted normally by the structure. Hypomobility results in restricted ROM.

joint capsule: A connective tissue structure that connects the bony components of a freely movable joint.

joint play: The involuntary movement that occurs between articular surfaces that is separate from the axial range of motion (ROM) of a joint produced by muscles. Joint play is an essential component of joint motion and must occur for the normal functioning of the joint.

least-packed position: A joint capsule at its most lax. Joints assume the least-packed position when they are inflamed.

loose-packed position: The position of a synovial joint in which the joint capsule is most lax and the joint is least stable. Joints tend to assume this position to accommodate the increased volume of synovial fluid when inflammation occurs.

open kinematic chain: A position in which the ends of the limbs or parts of the body are free to move without causing motion at another joint.

pathological range of motion: The amount of motion at a joint that fails to reach the normal physiological range or exceeds normal anatomical limits of motion of that joint.

physiological range of motion: The amount of motion available to a joint determined by the nervous system from information provided by joint sensory receptors. This information usually prevents a joint from being positioned such that injury could occur.

pivot joint: A bony projection from one bone fits into a ring formed by another bone and ligament structure to allow rotations around its own axis in one plane.

saddle joint: A joint that is convex in one plane and concave in the other, with the surfaces fitting together like a rider on a saddle.

suture: A synarthrotic joint in which two bony components are united by a thin layer of dense fibrous tissue.

symphysis: (SIM-fi-sis) A cartilaginous joint in which the two bony components are joined directly by fibrocartilage in the form of a disk or plate.

synarthrosis: (sin-ar-THRO-sis) A limited-movement, nonsynovial joint.

synchondrosis: (SIN-kond-ROE-sis) A joint in which the material connecting the two components is hyaline cartilage.

syndesmosis: (SIN-dez-mo-sis) A fibrous joint in which two bony components are joined directly by a ligament, cord, or aponeurotic membrane.

synovial fluid: (si-NO-vee-al) A thick, colorless, lubricating fluid secreted by the joint cavity membrane.

synovial joints: Freely moving joints that allow motion in one or more planes of action.

viscoelasticity: The combination of resistance offered by a fluid to a change of form and the ability of a material to return to its original state after deformation.

yellow elastic cartilage: Cartilage that is more opaque, flexible, and elastic than hyaline cartilage and is distinguished further by its yellow color. The ground substance is penetrated in all directions by frequently branching fibers.

LEARNING HOW TO LEARN

Kinesthetic learning is about using your body to learn to do something. This chapter is perfect for kinesthetic learning. Some activities ask you to move and to palpate, which reinforce learning. You cannot understand this information by reading alone; you have to do it. In addition, you can visualize the actions in your mind and read the words aloud. If you do all three—do, see, and hear—you will remember better.

This is the second chapter in the specific study of kinesiology and biomechanics. Chapter 7 describes the bones. Bones are a combination of structure and function, as with the rest of the human body. As mentioned in Chapter 7, the study of the skeletal system involves the study of joints. The purpose of most joints is to allow movement. Connective tissue that connects bones to create joints is an essential part of joint structure and function. Without connective tissue, the structural integrity of joints would not be maintained. Joints allow movement but require the contraction of muscle tissue to create movement. The human body is highly specialized. Its individual cells have developed specific jobs that can no longer function independently outside the community of the whole body. Each part needs the others.

JOINT OVERVIEW

SECTION OBJECTIVES

Chapter objectives covered in this section:

1. Describe the basic principles of joint design.
2. List the mechanical forces that act on the body.
3. Identify and describe three categories of joints.

After completing this section, the learner will be able to:

- Define articulation.
- Describe collagen and elastin.
- Define joint capsule, ligament, tendon, and bursae.
- Describe three types of cartilage.
- List joint categories.

Joints are where we bend and twist. Body movement depends on joints. Many systemic body functions, such as respiration and movement of blood and lymph, also depend on the mechanical pumping action of joint movement or muscle contraction alone. For example, lymph nodes often are located at jointed areas so that with every movement, the body massages the lymphatic system. The mechanical actions of breathing in and out depend on the movement of the ribs.

A firm understanding of the anatomy and physiology of jointed areas is necessary because massage therapists interact directly with the somatic structures of the body wall—muscles, connective tissue, joint structure, and bones—as the entry point to the entire body.

Joints are interdependent relationships:

- A joint cannot exist with only one bone; at least two must work together.
- Joints seldom operate independently of other joints. Instead, an orchestrated, synchronized network of links develops, which is similar to relationships within a family, friends, and work teams.
- Joints are passive and unable to function without the muscles. They can do nothing alone and depend on others to get the job done; again, this resembles the interactions of families, friends, and work teams.
- Joints and muscles need one another. Joints must move to be healthy, and function best in the way they are designed to move, while muscles need to function effectively to produce joint movement. (Chapter 9 provides additional information relating to muscle structure and function.)

The same can be said of us. Human beings need to be active and do their best when they work with their unique assortment of personal gifts. An elbow cannot operate as a knee, but an elbow is essential and no less important than the knee in the function of the body.

A joint, or **articulation**, connects parts of a structure. In the body, the structures joined are, of course, the bones. Joints illustrate the strong relationship between structure and function. The design of a joint depends on its function, and vice versa. Structure, such as bone shape and the way the bones attach to the joint, determines joint function in the body. For example, joints that require stability or are weight bearing are structured differently from joints that provide greater mobility. Also, each part of a joint has one or more specific functions essential for the overall performance of the joint. Any disruption or change in any of the parts affects the function of the whole joint.

Balance Between Joint Stability and Joint Mobility

Joints connect approximately 200 bones of many sizes and shapes in the human skeleton. Effective functioning of the total structure depends on the integrated action of many joints, some providing greater stability with less mobility and some providing mobility with less stability. Most joints serve a dual function of allowing mobility but maintaining stability. However, in general, stability must be achieved before mobility. As will be seen, structures associated with joints such as joint capsules, ligaments, and tendons stabilize joints.

Joint designs in the human body vary from simple to complex.

- The simplest human joints usually are less mobile and more stable.
- The more complex joints usually allow greater mobility and are less stable.

Box 8.1 Form and Force Stability

Form closure, which comes from the ligaments, bones, and other connective tissue that does not contract.

Force closure, which involves our tissues that contract, like muscles.

Stability and Mobility

- Form closure/stability is dependent on the shape of the bones of the joint and the way everything fits together.
- Force closure/stability is the action of muscle contraction to stabilize the joint.
- Excessive form stability results in a stuck or fixed joint.
- Excessive force stability can result in excess form stability by jamming the joint surfaces.
- Decreased form stability results in increased muscle contraction to produce force stability.
- Decreased force stability results in strain on the joint capsule.

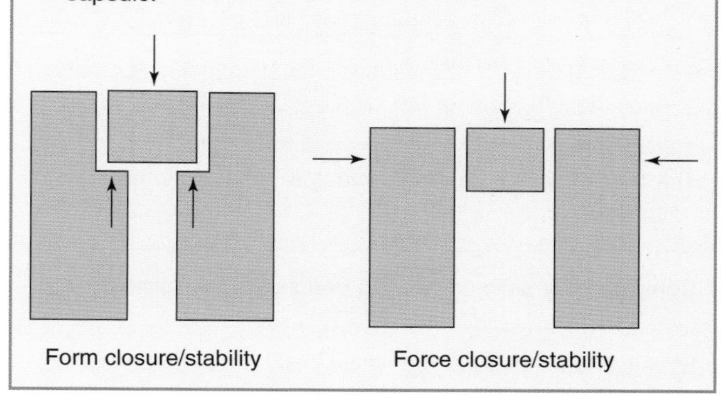

Figures modified from Vleeming A, Stoeckart R. *Movement, Stability, and Lumbopelvic Pain: Integration of Research and Therapy.* Elsevier; 2007, with permission from Elsevier.

Complex joints are more likely to be affected by injury, disease, or aging than simple joints. The complex joints have more parts and are subject to more wear and tear than simple joints (Box 8.1 and Activity 8.1).

Connective Tissue and Joint Structure

Connective tissue is used in the construction of human joints in the form of bones, ligaments, tendons, bursae, disks, plates, menisci, fat pads, and membranes. As discussed in Chapter 1, the structure of the connective tissue is characterized by a large extracellular matrix and a wide dispersion of cells. The extracellular matrix located between cells has a nonfibrous component, referred to as the *ground substance*, and a fibrous component.

The ground substance consists of proteins responsible for attracting and binding water. The concentration of these proteins in the extracellular matrix of bone, cartilage, membranes, tendons, or ligaments affects the water content and therefore the pliability of these structures. The nonfibrous component also plays a key role in protecting the connective tissue structure and strengthening it.

The fibrous component of the extracellular matrix contains two types of fibers: collagen and elastin.

Collagen

The primary fibrous component of the extracellular matrix in dense fibrous tissue is collagen (white fibrous tissue).

ACTIVITY 8.1

Assess what you already know about joints. Provide an example for each of the principles of joint design. It is ok if you do not get the "right" answer. The goal is to begin to think about how joints function. The first one is completed as an example.

Joints connect two or more bones.
The hip joint connects the pelvis and femur

Your turn
The design of a joint depends on its function.

___

Some joints provide greater stability than other joints.

___

Some joints provide greater mobility than other joints.

___

The structure of the joint determines the function of the joint.

___

Each part of the joint has a specific function that is essential to the whole function of the joint.

___

The breakdown of any joint structure affects the entire joint function.

___

Complex joints are more likely to malfunction than simple joints.

___

Effective functioning of the whole body depends on the integrated action of many joints working together.

___

Generally, stability must be achieved before mobility.

___

Most joints serve a dual function of allowing mobility and maintaining stability.

___

Simple joints provide more stability.

___

Complex joints provide more mobility.

___

Collagen has a tensile strength similar to that of steel and is responsible for the functional stability of connective tissue structures.

Collagen fibers are nonelastic but still provide limited mobility. In the relaxed position of some structures, collagen fibers assume a wavy configuration called *crimp*. The crimp or wave can be straightened, allowing for some flexibility in the structure.

Collagen has piezoelectric properties that generate small electrical currents when it is deformed; collagen oscillates or vibrates if electrical currents travel through it (Fig. 8.1A).

Elastin

Elastin, or yellow fibrous tissue, has elastic properties that allow fibers to return to their original condition after a stretching force has been applied (see Fig. 8.1B).

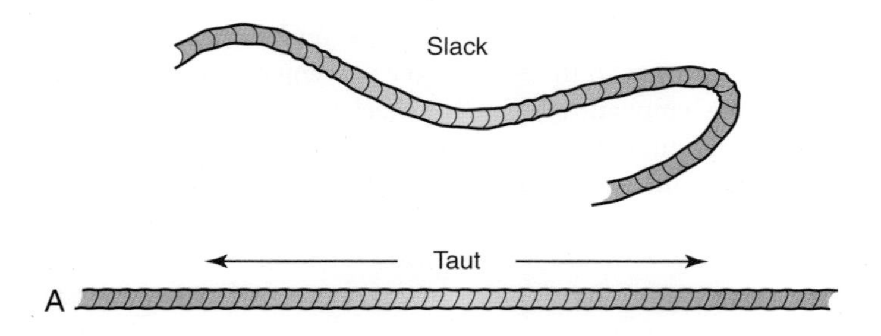

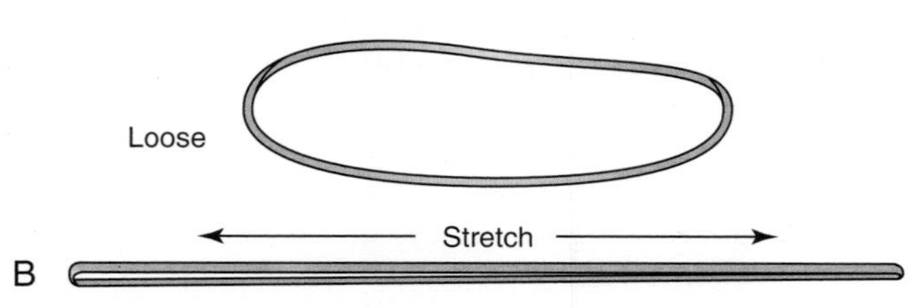

FIG. 8.1 (A) Collagen, like a rope. (B) Elastin, like a rubber band.

The arrangement of the collagen fibers, along with the collagen-to-elastin fiber ratio in various ligaments and tendons, determines the ability of these structures to provide stability and mobility for a particular joint.

The fibrous component of the extracellular matrix in ligaments contains greater collagen content than elastin content. However, the ratio of collagen-to-elastin fibers and their arrangement varies considerably among different ligaments.

Joint Capsule

The joint capsule is a dense fibrous connective tissue that is attached to the bone and forms a sleeve around the joint, sealing the joint space. It also provides passive stability by limiting movements. The capsule varies in thickness, is locally thickened to form capsular ligaments, and may also incorporate tendons. The section Diarthroses (Synovial Joints) later in the chapter presents more detailed information on the joint capsule.

Ligaments

The cells within ligaments are fibroblasts. Ligaments consist of 70% to 80% collagen, which gives the tissue tensile strength. Elastin fibers in the extracellular matrix provide some flexibility.

The extracellular fibers are arranged in the same direction, forming a regular arrangement.

Ligaments are avascular, meaning they do not have a blood supply, as do skin and organs. Ligaments obtain nourishment from the blood vessels in the membranes around the joint.

Extrinsic ligaments are found on the outside of the joint capsule and physically separate from the capsule. Intrinsic ligaments are thickenings of the articular capsule.

Tendons

Tendons, like ligaments, are composed of dense regular connective tissue. They connect bone to muscle. In addition to the usual connective tissue components associated with tendons, loose areolar connective tissue forms complete or partial sheaths around them. Double layers of connective tissue around the tendons at the wrist and hand form complete sheaths; these tendons sometimes are called *sheathed tendons.* The sheath protects the tendon and produces synovial fluid, which helps reduce friction.

Tendons help stabilize joints in that they pass across or around a joint to provide mechanical support; however, they can limit the range of movement in a joint.

Bursae

A bursa is a flat sac of synovial membrane in which the inner sides of the sac are separated by a fluid film. Bursae are located where moving structures are apt to rub against each other. Subcutaneous bursae are located between the skin and bones. Subtendinous bursae are located between tendons and bones. Submuscular bursae are located between muscles and bones. Although most of us have bursae in the same places, bursae can form as a response to demand if the body needs additional cushioning.

Cartilage

Cartilage usually is divided into three types: white fibrocartilage, yellow elastic cartilage, and hyaline cartilage.

- *White fibrocartilage:* White fibrocartilage consists primarily of collagen fibers and forms the cement in joints that permits little motion. This type of cartilage also forms the intervertebral disks and the menisci in the knees.
- *Yellow elastic cartilage:* Yellow elastic cartilage is found in the ears and epiglottis and differs from white fibrocartilage in that it has a higher ratio of elastin to collagen fibers. Yellow elastic cartilage is more opaque, flexible, and elastic than hyaline cartilage and is distinguished further by its yellow color. The ground substance is penetrated in all directions by frequently branching fibers.
- *Hyaline cartilage:* Hyaline cartilage forms a thin covering of articular cartilage on the ends of the bones in freely movable joints in the adult skeleton. Hyaline cartilage forms a smooth, resilient, low-friction surface for the articulation of one bone with another and disperses joint pressure over a wider area. Hyaline cartilage distributes any additional stresses applied to a joint and helps absorb some of the pressure imposed on the joint surfaces. These cartilaginous surfaces are capable of bearing and distributing weight over the lifetime of a person, assuming the individual has normal biomechanics, no injury, and no habits that wear down the cartilage. Water is the most abundant component of hyaline cartilage and, when combined with protein substances in the ground substance, forms a stiff gel (Fig. 8.2).

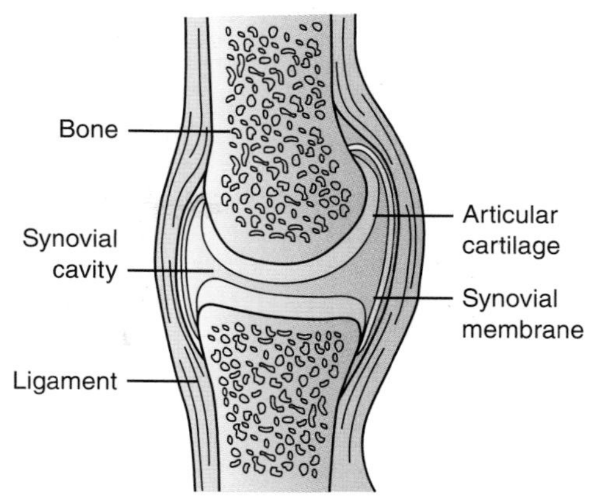

FIG. 8.2 Articular cartilage in the generic joint capsule. (Adapted from Barkauskas VH, et al. *Health and Physical Assessment*. 3rd ed. Mosby; 2002.)

Synovial Fluid

Synovial fluid is a thick, viscous, slippery fluid that contains hyaluronan (hyaluronic acid) a mucopolysaccharide (mucus-like) component of synovial fluid. Synovial fluid is secreted by fibroblast-like cells in the synovial membrane and interstitial fluid is filtered from the blood plasma. Synovial fluid is distributed during joint motion when the cartilage is compressed. The fluid flows back into the cartilage after motion or compression stops. Because hyaline cartilage in adults does not have blood vessels and nerves, its nourishment is derived from this back-and-forth flow of fluid. The free flow of fluid is essential for the survival of cartilage and as an aid in reducing friction.

The effects of immobilization, in which compression of joint surfaces is absent or diminished, can cause hyaline cartilage to degenerate. Viscosupplementation is a joint fluid therapy that involves the injection of gel-like hyaluronan into a joint to supplement the viscous (thick, slippery) properties of synovial fluid. This treatment is especially effective in the knee.

Bone

Bone is the hardest of all connective tissues found in the body. As with other forms of connective tissue, bone consists of a cellular component, a ground substance, and a fibrous component.

Viscoelasticity of Connective Tissue

Although connective tissue appears in many forms throughout the body, all connective tissue exhibits the common property of viscoelasticity. The behavior of viscoelastic materials is a combination of the properties of elasticity and viscosity:

- *Elasticity* refers to the ability of a material to return to its original state after being stretched.
- *Viscosity* refers to the resistance to a change of form offered by a fluid.

When a constant compressive or tensile force deforms connective tissue, the tissue moves in the direction of the force and then attempts to return to its original state. Under normal conditions viscoelastic materials initially modify in the direction of the force applied and then slowly return to their original state; this is called *creep*. If a connective tissue structure is held in a deformed position for an extended period, over days or weeks, the viscous creep pattern may become permanent, thus altering the structure and therefore the function of a joint.

Practical Application

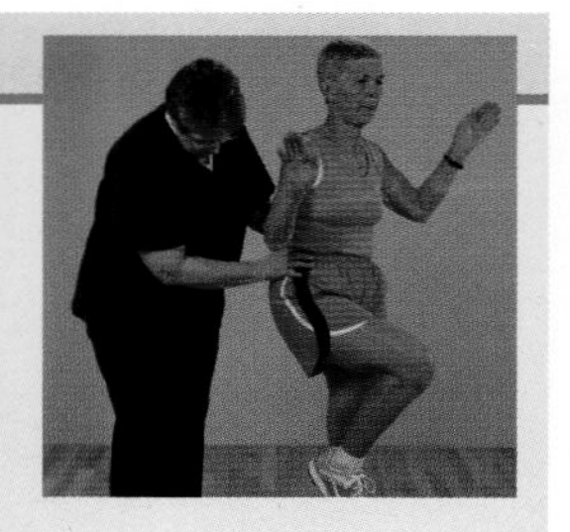

Movement is essential to joint health. Therapeutic massage can support joint function and, in some instances, replace movement to encourage the production and distribution of synovial fluid in the joint. Methods that use passive and active forms of joint movement are the methods of choice in these instances.

Plastic Range

Connective tissue subjected to sudden, prolonged, or excessive mechanical forces may exceed its elastic limits, and the tissue may enter the plastic range. In the plastic range, the tissue is permanently deformed and is no longer able to return to its original state after the removal of the deforming mechanical force. When the plastic range of connective tissue is exceeded by a mechanical force, a failure, such as a break or tear of the tissue, occurs:

- In the case of a ligament or tendon, the failure may occur in the middle of the structures, through tearing and disruption of the connective tissue fibers, and is called a *rupture.*
- Failure that occurs through a pulling off of part of the bone attached to the ligament is called *avulsion;* there is no injury to the ligament because it is still attached to a bony fragment.
- Failure that occurs in bony tissue is called a *fracture.*

Each type of connective tissue can undergo a certain percentage of deformation before failure. This percentage varies not only among the types of connective tissue, but also within the distinct types. Generally, tendons can deform more than ligaments, ligaments can deform more than cartilage, and cartilage can deform more than bone.

Two types of general pathological conditions develop with changes in elasticity and viscosity of connective tissue: laxity and shortening and stiffening.

Laxity. Ligament laxity places a joint at risk for injury because it compromises an important source of joint support and protection. Gymnastics, dancing, figure skating, and excessive use of stretching systems (e.g., yoga) can produce this condition. Connective tissue diseases also can cause joint laxity. Hypermobility spectrum disorders such as Marfan syndrome and Ehlers-Danlos syndrome (EDS) involve excessive flexibility resulting in instability. Remember that stability is established before mobility. When connective tissue is unstable around a joint, the muscles of the jointed area increase contraction to provide the necessary joint stability. This action pulls the bones of a joint together, reducing joint space, which may result in increased compression upon the bones of the joint. Although this is a good short-term strategy, other problems with joint function, such as a predisposition to osteoarthritis and osteoarthrosis, develop over the long term.

Massage approaches can be used to manage the muscle contractions around the joint and support the compensation pattern by keeping the muscle contractions appropriate to the need for stabilization and minimizing the excessive pulling together of the bones of the joint. A series of active joint movements using a pulsing action may increase stability around the joints. These movements do not stretch the tissues but rather mobilize the area through a gentle range of motion (ROM). The rehabilitation progresses to resistance exercises, used to challenge dynamic stabilizers of the joint to provide improved strength and ultimately stability of the joint. Stretching of unstable joints is avoided.

ACTIVITY 8.2

Return to Chapter 1 and review the information about connective tissue. Summarize the information on a separate sheet of paper.

Shortening/Stiffening. Connective tissue also tends to shorten, increase in density, and become less pliable and stiff. The result is pulling structures together and stiffening the area, thereby reducing mobility. This situation provides too much stability and tends to develop to compensate for changes in form and function. Should the body need to alter position for an extended period, such as a static position while working at a computer for hours at a time every day, connective tissue slowly alters to support that position. Connective tissue, particularly the ground substance, can thicken (densification) and shorten and become matted (fibrotic) if any inflammatory process does not resolve itself effectively.

Some restricted joint function develops from the tissues surrounding the joint instead of within and directly around the capsule itself. Because of this, it is necessary to assess the entire area for shortening. For example, shortening in the lumbodorsal fascia or pectoral fascia can limit the ROM of the shoulder joint. Over time, the reduction in movement causes pathological immobilization in the joint. Therefore any therapeutic massage or movement methods affecting joint function should address the entire body broadly (Activities 8.2 and 8.3).

Mechanical Forces Acting on the Body

- *External forces:* Forces that create loads on soft tissue by pushing or pulling on the body in a variety of ways. A belt around your waist creates an external compressive load. Gravity is an external force. Massage is an external force.
- *Internal forces:* Forces that create loads on soft tissue (e.g., misaligned joints or poor body mechanics) cause soft tissue to shorten, tighten, lengthen, and/or weaken, which may load surrounding tissue; for example, a tight muscle or tendon could compress a nerve running close by and cause pain or dysfunction. Increased pressure in the stomach from overeating also is an example of an internal force.
- *Tissue load:* Forces load soft tissues during massage application. Tissue load creates *stress* in tissues, and tissues exposed to force are considered to be loaded. During massage application (applied force), if there is

ACTIVITY 8.3

Develop a therapeutic intervention for a hypothetical joint dysfunction. First, define and describe the assessment procedures you would use. Then develop a therapeutic goal for the area. Finally, develop treatments based on the listed principles. Make plans for a hypermobile and hypomobile situation. Use the therapy modalities you are studying presently in your technique classes. Remember that the actual implementation of such a plan often would be supervised by the appropriate healthcare professional, who would approve the plan before it is implemented. The principles are listed next, followed by an example.

Assessment Principles

Hypermobility

- Joint stabilization structures become lax.
- Too much flexibility results in instability.
- Muscle splinting develops to stabilize the area.

Hypomobility

- The entire area must be assessed for shortening.
- Over time, the reduction in movement causes pathologic immobilization in the joint itself.
- Any therapeutic massage methods affecting joint function need to address the body broadly.

Therapeutic Goals

Hypermobility

- Support stability.
- Reduce excessive muscle tone surrounding the jointed area.

Hypomobility

- Restore pliability.
- Support normal muscle tone.

Treatment Principles

Hypermobility

- Manage the muscle contraction around the joint to support the compensation pattern by keeping the muscle contraction appropriate to the need for stabilization and minimizing the excessive pulling together of the joint cavity.

Hypomobility

Lengthen all muscle components to their available resting length.

Example

Situation: Hypermobile ankle from a bad sprain 3 years ago.

Assessment

- Assess the ankle for laxity in ligaments and other connective tissue structures by studying the range of motion (ROM).
- Assess for muscle splinting and shortening with palpation.

Therapeutic Goal

- Increase stability of the ankle to prevent future ankle sprains.

Treatment Principles

- Manage the muscle contraction around the joint with therapeutic massage.
- Encourage more specific rehabilitation protocols, including proprioception; active exercises are the only evidence-based approach to prevent reinjury. These activities include standing on one foot, using wobble boards, and walking on soft surfaces, such as a mat.

Your Turn

Hypermobility

Situation: ____________________

Assessment

Therapeutic Goal

Treatment Principles

Hypomobility

Situation: ____________________

Assessment

Therapeutic Goal

Treatment Principles

too much load, the tissue might fail and be injured; too little load and tissues may not respond as desired. The change in the shape of tissue (deformation) in response to the load is called the *strain*. Too much strain and tissues can be damaged. Not enough strain and the tissues may not respond and adapt.

Mechanical forces are actions that involve pushing and pulling. Every time we take a step, push against an object with our arms, or bend and twist, our bones and joints have to dissipate the stress of the mechanical forces imposed on them. When these forces meet an obstacle such as a bend or curve in a bone, the bone absorbs some forces and reflects others. Absorbed forces are transmitted to the soft tissues outside the bone, which helps dissipate excessive stress on joint surfaces. Tissue can be loaded by the mechanical forces of push or pull to stress the tissue in five distinct ways. Tissue types respond differently to different forces and stress. Bending stress seldom harms the soft tissues but will break bones. Tensile stresses seldom injure bone but often damage soft tissue. Massage therapy application consists of using mechanical forces to load tissue to produce therapeutic effects (Box 8.2).

The massage therapy leadership organizations worked together to develop entry-level massage educational standards. An important part of this work was to standardize massage terminology. To accomplish this task, massage applications are described by the way mechanical forces deform soft tissue. You can learn more at the website https://www.elapmassage.org.

The next five sections describe the types of mechanical force stresses and the potential injury and therapeutic application pertinent to therapeutic massage.

Box 8.2 Language Used in the Entry-Level Analysis Project Documents With Explanation

Anatomical tools: Palms, forearms, fingertips, knuckles, and so on are used to apply force to soft tissue.

Force: Something that internally or externally causes the movement of the body to change or soft-tissue structures to deform. In physics, a force is any external effort that causes an object to undergo a certain change, either concerning its movement, direction, or shape. For example, a muscle creates a force that is transferred to the tendon to pull on the bony attachment resulting in movement when it contracts. When a massage therapist moves joints passively, the massage therapist creates the force and the body part moved has changed direction. During massage, the massage therapist generates the force when the tissue is pressed, pushed, or pulled and has changed shape. There are several types of force, but for massage application, we need to understand mechanical/physical applied force. A mechanical/physical applied force (push or a pull) has both magnitudes (how much) and direction (which way). Its magnitude is measured in pounds (or in newtons). For example, a push against tissue might be 1 pound per square inch.

Key concept: A force is a push or a pull.

Friction: Friction is a force that acts in an opposite direction to movement. Friction is a force that holds back the movement of a sliding object. During massage, lubricants reduce friction, so the "anatomical tool" used to provide massage can slide. Too much lubricant equals too much slide. Not enough lubricant equals too much friction, and instead of sliding, the tissue is pushed or pulled. Most massage methods should move and change the shape of the tissue that occurs with pushing or pulling. If just the right amount of lubricant is used, then the tissues can be moved but the friction is not uncomfortable.

Pressure: In massage, we often use the word "pressure" to indicate magnitude. Light pressure equals small magnitude, and deep pressure equals increased magnitude. Pressure is the amount of force applied to the tissue. Pressure during massage is usually applied down into the client's body at an angle of 45 degrees to 90 degrees. Pressure applied within the 45-degree range will orient more horizontally, and pressure applied closer to the 90-degree range will be more perpendicular.

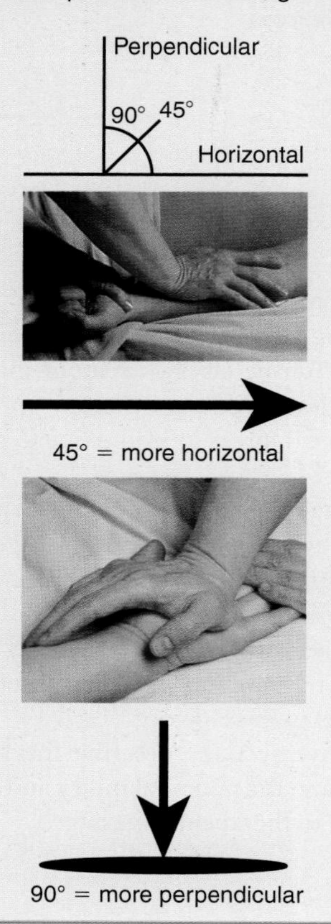

Pressure is also determined by the contact area. A large or broad contact used during massage (such as the forearm) distributes the force, and pressure is more comfortable than pressure applied with a narrow contact (such as the tip of the finger or elbow). The pressure applied in a small contact area concentrates force application, which is more specific and more apt to cause injury and pain sensations.

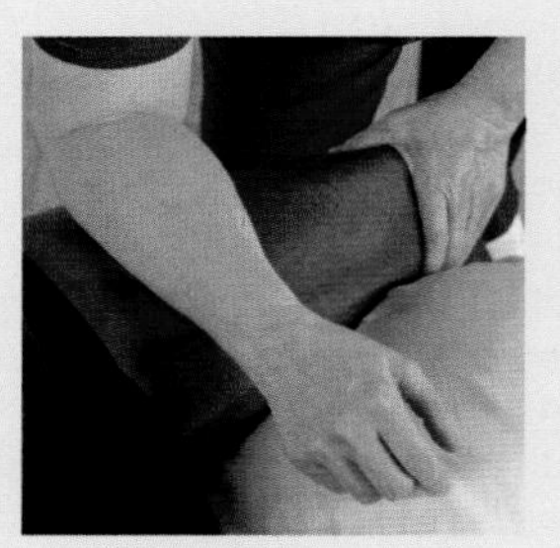

Broad base contact.

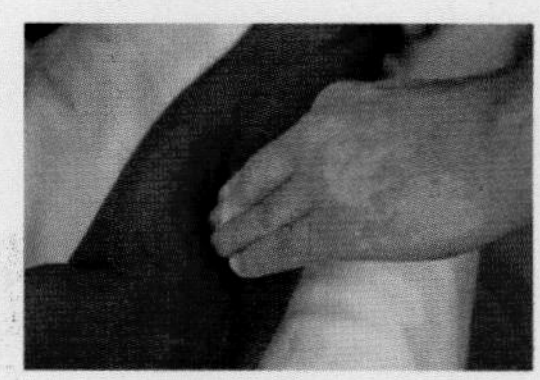

Narrow or small point of contact.

Key concept: During massage, the massage therapist applies the mechanical/physical force when we push or pull on the body tissues. We use methods to push or pull, such as gliding, kneading, twisting, stretching, and so on. When these methods slide on the tissue, there is friction. The intensity (magnitude) is dependent upon how strong the push or pull is and how much friction is resisting the motion. These two factors determine the amount of pressure.

Vector quantity: An important consideration with force is that it is a vector quantity. A vector quantity always has three variables:

1. Point of application
2. Magnitude
3. Direction

During massage application, the massage method will be modified by where (*point of application*) it is applied, how intense (*magnitude*), and the *direction* in relation to the tissues. Remember, an applied mechanical/physical force causes motion or a change in shape.

Key concept: If the force is applied to an object, it will move if it can move. If movement is not possible, then the object will change shape. During massage, we usually want the tissue to change shape, which means it cannot move while the massage method is applied. When tissue changes shape, it typically gets flatter, longer, twisted, or bunched up. Sometimes we want movement as well, such as when a joint is moved.

Box 8.2 Language Used in the Entry-Level Analysis Project Documents With Explanation—cont'd

External forces: Forces that create loads on soft tissue by pushing or pulling on the body in a variety of ways. A belt around your waist creates an external compressive load. Gravity is an external force. Massage is an external force.

Internal forces: Forces that create loads on soft tissue, such as misaligned joints or poor body mechanics cause soft tissue to shorten, tighten, lengthen, and/or weaken, which may load surrounding tissue. For example, a tight muscle or tendon could compress a nerve running close by and cause pain or dysfunction. Increased pressure in the stomach from overeating is also an example of an internal force.

Tissue load: Forces load soft tissues during massage application. Tissue load creates stress in tissues, and tissues exposed to force are considered to be loaded. During massage application (applied force), if there is too much load, the tissue might fail and be injured; if there is too little load, tissues may not respond as desired. The change in the shape of tissue in response to the load is called the *strain*. If there is too much strain, tissues can be damaged. If there is not enough strain, the tissues may not respond and adapt.

Example: The goal of the massage is to increase the length of the soft tissue in the calf. The massage therapist chooses an anatomical tool (forearm), to apply a force (push and pull) at the back of the leg just below the knee (point of application) using moderate pressure (magnitude) and push the tissue toward the ankle (direction). The applied force loads the tissue, causing stress, and the tissue changes shape due to the strain.

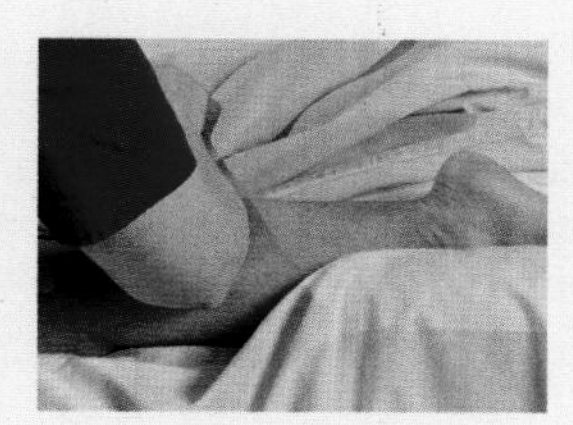

Categories of force load: The five types of loads that can act on soft tissue are tension, compression, shear, bending, and torsion. These five loads fall into two categories: simple loads and combined loads.

Simple loads: One specific type of load that results in one specific type of stress. The primary force load outcomes are compression stress, tension stress, and shear stress.

- *Compression stress* pushes or presses soft tissue making it shorter and thicker. Another way to understand compression is two pushing forces, directly opposing each other, that squeeze or press an object and try to squash it. For example, place a ball of clay on the table and squash it to make it flat. In this example, the clay is subjected to a compressive load. The result is compression stress. The flattening of the clay is the strain. Gravity is a force that is "pushing down" on the body while the reaction force of the chair, massage table, floor, and so on is "pushing up." Gravity creates compression stress.

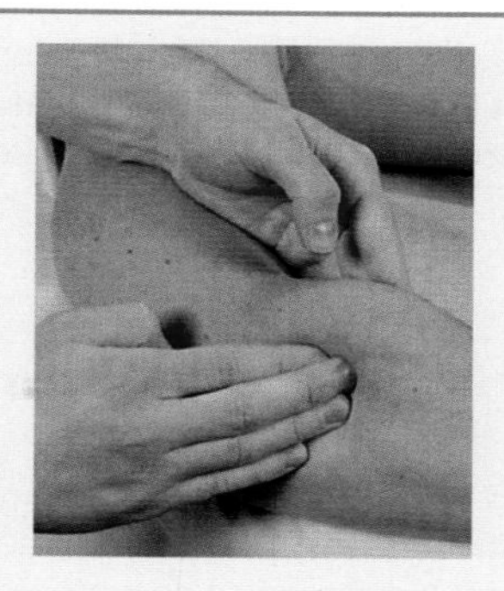

- *Tension stress* (or tensile stress) occurs when two forces pull on an object in opposite directions to stretch it make it longer and thinner and try to pull it apart. For example, stretching out a rubber band puts it in tension or "being subjected to a tensile load." The primary load that muscle tissue experiences is a tension load. When the muscle structure contracts, it pulls on the tendons at both ends, which stretch a little. So the tendons are under tensile stress.

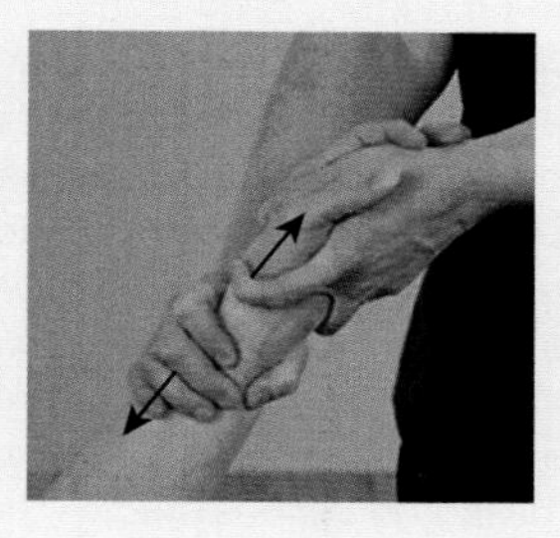

- *Shear stress* is two forces acting parallel to each other but in opposite directions so that one part of the tissue is moved or displaced relative to another part. Shear stress causes two objects to slide over one another. When an "anatomical tool" moves on the client's body during massage, there is shear stress. This sliding creates friction.

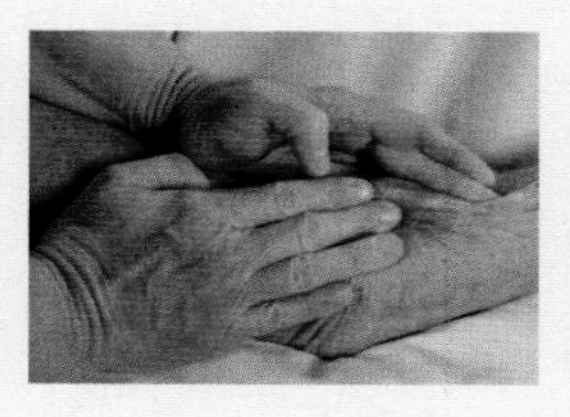

Combined loads: Different types of loads acting at the same time. The combined force load outcomes are torsion stress and bending stress.

- Torsional loading, which we usually just call *torsion*, is when forces cause a twist about its longitudinal axis. (Think about wringing water out of a sponge.) The stresses that occur during torsion include shear, compressive, and tensile stress. Torsion produces shear stresses inside the material.

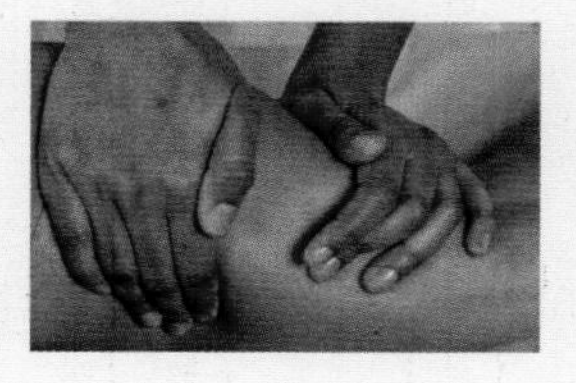

Continued

Box 8.2 Language Used in the Entry-Level Analysis Project Documents With Explanation—cont'd

- *Bending* loads produce tensile and compressive stresses. Think about bending a wire with both hands. You are creating compressive stress on one side and tensile stress on the other.

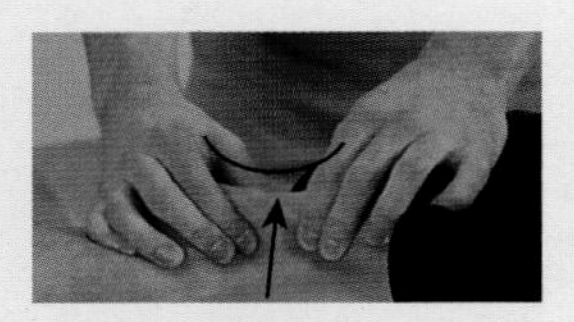

Soft-tissue deformation: *Deformation* means the tissue changes shape. As deformation occurs, internal forces in the material oppose the applied force. If the applied force is not too large, these internal forces may be sufficient to completely resist the applied force, allowing the substance to assume a different shape and return to its original shape when the load is removed. A larger applied force may lead to a permanent deformation of the substance or even to its structural failure. This is what happens when a bone breaks or a tendon is sprained. How much tissue deformation can occur is a function of the tissue properties, such as how stiff or pliable it is, time (or how long the force is applied), temperature (or if the tissue is cold or warm), and type of load (such as pulling to stretch). For example, bone is resistant to stretching but can break if bent. Depending on the magnitude of the applied stress and its duration, the deformation may become so large that the tissue is injured. During massage, we need to monitor the tissue to make sure that the force applied does not injure the tissue. One theoretical proposed mechanism for massage benefit is based on various studies that have looked at the plastic, viscoelastic, and piezoelectric properties of connective tissue. Sensory receptors of the nervous system are embedded in the soft tissue. These receptors are stimulated when tissues change shape, sending information to the spinal cord and brain about movement, position, and potential tissue damage. Vessels that carry blood and lymph are also embedded in the soft tissue, and movement and tissue shape changes will either support or interfere with fluid movement. Even though the concept of push-pull force application may seem simple, when thinking about the benefits of massage, it is amazing how much is affected by an intelligent and skilled mechanical force application.

Soft-Tissue Deformation Methods

The following sections give terminology and examples of the way that forces are applied during massage. Each of these methods has the potential to load tissue and create a variety of mechanical stresses, such as compression, tension, shear, torsion, and bending stress.

Compression Methods

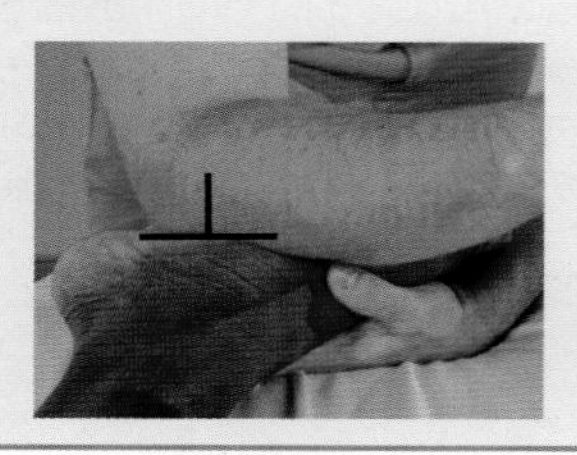

Examples: Approximation (pushing ends of tissues together), pushing tissue against another tissue, applying pressure into tissue

Direct pressure techniques: Often used interchangeably with static compression and ischemic compression

Gliding Methods

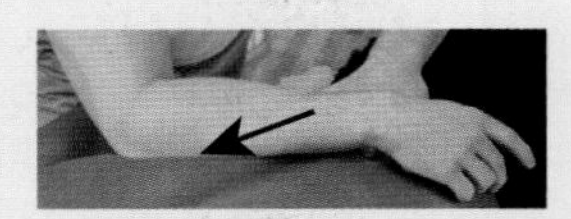

Examples: Stroking, Swedish/classical effleurage, a stroke applied in a smooth continuous motion that does not lose contact with the client's skin

Torsion/Twisting Methods

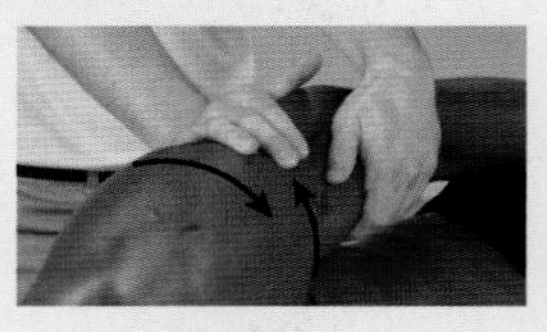

Examples: Kneading, skin rolling, fulling, wringing, fascial torquing, Swedish/classical pétrissage

Shearing Methods

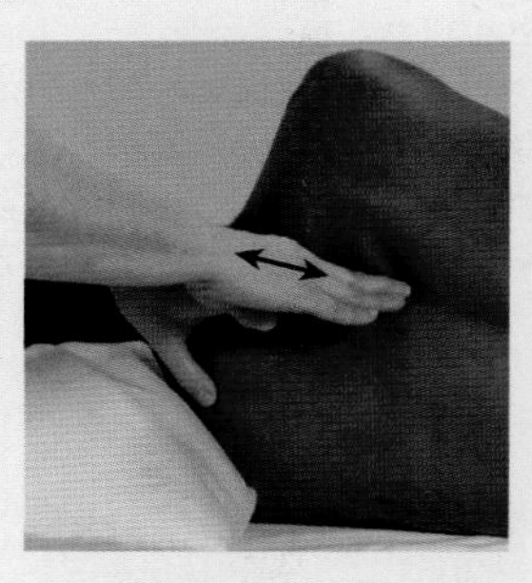

Examples: Superficial friction, linear friction, circular friction, cross-fiber friction, muscle layer separation

Elongation Methods

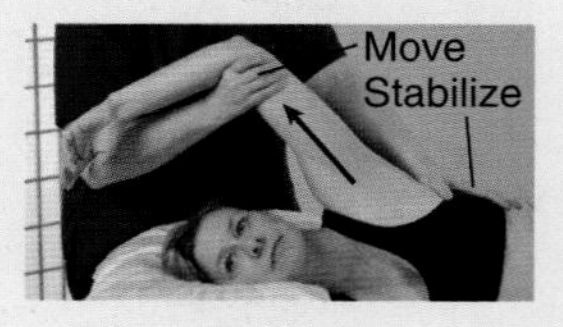

Examples: Crossed hands stretch, fascial spreading, pin and stretch, arm pulling, leg pulling, traction

Oscillating Methods

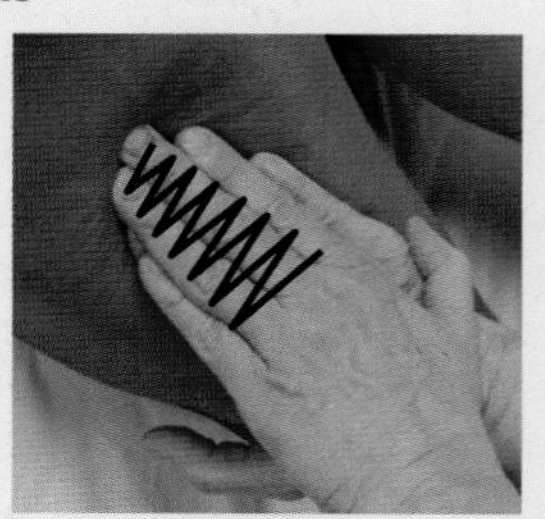

Examples: Vibration, rocking, jostling, or shaking

Box 8.2 Language Used in the Entry-Level Analysis Project Documents With Explanation—cont'd

Percussive Methods

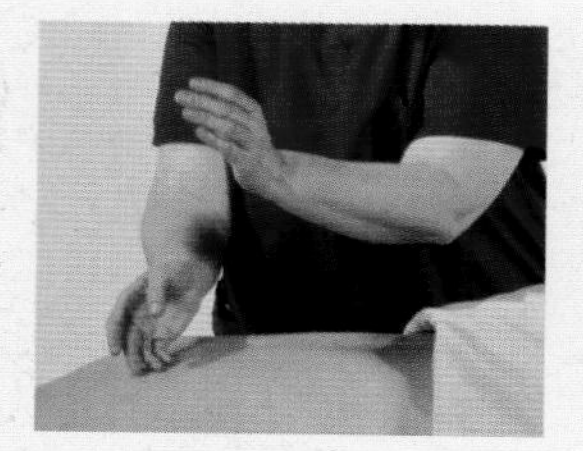

Examples: Tapping, hacking, cupping, slapping, beating, pounding, and clapping

Static Methods

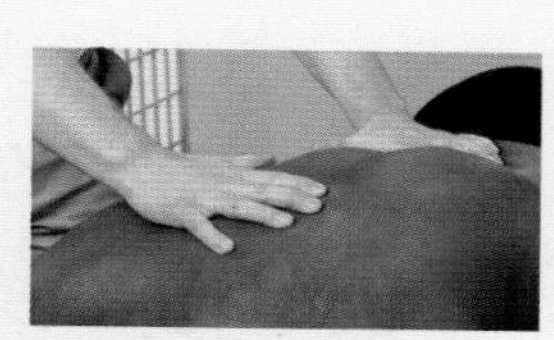

Examples: Holding, direct pressure

Movement Methods

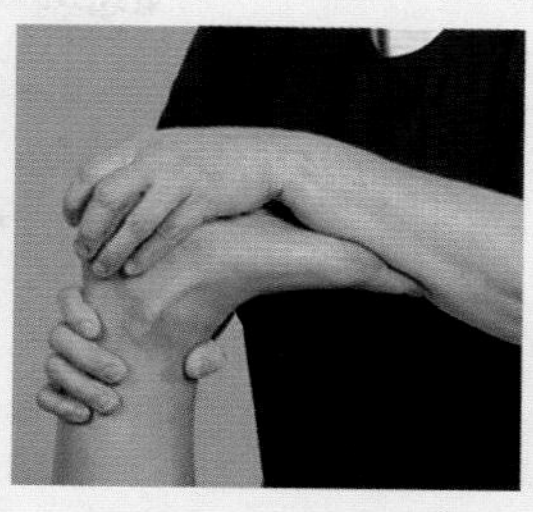

Examples: Active/passive joint movement, stretching

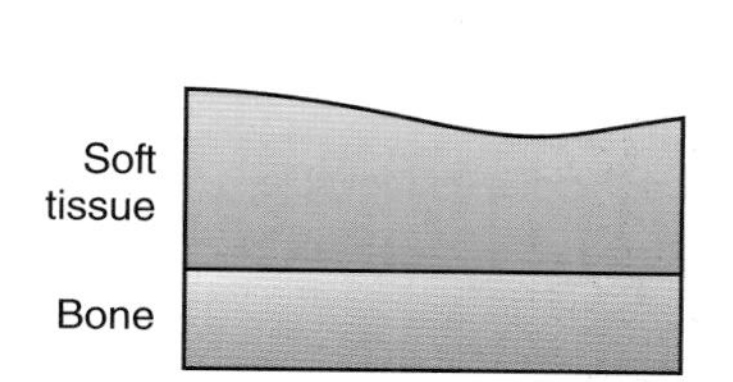

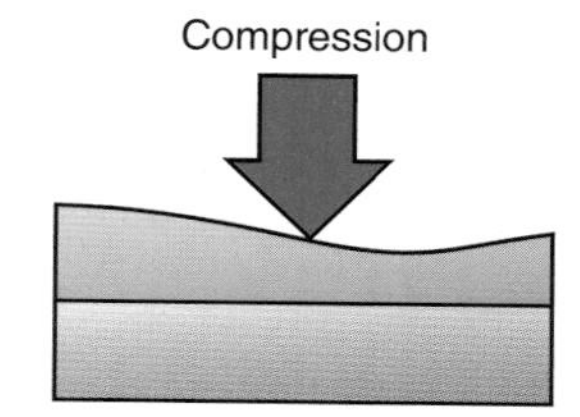

FIG. 8.3 Compression. (From Fritz S. Mosby's Fundamentals of Therapeutic Massage. 5th ed. Mosby/Elsevier; 2013.)

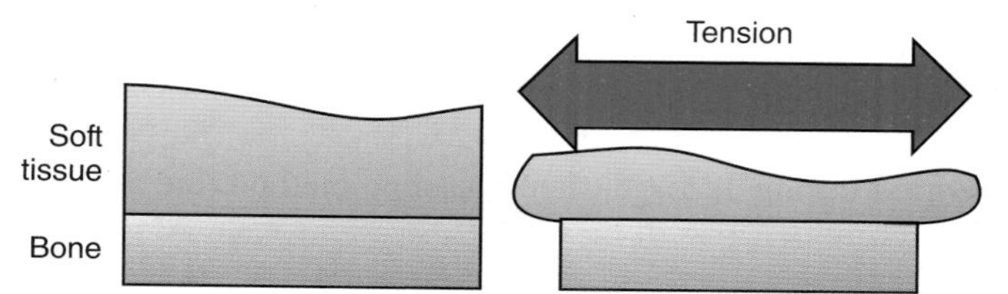

FIG. 8.4 Tension. (From Fritz S. *Mosby's Fundamentals of Therapeutic Massage*. 5th ed. Mosby/Elsevier; 2013.)

Compression

Compression stress occurs when two structures are pressed together (Fig. 8.3). Compression is a common way tissues become injured. Ligaments and tendons resist compressive injury. Muscle tissue, because of its extensive vascular structure, is not as resistant to compressive stress. Excessive compression ruptures or tears the integrity of the muscle tissue, causing bruising and connective tissue damage. Compression is a major mechanical force loading used in the application of massage to support circulation, stimulate nerve function, and restore connective tissue pliability. The massage therapist applies compression in such a way as to achieve benefits without damaging tissue, usually with the broad-based application of compression.

Tension

Tension stress, also called *tensile loading*, occurs when two ends of a structure are pulled away from each other (Fig. 8.4).

Bone resists tensile stress. However, tensile stress injuries are the most common way soft tissue is damaged. Examples of tensile stress injuries include avulsion (complete tearing of an attachment), muscle strains, ligament sprains, tendinitis, fascial pulling or tearing, and nerve traction injuries (sudden nerve stretching, such as those that occur in stingers). Tensile stress injuries are described as first degree (mild), second degree (moderate), and third degree (severe). Tensile stress is applied during massage, particularly during gliding and traction. Therapeutically, tensile stress supports the proper alignment of fiber structures and can increase pliability in connective tissue.

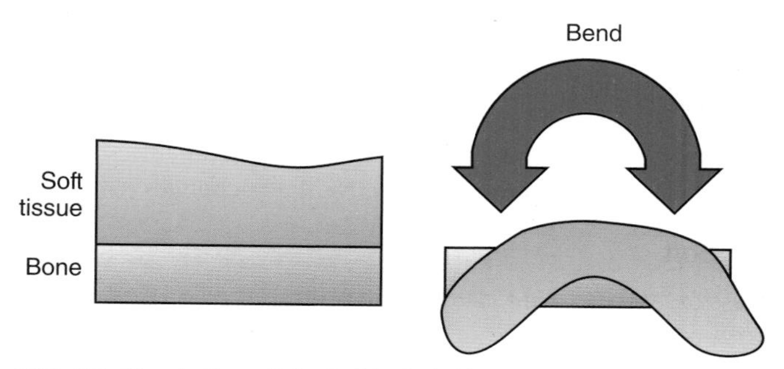

FIG. 8.5 Bend. (From Fritz S. *Mosby's Fundamentals of Therapeutic Massage*. 5th ed. Mosby/Elsevier; 2013.)

Bending

Bending stresses are a combination of compression and tension (Fig. 8.5). One side of a structure is exposed to compressive stress, whereas the other side is exposed to tensile stress. Bending stresses are a common cause of bone fractures and ligament injuries but seldom harm other soft tissues. Bending

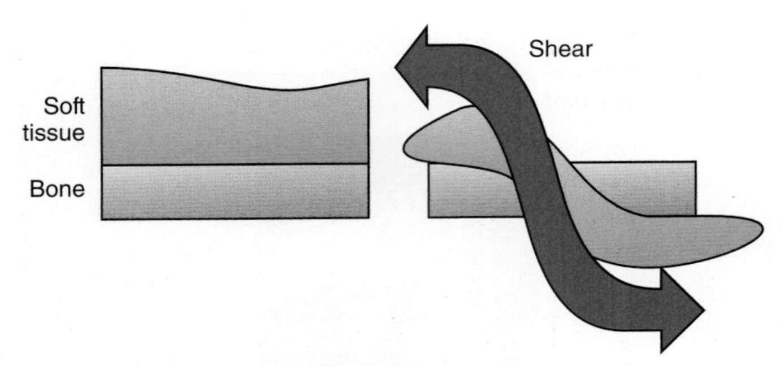

FIG. 8.6 Shear. (From Fritz S. *Mosby's Fundamentals of Therapeutic Massage*. 5th ed. Mosby/Elsevier; 2013.)

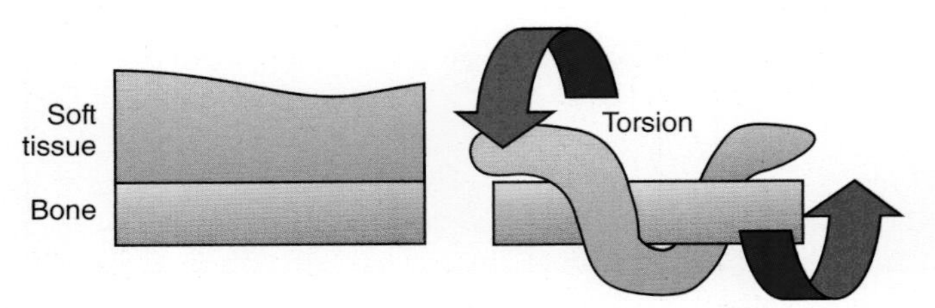

FIG. 8.7 Torsion. (From Fritz S. *Mosby's Fundamentals of Therapeutic Massage*. 5th ed. Mosby/Elsevier; 2013.)

is used during massage when kneading methods are applied. The proprioceptors in muscles and tendons respond to these forces. Bending stresses also affect connective tissues, especially the viscosity of the ground substance.

Shear

Shear is a sliding mechanical force with friction created between structures that are sliding against each other (Fig. 8.6). Excessive shearing force at a ligament or tendon creates an inflammatory irritation that leads to adhesion and fibrosis. Shear and friction, called *cross-fiber friction*, is a massage method that uses specific force to create therapeutic inflammation to reverse fibrotic connective tissue changes.

Torsion

Torsion stresses are twisting forces (Fig. 8.7). Torsion occurs with other types of loads, such as tension and shear. Torsion stress applied to a joint is likely to cause significant injury. Kneading massage methods introduce torsion stress into tissue and are especially effective in increasing the pliability of connective tissue.

Joint Categories

The joints of the human body are divided into three categories according to the type of motion allowed at the joint and the material connecting the joint. The three categories of joints (arthroses) are:

- **Synarthrosis:** Nonsynovial, *fibrous*, limited-movement joint
- **Amphiarthrosis:** Nonsynovial *cartilaginous* joint that is slightly movable
- **Diarthrosis:** *Synovial*, freely movable joint (most joints are diarthrosis)

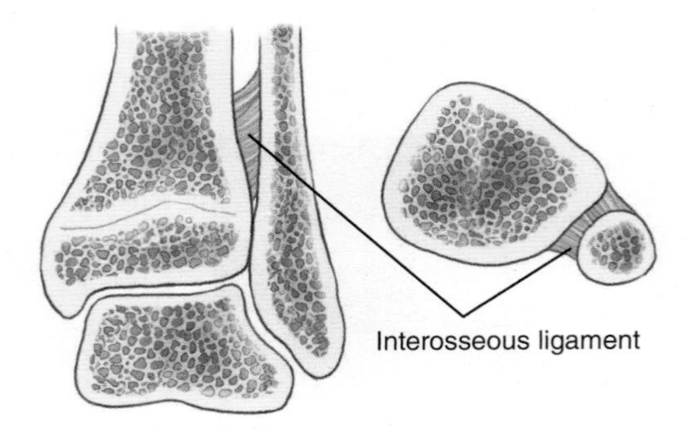

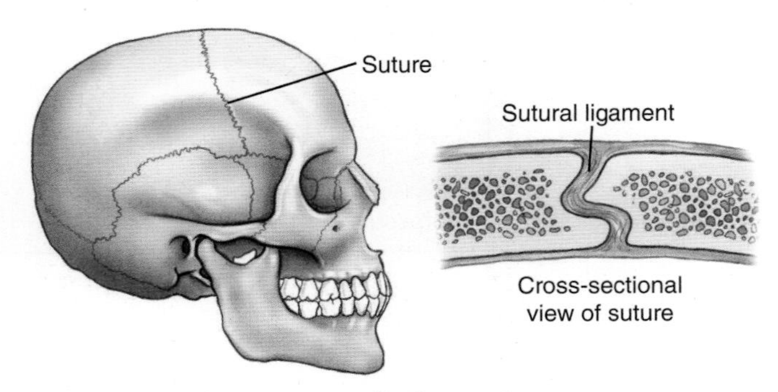

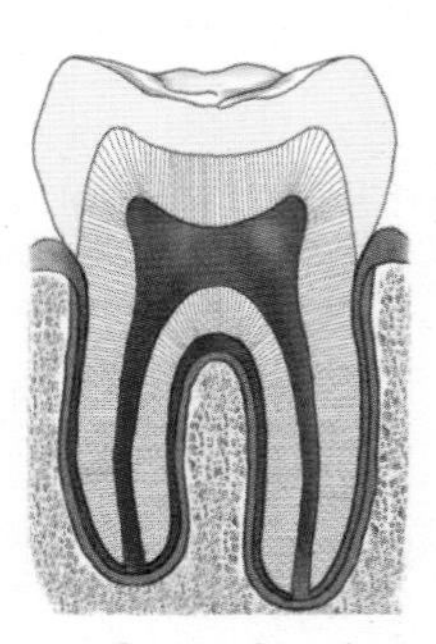

FIG. 8.8 Examples of the types of fibrous joints: (A) syndesmosis—amphiarthrodial (slightly movable); (B) suture—synarthrodial (immovable); (C) gomphosis—amphiarthrodial (only limited movement). (From Bontrager K, Lampignano J. *Textbook of Radiographic Positioning and Related Anatomy*. 8th ed. Mosby; 2014.)

Synarthroses (Fibrous Joints)

In fibrous joints the fibrous connective tissue directly connects bone to bone in a solid configuration that allows either an extremely small amount or no movement (Fig. 8.8). The material used to connect the bony components in synarthrodial joints is interosseous fibrous and cartilaginous connective tissues.

Three different types of fibrous joints are found in the human body: sutures, gomphoses, and syndesmoses.

- A **suture** is a joint in which two articulating bones are held together by a thin layer of dense fibrous tissue that is continuous with the periosteum. The ends of the bony components are grooved so that the edges interlock or overlap.

This type of joint is found only in the skull. Early in life, these sutures allow a small amount of movement. In adulthood, the bones slowly grow together to form a synostosis, or bony union, in which little or no motion is possible. The coronal suture is an example of a suture.

- A *gomphosis* is a joint in which the bony components fit together like a peg in a hole. The only gomphosis joint that exists in the human body is found between a tooth and the mandible or maxilla. In most adults, the loss of teeth mainly results from disease processes that affect the connective tissue cementing or holding the teeth. Under normal conditions in the adult, these joints do not permit motion.
- A **syndesmosis** is a fibrous joint in a ligament, cord, or aponeurotic membrane that joins the articulating bones. For example, a membrane joins the shaft of the tibia directly to the shaft of the fibula. A slight amount of motion at this joint accompanies movement at the knee and ankle joints.

Amphiarthroses (Cartilaginous Joints)

An amphiarthrosis is a slightly movable joint (Fig. 8.9). Fibrocartilage or hyaline growth cartilage holds the bony surfaces together. The two types of cartilaginous joints are symphyses and synchondroses:

- A **symphysis** is a joint in which thin layers of hyaline cartilage over each bone are separated from each other by fibrocartilage in the form of disks or plates. The symphysis pubis is the articulation of the two pubic bones. The structure of the symphysis pubis is quite stable, with the thick fibrocartilage providing a secure union between the two bones.
- A **synchondrosis** is a joint in which a thin layer of hyaline growth cartilage connects the two bones. The cartilage forms a bond between the two ossifying centers of bone. This type of joint permits bone growth while providing stability and allowing a small amount of movement. When bone growth is complete, these joints ossify and convert to bony unions. Sternocostal joints are synchondroses. Articular cartilage directly connects the adjacent surfaces of the rib and sternum.

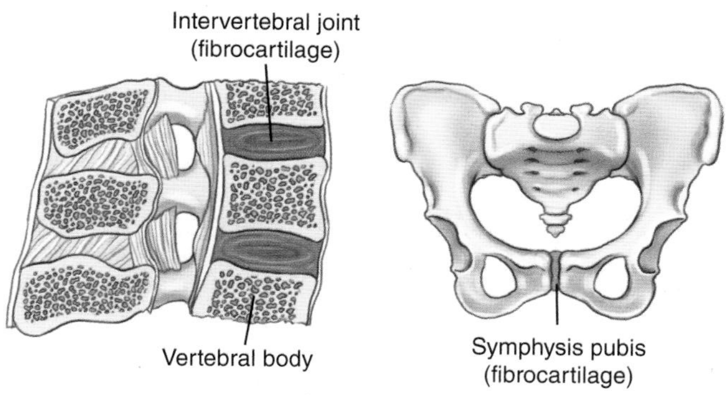

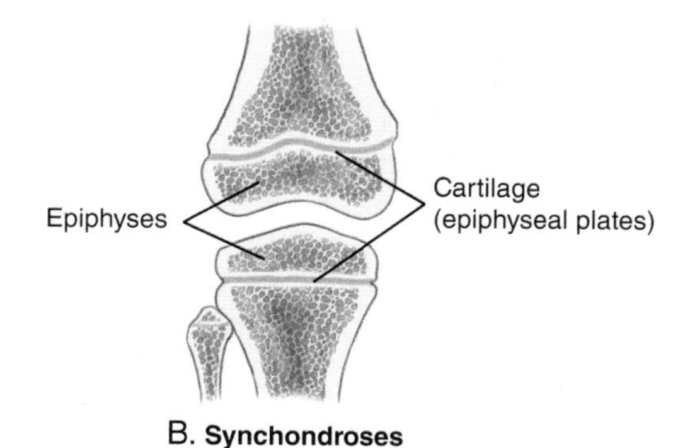

FIG. 8.9 Examples of the types of cartilaginous joints: (A) symphyses—amphiarthrodial (slightly movable); (B) synchondroses—synarthrodial (immovable). (From Bontrager K, Lampignano J. *Textbook of Radiographic Positioning and Related Anatomy*. 8th ed. Mosby; 2014.)

Diarthroses (Synovial Joints)

Most of our joints are **synovial joints**, which are freely movable. A smooth layer of articular cartilage protects the bone surfaces in freely movable joints (Fig. 8.10). All synovial joints are constructed similarly, with these features:

- A joint capsule formed of fibrous tissue surrounds the joint.
- The joint capsule encloses a joint cavity.
- A synovial membrane lines and forms the inner surface of the joint capsule.
- Synovial fluid is secreted by the synovial membrane into the joint cavity; it forms a lubricating film over the joint surfaces.
- Hyaline cartilage covers the joint surfaces.

In synovial joints the ends of the bony components move freely in relation to one another because no fibrous or cartilaginous tissue directly connects the bones. The bones in this type of joint have a space between them called the *joint* or *synovial cavity*, and the bony components connect indirectly to one another by means of a joint capsule, ligaments, and tendons. Ligaments and tendons play a key role in keeping joint surfaces connected and often assist in guiding motion. Although the bones are connected, some separation is necessary for the bones to be able to move. Separation of joint surfaces is limited by passive tension in ligaments, the joint capsule, and tendons. Active tension in muscles also limits the separation of joint surfaces.

The **joint capsule** consists of two layers: an outer layer, called the *stratum fibrosum*, and an inner layer, called the *stratum synovium*.

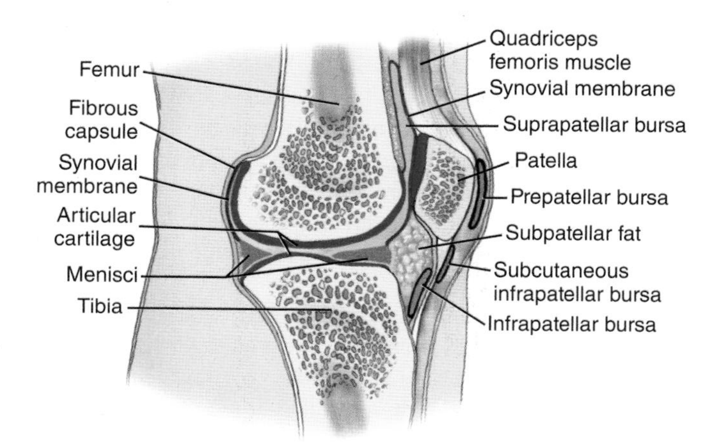

FIG. 8.10 Structures of the knee as a representation of a synovial joint. (From Muscolino JE. *Kinesiology: The Skeletal System and Muscle Function*. 2nd ed. Mosby/Elsevier; 2011.)

The stratum fibrosum, composed of dense fibrous tissue, surrounds the joint and is continuous with the periosteum of the adjoining bones. The outer layer is poorly vascularized but richly innervated by joint receptors. The receptors in and around the joint capsule can detect the rate and direction of motion, compression, tension, vibration, and pain. According to Hilton's law, a nerve trunk that supplies a joint also supplies the muscles of the joint and the skin over the attachment of the muscles. Therefore the stratum fibrosum is the source of extensive sensory data that affects the joints, muscles, and skin in the area.

The inner layer of the joint capsule, or stratum synovium, is highly vascularized but poorly innervated; it is insensitive to pain but undergoes vasodilation in response to heat and vasoconstriction in response to cold. The stratum synovium produces matrix collagen synovial fluid and serves as an entry point for nutrients and an exit point for waste materials. **Synovial fluid** is a thick, colorless fluid that resembles uncooked egg white. Synovial fluid lubricates the joint and provides nutrition to the tissues within the synovial cavity.

Section Summary

- Define articulation.
  - An articulation (i.e., joint) connects a minimum of two bones. Articulation structure is based on function. Some provide more stability with less mobility. Others provide more mobility with less stability.
- Describe collagen and elastin.
  - Collagen and elastin are the fibrous components of the extracellular matrix of connective tissue. Collagen is strong and provides stability. Elastin is elastic and provides mobility.
- Define joint capsule, ligament, tendon, and bursae.
  - A joint capsule is attached to bones, sealing the joint space. It consists of two layers; an outer layer of dense connective tissue and an inner layer called the *synovial membrane* (which produces synovial fluid to lubricate joints). A ligament is a collagen-dense connective tissue that connects the bones of joints (ligaments connect bone to bone). A tendon is a collagen-dense connective tissue that connects muscles to bones to move joints (tendons connect muscle to bone). A bursa is a flat sac filled with synovial fluid located where moving structures commonly rub against each other.
- Describe three types of cartilage.
  - *White fibrocartilage* is composed primarily of collagen fibers. *Yellow elastic cartilage* has a higher ratio of elastin to collagen fibers than does white fibrocartilage. *Hyaline cartilage* is predominantly water based; it lines the ends of bones in freely movable joints (diarthroses). Osteoarthritis results when this cartilage wears down.
- List joint categories.
  - *Synarthrosis (fibrous joints):* Nonsynovial, fibrous, limited movement. Types: suture, gomphosis, syndesmosis. *Amphiarthrosis (cartilaginous joints):* Nonsynovial, cartilaginous, slightly movable. Types: symphysis, synchondroses. *Diarthrosis (synovial joints):* Synovial, freely movable. Features: A joint capsule with an inner synovial membrane that secretes synovial fluid to lubricate joint surfaces covered in hyaline cartilage.

Practical Application

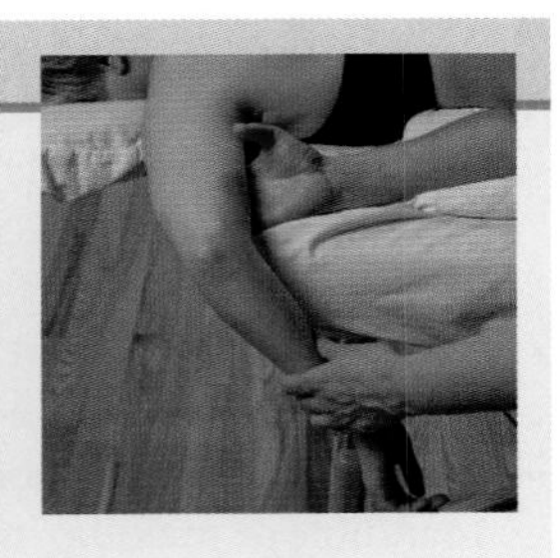

The joint design of our body not only helps provide stability for the joint but also permits motion. Small sacs called *bursae* are filled with synovial fluid and are located near some joints. As discussed earlier, bursae lie in areas subject to stress and help ease movement over and around the joints. In addition, synovial joints often have accessory structures, such as fibrocartilaginous disks and plates or menisci. Menisci, disks, and the synovial fluid help prevent excessive compression of opposing joint surfaces.

The same structures that hold joints together maintain joint space or hold joints apart. When these structures weaken and become worn, the joint cavity is not maintained as effectively, and the ends of bones begin to contact each other and rub together. Friction develops, and the production of synovial fluid increases in an attempt to reduce friction and maintain joint space. Deterioration commonly results in what is called "osteoarthritis," but is more accurately defined as *degenerative joint disease*. Massage application can be used to improve movement and reduce pain in diseased joints.

FOCUS ON PROFESSIONALISM

As a future massage therapist, you probably will work with healthcare providers who are experts in joint function and dysfunction. As a massage therapy professional, you need to be able to communicate accurately, understand what is being said to you or what is recorded in documentation, and understand the limits of massage training so that you can refer to experts when needed. Physicians in general, but especially orthopedists, physical therapists, and chiropractors, as well as athletic trainers, are joint function experts with whom you will need to interact. Massage therapy helps maintain joint health, manage joint pain, and support functional movement. However, joint function and dysfunction are complex, and massage therapy professionals must understand the limits of their education while also respecting the expertise of other highly trained and experienced individuals.

JOINT MOTION

SECTION OBJECTIVES

Chapter objective covered in this section:

4. Demonstrate the principles of joint motion.

After completing this chapter, the learner will be able to:

- Define arthrokinematics.
- Describe joint play.
- Define osteokinematics.
- Explain three categories of osteokinematic movement.
- Define end feel.
- Describe joint movements in the three planes of body movement.
- List joint movements specific to the forearm, wrist, ankle, spine, scapula, and pelvis.
- List the categories and subdivisions of synovial joints.
- Define kinematic chains.

Categories of Joint Movement

Joints are designed to permit body movement. The specifics of the design, including the size and shapes of the bones and the connective structure, influence the two types of movement of joints.

- *Arthrokinematic movement:* Small, involuntary movements that occur inside the joint capsule at the joint surfaces.
- *Osteokinematic movement:* This term describes the actual direction the bones move and includes extension, flexion, adduction, abduction, and internal and external rotation.

Arthrokinematics

The term arthrokinematics refers to movements of the articulating surfaces of the bones at joint surfaces. Most often, one of the joint surfaces is more stable than the other and serves as a base for the motion, whereas the other surface moves on this relatively fixed base.

The terms *roll, slide*, and *spin* describe the types of motion the moving part performs (Fig. 8.11):

- A *roll* refers to the rolling of one joint surface on another, similar to a bowling ball rolling down an alley. In the knee, the femoral condyles roll on the fixed tibial surface.
- *Sliding* refers to the gliding of one component over another, as when you slide on ice. When the scapula elevates and depresses, it slides on the underlying rib cage.
- *Spin* refers to a rotation of the movable component, as when a top spins. The head of the radius spins on the capitulum of the humerus during supination and pronation of the forearm.

Combinations of rolling, sliding, and spinning occur during the process of joint motion. A large amount of motion can occur in a confined space by combining motions. When a moving component in a joint alternately rolls in one direction while sliding in the opposite direction, the ROM available to the joint increases, and the opposing joint surfaces remain in contact with each other. Another method of increasing the range of available motion is by permitting both components to move at the same time. The humerus and the scapula move together during flexion and extension and abduction and adduction at the glenohumeral joint.

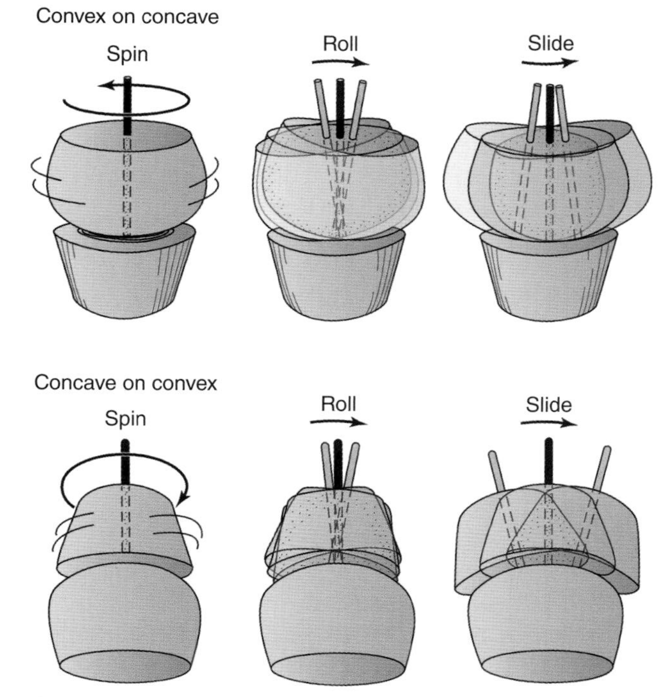

FIG. 8.11 Arthrokinematic movements. (From Malone TR, McPoil T, Nitz AJ. *Orthopedic and Sports Physical Therapy*. 3rd ed. Mosby; 1997.)

Joint Play

The involuntary movements that occur between articular surfaces, which have nothing to do with the ROM of a joint produced by muscles, are an essential component of joint motion and must occur for the joint to function normally. Called joint play, these small movements are essential for proper joint function.

The rolling and sliding movements of the articular surfaces are not usually visible or under voluntary control. An externally applied force, such as that applied by a therapist or physician, can move from one articular surface to another, and the amount of joint play can be assessed.

A door hinge is an excellent example. If you examine a door hinge, you will find that there are two plates, one attached to the door frame and one attached to the door. Between the two plates is a cylinder, and inside the cylinder is a pin. The pin fits inside the cylinder with just enough space around it so that the pin is free to rotate in the cylinder, allowing the door to swing. The distance the door swings is comparable to the ROM of a joint, whereas the amount of space in the cylinder that allows the pin to roll is comparable to joint play.

In an optimal situation, a joint has a sufficient amount of play to allow normal motion. For the human body, the amount of joint play is almost always approximately one-eighth inch, no matter which synovial joint is being examined or the amount of ROM of that joint. If the supporting joint structures are lax, the joint may have too much play and become unstable. If the joint structures are tight or if inflammation or degeneration is present, the joint has too little movement between the articular surfaces, the amount of joint play is reduced, and ROM may be restricted.

Osteokinematics

Osteokinematics refers to the movement of the bones by the action of the muscles rather than the movement of the articular surfaces. The amount of movement available through which a joint can be moved is called the *range of motion* of the joint. ROM is a measurement that determines the amount of movement allowed at a joint. Not everyone has the same ROM. Aging, disease, obesity, trauma, and injury all may affect a person's ROM. ROM is measured by active or passive movement of the joint. The anatomical position is considered the 0-degree point for measurement purposes.

Three categories of osteokinematic movement are anatomical, physiological, and pathological. **Anatomical range of motion** osteokinematic movement refers to the amount of motion available to a joint within its structural limits. Several factors determine the extent of the anatomical range, including the shape of the joint surfaces, the joint capsule, ligaments, muscle bulk, and surrounding musculotendinous and bony structures. Some joints have no bony joint limitations to motion, and the movement is limited only by soft tissue structures. For example, the knee joint has no bony limitations to motion. Flexion is limited by soft tissues, often muscles, whereas extension stops with ligament stretch. Other joints have definite bony restrictions to motion in addition to soft tissue limitations. The elbow joint is limited in extension (close-packed position) by bony contact of the ulna with the olecranon fossa of the humerus.

The anatomical motion may exceed the limits of available movement to a point where joint injury can occur. Therefore many joints have an established **physiological range of motion** set by the nervous system from information provided by joint sensory receptors. Physiological ROM is defined as "active ROM" (i.e., what the client can do). Usually, this physiological ROM is less than the anatomical ROM, preventing a joint from being positioned where injury could occur.

Pathological range of motion occurs when motion at a joint fails to reach the normal physiological range or exceeds normal anatomical limits of motion. The limits may be structural or functional. The two main pathological conditions are hypomobility and hypermobility.

Hypomobility

When the ROM is less than what normally would be permitted by the structure, the joint is hypomobile. **Hypomobility** may be caused by bony or cartilaginous blocks to motion or by the inability of the capsule, ligaments, or surrounding tissues to elongate sufficiently to allow a normal ROM. Contracture, which describes the shortening of soft tissue structures around a joint, is one cause of hypomobility.

Increased sensitivity and reactivity of joint receptors can cause the nervous system to increase muscle tension patterns, which in turn would limit ROM because muscles would not return to their normal resting length. The result would be hypomobility of joint movement even though nothing is dysfunctional in the joint itself. If this limited range is maintained, the joint capsule often alters tissue structure and becomes dysfunctional itself. These conditions are much more difficult to manage because of the complexities of dysfunctional patterns and compensation throughout the body.

Hypermobility

Hypermobility may be caused by a failure to limit motion by the bony or soft tissues, resulting in instability. Weak or flaccid muscles can contribute to hypermobility because they are less able to provide a stabilizing force to the joints. The joint may be subject to more trauma or damage because of excessive ROM, instability of the surrounding structures, or inability to withstand stresses. People with joint hypermobility syndrome have loose joints because they have weak ligaments. Flexible joints along with pain, stiffness, and other symptoms may be hypermobility spectrum disorders (HSDs). There are multiple causes. People with hypermobility issues may feel stiff and assessed as hypomobile because the connective tissues and muscles shorten to provide stability.

Practical Application

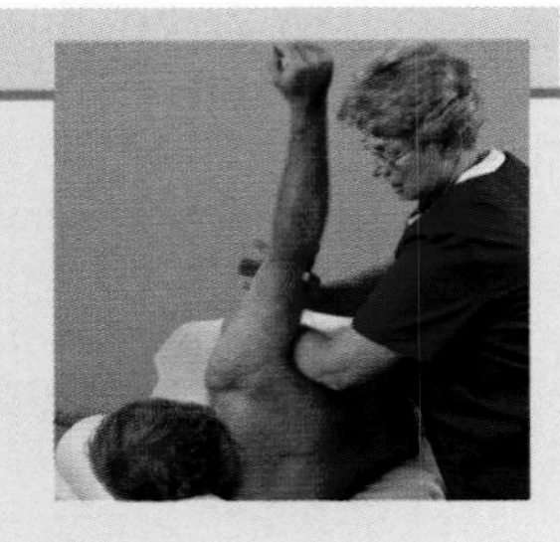

Hypermobility and hypomobility of a joint may have undesirable effects, not only at the affected joint, but also at adjacent joint structures, because the body develops compensation patterns to deal with the dysfunction.

Therapeutic massage methods can be used to increase or decrease the range of motion (ROM) for pathological joints to help return them to normal. By providing sensory stimulation to the joint nerve receptors, the abnormal tension patterns of surrounding muscles can be disrupted—restoring homeostasis and restoring ROM. Methods that address muscle tone and tolerance to stretch sensation can reverse some forms of hypomobility. Methods that support the strengthening of surrounding muscles can provide alternative stabilizing forces when the joint is lax. The practitioner can manage the splinting action of the muscle with therapeutic massage so that spasms do not cause pain and pull the joint capsule together.

Finding the right combination of therapeutic care is not a precise protocol, but more often an experimental decision-making process. Remember that any disruption to a part of the joint structure affects the entire joint function. When one joint is affected, the whole body must use compensation patterns to adjust. Over time, other joint movement patterns can become involved in dysfunction.

End Feel

The ability to palpate normal end feel and to distinguish changes from normal end feel is important in protecting joints during ROM assessment and massage application. The three major types of end feel are soft, hard or bony, and capsular.

Soft end feel of a joint is the normal sensation for most physiological limits of ROM. The joint moves in a normal arc and, when the range limit is reached, a small, pliable give remains if slightly more pressure is given. The space identified is the range between the physiological and anatomical barriers.

Bony or hard end feel is characterized by a hard and abrupt limit to joint movement. This occurs when bone contacts bone at the end of ROM. An example would be normal elbow extension. Usually, a hard end feel indicates a pathological condition.

Capsular end feel is characterized by a hard, leatherlike limitation of motion that has a slight give and occurs in full normal joint motion of the shoulder; otherwise, this type of end feel indicates dysfunction and is related to capsular restriction.

Two additional characteristics can quantify the limitation of joint motion: *springy block* and *approximation*.

Springy block is a rebound, or spring-back, movement at the end of ROM. This sensation occurs with internal derangement of a joint, such as when the cartilage is torn or connective tissue structures are binding.

Approximation is an asymptomatic limited ROM resulting from soft tissue approximation and occurs when the soft tissue of body segments prevents further motion, such as at normal terminal elbow flexion when the arm and forearm meet and the muscles touch.

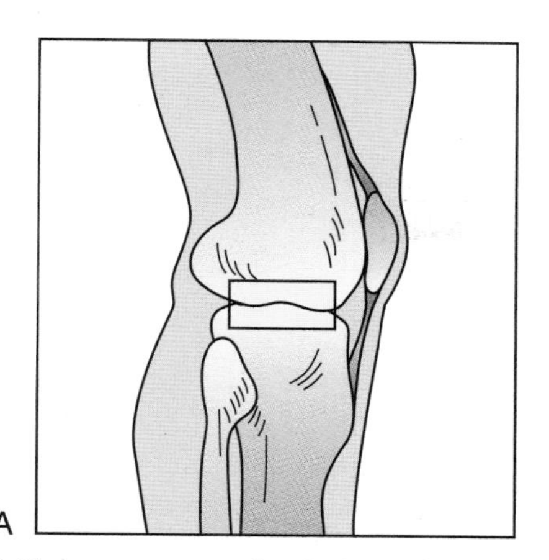

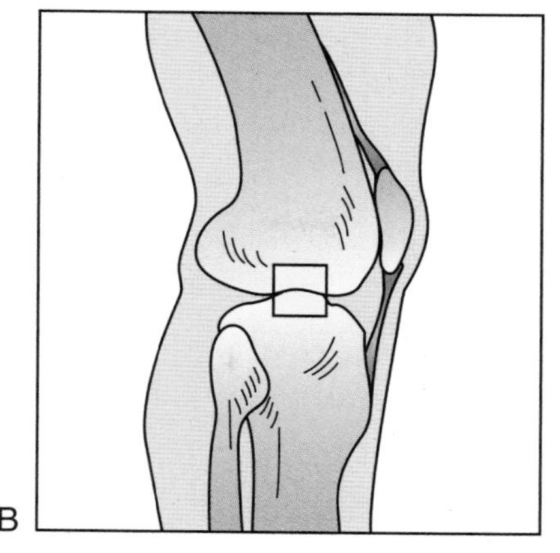

FIG. 8.12 The congruence of articular surfaces: (A) close-packed position and (B) loose-packed position.

Joint Positions and Stability

In most of our synovial joints, the ends of the articulating surfaces of the bones are opposite in shape to each other, usually convex and concave. All synovial joints have only one position in which the surfaces fit together and maximal contact between the opposing surfaces occurs. This is called the **close-packed position**, or locked position, and it allows no movement. The close-packed position is usually at the end of ROM, where the joint surfaces are compressed and the joint exhibits its greatest stability. The position of extension is the close-packed position for the elbow, knee, and interphalangeal joints. When not in this position, the joint is said to be in the **loose-packed position** also called open packed, or unlocked, where the amount of contact is reduced and movements of spin, roll, and glide may occur (Fig. 8.12). Joints tend to assume this position when inflammation occurs, to accommodate the increased volume of synovial fluid.

Movement into and out of the close-packed position is likely to have a beneficial effect on joint nutrition because the movement squeezes out the synovial fluid during each compression against the cartilage, and the fluid is reabsorbed when the compression is removed (Tables 8.1 and 8.2).

Table 8.1 Loose/Open-Packed Positions of Joints

Joint(s)	Position
Spine	Midway between flexion and extension
Temporomandibular	Mouth slightly open
Glenohumeral	55 Degrees abduction, 30 degrees horizontal adduction
Acromioclavicular	Arm resting by side in normal physiologic position
Sternoclavicular	Arm resting by side in normal physiologic position
Elbow	70 degrees flexion, 10 degrees supination
Radiohumeral	Full extension and full supination
Proximal radioulnar	70 degrees flexion, 35 degrees supination
Distal radioulnar	10 degrees supination
Wrist	Neutral with slight ulnar deviation
Carpometacarpal	Midway between abduction/adduction and flexion/extension
Thumb	Slight flexion
Interphalangeal	Slight flexion
Hip	30 degrees flexion, 30 degrees abduction, and slight lateral rotation
Knee	25 degrees flexion
Ankle	10 degrees plantar flexion, midway between maximum inversion or eversion
Subtalar	Midway between extremes of the range of movement
Midtarsal	Midway between extremes of the range of movement
Tarsometatarsal	Midway between extremes of the range of movement
Metatarsophalangeal	Neutral
Interphalangeal	Slight flexion

From Magee DJ. *Orthopedic Physical Assessment*. 5th ed. Saunders/Elsevier; 2008.

Movements of Joints

Cardinal Planes

Joint movement is named for the plane in which the movement occurs. Defining joint and segment motions and recording the location in space of specific points on the body both require a reference point (Fig. 8.13). In kinesiology, the three-dimensional, rectangular coordinate system is used to describe anatomical relationships of the body. Three imaginary planes are arranged perpendicular to each other through the body. These planes are called *the cardinal planes* of the body.

- The *frontal (coronal) plane* divides the body into front and back parts. Motions that occur in this plane are defined as right and left lateral flexion or as *abduction* and *adduction*. Right and left lateral flexions are side bending at the head, neck, or trunk. Abduction is a position or motion of the segment away from the midline, regardless of which segment moves. Abduction of the hip occurs when the thigh segment moves away from the midline or the pelvic segment approaches the thigh, as in tilting to the side while standing on one leg. Adduction is a position or motion toward the midline.
- The *sagittal plane* divides the body into right and left sides. Joint motions occurring in the sagittal plane are defined

Table 8.2 Close-Packed Positions of Joints

Joint(s)	Position
Spine	Extension
Temporomandibular	Clenched teeth
Glenohumeral	Abduction and lateral rotation
Acromioclavicular	Arm abducted to 30 degrees
Sternoclavicular	Maximum shoulder elevation
Elbow	Extension
Radiohumeral	Elbow flexed 90 degrees, forearm supinated 5 degrees
Proximal radioulnar	5 degrees supination
Distal radioulnar	5 degrees supination
Wrist	Extension with ulnar deviation
Carpometacarpal	Full flexion
Thumb	Full opposition
Interphalangeal	Full extension
Hip	Full extension and medial rotation[a]
Knee	Full extension and lateral rotation of the tibia
Ankle	Maximum dorsiflexion
Subtalar	Supination
Midtarsal	Supination
Tarsometatarsal	Supination
MTP	Full extension
Interphalangeal	Full extension

MTP, Metatarsophalangeal.
[a]Some authors include abduction.
From Magee DJ. *Orthopedic Physical Assessment.* 5th ed. Saunders/Elsevier; 2008.

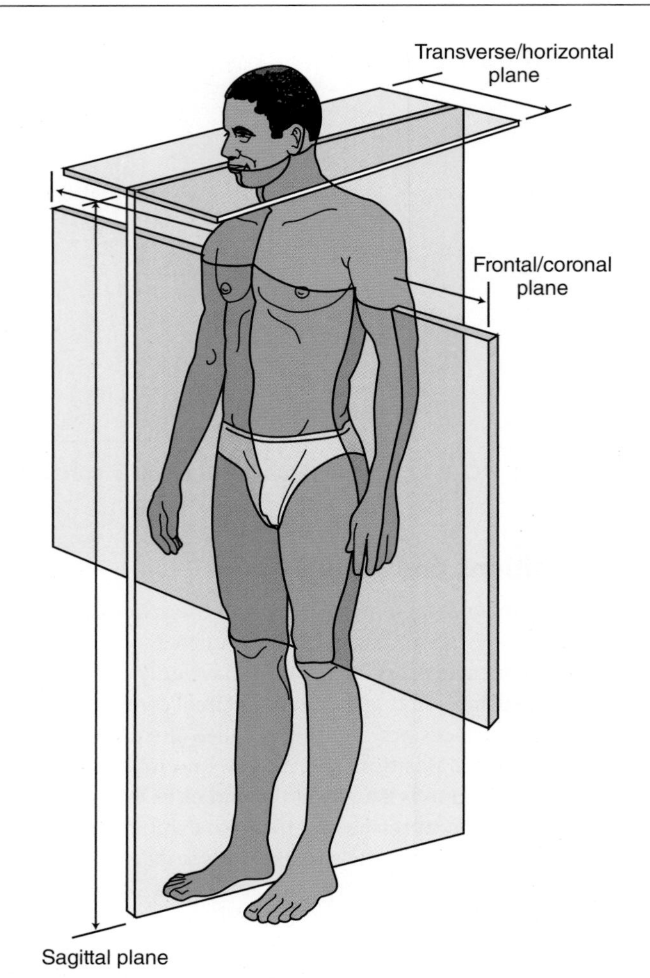

FIG. 8.13 The three imaginary planes of the body are called cardinal planes. (From Fritz S. *Mosby's Fundamentals of Therapeutic Massage*. 5th ed. Mosby/Elsevier; 2013.)

as *flexion* and *extension*. Flexion indicates that two segments approach each other; for example, flexion of the elbow may be accomplished by flexion of the forearm on the arm or by flexion of the arm on the forearm, as in a pull-up. Extension occurs when two segments move away from each other.

- The *horizontal/transverse plane* divides the body into upper and lower parts and is like a view from above. Rotations occur in this plane. Medial rotation, inward or internal rotation, is transverse rotation oriented to the anterior surface of the body. Medial rotation of the hip brings points marked on the anterior surface of the pelvis and femur closer together regardless of which of the segments moves. *Pronation* is the term for medial rotation of the forearm. Lateral rotation, outward or external rotation, is in the opposite direction and is oriented to the posterior surface of the body. *Supination* is a term used for the forearm and is the reference point for the anatomical position.

Sagittal, frontal, and transverse planes may be laid through any point of the body. For example, laying three planes through the center of a joint, such as the hip joint, may be convenient for determining body points in relation to such a joint. In the hand, the sagittal plane is centered through the third segment; in the foot, the sagittal plane is centered through the second segment.

Motion or position away from the reference segment is called *abduction*, and motion toward the segment is called *adduction*. At the wrist, the motion of abduction frequently is referred to as *radial deviation* (toward the radius), and adduction is called *ulnar deviation*. In the anatomical position, the foot is at a right angle to the dorsal aspect of the leg in the sagittal plane. Movement of the foot toward the tibia is called *dorsiflexion*, and movement of the sole away from the tibia is called *plantar flexion*.

The thumb is also a special case because it normally rotates 90 degrees from the plane of the hand. Thus, motions of flexion and extension occur in the frontal plane, and abduction and adduction occur in the sagittal plane.

Joint design permits many different types of movement. Some joints permit only flexion and extension. Others permit a wide range of movements, depending largely on the joint structure. Some movement terms may be used to describe motion at several joints throughout the body, whereas other terms are specific to a joint or group of joints. Motions or positions of flexion, abduction, and medial and lateral rotation are recorded as they move toward 180 degrees (Box 8.3; Figs. 8.14 and 8.15; and Activity 8.4). Most functions of daily living are multiplanar requiring movement in more than one plane at a time.

Box 8.3 Terms Describing Joint Movements

The following terms describe joint movements in general:

- **Flexion:** Bending movement that results in a decrease of the angle in a joint by bringing bones together. An example is the elbow joint when the hand is drawn to the shoulder.
- **Extension:** Straightening movement that results in an increase of the angle in a joint by moving bones apart. An example occurs when the hand is on the shoulder and moves away from the shoulder.
- **Abduction:** Lateral movement away from the midline of the trunk. An example is moving the arms or thighs out to the side.
- **Adduction:** Movement medially toward the midline of the trunk. An example is moving the arms to the side of the body or the thighs back to the anatomic position.
- **Diagonal abduction:** Movement by a limb through a diagonal plane directly across and away from the midline of the body. An example is moving the right arm from in front of the left hip to in front of the right shoulder.
- **Diagonal adduction:** Movement by a limb through a diagonal plane toward and across the midline of the body. An example is the return of the right arm from a flexed position to in front of the left hip.
- **Horizontal abduction:** Movement of the humerus in the horizontal plane away from the midline of the body. The movement also is known as horizontal extension or transverse abduction.
- **Horizontal adduction:** Movement of the humerus in the horizontal plane toward the midline of the body. The movement also is known as horizontal flexion or transverse adduction.
- **Circumduction:** Circular movement of a limb, combining the movements of flexion, extension, abduction, and adduction, to create a cone shape. An example is the shoulder joint moving circularly around a fixed point, as in doing arm circles.
- **Rotation:** Twisting or turning of a bone on its own axis. An example is turning the head from side to side to indicate "no."
- **Medial rotation:** Rotary movement around the longitudinal axis of a bone toward the midline of the body. The movement also is known as *inward rotation* or *internal rotation*. An example is turning the palms of the hands from the anatomic position to facing backward.
- **Lateral rotation:** Rotary movement around the longitudinal axis of a bone away from the midline of the body. The movement also is known as *outward rotation* or *external rotation*. An example is returning the palms from facing backward to the anatomic position so that they face forward.

The following terms describe movements specific to one of the following body parts: forearm, wrist, thumb, ankle, and foot:

- **Pronation:** Medial rotation of the radius where it lies diagonally across the ulna, resulting in the palm-down position of the forearm.
- **Supination:** Lateral rotation of the radius where it lies parallel to the ulna, resulting in the palm-up position of the forearm.
- **Radial deviation or wrist abduction:** Abduction movement at the wrist joint of the thumb side of the hand toward the forearm.
- **Ulnar deviation or wrist adduction:** Adduction movement at the wrist joint of the little finger side of the hand toward the forearm.
- **Opposition of the thumb:** Diagonal movement of the thumb across the palmar surface of the hand to contact the fingers.
- **Eversion:** Turning off the sole outward or laterally. An example is moving the body weight to the inner edge of the foot.
- **Inversion:** Turning off the sole inward or medially. An example is moving our body weight to the outer edge of the foot.
- **Dorsiflexion (or dorsal flexion):** Movement of the ankle that results in the top of the foot moving toward the anterior tibia. An example of this is pointing the toes up.
- **Plantar flexion:** Movement of the ankle that results in the foot or toes moving away from the anterior fibula. An example of this is pointing the toes down.

The following terms describe movements of the shoulder girdle and shoulder joint:

- **Elevation:** Movement of the shoulder girdle to become closer to the ears. Such movement occurs in shrugging of the shoulders.
- **Depression:** Inferior movement of the shoulder girdle. An example is returning to the normal position from a shoulder shrug.
- **Protraction:** Forward movement of the shoulder girdle away from the spine, also known as *abduction*.
- **Retraction:** Backward movement of the shoulder girdle toward the spine, also known as *adduction*.
- **Downward rotation:** Rotary movement of the scapula such that the glenoid fossa orients downward (the inferior angle of the scapula moves medially). The movement occurs when the acromion process moves down.
- **Upward rotation:** Rotary movement of the scapula such that the glenoid fossa orients upward (the inferior angle of the scapula moves laterally). The movement occurs when the acromion process moves up.

The following terms describe movements of the spinal and pelvic girdle joints:

- **Lateral flexion (side bending):** Movement of the head, neck, or trunk laterally to the side.
- **Nutation (posterior pelvic tilt):** Forward motion of the base of the sacrum into the pelvis (tuck your tail) or the backward rotation of the ilium on the sacrum.
- **Counternutation (anterior pelvic tilt):** Backward motion of the base of the sacrum out of the pelvis (wag your tail) or forward rotation of the ilium on the sacrum.
- **Iliosacral motion:** This is ilium movement on the sacrum. Movements of the ilium include anterior/posterior rotation, superior/inferior movement, and medial/lateral flaring.
- **Sacroilial motion:** This is sacral movement on the ilium. Movements of the sacrum include flexion/extension and rotation.

Continued

Box 8.3 Terms Describing Joint Movements—cont'd

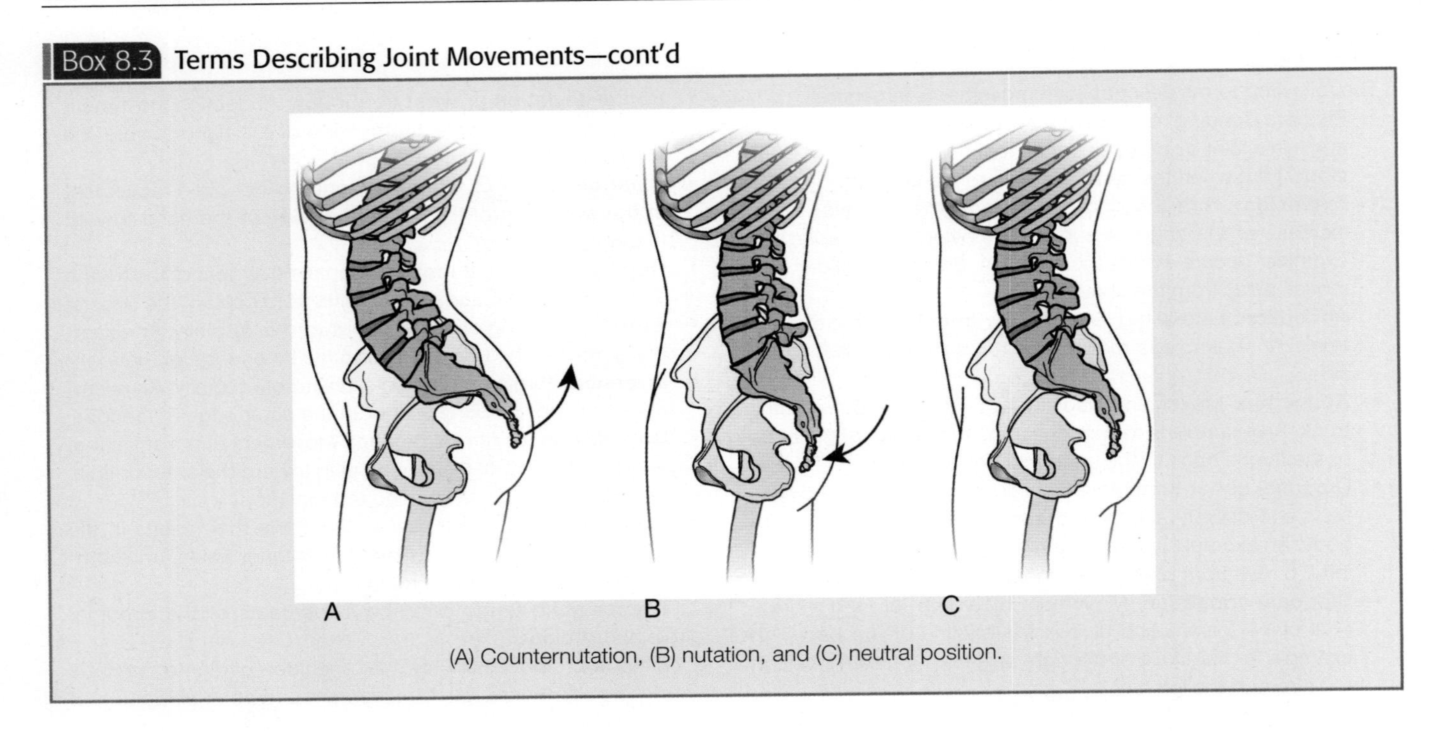

(A) Counternutation, (B) nutation, and (C) neutral position.

Classification of Synovial Joints by Movements

Traditionally, synovial joints have been divided into three main categories based on the number of axes of rotation around which motion occurs. An axis is a stationary point around which movement occurs. The three main categories are uniaxial, biaxial, and triaxial. A further subdivision of the joints is made according to the shape and configuration of the ends of the bony components.

A *uniaxial joint* is constructed so that motion of the bony components is allowed in only one of the planes around a single axis. The two types of joints in this category are hinge joints and pivot joints:

- A **hinge joint** allows flexion and extension in one direction, changing the angle of the bones at the joint, as in a door hinge. Examples are the elbow and interphalangeal joints.
- A **pivot joint** allows rotation around the length of the bone. A pivot (trochoid) joint is a type of joint constructed so that one component is shaped like a ring and the other component is shaped so that it can rotate within the ring. Examples are the joint between the first and second cervical vertebrae and the joint at the proximal ends of the radius and the ulna.

Biaxial joints allow movement in two planes around two axes. The two types of joints in this category are condyloid joints and saddle joints:

- A **condyloid (condylar) joint**, also called an *ellipsoid joint*, allows movement in two directions, but one motion dominates. The joint surfaces in a condyloid joint are shaped so that one bony surface is concave and the other is convex. The movements allowed are flexion, extension, abduction, and adduction. Examples are the wrist joint, metacarpophalangeal (MCP) joints, metatarsophalangeal (MTP) joints, and the atlantooccipital joint.
- In a **saddle joint**, each joint surface is convex in one plane and concave in the other, and these surfaces fit together similarly to a rider on a saddle. Movements allowed are flexion, extension, abduction, adduction, and a small degree of axial rotation. Examples are the joint between the wrist and the metacarpal bone of the thumb (first carpometacarpal joint) and the sternoclavicular joint.

Multiaxial/Triaxial joints are joints in which the bony components are free to move in three planes around three axes. Motion at these joints may also occur in oblique planes. The two types of joints in this category are ball-and-socket joints and plane or gliding joints.

- A **ball-and-socket joint** allows movement in many directions around a central point. Ball-and-socket joints are formed when a ball-shaped convex surface is fitted into a concave socket. Movements allowed are flexion, extension, abduction, adduction, and rotation. This type of joint gives the greatest freedom of movement but also is the easiest to dislocate. Examples are the hip and shoulder joints.
- A **gliding joint**, also called a *synovial plane joint*, permits gliding between two or more bones. This joint allows only a gliding motion in various planes. Examples are the superior tibiofibular joint, acromioclavicular joint, costovertebral joints, and zygapophyseal joints between the vertebral arches (Fig. 8.16).

Kinematic/Kinetic Chains

The kinematic chain/kinetic chain is an engineering concept used to describe human movement. The terms kinematic chain and kinetic chain are technically different but used interchangeably. Kinematics is the analysis of the geometric aspects of motion without the forces causing it. It describes movement

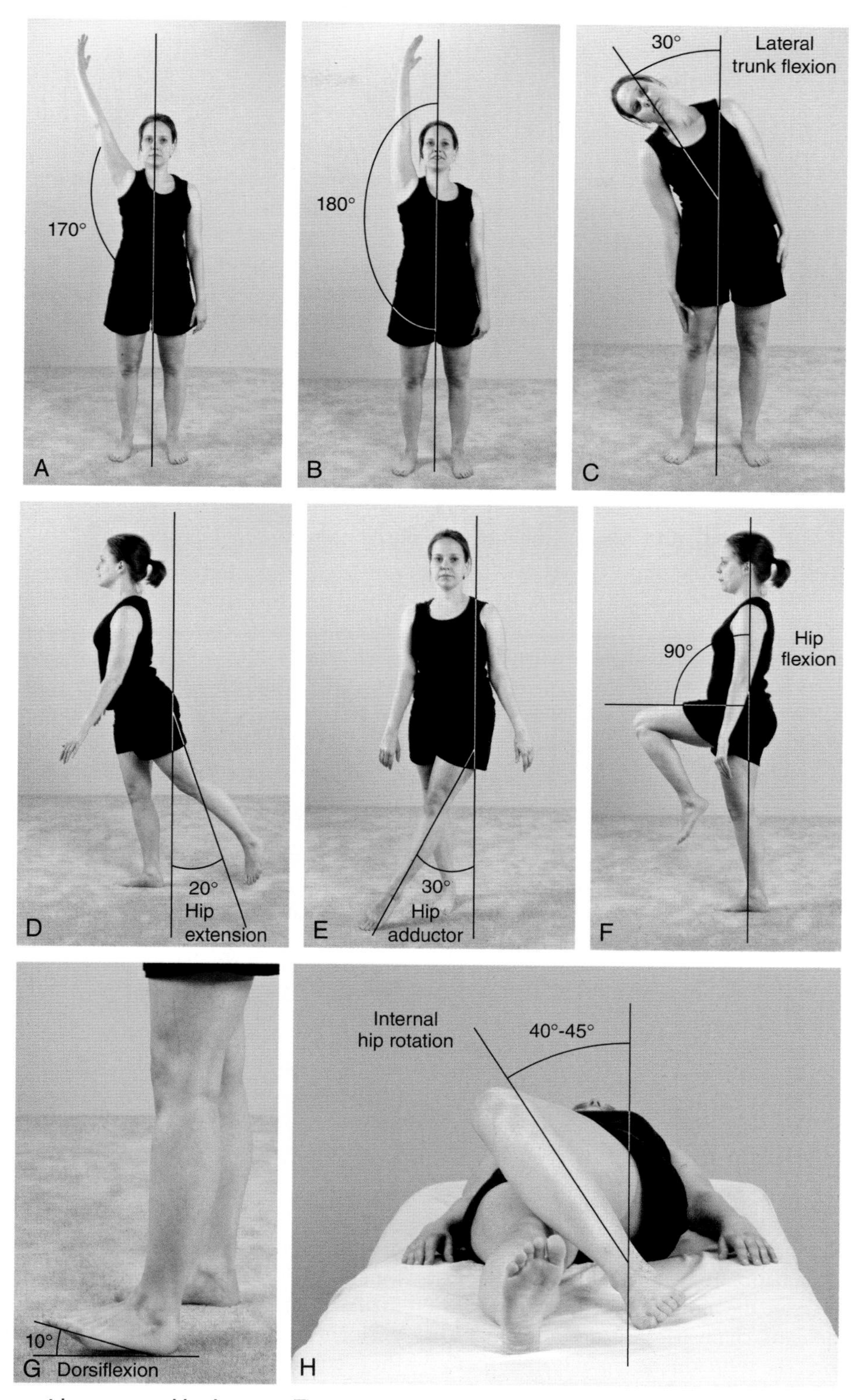

FIG. 8.14 Joint movement is measured in degrees. The system presented in this book uses 0 degrees as the reference point for the standard anatomic position. Motions or positions of flexion, extension, abduction, and medial and lateral rotation are recorded as they move toward 180 degrees. (A) 170 degrees; (B) 180 degrees; (C) 30 degrees, lateral trunk flexion; (D) 20 degrees, hip extension; (E) 30 degrees, hip adductor; (F) 90 degrees, hip flexion; (G) 10 degrees, dorsiflexion; (H) 40–45 degrees, internal hip rotation.

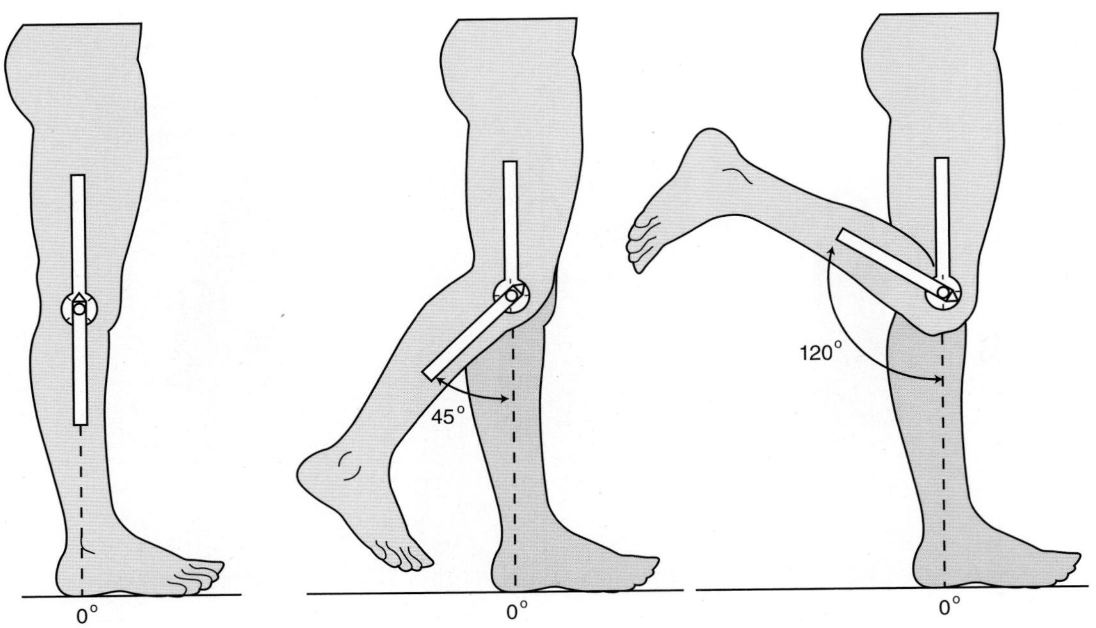

FIG. 8.15 Measurement of knee positions in the sagittal plane.

ACTIVITY 8.4

Find the definitions of the joint movements in Chapter 3 and compare them to the ones you just studied in this chapter. Then, using both definitions, design a joint movement sequence that moves all the synovial joints in your body. An example is provided to get you started.

Example

Flexion

Drop the chin to chest, make a fist, bend elbows so that hands touch the shoulders, bring a knee to the chest, and then repeat with another knee, bring the heel to the buttocks, and then repeat with another heel, curling toes toward the sole.

Your Turn

Abduction
Adduction
Extension
Horizontal abduction
Horizontal adduction
Circumduction
Rotation (right or left)
Rotation (medially or laterally)
Pronation
Supination
Elevation
Depression
Protraction
Retraction
Downward rotation
Upward rotation
Radial deviation
Ulnar deviation
Opposition of the thumb
Eversion
Inversion
Dorsiflexion
Plantar flexion
Lateral flexion (right or left; side bending)
Nutation
Counternutation

patterns and joint angles in relation to one another. Analyzing gait mechanics is a kinematic study. Kinetics is about the forces and torques that create the motion of a body with mass. Engineers use the kinematic chain because it is the technically correct description. The term kinetic chain is used more often when describing human movement but is interchangeable with kinematic chain. Regardless the terms describe how motions of multiple joints are coupled.

A *kinematic/kinetic chain* is a system of rigid bodies, or bones, connected by joints and describes the association between joints as they operate in relation to one another. The concept of kinematic/kinetic chains is useful for analyzing human motion and the effects of injury and disease on the joints of the body. Anatomically, the kinematic/kinetic chain describes the interrelated groups of body segments, connecting joints, and muscles working together to perform movements and the portion of the spine to which they connect. The upper chain consists of the fingers, wrists, forearms, elbows, upper arms, shoulders, shoulder blades, and spinal column. The lower chain includes the toes, feet, ankles, lower legs, knees, upper legs, hips, pelvis, and spine. In both chains, each joint is independently capable of a variety of movements but if the distal end of the chain is fixed then the structures function together. Two types are closed kinematic/kinetic chains and open kinematic/kinetic chains.

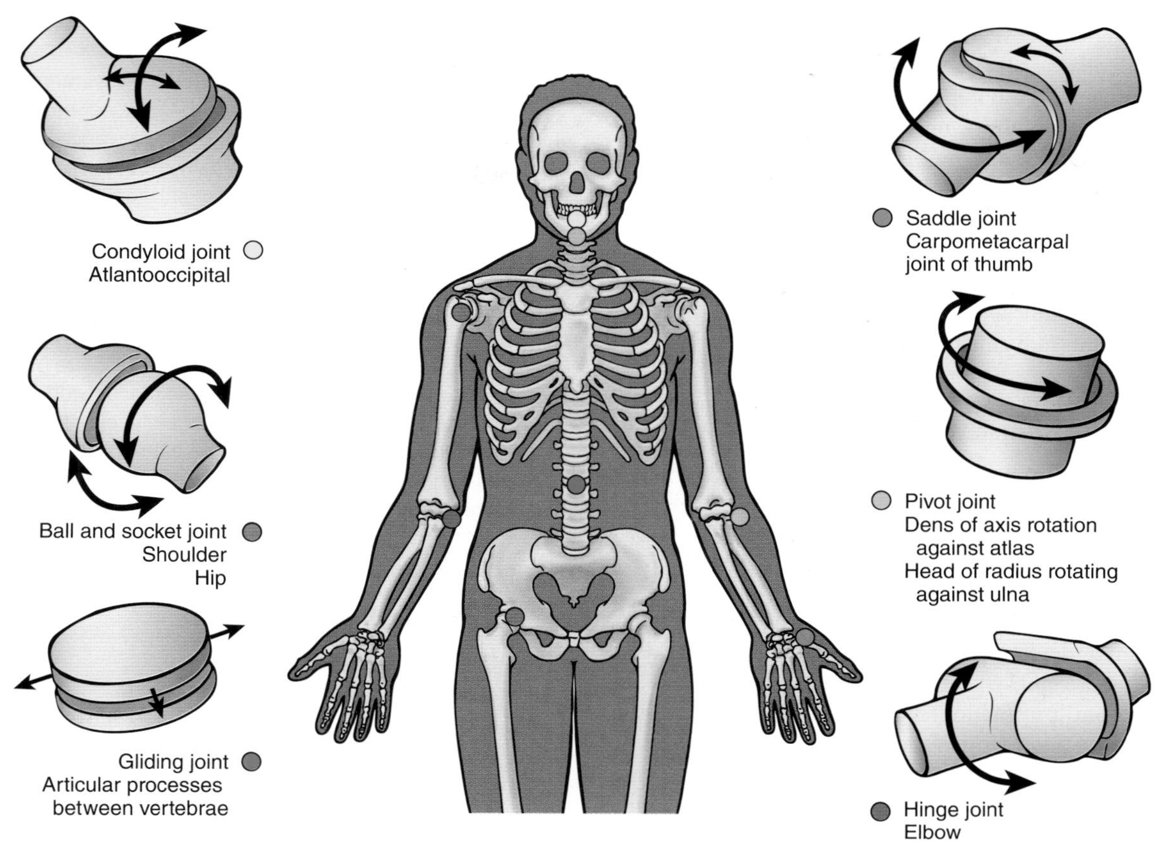

FIG. 8.16 Synovial joint types.

Closed Kinematic/Kinetic Chain

Some joints of the human body are linked in a series in which motion at one of the joints is accompanied by motion at an adjacent joint. This is called a closed kinematic/kinetic chain. For instance, when a person is standing erect and bends both knees, simultaneous motion must occur at the ankle and hip joints. The interaction between joints in the chain is predictable in terms of linked movement because the joints are interdependent. A change in the structure or function of one joint in the chain usually causes a change in the function of a joint immediately adjacent to the affected joint or at a distal joint. For example, if ROM at the knee was limited, the hip and ankle joints would have to compensate so that the foot could clear the floor to avoid stumbling when a person walks. A closed kinematic chain occurs when the foot is on the floor or the hand grasps an immovable object. If the hand applies a compressive force to a fixed object, a closed kinematic chain is created.

Open Kinematic/Kinetic Chain

When the ends of the limbs or parts of the body are free to move without causing motion at another joint, the system is referred to as an open kinematic chain.

The ends of our limbs often are not fixed but are free to move without necessarily causing motion at another joint. When a person lifts the lower limb from the ground, the knee is free to bend without causing or changing motion at the hip or ankle. The motion of waving the hand may occur at the wrist without causing motion of the elbow or shoulder. In an open kinematic chain, motion does not occur in a predictable fashion because joints may function independently (i.e., in unison). For example, you can wave your whole upper limb by moving your arm at the shoulder or by moving only at the wrist.

Closed and open kinematic/kinetic chains influence ergonomics, exercise, rehabilitation, prosthetic design, and interestingly, robot design.

Section Summary

- Define arthrokinematics.
    - Arthrokinematics: Movement based on the articulating surface/shape of bones.
- Describe joint play.
    - Joint play: Involuntary movement between articular surfaces. Articular surfaces need sufficient space to allow motion. Not associated with ROM. Example: A door hinge consisting of two plates with a cylinder and pin. The door swing is ROM. The space in the cylinder which allows for pin rotation is joint play.
- Define osteokinematics.
    - Osteokinematics: Movement based on the action of muscles.
- Explain three categories of osteokinematic movement.
    - Anatomical ROM: The structural limits of joint motion, determined by bone shape and fit (hard end feel).

Physiological ROM: The soft tissue limits of joint motion (provided by sensory receptors to prevent joint injury) (soft end feel). Pathological ROM: Too little physiologic ROM (hypomobility), or too much physiological/anatomical ROM (hypermobility) (usually hard/capsular end feel).

- Define end feel.
  - End feel is the assessed sensation of joints when taken to the end range, divided into three major types: soft, hard (i.e., bony), and capsular.
- Describe joint movements in the three planes of body movement.
  - Joint movements occur in the three cardinal planes of the body. Sagittal plane: flexion, extension. Frontal plane: adduction, abduction, right/left lateral flexion. Transverse/horizontal plane: medial/internal rotation, lateral/external rotation.
- List joint movements specific to the forearm, wrist, ankle, spine, scapula, and pelvis.
  - Forearm: pronation/supination. Wrist: radial deviation/ulnar deviation. Ankle: dorsiflexion/plantar flexion. Spine: right/left lateral flexion. Scapula: elevation, depression, protraction, retraction. Pelvis: elevation, depression, anterior/posterior tilt.
- List the categories and subdivisions of synovial joints.
  - Category: uniaxial (one plane). Subdivisions: hinge, pivot. Category: biaxial (two planes). Subdivisions: condyloid, saddle. Category: multiaxial/ triaxial (three planes). Subdivisions: ball-and-socket, gliding.
- Define kinematic/kinetic chains.
  - Kinematic/kinetic chains are systems of rigid bodies (bones) connected by joints. They describe how joints operate in relation to one another. Closed chains: movement at one joint moves an adjacent joint. Open chains: movement at one joint does not move an adjacent joint.

Practical Application

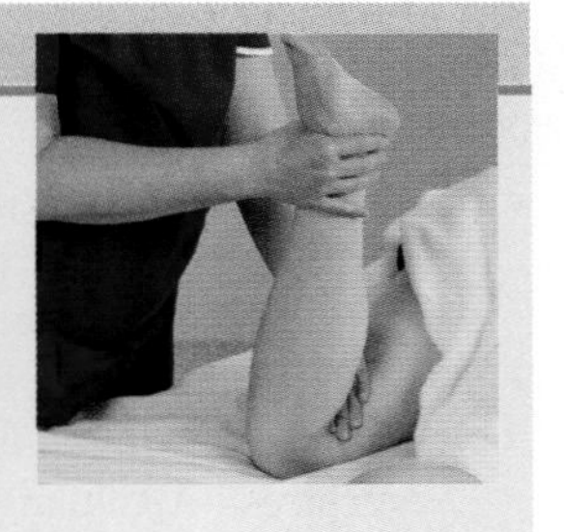

An understanding of joint movement is fundamental to any therapeutic massage system. Many systems, particularly movement modalities, are based on body movement patterns provided by joints. A comparison of these systems (e.g., yoga, tai chi, or Feldenkrais) reveals the intricate and interactive interplay of the joint moved alone or in a dynamic combination of movements.

All types of athletes depend on the proper functioning of their joints, as do dancers and others who purposefully move their bodies, including massage therapists. These people often seek out therapeutic massage to enhance their performance and maintain or restore optimal functioning. Especially when working with closed kinematic chains, the practitioner must address all joints in the pattern for proper function to be restored in any particular area.

MENTORING TIP

The joints are where movement occurs. Movement is caused by the pulling action of muscles when they contract and distribute the pulling forces into the fascia, tendons, and joint capsule. No one muscle specifically moves a particular joint. Muscle tissues are triggered to shorten when the motor nerves respond to messages sent from the sensory receptors of the nervous system. Muscle fibers are embedded in the fascial elements of the muscle tissues, and the mechanical force to move is generated when muscle cells are triggered to contract. Muscle cells are bundled together into muscles, which are bundled into muscle groups, which are bundled into deep fascial compartments. All these pieces work together in chain reactions of cause and effect. Muscle shortening creates tension on connective tissue elements, which pulls on bones to move joints. It is a series of events that includes posture, stability, balance, and more. Amazing.

IDENTIFICATION AND PALPATION OF SPECIFIC JOINTS

SECTION OBJECTIVES

Chapter objectives covered in this section:

5. Identify and palpate individual joints of the skull, shoulder, elbow, wrist, and hand.
6. Identify and palpate individual joints of the pelvis and hip, knee, ankle and foot, spine, and thorax.

After completing this section, the learner will be able to:

- Palpate and describe these jointed areas: joints of the: skull, shoulder, elbow, wrist and hand, pelvis and hip, knee, ankle and foot, spine and thorax.

As massage therapists, we touch and move the body during massage for both assessment and massage intervention. When we are touching the body to gather assessment information, we are palpating, which is an essential assessment skill. Joint movement is also an assessment skill that is necessary to learn. The information and activities in this section will help you develop palpation and joint movement assessment skills.

Joints of the Skull

The joints of the skull are the cranial sutures and the temporomandibular joint (TMJ).

Cranial Sutures

Recall from Chapter 7 that the four cranial sutures are:

- Coronal: Between the frontal and parietal bones
- Sagittal: Between the two parietal bones
- Squamous: Between the parietal and temporal bones
- Lambdoidal: Between the occipital and parietal bones

Palpation

Palpate the sutures of the skull as follows:

1. Place your fingertips on your eyebrows and slide them firmly up your forehead to the top of your skull to where you feel the first indentation; this is the coronal suture.
2. Pressing your finger firmly into the suture, follow the indentation down on either side to where the suture ends, about midway between the top of the ear and the eye.

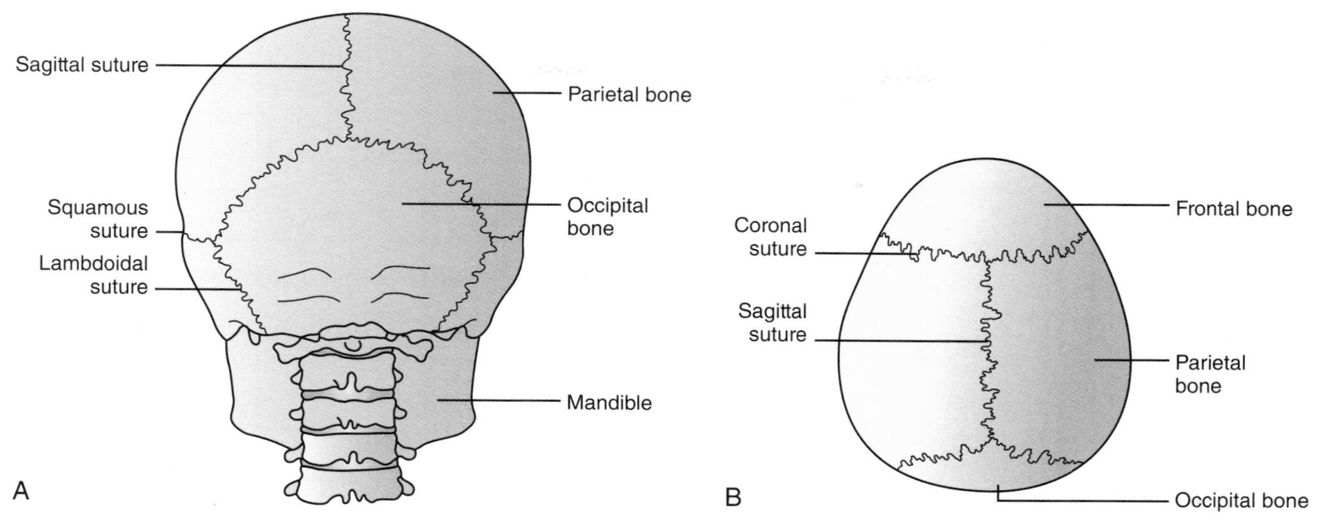

FIG. 8.17 Sutures of the skull. (A) Posterior skull. (B) Top view of skull.

3. Move posteriorly along the next indentation that arcs over your ear; this is the squamous suture.
4. Behind the ear, just above the mastoid process, palpate the indentation that moves in an arc superiorly and posteriorly; this is the lambdoidal suture.
5. At the midway point of the lambdoidal suture, find the indentation that travels superiorly and anteriorly along the middle of the skull to join with the coronal suture; this is the sagittal suture (Fig. 8.17).

Temporomandibular Joint

The TMJ consists of these structures:

- *Articulating bones:* Temporal bone and mandible
- *Joint type:* Synovial modified hinge joint
- *Ligaments:* Lateral temporomandibular ligament from the zygomatic arch to the mandible; sphenomandibular ligament from the sphenoid to the mandible (not pictured in Fig. 8.18); and the stylomandibular ligament from the styloid process to the mandible

The TMJ is one of the strongest joints in the body and the only biarticular joint. This means that the joint has two separate cavities. This construction requires a balanced action in the joint so that both jointed areas work freely. When this is not the case, the result is TMJ dysfunction.

The TMJ allows five movements—depression, elevation, protraction, retraction, and lateral deviation to the left and right.

Palpation

Palpate the joint just in front of each ear while opening and closing the jaw (see Fig. 8.18 and Activity 8.5).

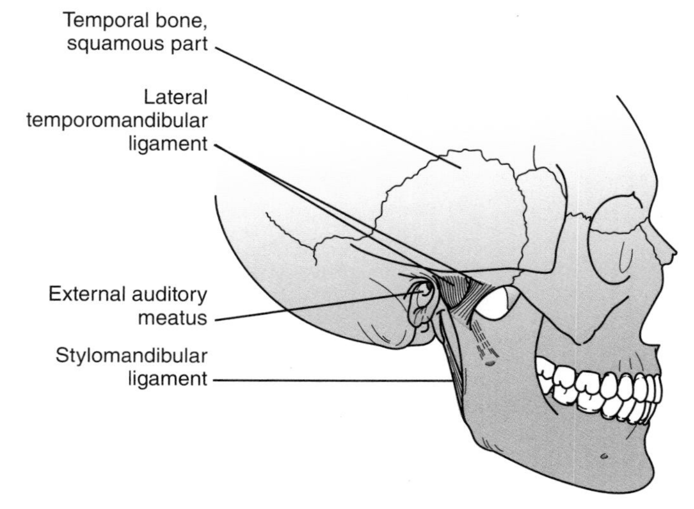

FIG. 8.18 Temporomandibular joint.

> **ACTIVITY 8.5**
>
> Move your temporomandibular joint (TMJ) through each of the five movement patterns.

Joints of the Shoulder

The shoulder joints include the glenohumeral, sternoclavicular, and acromioclavicular joints and the scapulocostal junction.

Glenohumeral Joint

The glenohumeral joint consists of these structures:

- *Articulating bones*: Humerus and scapula
- *Joint type*: Synovial ball and socket
- *Ligaments*: Glenohumeral: Inferior, middle, and superior, from the glenoid cavity of the scapula to the head of the humerus; coracohumeral ligament from the coracoid process to the greater and lesser tuberosity of humerus (not pictured in Fig. 8.19). The glenohumeral joint is the main joint of the shoulder and the most mobile joint in the body. The joint is shallow, which allows for its high degree of mobility but also accounts for its reduced stability. Because of this decrease in stability, it can be easily injured. Most of the support for this joint is provided by the muscles of the joint (especially the rotator cuff muscles, which are discussed in Chapter 9). The shoulder joint does get considerable stability from the glenoid

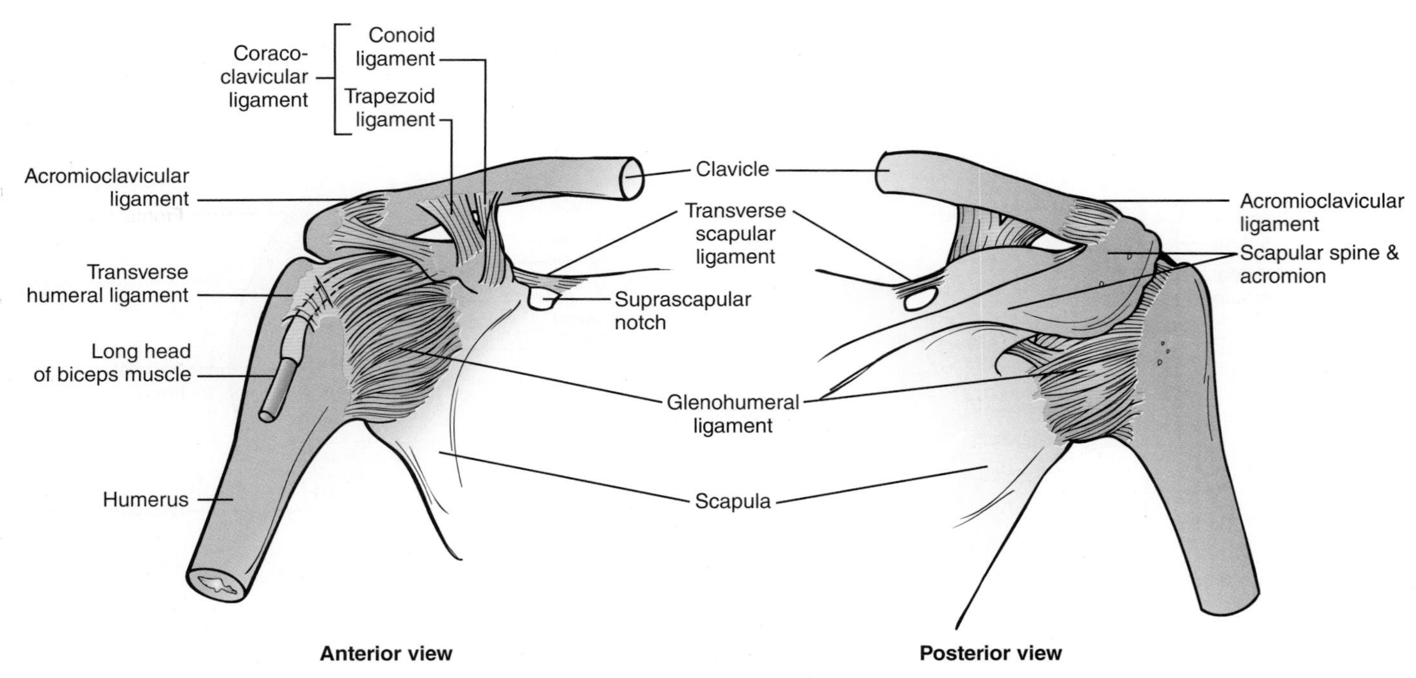

FIG. 8.19 Ligaments of the shoulder.

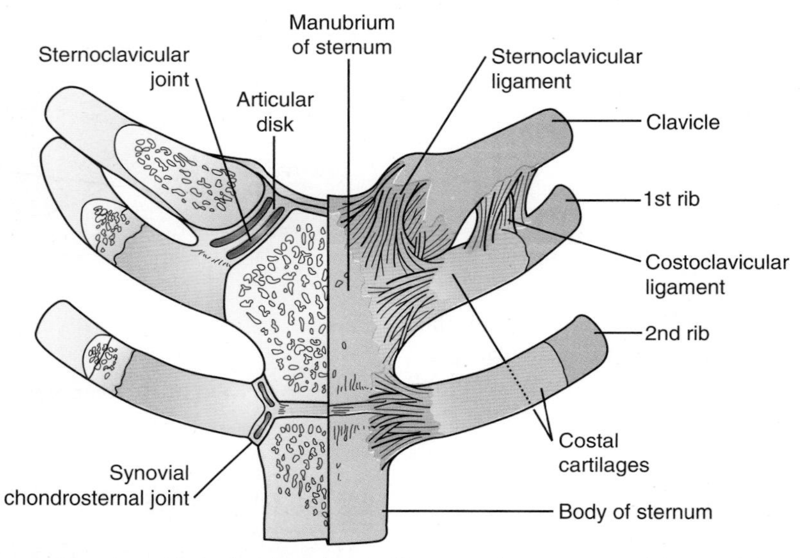

FIG. 8.20 Joints of the sternum. The sternoclavicular joint is located between the sternum and the medial end of the clavicle. The sternoclavicular joint contains an articular disk.

labrum, which acts as a lip to the shallow fossa, deepening it. Some further support is provided by the ligaments and a loose joint capsule, with little support from the bony structures themselves. The tendons of the rotator cuff muscles provide additional stability (Fig. 8.19).

The glenohumeral joint allows these movements—flexion, extension, abduction, adduction, medial (internal) rotation, and lateral (external) rotation.

Sternoclavicular Joint

The sternoclavicular joint consists of these structures:

- *Articulating bones:* Clavicle and manubrium of the sternum
- *Joint type:* Synovial saddle joint
- *Ligaments:* Anterior and posterior sternoclavicular ligament from clavicle to sternum; interclavicular ligament joining both clavicles; costoclavicular ligament from clavicle to first rib; and a fibrocartilaginous (articular) disk located within the joint

The movements of the sternoclavicular joint follow the movements of the scapula and clavicle because no muscle works directly on this joint. A decrease or loss of mobility in this joint directly affects shoulder movement. This joint is the only direct connection between the axial skeleton and the shoulder girdle and arm (Fig. 8.20).

The sternoclavicular joint allows these movements—elevation, depression, protraction, retraction, upward rotation, and downward rotation.

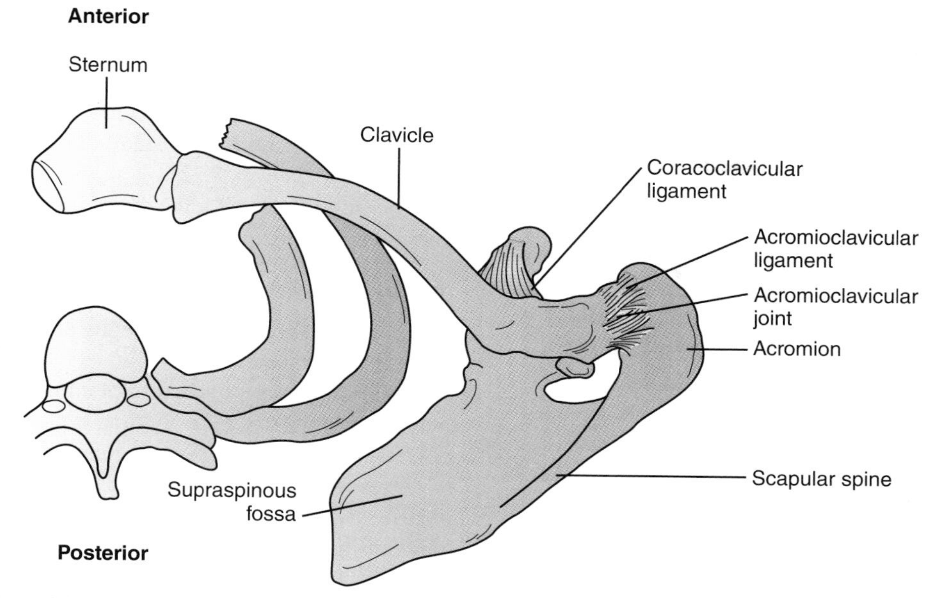

FIG. 8.21 Superior view of the acromial clavicular joint of the shoulder girdle. This view illustrates the attachments of the lateral end of the clavicle, especially to the acromion and coracoid process.

Box 8.4 Scapulocostal Junction

Although not a true structural joint because it does not involve bone-to-bone contact, the scapula moves across the rib cage (thorax), creating a functional joint. Much of the movement results from sternoclavicular action, with the rest of the action provided by movement in the acromioclavicular joint. If the scapula is limited in its movement, all shoulder movement is restricted, although one can compensate for restrictions in retraction most easily. The movements of the scapulocostal junction include elevation, depression, protraction, retraction, and upward and downward rotation.

Acromioclavicular Joint

The acromioclavicular joint consists of these structures:

- *Articulating bones:* Clavicle and scapula
- *Joint type:* Synovial gliding
- *Ligaments:* Acromioclavicular ligament from the acromion process to the clavicle and coracoclavicular ligament from the coracoid process to the clavicle

The acromioclavicular joint may contain a fibrocartilaginous disk. Note that some people do not have an acromioclavicular joint because the bones have fused.

Although a small joint, the acromioclavicular joint is important for shoulder movements (Fig. 8.21).

The acromioclavicular joint allows these movements—anterior and posterior gliding, upward and downward rotation, and elevation and depression. Movements that separate the joint are also possible (Box 8.4).

Palpation

Palpate the shoulder as follows:

1. The position of three major points—the tip of the acromion, the greater tubercle of the humerus, and the coracoid process—provide clues as to the exact position of the shoulder.
2. Beginning at the jugular notch of the manubrium, move slightly laterally to locate the sternoclavicular joint. To confirm the location of the joint, hold lightly while moving the same-side arm into flexion and extension. Compare this joint movement with the direction of the scapular movements.
3. Continue along the clavicle, following the convex curve of the medial two-thirds and the concave curve of the lateral third.
4. Reach back to the spine of the scapula and follow it laterally; at its end, move superiorly and anteriorly, where it becomes the acromion (the high point of the shoulder). This is a large flat area, with a slight concavity.
5. Find the anterior tip of the acromion and move slightly medially; the elevated ridge marks the start of the acromioclavicular joint.
6. Move back to the top of the acromion, then laterally and inferiorly to the outer edge of the greater tubercle of the humerus.
7. Moving anteriorly and medially, locate the lesser tubercle.
8. Continuing medially onto the soft tissues of the anterior chest, press in to locate the coracoid process of the scapula just below the concave portion of the lateral clavicle.
9. The glenohumeral joint, where the arm connects to the body, is easiest to palpate when the arm is in passive extension or actively moving through circumduction.
10. The fibrous capsule of the rotator cuff (muscles and tendons that surround the joint) often makes feeling the bony structures difficult.

ACTIVITY 8.6

Move your shoulder joints, individually and (if possible) together, through the ranges of motion.

11. Of the four muscles of the rotator cuff, three—the supraspinatus, infraspinatus, and teres minor—attach on the greater tubercle of the humerus, and their attachments are easiest to palpate.
12. The fourth, the subscapularis, inserts on the lesser tubercle and is not palpated easily (Activity 8.6).

Joints of the Elbow

The joints of the elbow joint region are the ulnohumeral, radiohumeral, and proximal radioulnar joints.

Ulnohumeral and Radiohumeral Joints

The ulnohumeral and radiohumeral joints consist of these structures:

- *Articulating bones:* Humerus with the ulna and humerus with the radius
- *Joint type:* Synovial hinge (ulnohumeral)
- *Ligaments:* Medial (ulnar) collateral: Anterior, posterior, transverse fibers from the medial epicondyle of the humerus and olecranon process of the ulna to the coronoid process of the ulna; radial collateral from the lateral epicondyle of the humerus to the annular ligament; and annular ligament from the anterior portion of radial notch around to the posterior margin of radial notch

Because of its bony structure and the support of muscles and ligaments, the elbow is a stable joint. Most elbow action involves the ulnohumeral joint, even though the radius also interacts with the humerus. During flexion, the trochlear notch of the ulna slides on the humeral trochlea, whereas the head of the radius slides on the capitulum. In extension, the movements are reversed and stop when the olecranon process reaches its anatomical barrier at the olecranon fossa. The elbow is one of the few areas in the body where a hard end feel and anatomical barrier occurs. Hyperextension is possible in individuals who have a small olecranon process or a large olecranon fossa (Fig. 8.22).

The ulnohumeral and radiohumeral joints allow these movements—flexion and extension.

Radioulnar Joints

The three radioulnar joints are the proximal, middle, and distal radioulnar joints.

The proximal radioulnar joint consists of these structures:

- *Articulating bones*: Radius and ulna
- *Joint type*: Synovial pivot (proximal radioulnar joint)
- *Ligaments*: Annular ligament (see the previous joint)

The proximal radioulnar joint articulates at the proximal ends of the radius and ulna and is listed as part of the elbow complex because it has the same soft tissue support as the elbow joint and most of the actions occur in this area (see Fig. 8.22). The head of the radius moves clockwise and counterclockwise around the ulna at the proximal end. During pronation, the distal cut of the radius crosses the ulna and ends diagonal to the ulna, allowing the palm to face down. Supination returns the radius and ulna to parallel positions, with the palm facing up, as in holding a bowl of soup (soup = supination, or up as in sUPination—a clue to remembering the position).

The interosseous membrane forms the middle radioulnar joint and connects the shafts of the ulna and radius; its fibers run in a diagonal pattern perpendicular to one another. This membrane is taut during supination and relaxed in pronation. The distal radioulnar joint is located between the distal ends of the radius and ulna (Fig. 8.23).

The proximal radioulnar joint allows these movements—pronation and supination.

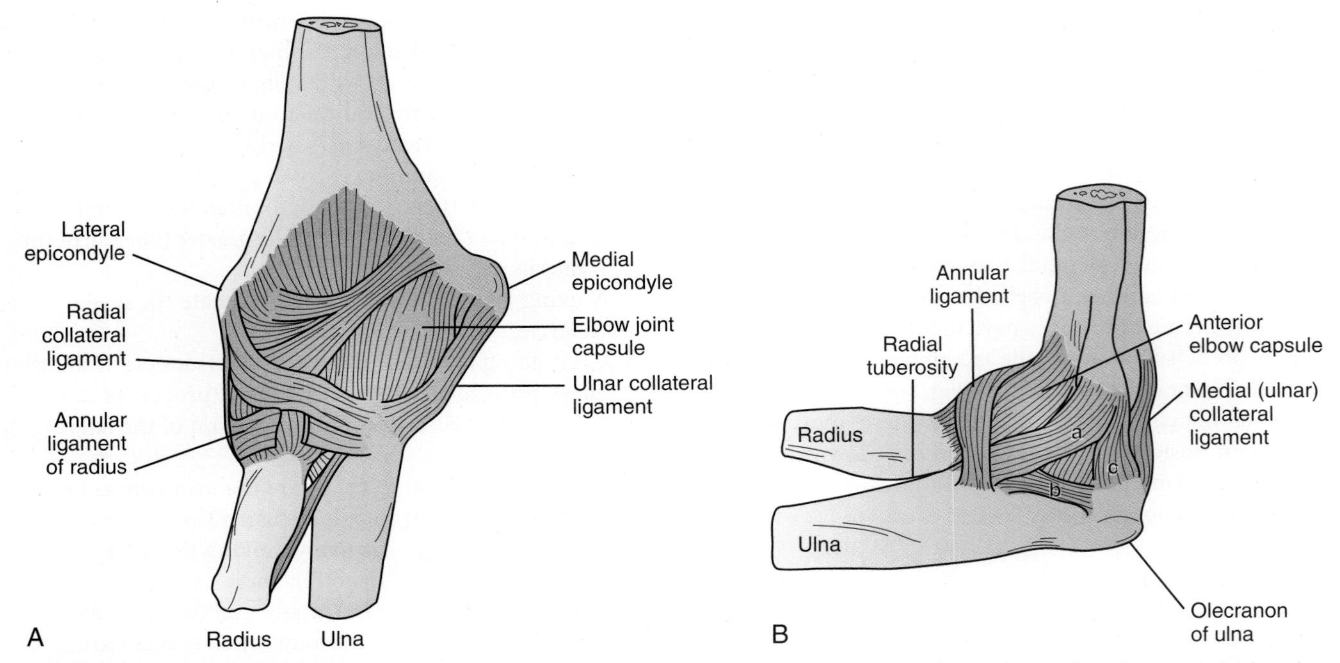

FIG. 8.22 Ligaments of the elbow joint: (A) Anterior view and (B) medial view. *a*, Anterior band; *b*, transverse band; *c*, posterior band.

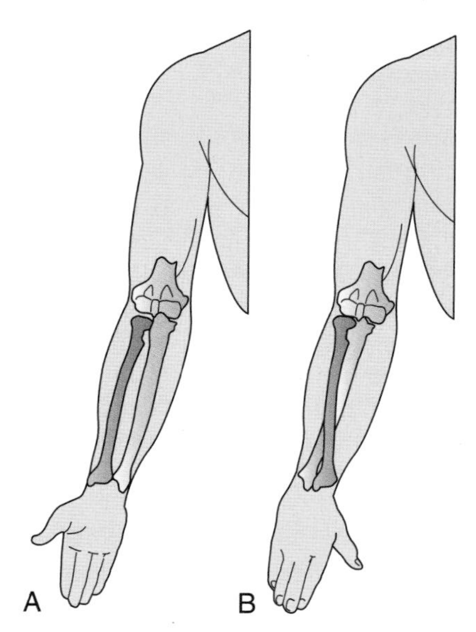

FIG. 8.23 (A) Supination and (B) pronation.

Palpation

Palpate the elbow as follows:

1. Locate the medial and lateral epicondyles of the humerus and the olecranon process of the ulna.
2. A bursa lies between the olecranon process and the skin. The bursa will feel like a small bubble.
3. The synovial membrane is most accessible to examination between the olecranon and the epicondyles. You can trace the ulna by following the bony ridge toward the wrist from the olecranon.
4. The area between the medial epicondyle and olecranon may be sensitive because of the proximity of the ulnar nerve.
5. Supinate and pronate the forearm at the radioulnar joint, and feel the radius rotate on the ulna (Activity 8.7).

ACTIVITY 8.7

Move your elbow joint through the range of motion (ROM) positions.

Joints of the Wrist and Hand

The joints of the wrist and hand include the radiocarpal and carpometacarpal joints.

Radiocarpal (Wrist) Joint

The radiocarpal joint consists of these structures:

- *Articulating bones:* Radius, scaphoid, and lunate, with some triquetral bone involvement
- *Joint type:* Synovial condyloid
- *Ligaments:* Palmar radiocarpal ligament from the radius to the scaphoid, lunate, and triquetral bones; palmar ulnocarpal ligament from the ulna to the scaphoid, lunate, and triquetral bones; and dorsal radiocarpal ligament from the radius to the scaphoid, lunate, and triquetral bones

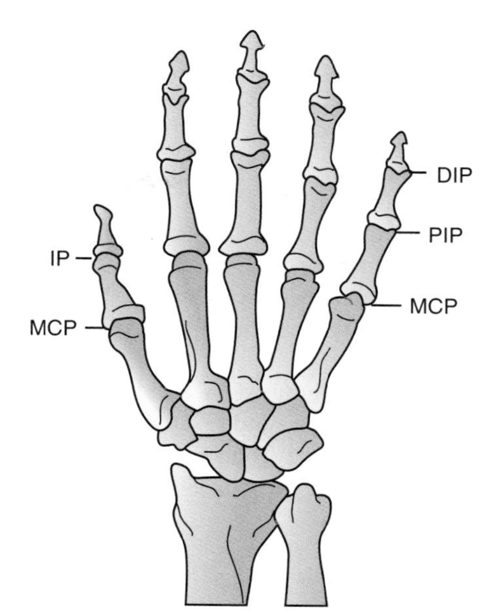

FIG. 8.24 Hand joints. *DIP*, Distal interphalangeal; *IP*, interphalangeal; *MCP*, metacarpophalangeal; *PIP*, proximal interphalangeal.

The wrist is called the *radiocarpal joint* because the radius alone articulates with the carpal bones. The ulna joins the wrist indirectly by a disk that articulates with the carpal bones. This allows forearm pronation and supination to take place without affecting any wrist movements. The joint capsule of the wrist is loose in the anterior and posterior directions, allowing easy flexion and extension, but it is tight laterally and medially, allowing for minimal ulnar deviation and radial deviation.

The radiocarpal joint allows these movements—flexion, extension, and radial and ulnar deviation.

Hand Joints

The intricate pattern of hand joints is where all the movements involving the fingers take place. The hand is capable of a variety of functions that vary from the precise handling of objects to acts of great strength. The opposable thumb allows us to grasp and manipulate objects. Because the thumb in the resting position is rotated relative to the rest of the fingers, the thumb faces the other fingers.

The first carpometacarpal joint of the thumb consists of these structures:

- *Articulating bones:* First metacarpal with trapezium
- *Joint type:* Synovial saddle
- *Ligaments:* Radial and ulnar collateral and anterior and posterior oblique ligaments of the thumb, with assistance from the articular capsule

The MCP joints between the metacarpals of the palm and the phalanges of the fingers form condyloid joints that allow flexion, extension, abduction, and adduction of the fingers.

Joints between phalanges are hinge joints that permit flexion and extension. These joints are called *proximal interphalangeal (PIP) joints* and *distal interphalangeal (DIP) joints* (Fig. 8.24).

The first carpometacarpal joint allows these movements—opposition (abduction, flexion, and medial rotation) and repositioning (adduction, extension, and lateral rotation).

Palpation

Palpate the wrist and hand as follows:

1. At the wrist, locate the bony tips of the radius (laterally) and the ulna (medially).
2. On the dorsum of the wrist, palpate the groove of the radiocarpal or wrist joint.
3. Each carpal bone within the hand cannot be identified readily, so instead palpate the carpal structure while moving the wrist. Palpate each of the five metacarpals and the proximal, middle, and distal phalanges and connecting joints.
4. Remember that the thumb lacks a middle phalanx.
5. Partially flex your fingers and find the groove marking the MCP joint of each finger. The joint is located at the first knuckle and is palpated best on either side of the extensor tendon (Activity 8.8).

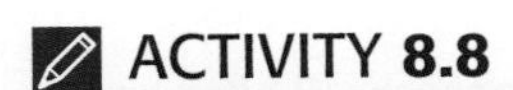

Move your hand and fingers through the ranges of motion.

Joints of the Pelvis and Hip

The joints of the hip and pelvis include the sacroiliac joint, symphysis pubis, and hip joints (Box 8.5).

Sacroiliac Joint

The sacroiliac joint consists of these structures:

- *Articulating bones:* Sacrum and the two ilia
- *Joint type:* Part synovial (anterior half) and part fibrous
- *Ligaments:* The anterior sacroiliac ligament covers the anterior and inferior aspects of the joint; the interosseous sacroiliac ligament links the sacrum and the ilium; and the dorsal sacroiliac ligament covers the posterior aspect of the joint. The sacrotuberous ligament connects the sacrum with the ischial tuberosity, and the sacrospinous ligament connects the sacrum to the ischial spine.

The sacroiliac joints connect the ilia to the spine, transfer the weight of the body to the hip, and work as shock absorbers during walking and running. Ligaments provide much support. They are more relaxed in the female. This laxity increases with hormones released during menstrual cycles and especially during pregnancy.

Box 8.5 The Complex Pelvis

The pelvis comprises three bones arranged in a ring. The pelvis has three principal functions:

1. Transmits weight from the axial skeleton to the lower limbs in the standing position or to the ischial tuberosities when sitting.
2. Provides proximal attachments for muscles that insert onto and move the legs.
3. Protects the lower structures of the digestive and urinary tracts and the reproductive systems.

During the birth of a baby, the head of the infant must pass through the ring (pelvic outlet) of the pelvic girdle.

The pelvis is connected to the skeleton of the upper body at the sacroiliac joint. The sacrum and the coccyx also have a connection to the pelvis.

The joints of the pelvis are capable of tiny movement. Much of this movement occurs at the sacroiliac joint.

- Nutation/counternutation describes sacral movement in relationship to the movement of the ilium.
  - Nutation is the forward motion of the base of the sacrum into the pelvis (tuck your tail) or the backward rotation of the ilium on the sacrum.
  - Counternutation is the opposite movement of nutation. A lordotic position or anterior pelvic tilt is created by the rotation of the ilium on the sacrum or backward motion of the base of the sacrum out of the pelvis (wag your tail).
- Iliosacral movement is ilium movement on the sacrum—anterior/posterior rotation, superior/inferior movement, and medial/lateral flaring.
- Sacroiliac motion is sacral movement on the ilium—flexion/extension and rotation.
- Symphysis pubis joint motion may be either superior or inferior. There is only approximately 2 mm of motion possible at this joint.

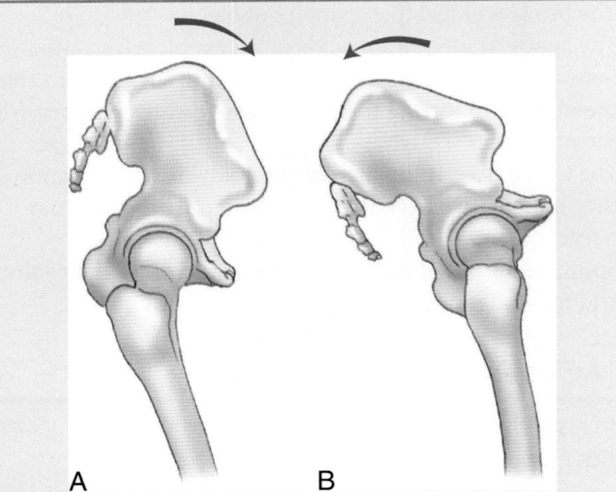

(A) Anterior tilt of the pelvis. Counternutation: Anterior superior iliac spine (ASIS) down and posterior superior iliac spine (PSIS) up. This rotation closes or compresses the sacroiliac joint. (B) Posterior tilt of the pelvis nutation. ASIS is up and the PSIS is down. This rotation opens or gaps the sacroiliac joint. (From Muscolino JE. *Kinesiology: The Skeletal System and Muscle Function.* 2nd ed. Mosby/Elsevier; 2011.)

- *Outflare* is the external (outward) rotation of the ilium on the sacrum. This movement closes the sacroiliac joints and opens the pubis.
- *Inflare* is the internal rotation of the ilium on the sacrum. This will open the sacroiliac joint in the back and close the pubis joint in the front.

All these tiny movements can become very confusing. They all relate to the sacroiliac joint movement and the way the symphysis pubis moves. When these integrated but independent movements are disrupted, many pain patterns result.

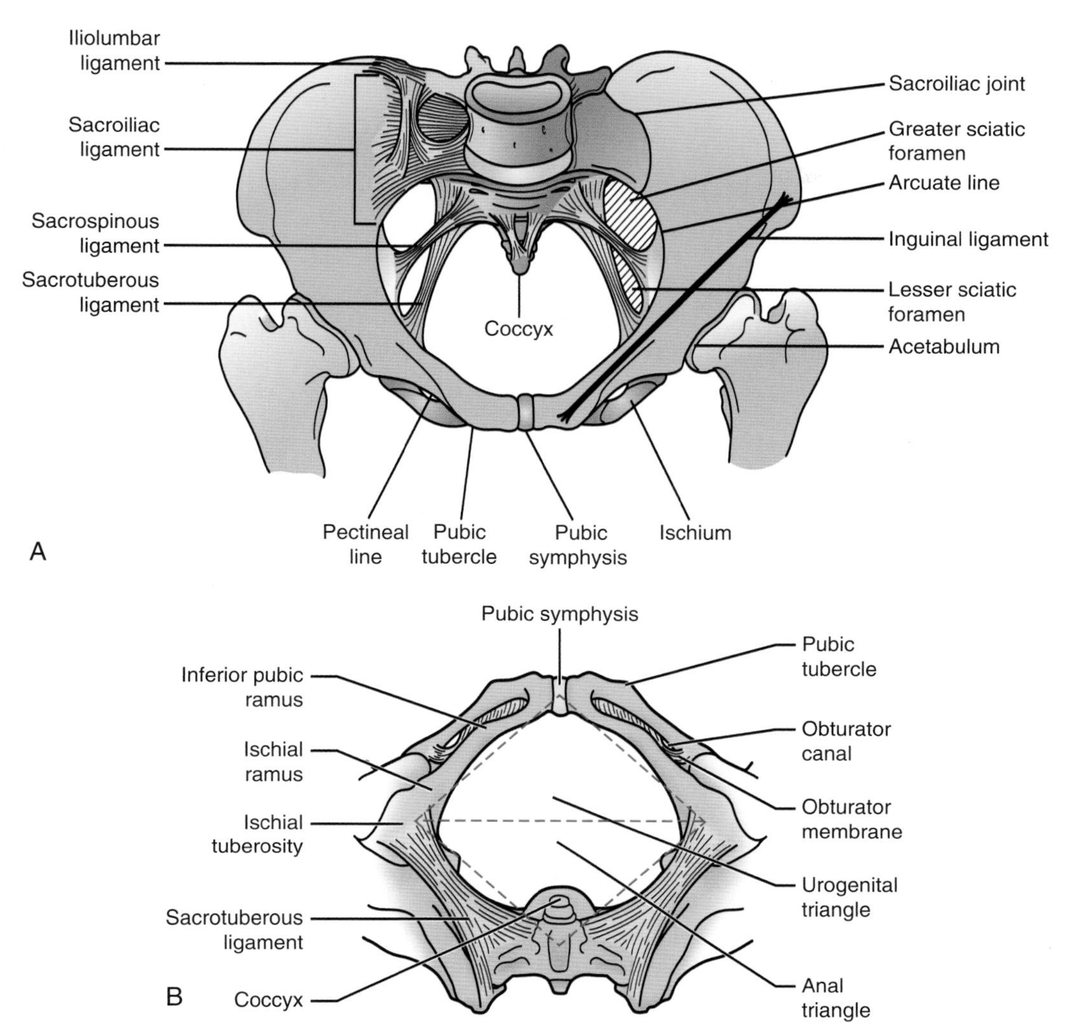

FIG. 8.25 (A) Pelvic ligaments, anterior view. These important ligaments give the pelvis its strength. (B) Ligaments of the symphysis pubis.

The movement allowed is a small but important anterior, posterior, lateral, and medial rotation in a side-lying, figure-eight pattern. This rotary movement of the pelvis allows the vertebral column to remain relatively still as we walk. When the sacroiliac joint does not move, the sacral lumbar junction compensates for the lack of rotation, putting strain on the spine. No direct muscle action occurs at the sacroiliac joint. Instead, the sacroiliac joint moves as a result of other joint movements in the area.

Symphysis Pubis

The symphysis pubis (also called *pubic symphysis*) consists of these structures:

- *Articulating bones*: The two pubic bones
- *Joint type*: Cartilaginous
- *Ligaments*: The superior pubic ligament supports the anterior, posterior, and superior aspects, and the arcuate (inferior) pubic ligament supports the inferior aspect (not pictured in Fig. 8.25).

The stability of this joint is important. The joint connects the left and right coxal or hip bones anteriorly. Should this joint become misaligned, which can happen during childbirth or trauma such as a fall, the stability of the pelvis is compromised, and many postural and soft tissue problems can result (see Fig. 8.25).

The symphysis pubis allows for independent motion of each side of the pelvis, which is important when walking. Symphysis pubis motion is especially important during pregnancy and delivery.

Hip Joint

The hip joint consists of these structures:

- *Articulating bones:* Acetabulum of the pelvic bone (formed by the ilium, pubis, and ischium) and the femur
- *Joint type:* Synovial ball and socket
- *Ligaments:* Iliofemoral ligament from the anterior superior iliac spine (ASIS) to the intertrochanteric line of the femur; ischiofemoral ligament from the ischium to the femur on the posterior side; pubofemoral ligament from the pubis to the intertrochanteric line of the femur; and the ligamentum teres, also known as the *ligament of the head of the femur*, from the head of the femur to the acetabulum (Fig. 8.26)

A fibrocartilaginous ring called the *labrum* attaches around the edge of the acetabulum and is reinforced by the transverse acetabular ligament. This ring helps hold the femoral head in

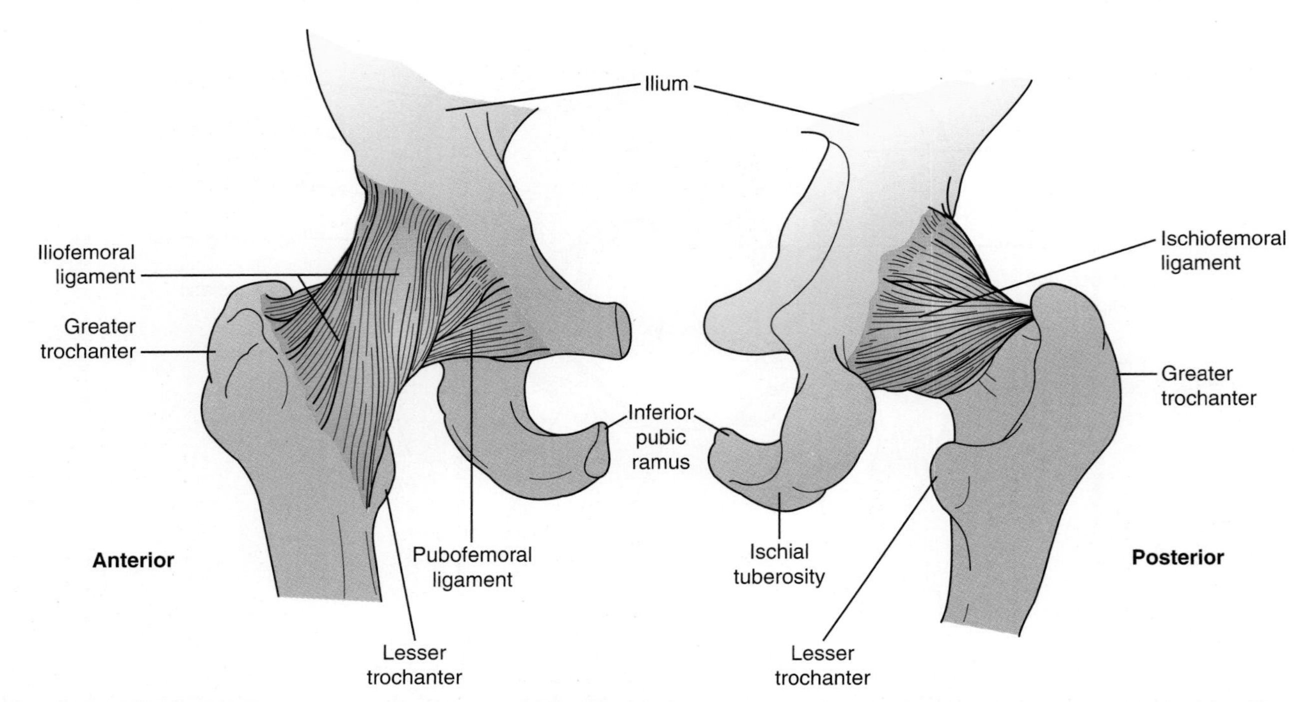

FIG. 8.26 Ligaments of the hip joint. The three principal hip joint ligaments are arranged in a continuum that surrounds the joint. The iliofemoral ligament is especially important in limiting the extension of the hip.

place by increasing the depth of the acetabulum (not pictured in Fig. 8.26).

The hip joint is a massive joint. Although it is a mobile ball-and-socket joint, the hip joint is less mobile than the shoulder joint because the round head of the femur fits into the deep socket of the acetabulum of the pelvis. This structure provides stability. Therefore the hip joint is less susceptible to injury than the shoulder joint. In anatomical position, the femoral head is not fully in the hip socket. A better fit is when the femur is flexed to 90 degrees, slightly abducted, and laterally rotated. The most relaxed position is flexion, abduction, and lateral rotation (e.g., such as when sitting in a relaxed position with the leg falling to the side).

The joint capsule is large. The capsule is looser in flexion than in extension.

Usually, the thigh moves on the pelvis, but the pelvis can move on the thigh if the thigh is fixed. The pelvis can move forward. This motion is called *anterior tilt* and tends to increase the lordosis of the lumbar spine. Posterior tilt, the opposite movement, decreases lumbar lordosis. The pelvis can also elevate, depress, and rotate to the right or left.

The hip joint allows the following movements: flexion, extension, abduction, adduction, medial rotation, and lateral rotation.

Palpation

Palpate the pelvic and hip joint region as follows:

1. The hip joint itself lies deep within the body and is not directly palpable.
2. The posterior edge of the greater trochanter of the femur is easiest to locate and can be felt about a palm's width below the iliac crest.
3. The superficial trochanteric bursa lies on the posterolateral surface of the greater trochanter.
4. At the same level as the greater trochanter, locate the pubic tubercles.
5. The symphysis pubis can be palpated at the anterior midline of the body.
6. The sacroiliac joint is located just inferior to the posterior superior iliac spine (PSIS) near the dimples of the gluteal area. It is not directly palpable because it is covered with ligaments, but movements can be felt there. A small degree of motion can be felt if the finger or thumb is held in this area while a person is walking or marching in place. You may also feel nutation/counternutation (Activity 8.9).

ACTIVITY 8.9

Move your pelvis and hip through the ranges of motion.

Joints of the Knee

The tibiofemoral joint is located between the femur and tibia. The patellofemoral joint is found between the patella and the trochlear groove of the femur. These two joints consist of these structures:

- *Articulating bones:* Femur, tibia, and patella
- *Joint type:* Synovial modified hinge
- *Ligaments:* The patellar ligament runs from the patella to the tibial tuberosity (the quadriceps femoris tendon also provides stability to the patella); the oblique popliteal ligament joins the lateral aspect of the fibrous capsule to the lateral condyle of the femur; the tibial (medial) collateral ligament joins the medial epicondyle of the femur to the

Box 8.6 The Complex Knee

The knee joint is the most complicated in the body, is not as stable as other joints, and yet is one of the most frequently used joints. Prolonged standing while the knee is in a slightly flexed position, instead of the normal locked extension position, puts stress on the articular surfaces of the condyles and can damage the cartilage.

The medial condyle is more curved than the lateral condyle, which contributes to the automatic rotation of the knee during flexion and extension when the knee joint is near full extension. The femoral condyle first rolls off the tibial condyle and then glides, producing a combined rolling-gliding movement. The opposite action occurs in the extension of the knee: first a glide and then rolling.

In males, the acetabulum is located almost directly above the knee, which allows for an even distribution of weight-bearing forces during movement. In contrast, the wider female pelvis results in the knee being medial to the acetabulum. This arrangement puts strain on the female knee during movement. Female knees are not as well equipped to handle the strain of running and repetitive impact activities of the lower extremities.

The fibrocartilaginous menisci provide more surface contact on the tibia for the femur, which allows for stability between the rounded femoral condyles, which sit on an almost flat tibia. The menisci are attached to muscles and connected by ligaments to each other and the bones. These shock absorbers protect bone and cartilage and increase the movement of synovial fluid. The menisci move in the joint capsule, depending on the forces imposed on them. If the movement against the menisci is too abrupt or quickly changes direction such that they cannot shift position, the menisci can be crushed or torn.

The joint capsule is slack anteriorly and taut posteriorly in extension and just the opposite in flexion. The posterior knee capsule is thick and consists of two strong bands connecting the femoral and tibial condyles. These ligaments resist hyperextension of the joint and provide stability in the standing position in normal extension. In normal extension, all the ligaments are taut, and one can stabilize the joint passively without any muscular action. Extension is the most stable position for the knee.

The patella protects the knee joint from external impacts, such as falling forward onto the knees. The patella moves in a groove between the femoral condyles by the contraction of the quadriceps femoris muscles. The more flexion, the greater the pull on the patella. The contraction of the quadriceps femoris tends to pull the patella laterally during active extension. The position of the patella becomes somewhat unstable in this position. The patella provides an increased mechanical advantage for the quadriceps femoris muscles when contracting to move the knee into extension. The knee is prone to injury because it relies on soft tissue for much of its support when in a flexed position.

medial condyle of the tibia; the anterolateral ligament joins the femur and tibia; the fibular (lateral) collateral ligament joins the lateral epicondyle of the femur to the fibula; the anterior cruciate ligament joins the anterior medial intercondylar area of the tibia to the posteromedial surface of the lateral condyle of the femur; the posterior cruciate ligament joins the posterior intercondylar area of the tibia to the anteromedial condyle of the femur; the posterior meniscofemoral ligament attaches the lateral meniscus to the posterior surface at the femur; the transverse ligament joins the medial meniscus to the lateral meniscus (Box 8.6 and Fig. 8.27).

The knee joints allow these movements—flexion, extension, medial rotation, and lateral rotation.

Palpation

Palpate the knee joint as follows:

1. Landmarks in and around the knee help orient you to this complicated joint.
2. Locate the flat medial surface of the tibia, the shin.
3. Follow its anterior border upward to the tibial tuberosity.
4. Move medially and follow the medial border of the tibia upward until it merges into a bony prominence, the medial tibial condyle, which is higher than the tibial tuberosity.
5. In a comparable location on the other side of the knee, find a similar prominence, the lateral condyle of the tibia.
6. Just below the level of the lateral tibial condyle, find the head of the fibula.
7. Now identify three parts of the distal femur. Bring your fingertips firmly down the medial surface of the thigh along a line where the inner seam of your pant leg would be.
8. Your fingers will run up against an abrupt bony prominence, the adductor tubercle.
9. Just below this is the medial epicondyle.
10. The lateral epicondyle of the femur is found in a similar area on the other side.
11. The patella rests on the anterior articulating surface of the femur, roughly midway between the epicondyles, and lies within the tendon of the quadriceps femoris muscles.
12. This structure continues below the knee joint as the patellar ligament and attaches to the tibial tuberosity.
13. Two collateral ligaments, one on each side of the knee, give medial and lateral stability to the joint.
14. To feel the lateral collateral ligament, cross one leg so that your ankle rests on the opposite knee.
15. Find the firm cord that runs from the lateral epicondyle of the femur to the head of the fibula.
16. The medial collateral ligament can usually be palpated on the medial side.
17. Two cruciate ligaments cross obliquely within the knee joint giving it anteroposterior stability and cannot be palpated.
18. With the knee joint flexed to about 90 degrees, you can press your thumbs—one on each side of the patellar ligament—into the groove of the tibiofemoral joint. Note that the patella lies just proximal to this joint line.
19. As you press your thumbs downward, you can feel the edge of the proximal surface of the tibia. Follow it medially, then laterally until you are stopped by the converging femur and tibia.

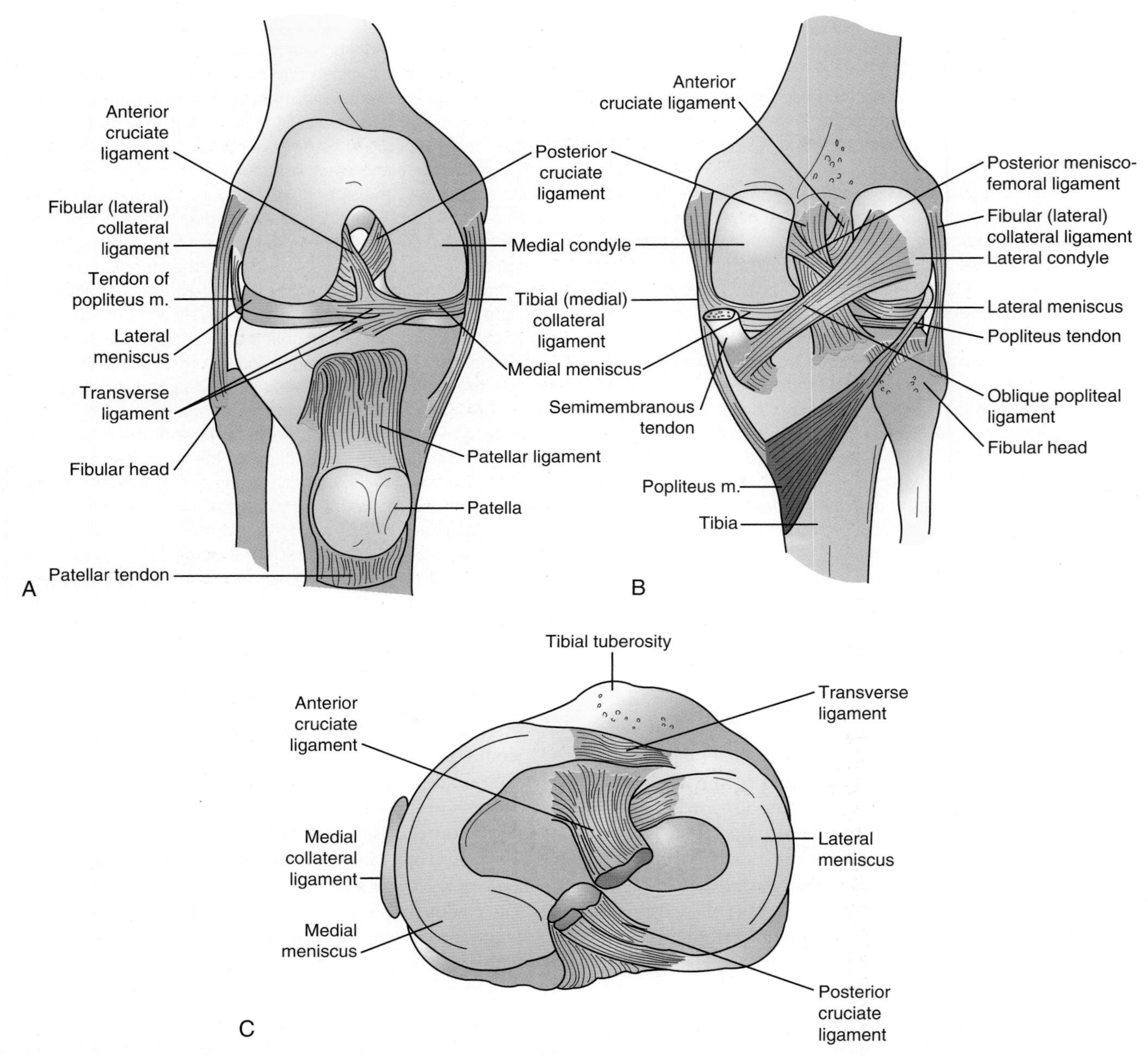

FIG. 8.27 Knee joint opened; anterior, posterior, and proximal views. (A) Anterior view of the knee joint, opened by folding the patella and patellar ligament inferiorly. On the lateral side is the fibular collateral ligament, separated by the popliteal tendon from the lateral meniscus. On the medial side, the tibial collateral ligament is attached to the medial meniscus. The anterior and posterior cruciate ligaments are seen between the femoral condyles. (B) Posterior view of the opened knee joint with a more complete view of the posterior cruciate ligament. (C) The femur is removed, showing the proximal (articular) end of the right tibia. On the medial side is the gently curved medial meniscus; on the lateral side is the more tightly curved lateral meniscus. The anterior end of the medial meniscus is anchored to the surface of the tibia by the transverse ligament. The cut ends of the anterior and posterior cruciate ligaments are shown, as well as the meniscofemoral ligament.

20. The medial and lateral menisci, crescent-shaped fibrocartilaginous pads that lie on the tibial plateaus, form cushions between the tibia and femur. They can be palpated in the space between the tibia and femur on either side of the midline.
21. The soft tissue in front of the joint space, on either side of the patellar ligament, is the infrapatellar fat pad.
22. Several bursae lie near the knee. The prepatellar bursa lies between the patella and the overlying skin, whereas the superficial infrapatellar bursa lies anterior to the patellar ligament.
23. Observe the concavities that are usually evident at each side and above the patella. In these areas is the synovial cavity of the knee joint. Although the synovium is not normally detectable, these areas may become swollen and tender when the joint is inflamed. You may also see the swelling from the protrusion of the fat pad, which is often confused with effusion (fluid in the capsule) (Activity 8.10).

ACTIVITY 8.10

Move your knee joint through the range of motion (ROM) positions.

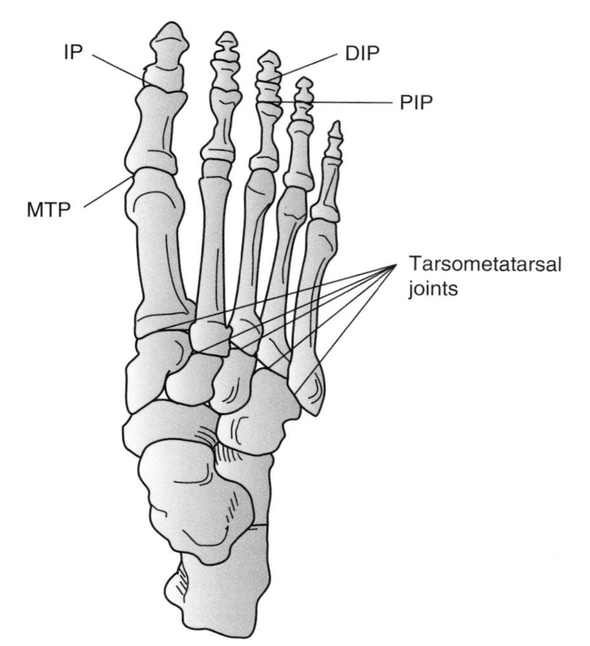

FIG. 8.28 Foot joints. *DIP*, Distal interphalangeal; *IP*, interphalangeal; *MTP*, metatarsophalangeal; *PIP*, proximal interphalangeal.

Joints of the Ankle and Foot

The joints of the ankle and foot include the talocrural, distal tibiofibular, subtalar (talocalcaneal joints), intertarsal, tarsometatarsal, MTP joints, and interphalangeal joints (Fig. 8.28).

Talocrural Joint

The talocrural joint (the ankle joint) consists of these structures (Box 8.7):

- *Articulating bones:* Tibia, fibula, and talus
- *Joint type:* Synovial hinge
- *Ligaments:* Medial collateral or deltoid from the medial malleolus to the navicular, calcaneus, and talus; talofibular ligaments from the lateral malleolus to the talus; and calcaneofibular from the fibula to the lateral calcaneus

The metatarsals make up the body of the foot, and the phalanges make up the toes (see Fig. 8.28; also Fig. 8.29).

The talocrural joint allows these movements—dorsiflexion (extension) and plantar flexion (flexion).

Distal Tibiofibular Joint and Subtalar/Talocalcaneal Joint

The distal tibiofibular joint is a fibrous syndesmosis joint that holds the tibia and fibula together. The ankle (talocrural) joint is formed by the distal ends of the tibia and fibula meeting the talus.

Immediately distal to the ankle joint is the talocalcaneal joint, or the articulation of the talus with the calcaneus. This joint is often referred to as the *subtalar joint*. It is reinforced by the joint capsule and interosseous ligaments. No muscles attach to the talus, which is moved indirectly by the structures surrounding it. The subtalar joint is most stable when in a supinated position (the major component of supination is inversion). It is least stable when pronated (the major component of pronation is eversion).

Motions of the ankle joint itself are limited to dorsiflexion and plantar flexion, as previously stated. Inversion and eversion of the foot are functions of the subtalar and transverse tarsal joints (see Fig. 8.29).

Box 8.7 Why Plantar Flexion and Dorsiflexion?

A transverse axis through the ankle joint allows a pair of actions similar to flexion and extension at the wrist joint.

The analogous action to wrist flexion would tip the sole downward, increasing the angle between the foot and leg. The usual term for the increase in such an angle would be *extension*, but to emphasize the relation between foot and hand, this action is instead termed *plantar flexion*.

The action similar to extension at the wrist would be a tipping of the upper surface (dorsum) of the foot toward the anterior surface of the leg.

However, this would decrease the angle between the body segments, an action usually termed *flexion*. Because the term *plantar flexion* has been used for the opposite action, this is now referred to as *dorsiflexion*.

Foot Joints

The joints of the foot are:

- Intertarsal: Between the tarsal bones
- Tarsometatarsal: Between the tarsals and the metatarsals
- MTP: Between the metatarsals and the phalanges
- Interphalangeal: Between the proximal, middle, and distal phalanges

The MTP joints are condyloid. The great toe has one interphalangeal joint. The remaining toes have two interphalangeal joints each. The more proximal joint is the PIP joint, and the distal joint is the DIP joint. The interphalangeal joints are hinge joints. The design of the foot bones and joints creates curved structures called *arches*. The foot has three arches: a medial arch, a lateral longitudinal arch, and a transverse arch.

The medial longitudinal arch is the highest and is composed of the calcaneus, talus, navicular, cuneiforms, and the first three metatarsals. The lateral longitudinal arch is lower and flatter than the medial arch. It is composed of the calcaneus, cuboid, and fourth and fifth metatarsals. The *transverse arch* is composed of the cuneiforms, the cuboid, and the metatarsals.

Palpation

Palpate the ankle and foot joint as follows:

1. Identify the landmarks of the ankle, which are the medial malleolus, the bony prominence at the distal end of the tibia, and the lateral malleolus, at the distal end of the fibula.
2. Ligaments extend from each malleolus into the foot.
3. The heads of the metatarsals are palpable in the ball of the foot. These and the associated MTP joints are proximal to the webs of the toes.

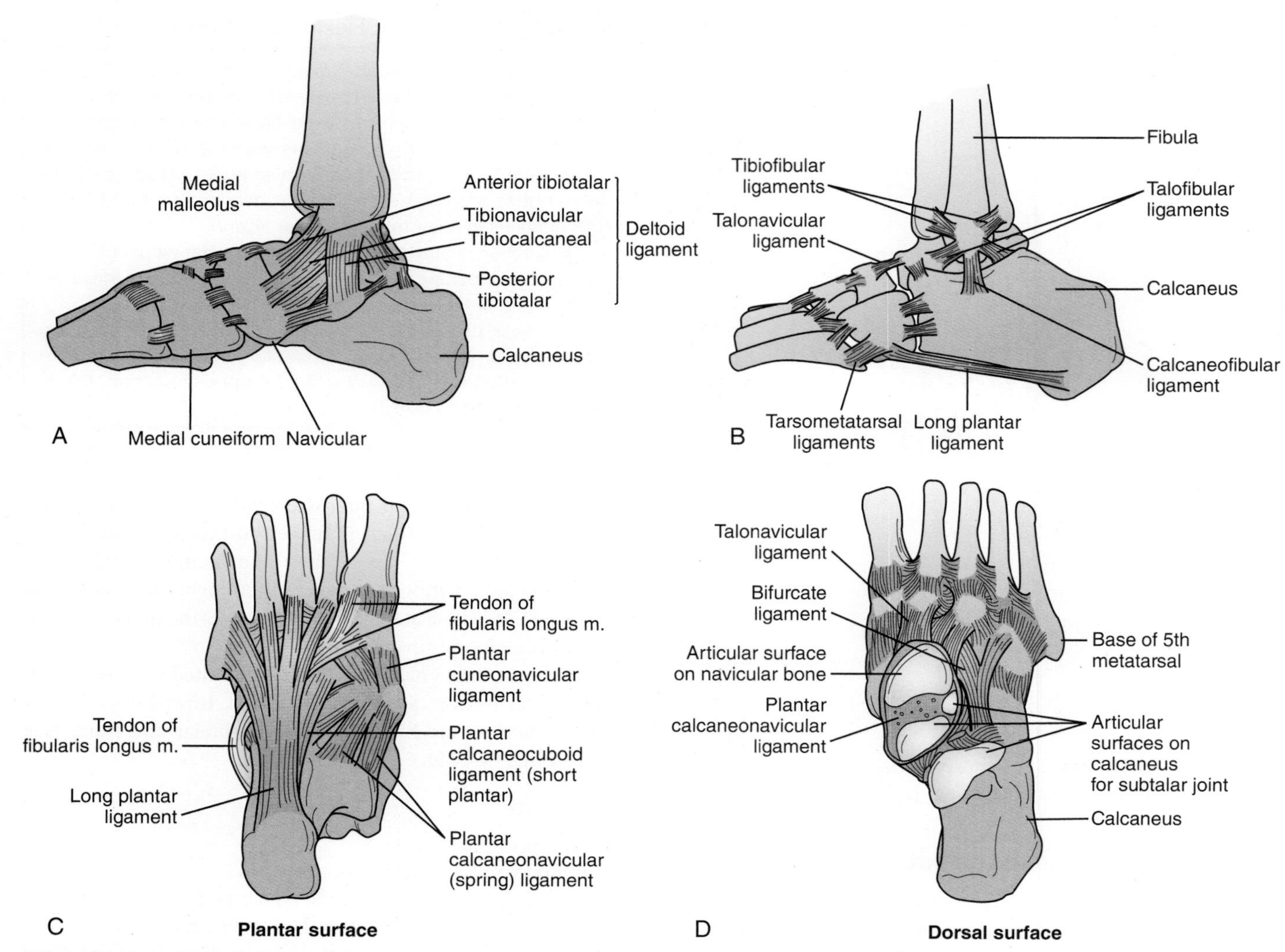

FIG. 8.29 (A) Medial view. The deltoid ligament attaches the medial malleolus of the tibia to several underlying bones. The deltoid ligament consists of anterior tibiotalar, tibionavicular, tibiocalcaneal, and posterior tibiotalar portions. (B) Lateral view of ligaments of the ankle. (C) Plantar view of plantar ligaments of the foot, including the long plantar, short plantar, and spring ligaments. (D) Dorsal view with the talus removed, showing the rounded socket in which it articulates (the talocalcaneonavicular joint). The bifurcate and talonavicular ligaments help stabilize the bones forming this articulation.

ACTIVITY 8.11

Move your ankles and feet through the ranges of motion.

4. From the base of the large toe to the heel, palpate the medial longitudinal arch.
5. Beginning at the base of the little toe and moving to the heel, palpate the lateral longitudinal arch.
6. The transverse arch is palpated by beginning just below the base of the large toe and moving across the foot to the base of the little toe (Activity 8.11).

Joints of the Spine and Thorax

The spine and thorax joints consist of the atlantooccipital, atlantoaxial, intervertebral disk, zygapophyseal, costospinal (costovertebral and costotransverse), and sternocostal (costochondral and chondrosternal) joints (Fig. 8.30).

Joints of the Spine

Atlantooccipital Joint

- *Articulating bones:* Atlas (C1) and occipital bone at the occipital condyles
- *Joint type:* Synovial condyloid (ellipsoid)

The atlantooccipital joint allows these movements—flexion, extension, right lateral flexion, and left lateral flexion.

Atlantoaxial Joint

- *Articulating bones:* Atlas (C1) and axis (C2)
- *Joint type:* Synovial

The atlantoaxial joint allows these movements—right and left rotation.

Intervertebral Disk Joints

- *Articulating bones*: Adjacent vertebrae
- *Joint type*: Cartilaginous symphysis

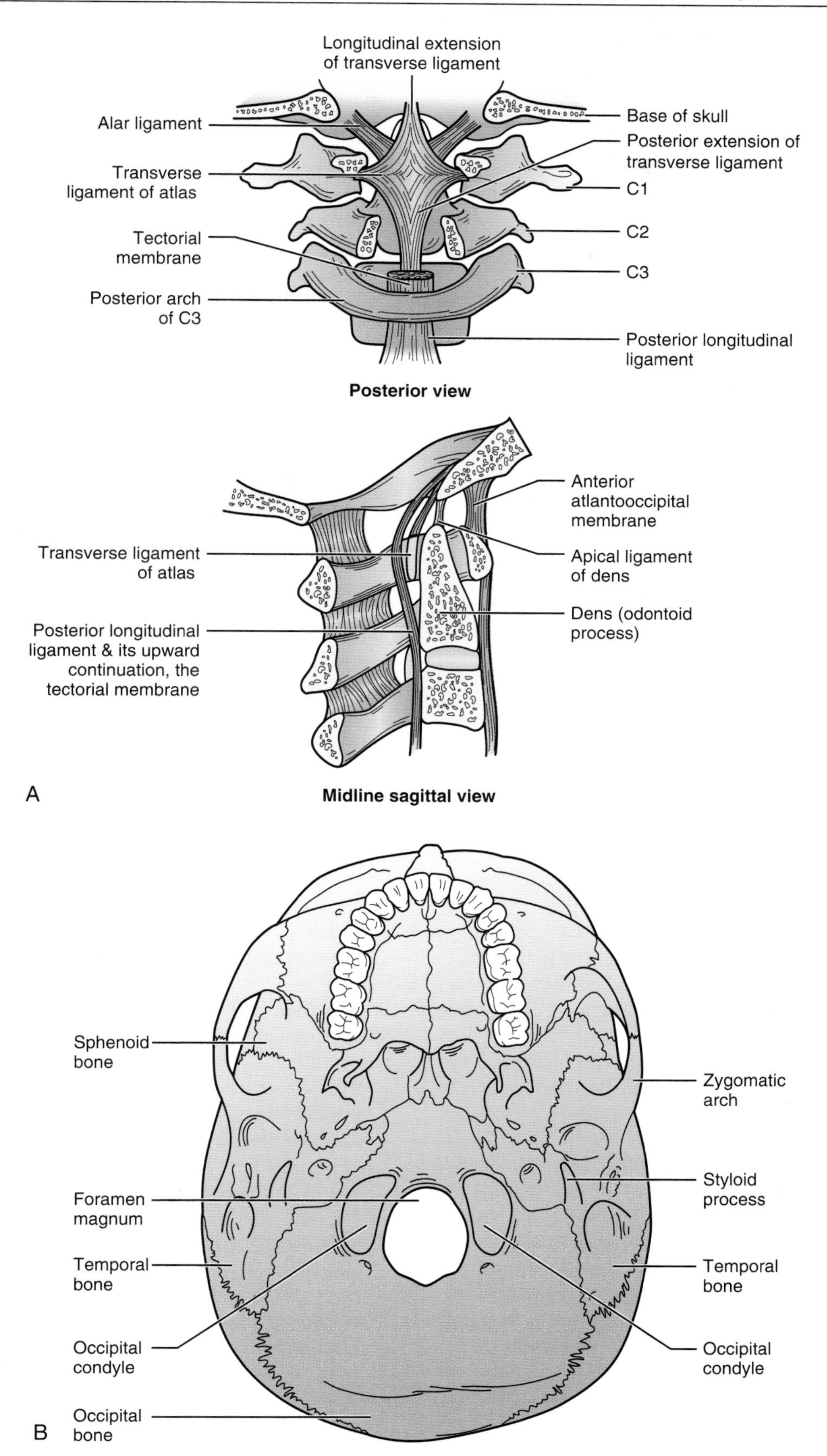

FIG. 8.30 (A) Ligaments connecting the skull and vertebral column. Both C1 and C2 vertebrae are separately attached to the base of the skull to ensure maximal stability. The transverse ligament of the atlas prevents the dens from moving posteriorly and crushing the spinal cord as it passes through the foramen of the C1 vertebra. With its upward and downward extensions, the transverse ligament forms the cruciform ligament. (B) Base of the skull. In this view, the large occipital condyles are shown. These are the surfaces at which the skull articulates with the C1 vertebra, the atlas.

Individual intervertebral disk joints allow minimal movement; movement of the spine as a unit is much greater.

Zygapophyseal (Facet) Joints

- *Articulating bones:* Superior and inferior articulating facets of adjacent vertebrae
- *Joint type:* Synovial gliding

The zygapophyseal joints allow these movements—flexion, extension, right and left lateral flexion, right and left rotation, and gliding.

Ligaments

The supraspinous ligament and interspinous ligaments run along the ends of the spinous processes of each vertebra; the supraspinous ligament enlarges in the cervical region and becomes the ligamentum nuchae in the cervical area; intertransverse ligaments connect the transverse processes; ligamenta flava connect adjacent laminae; the anterior longitudinal ligament, which connects the anterior vertebral body and disk to the anterior vertebral body and disk located directly above, runs the entire length of the spine; and the posterior longitudinal ligament, which connects the posterior vertebral body and disk to the above posterior vertebral body and disk, runs the entire length of the spine.

Movements of individual vertebrae are slight, but the cumulative effect of main movements occurs at C7 to T1, the cervical thoracic junction; T12 to L1, the thoracolumbar junction; and L5 to S1, the sacral lumbar junction. These areas, where one curve ends and another begins, are more flexible and more prone to injury. In flexion, the body of the vertebra moves forward, compressing the disk anteriorly and expanding it posteriorly. The fluid nucleus pulposus moves toward the back, and the posterior ligaments stabilize. In extension, the opposite occurs.

Lateral flexion creates a similar pattern. Compression on the side of the lateral flexion increases pressure in the disk on the opposite side. The action of the disks and the ligaments is more involved in movement than the actual bony components of the spine.

Viewed laterally, the spine has cervical and lumbar lordoses and a thoracic kyphosis. The sacral curve forms a second kyphosis.

The most mobile portion of the spine is the neck. Flexion and extension occur chiefly between the head and the first cervical vertebra, rotation occurs primarily between the first and second vertebrae, and lateral bending involves the cervical spine from the second to the seventh vertebra.

Movements of the rest of the spine (i.e., from the sacrum to the base of the neck) are more difficult to measure than those in the neck and are subject to considerable individual variation. The most mobile areas are at the thoracolumbar junction of T11 to T12, T12 to L1, L4 to L5, and the lumbosacral joint (L5 to S1). The angle at the lumbosacral joint is tipped anteriorly so that when the lumbar vertebra wants to slide forward, contact between the superior articular processes of S1 and the inferior articular process of L5 prevents the movement. What looks like spinal flexion takes place partly at the hip joints. For this reason, and because the length of the limbs varies so much among individuals, flexion cannot be estimated accurately by noting the distance of our fingertips from the floor when we bend over. On forward flexion, watch the lumbar area; its normal lordosis should flatten (Figs. 8.31–8.33).

Palpation

Palpate the spinal joints as follows:

1. Beginning just below the skull, palpate the spinous processes of the cervical vertebrae.
2. The spinous processes of C2, C7, and often T1 are usually larger and more prominent.
3. Continue along the thoracic spine, noticing the bony prominences of each vertebra.
4. A line drawn between the iliac crests runs between the spinous processes of L4 and L5. This point is used often as a reference to locate the other vertebrae.
5. Palpate each of the vertebrae, locating each spinous process.
6. Then palpate again during rotation of the spine, and identify the thoracolumbar junction of T11 to T12, T12 to L1, L4 to L5, and the lumbosacral joint.

Joints of the Thorax

The costospinal joints consist of costovertebral and costotransverse joints.

Costospinal Joints

- *Articulating bones:* Rib with facets and hemifacets on adjoining vertebrae
- *Joint type:* Synovial plane
- *Ligaments:* Costotransverse ligaments from the rib to the transverse process and radiate ligaments from the rib to the vertebral bodies

The costospinal joints allow gliding (Fig. 8.34).

Sternocostal Joints

Sternocostal joints consist of costochondral and chondrosternal joints.

- *Articulating bones:* Costochondral joints: The first through the seventh ribs articulate with costal cartilage. Chondrosternal joints: The cartilage articulates with the sternum.
- *Joint type:* Cartilaginous and synovial
- *Ligaments:* Costochondral joints are synchondroses and have no ligaments for support; chondrosternal joints are synovial and are supported by an intraarticular ligament and a thin capsule.

The sternocostal and costospinal joints allow this movement—Similar to the movement of a handle on a bucket, movement of the thoracic cage occurs during respiration. Small movement of the ribs at the costospinal joints produces large movements anteriorly of the sternum and laterally of the rib shafts. The result is a change in the diameter of the thoracic cage that shifts intrathoracic pressure and enables inspiration to occur (Fig. 8.35).

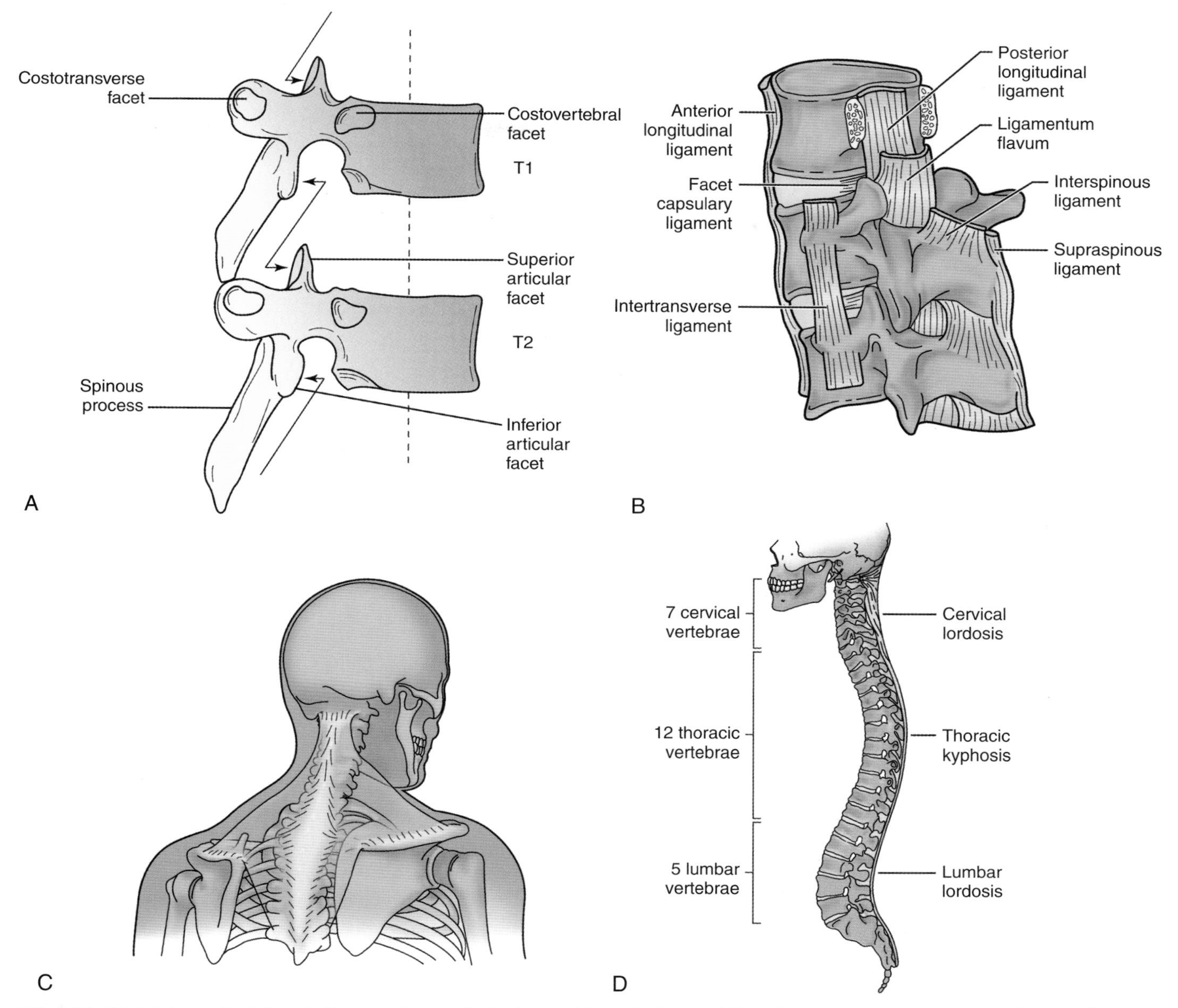

FIG. 8.31 (A) Vertebral articulations in the frontal plane. (In lumbar vertebrae [*not shown*] the articular facets are in the sagittal plane.) The *vertical dashed line* indicates the articulation of adjacent vertebral bodies. The *jagged lines* indicate the way articular facets align with one another. (B) Ligaments of the spine. (C) Ligamentum nuchae. (D) Cervical and lumbar lordoses and thoracic kyphosis. The sacral curve forms a second kyphosis.

Palpation

Palpate the joints of the thorax as follows:

1. In the thoracic region, follow each rib from its costospinal joints to the costal cartilage.
2. Feel for the bucket-handle motion of the ribs during breathing (Activity 8.12).

Section Summary

- Palpate and describe the following jointed areas: joints of the skull, shoulder, elbow, wrist and hand, pelvis and hip, knee, ankle and foot, spine and thorax.
  - *skull* (joints: cranial sutures, temporomandibular joint [TMJ]) Figs. 8.17, 8.18, Activity 8.5; *shoulder* (joints: glenohumeral, sternoclavicular, acromioclavicular, scapulocostal junction) Figs. 8.19–8.21, Activity 8.6; *elbow* (joints: ulnohumeral, radiohumeral, radioulnar) Figs. 8.22, 8.23, Activity 8.7; *wrist* and *hand* (joints: radiocarpal, carpometacarpal) Fig. 8.24, Activity 8.8; *pelvis* and *hip* (joints: sacroiliac, symphysis pubis, hip) Figs. 8.25, 8.26, Activity 8.9; *knee* (joints: tibiofemoral, patellofemoral) Fig. 8.27, Activity 8.10; *ankle* and *foot* (joints: talocrural, tibiofibular, subtalar, intertarsal, tarsometatarsal, MTP, interphalangeal) Figs. 8.28, 8.29, Activity 8.11, *spine* and *thorax* (joints: atlantooccipital, atlantoaxial, intervertebral disk, zygapophyseal [facet], costospinal [costovertebral and costotransverse], sternocostal [costochondral and chondrosternal]) Figs. 8.30–8.35, Activity 8.12.

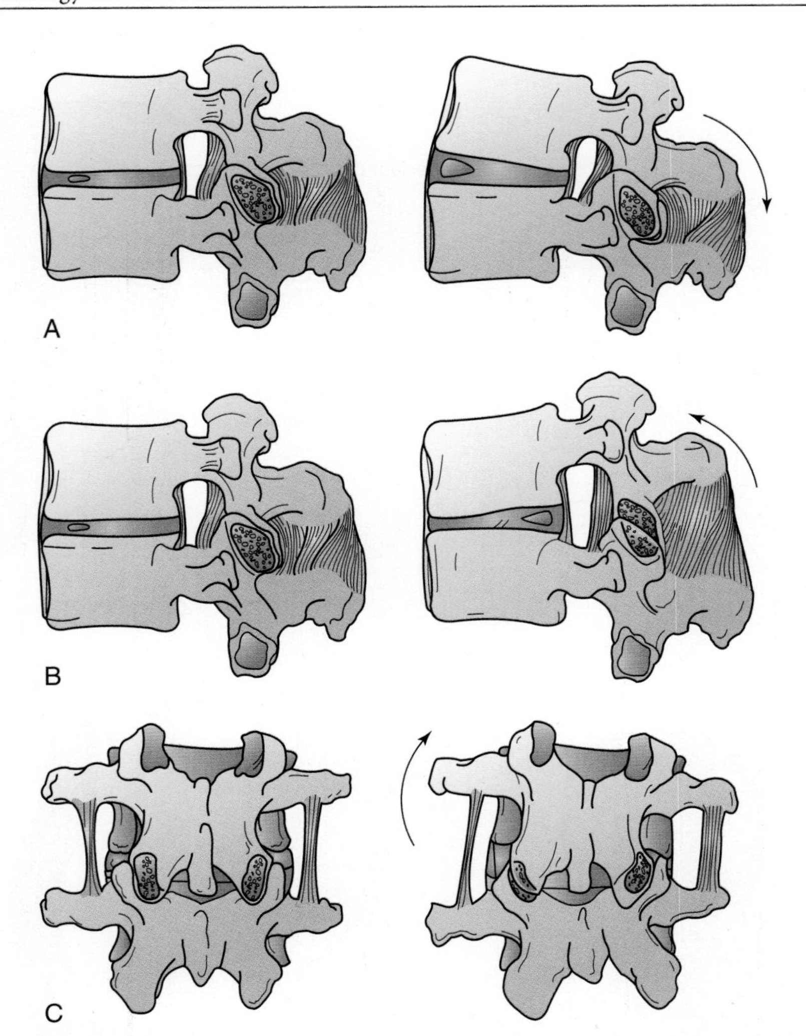

FIG. 8.32 Motion between adjacent vertebrae. (A–C) *Left*, Vertebrae in their neutral positions. (A) *Right*, Vertebra in extension. The anterior longitudinal ligament is becoming taut. (B) *Right*, Vertebra in flexion. Notice that the interspinous and supraspinous ligaments, as well as the ligamentum flavum, are being stretched. (C) *Right*, Vertebra in right lateral flexion. The left intertransverse ligament is becoming taut.

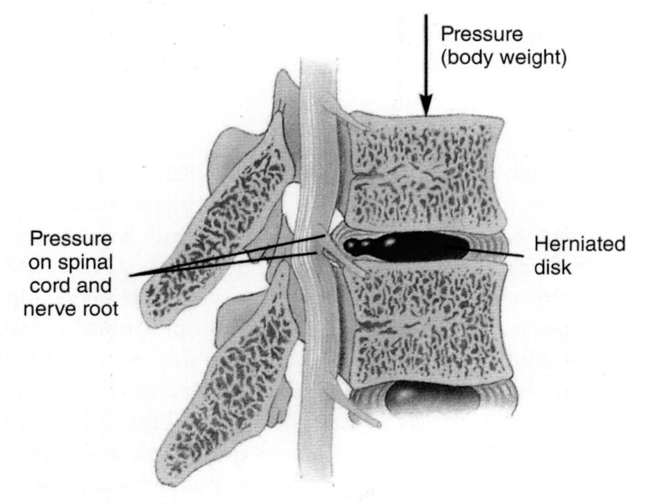

FIG. 8.33 Herniated disk. (From Thibodeau GA, Patton KT. *Anatomy & Physiology*. 6th ed. Mosby/Elsevier; 2007.)

INTEGRATING JOINT MOVEMENT INTO MASSAGE

SECTION OBJECTIVES

Chapter objective covered in this section:

7. Design a joint movement sequence for the body.

After completing this section, the learner will be able to:

- Explain why joint movement is important to massage application.
- Define active and passive joint movement.

Joint movement is how we move an area to measure joint range of motion (ROM). We also use joint movement to position an area for the application of muscle energy techniques to lengthen muscles and for stretching methods to elongate connective tissues. For this reason, the massage professional should concentrate on developing the ability to use joint movement efficiently and effectively.

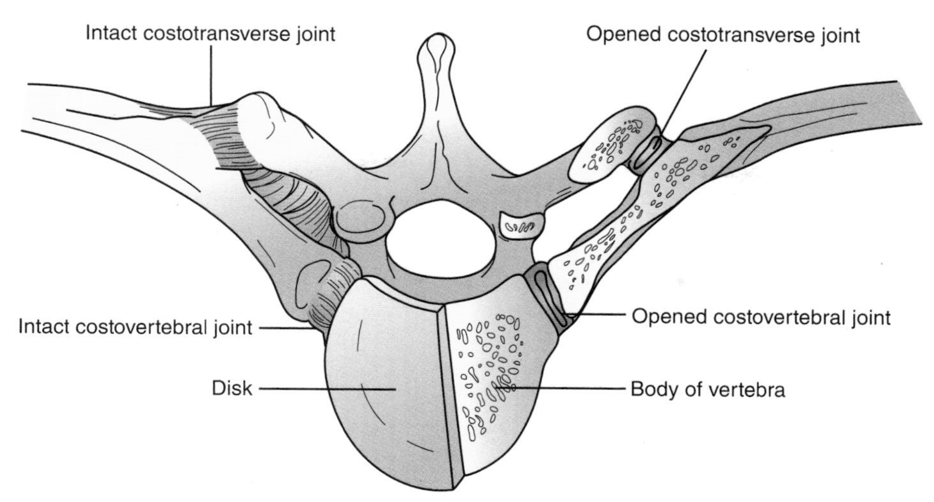

FIG. 8.34 Costospinal joints between the ribs and spine. On the *left* are shown the intact costovertebral and costotransverse joints, reinforced by ligaments. On the *right*, the joints have been opened, revealing the synovial spaces within them.

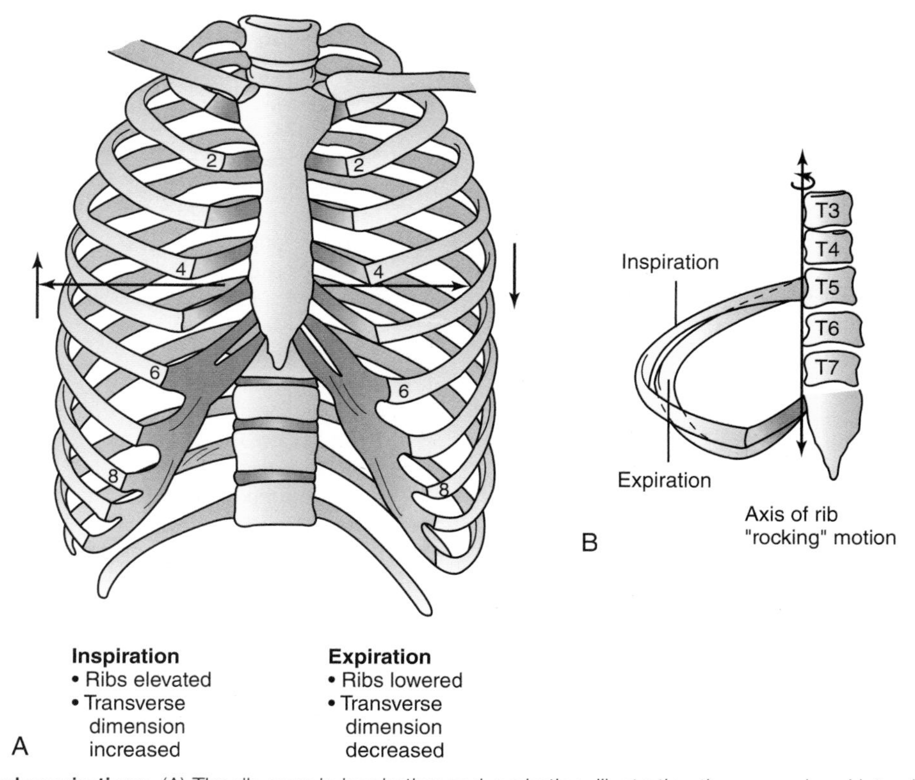

FIG. 8.35 Rib cage and respirations. (A) The rib cage in inspiration and expiration, illustrating the upward and lateral excursion that takes place at inspiration. This results in an increase in intrathoracic volume and the movement of air into the tracheobronchial tree. (B) The "bucket-handle" motion of a sample single rib during inspiration and expiration.

ACTIVITY 8.12

Move your spine and thorax through the ranges of motion.

Joint movement is effective because it provides a means of controlled stimulation to the joint mechanoreceptors. Movement initiates muscle tone readjustment through the reflex center of the spinal cord and lower brain centers. As positions change, the supported movement gives the nervous system an entirely different set of signals to process. The joint sensory receptors can learn not to be so hypersensitive. As a result, any protective spasms and movement restrictions may lessen.

The joint movement also encourages lubrication of the enhanced joint and contributes an important addition to the lymphatic and venous circulations. Much of the pumping action that moves these fluids in the vessels results from compression against the lymph and blood vessels during joint movement and muscle contraction.

The tendons, ligaments, and joint capsule are warmed from the movement. This mechanical effect helps keep these tissues pliable.

Determining Range of Motion

The most important aspect of joint movement is that it is used to assess whether a joint area is functioning effectively. Recall that ROM is the angle through which a joint moves from the anatomical position to the ends of its motion in a particular direction. It is measured in degrees. There is a normal ROM for each joint. Assessment methods that move a joint can determine if a joint can move within a normal ROM. If the joint moves less than the normal range or more than the normal range, a problem may exist. Remember that individuals may vary from "normal or average" without having a problem. Compare each individual ROM to the other side if there is a paired joint. The findings should be similar. If there is a discrepancy from side to side, this is a more accurate assessment than a comparison to "textbook normal."

By comparing what is considered normal ROM for a joint to what the massage client can do, the massage therapist may be able to determine indications for massage intervention or possible referral (Box 8.8).

The range or amount of movement at a joint is determined by these factors:

- The shape of the bones that form the joint
- The tautness or laxness of the ligament and capsule structure of the joint
- The length of the soft tissue structure that supports and moves the joint
- Whether the joint is moving independently of other joints (open chain) or links to other joints in a combined movement (closed chain)

Box 8.9 reviews joint movement.

Box 8.8 Normal Range of Motion for Each Joint

Remember that each person is unique, and many factors influence the available range of motion (ROM). Just because a joint does not have the textbook ROM does not mean that what is displayed is abnormal. Abnormality is indicated by nonoptimal function. This can be either a limit or an exaggeration in the "textbook normal" ROM.

Available ROM is measured from the neutral anatomic position (0). Note: If 0 is listed first, this means movement is away from neutral; if 0 is listed second, it means the joint is moving toward neutral.

Normal values (in degrees):

- Hip flexion: 0–125
- Hip extension: 115–0
- Hip hyperextension: 0–15
- Hip abduction: 0–45
- Hip adduction: 45–0
- Hip lateral (external) rotation: 0–45
- Hip medial (internal) rotation: 0–45
- Knee flexion: 0–130
- Knee extension: 120–0
- Ankle plantar flexion (movement downward): 0–50
- Ankle dorsiflexion (movement upward): 0–20
- Foot inversion (turned inward): 0–35
- Foot eversion (turned outward): 0–25
- Shoulder flexion: 0–90
- Shoulder extension: 0–50
- Shoulder abduction: 0–90
- Shoulder adduction: 90–0
- Shoulder lateral (external) rotation: 0–90
- Shoulder medial (internal) rotation: 0–90
- Elbow flexion: 0–160
- Elbow extension: 145–0
- Elbow pronation: 0–90
- Elbow supination: 0–90
- Wrist flexion: 0–90
- Wrist extension: 0–70
- Wrist abduction: 0–25
- Wrist adduction: 0–65

Elements That Can Cause Joint Dysfunction

Joints have various degrees of ROM. There are anatomical, physiological, and pathological barriers to motion. A barrier is a point of resistance and can feel hard, such as when bone contacts bone or during binding, when soft tissue is short.

Anatomical barriers are determined by the shape and fit of the bones at the joint. The anatomical barrier is seldom reached because the possibility of injury is greatest in this position. Instead, the body protects the joint by establishing physiological barriers.

Physiological barriers are the result of the limits in ROM imposed by protective nerve and sensory function to support optimal function. The sensation at the barrier is soft and pliable.

An adaptation in a physiological barrier that causes the protective function to limit instead of support optimal functioning is called a *pathological barrier*. Pathological barriers often are manifested as stiffness, pain, or a "catch."

Factors that contribute to the pathological condition can occur in these ways:

- If the ligaments and connective tissue that make up the joint capsule are not firm enough to maintain joint space, the joint play is lost.
- If the capsule is too tight, joint play is lost as well. Muscles around a joint can shorten, pulling the bone ends together and affecting joint play.
- If the ligaments and joint capsule are not pliable, flexibility is lost.
- If the ligaments and joint capsule do not support the joint, the fit is disrupted.
- Muscle contraction may pull the joint out of alignment. Muscle groups that flex and adduct the joints are about 30% stronger and have more mass than the extensors and abductors.
- If the body uses muscle contraction to stabilize a joint, the uneven pull between flexors and extensors and adductors and abductors disturbs the fit of the bones at the joint.

Types of Joint Movement Methods

Joint movement involves moving the jointed areas within the client's physiological limits of ROM. The two types of joint movement are active joint movement and passive joint movement:

Box 8.9 Review of Joint Movement

Joints allow us to move. Joint position and velocity receptors inform the central nervous system where and how the body is positioned in gravity and how fast it is moving. These sensory data are the major determining factors for muscle motor tone patterns.

Joint movement techniques focus on the *synovial*, or freely movable, joints in the body. To a lesser extent, these methods can address the joints of the vertebral column, hand, and foot, as well as the facet joints of the ribs, the sacroiliac joint, and the sternoclavicular joint. These joints are not directly influenced by muscles but rather move through indirect muscle action.

We can control some joint movements voluntarily; we can move our limbs through various motions, such as flexion, extension, abduction, adduction, and rotation. These are referred to as *physiologic movements* or *osteokinematic movements*.

For normal physiologic movement, other types of movements (*accessory movements* or *arthrokinematic movements*) must occur as a result of the inherent laxity, or joint play, which exists in each joint. This laxity allows the ends of the bones to slide, roll, or spin smoothly on each other inside the joint capsule. These essential movements occur during movement of the joint and are not under voluntary control.

A good example of joint motion is found on a door:

- The hinge holds the door both to the casing and away from the casing.
- For the door to open and close efficiently (*osteokinematic movement*), the space between the door and the door casing must be maintained and the fit must be correct.
- If the fit of the door in the door casing is incorrect or if the space is not maintained, the door will not open and close correctly.
- Ligaments act as the hinges in the body.
- The door hinge must be oiled. In the joint, the synovial membrane secretes synovial fluid, produced on demand by joint movement.
- If a joint does not move or is not moved, it will lock up like a rusty door hinge, and movement will be restricted or lost.
- If you look closely at a door hinge, you will notice the space around the pin in the hinge.
- If you move the hinge back and forth (not swing the door), the hinge and pin mechanism moves a little *(arthrokinematic movement)*.
- This little movement can be likened to joint play.

Box 8.10 Variations for Joint Movement

Active Joint Movement

In active joint movement, the client moves the area without any type of interaction by the massage practitioner. This is a good assessment method and should be used before and after any type of soft-tissue work, because it provides information about the limits of range of motion (ROM) and the improvement after the work is complete. Active joint movement is also great to teach as a self-help tool.

There are two variations of active joint movement methods: active assisted and active resistive:

- **Active assisted joint movement:** In active assisted joint movement, the client moves the joint through the ROM, and the massage practitioner helps or assists the movement. This approach is especially useful in cases of weakness or pain with movement. The action remains within the comfortable limits of movement for the client. The focus is to create movement within the joint capsule, encouraging synovial fluid lubrication to warm and soften connective tissue and support muscle function.
- **Active resisted (resistive) joint movement:** In active resisted joint movement, the massage practitioner firmly grasps and holds the end of the bone just distal to the affected joint. The massage practitioner leans back slightly to place a small traction on the limb to take up the slack in the tissue. Then the practitioner instructs the client to push slowly against a stabilizing hand or arm while moving the joint through its entire ROM. A tap or light slap against the limb to begin the movement works well to focus the client's attention. The counterforce applied by the massage practitioner does not exceed the pushing or pulling action of the client, but rather matches it and then allows movement.
- **Passive joint movement:** If a client is paralyzed or ill, only passive joint movement may be possible. Some clients do not wish to participate in active joint movement and prefer to take a very passive role during the massage. Client participation is not necessary.

- In *active joint movement* the client moves the joint by active contraction of muscle groups. The two variations of active joint movement are *active assisted movement*, which occurs when both the client and the massage practitioner move the area, and *active resistive movement*, which occurs when the client actively moves the joint against resistance provided by the massage practitioner.
- In *passive joint movement* the client's muscles remain relaxed and the massage practitioner moves the joint with no assistance from the client. When doing passive joint movement, the massage practitioner should feel for the soft or hard end feel of the joint ROM (Box 8.10).

Whether active or passive, joint movements are always done within the comfortable limits of the client's ROM. The client's body must always be stabilized; only the joint being addressed should be allowed to move. Occasionally, the entire limb is moved to allow for coordinated interaction among all the joints of the area, but the rest of the body is stabilized. It is essential to move slowly, because quick changes or abrupt moves may cause the muscles to initiate protective contractions.

Joint-specific work, including any type of high-velocity thrust manipulation, is beyond the scope of practice of the massage professional. Because of the interplay among the joint proprioceptors, muscle tone, innervation of the joint, and surrounding muscles by the same nerve pattern, any damage to a joint can cause long-term problems. Working within the physiological ranges of motion for the particular client is within the scope of practice of the massage professional. Specific corrective procedures for pathological ROM are best applied in a supervised healthcare setting.

Applying Joint Movement Methods

When massage therapists use joint movement techniques, they must remain within the physiological barriers. If a pathological barrier exists that limits motion, techniques are used to gently and slowly encourage the joint structures to increase the limits of ROM to the physiological barrier. If a pathological barrier exists where there is excessive joint motion, techniques are used to gently and slowly encourage the joint structures to reduce the limits of ROM to the physiological barrier.

Hand placement with joint movement is important. Make sure the area is not squeezed, pinched, or restricted in its movement pattern. One hand should be placed close to the joint to act as a stabilizer and allow evaluation. As an alternative method of positioning the stabilizing hand, the jointed area can be moved without stabilization while the massage practitioner observes where the client's body moves most in response to the ROM action. The stabilizing hand then is placed at this point. The other hand is placed at the distal end of the bone; this is the hand that provides the movement. The stabilizing hand must remain in contact with the client and must be placed near the affected joint.

The movements are rhythmic, smooth, slow, and controlled. It is neither necessary nor desirable to have the client's limbs flailing about. During a massage session, strive to move every joint. Joint movement should be incorporated into every massage when possible.

Section Summary

- Explain why joint movement is important to massage application.
  - Joint movement during massage application has many benefits and effects, including assessment of joint ROM, muscle energy technique/stretching positioning, stimulation of joint mechanoreceptors to reduce hypersensitization and muscle guarding, synovial fluid secretion for lubrication, lymph and blood circulation, tendon/ligament/joint capsule pliability. Review Box 8.9.
- Define active and passive joint movement.
  - *Active joint movement:* The client moves the joint. Variations: Active assisted joint movement (both the client and therapist move the joint), active resisted joint movement (the client moves the joint against resistance applied by the therapist). *Passive joint movement:* The therapist moves the joint.

PATHOLOGICAL CONDITIONS OF JOINTS

SECTION OBJECTIVES

Chapter objective covered in this section:

8. Identify pathological conditions of joints and describe general treatment protocols used for intervention.

After completing this section, the learner will be able to:

- Categorize joint pathology based on similar causal factors.
- Describe types of joint injury.
- Define effusion and edema.
- Define seven types of abnormal spinal curvatures.
- List conditions related to backache.

Any process or event that disturbs the normal function of a specific joint usually sets up a chain of events that eventually affects every part of a joint and its surrounding structures. Joint conditions can result from repetitive overuse, inflammatory joint diseases, injuries, and structural deviations, such as kyphosis, lordosis, and scoliosis.

Conditions Caused by Movement

Repetitive Overuse

Constant static stress on the joints, such as occurs in prolonged standing, sitting, or squatting, can damage joint structures. Ligaments subjected to constant tensile loads creep and can undergo excessive lengthening.

Cartilage subjected to constant compressive loading also can creep and may undergo excessive deformation. Joints and their supporting structures subjected to repetitive loading can be injured and fail because they do not have time to recover their original dimensions before they are subjected to another loading cycle. These types of injuries are common in massage therapists, athletes, dancers, musicians, and factory and office workers.

Bursitis

Bursitis is one of the most common causes of joint pain. Inflammation of the bursae—especially those located between the bony prominences and a muscle or tendon, such as in the shoulder, elbow, hip, or knee—usually results from trauma. Repetitive overuse or rheumatoid or gouty arthritis also may cause bursitis. A common treatment includes the use of rest during the acute phase but only for a short time to avoid pathological immobilization. Analgesics and local injections of antiinflammatory medications also can be helpful. Ice can reduce inflammation and pain. Massage that reduces any muscle tension contributing to the development of inflammation and a readjustment of activities to reduce strain on the bursa are beneficial. Often, a postural deviation changes the angle of function at a joint, resulting in irritation at an area of a bursa. Restoring normal postural alignment alleviates the irritation, and the bursitis may resolve itself.

Lateral Epicondylitis (Epicondylosis)

Lateral epicondylitis (tennis elbow) follows the repetitive extension of the wrist or pronation-supination of the forearm. Pain and tenderness develop at the lateral epicondyle and possibly in the proximal extensor muscles. When the wrist is extended against resistance, pain increases. Treatment is for bursitis.

Medial Epicondylitis (Epicondylosis)

Medial epicondylitis (golfer's or pitcher's elbow) follows repetitive wrist flexion, as in throwing. Tenderness is maximal at the medial epicondyle. Wrist flexion against resistance increases the pain. Again, treatment is for bursitis.

INDICATIONS/CONTRAINDICATIONS for Therapeutic Massage

Rest, rehabilitative exercise, ergonomically correct equipment, education, and other similar methods often are used to treat and manage overuse syndromes. Massage can restore and manage some types of connective tissue dysfunctions. Movement modalities, such as active and passive joint movement, can be used to balance movement function and reduce tension patterns.

Inflammatory Joint Disease (Arthritis)

The most common type of joint disorder is termed *arthritis*, which means "inflammation of the joint." Several different kinds of arthritis can occur (Fig. 8.36). The four types of inflammatory joint disease (arthritis) are physical stress-induced, immune-related, crystal-induced, and infectious.

Physical Stress–Induced Arthritis: Degenerative Joint Disease (Osteoarthritis)

Osteoarthritis, or degenerative joint disease, usually first occurs in middle age and progresses with the aging process as a result of normal wear and tear. Although osteoarthritis appears to be a natural result of aging, factors such as obesity, repeated physical stressors, and previous injury without restoration to normal function can help bring it about earlier and more intensely. Osteoarthritis may be a genetic disorder. Although some inflammation may be present, it results from the degenerative process. The disease process involves the growth of new bone (called *spurs* or *osteophytes*) at the edges of the articular surfaces, thickening of the synovial membrane, atrophy of the cartilage, and calcification of the ligaments. Friction increases between the joint surfaces, further increasing the degenerative process. Pain is usually less intense in the morning and steadily worsens throughout the day. Osteoarthritis occurs mostly in joints used in weight bearing, such as the hips, knees, and spinal column, but it can occur in any joint. Previously injured joints tend to develop some arthritis later in life.

In the hands, nodules on the dorsal lateral aspects of the DIP joints, called *Heberden nodes*, result from the bony overgrowth of osteoarthritis. Flexion and deviation deformities may develop. Usually hard and painless, Heberden nodes affect the middle-aged or elderly and often are associated with arthritic changes in other joints.

Methods of treatment include the use of nonsteroidal antiinflammatory drugs (NSAIDs) and pain medications. Nonpharmaceutical interventions include moderate exercise that does not cause pain, the use of ice, and topical counterirritant ointments, such as capsicum-based preparations.

INDICATIONS/CONTRAINDICATIONS for Therapeutic Massage

Therapeutic massage can manage excessive protective muscle spasms that may develop. Gentle traction or distraction methods can provide temporary relief. General systemic changes in the neurotransmitters and hormones that accompany exercise and many forms of massage therapy can elevate mood and thus reduce pain perception.

Immune-Related Arthritis: Rheumatoid and Psoriatic Arthritis

Rheumatoid arthritis is the most common immune-related form of inflammatory joint disease. Rheumatoid arthritis has many characteristics similar to other autoimmune disorders in which antibodies attack normal body tissues. The disease is a crippling condition characterized by swelling of the joints in the hands, feet, and other parts of the body as a result of inflammation and

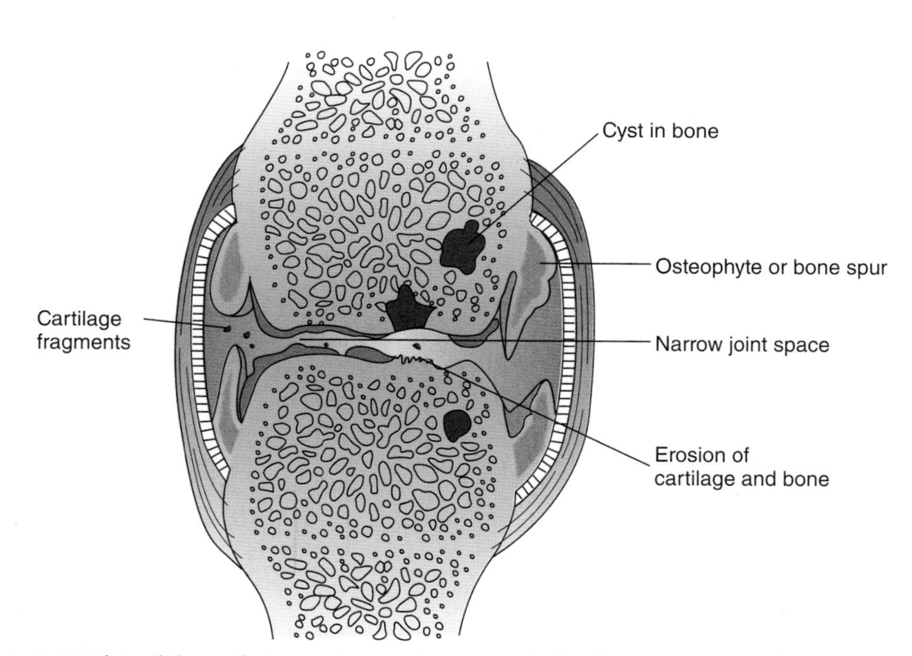

FIG. 8.36 Schematic presentation of the pathologic changes in osteoarthritis. Fragmentation and loss of cartilage denude the subchondral bone, which undergoes sclerosis and cystic change. Osteophytes form on the lateral sides and protrude into the adjacent soft tissues, causing irritation, inflammation, and fibrosis. (From VanMeter KC, Hubert RJ. *Gould's Pathophysiology for the Health Professions*. 5th ed. Elsevier; 2014.)

overgrowth of the synovial membranes and other joint tissues. The disease process changes the composition and quantity of the synovial fluid, altering the lubrication of the joint. The articular cartilage gradually is destroyed, the joint cavity develops adhesions, and the surfaces become stuck together. The joints stiffen and may eventually become useless. The cause of rheumatoid arthritis is uncertain, and the interaction of multiple agents is probable. Genetic factors may influence susceptibility. Psoriatic arthritis occurs when the immune system attacks healthy cells and tissue. The immune response causes inflammation in joints as well as overproduction of skin cells.

Treatment includes the use of various NSAIDs. Disease-modifying antirheumatic drugs (DMARDs) and biologic agents are the standard of care in rheumatoid and psoriatic arthritis and should be used early in the process. The administration of steroids may provide some relief in severe conditions. Localized injection of steroids can reduce severe acute localized symptoms. The use of steroids is controversial, and the benefits do not always outweigh the risks of long-term use.

INDICATIONS/CONTRAINDICATIONS for Therapeutic Massage

Because the progression and flare-ups of the disease are often stress-related, the generalized gentle stress-reduction methods provided by massage therapy may be beneficial in the long-term management of the condition, if supervised as part of a total care program. The practitioner should refrain from performing friction techniques or any other forms of massage therapy that cause inflammation. General systemic changes in the neurotransmitters and hormones that accompany exercise and many forms of massage therapy can elevate mood and thereby reduce pain perception.

Crystal-Induced Arthritis

Gout is a form of arthritis caused by a disturbance of metabolism or underexcretion of uric acid in patients with a relatively normal serum concentration. One of the by-products of metabolism is uric acid, which normally is excreted in the urine. If an overproduction of uric acid occurs or for some reason, an insufficient quantity is excreted, the accumulated uric acid forms crystals, which are deposited as masses around the joints and other parts of the body. Gout is characterized by a painful and tender, hot, dusky-red swelling that extends beyond the margin of the joint. Gout is easily mistaken for cellulitis. Any joint can be involved, but the one most commonly affected is the MTP joint of the great toe. Most victims of gout are men past middle age. Treatment includes dietary modifications and several medications to increase the excretion of uric acid by the kidneys.

INDICATIONS/CONTRAINDICATIONS for Therapeutic Massage

Massage therapy is regionally contraindicated.

Infectious Arthritis

Infectious arthritis can be brought on by infections, such as rheumatic fever, gonorrhea, and tuberculosis. Gonorrheal arthritis is becoming widespread because of the tremendous increase in the number of cases of gonorrhea.

The joints and bones themselves are subject to attack by the tuberculosis organism, and the result may be the gradual destruction of parts of the bone near the joint. The organism is carried by the bloodstream, usually from the lungs or lymph nodes, and may cause considerable damage before being discovered. Several vertebrae sometimes are affected, or one hip or other single joint may be diseased. The client may complain only of difficulty walking, and diagnosis is difficult unless an accompanying lung tuberculosis has been found. This disorder is most common in children. Referral for proper diagnosis is important.

INDICATIONS/CONTRAINDICATIONS for Therapeutic Massage

Infectious disease is a contraindication to massage unless appropriate healthcare professionals directly supervise the massage practitioner.

Conditions Caused by Injury

Joint injuries usually are classified as dislocations and sprains. A *dislocation* is a dislodging of the joint parts. A *sprain* is the wrenching of a joint with rupture or tearing of the ligaments, the joint capsule, or both.

Injury, such as the tearing of a ligament or joint capsule, results in a lack of support for the joint (Fig. 8.37). Instability causes the separation of the articulating bones, with wobbling or deviation from the normal alignment of the bones of the joint. These changes in alignment create an abnormal joint distraction on the side where a ligament is torn. As a result, the other ligaments, tendons, and the joint capsule may become excessively stretched in the area of the injury.

Injury on one side of the joint also can affect the other side by subjecting it to abnormal compression during weight bearing or movement. Compensation in movement patterns,

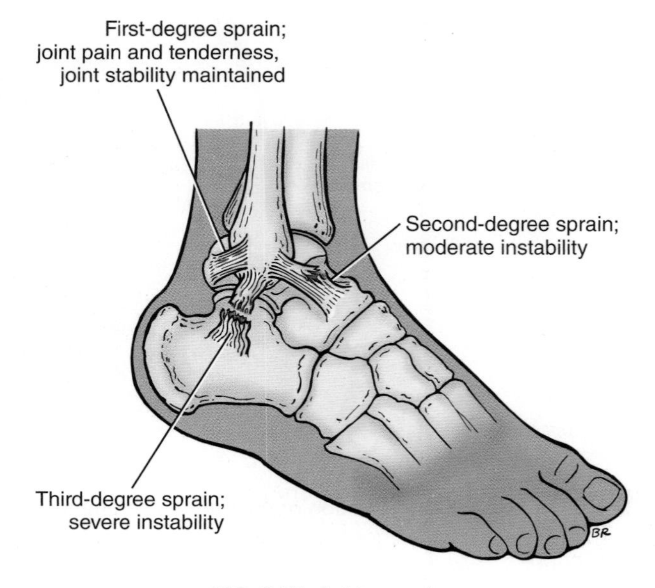

FIG. 8.37 Ankle sprains.

from instability and pain, can result in uneven pressure on the joint. Protective muscle spasms develop, which limit movement. In the short-term acute phase of injury, this action provides effective splinting of the area, but if the restriction in ROM continues, immobilization can result.

Joint injury usually is measured in this way:

- *First degree:* A partial tear (5%) with pain and swelling but with the ability to bear weight and move through the normal ROM.
- *Second degree:* Larger tearing of structures with pain and swelling and inability to bear weight without pain and weakness that compromises ROM. Assessment reveals increased laxity compared with the other side but still has a firm endpoint.
- *Third degree:* Extensive injury to joint structures, including full ligament tears and the inability to bear weight and loss of normal ROM; no obvious endpoint with increased laxity.

Immobilization

Immobilization is detrimental to joint structure and function, and it can be caused by a cast or other form of external restraining mechanism, muscle splinting, as a reaction to pain and inflammation, or paralysis. Immobilization affects the surrounding soft tissues, the articular surfaces of the joint, and the underlying bone. The detrimental effects of immobilization include the development of fibrofatty connective tissue within the joint space; adhesions between the folds of the synovium; atrophy of cartilage; regional osteoporosis; weakening of ligaments at attachment sites; and a decrease in the water content of articular cartilage, tendons, ligaments, and the joint capsule. Swelling or immobilization of a joint also inhibits and weakens the muscles surrounding the joint; therefore the joint is unable to function normally and is at elevated risk for additional injury.

An injured joint subjected to inflammation and swelling assumes a least-packed position of comfort to minimize the pressure within the joint space. Pain decreases in this position. If the joint movement is restricted for a few weeks in the position of comfort, contractures can develop in the surrounding soft tissues and the joint capsule. As a result, the normal range of joint motion is compromised.

Joint Swelling/Effusion and Edema

Swelling is due to fluid accumulation (edema, effusion) or blood accumulation (ecchymosis, bruising). Swollen joints happen when fluid increases in the tissues that surround the joints. Joint swelling is common with different types of arthritis, infections, and injuries. **Effusion** is the term for the accumulation of fluid in a body cavity. The space between the bones enclosed by the joint capsule is a cavity. Therefore, swelling within a joint capsule is effusion. In most cases, this is due to the collection of synovial fluid, but sometimes pus or blood may be within the joint space. The excess fluid hampers normal joint movement as a result of the increased intraarticular pressure caused by joint swelling. The knee is most commonly affected. This fluid can be drained, usually with needle aspiration.

Edema is swelling that occurs outside a joint. Fluid accumulates between the cells (intercellular) and within the tissues. Treatment for edema includes:

- Movement: Moving the legs, especially, may help pump the excess fluid back toward the heart. Elevation: Hold the swollen area above the level of the heart.
- Massage: Stroking the affected area toward the heart using firm but not painful pressure may help move the excess fluid out of the area.
- Compression: Wraps and pressure garments prevent fluid from collecting in the tissue.

INDICATIONS/CONTRAINDICATIONS for Therapeutic Massage

Any type of swelling is an indication of some sort of pathology. The reason for the swelling needs to be determined by a medical professional. It is unlikely that massage can address effusion so it is considered a local caution. Massage may help manage edema. While there are massage methods specialized for managing tissue fluid accumulation, a general massage application is likely sufficient to assist fluid movement.

Temporomandibular Joint and Muscle Disorders

TMJ and muscle disorders are problems that affect the chewing muscles and joints that connect the lower jaw to the skull. Dysfunction with the joint and muscles around it may cause pain and stiffness in the face, jaw, or neck, reduced movement, locking of the jaw, and painful clicking or popping in the jaw. The disk in the joint may be involved. Internal derangement of the joint involves a displaced disk. Injury to the condyles on the mandible may be involved. Trauma to the jaw or TMJ appears to be the cause of TMJ disorders; however, researchers have not identified the exact cause.

INDICATIONS/CONTRAINDICATIONS for Therapeutic Massage

Massage can be used to reduce the stiffness in the muscles and related soft tissue that affect the joint, including tissues of the head, face, cervical area, and shoulders. Caution is required because the area is highly innervated and methods that are too aggressive may increase symptoms. Caution is also necessary to avoid passive movement of the joint, especially lateral deviation to the left and right.

Casts and Splints

Immobilization, such as with casts and splints, is more difficult to handle. Physicians recognize that prolonged immobilization is undesirable and have developed forms of external stabilization that allow mobility. Dynamic movable splinting devices such as air casts and continuous passive motion devices that are capable of moving joints passively and repeatedly through a specified ROM have been beneficial in reducing immobilization in joints.

INDICATIONS/CONTRAINDICATIONS for Therapeutic Massage

Therapeutic massage can be used to maintain pliability in accessible musculature and connective tissue structures. Therapeutic massage methods and movement approaches are beneficial in assisting a return to normal function after the removal of the splinting.

Massage therapy also can aid management of compensatory patterns that develop because of casting and other forms of immobilization. Although direct work over an area that is actively healing is contraindicated unless the massage practitioner is supervised, massage and other forms of soft tissue work, coupled with movement therapies, can manage the tension and possible pain that the rest of the body may develop from the changes in movement; sleeping positions; and other issues caused by the casting, immobilization process, gait changes, and compensation patterns.

Paralysis

In conditions involving paralysis, therapeutic massage helps maintain and in some instances restore the pliability of connective tissues. Joint movement applications can passively replace lost joint movement and mimic compressive forces on the bones and jointed areas, helping prevent contracture and any other detrimental effects of immobilization. Massage intervention for those with paralysis must be supervised as part of a total treatment program. The practitioner must exercise caution when applying pressure and intensity because normal feedback mechanisms are disrupted.

Adhesive Capsulitis (Frozen Shoulder)

Adhesive capsulitis refers to mysterious fibrosis of the glenohumeral joint capsule, manifested by a diffuse, dull, aching pain in the shoulder and progressive restriction of motion but usually no localized tenderness. The condition is usually unilateral and most often occurs in those 50 to 70 years of age, specifically people with diabetes. The onset often is preceded by some sort of pathological condition, resulting in the joint being immobilized. Pathological immobilization sets in. The course is chronic, lasting months to years, but the disorder often resolves itself spontaneously, at least partially. Treatment is with physical therapy, including ROM exercises.

Conditions Caused by Structural Deviations

Abnormal Spinal Curvatures

Abnormal spinal curvatures result from postural deviation. Several types can occur.

- Flattening of the lumbar curve (hypolordosis) accompanied by muscle spasm in the lumbar area and decreased spinal mobility is a combination of signs suggesting the possibility of a herniated lumbar disk or, especially in men, *ankylosing spondylitis.*
- *Hyperlordosis* is an accentuation of the normal lumbar lordotic curve that develops as a result of an excessively anteriorly tilted pelvis. Hyperlordosis also may compensate for a thoracic hyperkyphosis or flexion deformities of the hips.
- *Hyperkyphosis (also called kyphosis)*, a rounded thoracic convexity, is common in aging and occurs, especially in females.
- *Gibbus* is an angular deformity of a collapsed vertebra. Causes include metastatic cancer and tuberculosis of the spine.
- *List* is a lateral tilt of the spine. When a plumb line dropped from the spinous process of T1 falls to one side of the gluteal cleft, a list is present. Causes include a herniated disk and painful spasms of the paravertebral muscles.
- *Scoliosis* is a lateral S or C curvature of the spine and is associated with lateral flexion and rotation of the vertebrae on one another, and the rib cage is deformed accordingly. Structural scoliosis is seen when the client bends forward. On the side of the thoracic convexity, the ribs bulge posteriorly and are separated widely. On the opposite side, the ribs are displaced anteriorly and are close together.
- *Functional scoliosis* compensates for other abnormalities, such as unequal lower limb lengths. The scoliosis disappears with forward flexion.

Conditions Caused by Hypermobility

Hypermobility Spectrum Disorders

Hypermobility spectrum disorders (HSDs) are a collection of connective tissue disorders characterized by joint instability and chronic pain. Fatigue and other systemic symptoms that affect daily functioning may occur, as well. HSDs are diagnosed after other possible conditions have been excluded, such as any of the Ehlers-Danlos syndromes (EDS). The Beighton score is used to identify and diagnose hypermobility. Hypermobility is only considered a disorder when it causes adverse symptoms that affect the quality of life. People with HSDs may experience

- Joint "popping" or "cracking"
- Flat feet
- Frequent ankle sprains
- Back pain
- Widespread aching pain or fibromyalgia
- Osteoarthritis
- Problems with healing (thin scars) or fragile skin
- Easy bruising
- Varicose veins
- Low blood pressure, dizziness when standing up
- Fatigue

Ehlers-Danlos Syndromes

Ehlers-Danlos syndrome, hypermobility type, is a condition that affects the joints. A defect in collagen causes this syndrome.

Marfan Syndrome

Marfan syndrome results from a defect in the gene responsible for building connective tissue fibrillin and elastic fibers. Marfan syndrome includes heart problems, especially those related to the aorta, the large blood vessel that carries blood away from the heart to the rest of the body. Other signs can include sudden lung collapse and eye problems, including severe nearsightedness, dislocated lenses, detached retina, early glaucoma, and early cataracts.

INDICATIONS/CONTRAINDICATIONS for Therapeutic Massage

Hypermobility spectrum disorders are complex and should be managed by an interdisciplinary team. Massage therapy can be helpful. Carefully applied techniques can help manage pain and stiffness without stressing the joints. Avoid stretching beyond the typical joint range of motion. The joints of individuals with hypermobile soft tissues are inherently less stable and require an increased focus on protective stabilization from myofascial structures. General, moderate pressure massage application using a broad-based contact and working across the muscle structures rather than along the fiber direction may provide a sense of tissue lengthening without compromising stability. Bolster to prevent hyperextension. Especially bolster under the abdomen to maintain a neutral position of the spine when in the prone position.

Other Conditions of the Joints

Backache

Backache is a common complaint. Although lower back pain is the most common complaint, neck or cervical pain is also common. The usual cause is muscular and will be discussed in Chapters 9 and 10.

In disorders of the intervertebral disks, pain may be severe, with muscle spasms and the resulting nerve impingement extending symptoms along the course of the nerve to the legs and groin. The condition can degenerate into a ruptured disk, which is most commonly a posterior or posterolateral protrusion of the nucleus pulposus through a tear in the annulus fibrosus, placing pressure on nerves.

Abnormalities of the vertebrae or ligaments and other supporting structures include:

- Strains on the lumbosacral joint (where the lumbar region joins the sacrum) or strains on the sacroiliac joint (where the sacrum joins the ilium).
- Spondylolisthesis, or the moving forward of one vertebra on another, usually occurs at the L5/S1 junction.
- Spondylitis, or inflammation of more than one vertebra.
- Ankylosing spondylitis, or rheumatoid inflammatory disorder, in which the articular hyaline cartilage is destroyed, the bones fuse, and the spinal ligaments ossify. The disease tends to begin in the sacroiliac joints and progress up the spine.
- Spondylosis, or degenerative joint disease (osteoarthritis) of the spine, induces the formation of bony spurs at the disk margin of the vertebral bodies. The disease causes degenerative changes in the intervertebral disks.

INDICATIONS/CONTRAINDICATIONS for Therapeutic Massage

Most backaches are preventable. The back muscles should not be used for lifting. Instead, you should bring the weight close to the body, above the hips if possible, and allow the legs to do the actual lifting. An adequate exercise program is also important.

Massage therapy modalities are effective in managing backache. The benefits derive from a reduction in protective muscle spasm compensation (guarding) and generalized pain-modulating effects. The practitioner should be aware that a protective spasm provides stabilization. The goal is not to eliminate protective spasms totally, but rather to support the body in managing dysfunctional patterns. Complex backache involving the joint structures requires that therapeutic massage be incorporated into a total treatment program, with supervision by the appropriate healthcare professional.

Therapeutic massage can be a beneficial adjunct treatment, especially with the symptomatic management of pain in supporting an increase in ROM.

Ganglia

Ganglia are cystic, round, usually nontender swellings located along tendon sheaths or joint capsules. The dorsum of the hand and wrist is a frequent site of involvement. Flexion of the wrist makes ganglia more prominent, whereas extension tends to obscure them. Ganglia also may develop elsewhere on the hands, wrists, ankles, and feet.

INDICATIONS/CONTRAINDICATIONS for Therapeutic Massage

Massage methods are regionally contraindicated.

JOINT SURGERY AND PROCEDURE OPTIONS

Arthroscopy

Arthroscopy involves small incisions, specialized instruments, and a tiny camera. It is indicated for tears in soft tissues around the knee, hip, shoulder, and other joints. It can be used to repair damaged cartilage and remove broken, free-floating cartilage pieces.

Joint Resurfacing

In joint resurfacing, surgeons replace only one of the three compartments of the knee—the medial (inside), lateral (outside), or patellofemoral (front) compartment—with an implant. In the hip, surgeons replace the hip socket with a metal cup, and the damaged hip ball is reshaped and capped with a metal, dome-shaped prosthesis.

Synovectomy

In conditions involving inflammatory arthritis, the lining of the joints (synovium) becomes inflamed, and overgrowth damages the surrounding cartilage and joints. Surgeons remove most or all of the affected synovium.

Arthrodesis, or Fusion

Surgeons use pins, plates, rods, or other hardware to join two or more bones in the ankles, wrists, thumbs, fingers, or spine, making one continuous joint. Over time the bones grow together and lock the joint in place.

Total Joint Replacement

The damaged joint is replaced with an implant made of combinations of metal, plastic, and/or ceramic components that mimic the motion of the natural joint. Hip and knee joint replacements are most common. Other joints that can be replaced include the shoulders, fingers, ankles, and elbows.

Stem Cells

Mesenchymal stem cells (MSCs) from bone marrow can become cartilage. Treatment involves injecting or implanting the patient's bone marrow concentrate, a rich source of stem cells and growth factors, into damaged areas.

Platelet-Rich Plasma

Platelets are separated from the person's blood, concentrated, and injected into damaged areas, where they reduce inflammation and promote tissue repair. PRP is safe and effective for cartilage tears and relief of osteoarthritis-related knee pain.

Joint Injections or Aspirations

Joint injection is used to place a therapeutic substance into the joint. Joint aspiration is to remove joint fluid from a swelling joint.

Commonly injected substances include:

- Corticosteroids: Antiinflammatory agents that slow down the accumulation of cells responsible for producing inflammation and pain within the joint space
- Hyaluronic acids: Viscous substances that mimic the actions of synovial fluid and may relieve symptoms up to 6 to 12 months

INDICATIONS/CONTRAINDICATIONS for Therapeutic Massage

Avoid the surgical/procedure site during the acute healing phase. Have the client demonstrate the available movement of a replaced, repaired, or treated joint. Do not attempt to increase the joint range of motion with stretching methods. This is especially important with joint replacement. Scar tissue management can begin when the incision area is closed. Do not massage areas where injections have been performed since the injected substance works by being in contact with the joint surfaces.

Section Summary

- Categorize joint pathology based on similar causal factors.
  - *Movement:* Repetitive overuse, bursitis, lateral epicondylitis (tennis elbow), medial epicondylitis (golfer's elbow). *Inflammatory joint disease (arthritis)* (see Fig. 8.36). osteoarthritis (degenerative disc disease), rheumatoid and psoriatic arthritis (immune-related), crystal-induced arthritis (gout), infectious arthritis. *Immobilization:* Swelling, development of fibrofatty connective tissue within the joint space, synovium adhesions, cartilage atrophy, regional osteoporosis, weakening of ligaments, water content decrease of articular cartilage/tendons/ligaments/joint capsule.
- Describe types of joint injury (see Fig. 8.37).
  - *Dislocations:* A dislodging of the joint parts. *Sprain:* Wrenching of a joint with rupture/tearing of the ligaments/joint capsule. Usually measured from mild to severe as first degree, second degree, or third degree.
- Define effusion and edema.
  - *Effusion:* Swelling (fluid accumulation) inside the joint capsule (or body cavity). *Edema:* swelling in soft tissues outside the joint capsule.
- Define seven types of abnormal spinal curvatures.

  (1) *Hypolordosis* (flatback): Flattening/too little lumbar curve. (2) *Hyperlordosis* (swayback): Accentuation/too much lumbar curve. (3) *Hyperkyphosis* (humpback): Rounded/too much thoracic curve. (4) *Gibbus:* Angular deformity of collapsed vertebra. (5) *List:* Lateral tilt of the spine. (6) *Scoliosis:* Lateral S or C curve of the spine. (7) *Functional scoliosis:* Compensation for other abnormalities. Recognize hypermobility spectrum disorders
- Adapt massage to manage stiffness and pain without stressing lax joint structures.
- List conditions related to backache.
  - Degenerated or ruptured disks, lumbosacral or sacroiliac strain, spondylolisthesis (forward movement of vertebra), spondylitis (vertebra inflammation), ankylosing spondylitis (rheumatoid inflammatory disorder), spondylosis (degenerative joint disease/osteoarthritis).

SUMMARY

A comprehensive understanding of joint structure and function is necessary for the effective practice of therapeutic massage for the joints. The massage practitioner can use methods to support joint health and provide benefits in managing joint dysfunction.

The health and strength of joint structures depend on a certain amount of stress and strain. Cartilage and bone nutrition and growth depend on joint movement and muscle contraction. Cartilage nutrition depends on joint movement through a full ROM to ensure that all the articular cartilage receives the nutrients necessary for health. Ligaments and muscles (and their tendons) depend on a normal amount of stress and strain to maintain and increase strength. Bone density and strength increase after the stress and strain created by muscle and joint activity. Bone density and strength decrease when stress and strain are absent.

Without stress and strain, the joints do not function well, but with too much stress and strain a pathological condition may develop. Human beings are similar in that we need to be exposed to challenges in life but attempting to deal with too much can be overwhelming. The concept of balance is illustrated again in joint health and personal well-being.

The author would like to thank Joseph E. Muscolino for his special contributions to this chapter.

Visit the Evolve website: https://evolve.elsevier.com/Fritz/essential/

The Evolve website provides support for the review of the chapter content and chapter quizzes to help you prepare for the MBLEx or other massage therapy certification or licensing exams. End-of-chapter questions for discussion and review answer key and rationales and author's responses to critical thinking and clinical reasoning scenarios are on the Evolve site.

CRITICAL THINKING/CLINICAL REASONING

Each chapter will feature a critical thinking and clinical reasoning application of the content related to massage therapy practice. A client scenario will be presented with recommendations for additional research often using MedlinePlus or PubMed. Relevant questions based on the chapter content outline are provided to guide the discussion. There are no specific current answers to the questions. However, responses should be supportive of evidence-informed practices and based on biological plausibility if sufficient research is not available. The author's decision-making process related to the scenario and questions is on the Evolve site. Compare and contrast your thoughts and discussion with the author and determine where you agree or disagree.

Scenario

The client is a 52-year-old carpenter. The client fell off a roof 15 years ago injured their pelvis and dislocated their right shoulder. Two years ago, the client had right hip replacement surgery and was doing okay. Their knees bother them from being on ladders and working while kneeling. The left knee is worse and has been getting hyaluronic acid injections that are providing moderate relief. Their right elbow bothers them likely from using various carpentry tools. Their low back aches. Three days ago, the client tripped and sprained their left ankle and is walking on it. They have had repeated sprains in the same ankle over the years and the joint is hypermobile. The client hopes that massage therapy will help them be less achy and stiff.

Explore These Sites

- MedlinePlus: *Search terms—osteoarthritis, hip replacement surgery, shoulder dislocation, joint injuries*
- PubMed: *Search terms—regenerative medicine strategies for joints, osteoarthritis and massage therapy*

Discuss These Points

- What are the factors that have predisposed to joint dysfunction?
- What is a logical reason the shoulder joint dislocated during the fall and the hip joint did not?
- When the client fell and injured their pelvis, what would have likely occurred? How would you categorize the type of mechanical force and what type of mechanical stress occurred that eventually led to the hip replacement surgery?
- Both the shoulder and the hip joint were injured during the fall. Which one may assess as hypomobile but more likely is hypermobile and why?
- When the elbow is assessed, tender areas are palpated on both the lateral and medial epicondyle. Where are these landmarks? What are two common joint pathologies related to these areas?
- During the palpation assessment, the client indicated tenderness just inferior to the posterior superior iliac spine. What joint is located in this area and how might dysfunction in this joint relate to the low back aching?
- How are standing on the ladder and swinging a hammer similar in causing joint injury?
- In a joint movement sequence on the left lower limb, what joints are being moved, and what movements are occurring at those joints?
- How might the assessment of joint movement differ on the left lower limb versus the right lower limb?
- What cautions are needed for working on the right hip?
- What is the purpose of the knee injections?
- Which of the conditions the client is experiencing would be considered an acute injury?
- Palpation just distal to the left tibiofibular joint indicates some edema and tenderness. What would be the logical reason for this finding, and are any adaptations to massage indicated?

MULTIPLE-CHOICE QUESTIONS FOR REVIEW AND DISCUSSION

The answers, with rationales, can be found on the Evolve site.

These questions are used for review and discussion. It is as important to understand why wrong answers are wrong as it is to know why the correct answer is correct. The answers to the questions, with rationales and explanations about why the correct answer is correct and why wrong answers are wrong, can be found on the Evolve site. Guidance also is provided on how questions are developed and how the textbook content can be presented in a multiple-choice question format. At the end of the question section here in the textbook, you will find an Exercise that asks you to write more questions. Use the various questions in the chapter as examples. This is one of the best study strategies for test taking.

It is important to understand that the actual licensing exam you take may not contain any of the specific questions found in this textbook or the review material and practice tests on the Evolve site. Therefore, just because you can answer any of these questions correctly does not mean you will pass the licensing exam. The questions are content and style examples to help you prepare—this is why understanding why wrong answers are wrong is just as important as identifying the correct answer. Also, make sure you understand all the terminology used in the questions and possible answers in the review and discussion questions. Look up words you do not understand.

1. Massage methods that move the body most influence which of the following?
   a. Synarthrosis joints
   b. Synchondrosis joints
   c. Synovial joints
   d. Interosseous ligaments
2. A client reports spraining a knee when hit on the lateral side, resulting in a convex position of the medial collateral ligament. Which of the following stresses best describes the injury to the ligament?
   a. Shear
   b. Compression
   c. Tension
   d. Torsion
3. Which of the following would describe the movement of the ribs during inspiration?
   a. The ribs are rotated.
   b. The ribs are depressed.

c. The ribs are fixed.
d. The ribs are elevated.

4. Joint function is a relationship between ______.
a. Bones and landmarks
b. Stability and mobility
c. Articulations and diarthroses
d. Synovial fluid and pathological range of motion

5. Joints in which stability is reduced because of increased laxity of supportive ligaments also have an increase in ______.
a. Joint play
b. Hypomobility
c. Muscle relaxation
d. Plasma membrane

6. A client sprained a joint in one finger. What is going to be the most comfortable position for the joint and why?
a. The closed-packed position is the most stable position of the joint
b. The loose-packed position so that movement can occur most easily
c. The loose-packed position to accommodate swelling
d. The closed-packed position to accommodate increased synovial fluid

7. During the massage session, passive joint movement is used for assessing the range of motion of the arm during circumduction. Which of the following best describes the action used during this process?
a. Bending movement that reduces the angle of a joint
b. Movement of the arm medially toward the midline of the body
c. Twisting and turning of a bone on its own axis
d. Combined movements of flexion, extension, abduction, and adduction to create a cone shape

8. During assessment you want the client to rotate the hip externally. What instructions would you give the client?
a. Please move your leg so that you cross it over the other leg at the ankles.
b. Please straighten your legs and turn the entire leg so that you point your toes toward each other.
c. Please straighten your legs and turn the entire leg so that you point your toes away from each other.
d. Please bring your knee toward your chest.

9. If an injury to the sternoclavicular joint limits its range of motion, what other structure will be affected?
a. Radius
b. Olecranon
c. Scapula
d. Deltoid ligament

10. A client continues to sprain the ankles. You notice that the client wears boots with a 2-inch heel. How would this contribute to injury potential?
a. The heel positions the ankle in dorsiflexion, making the ankle joint less stable.
b. The heel positions the ankle in plantar flexion, making the ankle joint less stable.
c. The weight is shifted to the ball of the foot, creating an open kinematic chain.
d. The inferior tibiofibular joint is extended when the heel is raised, creating instability.

11. Which movement of the vertebral joints is most stabilized by the anterior longitudinal ligament?
a. Extension
b. Flexion
c. Rotation
d. Lateral flexion

12. The loose-packed position of the hip joint is _____.
a. Flexion, abduction, and lateral rotation
b. Extension, adduction, and medial rotation
c. Flexion, adduction, and lateral rotation
d. Extension, abduction, and lateral rotation

13. If the leg is fixed and does not move and the pelvis moves forward into anteversion, what is the result?
a. Increased kyphosis
b. Increased lordosis
c. Decreased lordosis
d. Decreased scoliosis

14. The most stable position of the knee joint is ______.
a. In slight flexion
b. In full hyperextension
c. In locked extension
d. In locked flexion

15. A client playing football was tackled. Pressure was put on the lateral side of the left knee. Which ligament would receive the most extension strain?
a. Lateral collateral
b. Medial collateral
c. Posterior cruciate
d. Posterior meniscofemoral

16. Which of the following pathological conditions of the joints responds most positively to massage?
a. Dislocation
b. Rheumatoid arthritis
c. Lateral epicondylitis
d. Kyphosis

17. A client has been participating in a stretching program for more than a year. Initially, the program was helpful, but during the last 3 months the program has become more aggressive and the client is complaining of joint pain. Which alteration in connective tissue may explain what has occurred?
a. The client has experienced a rupture in the connective tissue structures and has developed lax ligaments.
b. The client has exceeded the limits of the elastic range of the tissue, consistently deformed the tissue in the plastic range, and developed lax ligaments.
c. An avulsion failure of connective tissue has occurred, creating a decrease in mobility.
d. The tissue has become dehydrated, increasing creep tendency and contributing to the stability provided by muscle contraction.

18. A client complains of a feeling of shortening and pulling in the area of the lower back and sacroiliac joints. Assessment indicates decreased pliability in the connective tissue structures in this area. Which of the following massage applications is most appropriate to achieve an increase in short-term mobility without compromising stability or creating a remodeling process of the tissue?
    a. Application of massage methods that slowly introduce creep, increasing pliability at the plastic range of the tissue
    b. Application of therapeutic inflammation coupled with stretching to exceed the plastic range of the tissue
    c. Application of elongation stretching to breach the plastic range of the tissue, creating inflammation to restore an appropriate creep pattern
    d. Application of abrupt bending of the connective tissue to support the increase in ligament laxity, thereby increasing mobility
19. A client has been diagnosed with a hypermobile knee joint. Which of the following would be part of an appropriate treatment plan?
    a. Extend the elastic range of connective tissue structures by altering the plastic range
    b. Elongate the plastic component of connective tissue in the direction of the shortening
    c. Restore pliability using stretching at the joint end range.
    d. Manage muscle contraction around the joint using standard massage methods
20. A client is experiencing muscle spasms and reduced mobility around a shoulder joint that has a history of dislocation. Which of the following applications of massage would be best in assisting this client?
    a. Increase the plastic range of the ligament structures and stretched tense muscles
    b. Use friction on tendons and ligaments, and then incorporate a stretching program to increase flexibility
    c. Reduce muscle spasms to the point that mobility is supported but stability is not compromised
    d. Use massage methods and stretching to eliminate muscle spasms

CHAPTER 9 Muscles

https://evolve.elsevier.com/Fritz/essential/

CHAPTER OBJECTIVES

After completing this chapter, the learner will be able to:

1. Explain the various terminologies used to describe muscles.
2. Describe the relationship between the structure and the function of muscles.
3. Describe the anatomy and physiology of skeletal muscle fibers.
4. List the components of myotatic units.
5. Identify the different muscle shapes and fiber arrangements.
6. Describe the response of proprioceptors to stimuli and the most common reflexes.
7. Identify the energy source for muscle contraction.
8. Describe the integrated connective tissue structure of muscle.
9. Explain and demonstrate the three types of muscle actions.
10. Describe how muscles are named.
11. Learn how to palpate individual muscles.
12. Identify the attachments, actions, synergists, and antagonists of individual muscles.
13. Identify common pathology related to muscles and explain indications and contraindications for massage.

CHAPTER OUTLINE

KEY TERMS

agonist: (AG-on-ist) A muscle that causes or controls joint motion through a specified plane of motion; also known as a ***mover***.

all-or-none response: The property by which a muscle fiber (cell), when stimulated to contract, contracts to its full ability or does not contract at all.

antagonist: (an-TAG-a-nist) A muscle usually located on the opposite side of a joint from the mover (agonist) and having the opposite action. The antagonist must lengthen when the mover contracts and shortens.

aponeurosis: (a-po-new-RO-sis) A broad, flat sheet of fibrous connective tissue.

biotensegrity: A concept that the bones of the skeletal system are held together by tension forces produced from interrelated muscular and fascial chains.

concentric action: (kon-SEN-trik) A contraction in which the muscle shortens with tone because its contractile force is greater than the opposing force at the attachments of the muscle. Concentric contractions are contractions of a mover (agonist) wherein it creates the movement of a body part.

contractility: (kon-trak-TIL-i-tee) The ability of a muscle to shorten forcibly with adequate stimulation. This property sets muscle apart from all other types of tissue.

deep fascia: (FAY-shee-a) A coarse sheet of fibrous connective tissue that binds muscles into functional groups and forms partitions, called ***intermuscular septa***, between muscle groups.

dynamic force: Force applied to an object that produces movement in or of the object.

eccentric action: (ek-SEN-trik) A contraction in which the muscle lengthens with tone because its contractile force is less than the opposing force at the attachments of the muscle. Eccentric contractions are contractions of an antagonist that usually restrain or control the action of the prime mover. Eccentric contractions sometimes are described as negative contractions.
elasticity: The ability of a muscle to recoil and resume its original resting length after being stretched.
excitability: The ability of a muscle to receive and respond to a stimulus.
extensibility: (eks-ten-si-BIL-i-tee) The ability of a muscle to be stretched or extended.
fascia: (FAY-shee-a) A fibrous or loose type of connective tissue; a fibrous membrane covering, supporting, and separating muscles; the subcutaneous tissue that connects the skin to the muscles.
fixator: (FIK-say-tor) A stabilizing muscle located at a joint or body part that contracts to fix, or stabilize, the area, enabling another limb or body segment to exert force and move. The fixator also may be described as a muscle (or other force) that stops one attachment of a muscle from moving so that the other attachment of the muscle must move.
insertion: The attachment of a muscle that moves (or usually moves) when the muscle contracts. The insertion of a muscle is usually the distal attachment of the muscle. For muscles located on the axial body, the insertion is usually the superior attachment of the muscle or the part of the muscle that attaches farthest from the midline, or center, of the body.
isometric action: (i-so-MET-rik) A contraction in which the muscle stays the same length with tone because its contractile force equals that of the opposing force at the attachments of the muscle. The muscle tenses but does not produce movement. Isometric contractions are usually contractions of a fixator/stabilizer muscle (or neutralizer muscle) that acts to stabilize or fix a body part in position while another joint action is occurring.
isotonic action: (i-so-TON-ik) The action of the muscle that occurs when tension develops in the muscle while it shortens or lengthens.
loading: The application of a mechanical load or force.
maximal stimulus: The point at which all motor units of a muscle have been recruited and the muscle is unable to increase in strength.
mechanotransduction: (me-can-o-trans-DUC-shun) The ability to convert mechanical force into neurochemical signals, forming a body-wide communication network.
motor unit: A motor neuron and all the muscle fibers it controls.
muscle synergies: The coordinated recruitment of a group of muscles.
myofascia: Integrated fascial, extracellular matrix, and muscle tissue organized as an interconnected structure that surrounds groups of muscles, the limbs, and the entire body.
myoglobin: (MI-oh-glo-ben) A red pigment similar to hemoglobin that stores oxygen within the muscle cells.
origin: The attachment of a muscle that does not move (or usually does not move) when the muscle contracts. The origin of a muscle is usually the proximal attachment of the muscle. For muscles located on the axial body, the origin is usually the inferior attachment of the muscle or the part of the muscle that attaches closest to the midline, or center, of the body.
oxygen debt: The extra amount of oxygen that must be taken in to remove the buildup of lactic acid from anaerobic respiration of glucose (to convert lactic acid to glucose or glycogen).
resting tone: The state of tension in resting muscles.
reverse action: An action in which a muscle contracts and the attachment that normally stays fixed (the origin) moves, and the attachment that usually moves (the insertion) stays fixed.
sliding filament mechanism: The process describing skeletal muscle contraction in which the thick and thin filaments slide past one another.
static force: Force applied to an object in such a way that it does not produce movement.
synergist: (SIN-er-jist) Movers of a joint other than the prime mover(s); that is, assistant, secondary, or emergency movers. A synergist may be more broadly defined as any muscle that helps the action occur (i.e., also may be a fixator, neutralizer, or support muscle, as well as other movers).
threshold stimulus: The stimulus at which the first observable muscle contraction occurs.
trigger point: A hyperirritable locus (point or place) within a taut band of skeletal muscle, located in the muscular tissue or its associated fascia. The spot is painful on compression and can evoke characteristic referred pain and autonomic phenomena.

LEARNING HOW TO LEARN

Volumes have been written about the intricacies of soft tissue structure and function. This text, by necessity, limits itself to the most functionally practical information related to the methods used by massage therapists. As a massage student (and, subsequently, a practitioner) you will find it helpful to continue both formal study and self-study of this material.

According to the learning theory of Bloom's Taxonomy, we go through a learning process:

- First we learn to remember.
- Next, we learn the same information to understand.
- Once we understand, we can apply what we have learned.
- Understanding allows us to analyze, evaluate, and create.

We must be patient while learning about muscles. Repetition is the key, and each time we repeat the content, we move closer to understanding and applying the information.

Muscles and their associated connective tissue make up the soft tissues of our bodies. Using artistic terms, you could say that muscles and connective tissue are the art medium of massage practitioners. Just as a sculptor needs to understand clay, the massage therapist needs to understand muscles. Because soft tissue accounts for about half the tissue mass of the body and most pain patterns find themselves connected to soft tissue dysfunction of various types, careful study of this area of anatomy and physiology obviously is important.

When studying anatomy and physiology, we must continue to see the body as a whole, in structure and function, and this is especially true in the study of the muscles. Physiologically, one muscle does not operate independently of others. Structural design knits together the muscles, bones, and connective tissue structures into intertwining spans that are necessary for stability and mobility. To assist you in learning about muscles, this chapter breaks the anatomy into isolated segments. Chapter 10 then puts all these pieces back together so that you can better understand how to apply the information in massage therapy treatments.

The body has three types of muscle tissue: skeletal muscle, cardiac muscle, and smooth muscle. This chapter focuses on skeletal muscle tissue and provides a brief overview of cardiac and smooth muscle. In addition, there is a focus on the importance of connective tissue, especially the fascial relationship to muscle structure and function. Terminology is important and sometimes confusing, so the chapter begins with that discussion.

TERMINOLOGY

SECTION OBJECTIVES

Chapter objective covered in this section:

1. Explain the various terminologies used to describe muscles.

After completing this section, the student will be able to:

- Explain the importance of the Terminologia Anatomica.
- Use muscle attachment terminology based on both anatomy and physiology.

Anatomical terminology for muscle names and attachments is sometimes confusing. Terminology used for the muscular system is not always consistent. Multiple names and spellings for muscle names, and duplicate terminology to describe the location of muscles, exist. Additionally, muscular terminology can vary from country to country, depending on the language (Box 9.1).

Box 9.1 Why It Is Confusing

The following are just a few examples of the ways terminology can become confusing.

Muscle Name Variations

Musculus deltoideus (derived from Latin and German)
Deltoid (English)
Which is correct: deltoideus or deltoid?

Multiple Names for the Same Muscles

Peronealis (derived from Latin and German)
Fibularis (derived from Latin and German)
Peroneal (English)
Fibular (English)
Which is correct: peronealis, peroneal, fibularis, or fibular?
Venter frontalis musculus occipitofrontalis (derived from Latin and German)
Venter frontalis musculi occipitofrontalis (derived from Latin and German)
Frontal belly of occipitofrontalis (English)
Frontalis (English)
Frontal part of occipitofrontalis
Which is correct? There are five different names.

Word Sequence Issues

Musculus serratus posterior inferior (derived from Latin and German)
Serratus posterior inferior (English)
Inferior serratus posterior (English)
Which is correct: inferior at the beginning or at the end, and posterior in the middle or at the end?

Muscle Attachment Terminology

Origin/insertion
Proximal/distal
Arises from/attaches to
From/to
Which is correct? Consultation with anatomy experts yielded this response: "It depends." All the terms are correct, even if confusing.

International Anatomical Terminology

The *Terminologia Anatomica* (TA) is the international standard on human anatomical terminology. The revision of modern anatomical terminology was initiated in 1887. More than 100 years later, the *Terminologia Anatomica: International Anatomical Terminology* was finally accepted by the International Federation of Associations of Anatomists in 1997 and published in 1998 and revised in 2019 (FIPAT, 2019). This means that all medical practitioners (traditional and complementary) in every country around the world now have a common terminology. The problem is that the common terminology is not used consistently. Anatomical terminology is the foundation of medical terminology, and Latin is the international anatomical language. Only Latin is the international basis for creating equivalent terms in other languages. English is not the basis for terminology in other languages, yet many commonly used terms are English.

The International Federation of Associations of Anatomists (IFAA) website can be informative (https://ifaa.net/).

TERMINOLOGIA ANATOMICA The Federative International Programme for Anatomical Terminology is found at: https://fipat.library.dal.ca/TA2/.

Muscle Attachment Terminology

Muscles and associated connective tissues must be attached directly or indirectly to bone to produce movement. The terms most commonly used in the past to describe muscle attachments to the bone or other tissue are **origin** and **insertion**. Classically, the *origin* of a muscle has been defined as the attachment that does not move when the muscle contracts; he rigin is usually the proximal attachment or the attachment closer to the midline or center of the body. The *insertion* has been defined as the attachment that does move when the muscle contracts; the insertion is usually the distal attachment or the attachment farther from the midline or center of the body. Origin and insertion terminology is a *physiological description* of a muscle's attachments because it names an attachment on the basis of whether or not it moves

Unfortunately, this terminology can lead to confusion about the structural locations of muscles and the ways in which muscles really function. The problem with this terminology is that it can create an impression that one attachment of a muscle is always fixed and that the other attachment always moves. Origins and insertions of muscles often switch; that is, the insertion could stay fixed while the origin moves. When this situation occurs, the movement is called a **reverse action**. Simple examples of reverse actions are when the biceps brachii contracts and causes the arm to move toward the forearm (instead of the forearm moving toward the arm), as when a person is doing a chin-up; or when the quadriceps femoris group contracts and causes the thigh to move toward the leg (instead of the leg moving toward the thigh), as when standing up from a seated position.

In an effort to simplify the learning and understanding of muscles, their attachments and actions, a simpler terminology is slowly becoming more widespread and accepted; this involves naming the attachments of a muscle by the locations of the attachments. This system would be an *anatomical naming system*. For example, the attachments of the biceps brachii on the scapula would be called the *proximal attachments*, and the attachment onto the forearm would be called the *distal attachment*. There has also been an attempt to use "arises from" and "attaches to" or, even more simply, "from" and "to."

Based on this information, muscle attachments can be stated in this way:

- Origin/insertion: Based on physiology or function
- Fixed end/mobile end: Based on physiology or function
- Proximal/distal: Based on anatomy or structure
- Arises from/attaches to: Based on anatomy or structure

This textbook includes all the ways attachments can be stated. It may be cumbersome, but it is the only way to be accurate. The most proximal (origin) attachment is typically listed first. Here is how the attachment terminology appears in the individual muscle sections that follow:

- Origin, fixed end, proximal attachment, arises from
- Insertion, mobile end, distal attachment, attaches to

Section Summary

- Explain the importance of the *Terminologia Anatomica*.
  - The TA creates a standard common terminology for all medical practitioners (traditional and complementary).
- Use muscle attachment terminology based on both anatomy and physiology.
  - Tendons attach muscles to bones. These attachments have multiple names based on their physiology/function, or anatomy/structure. (Origin/insertion: physiology/function). (Fixed end/mobile end: physiology/function). (Proximal/distal: anatomy/structure). (Arises from/attaches to: anatomy/structure). Correlated terms: (Origin—fixed end, proximal attachment, arises from), (Insertion—mobile end, distal attachment, attaches to).

FOCUS ON PROFESSIONALISM

Change often happens slowly. Terminology is an example. The terms "origin" and "insertion" have not been recommended by the *Terminologia Anatomica* since the late 1990s. Yet these terms, used to identify attachment points for muscles, persist. The only way this author has found to deal with this issue is to list all the terms in use. This is tedious but the most accurate approach. For muscle attachment terminology, this means all of the following terms are correct: proximal/distal, fixed end/mobile end, origin/insertion, arises from/attaches to. Generally (but not always) proximal, fixed end, origin and arises from can be used interchangeably. Distal, mobile end, insertion and attaches to can also be used interchangeably.

Actually, terminology is problematic in many areas. Recommended massage therapy terminology has also changed. The Entry Level Analysis Project (ELAP) has recommended a more generic terminology. You can read more at the ELAP website (www.elapmassage.org). So, what do we do? As a massage therapy professional, you need to remain current when terminology changes and be patient while the shift in usage occurs. Sometimes we need to speak multiple "terminology languages."

MUSCLE STRUCTURE AND FUNCTION

SECTION OBJECTIVES

Chapter objectives covered in this section:

2. Describe the relationship between the structure and the function of muscles.
3. Describe the anatomy and physiology of skeletal muscle fibers.
4. List the components of myotatic units.
5. Identify the different muscle shapes and fiber arrangements.
6. Describe the response of proprioceptors to stimuli and the most common reflexes.
7. Identify the energy source for muscle contraction

After completing this section, the student will be able to:

- List the three types of muscle.
- List and describe the major functions of muscle.
- Describe types of muscle actions.
- Identify the energy source for muscle contraction.
- Explain the difference between red slow-twitch and white fast-twitch muscle fibers.
- List the components of myotatic units.
- Describe reflexes related to muscle function.

A prominent functional characteristic of muscle tissue is its ability to transform chemical energy from adenosine triphosphate (ATP) into mechanical energy. When this happens, muscle cells can exert force. Recall that force is energy applied in such a way that it initiates motion, changes the speed or direction of a motion, or alters the size and shape of an object.

Energy is defined technically as the capacity to do work. When a muscle contracts, muscle tissue transforms one form of energy into another and is able to produce force. **Dynamic force** creates movement and change; **static force** produces no movement or noticeable change but still expends energy.

The Muscle Organ

The muscular system is a body organ system. Recall that chemicals combine to make molecules, molecules combine to make cells, cells combine to make tissues, tissues combine to make organs, organs combine to make systems, and systems combine to make us. A whole skeletal muscle is considered an organ of the muscular system. Each muscle organ consists of skeletal muscle tissue, connective tissue, nerve tissue, and blood or vascular tissue. The correct terminology for an individual skeletal muscle would be *muscle organ*, but it is usually shortened to the term *muscle*. Skeletal muscles vary considerably in size, shape, and arrangement of fibers. They range from extremely tiny strands (e.g., the stapedium muscle of the middle ear) to large masses (e.g., the muscles of the thigh). Some skeletal muscles are broad in shape, and some are narrow. In some muscles the fibers are parallel to the long axis of the muscle; in some muscles they converge to a narrow attachment; and in some muscles they are oblique.

The Three Types of Muscles and Their Functions

The functions of the three muscle types—smooth, cardiac, and skeletal—are integral to the maintenance of homeostasis of the whole body. Skeletal, cardiac, and smooth muscles produce movement, such as that involved in breathing, the heartbeat, digestion, and elimination. All three types of muscle tissue produce the movement necessary for survival. Skeletal muscle moves the skeleton at the joints so that we can seek shelter, gather food, and protect ourselves.

Function of Skeletal Muscle

The four major functions of skeletal muscle are to:

- Produce movement
- Stabilize joints
- Maintain posture
- Generate heat

Stabilization of joint structures is an often-overlooked function of muscle. The dynamic and static contraction of muscles surrounding the joint provides external stability, supporting the structures of the joint. This is especially true of the more mobile joints, which by nature have a loose structural design. To maintain stable body posture, the dynamic tension of muscle contraction opposes the force of gravity. The relative constancy of the internal temperature of the body is maintained in a cool external environment by the heat generated as a by-product of muscle tissue contraction.

Muscle as an Endocrine Organ

Skeletal muscle, triggered by exercise, behaves as an endocrine organ. Several molecules, secreted by muscle (myokines) and adipose tissues (adipokines) in response to exercise, are involved in bone metabolism. Myokines released by contracting skeletal muscles interface with inflammatory and antiinflammatory networks and support a systemic antiinflammatory response. Myokines affect visceral fat and glucose and lipid metabolism. This may be part of the reason exercise produces beneficial effects (Lombardi et al., 2016; Chung and Choi, 2018; Pratesi et al., 2018; Yang et al., 2022).

Function of Cardiac and Smooth Muscle Tissue

Cardiac and smooth muscle tissues operate by mechanisms similar to those in skeletal muscle tissues.

Cardiac Muscle

Cardiac muscle (Fig. 9.1A), also known as *striated involuntary muscle*, is found in only one organ of the body—the heart. Forming the bulk of the wall of each heart chamber, cardiac muscle contracts rhythmically and continuously to provide the pumping action necessary to maintain a consistent blood flow through our internal environment.

The functional anatomy of cardiac muscle tissue resembles that of skeletal muscle but has specialized features related to the role of pumping blood continuously. Each cardiac muscle fiber contains parallel myofibrils composed of sarcomeres that give the whole fiber a striated appearance. However, the cardiac muscle fiber does not taper, as does a skeletal muscle fiber; rather, it forms strong, electrically coupled junctions (intercalated disks) with other fibers.

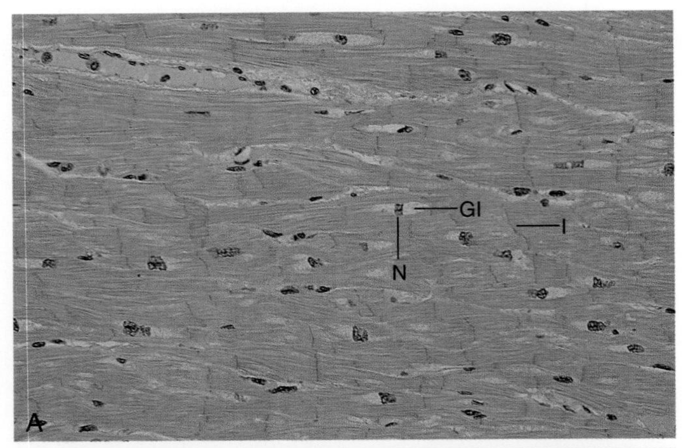

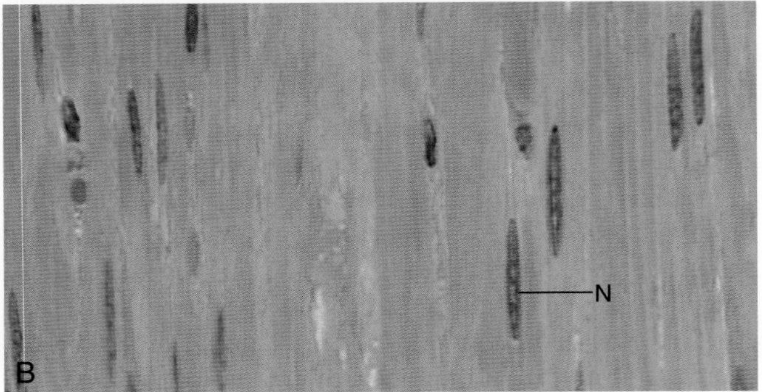

FIG. 9.1 (A) Micrograph of cardiac muscle. The intercalated disks *(I)* are characteristic of cardiac muscle. *N*, nuclei. *GI*, glycogen deposits. (B) Micrograph of smooth muscle. The central placement of nuclei *(N)* in the spindle-shaped smooth muscle fibers is notable. (From Gartner LP, Hiutt JL. *Color Textbook of Histology*. 3rd ed. Saunders; 2007.)

The cardiac muscle forms a continuous contractile band around the heart that conducts a single impulse across a continuous sarcolemma, allowing for an efficient, coordinated pumping action. This means that even though many adjacent cardiac muscle cells contract simultaneously, they have a prolonged contraction rather than a rapid twitch. Cardiac muscle does not normally run low on ATP and thus does not experience fatigue. This characteristic of cardiac muscle is vital for keeping the heart pumping continuously.

Unlike skeletal muscle, in which a nervous impulse is necessary to excite the sarcolemma to produce its impulse, cardiac muscle can be self-exciting. Cardiac muscle cells can have a continuing rhythm of excitation and contraction on their own, although the rate of self-induced impulses is usually too slow to allow for strenuous activity. Central nervous system control of the heart is normal and is necessary for strenuous activity and for generally altering the rate of heart contractions to meet the demands placed on the heart.

Smooth Muscle. Smooth muscle comprises small, tapered cells with single nuclei (see Fig. 9.1B). Smooth muscle fibers lack striations because the thick and thin myofilaments are arranged differently from skeletal or cardiac muscle fibers. These arrangements of myofilaments crisscross the cell and attach at their ends to the plasma membrane of the cell.

When cross-bridges pull the thin filaments together, the muscle balls up and thus contracts the cell. Because the myofilaments are not organized into sarcomeres, they have more freedom of movement and can contract a smooth muscle fiber to shorter lengths than in skeletal and cardiac muscle.

The two types of smooth muscle tissue are visceral muscle and multiunit muscle. In visceral or single-unit muscles, gap junctions join individual smooth muscles into large, continuous sheets, much like the fibers observed in cardiac muscle. Visceral muscle is the most common type of smooth muscle and forms the muscular layer in the walls of many hollow structures, such as in the digestive, urinary, and reproductive tracts.

Similar to cardiac muscle, visceral smooth muscle commonly has a rhythmic self-excitation, or autorhythmicity (meaning self-rhythm), that spreads across the entire tissue. When these rhythmic, spreading waves of contraction become strong enough, they can push the contents of a hollow organ progressively along its lumen (the interior of a tubular structure). This type of contraction, called *peristalsis*, moves food along the digestive tract, assists the flow of urine to the bladder, and pushes a baby out of the uterus during labor. Such contractions also can be coordinated to produce mixing movements in the stomach and other organs.

Multiunit smooth muscle tissue does not function as a single unit as does visceral muscle; instead, it is composed of many independent, single-cell units. Each independent fiber does not generate its own impulse, but rather responds only to nervous input. Although this type of smooth muscle can form thin sheets, as in the walls of large blood vessels, it more often is found in bundles (e.g., the erector pili muscles of the skin) or as single fibers, such as those surrounding small blood and lymph vessels.

Functional Characteristics of Muscles

Muscles have four functional characteristics (Activity 9.1).

1. **Excitability** is the ability to receive and respond to a stimulus. A stimulus is a change in the internal or external environment. One of the major reasons massage applications are beneficial is that they provide specific forms of stimulus to the muscles through the application of mechanical forces and with movement, which help maintain homeostasis.
2. **Contractility** is the ability to shorten forcibly with adequate stimulation. This property sets muscle apart from all other types of tissue. As mentioned earlier, muscle tissue interacts with all body systems, but it makes a unique contribution. The ability to contract allows the entire body to move, as well as certain parts of the body, such as the digestive tract.
3. **Extensibility** is the ability to be stretched or extended. In a typical movement pattern, one group of muscles contracts (concentrically shortens), whereas the group that has opposing actions lengthens. Because of this, the integrated functions of stability, balance, and the ability to return to a neutral position occur.
4. **Elasticity** is the ability to recoil and resume the original resting length after being stretched.

A number of systems support muscle tissue functions.

- The nervous system directly controls the contraction of skeletal muscle and smooth muscle and also influences the rate of rhythmic contraction in cardiac muscle and visceral smooth muscle.
- The endocrine system produces hormones that promote repair of muscle tissue and assist the nervous system in regulating muscle contraction throughout the body.
- The blood delivers nutrients and carries away waste products.
- Nutrients for the muscles come from the digestive system. For example, the energy for muscle contraction is ATP; glucose is the fuel for the manufacture of ATP. Potassium and insulin are required for glucose to enter the muscle cell.
- The digestive, respiratory, and urinary systems eliminate the waste products of muscle metabolism. Lactic acid, an end product of intense muscle activity, can be broken down within the muscle cell by the Krebs cycle or can be transported by the bloodstream to the liver to be converted back to glucose. These processes use oxygen.
- The immune system helps defend muscle tissue against infection and cancer, as it does for all body tissues.

ACTIVITY 9.1

On a separate piece of paper, using the functional characteristics of muscle as an analogy, provide examples of the ways in which your learning thus far has functioned like a muscle. Examples are provided to get you started.

Examples

Excitability: The ability to receive and respond to a stimulus.
Learning the names of the muscles is a new stimulus.

Contractility: The ability to shorten forcibly and produce movement when adequately stimulated.
Using the information about the endocrine system has helped me better understand mood so that I can move more deliberately from one mood to another.

Extensibility: The ability to be stretched or extended.
Seeking to understand the Eastern concepts in this text has stretched my belief system.

Elasticity: The ability to recoil and resume the original resting length after being stretched.
My self-awareness has been reinforced by acquiring knowledge about my body.

Your Turn

Excitability: The ability to receive and respond to a stimulus.

Contractility: The ability to shorten forcibly and produce movement when adequately stimulated.

Extensibility: The ability to be stretched or extended.

Elasticity: The ability to recoil and resume the original resting length after being stretched.

Types of Muscle Actions

As with changes in attachment terminology, a change is occurring in descriptive terms for muscle function (Box 9.2). The word *action* is replacing *contraction*. Muscles can contract (produce actions) in different ways, depending on the demand. Contraction and action are used interchangeably and both are considered correct.

Box 9.2 Names of Muscles by Function

Mover (agonist) A muscle or muscles using concentric contractions that are the main force causing a joint motion through a specified plane of motion; the mover or movers most responsible for the action can be called the *prime mover(s)*.

Antagonist A muscle that has the opposite action to the mover and usually is located on the opposite side of the joint and eccentrically contracts and lengthens, restraining and controlling an opposite force (usually a force external to the body, such as gravity).

Fixator (stabilizer) A muscle that surrounds the joint or body segment and isometrically contracts to support or stabilize one attachment of the mover (or antagonist), enabling the other attachment of the mover (or antagonist) to work effectively. Usually, the fixator establishes a firm base for the more distal attachment to carry out movements.

Neutralizer A muscle that stops an unwanted action of the mover (or antagonist) at the attachment of the mover (or antagonist) that is moving. Like fixators, neutralizers work by way of isometric contractions.

Support muscle A muscle that acts at a joint other than where the action in question is occurring to hold a body part in position while the action in question is occurring. Support muscles generally work by way of isometric contractions.

Synergist A helper mover (assistant mover or emergency mover) of the action that is occurring, more broadly defined as any muscle that helps an action occur. Synergists are sometimes known as *guiding muscles*.

Mover and antagonist muscles can contract at the same time in what is called a *co-contraction*. The result is no movement because the forces generated resist each other. Isometric contraction occurs, providing stability.

Muscle tension is often mentioned in discussions of a "tight" muscle. However, a muscle can be "tight" for several reasons: because it is shortened, because it is lengthened and taut, or because it has increased fluid (hydrostatic pressure). With regard to muscle action, tension occurs because the muscle fibers are shortening.

Isometric and Isotonic Actions

Muscle actions are classified as isometric or isotonic.

Isometric

An **isometric action** (contraction) occurs when tension develops within a muscle but no appreciable change occurs in the joint angle or the length of the muscle. In other words, muscle tension increases, but no movement occurs. Isometric actions are static actions because large amounts of tension develop in the muscle to maintain the joint angle in a static or stable position, such as upright posture. Fixing or stabilizing a proximal joint so that a distal joint can move is an example of the way the body uses isometric functions (Fig. 9.2A).

Isotonic

Isotonic action occurs when tension develops in the muscle while it shortens or lengthens. Isotonic actions are dynamic contractions because the varying degrees of tension in the muscle cause the joint angles to change. Isotonic contractions produce movement. Isotonic muscle actions can be classified as concentric or eccentric, depending on whether shortening or lengthening occurs.

In a **concentric action**, the muscle develops tension as it shortens, and the contraction develops enough force to overcome any applied resistance. Concentric actions cause movement against gravity or resistance and are described as being positive contractions. Concentric actions occur as the angle of the joint decreases. An example is the biceps brachii curl, in which one lifts a weight toward the shoulder by moving the forearm toward the arm by bending the elbow (see Fig. 9.2B).

Eccentric actions take place when the muscle lengthens while under tension and changes in tension to control the

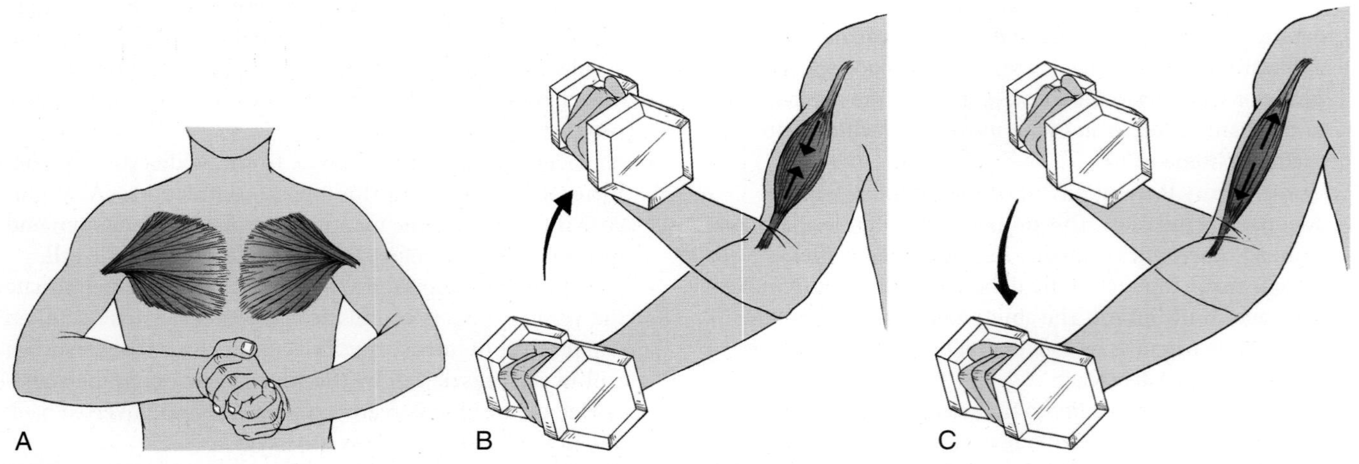

FIG. 9.2 (A) Isometric exercise is muscle activity with no change in length. No work is performed. (B) Concentric muscle activity. Muscle shortens during tension production. (C) Eccentric muscle activity. Muscle lengthens during tension production. (From Greenstein GM. *Clinical Assessment of Neuromusculoskeletal Disorders*. Mosby; 1997.)

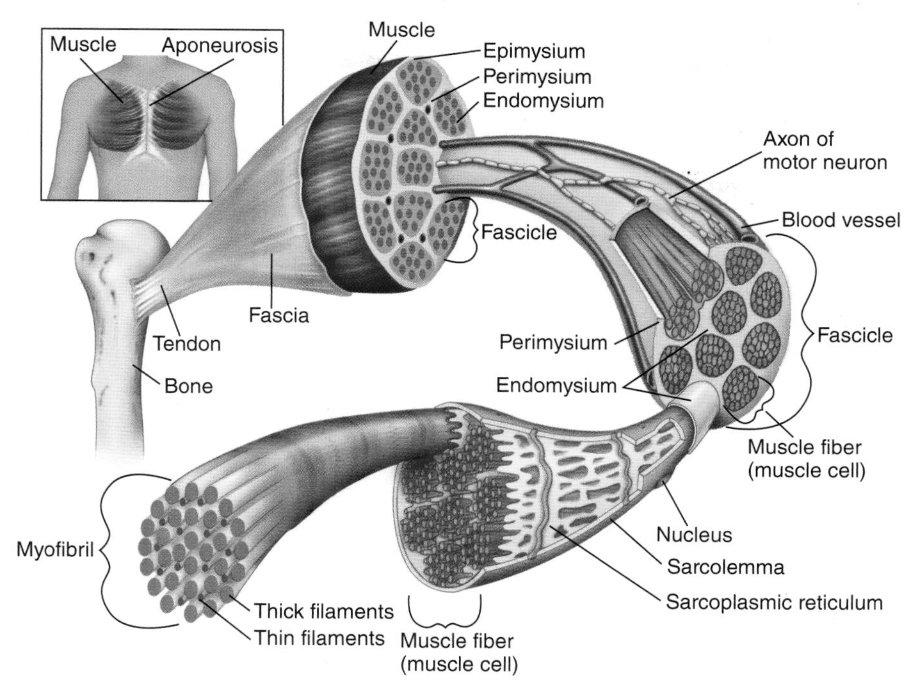

FIG. 9.3 Structure of a muscle organ. The connective tissue coverings—the epimysium, perimysium, and endomysium—are continuous with each other and with the tendon. Muscle fibers are held together by the perimysium in groups called *fascicles*. (From Thibodeau GA, Patton KT. *Anatomy and Physiology*. 5th ed. Mosby; 2003.)

descent of the resistance. Eccentric actions control movement with gravity or resistance. Typically, eccentric actions happen as an **antagonist** lengthens in a controlled fashion in response to a force (usually a force external to the body) that is moving a body part at the joint in the opposite direction. The muscle slowly yields to resistance, allowing it to be lengthened. Eccentric actions occur as the angle of the joint increases. An example is the reverse of the biceps curl, such as when one lowers a weight from the shoulder by extending the forearm at the elbow joint (see Fig. 9.2C). Gravity, which is the prime mover, creates the action while the eccentric action of the biceps brachii keeps the movement under control. The amount of tension in the muscle may increase or decrease, depending on the weight of the object providing the resistance to gravity. Using the previous example, if the object is light, the biceps brachii decreases in tension as it lengthens. If the weight is substantial, the biceps brachii increases in tension.

Anatomy and Physiology of Muscle Fibers

Each skeletal muscle is an individual organ made of hundreds or thousands of muscle fibers (or cells), large amounts of connective tissue and nerve fibers, and many blood vessels (Fig. 9.3).

- Skeletal muscle fibers are long, cylindric, tapered cells that have cross-striations created by the contractile structure inside.
- The sarcolemma is the plasma membrane that covers muscle cells. Numerous nuclei lie beneath the sarcolemma.
- The sarcoplasm of a muscle fiber is similar to the cytoplasm of other cells but contains large amounts of stored glycogen and a unique oxygen-binding protein called *myoglobin.*
- **Myoglobin** is a red pigment similar to hemoglobin that stores oxygen within the muscle cells.
- Sarcomeres are the structural units of contraction in skeletal muscle fibers.
- Myofibrils, which are chains of sarcomeres, are packed side by side within the sarcoplasm.

The functional units of skeletal muscles are small portions of the myofibrils, and each myofibril is a chain of sarcomere units laid end to end. These structures are held together by various layers of connective tissue. When a muscle cell contracts, its individual sarcomeres shorten. Within a neuromuscular unit, once a contraction has been initiated, it cannot be stopped, and the muscle fibers contract to their full ability or do not contract at all. This is called the **all-or-none response**.

In muscle contraction, shortening of a sarcomere occurs because of the two types of filaments found within the myofibril. The thick filaments are myosin, and the thin filaments are actin. The actin and myosin filaments slide over one another, shortening the myofibrils. This is called the **sliding filament mechanism**. The contraction sequence is:

1. The nervous system activates muscle fibers by stimulating the motor neuron.
2. The neurotransmitter acetylcholine crosses the synapse between the motor neuron and the muscle cell.
3. Myosin attaches to active sites on the actin subunits of the filaments, forming cross-bridges, and the sliding begins.
4. Each cross-bridge attaches and detaches several times during a contraction, working like a tiny ratchet to generate tension and pull the thin actin filaments toward the center of the sarcomere. In this way the actin "crawls" along the myosin.

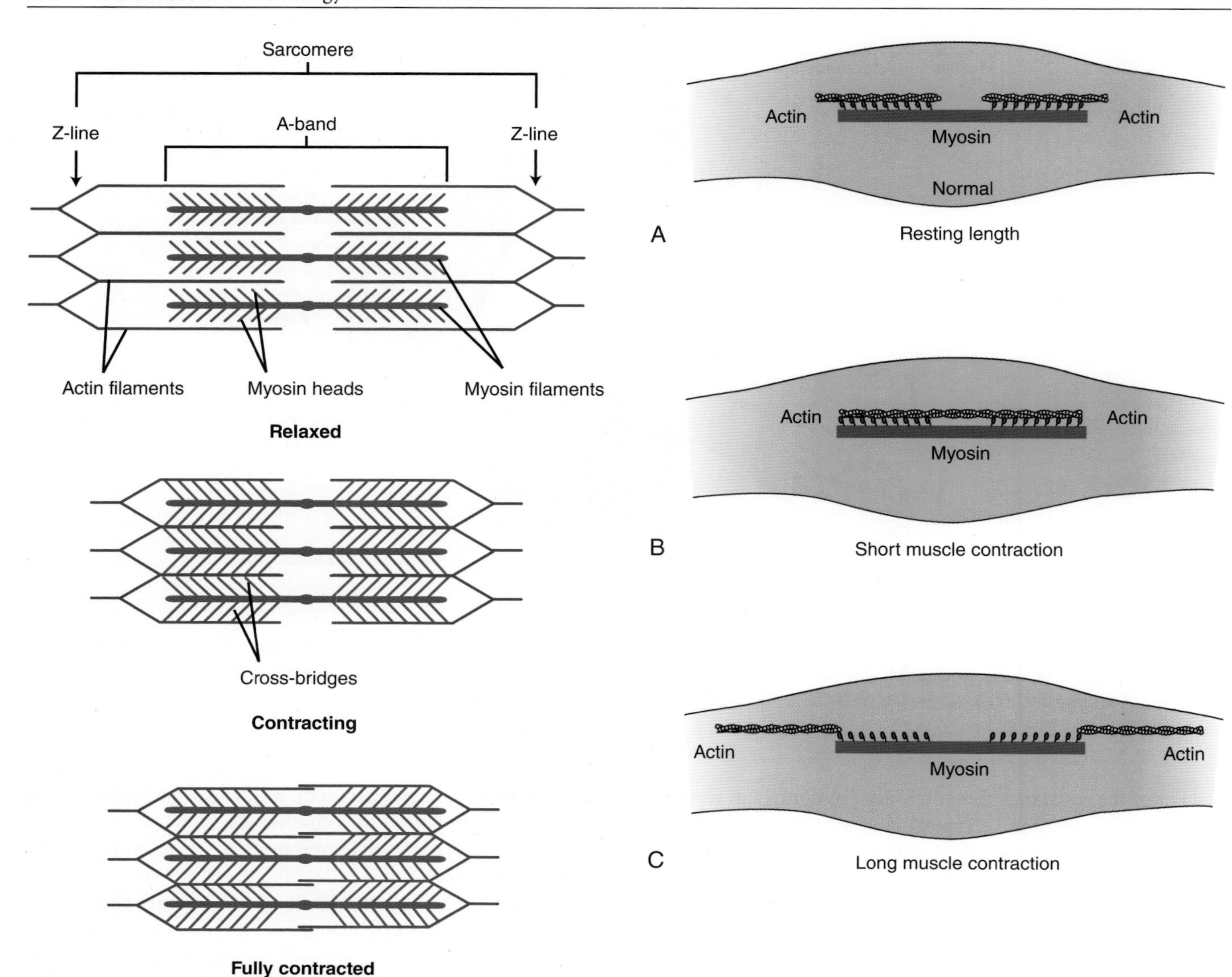

FIG. 9.4 Relaxed/contracted muscle. (From Muscolino JE. *Kinesiology: The Skeletal System and Muscle Function*. 2nd ed. Mosby; 2011.)

5. As this event occurs simultaneously in the sarcomeres throughout the cell, the muscle cell shortens (Fig. 9.4).

The attachment of myosin cross-bridges to actin requires calcium, and the nerve impulse leading to contraction causes an increase in calcium ions within the muscle cell. Sliding of these filaments continues as long as the calcium signal and ATP are present. Relaxation occurs when the nerve impulse no longer stimulates calcium release and the myosin can no longer grip the actin, and so the sliding reverses.

Length-Tension Relationship

A direct relationship exists between tension development in a muscle and the length of the muscle (Fig. 9.5). An optimum length exists at which the muscle is capable of developing maximal tension. Muscles can develop maximal tension because the actin and myosin filaments are positioned to form the maximum number of cross-bridges. If the muscles are shortened or lengthened beyond the optimum length, the amount of tension the muscle is able to generate decreases. A muscle that is too short cannot create a pulling force, because there is little or no "crawl" space for the actin and myosin. If the muscle is too long, it cannot contract much because the actin and myosin are positioned too far apart to create an effective "crawl" action for muscle contraction.

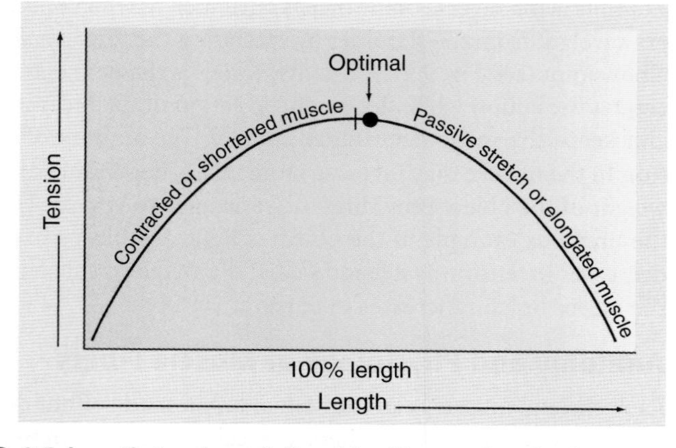

FIG. 9.5 Length-tension relationship: (A) normal resting length, (B) short muscle contraction, (C) long muscle contraction, and (D) optimal length-tension relationship.

In addition to the contractile components of the actin and myosin cross-bridge structures, elastic connective tissue elements of muscles influence the length-tension relationship. The elastic component of the muscle connective tissue coverings (i.e., epimysium, perimysium, or endomysium) and the tendon limit the length of the muscle structure.

Innervation

The autonomic division of the peripheral nervous system innervates the cardiac and smooth muscles. The somatic division of the peripheral nervous system innervates the skeletal muscles. Motor nerves stimulate the skeletal muscles to contract. The area of contact between the motor nerve and the muscle is the motor end plate, or myoneural (neuromuscular) junction. The motor end plate is a modified synapse consisting of a terminal bud of a nerve cell axon and a muscle fiber. When the nerve is stimulated, the terminal bud releases acetylcholine, and contraction follows.

A motor point is the location at which the motor neuron enters the muscle, and a visible contraction can be elicited with a minimal amount of stimulation. Motor points most often are located in the belly of the muscle. Muscles with a large belly may have more than one motor point. The motor point works in the same way a pilot light does in a gas furnace. Even though all the burners in the furnace are not on (much as with a muscle at rest), because of the pilot light, the furnace can respond quickly to the signal of the thermostat for more heat, causing more burners to light.

A single motor neuron innervates many muscle fibers, delivering stimuli to each one and making them all contract as a group; such a group is called a **motor unit** (Fig. 9.6). The muscle fibers in a single motor unit are not clustered together, but rather are spread throughout the muscle; thus the stimulation of a single motor unit causes a weak contraction of the entire muscle. The more strength that is needed, the more motor units are recruited. The size of the motor units determines whether a muscle contracts forcefully or minimally. Large motor units with 700 fibers are found in the quadriceps femoris and other large, strong muscles that participate in running and walking. At the other extreme, 5 to 10 fibers per motor unit provide the extrinsic muscles of the eyeball with the ability to produce fine eye motions.

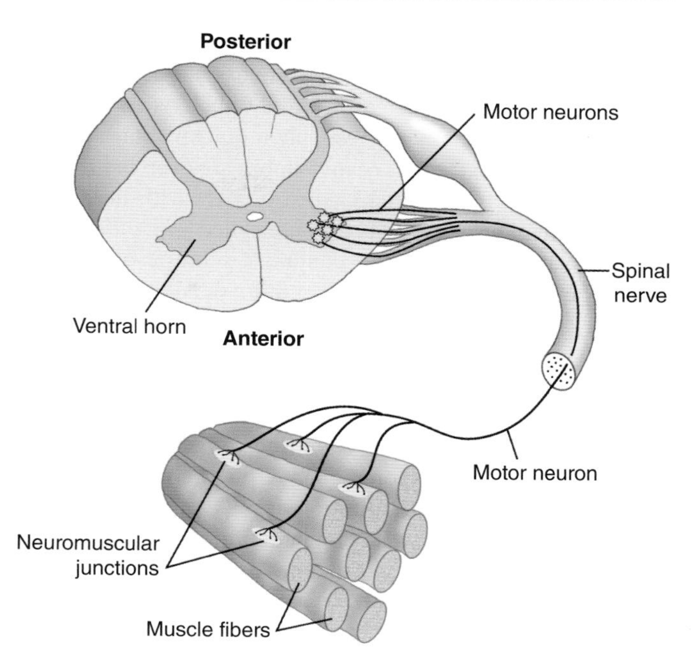

FIG. 9.6 Motor unit. (From Muscolino JE. *Kinesiology: The Skeletal System and Muscle Function*. 2nd ed. Mosby; 2011.)

Resting Muscle Tone

When the synapses in normal muscles stop firing, the muscles relax. Even so, they maintain a certain amount of contraction that keeps them ready to respond; this minimal amount of tautness is known as **resting tone**. Resting tone maintains the natural firmness of our muscles and their state of ready responsiveness. Appropriate amounts of resting tone help stabilize our joints and maintain our posture. Resting muscle tone is controlled by small signals from the spinal cord, brain, and spindles of the individual muscles. Because the stimulation occurs alternately to different sets of motor units within the muscle itself, some parts of the muscle contract while others relax. This keeps the muscle, especially postural muscles, from fatiguing.

This changeover in the signaling, which maintains resting muscle tone, can easily be demonstrated. Hold a heavy book in your hand as you slowly start to flex your forearm at the elbow joint. The small twitch in the muscle occurs with a changeover in motor units. Sometimes it feels like a small loss of strength that quickly returns.

Threshold Stimulus and Treppe

The stimulus at which the first noticeable muscle contraction occurs is called the **threshold stimulus**. Beyond this point the muscle contracts more vigorously as the intensity of the stimulus increases. The stimulus intensity beyond which the muscle fails to increase in strength is called the **maximal stimulus**, or the point at which all the motor units of the muscle have been recruited. Thus the same muscle can apply a gentle stroke or a firm slap, depending on the intensity of the stimulus.

The first contraction of a muscle unit may be as little as one half the strength of those that occur in succession after it; this is called *treppe*. Many factors cause this stair-step effect; for example, as the muscle begins work and produces heat, the muscle enzyme systems become more efficient, releasing more calcium ions, and this produces a stronger contraction with each successive twitch during the beginning phase of muscle activity. Treppe is one reason warming up before exercise is important.

Energy Source for Muscle Contraction

The energy required for muscular contraction comes from adenosine triphosphate (ATP). Efficient contraction of muscle fibers requires glucose and oxygen. Some muscle fibers store glucose in the form of glycogen, which is then broken down into glucose as the muscle fiber needs it. Glucose is a nutrient molecule that contains many chemical bonds. The potential energy stored in these chemical bonds is released during catabolic reactions in the sarcoplasm and mitochondria. Oxygen is needed for the catabolic process known as *aerobic respiration*.

Myoglobin contains iron groups that attract oxygen molecules and hold them temporarily. When the oxygen concentration inside a muscle fiber decreases rapidly, such as occurs during exercise, myoglobin can resupply it quickly. Muscle fibers that contain large amounts of myoglobin are deep red and are called *red fibers* (slow twitch). Muscle fibers with little myoglobin in them are light pink and are called *white fibers* (fast twitch). Most muscle tissues contain a mixture of red and white fibers. These are discussed in more detail in the section on the types of muscle fibers.

When the oxygen concentration is low, muscle fibers can shift use to another catabolic process called *anaerobic respiration*, which does not require the immediate use of oxygen. Muscle fibers having difficulty getting oxygen or fibers that generate a great deal of force quickly may rely on anaerobic respiration. Anaerobic respiration results in the formation of lactic acid, which may accumulate in muscle tissue during activity in which insufficient oxygen is available. The lactic acid then can be broken down by way of aerobic respiration if oxygen becomes present or can diffuse into the blood and be taken to the liver, where it is converted back to glucose.

These processes require oxygen. After heavy exercise, the lack of oxygen in some tissues is called *oxygen debt*. **Oxygen debt** is defined as the extra amount of oxygen that must be taken in to break down or convert the lactic acid. A person may continue to breathe heavily to repay the oxygen debt and process the lactic acid by way of aerobic respiration in the muscle cell or in the liver. Lower levels of oxygen in the blood and the correspondingly higher levels of carbon dioxide and lactic acid (by-products of metabolism from muscle action) signal the brainstem to increase the rate of breathing to compensate for the oxygen debt. When the oxygen debt has been paid, lactic acid has been converted, oxygen levels rise back to normal levels, and breathing returns to normal.

Heat is a by-product of muscle activity. Several homeostatic mechanisms, such as radiation of heat from the skin surface and sweating, prevent heat buildup from reaching dangerous levels. When the external environment is cold, shivering causes muscle contraction, which produces more heat.

Muscle Fatigue

Muscle fatigue is a state of exhaustion (a loss of strength or endurance) produced by strenuous muscular activity. Two types of muscle fatigue are physiological and psychological. Low levels of ATP cause physiological muscle fatigue, and the myosin cross-bridges become incapable of producing the force required for further muscle contractions. The lack of ATP that produces fatigue may result from a depletion of oxygen or glucose in muscle fibers or from the inability to regenerate ATP quickly enough. Acidic metabolic waste products alter the normal pH balance and also contribute to physiological fatigue. Complete physiological fatigue seldom occurs. Usually, psychological fatigue is what produces the exhausted feeling that stops us from continuing a muscular activity. We feel tired and do not want to continue an activity. The mechanism is protective and keeps the body from continually functioning at maximal levels and producing physiological fatigue that is stressful and draining on the whole body.

ACTIVITY 9.2

Do you think the statement "Where there is pain, I rub" is a valid therapeutic approach? Use the clinical reasoning model to formulate your position.

What are the facts?
What is considered normal or balanced function?
What has happened?
What caused the imbalance?
What was done or is being done?
What has worked or not worked?
What are the possibilities?

What does my intuition suggest?

What are the possible patterns of dysfunction?
What are the possible contributing factors?
What are possible interventions?
What might work?
What are other ways to look at the situation?
What do the data suggest?
What is the logical progression of the symptom pattern, contributing factors, and current behaviors?
What are the logical consequences of each intervention identified as a possibility?
What are the pros and cons of each intervention suggested?
What are the consequences of not acting?
What are the consequences of acting?
In terms of each intervention considered, what would be the impact on the persons involved: client, practitioner, and other professionals working with the client?
How does each person involved feel about the possible interventions?
Does the practitioner feel qualified to work with such situations?
Does a feeling of cooperation and agreement exist among all parties involved?

Summarize your reasons for determining the validity or invalidity of the statement "Where there is pain, I rub."

Blood Supply

Contracting muscle fibers use tremendous amounts of oxygen and nutrients and give off large amounts of metabolic waste. The blood delivers oxygen and nutrients and takes away waste products. Muscle tissue is highly vascularized, and the structure of capillaries in muscle has been modified so that they are long and winding. Thus when a muscle stretches, the capillaries can easily accommodate the change in shape (Activity 9.2).

Types of Muscle Fibers

Muscles contain fast-, slow-, and intermediate-twitch fibers, which contract at different rates and with different characteristics, allowing muscles a wide range of action.

- *Fast-twitch (white) fibers* contract more rapidly and forcefully, are larger than red fibers, and belong to larger motor units that activate when the nervous system demands rapid, powerful motion. They fatigue quickly and are considered anaerobic because they do not require much oxygen to contract. Muscles that need to respond quickly for short range of motion movements predominantly have fast-twitch fibers. Because white fibers are anaerobic, they fatigue more easily because the lactic acid accumulates and interferes with contractions. As previously mentioned, the liver needs oxygen to convert the lactic acid to glucose or glycogen.

- *Slow-twitch (red) fibers* are smaller; contract more slowly and with less intensity; and belong to smaller motor units that respond during slower, finer movements. These fibers contain much larger amounts of myoglobin and are classified as aerobic because they require oxygen for contraction. Some texts divide red fibers into fast and slow types. Because of their aerobic quality, red fibers do not produce lactic acid. For this reason postural muscles, which are composed mainly of red fibers, can sustain a contraction longer without fatiguing.
- *Intermediate-twitch fibers* combine the qualities of red and white fibers to provide a rapid, moderately forceful contraction with moderate fatigue resistance. Muscles of the limbs are an example.

Although the fiber composition varies from muscle to muscle, on average 50% of the fibers in a muscle are red, 35% are intermediate, and 15% are white. As many as 90% of the fibers in postural muscles are red, whereas leg muscles contain a higher proportion of white and intermediate fibers.

Genetics greatly determines the fiber configuration, but this can change as a result of demands made on the muscles. For example, the most successful sprinters are born with more white fibers in their leg muscles. Sometimes others can be trained to be sprinters because their fiber configuration adjusts well to the demands of sprinting.

Repair of Muscle

Most of an adult's muscle cells are already in place at birth. As we grow, existing muscle fibers enlarge (hypertrophy) by as much as 30% of their original size. An injured muscle often is repaired with connective tissue. The body has a specific repair process for regenerating muscle cells. Within hours of an injury, enzymes in the body begin to digest the damaged cell portion. Satellite cells, which are inactive during normal muscle activity, begin to form the new fibers by creating myotubes, which combine to form myofibrils. These new cells take on the characteristics of muscle fibers. Exercise influences the growth of satellite cells and aids in maintaining plasticity of connective tissue. Cardiac muscle has no satellite cells, and its damaged cells are replaced with fibrous connective tissue. Smooth muscle is able to regenerate itself throughout life.

Myotatic Units (Functional Muscle Groups)

Myotatic units are functional muscle groups. They are interconnected neurologically so that movement occurs smoothly, sequentially, and in a coordinated manner. Only rarely does any muscle act independently. Most muscles play a part in a movement pattern, just as actors do in a play. Roles can change, depending on the response required. A muscle can be the star, or prime mover, and in the next instant become one of the supporting cast. A moment later the same muscle can assume the opposite role. As previously described, three types of muscle actions exist: (1) concentric, in which the muscle shortens (acceleration) and the joint angle decreases; (2) eccentric, in which the muscle maintains a controlled lengthening (deceleration) response as the joint angle increases; and (3) isometric, in which the muscle shortens but produces no movement. The terms *mover* (**agonist**), *prime mover, antagonist,* **fixator** *(stabilizer), neutralizer, support,* and **synergist** describe the function of muscles in a complete movement pattern.

Because the central nervous system processes movement patterns, understanding the interaction of muscles in functional units is important. This integrated function often is called the *kinetic chain* and is explained in depth in Chapter 10.

The mover/antagonist interaction is easy to visualize in muscle pairs, such as the biceps brachii, which flexes the elbow joint, and triceps brachii, which extends the elbow joint. However, the interaction becomes more complex when we consider that the deltoid and quadriceps femoris and the adductors and hamstrings form a functional unit because of our gait (walking pattern). The various functional units that require muscles to cooperate in producing body-wide movements (e.g., walking, maintaining balance) need sophisticated reflex control by the nervous system. Recall that reflex arcs are covered in Chapter 4; it may be helpful to review this information. When the role of stabilization is factored into a movement pattern, the functional (or myotatic) muscle group interaction becomes quite complex. Whenever maintaining posture is part of the pattern, a body-wide process is involved. Chapter 10 presents more information on biomechanics.

Muscle Shapes

The bundles of muscle fibers known as *fascicles* form different patterns in muscles, resulting in the different shapes of

Practical Application

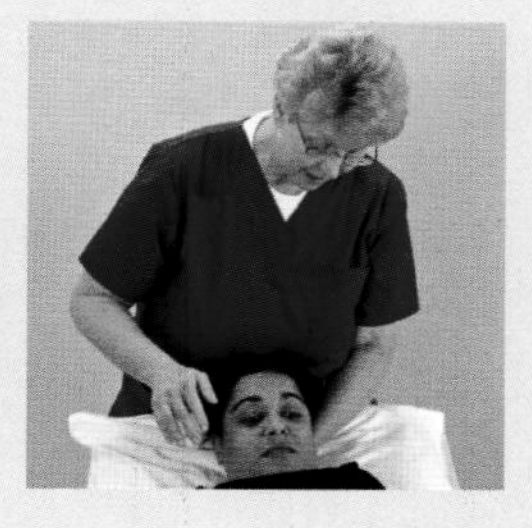

When considering myotatic units and the development of patterns of compensation to any change in the body, one may assume logically that any alteration in musculoskeletal function has a body-wide effect. For example, the arm and thigh muscles are connected in agonist/antagonist patterns through the gait reflex, and the neck and trunk muscles interact together through the ocular/pelvic and righting reflexes that keep us upright with eyes forward. Because the components of the body are interdependent, everything affects everything else. Often, effective applications of massage depend on unraveling complex functional groups of muscles. In many cases, addressing the entire body during each session in what is called a *general constitutional approach* is just as effective. Spot work or addressing an isolated area and excluding the rest of the body, is less effective.

muscles (Fig. 9.7). These fascicle forms affect function, primarily the strength and direction of movement. The next sections describe the more common patterns of fascicle arrangement.

Parallel

The fascicles are long and oriented parallel with the longitudinal axis of the muscle. Some of these muscles are straplike (e.g., the sartorius), and others are fusiform with an expanded belly (e.g., the biceps brachii).

Convergent

The fascicle pattern begins with a broad origin and converges to blend with a much smaller tendon. The result is a triangular muscle (e.g., the pectoralis major).

Pennate

The fascicles are short, lie at an angle to the muscle, and attach to one or more tendons running the length of the muscle. A unipennate muscle (e.g., the extensor digitorum longus) has fascicles that insert on only one side of the tendon. A bipennate muscle (e.g., the rectus femoris) has fascicles that insert into the tendon from both sides; the result looks like a feather. A muscle resembling many feathers, all inserted into one large tendon, is called a *multipennate muscle*.

Circular

The fascicles are arranged in concentric rings around external body openings. These muscles, which contract to close the openings, are called *sphincters*.

The various patterns of fascicle arrangement determine the strength and amount of movement a muscle provides. Skeletal muscles can shorten to about 50% of their resting length when contracted. The longer and more parallel the muscle fibers to the long axis of the muscle, the greater the muscle shortening. Parallel muscles shorten as a direct result of the shortening of their fibers; these muscles produce the greatest amount of shortening. The fibers do this at the expense of strength; parallel muscles are not powerful. The fibers of pennate muscles rotate around their tendon attachments. Pennate muscles can pack more fibers into the same amount of space as parallel fibers and thus can produce the stronger contraction, albeit over a shorter range of motion (Activity 9.3).

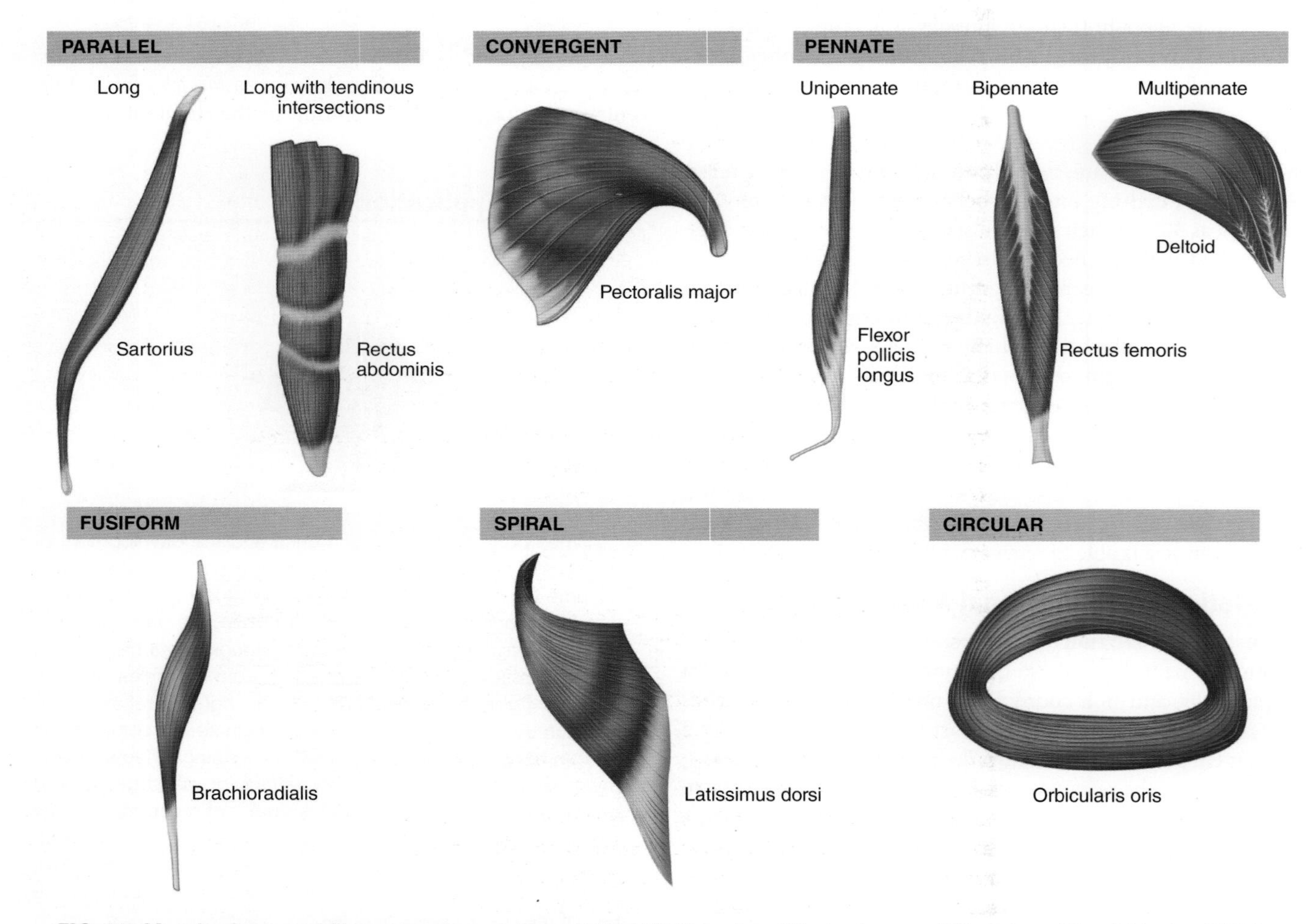

FIG. 9.7 Muscle shape and fiber arrangement. (From Patton KT, Thibodeau GA. *Anatomy and Physiology*. 7th ed. Mosby; 2010.)

ACTIVITY 9.3

Draw the following muscle shapes on a separate sheet of paper:

Parallel
Pennate
Convergent
Circular

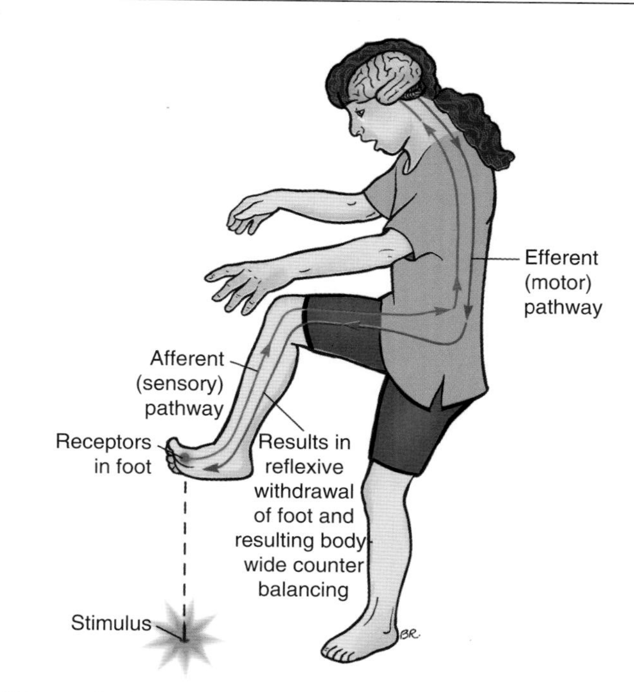

FIG. 9.8 Reflex response. Local stimulation of a few specific receptors leads to a large number of outgoing impulses, which affect many muscles. (From Fritz S. *Mosby's Fundamentals of Therapeutic Massage*. 5th ed. Mosby; 2013.)

Proprioceptors and Reflexes

The central nervous system coordinates motion by being constantly aware of any muscle action. Recall from Chapter 5 that proprioceptors are sensory receptors that provide the central nervous system with information about position, movement, muscle tension, joint activity, and equilibrium. Methods that move, stretch, and apply tension to the muscles and joints stimulate these receptors:

- Muscle spindles: Respond to sudden and prolonged stretch.
- Tendon organs: Respond to tension in the muscle that is relayed to the tendon. Ligaments contain receptors that respond to strain at the joint and feedback information to adjust the tension patterns of associated muscles.
- Joint kinesthetic receptors in the joint capsule: Respond to pressure, acceleration, and deceleration of joint movement. The two main types of joint kinesthetic receptors are type II cutaneous mechanoreceptors and lamellated (pacinian) corpuscles.

Somatic reflex arcs interpret and process stimulation of nervous system receptors (Fig. 9.8). The reflexes most often stimulated are the stretch reflex, tendon reflex, flexor reflex, and crossed extensor reflex.

Stretch Reflex

The sensitivity of muscle spindles to stretching sets the level of muscle tone throughout the body. The muscle spindles activate the stretch reflex when a muscle is subjected to sudden or prolonged stretching. This activation causes a reflexive contraction of the same muscle. As was explained in Chapter 5, a muscle spindle produces nerve impulses that it sends by way of a sensory neuron to the dorsal root of the spinal cord, where an impulse synapses with a motor neuron. The motor neuron carries the impulse to the stretched muscle, generating a muscle action potential and causing the muscle and its synergists to contract. Muscle contraction stops spindle cell discharge unless the muscle is held in a lengthened state, and a small amount of stretch reflex continues to be generated. The effect of the muscle fiber length stimulates the stretch reflex, resulting in facilitation and concentric shortening of the muscle.

The principle of reciprocal inhibition comes into play during the stretch reflex. At the same time the original muscle is stimulated to contract, sensory signals synapse with association neurons to its antagonist(s), inhibiting any signal through the motor neurons to the antagonists; this results in relaxation of the antagonist. To simplify, when one muscle contracts, its antagonist or opposing muscle group must lengthen to allow movement. The massage practitioner can initiate the pathway of this inhibition circuitry (reciprocal innervation) therapeutically to assist in muscle relaxation.

Tendon Reflex

The tendon reflex operates as a feedback mechanism that monitors and controls muscle tension by inducing muscle relaxation. This reflex is mediated by the tendon organs that detect and respond to changes in muscle tension caused by a sudden or intense muscle contraction. When the tendon organ is stimulated, it sends a signal along a sensory neuron to the spinal cord, where it synapses with an inhibitory association neuron, which inhibits the motor neurons that innervate the original muscle. This inhibition causes the muscle to relax.

At the same time the original muscle is inhibited from acting, a small increase occurs in the signal sent to the antagonist. The opposite of reciprocal inhibition, this signal causes a small contraction to take place in the antagonist. It is possible to initiate this signal therapeutically to assist in relaxing a tense muscle and in stimulating its antagonist.

Flexor Reflex and Crossed Extensor Reflex

The flexor (withdrawal) and crossed extensor reflexes are polysynaptic reflex arcs. A single sensory neuron, most likely located in the skin, can activate several motor neurons. Stimulation of these reflexes affects both sides of the body through intersegmental reflex arcs. The flexor reflex withdraws the limb from an unpleasant or painful stimulus, whereas the crossed extensor reflex extends the limb on the opposite side of the spinal cord to maintain balance. The circuitry of contralateral reflex arcs synchronizes control over the contracting and inhibited muscles. These reflexes also explain why tension patterns are seldom found on only one side of the body. As with the stretch reflex, the principle of reciprocal inhibition is active in flexor and extensor reflexes.

Postural Reflexes

In addition, a series of reflexes maintain posture and the position of the head so that the eyes remain in the horizontal plane and oriented forward. These righting and tonic neck reflexes, together with oculopelvic reflexes, coordinate position and function of the neck, trunk, and pelvic muscles. Looking back over the head or tipping the head back activates the extensors and inhibits the flexors. Looking down toward the navel or tipping the head down activates the flexors and inhibits the extensors. Looking left or turning the head to the left activates muscles that would rotate the body left and inhibits those that would rotate the body right. Losing postural balance during eye and head movement causes the opposite reaction, returning the body to an upright position in gravity.

Section Summary

- List the three types of muscle.
  - Skeletal, cardiac, smooth.
- List and describe the major functions of muscle.
  - Muscles produce movement, stabilize joints, maintain posture, produce heat. Skeletal muscle moves/stabilizes bones/joints. Cardiac muscle (found only in the heart) pumps blood. Smooth muscle (divided into multiunit and visceral muscle) moves fluid in blood/lymph vessels (multiunit), and fluid/waste via peristalsis in digestive/urinary/reproductive organs (visceral).
- Describe types of muscle actions.
  - Muscle actions (i.e., contractions) are classified as isometric or isotonic. Isometric: muscle tension increases but no movement occurs. Isotonic: muscle tension increases, producing movement (concentric shortening or eccentric lengthening). Concentric: muscle tension increases as it shortens, decreasing the joint angle. Eccentric: muscle tension increases or decreases (depending on demand) as it lengthens, increasing the joint angle.
- Identify the energy source for muscle contraction.
  - ATP is the energy source for muscle contraction. Glucose is the fuel for the manufacture of ATP. Calcium is required for the attachment of cross-bridges from myosin to actin, the contractile filaments within myofibrils, chains of sarcomeres, and the contractile units in skeletal muscle.
- Explain the difference between red slow-twitch and white fast-twitch muscle fibers.
  - Red fibers (slow-twitch) contain large amounts of myoglobin (considered aerobic). White fibers (fast twitch) contain small amounts of myoglobin (considered anaerobic). Intermediate-twitch fibers combine qualities of red and white fibers. Myoglobin is a protein containing iron groups that attract oxygen molecules and hold them temporarily. Myoglobin resupplies oxygen to muscle during strenuous activity. Aerobic respiration is the catabolic process requiring oxygen. Anaerobic respiration is the catabolic process not requiring oxygen, producing lactic acid. Lactic acid is converted into glucose or glycogen by the liver.
- List the components of myotatic units.
  - Agonist (mover), synergist (agonist helper), antagonist (agonist opposer), and fixator (stabilizer). Myotatic units (neurologically connected functional muscle groups) coordinate smooth, sequential movement.
- Describe reflexes related to muscle function.
  - Stretch reflex: activated by muscle spindle receptors when a muscle is subjected to sudden or prolonged stretch, causing a reflexive contraction of the muscle. Tendon reflex: activated by tendon organ receptors when a muscle suddenly or intensely contracts, causing the muscle to relax. Flexor reflex and crossed extensor reflex: the flexor reflex causes a limb to withdraw from unpleasant/painful stimuli, while the crossed extensor reflex causes extension of the opposing limb to maintain balance. Postural reflexes: coordinate the position of the neck, trunk, and pelvic muscles to maintain posture and head position so that the eyes remain level (see Fig. 9.8).

FASCIA AND THE MYOFASCIAL STRUCTURE AND FUNCTION

SECTION OBJECTIVES

Chapter objective covered in this section:

8. Describe the integrated connective tissue structure of muscle.

After completing this section, the student will be able to:

- Define fascia.
- Define biotensegrity and myofascial continuity.
- Explain pathological connective tissue changes.

Recall from Chapter 1 that the connective tissue matrix, which consists of the ground substance and the fibers, ranges from a fluid to a semisolid or gel and is composed mostly of polysaccharides (protein and sugar). Aside from cells and fibers, matrix also contains many blood vessels and nerves.

Recall that **fascia** is one form of connective tissue and makes up one integrated and totally connected network, from the attachments on the inner aspects of the skull to the fascia in the soles of the feet, and from the skin to the innermost center of the body. If any part of a fascial structure becomes deformed or distorted, adverse effects can occur on any of the interconnected structures within the network. Chapters 1 and 8 previously discussed connective tissue structure and function in relationship to tissue types and joint structure and function. Fascia will now be discussed in relationship to muscles (Box 9.3).

- Each muscle fiber is surrounded by a fine sheath of collagenic connective tissue called the *endomysium*.
- Several muscle fibers are wrapped together in side-by-side bundles, called *fascicles*.
- Fascicles are wrapped in a collagenic sheath called the *perimysium*.

Box 9.3 Various Definitions of Fascia

There are different views and scientific understanding of fascia. As a result, currently there is no official definition of fascia. The fascia is a complex, fibrous tissue that encompasses, interlinks, and encases various subsystems within the cranium, thoracic and abdominal cavities, and limbs.

There appears to be general agreement that fascial tissue is found throughout the body. The fascia creates different interdependent layers with several depths, from the skin to the periosteum. There is a layer of lubricant, primarily hyaluronan, produced by cells called *fasciacytes*. The hyaluronan fills the cell spaces, allowing for sliding of different tissue layers and structures, such as nerves, blood vessels, adjacent tissues, and structures within compartments. Fascia can wrap, combine with other tissues, support, and form structural elements of the bloodstream, bone tissue, meningeal tissue, organs, and muscles. The fascia is innervated, especially with sensory nerves.

According to the Federative Committee on Anatomical Terminology, the superficial fascia (fascia superficialis) is a "whole loose layer of subcutaneous tissue lying superficial to the denser layer of fascia profunda." The deep fascia (fascia profunda) lies below the superficial fascia.

Fascia is "a sheath, a sheet, or any other dissectible aggregations of connective tissue that forms beneath the skin to attach, enclose, and separate muscles and other internal organs."

According to the Fascia Nomenclature Committee, the fascial system consists of the three-dimensional continuum of soft, collagen-containing, loose and dense fibrous connective tissues that permeate the body. It incorporates elements such as adipose tissue, adventitia and neurovascular sheaths, aponeuroses, deep and superficial fasciae, epineurium, joint capsules, ligaments, membranes, meninges, myofascial expansions, periosteum, retinacula, septa, tendons, visceral fasciae, and all the intramuscular and intermuscular connective tissues including endoperiepimysium. The fascial system interpenetrates and surrounds all organs, muscles, bones, and nerve fibers, endowing the body with a functional structure, and providing an environment that enables all body systems to operate in an integrated manner.

From Scarr G, Blyum L, Levin SM, de Solórzano SL. "Moving beyond Vesalius: Why anatomy needs a mapping update." *Med Hypotheses* 2024;183: 111257; Kumka M, Bonar J. Fascia: a morphological description and classification system based on a literature review. *J Can Chiropr Assoc.* 2012;56(3); Schleip R, Jäger H, Klingler W. What is "fascia"? A review of different nomenclatures. *J Bodywork Ther.* 2012;16(4):496–502; Thalhamer C. A fundamental critique of the fascial distortion model and its application in clinical practice. *J Bodywork Move Ther.* 2018;22(1):112–117.

- The fascicles are bound together with more dense, fibrous connective tissue called the *epimysium*.
- The epimysium surrounds the entire muscle.
- External to the epimysium is the **deep fascia**, an even coarser sheet of fibrous connective tissue that binds muscles into functional groups.
- The deep fascia forms partitions between muscle groups called *intermuscular septa*.

All these connective tissue sheaths are continuous with one another. Near the ends of muscles, the actual muscle fiber ends, but the connective tissue continues and converges to become the tendons and aponeuroses that join muscles to bones or other connective tissue structures. Tendons and aponeuroses are the continuation of the endomysium, perimysium, and epimysium minus the muscle fibers, which attach muscle to bone. The point where the muscle fiber ends and the tendon begins is called the *musculotendinous junction*. The difference between a tendon and an aponeurosis is one of shape. A tendon by definition is round and cordlike; an **aponeurosis** is a broad, flat sheet.

The tendon or aponeurosis blends and wraps into the connective tissue coverings and structures, including ligaments and other tendons, or into a seam of fibrous connective tissue, called a *raphe*, at the attachment site. Muscle attachments do not stick on bone but wrap around the bone such that the muscles can lift the bone when they contract. The middle of the muscle or the area with the largest and broadest concentration of muscle fibers is the belly of the muscle (Fig. 9.9). When muscle fibers contract, they pull on the connective tissue sheaths, which transmit the force to the bone to be moved. As the muscle contracts, fibers get thicker, forcing the fascial tubular layers surrounding the muscle (endomysium, perimysium, and epimysium) to expand in diameter and shorten in length, contributing to the pulling force.

Because the individual skeletal muscle fibers are fragile, the connective tissue supports each cell, reinforces the muscle as a whole, and gives muscle tissue its natural elasticity. These sheaths also provide entry and exit routes for the blood vessels and nerve fibers that serve the muscles, as well as a vast surface area for muscular attachment.

The fascial components of the connective tissue network form one structure. Nerves and blood vessels do not just pass through holes in the fascia; rather, they are contained and supported in wrappings of this connective tissue type that intertwine into the entire fascial network. Movement of any one body part creates a force that can be transmitted along fascial planes throughout the body.

Fascia provides a supporting matrix for more highly organized structures and attaches extensively to and invests into muscles.

- The superficial fascia, which forms the adipose tissue, allows for the storage of fat and also provides a surface covering that aids in the conservation of body heat. It is connected to the deep fascia by tiny fibers that are crimped and wavy to allow sliding of one layer over the other.
- Deep fascia wraps and preserves the shape of the limbs and promotes circulation in the veins and lymphatic vessels.
- Connective tissue sheaths cover and define muscle groups and individual muscle structures.
- The layer of deep fascia, as well as intermuscular septa and interosseous membranes, wrap to cover and enclose as well as separate structure layers, thus providing surface areas used for muscular attachment.
- Fascia supplies restraining mechanisms in the form of retention bands and fibrous pulleys, thereby assisting in the coordination of movement.
- Where connective tissue has a loose texture, it allows movement between adjacent structures and, by the formation of bursal sacs, reduces the effects of pressure and friction.
- Fascia is able to contract in a smooth, muscle-like manner because of the presence of myofibroblasts.

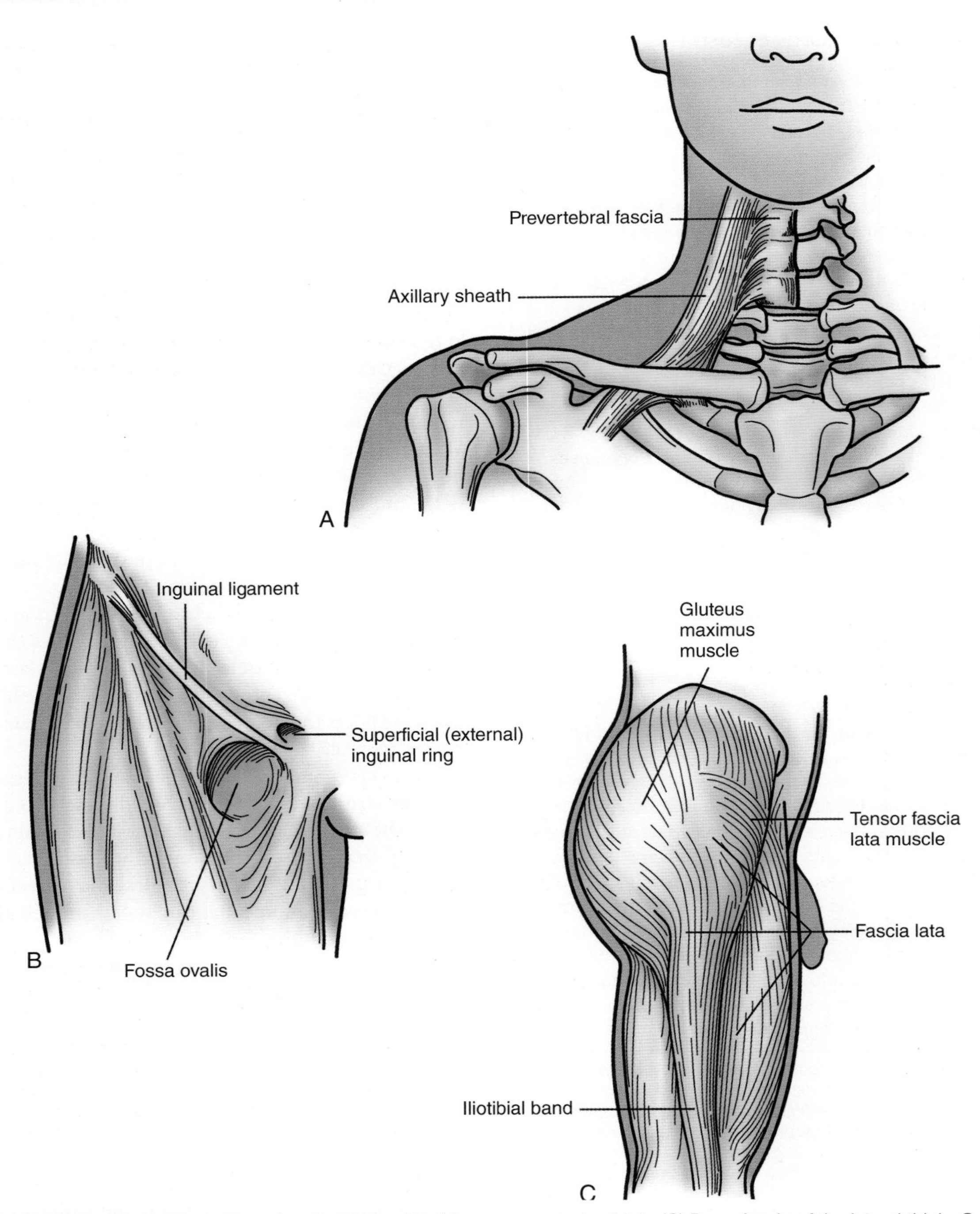

FIG. 9.9 (A) Cervical fascia and the axillary sheath. (B) Fascia of the upper anterior thigh. (C) Deep fascia of the lateral thigh. On the lateral side of the thigh, the fascia lata thickens to form the elongated iliotibial band. (Adapted from Mathers LH, Chase RA, Dolph J, et al. *Clinical Anatomy Principles*. Mosby; 1995.)

- Because connective tissue contains embryonic-like mesenchymal cells, it is capable of developing into more specialized elements.
- Connective tissue provides (by its fascial planes) pathways for nerves and blood and lymphatic vessels and structures.
- Many of the neural structures in fascia are sensory.
- Fascia has the ability to convert mechanical force into neurochemical signals forming a body-wide communication network called **mechanotransduction**.
- The mesh of loose connective tissue contains the tissue fluid and provides an essential medium through which to bring the cellular elements of other tissues into functional contact with blood and lymph. Connective tissues were recently found to be interconnected fluid-filled spaces, supported by a lattice of thick collagen "bundles, through which interstitial fluid flows around the body" (Benias et al., 2018). These fluid-filled spaces collectively are called the *interstitium* and were recently identified in connective

tissues all over the body, including below the skin's surface; lining the digestive tract, lungs and urinary systems; and surrounding muscles.
- Connective tissue has a nutritive function and contains about a quarter of all body fluids.
- Chemical (nutritional) factors influence the strength of connective tissue coverings of muscles and bones.
- Because of its fibroblastic activity, connective tissue aids in the repair of injuries by generating collagenous fibers, creating scar tissue.
- Fascia is a major location of inflammatory processes.
- Fluids and infectious processes often travel along fascial planes and interstitium.
- A histiocyte is a type of immune cell that eats foreign substances in an effort to protect the body from infection. The histiocytes of connective tissue comprise part of an important defense mechanism against bacterial invasion by their phagocytic activity. Histiocytes also play a part as scavengers in removing cell debris and foreign material.
- Connective tissue represents an important neutralizer or detoxifier to endogenous waste (those produced in the body from physiological processes) and exogenous toxins (from outside the body).
- The mechanical barrier presented by fascia has important defensive functions in cases of infectious pathogen invasion.

In therapeutic terms, trying to consider muscle as a separate structure, as shown in Fig. 9.10, from fascia is illogical because the two are related so intimately. Without connective tissue structure, muscle would be a jellylike mass without form or functional ability (Boxes 9.4 and 9.5). Fascial tissues are seen as one interconnected tensional network that adapts its fiber arrangement and matrix density based on local tensional demands.

Biotensegrity and Myofascial Continuity

In the body the bones, muscle, and fascia create a tensegric structure. The bones supply compression elements, and the myofascia supplies tension elements to create a body-wide tensegrity system using the resting muscle tone of numerous viscoelastic muscular chains to maintain constant tension for stability. A tent made of canvas, poles, and tension supplied by ropes is a good example.

The stability of a tensegric structure is less stiff and more resilient than the continuous compression structure in which one structure is piled on another like a brick wall. Load one "corner" of a tensegric structure, and the whole structure gives a little to accommodate. Load the structure too much, and the structure ultimately breaks, but not necessarily anywhere near the load. Because the structure distributes strain throughout the structure along the lines of tension, the tensegric structure may give at some weak point away from the area of applied strain. A principle of massage application that supports this process is to identify the symptoms (the weak part) and look elsewhere for the cause (origin of the strain).

All the interconnected structural elements of a tensegric model rearrange themselves in response to a local stress. As the applied stress increases, more of the components come to lie in the direction of the applied stress, resulting in a linear stiffening of the material. In other words, tensegric structures show resiliency, becoming more stable as the load increases, up to a certain point. Based on tensegrity concepts, a system or interconnected view of body structure and function can be envisioned, with the body construed as an integrated system. An injury at any given site often can be caused by long-term strain in other parts. Discovering these pathways and easing

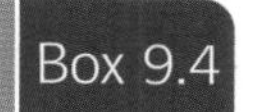

Box 9.4 Biomechanical Laws: The Influence on the Fascia and Muscle Unit

Basic laws govern the mechanical principles influencing the body neurologically and anatomically.

Wolff's law states that biological systems (including soft and hard tissues) deform in relation to the lines of force imposed on them.

Hooke's law states that deformation (resulting from strain) imposed on an elastic body is in proportion to the stress (force load) placed on it.

Newton's third law states that when two bodies interact, the force exerted by the first on the second is equal in magnitude and opposite in direction to the force exerted by the second on the first.

Arndt-Schultz's law states that weak stimuli excite physiological activity, moderately strong ones favor it, strong ones retard it, and very strong ones arrest it.

Hilton's law states that the nerve supplying a joint also supplies the muscles that move the joint and the skin covering the articular insertion of those muscles.

These biomechanical laws influence the behavior of the fascia/muscle fiber unit—the myofascial complex. Application of massage must respect these laws for massage to be effective. Appropriate application of force introduced into the tissue by massage is the key. Depth of pressure and direction, coupled with drag and duration, are qualities of massage application that determine the type of force introduced. Wolff's law, Hooke's law, and Newton's law in particular describe how forces interact. For example, if a client shows a connective tissue shortening in a diagonal pattern from the top of the shoulder at the acromioclavicular joint to the lumbar dorsal fascia, the forces imposed by the massage have to interact with that same directional line.

Muscle and fascia are anatomically inseparable. Therefore fascia moves during muscular activities acting on bone, joints, ligaments, and tendons. Sensory receptors of the nervous system exist in fascia and relate to proprioception and pain reception.

Fascia is colloidal, as is most of the soft tissue of the body. A colloid consists of particles of solid material suspended in fluid (e.g., wallpaper paste); the colloid conforms to the shape of the container it is in and responds to pressure in predictable ways. The amount of resistance colloids offer to pressure applied to the tissues increases proportionally to the velocity (speed) of the force applied to them. This response makes a slow touch a fundamental requirement of massage application; it is necessary to avoid resistance when attempting to produce a change in, or release of, restricted fascial structures.

Adapted from Chaitow L, DeLany J. *Clinical Applications of Neuromuscular Technique.* Vol. 2. Churchill Livingstone; 2008.

Box 9.5 Biomechanical Terms Relating to Fascia

Creep Continued deformation (increasing strain) of a viscoelastic material under constant load (traction, compression, twist).
Hysteresis The process of energy loss caused by friction when tissues are loaded and unloaded.
Load The degree of force (stress) applied to an area.
Strain A change in shape as a result of stress.
Stress Force (load) normalized over the area on which it acts. (All tissues exhibit stress-strain responses.)
Thixotropy A quality of colloids in which the more rapidly force is applied (load), the more rigid the tissue response.
Viscoelastic The potential to deform elastically when load is applied and to return to the original nondeformed state when load is removed.
Viscoplastic A permanent deformation resulting from the elastic potential having been exceeded or pressure forces sustained.

Adapted from Chaitow L, DeLany J. *Clinical Applications of Neuromuscular Technique*. Vol. 2. Churchill Livingstone; 2008.

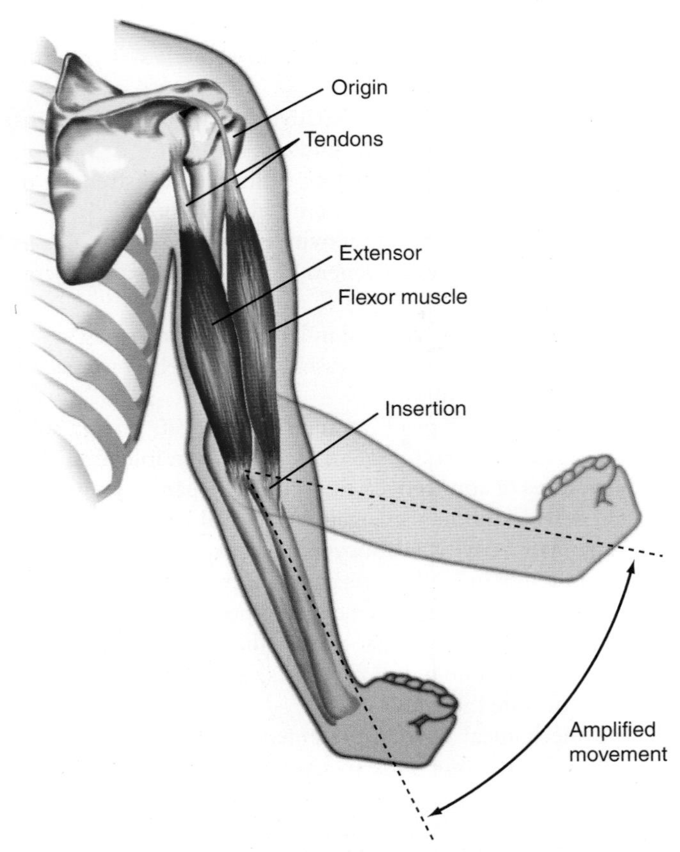

FIG. 9.10 Attachments of a skeletal muscle. A muscle attaches at a relatively stable part of the skeleton (proximal attachment—origin) and inserts at the skeletal part that is moved when the muscle contracts (distal attachment—insertion). (From Koeppen BM, Stanton BA. *Berne & Levy Physiology*. 6th ed. Mosby; 2010.)

chronic strain at some point removes the painful portion and then becomes a natural part of restoring systemic ease and preventing future injuries. Full-body massage applications best address the tensegric nature of the body. Full-body massage that addresses these areas of strain creates ease in the tensegrity system. Spot work often is directed at the symptom and not the cause and therefore is less effective.

The term **biotensegrity** structure suggests that when human movement occurs, the entire musculoskeletal system constantly adjusts during this movement (Swanson, 2013). Muscles can no longer be viewed as independent anatomical structures that simply connect one bone to another bone. Instead, the body consists of numerous muscles connected in series, end to end, spanning the entire musculoskeletal system, creating long viscoelastic myofascial chains that cross multiple joints (Dischiavi et al., 2018).

Myofascial continuity describes the connection between structures forming the myofascial chains. The concept of myofascial continuity suggests that muscles activate along kinematic chains with common fascial coverings. Muscles play a valuable role in managing the mechanical tension. The transmission of the mechanical force when muscles activate is ensured by the fascial integrity (Ingber, 2018; Ermakov, 2018). One of the fundamental characteristics of the fascia is the ability to adapt to mechanical stress and adapt based on relationships between structure and function. Muscles operate across functionally integrated body-wide continuities within the fascial network. Points of integration are where tension elements and compression come together. These points are often where changes in myofascia are identified. Strain, tension, fixation, compensations, and most movements are distributed along these lines. Circles represent points of integration and a common point for intervention (Figs. 9.11 to 9.13) (Wilke et al., 2016; Palomeque-del-Cerro et al., 2017; Zheng et al., 2018; Vulfsons et al., 2018; Ajimsha et al., 2020).

Muscle Synergies

Muscle synergy occurs when individual muscles, working together based on a nervous system sequence, produce coordinated movements of the whole organism.

The most basic functional movements produced by skeletal muscles are standing and walking. Synergistic coordination occurs to efficiently accomplish tasks such as reaching, grasping, lifting, running, and so forth. Each muscle synergy pattern consists of co-activation of multiple muscles in an efficient sequence. However, just how the nervous system integrates the concurrent control of locomotion and balance function remains unclear. Myofascial chains correlate to organized muscle synergies, which is interesting. The idea of the musculoskeletal system functioning as interconnected muscular chains coordinated through the nervous system questions the idea of numerous isolated muscles, which reflects the current interpretation of the muscle system (Berniker et al., 2009; Trech and Jark, 2009; Bizzi, and Cheung, 2013; Singh et al., 2018).

The pattern of synergy contraction typically involves this sequence: Agonist is supported by synergists, fixators, and co-contraction of antagonist, and neutralizers. Support muscles in other body areas also act to integrate the movement

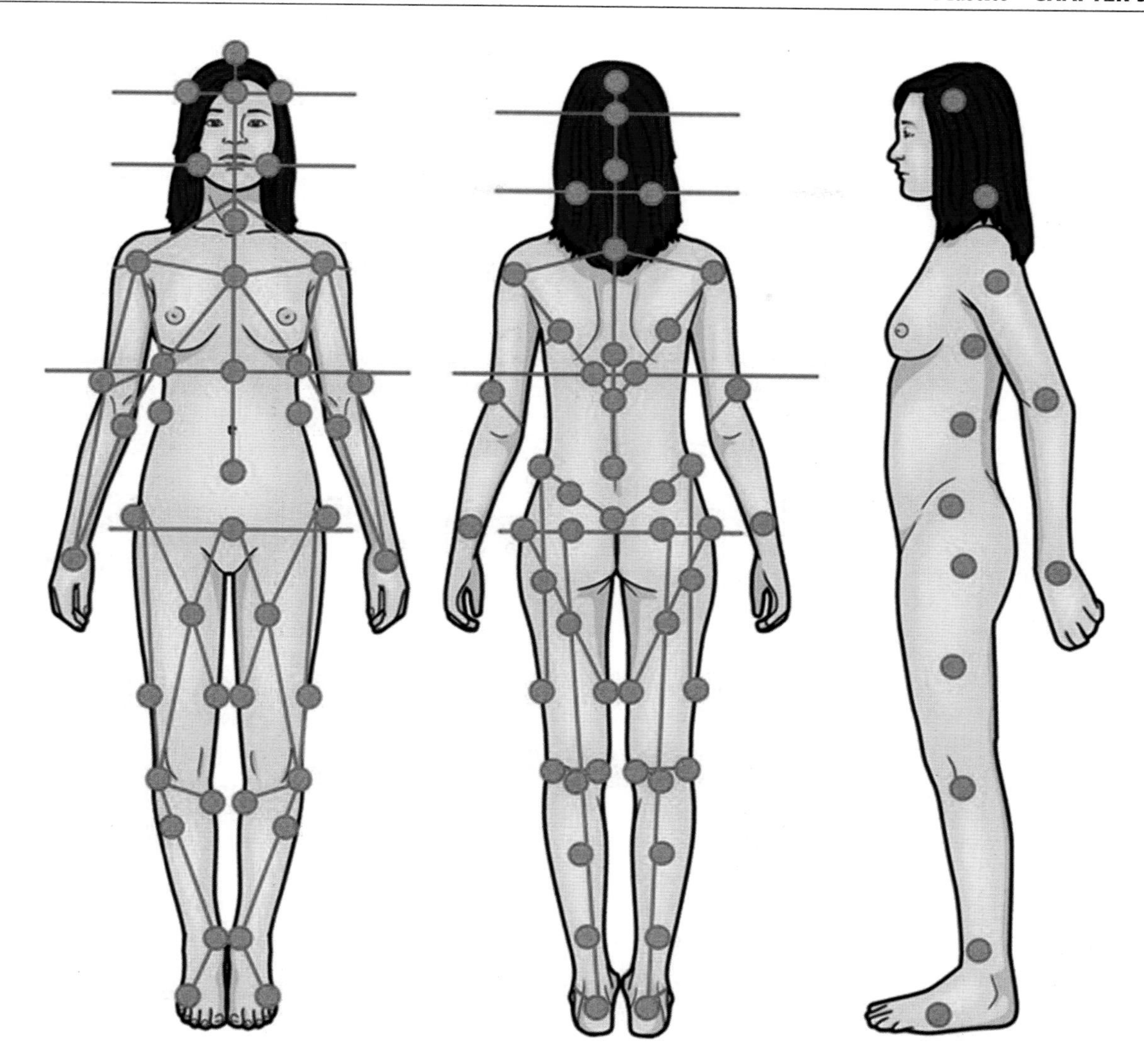

FIG. 9.11 Points of integration. Points of integration are where tension elements and compression come together. Concentrate massage application relative to these areas of the body. Strain, tension, fixation, compensations, and most movements are distributed along these lines. Circles represent points of integration and common point for intervention.

body-wide. This pattern is general. Exceptions occur, but the pattern provides a framework for understanding muscle interaction.

Disruption of the activation sequence causes labored movement, resulting in muscle fatigue. In clinical practice these muscle synergies of motor function are called *muscle activation sequences* or *muscle firing patterns*. Chapter 10 provides more discussion on using muscle activation sequences for assessment and intervention during the massage session.

Fascial Response to Mechanical Forces

The body is exposed to mechanical forces all the time. Every time we sit, stand, lift, push, and so on the fascia is exposed to external mechanical forces. Every time we breathe, our heart beats, and food moves through the digestive system, we are exposed to internal mechanical forces.

Mechanical forces are important regulators of connective tissue homeostasis. This tissue is designed to move, and lack of movement creates dysfunction. Fibroblasts sense force-induced deformations (strains) in the extracellular matrix. Changes in cell shape are well-established factors regulating a wide range of cellular functions, including signal transduction, gene expression, and matrix adhesion. The extracellular matrix plays a key role in the transmission of mechanical forces generated by muscle contraction or externally applied mechanical forces, such as those used during massage application (Petersen, 2012). Applying force is called **loading**, and releasing force is called *unloading*. Theoretically, when a mechanical force is gradually applied to fascia, it has an elastic reaction in which a degree of slack is allowed to be taken up, and the tissue begins to creep because of its viscoelastic nature.

Daily activities, repetitive strain, or a traumatic event can influence how mechanical forces affect body function. This can lead to a process of progressive deterioration. The adaptive strain affects multiple systems, including the nervous and endocrine systems (Schwartz et al., 2018a,b). Therapeutically

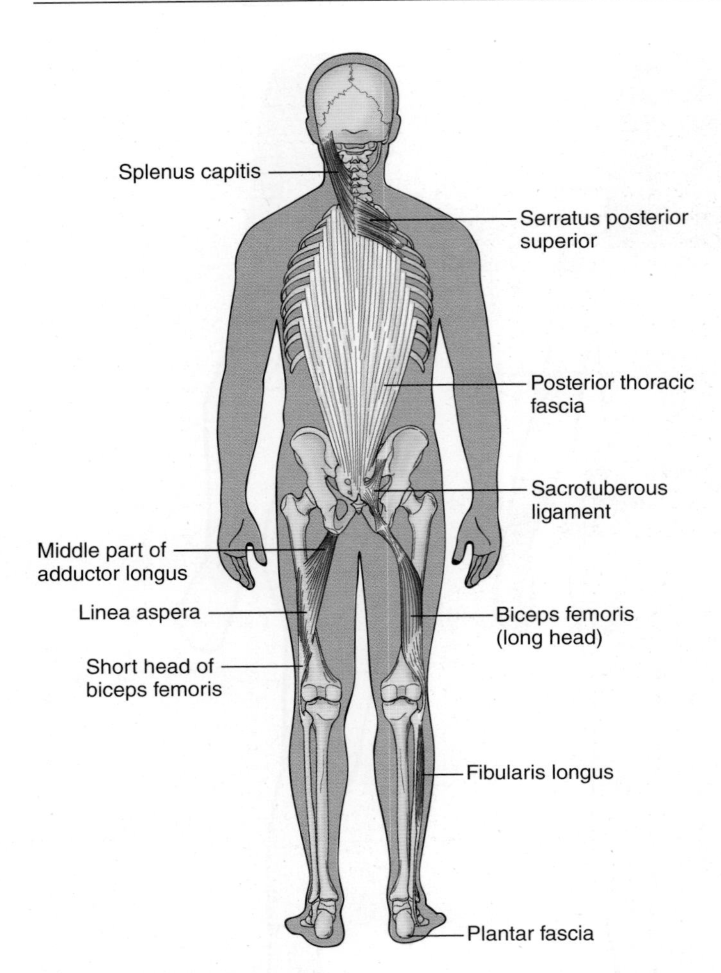

FIG. 9.12 Myofascial continuity. The body is an interconnected system. This example shows an anatomical connection from the skull to the bottom of the foot. This muscle/fascia joining is necessary for the body to function as an integrated unit. (Adapted from Myers T. *Anatomy Trains: Myofascial Meridians for Manual and Movement Therapists*. Churchill Livingstone; 2002.)

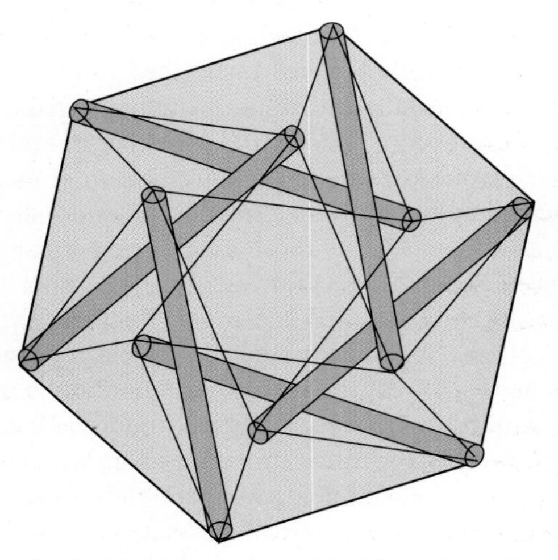

FIG. 9.13 An abstract image of a cell that is kept together by tensegrity.

applied mechanical force may support homeostasis (Ault et al., 2017; Simmons et al., 2018; Langevin et al., 2018; Do and Yim, 2018; Nedelec et al., 2018). However, many claims regarding the effects of massage techniques targeted toward fascia are not supported by research (Laimi et al., 2018).

Pathological changes in connective tissue result in alterations, such as thickening, shortening, calcification, and erosion. These changes may result from sudden or sustained torsion, tension, compression, and bend and shear mechanical forces, as well as lack of proper movement. Sustained inappropriate forces cause the fascia to adapt and result in reduced pliability and may lead to varying degrees of fascial entrapment of nerve structures and consequently a wide range of symptoms and dysfunctions. Nerve receptors within the fascia report to the central nervous system as part of any adaptation process. The lamellated (pacinian) corpuscles are particularly important because they inform the central nervous system about the rate of movement acceleration taking place in the area. This involvement can affect reflex responses. Other sensory input in response to biomechanical stress involves fascial structures, such as tendons and ligaments, which contain highly specialized and sensitive mechanoreceptor and proprioceptor reporting stations. Fascial changes adversely influence many of these sensing receptors, which are implicated in pain syndromes.

Fascial stiffness might be influenced and regulated by the state of the autonomic nervous system. Thus, intervention in the fascial system may affect the autonomic nervous system and organs it influences. For example, an increased breathing rate can cause an increase in fascial tone, which in turn may create added stabilization and stiffness of the low back. Muscle stiffness can be evaluated in either the relaxed (passive) state or the contracted state; the mechanisms involved in each state are different. Muscle resistance to passive stretching comes primarily from two sources: titin and the extracellular matrix (ECM).

Based on ongoing investigation, massage therapy influences on fascia could be clarified based on distribution of the slippery substance hyaluronan (hyaluronic acid), managing densification and fibrotic changes, including scar tissue, and specifically working with the myofascial trigger point phenomena (Pavan et al., 2014; Bordoni and Zanier, 2014; Kwong and Findley, 2014). It is biologically plausible that massage can be adapted to therapeutically affect these tissues based on client-reported outcomes, such as less stiffness, reduced pain perception, and increased function (Box 9.6).

Section Summary

- Define fascia.
  - Fascia is a body-wide connective tissue which supports, separates, and attaches tissue layers from visceral to superficial. Superficial fascia: loose areolar connective tissue that connects the skin to deep fascia and includes adipose tissue. Deep fascia: dense connective tissue surrounding individual muscles and muscle groups.
- Define biotensegrity and myofascial continuity.
  - Biotensegrity: using a tent as an analogy—the bones are poles supplying compression; muscles/tendons/ligaments are ropes supplying tension; and fascia is the canvas

Box 9.6 What Are Myofascial Massage Approaches?

There is no unified definition of myofascial approaches. However, the methods typically include techniques that apply prolonged light pressure with specific directions into the fascial system in order to relieve pain and release restrictions. Myofascial release (MFR) is a common and confusing term used to describe multiple techniques that slowly apply an external mechanical load designed to actively move the fascia and underlying soft tissue in areas of decreased fascial mobility.

Methods also include suction to lift the skin and superficial fascia, typically called cupping. Negative pressure causes stretching of the skin and underlying tissue and dilation of the capillaries. If the suction is left in place too long, capillary rupture and ecchymosis occur, resulting in the red, round circles commonly seen when suction cups are removed. Ecchymosis occurs when blood leaks from a broken capillary into surrounding tissue under the skin. This causes discoloration. These red circles are not bruises. Bruises are typically caused by a compressive injury, such as a fall or a knock. Ecchymosis is not always a result of trauma and not necessarily related to compression trauma (Lowe, 2017).

Lowe DT. Cupping therapy: an analysis of the effects of suction on skin and the possible influence on human health. *Complement Ther Clin Pract.* 2017;29:162–168. https://doi.org/10.1016/j.ctcp.2017.09.008.

under/distributing tension to hold everything together. This means strain of one part is distributed body-wide (explaining compensation patterns). Myofascial continuity: the principle that muscles activate and transmit force along kinematic chains with common fascial coverings.

- Explain pathological connective tissue changes.
  - Pathological connective tissue changes, such as thickening, shortening, calcification, and erosion, may result from adaptation to sudden or sustained mechanical forces, as well as reduced or improper movement. This results in reduced pliability and may lead to fascial entrapment of nerve structures. Densification: when the ground substance of fascia (mostly composed of water) thickens/loses pliability. Fibrosis: when the fibers (collagen/elastin) of fascia shorten, such as with scar tissue.

Practical Application

Recall from Chapter 8 that creep is the term for the slow, delayed, and continuous deformation that occurs in response to a sustained, slowly applied load. Therapeutically the goal is to produce creep to elongate shortened and binding tissue to a more functional position. Theoretically the mechanical forces created by massage application may produce creep and must be applied with slow and appropriate pressure with sustained drag and without causing injury. Many soft tissue methods, including massage, consider creep a mechanism that results in tissue change. However, the available research does not totally support this premise.

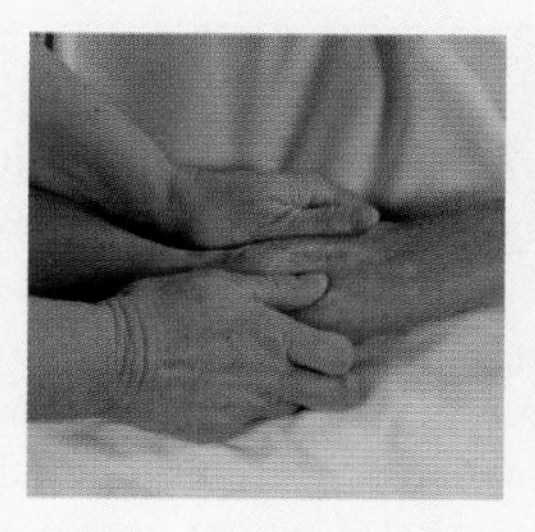

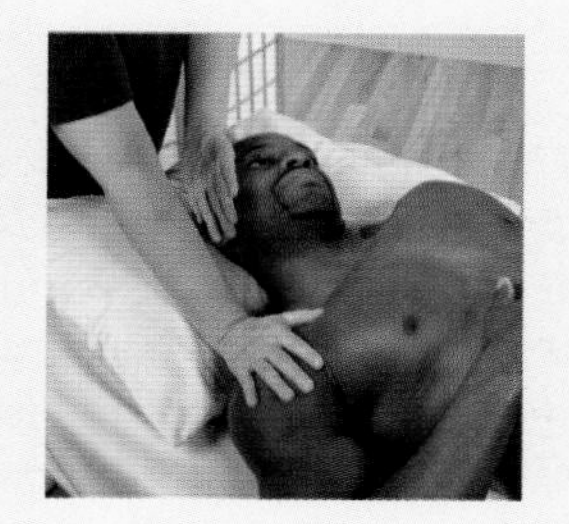

Thixotropy relates to the quality of gelatinous substances called *colloids* in which the more rapidly the force is applied (load), the more rigid and the less pliable the tissue response will be. Muscle tissue that is rigid or feels dense may have undergone thixotropic changes. If the practitioner gradually applies force, as described previously, it is thought that the tissues absorb and store energy. Expanding on this theory to influence connective tissue pliability, massage application must not be abrupt or the tissue will respond by becoming more rigid.

Hysteresis describes the process of energy loss because of friction and tiny structural damage that occurs when tissues are loaded and unloaded repetitively. The tissues produce heat as they are loaded and unloaded, which occurs with on-and-off pressure application. Creating hysteresis may reduce stiffness and improve the way the tissue responds to subsequent load application.

The properties of hysteresis and creep provide the basis for myofascial release techniques. But again, new research is questioning these theories and offering new possibilities. One of the most plausible is that loading and unloading fascia changes the water content of the tissue, which in turn changes the pliability. Still another is that the fascia is a communication network wherein loading and unloading the tissue changes the shape of the cells, resulting in a chemical change. According to yet another theory, myofibroblast contraction produces fascial tone—thus the influence of manual force on myofibroblasts changes fascial tone.

Something happens when massage therapy application is adapted to target the connective tissue network. Typically, approaches include slowly applied loads which result in slow continuous deformation of tissue. The research has not been able to provide objective information why changes occur.

The same situation exists for the myofibroblasts, which are like tiny smooth muscle cells that evolve from fibroblasts and are found imbedded in connective tissues. These cells are especially active during wound healing, helping to pull tissue together. However, myofibroblasts are found in fascial tissues that are not injured. Researchers know they exist, know that the autonomic nervous system exerts some control and that the myofibroblasts are part of the mechanism of maintaining fascial tautness (tone). How massage may affect fascial tone is still based on interesting speculation and not fact. Any contraction of the muscles results in a simultaneous stretch of the fascial tissue. How might this information explain methods, such as muscle energy techniques, that involve an active muscle contraction to support soft tissue elongation? Fascia contains free nerve endings, mechanoreceptors, and other sensory and motor nerves. Researchers have found these neurostructures.

This research demonstrates how fibroblasts can cause or contribute to the maintenance of fascial binds by increasing their own prestress and thus increasing prestress within the fascia. Also, the release that occurs during the application of myofascial release techniques may result from fibroblasts sensing the mechanical forces being applied by means of mechanotransduction. The mechanotransduction could then lead to changes in fibroblast prestress, which would decrease the prestress within the fascia. Further, cell-to-cell communication between fibroblasts within the fascia could potentially contribute to numerous fibroblasts changing their level of prestress, which would then cause a more robust change in the prestress within the fascia, leading to a palpable release. With the bind released, the normal physiological motion would be restored within the tissue and the fibroblasts would then return to their normal resting prestress. Research has not specifically determined that massage application affects nerves and receptors in the fascia—but research in massage mechanisms has not eliminated the possibility of an effect on the sensory and motor function either. We don't know. This type of information does add to critical thinking and clinical reasoning in support of the concept of "mimic normal" when adapting massage to focus on specific outcomes, such as fascial pliability. This is where the concept of biological plausibility comes in. When we don't know for sure (a fact) but a logical justification can be made based on what is known, we are speaking intelligently.

FOCUS ON PROFESSIONALISM

Research is providing exciting information about connective tissue structures, fascia in particular. *However*, this information does not necessarily support all claims made related to massage methods targeting connective tissue, especially the fascia. It is important not to generalize the specific nature of a research finding. Just because something happens with bioengineered tissue in a lab experiment does not necessarily mean that information translates into therapeutic practice.

The ground substance of fascia consists mainly of water, but not ordinary water as we think of it. This water is stabilized by a complex of glycosaminoglycans (GAGs), proteoglycans, and glycoproteins. The effect of GAGs in water is similar to that of gelatin. Mixing a package of gelatin in water transforms the water from a flowing liquid into a solid mass, or gel. Because of the presence of proteins bound to the water, water in our bodies is in more of a gel-like state. The concept of a liquid crystalline, or gel-like, state of water is not new (Pollack, 2018). The gel can become thicker or thinner. If it thickens too much, it becomes dense, loses pliability, and is experienced as stiffness. This affect is called *densification*. Also, the fibers in connective tissue matrix can shorten and pull. The fibers can also mat, tangle, and shorten. This is called *fibrosis*. Fibrosis or fibromatosis often occurs related to a chronic localized inflammatory response of tissue trauma, including scar tissue formation. Over time, densification can develop into fibrosis. It is more plausible to think that massage might help restore pliability to dense ground substance than to think massage can reverse fibrosis.

Densification is related to the water content of fascia, which partially determines its stiffness. It is logical that pulling or pressing fascia (as occurs during almost all manual therapies), causes water to be extruded (like a sponge), making the tissues more pliable. As water in the fascia is squeezed out during tissue compression and elongation, tissues can be mobilized and lengthened more effectively and comfortably than if they were still densely packed with water. The change in water content of fascia increases the tolerance to the uncomfortable sensation in muscle tissues when elongation occurs. Because the client is more comfortable, the myofascial unit can be lengthened more effectively.

Elongation of muscle tissue straightens out the wavy collagen fibrils in connective tissue. However, it is unlikely that enough force can be put on collagen to actually change the length of the collagen fibers. When the force creating the elongation on the connective tissues stops, the collagen fibers return to the wavy crimped configuration.

All sorts of ideas come to mind about the implications for massage. Massage application has the rhythmic squeezing component as an aspect of many applications, such as kneading and elongation. It is easy to speculate and conclude that a reason massage makes tissue longer and more pliable is because of the shifting of water into and out of collagen, which is a major component of fascia. However, caution is necessary. Research has not proved this. Nor has research disproved it. Therefore, we don't know and cannot state our speculations as a fact (Thalhamer, 2018).

INDIVIDUAL MUSCLES

SECTION OBJECTIVES

Chapter objectives covered in this section:

9. Explain and demonstrate the three types of muscle actions.
10. Describe how muscles are named.
11. Learn how to palpate individual muscles.
12. Identify the attachments, actions, synergists, antagonists, and common trigger points of individual muscles.

After completing this section, the student will be able to:

- Explain the three types of muscle actions.
- Describe how muscles are named.
- Apply knowledge of the muscular system to therapeutic massage application.

MENTORING TIP

Based on the previous section related to the continuity, synergy, and integrated nature of function, it can seem odd to study individual muscles because in truth, no muscle functions individually. However, there is value in the anatomical study of individual muscles so long as the relationship of functional units is understood and related to massage therapy application. To assist this, the following section is organized by anatomical regions, and the muscles of each region are listed from superficial to deep. This correlates with massage application. As we massage each region, we first address the superficial layers of muscle, then work deeper. Each individual muscle structure is described in context with the functional muscle groups. Although we understand that the body operates as a unit, the massage practitioner must know the individual parts making up that unit.

The following section describes the individual muscles most often discussed by massage professionals. We discuss their primary function or functions; attachments; innervation; synergists; antagonists; and, if applicable, common trigger point areas and referred pain patterns.

This section contains a great deal of information. One way to study it is to get to know the muscles as you would get to

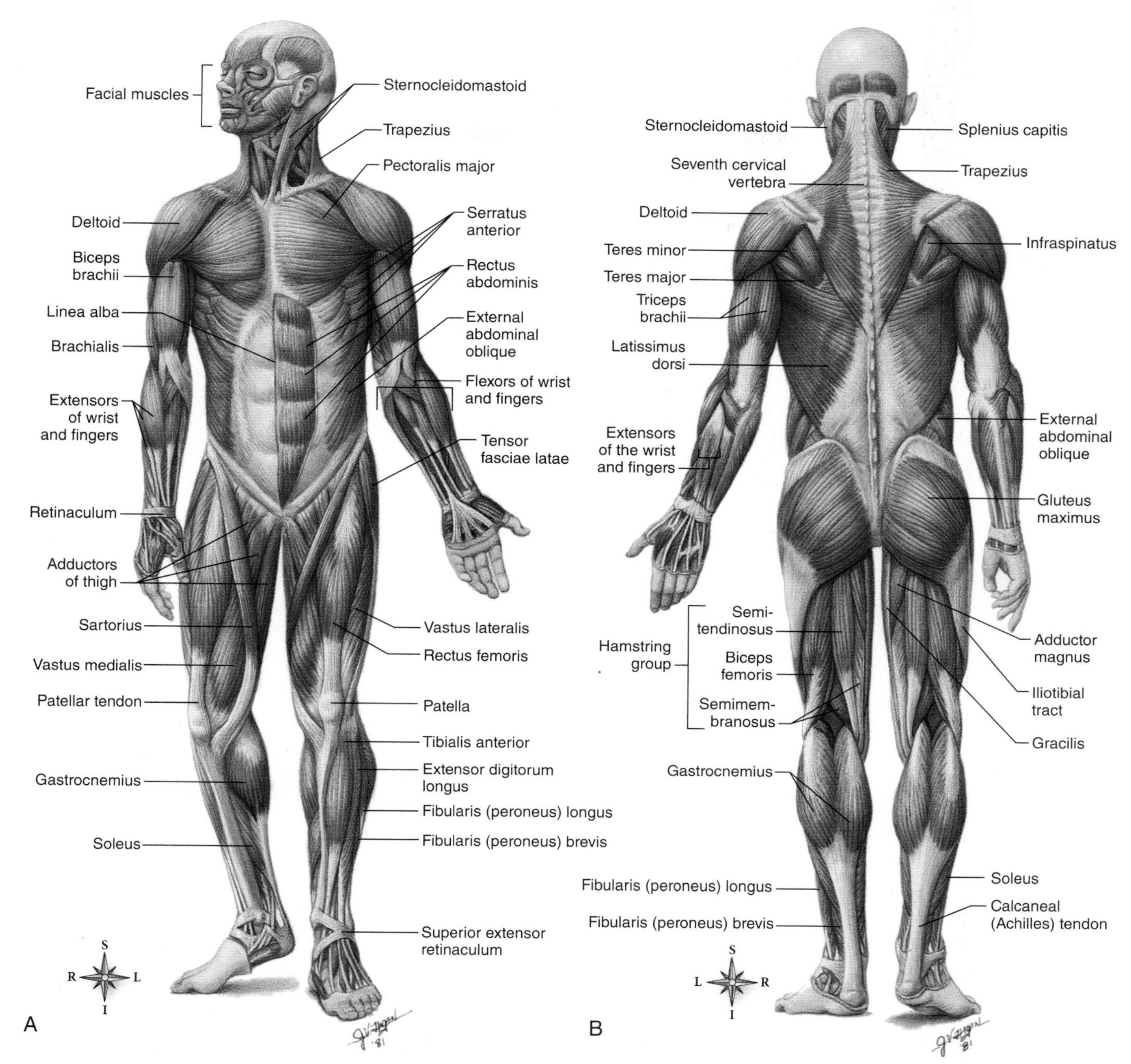

FIG. 9.14 Muscles of the body: (A) anterior view, (B) posterior view, and (C) lateral view. (From Patton KT, Colrus B, Kulka J. *Survival Guide for Anatomy & Physiology*. 2nd ed. Elsevier; 2014.)

know a new friend. Knowing where to find them, what they do, who their friends are, and what bothers them is helpful. Activities (e.g., palpation and movement; coloring, drawing, and labeling the attachment points; and locating common trigger points) reinforce your knowledge of the structure and function of individual muscles and groups of muscles.

To appreciate friends as individuals, you do not need to know every detail of their lives. If you need to know more about a muscle, you can always ask questions and look up additional material in reference texts as needed. Note that not all authors agree about specific details, and different references list slightly different attachment sites, functions, and so forth. As with most differing opinions, the answer is not always black or white but somewhere in between.

As you study individual muscles, keep these points in mind:

- Muscles are arranged in layers, and most body areas have three to five layers of muscles. This text lists muscles from the superficial to deepest layers.
- Those muscles considered deep lie closest to the bone, and those considered superficial lie closest to the skin (Fig. 9.14).
- Muscles with similar functions are bundled together by deep fascia into compartments (e.g., the anterior, medial, and posterior compartments of the thigh).
- Compartments of bundled muscles function to move joints, and joints move in the sagittal plane (flexions and extensions), frontal plane (abductions and adductions), and transverse plane (internal and external rotations).
- Muscle shape and fiber direction can also indicate function.

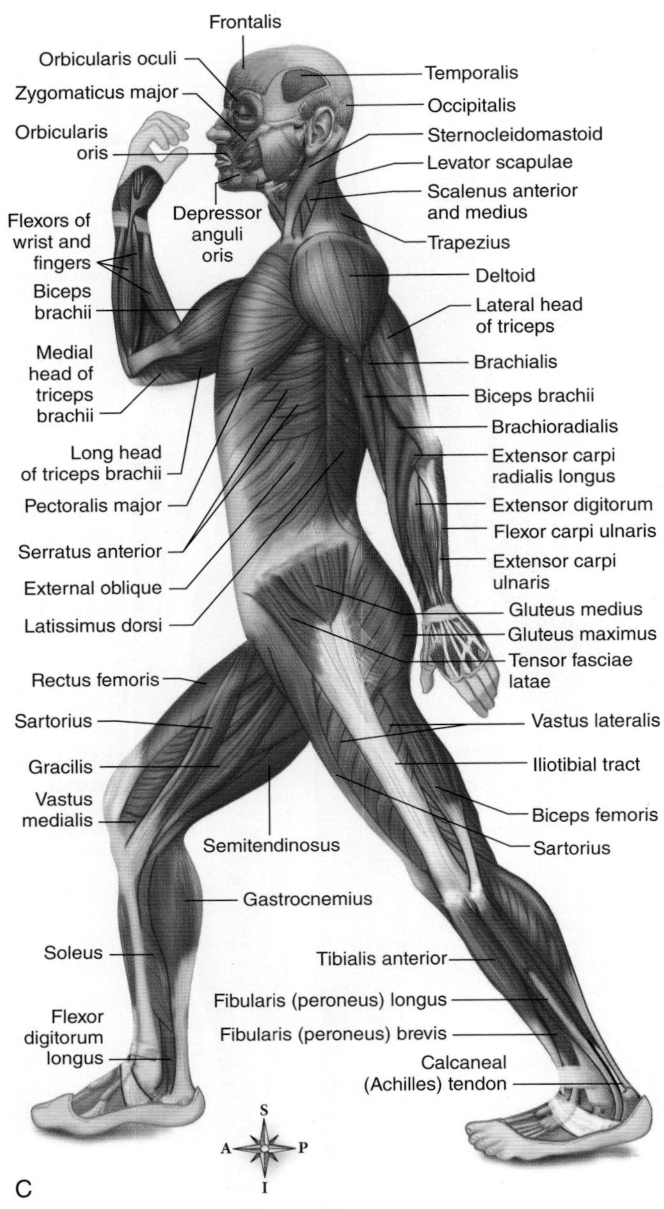

FIG. 9.14, cont'd

- Muscles shaped like cylinders with vertical fibers typically function on the sagittal plane, are movers and sometimes stabilizers (as well as flexors and extensors) and are located on the front and back of the body.

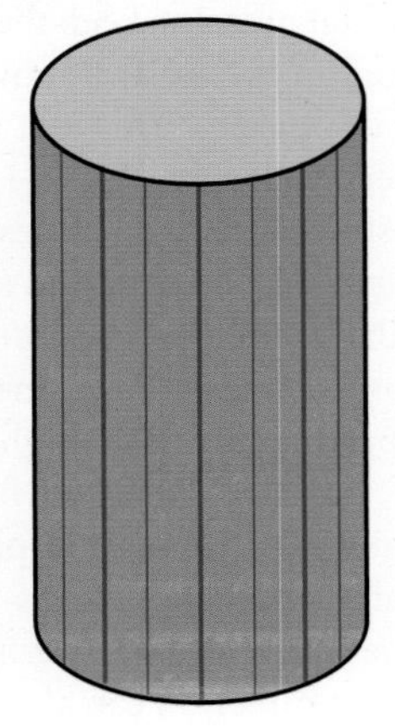

- Muscles shaped like triangles with diagonal fiber direction typically function in the frontal plane and are stabilizers and sometimes movers, as well as abductors and adductors. These muscles are located on the lateral or medial side of the body,

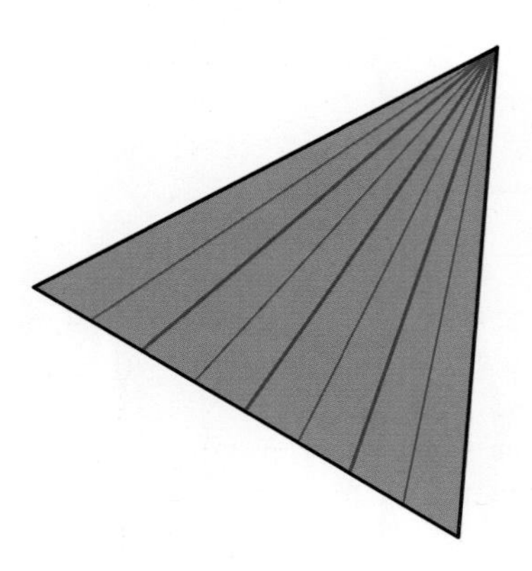

- Muscles shaped like rectangles with horizontal fiber direction function in the transverse plane, are stabilizers and rarely movers, but can produce internal and external rotation.

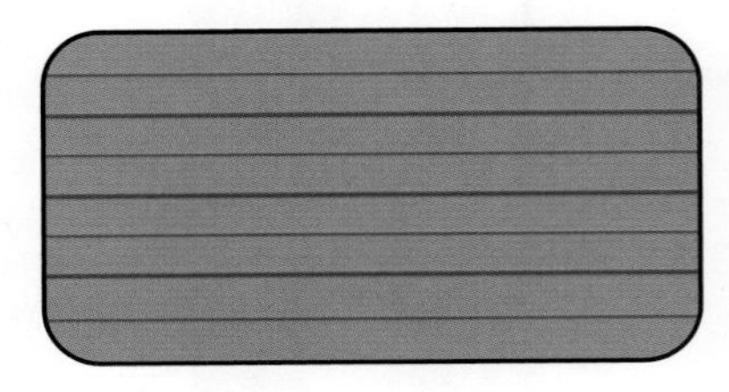

- The length of the muscle fiber determines the distance a muscle can contract to a shorter length or stretch to a longer length. Generally, muscle fibers can contract or stretch 50% of their resting lengths.
  - Shorter muscles (shorter fiber lengths) contract less distance (excursion) than longer muscles.
- Muscles have three main actions:
  1. **Concentric action**, in which the muscle fibers shorten as a result of the neurological and chemical response of actin and myosin. The muscle contraction pulls and moves a bone that is part of a joint, and the joint moves. This movement is typically considered the muscle's primary function. When a muscle is functioning during concentric action, it is called the *prime mover* or *agonist*. The muscle is producing acceleration (increase of motion or action).
  2. **Eccentric action** restrains/controls (especially rapid movement) and controls movement produced by the agonist by lengthening while at the same time maintaining muscle fiber shortening. The eccentric action is as important as the concentric action and even more important in terms of muscle dysfunction. When a muscle is functioning eccentrically, it is usually called

the *antagonist*. The muscle is producing deceleration (decrease of motion or action).

3. Isometric action occurs when the muscle fibers shorten and attempt to pull on a bone but the actual movement is prevented at the joint. The tissue stiffens and becomes contracted when the muscle is acting as a *stabilizer (fixator)* and *neutralizer*. Stabilization and guiding of movement are essential for proper function.

- Each muscle can perform these three actions, and they are all important. However, a muscle can efficiently perform only one action at a time. Dysfunction can occur when these muscle actions are not used efficiently (e.g., if a muscle tries to produce movement when what is really needed is stabilization, or the muscle attempts to create a movement but at the same time is opposing the movement).
- Muscles work in functional units, never alone. Functional units consist of three or more muscles, bundled into compartments, alternating among concentric, eccentric, and isometric actions and integrated within myofascial continuity.

When these functions of muscles are specifically important to the massage profession, we discuss them as well. When studying the individual muscles, pay attention to all elements provided for each muscle. Also pay attention to referred pain patterns, because these are the symptoms clients will complain about if dysfunction with the muscle occurs.

How Muscles Are Named

Muscle names seem more logical and easier to learn when the reasons for the names are clear. Many of the muscles of the body are named using one or more of these features:

- *Location:* Many muscles are named for their location using medical terminology. The brachialis (arm muscle) and gluteus (buttock) muscles are examples.
- *Function:* The function of a muscle is frequently a part of its name. The adductor muscles of the thigh adduct or move the thigh at the hip joint toward the midline of the body.
- *Shape:* Shape is a descriptive feature used for naming many muscles. The deltoid (triangular) muscle covering the shoulder is shaped like a delta or triangle.
- *Direction of fibers:* Muscles may be named according to the orientation of their fibers. The term *rectus* means "straight." The fibers of the rectus abdominis muscle run straight up and down (vertically) and are parallel to one another.
- *Number of heads or divisions:* The number of divisions or heads (points of attachment) may be used to name a muscle. The word part *-cep* means "head." The biceps (two), triceps (three), and quadriceps (four) refer to multiple heads or points of attachment. The *biceps brachii* is a muscle having two heads located in the arm.
- *Points of attachment:* A muscle attaches from one site to another site. These attachment sites may be used to name a muscle. For example, the sternocleidomastoid has an attachment on the sternum and clavicle and another attachment on the mastoid process of the temporal bone.
- *Size of the muscle:* The size of a muscle can be used to name a muscle, especially if it is compared with the size of nearby muscles. For example, the gluteus maximus is the largest muscle of the gluteal (Greek *glautos*, meaning "buttock") region. Nearby is a small gluteal muscle, gluteus minimus, and a midsize gluteal muscle, gluteus medius.

Muscle Attachment Terminology

As discussed previously, unless terminology is consistent, it can be confusing. Terminology used for the muscular system is not consistent. There are multiple names and spellings for muscle names and duplicate terminology to describe the location of muscles. The attachment terminology appears as follows in the individual muscle sections:

- Origin, fixed end, proximal attachment, arises from
- Insertion, mobile end, distal attachment, attaches to

The repetition of attachment terminology variations will prepare you to understand information presented in other textbooks and various exams.

How to Palpate Muscles

Massage is palpation, and palpation is assessment; both are part of an intervention process. It is essential that you feel the muscle and associated connective tissues during massage. It is essential to understand the tissue you massage. Practice, practice, and practice palpation.

You can palpate muscles that are relaxed or contracted as follows:

- Distinguishing whether you are palpating the correct muscle is difficult at times, because many structures (e.g., tendons, fascia, and ligaments) can attach in the same place.
- With relaxed muscles, locating the muscle depends on anatomical knowledge and the ability to identify bony landmarks.
- To palpate muscles when they are relaxed, read the attachment descriptions carefully and place your hand on the location described. Then trace the path of the muscle between the attachments.
- Notice the fiber direction, which determines the angle of pull when the muscle shortens.
- The largest area of the muscle is usually near the middle of the muscle and is called the *belly*.
- To identify a specific muscle, first identify the attachments and belly of the muscle while the muscle is relaxed, and then have the client actively contract the muscle.
- You can do this by placing the muscle in the concentric action position and then having the client hold that position or move the muscle a bit between concentric and eccentric patterns.
- While the client holds the position or slightly contracts the specific muscle, you should be able to feel the muscle tensing, bunching up, or pushing out.
- Remember that three or more layers of muscles cover each area and are bundled into compartments.
- A compartment is easiest to palpate. The more superficial muscles in a compartment are easier to palpate than the deeper muscles.

- Identifying the deeper muscle layers is more difficult. The deeper muscles usually have smaller movement patterns, so using a slight contraction to initiate a tiny movement to differentiate the smaller deeper layers is helpful.
- Then initiate a larger or stronger contraction to identify the more superficial layers of the muscle.
- Palpation of deeper muscles requires more pressure but should not feel painful or abrupt to the massage client.

Organization of This Section

The muscles are organized by body area, beginning with the face and head, and are listed from superficial to deep. At the beginning of each body area an overview description of the muscles and function is provided. Before each specific body section is a series of illustrations that form a mini atlas. These illustrations are borrowed from *Gray's Anatomy for Students* (2014). The intent of each mini atlas is to provide visual orientation of muscle locations and relationships to one another. The mini atlas provides a visual orientation for references when studying each of the individual muscles in that section. The more realistic illustration provided by each mini atlas is coupled with the more graphic view of individual muscles. Although the mini atlases can provide excellent overview and orientation, it is not possible to display each muscle because of the overlapping structure of muscle layers.

Individual Muscles Grouped by Body Area

Directly after the mini atlas is a series of illustrations of individual muscles. Each individual muscle is described, providing this information:

- Muscle name and pronunciation
- What the muscle name means
- Concentric action
- Eccentric action
- Isometric action
- Origin, fixed end, proximal attachment, arises from
- Insertion, mobile end, distal attachment, attaches to
- Innervation
- Major synergists
- Major antagonists
- Tender/trigger points
- Common symptom/Common symptom/Referred pain pattern

Special Note on Tender/Trigger Points and Referred Pain Patterns

Trigger points as soft tissue pathology are somewhat controversial. There are many theories about what trigger points are and what causes them. The evidence based on research evolves, but no clear data can confirm or deny the existence of trigger points. Regardless, the concept of a focal point in muscles that is linked to identifiable pain patterns is useful in the clinical application of massage and helps frame the symptoms a client experiences. The trigger point hypothesis continues to be researched. These point locations are now used as sites for dry-needling applications. The points correlate with the traditional acupuncture point locations. In this edition the terminology has been expanded to tender/trigger points and common symptom/referred pain pattern in an attempt to broaden the understanding of the point relationship to muscle-related pain symptoms. Someday, evidence may be sufficient to figure out just what is going on with the "trigger point phenomena." Until then, remember that trigger points are hypothetical, not fact. They are useful as a concept but not totally understood, and massage can often help the client feel better for a while.

Individual Muscle Drawing Activities

Skeletal pictures are provided in this chapter to be used as coloring/drawing activities. Use these pictures to draw individual muscles or muscle groups. If the activity requires more than one muscle to be drawn on the same picture, you should make each muscle a different color. Label the attachment sites with different colors and use those colors consistently throughout all the activities. Mark the trigger point or points in yet another color and be consistent throughout the activities. Fine-point colored pencils work best for these activities. This type of kinesthetic learning is effective for memory retention. Do not become overly concerned with your artistic ability. The learning occurs in the doing, not the result. The drawing activities include exercises such as this:

Draw and color the ___________(muscle name) in the spaces provided. For each muscle:

1. Label the proximal attachment/origin and distal attachment/insertion locations: *O* for origin; *I* for insertion.
2. Place an X on the location of the trigger points. (NOTE: The term trigger point is used in the drawing activities to indicate tender/trigger points.)
3. Palpate this muscle; identify the attachment points and the bellies of the muscles.
4. Move these muscles on yourself.

Make sure to palpate the muscles on yourself, or even better another person such as a family member or classmate and move the muscle. The combined drawing, labeling, palpation, and movement activities provide an excellent system for learning muscles.

Muscles of the Face and Head

The superficial muscles of the head, including those of the scalp and face, produce movement for facial expressions, which are vital to nonverbal communication (Fig. 9.15). The muscles vary in shape and strength. Many adjacent muscles tend to be fused together. Unlike most skeletal muscles, which attach onto bones of the skeleton, many muscles of facial expression attach into skin or other muscles. Muscles of the head and face lift our eyebrows, flare our nostrils, and open and close our eyes and mouth. Many of these muscles are implicated in headaches and tend to tense when a person is stressed, especially if in pain. Careful massage to the area can be soothing and effective in managing tension headaches.

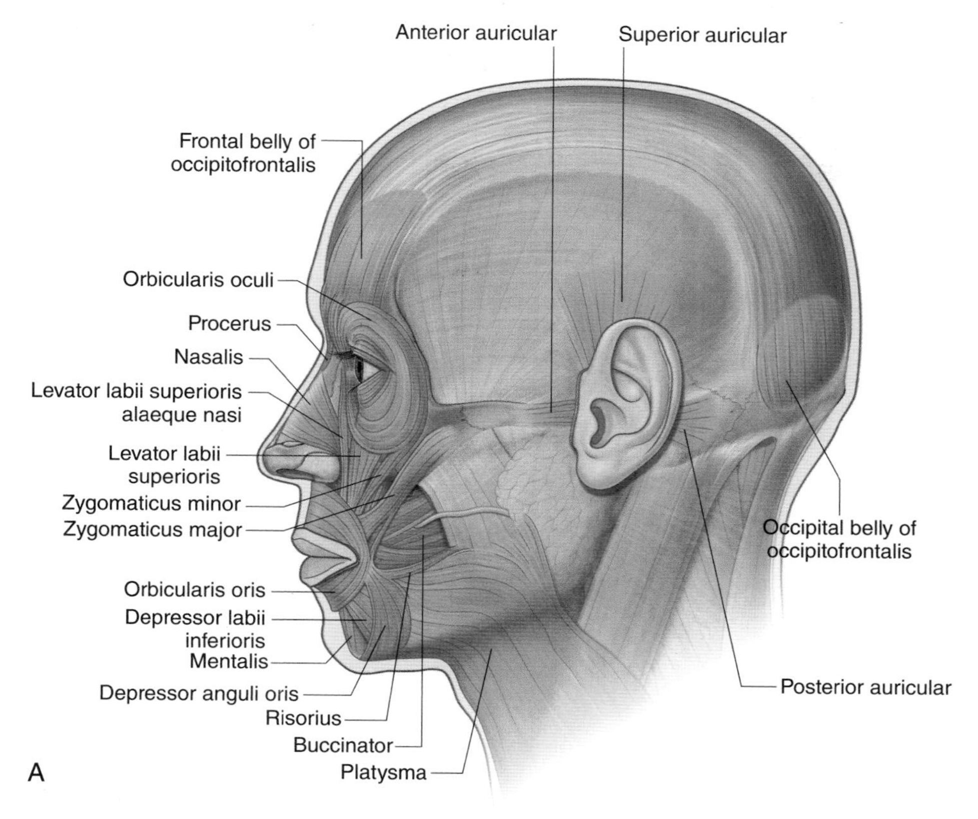

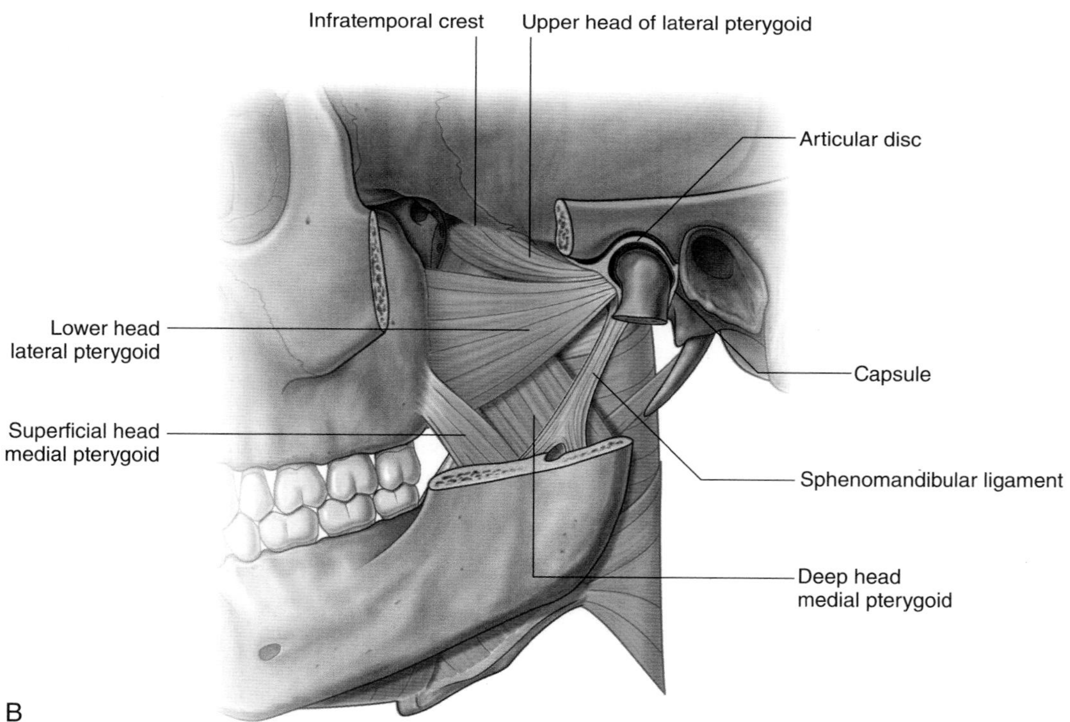

FIG. 9.15 (A) Facial muscles. (B) Lateral pterygoid muscles. (From Drake RL, Vogl W, Mitchell WM. *Gray's Anatomy for Students*. 2nd ed. Churchill Livingstone; 2010.)

Facial Expression Muscles

Occipitofrontalis (ok-SIP-ih-toe-fron-TAL-iss)

Also called the *epicranius, occipitofrontalis* means "back of the head and related to the forehead." The muscle sometimes is described as separate muscles—the occipitalis and the frontalis.

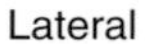

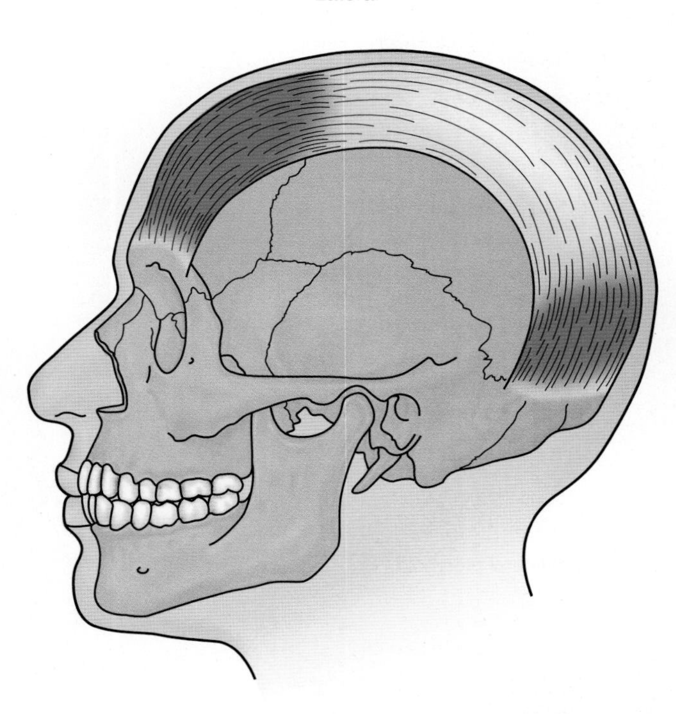

- *Concentric action:*
  - Draws the scalp anteriorly and posteriorly, elevates the eyebrows, and wrinkles the forehead
- *Origin, fixed end, proximal attachment, arises from:*
  - Occipital belly—lateral two-thirds of the highest nuchal line of the occipital bone and the mastoid area of the temporal bone
  - Frontal belly—galea aponeurotica near the coronal suture
- *Insertion, mobile end, distal attachment, attaches to:*
  - Occipital belly—galea aponeurotica
  - Frontal belly—fascia and skin superior to the eye and nose
- *Innervation:*
  - Occipitalis—posterior auricular branch of the facial nerve (cranial nerve VII)
  - Frontalis—temporal branches of the facial nerve (cranial nerve VII)
- *Major synergists:*
  - Occipitalis—no major synergists
  - Frontalis—no major synergists
- *Major antagonists:*
  - Occipitalis—frontalis
  - Frontalis—occipitalis, corrugator supercilii, and procerus
- *Tender/trigger points:*
  - Occipitalis—near attachment at the galea aponeurotica
  - Frontalis—belly of the muscle superior to the eyebrow
- *Referred pain patterns:*
  - Eye, ear, and the scalp superior to the ear and deep occipital pain

Procerus (pro-SEHR-us)

Procerus means "tall."

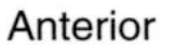

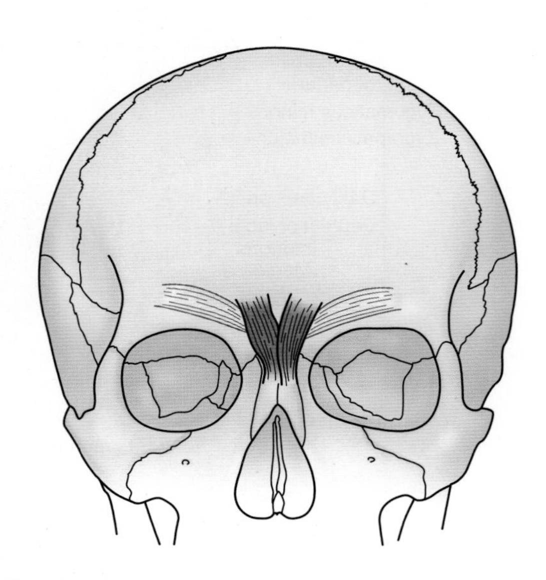

- *Concentric action:*
  - Draws medial angle of the eyebrow downward and produces transverse wrinkles over the bridge of the nose
- *Origin, fixed end, proximal attachment, arises from:*
  - Fascia covering the inferior part of the nasal bone and the superior part of the lateral nasal cartilage
- *Insertion, mobile end, distal attachment, attaches to:*
  - Skin over the lower forehead between the eyebrows
- *Innervation:*
  - Superior buccal branch of the facial nerve (cranial nerve VII)
- *Major synergist:*
  - Corrugator supercilii
- *Major antagonist:*
  - Occipitofrontalis
- *Tender/trigger point:*
  - No common tender/trigger points identified. Tender/trigger points that form are likely located in the belly of the muscles.

Corrugator supercilii (kor-u-GA-tor su-per-SIL-ee-eye)

Corrugator supercilii means "to wrinkle the eyebrows."

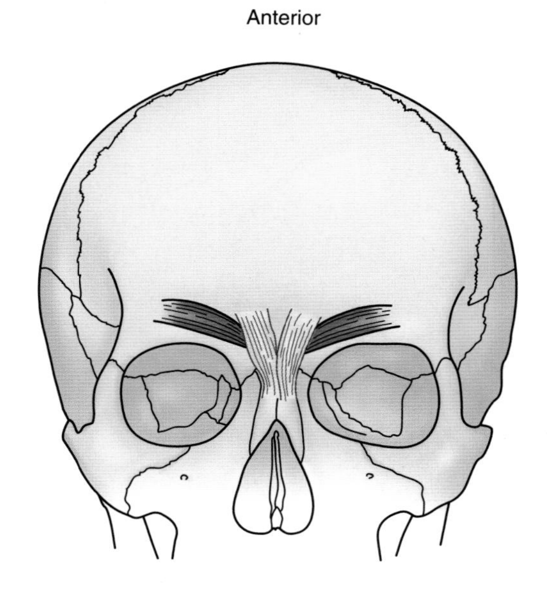

- *Concentric action:*
  - Draws the eyebrow inferiorly and medially
- *Origin, fixed end, proximal attachment, arises from:*
  - Medial end of the superciliary arch of the frontal bone
- *Insertion, mobile end, distal attachment, attaches to:*
  - Skin deep to the medial portion of the eyebrow
- *Innervation:*
  - Temporal branch of the facial nerve (cranial nerve VII)
- *Major synergist:*
  - Procerus
- *Major antagonist:*
  - Occipitofrontalis
- *Tender/trigger points:*
  - No common tender/trigger points identified. Tender/trigger points that form are likely located in the belly of the muscles.

Nasalis (nay-SAL-iss)

Nasalis means "related to the nose."

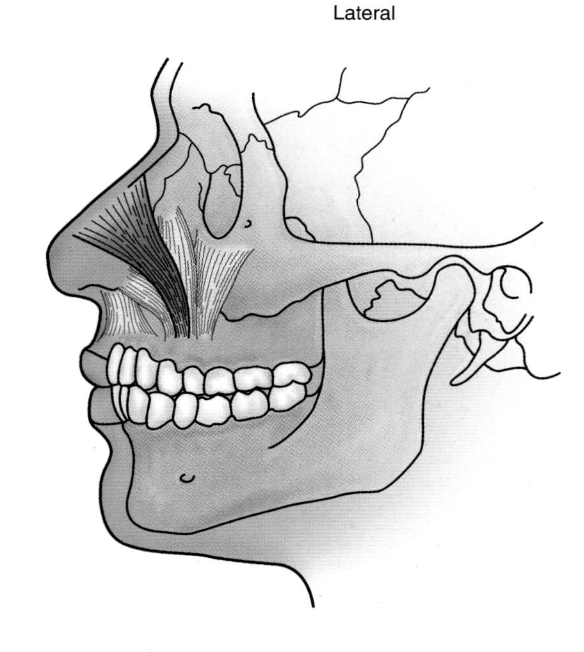

- *Concentric action:*
  - Flares the nasal aperture
- *Origin, fixed end, proximal attachment, arises from:*
  - Transverse part—maxilla, lateral to the nose
  - Alar part—nasal notch of the maxilla and lesser alar cartilage
- *Insertion, mobile end, distal attachment, attaches to:*
  - Aponeurosis of the procerus and the same muscle on the opposite side and cartilage of the nose
- *Innervation:*
  - Superior buccal branch of the facial nerve (cranial nerve VII)
- *Major synergist:*
  - Levator labii superioris alaeque nasi
- *Major antagonist:*
  - Depressor septi nasi
- *Tender/trigger points:*
  - No common tender/trigger points identified. Tender/trigger points that form are likely located in the belly of the muscles.

ACTIVITY 9.4

Draw and color the *facial expression muscles* in the spaces provided. For each muscle:

1. Label the origin and insertion attachment points: *O* for origin; *I* for insertion.
2. Place an X on the trigger points.
3. Palpate these muscles; identify the attachment points and the bellies of the muscles.
4. Move these muscles on yourself.

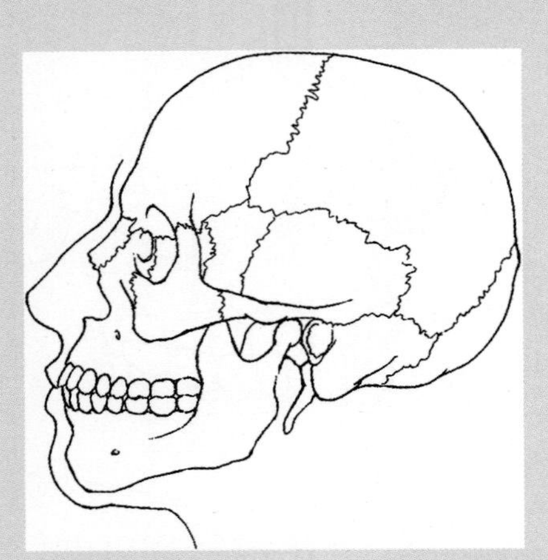

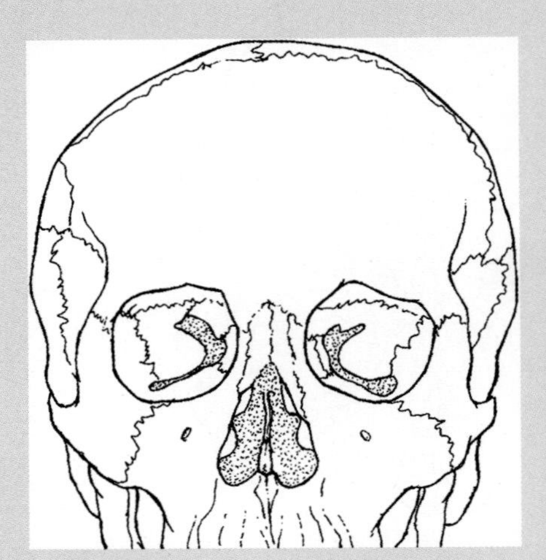

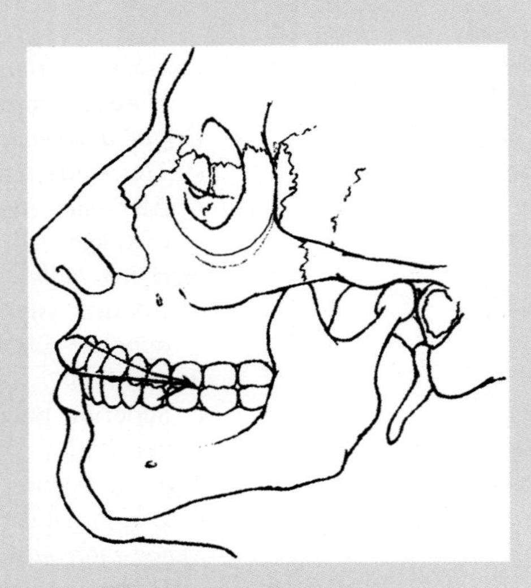

Ear Muscles

Auricularis (aw-RIK-u-lar-iss) posterior

Lateral

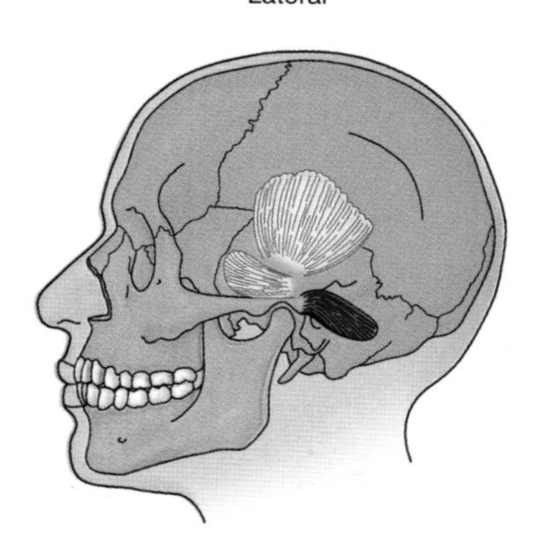

- *Concentric action:*
  - Draws the ear posteriorly
- *Origin, fixed end, proximal attachment, arises from:*
  - Mastoid area of the temporal bone
- *Insertion, mobile end, distal attachment, attaches to:*
  - Inferior part of the cranial part of the conchae of the ear
- *Innervation:*
  - Posterior auricular branches of the facial nerve (cranial nerve VII)

Auricularis (aw-RIK-u-lar-iss) superior

Lateral

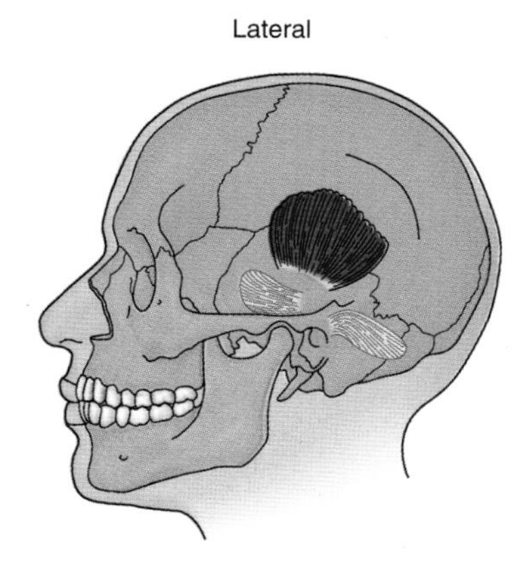

- *Concentric action:*
  - Elevates the ear and tightens and moves the scalp
- *Origin, fixed end, proximal attachment, arises from:*
  - Galea aponeurotica
- *Insertion, mobile end, distal attachment, attaches to:*
  - Superior part of the cranial surface of the ear
- *Innervation:*
  - Temporal branches of the facial nerve (cranial nerve VII)
- *Major synergist:*
  - Temporoparietalis
- *Major antagonists:*
  - Auricularis anterior and auricularis posterior
- *Tender/trigger points:*
  - No common tender/trigger points identified. Tender/trigger points that form are likely located in the belly of the muscles.

Auricularis (aw-RIK-u-lar-iss) anterior

The auricularis muscles, as a group, move the ear. *Auricularis* means "belonging to the ear."

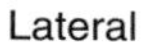

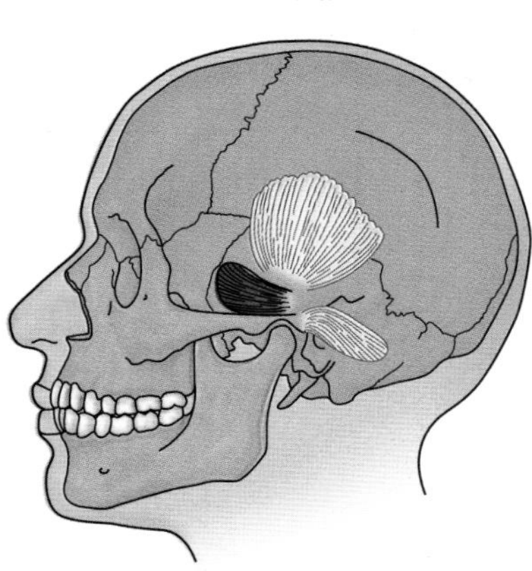

- *Concentric action:*
  - Draws the ear anteriorly and tightens and moves the scalp
- *Origin, fixed end, proximal attachment, arises from:*
  - Lateral edge of the galea aponeurotica
- *Insertion, mobile end, distal attachment, attaches to:*
  - Spine of the helix of the ear
- *Innervation:*
  - Temporal branches of the facial nerve (cranial nerve VII)
  - Trigger points that form are likely located in the belly of the muscles.

ACTIVITY 9.5

Draw and color the *ear muscles* in the spaces provided. For each muscle:

1. Label the origin and insertion attachment points: *O* for origin; *I* for insertion.
2. Palpate these muscles; identify the attachment points and the bellies of the muscles.
3. Move these muscles on yourself.

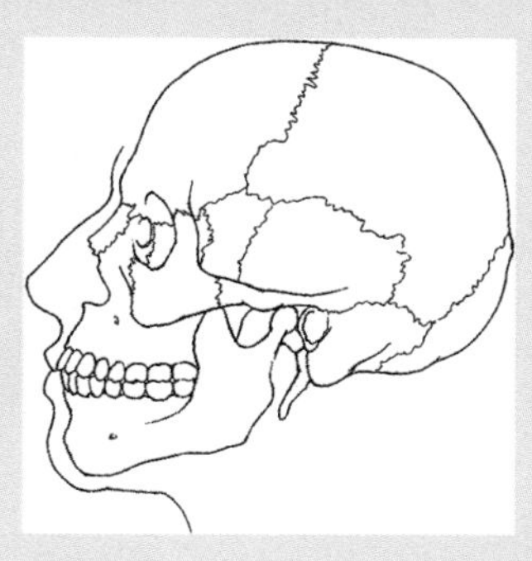

Eye Muscle

Orbicularis oculi (or-BIK-you-LAR-iss OK-you-li)

Orbicularis oculi means "a small disk belonging to the eye." This muscle is a sphincter muscle of the eye and has three parts: orbital, palpebral, and lacrimal.

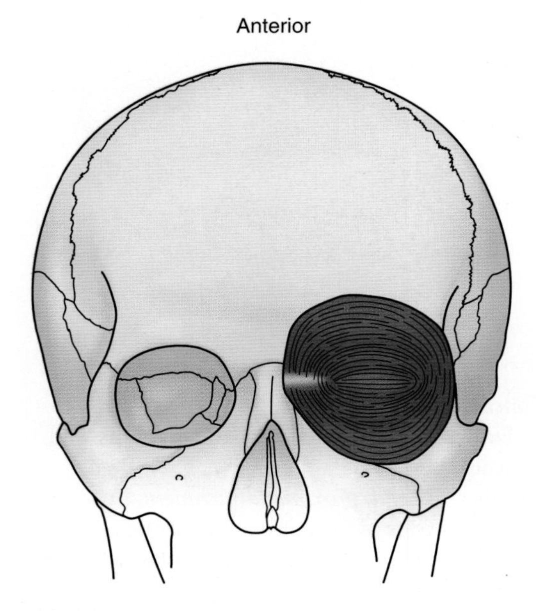

- *Concentric action:*
  - Closes and squints the eye, depresses the upper eyelid, and elevates the lower eyelid
- *Origin, fixed end, proximal attachment, arises from:*
  - Orbital portion—medial orbital margin
  - Palpebral (eyelid) portion—medial palpebral ligament
  - Lacrimal portion—lacrimal bone
- *Insertion, mobile end, distal attachment, attaches to:*
  - Orbital portion—medial orbital margin (this muscle returns to attach to the same place from which it originated)
  - Palpebral portion—lateral palpebral ligament
  - Lacrimal portion—medial palpebral raphe
- *Innervation:*
  - Temporal and zygomatic branches of the facial nerve (cranial nerve VII)
- *Major synergists:*
  - No major synergists
- *Major antagonist:*
  - Levator palpebrae superioris
- *Tender/trigger point:*
  - Orbital area superior to the eyelid
- *Common symptom/Common symptom/Referred pain pattern:*
  - To the nose

ACTIVITY **9.6**

Draw and color the *eye muscle* in the space provided:

1. Label the origin and insertion attachment points: *O* for origin; *I* for insertion.
2. Place an X on the trigger point.
3. Palpate this muscle; identify the attachment points and the belly of the muscle.
4. Move this muscle on yourself.

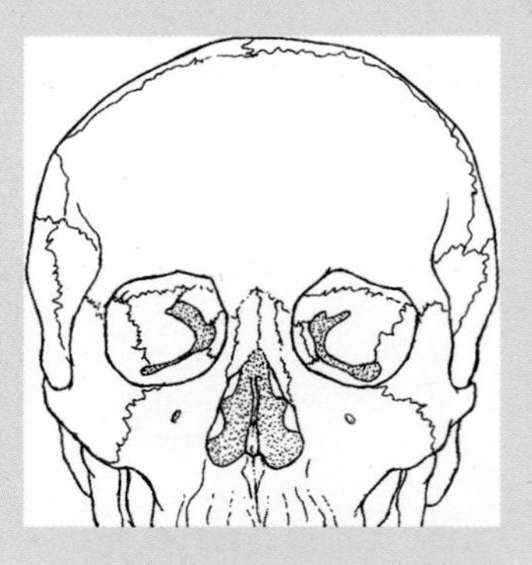

Muscles That Move the Mouth

Orbicularis oris (or-BIK-you-LAR-iss OR-iss)

Orbicularis oris means "a small disk belonging to the mouth."

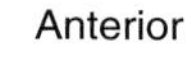

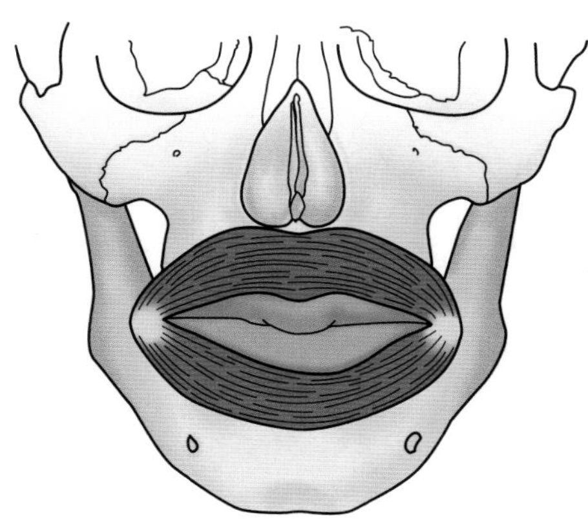

- *Concentric action:*
  - Closes the mouth, protracts the lips (causes the lips to protrude anteriorly), and draws the angle of the mouth medially
- *Origin, fixed end, proximal attachment, arises from:*
  - Modiolus, a fibromuscular mass at the corners of the mouth
- *Insertion, mobile end, distal attachment, attaches to:*
  - Skin and fascia of the lips and tissue surrounding the lips
- *Innervation:*
  - Lower buccal and mandibular branches of the facial nerve (cranial nerve VII)
- *Major synergist:*
  - Mentalis
- *Major antagonists:*
  - Depressor labii inferioris, platysma, and levators of the upper lip
- *Tender/trigger points:*
  - No common tender/trigger points identified.

Depressor anguli oris (de-PRESS-or ANG-you-li OR-iss)

Depressor anguli oris means "to press down the corner belonging to the mouth."

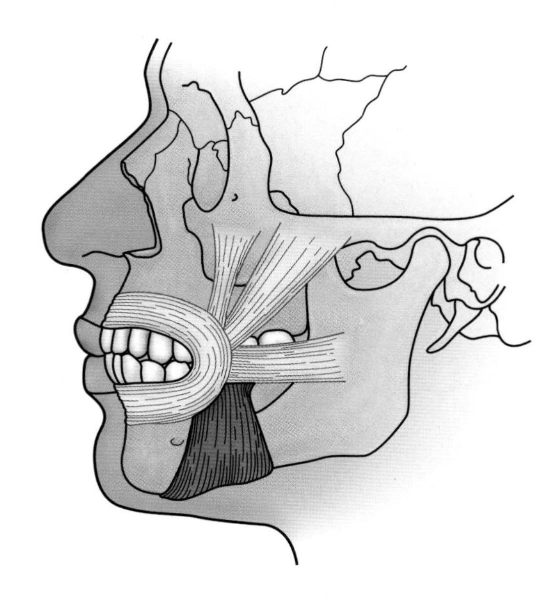

- *Concentric action:*
  - Draws the angle of the mouth downward and laterally (This muscle is involved in opening the mouth and in expressions of sadness.)
- *Origin, fixed end, proximal attachment, arises from:*
  - Oblique line of the mandible, inferior and lateral to the depressor labii inferioris
- *Insertion, mobile end, distal attachment, attaches to:*
  - Angle of the mouth
- *Innervation:*
  - Mandibular branch of the facial nerve (cranial nerve VII)
- *Major synergists:*
  - Risorius and zygomaticus major
- *Major antagonists:*
  - Levator anguli oris and zygomaticus major
- *Tender/trigger points:*
  - No common tender/trigger points identified. Tender/trigger points that form likely are located in the belly of the muscle.

Risorius (rih-ZOR-ee-us)

Risorius means "to cause one to laugh."

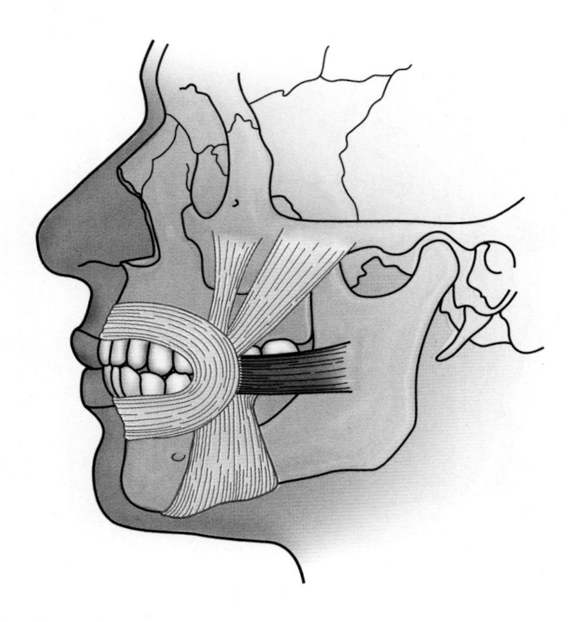

- *Concentric action:*
  - Draws the angle of the mouth laterally
- *Origin, fixed end, proximal attachment, arises from:*
  - Parotid fascia superficial to the masseter muscle
- *Insertion, mobile end, distal attachment, attaches to:*
  - Fascia at the lateral angle of the mouth
- *Innervation:*
  - Mandibular branches of the facial nerve (cranial nerve VII)
- *Major synergists:*
  - Zygomaticus major and depressor anguli oris
- *Major antagonist:*
  - Orbicularis oris
- *Tender/trigger points:*
  - No common tender/trigger points identified. Tender/trigger points that form likely are located in the belly of the muscle.

Zygomaticus major (ZYE-go-MAT-ik-us)

Zygomaticus means "connected to the yoke or connector;" *major* means "larger."

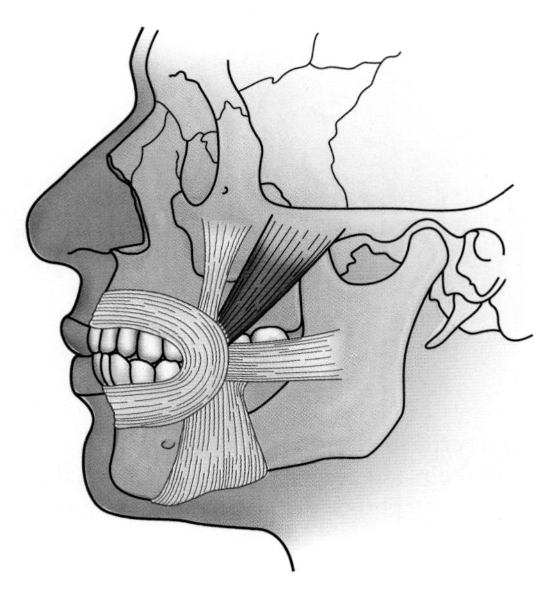

- *Concentric action:*
  - Elevates and draws the angle of the mouth laterally (as in laughing)
- *Origin, fixed end, proximal attachment, arises from:*
  - Zygomatic bone anterior to the zygomaticotemporal suture
- *Insertion, mobile end, distal attachment, attaches to:*
  - Angle of the mouth, blending with the levator anguli oris and the orbicularis oris
- *Innervation:*
  - Buccal branches of the facial nerve (cranial nerve VII)
- *Major synergist:*
  - Levator anguli oris
- *Major antagonist:*
  - Depressor anguli oris
- *Tender/trigger points:*
  - No common tender/trigger points identified. Tender/trigger points that form likely are located in the belly of the muscle.

Zygomaticus minor (ZYE-go-MAT-ik-us)

Zygomaticus means "connected to the yoke or connector;" *minor* means "smaller."

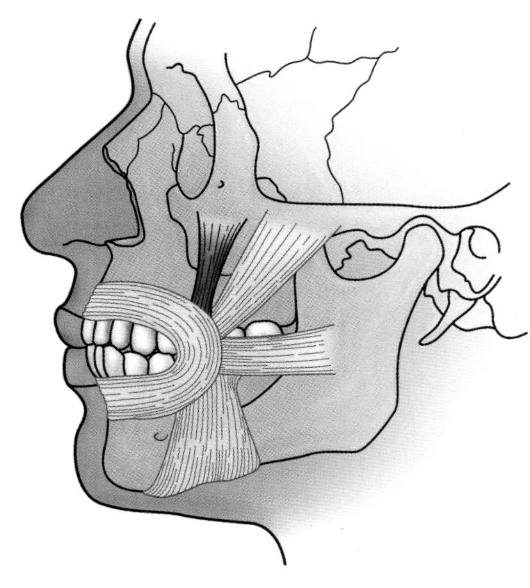

- *Concentric action:*
  - Elevates and everts the upper lip and produces the nasolabial sulcus
- *Origin, fixed end, proximal attachment, arises from:*
  - Lateral surface of the zygomatic bone, immediately posterior to the zygomaticomaxillary suture
- *Insertion, mobile end, distal attachment, attaches to:*
  - Angle of the mouth, blending with the levator labii superioris
- *Innervation:*
  - Buccal branches of the facial nerve (cranial nerve VII)
- *Major synergists:*
  - Levator labii superioris and levator labii superioris alaeque nasi
- *Major antagonist:*
  - Orbicularis oris
- *Tender/trigger points:*
  - No common tender/trigger points identified. Tender/trigger points that form likely are located in the belly of the muscle.

Levator labii superioris (le-VAY-tor LAY-bee-eye su-PEER-ee-OR-iss)

Levator labii means "one that raises the lip;" *superioris* means "above" or "upper."

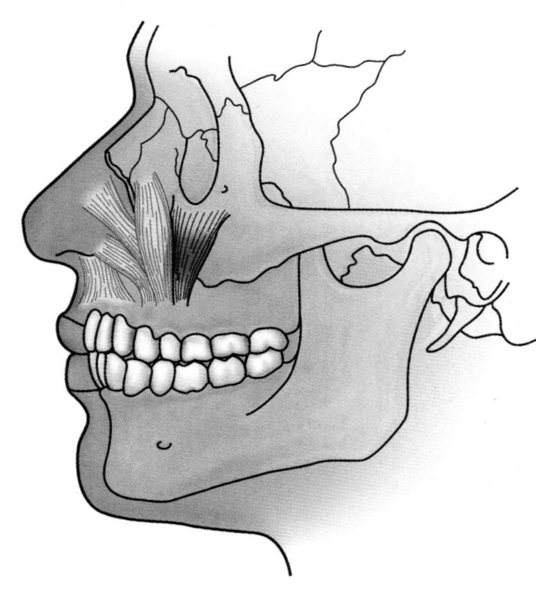

- *Concentric action:*
  - Elevates and everts the upper lip
- *Origin, fixed end, proximal attachment, arises from:*
  - Maxilla and zygomatic bone, from the lower margin of the orbital opening immediately superior to the infraorbital foramen
- *Insertion, mobile end, distal attachment, attaches to:*
  - Muscular substance of the lateral part of the upper lip
- *Innervation:*
  - Buccal branches of the facial nerve (cranial nerve VII)
- *Major synergists:*
  - Levator labii superioris alaeque nasi and zygomaticus minor
- *Major antagonist:*
  - Orbicularis oris
- *Tender/trigger points:*
  - No common trigger points identified. Trigger points that form likely are located in the belly of the muscle.

Levator labii superioris alaeque nasi (le-VAY-tor LAY-bee-eye su-PEER-ee-OR-iss AL-ek-wee NAY-see)

Levator labii and *alaeque nasi* mean "one that raises the lip" and "belonging to the wing of the nose," respectively; *superioris* means "above" or "upper."

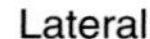

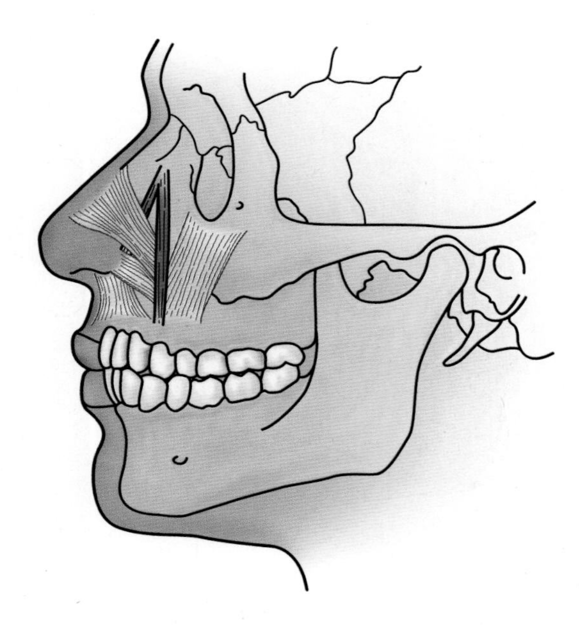

- *Concentric action:*
  - Elevates and everts the upper lip and flares the nostril
- *Origin, fixed end, proximal attachment, arises from:*
  - Frontal process of the maxilla
- *Insertion, mobile end, distal attachment, attaches to:*
  - The muscle divides into the lateral slip, which inserts into the lateral part of the upper lip, and the medial slip, which inserts into the greater alar cartilage and the skin of the nose
- *Innervation:*
  - Buccal branches of the facial nerve (cranial nerve VII)
- *Major synergists:*
  - Levator labii superioris and zygomaticus minor
- *Major antagonists:*
  - Orbicularis oris and depressor septi nasi
- *Tender/trigger points:*
  - No common tender/trigger points identified. Tender/trigger points that form likely are located in the belly of the muscle.

Depressor labii inferioris (de-PRESS-or LAY-bee-eye in-FEAR-ee-or-iss)

Depressor labii means "to press down the lip;" *inferioris* means "lower" or "beneath."

Anterior

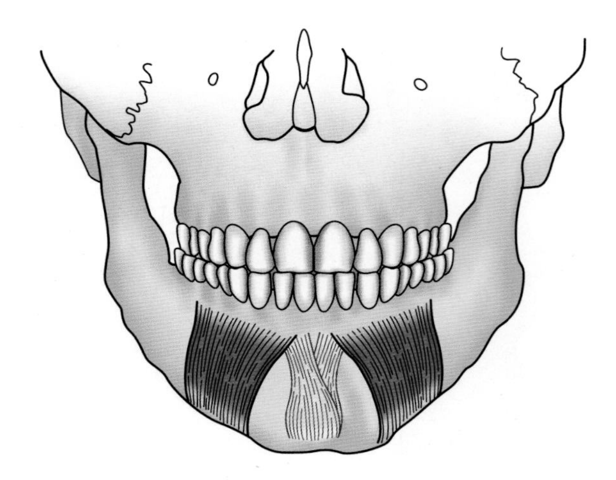

- *Concentric action:*
  - Depresses, everts, and draws the lower lip laterally
- *Origin, fixed end, proximal attachment, arises from:*
  - Oblique line of the mandible, between the symphysis menti and the mental foramen
- *Insertion, mobile end, distal attachment, attaches to:*
  - Skin of the lower lip, blending with the orbicularis oris
- *Innervation:*
  - Buccal branches of the facial nerve (cranial nerve VII)
- *Major synergist:*
  - Platysma
- *Major antagonists:*
  - Mentalis and orbicularis oris
- *Tender/trigger points:*
  - No common tender/trigger points identified. Tender/trigger points that form likely are located in the belly of the muscle.

Mentalis (men-TAL-iss)

Mentalis means "related to the chin."

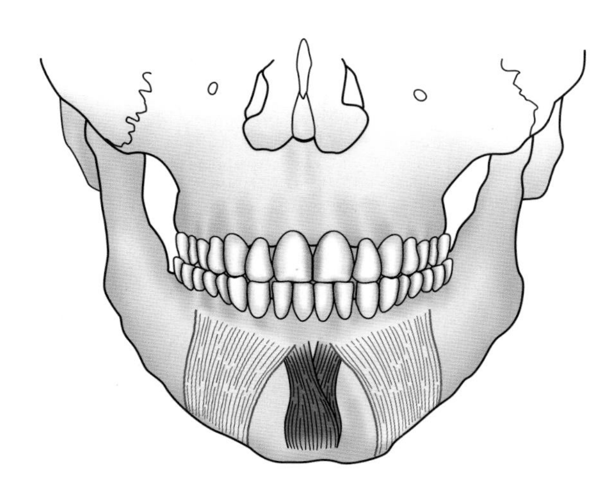

- *Concentric action:*
  - Elevates, everts, and protracts the lower lip and wrinkles the skin of the chin
- *Origin, fixed end, proximal attachment, arises from:*
  - Incisive fossa of the mandible
- *Insertion, mobile end, distal attachment, attaches to:*
  - Skin of the chin
- *Innervation:*
  - Mandibular marginal branch of the facial nerve (cranial nerve VII)
- *Major synergists:*
  - Orbicularis oris and depressor labii inferioris
- *Major antagonists:*
  - Platysma and depressor labii inferioris
- *Tender/trigger points:*
  - No common tender/trigger points identified. Tender/trigger points that form likely are located in the belly of the muscle.

Levator anguli oris (le-VAY-tor ANG-you-li OR-iss)

Levator anguli oris means "one that raises the corner of the mouth."

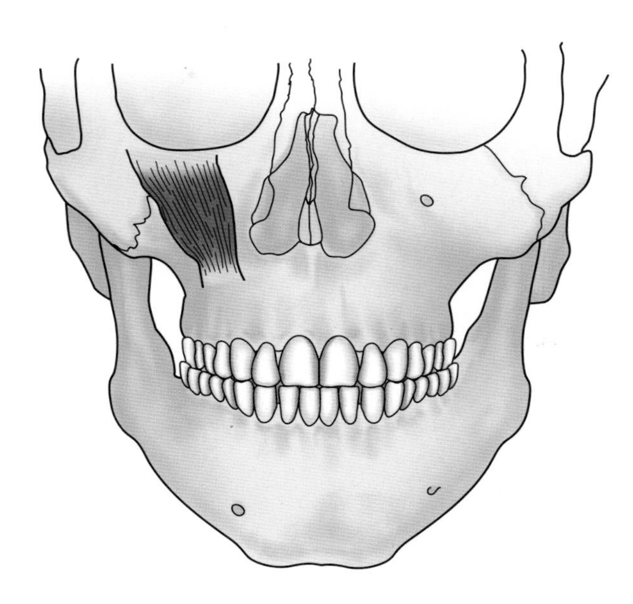

- *Concentric action:*
  - Elevates the angle of the mouth and produces the nasolabial sulcus
- *Origin, fixed end, proximal attachment, arises from:*
  - Canine fossa of the maxilla, just inferior to the infraorbital foramen
- *Insertion, mobile end, distal attachment, attaches to:*
  - Angle of the mouth, blending with the zygomaticus major, depressor anguli oris, and orbicularis oris
- *Innervation:*
  - Buccal branches of the facial nerve (cranial nerve VII)
- *Major synergist:*
  - Zygomaticus major
- *Major antagonist:*
  - Depressor anguli oris
- *Tender/trigger points:*
  - No common tender/trigger points identified. Tender/trigger points that form likely are located in the belly of the muscle.

Buccinator (BUK-sin-ate-or)

Buccinator means "trumpeter."

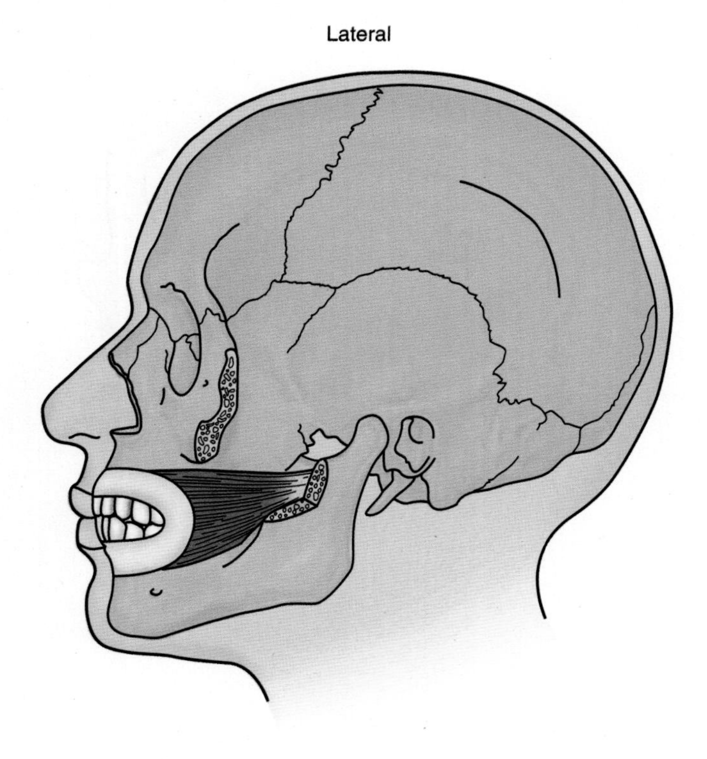

- *Concentric action:*
  - Compresses the cheek against the teeth (This muscle aids in mastication and forcing air out between the lips.)
- *Origin, fixed end, proximal attachment, arises from:*
  - Alveolar processes of the maxilla and mandible and the pterygomandibular raphe
- *Insertion, mobile end, distal attachment, attaches to:*
  - Angle of the mouth
- *Innervation:*
  - Lower buccal branches of the facial nerve (cranial nerve VII)
- *Major synergists:*
  - No major synergist
- *Major antagonists:*
  - No major antagonist
- *Tender/trigger points:*
  - No common tender/trigger points identified. Tender/trigger points that form likely are located in the belly of the muscle.

Platysma (PLAH-tiz-ma)

Platysma means "a flat plate."

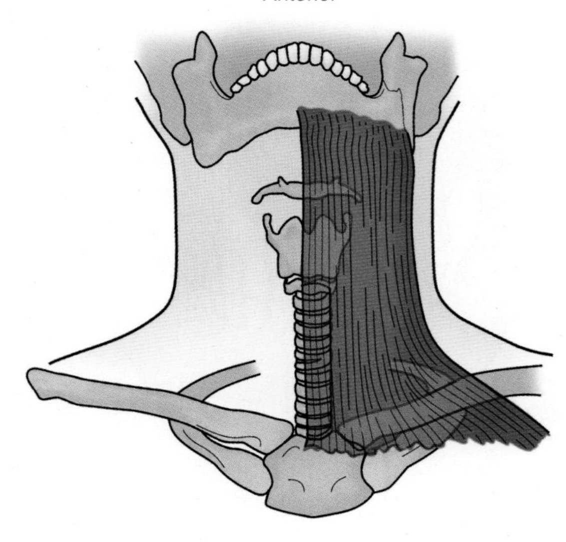

- *Concentric action:*
  - Draws up the skin of the superior chest and neck, creating ridges of skin in the neck; depresses and draws the lower lip laterally; and depresses the mandible at the temporomandibular joint
- *Origin, fixed end, proximal attachment, arises from:*
  - Fascia covering the superior parts of the pectoralis major and deltoid
- *Insertion, mobile end, distal attachment, attaches to:*
  - Mandible and the fascia of the lower face (blending with the contralateral platysma and many other muscles of facial expression)
- *Innervation:*
  - Cervical branch of the facial nerve (cranial nerve VII)
- *Major synergists:*
  - Depressor labii inferioris and depressors of the mandible
- *Major antagonists:*
  - Mentalis, orbicularis oris, and elevators of the mandible
- *Tender/trigger points:*
  - No common tender/trigger points identified. Tender/trigger points that form likely are located in the belly of the muscle.

Muscles of Mastication (Chewing)

Four main pairs of muscles are involved in mastication (chewing) because they move the TMJ. These muscles are powerful. The masseter and temporalis muscles are the prime movers of jaw closure (elevation of the mandible at the TMJ). The medial and lateral pterygoid muscles provide side-to-side grinding movements. Tension and tone imbalance in these groups of muscles are common causes of TMJ dysfunction. The buccinator muscles keep the cheeks close to the teeth to help us chew. The tongue is composed of specialized muscle fibers that curl, squeeze, and fold the tongue.

ACTIVITY 9.7

Draw and color the *muscles that move the mouth* in the spaces provided. For each muscle:

1. Label the origin and insertion attachment points: *O* for origin; *I* for insertion.
2. Palpate these muscles; identify the attachment points and the bellies of the muscles.
3. Move these muscles on yourself.
   Note: Levators help us smile. Depressors help us frown.

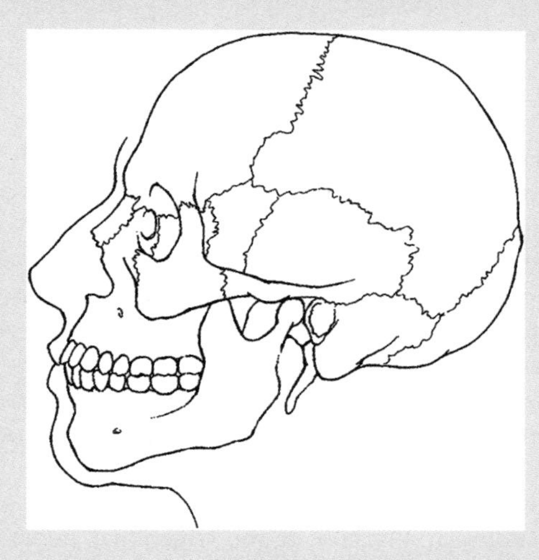

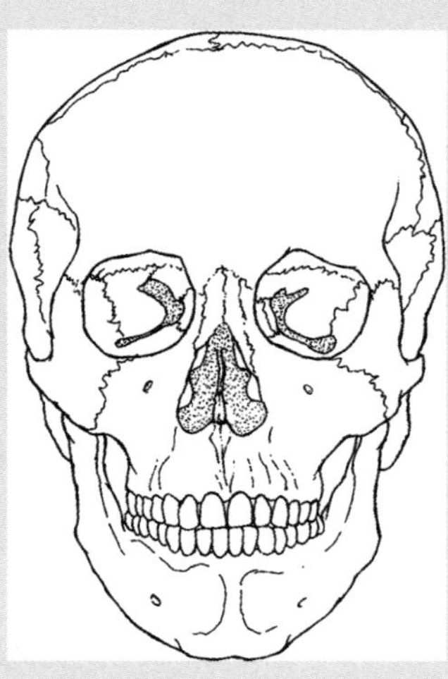

Masseter (MAS-sit-er)

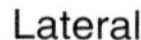

Masseter means "one who chews."

Lateral

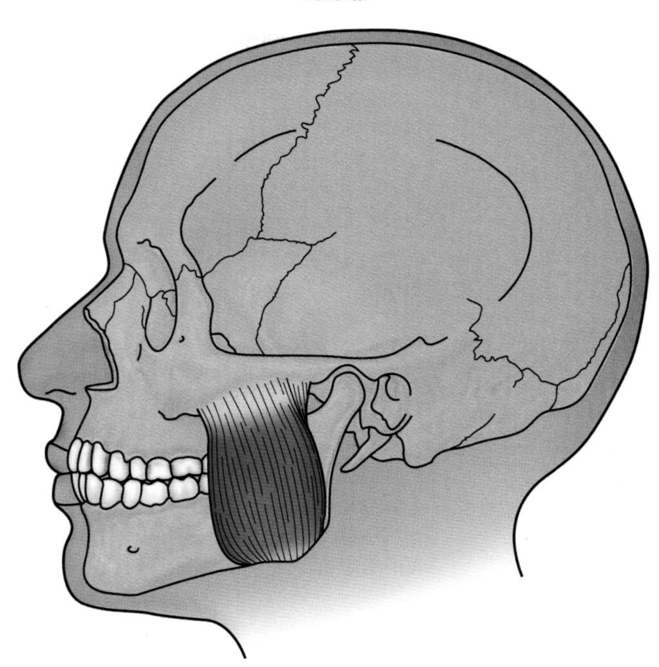

- *Concentric action:*
  - Elevates the mandible at the TMJ
- *Eccentric action:*
  - Restrains/controls (especially rapid movement) depression of the mandible
- *Origin, fixed end, proximal attachment, arises from:*
  - Superficial portion—anterior two-thirds of the inferior border of the zygomatic arch
  - Deep portion—medial surface of the zygomatic arch
- *Insertion, mobile end, distal attachment, attaches to:*
  - Coronoid process, ramus, and angle of the mandible
- *Innervation:*
  - Mandibular division of the trigeminal nerve (cranial nerve V)
- *Major synergists:*
  - Temporalis and medial pterygoid
- *Major antagonists:*
  - Suprahyoid muscles
- *Tender/trigger points:*
  - Superior at the tendinous junction near the zygomatic arch and in the belly of the muscle
- *Referred pain patterns:*
  - Upper jaw (maxillary region) and lower jaw (mandibular region), the ear, and the eyebrow

Temporalis (temp-or-AL-iss)

Temporalis means "related to the temple of the head."

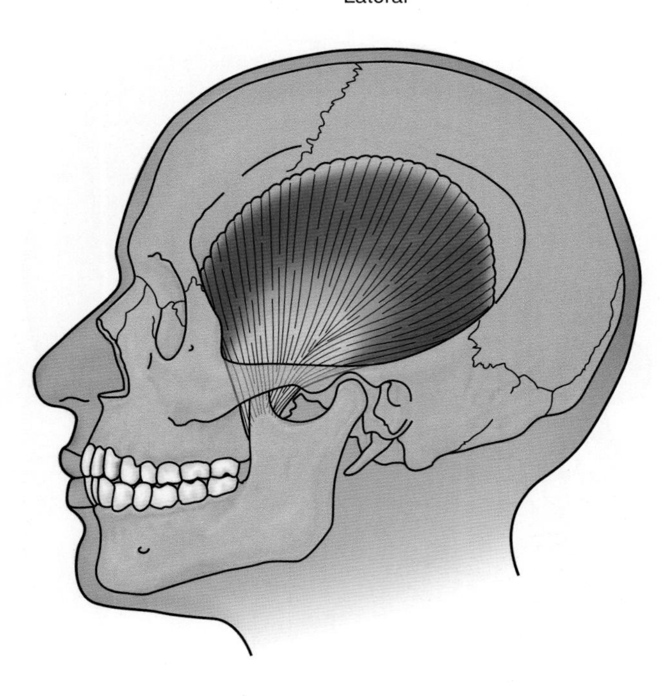

- *Concentric action:*
  - Elevates the mandible at the TMJ
- *Eccentric action:*
  - Restrains/controls (especially rapid movement) depression of the mandible
- *Origin, fixed end, proximal attachment, arises from:*
  - Temporal fossa and deep surface of the temporal fascia
- *Insertion, mobile end, distal attachment, attaches to:*
  - Ramus of the mandible and medial surface and anterior border of the coronoid process
- *Innervation:*
  - Anterior and posterior deep temporal nerve from the mandibular portion of the trigeminal nerve (cranial nerve V)
- *Major synergists:*
  - Masseter and medial pterygoid
- *Major antagonists:*
  - Suprahyoid muscles
- *Tender/trigger points:*
  - Anterior, medial, and posterior along the inferior aspect of the muscle near the tendinous junction at the coronoid process of the mandible
- *Referred pain patterns:*
  - Temporal region, eyebrow, and upper teeth

Lateral (external) pterygoid (TER-ih-goyd) (pterygoideus lateralis)

Pterygoid means "wing shaped;" *lateral* means "to the side."

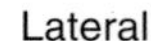

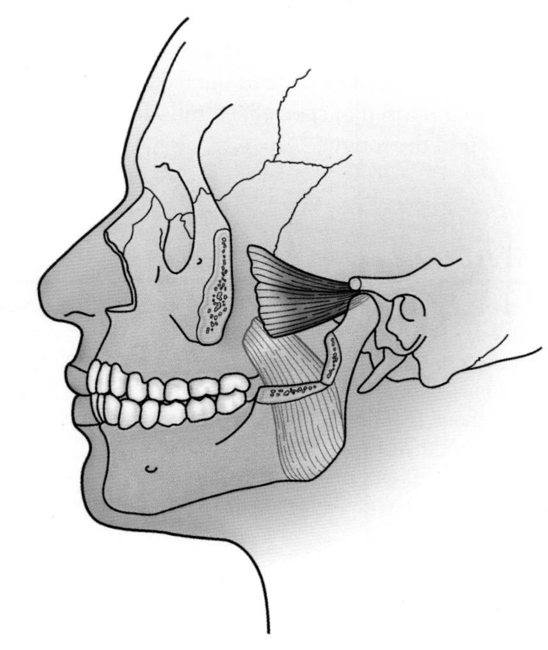

- *Concentric actions:*
  - Protraction and contralateral deviation (movement to the opposite side) of the mandible at the TMJ
- *Origin, fixed end, proximal attachment, arises from:*
  - Superior head—greater wing of the sphenoid bone
  - Inferior head—lateral surface of the lateral pterygoid plate of the sphenoid bone
- *Insertion, mobile end, distal attachment, attaches to:*
  - Anterior surface of the neck of the mandible and articular capsule and disk of the TMJ
- *Innervation:*
  - Mandibular division of the trigeminal nerve (cranial nerve V)
- *Major synergist:*
  - Medial pterygoid
- *Major antagonists:*
  - Opposite-sided lateral and medial pterygoid muscles
- *Tender/trigger points:*
  - Belly of both divisions of the muscle
- *Common symptom/Common symptom/Referred pain pattern:*
  - Cheek and TMJ

The student should note that the lateral pterygoid is palpated from inside the mouth.

Medial (internal) pterygoid (TER-ih-goyd) (pterygoideus medialis)

Pterygoid means "wing shaped;" *medial* is means "related to the middle."

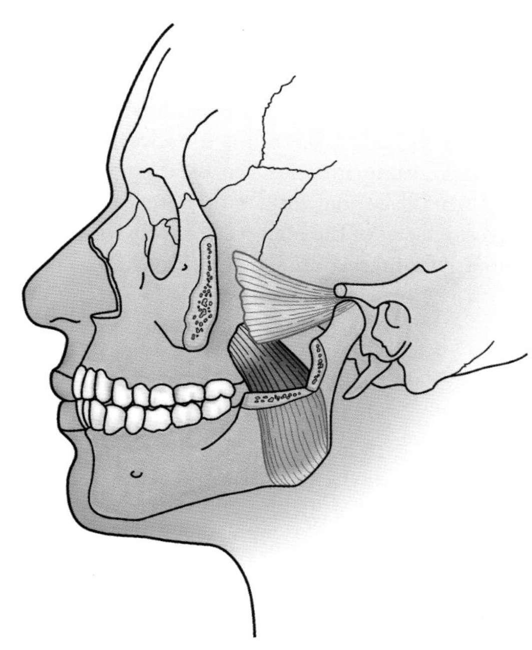

- *Concentric action:*
  - Elevation, protraction, and contralateral deviation (movement to the opposite side) of the mandible at the TMJ
- *Origin, fixed end, proximal attachment, arises from:*
  - Medial surface of the lateral pterygoid plate of the sphenoid bone, pyramidal surface of the palatine bone, and tuberosity of the maxilla
- *Insertion, mobile end, distal attachment, attaches to:*
  - Internal surface of the angle and inferior ramus of the mandible
- *Innervation:*
  - Mandibular division of the trigeminal nerve (cranial nerve V)
- *Major synergists:*
  - Lateral pterygoid, temporalis, and masseter
- *Major antagonists:*
  - Suprahyoid muscles and opposite-sided lateral and medial pterygoid muscles
- *Tender/trigger points:*
  - Belly of the muscle, with best access from inside the mouth
- *Common symptom/Common symptom/Referred pain pattern:*
  - Back of the throat and into the ear

ACTIVITY 9.8

Draw and color the *mastication muscles* in the spaces provided. For each muscle:

1. Label the origin and insertion attachment points: *O* for origin; *I* for insertion.
2. Place an X on the trigger points.
3. Palpate this muscle; identify the attachment points and the bellies of the muscles.
4. Move these muscles on yourself.

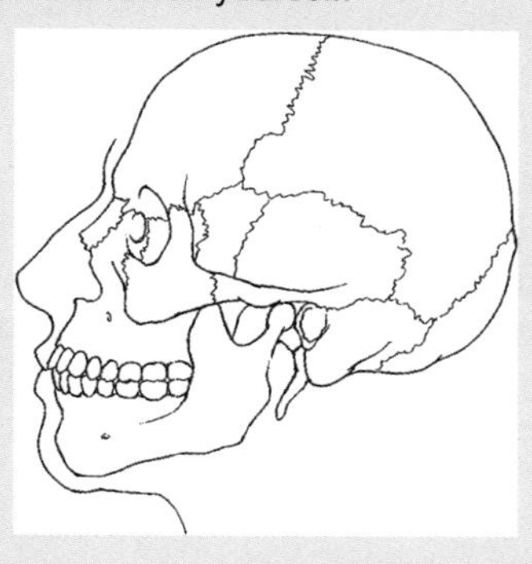

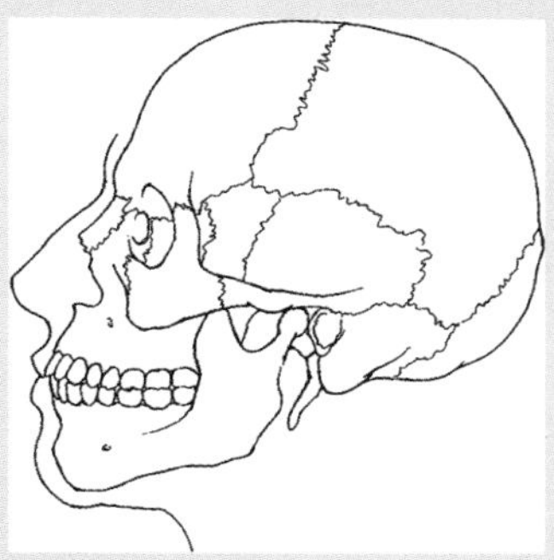

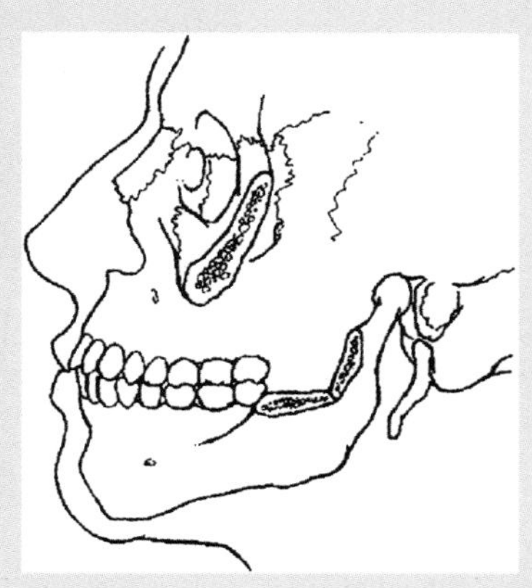

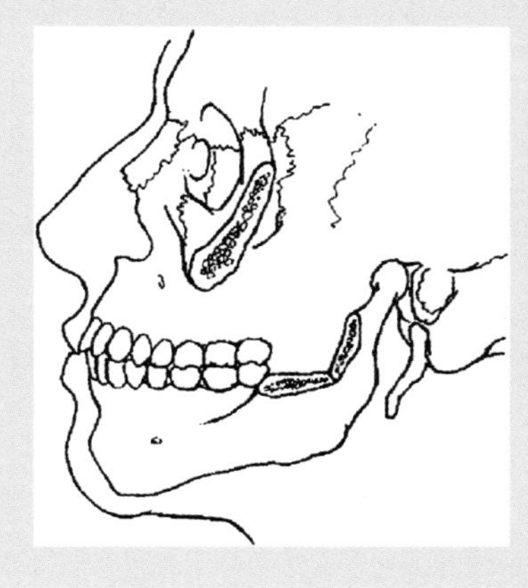

Muscles of the Neck

The sternocleidomastoid muscles divide the neck into the anterior and posterior triangles. Muscles of the neck move the neck at the cervical spinal joints. Most of the muscles of the anterior neck also assist in swallowing. Muscles of the neck that attach to the head provide movements of the head on the neck at the atlantooccipital joint. The sternocleidomastoid muscles are the major neck flexors. The sternocleidomastoid and deeper neck muscles, including the scalene muscles, and several straplike muscles of the vertebral column at the back of the neck provide lateral flexion of the neck. The posterior muscles of the neck, including the upper trapezius and other deeper musculature, provide extension of the neck. The sternocleidomastoid assists in head extension if the neck is stabilized. Tension and muscle imbalances of the neck muscles are a major cause of headaches and arm and shoulder pain and dysfunction because of impingement of the cervical and brachial plexuses of nerves. These muscles do more than just provide head movement. These muscles isometrically act to stabilize and balance the head in an upright, eyes-forward position and therefore are involved in righting and postural reflexes. They often act in sequence with trunk flexors and extensors. Therefore neck muscle problems are a common finding with low back pain and with hamstring and quadriceps dysfunction. Because the head is so heavy, these muscles often become short and increase in tension, especially with a postural imbalance.

Because many of these muscles attach to the upper ribs, they function as accessory breathing muscles and can become dysfunctional if these muscles are used excessively during breathing. In massage that targets this area, the practitioner must address muscles of the region effectively while being cautious of underlying nerves and vessels (Fig. 9.16).

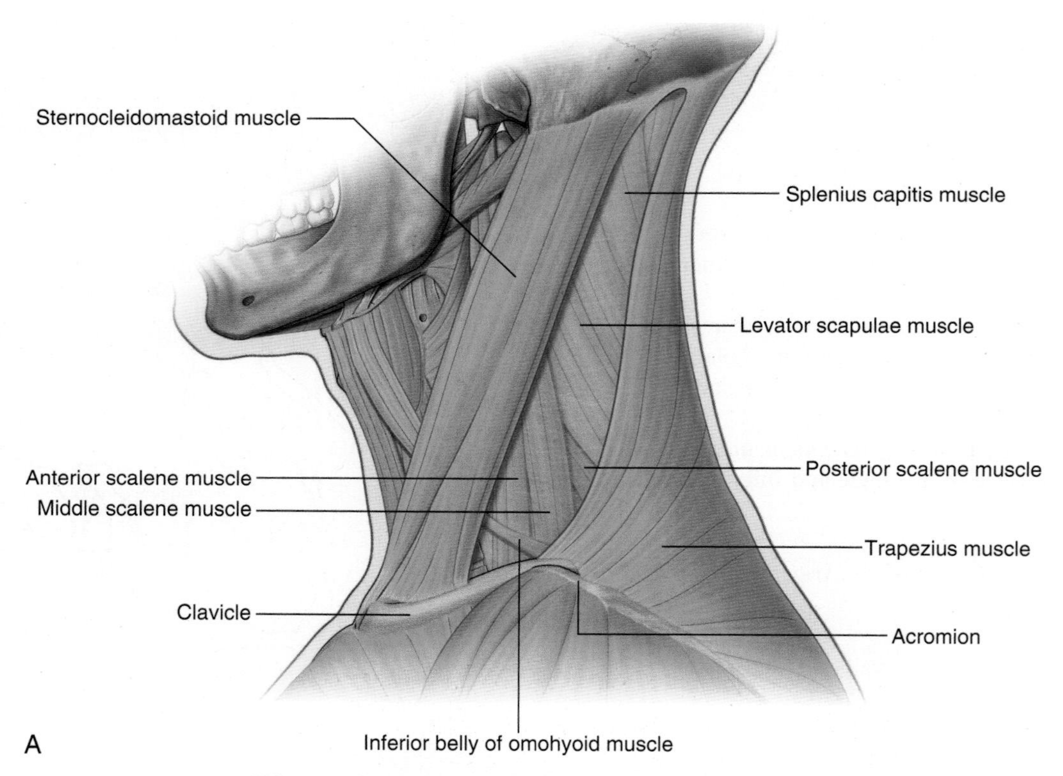

FIG. 9.16 (A) Muscles of the posterior triangle of the neck.

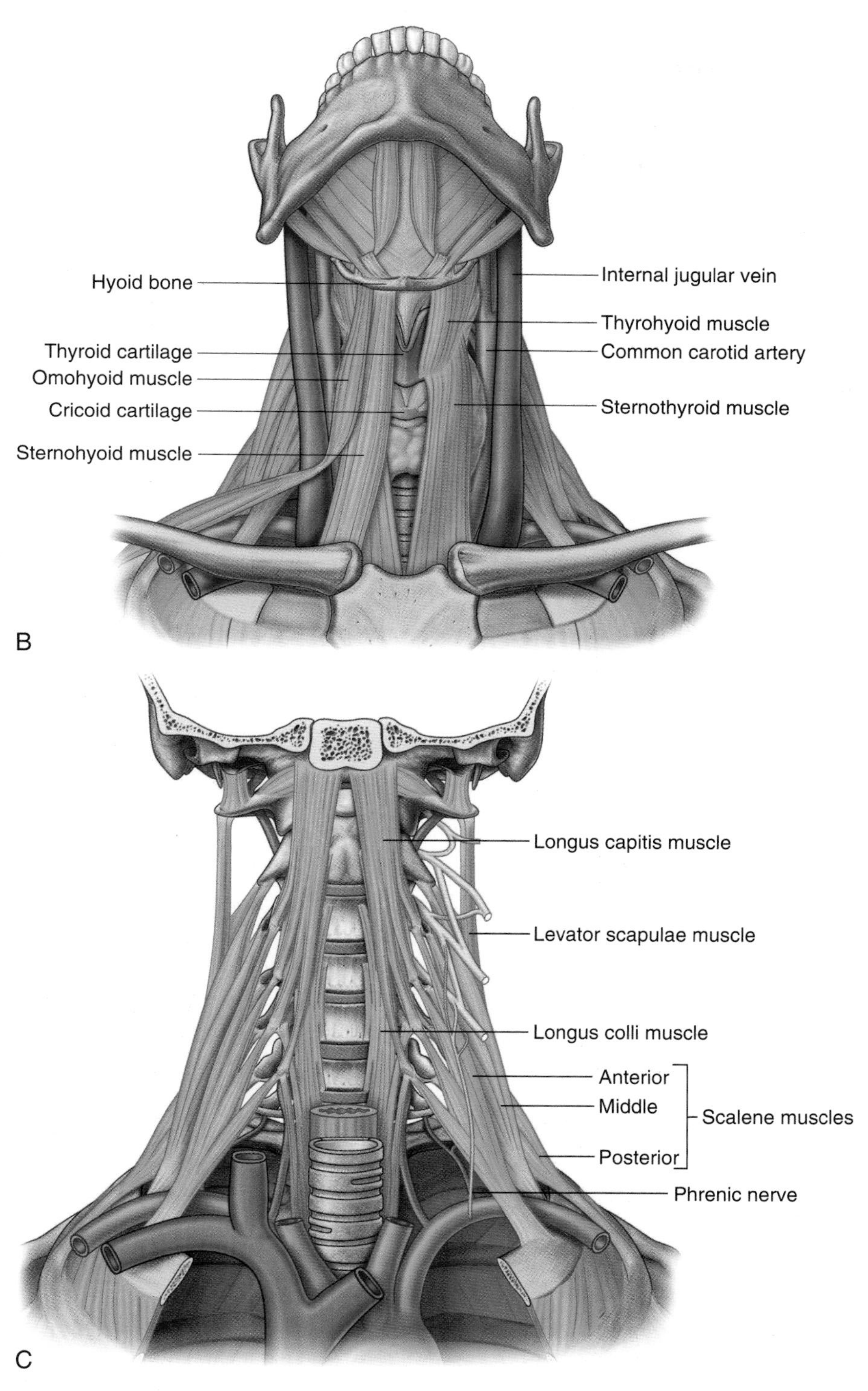

FIG. 9.16, cont'd (B) Anterior neck/hyoid muscles.)(C) Prevertebral and lateral vertebral muscles supplied by the cervical plexus. (From Drake RL, Vogl W, Mitchell WM. *Gray's Anatomy for Students*. 2nd ed. Churchill Livingstone; 2010.)

Sternocleidomastoid (STER-no-CLY-do-mas-toyd) (sternocleidomastoideus)

Sternocleidomastoid means "connecting to the sternum, clavicle, and mastoid process of the skull."

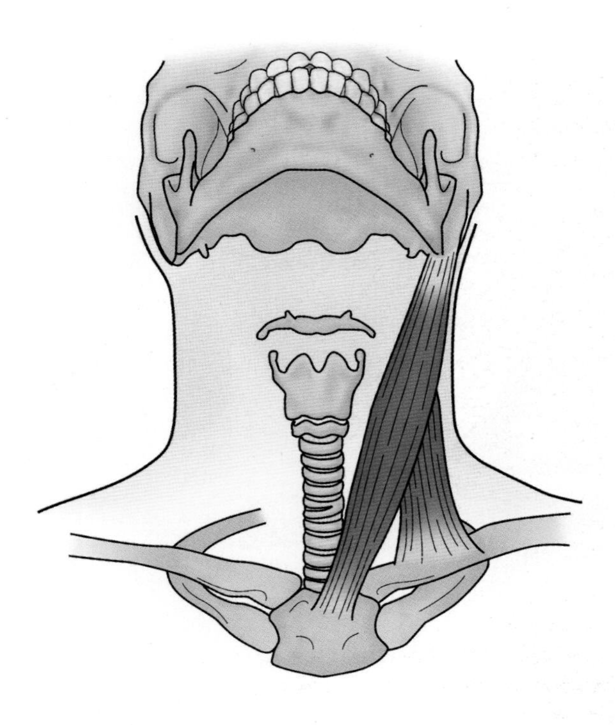

- *Concentric action:*
  - Flexion of the neck at the spinal joints, lateral flexion and contralateral rotation of the neck and the head at the spinal joints, and extension of the head at the atlantooccipital joint
- *Eccentric action:*
  - Restrains/controls (especially rapid movement) extension of the neck, contralateral lateral flexion of the neck and head, ipsilateral rotation of the neck and head, and flexion of the head
- *Isometric action:*
  - Assists in stabilizing the head in space when the mandible moves
- *Origin, fixed end, proximal attachment, arises from:*
  - Sternal head—superior aspect of anterior surface of manubrium of the sternum
  - Clavicular head—superior border of the anterior surface of the medial third of the clavicle
- *Insertion, mobile end, distal attachment, attaches to:*
  - Superior surface of the mastoid process and lateral half of the superior nuchal line of occiput
- *Innervation:*
  - Spinal accessory nerve (cranial nerve XI) and ventral rami of second and third cervical spinal nerves
- *Major synergists:*
  - Scalene muscles, opposite-sided splenius capitis, and suboccipital muscles
- *Major antagonists:*
  - Upper trapezius and semispinalis capitis (opposite-sided sternocleidomastoid)
- *Tender/trigger points:*
  - Several points along the entire length of both divisions of the muscle
- *Common symptom/Common symptom/Referred pain pattern:*
  - Head and face, particularly the occipital region, ear, and forehead. Autonomic nervous system phenomena and proprioceptive disturbances are common.

ACTIVITY 9.9

Draw and color the *sternocleidomastoid muscle* in the space provided.

1. Label the origin and insertion attachment points: *O* for origin; *I* for insertion.
2. Place an X on the trigger point.
3. Palpate this muscle; identify the attachment points and the belly of the muscle.
4. Move this muscle on yourself.

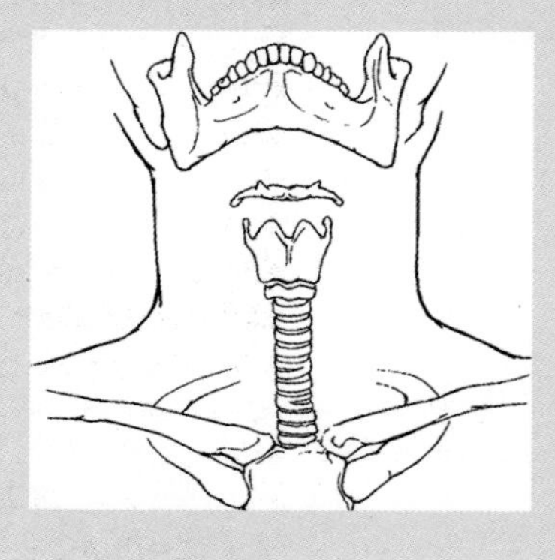

Anterior Triangle of the Neck

As a group, the suprahyoid muscles are located superior to the hyoid bone. These muscles can elevate the hyoid bone, which affects the movement of the tongue and other movements necessary for swallowing. If the mandible and hyoid bone are stabilized, this group of muscles can function as weak accessory flexors of the neck at the spinal joints.

Digastric (dye-GAS-trik) (digastricus)

Digastric means "two bellies."

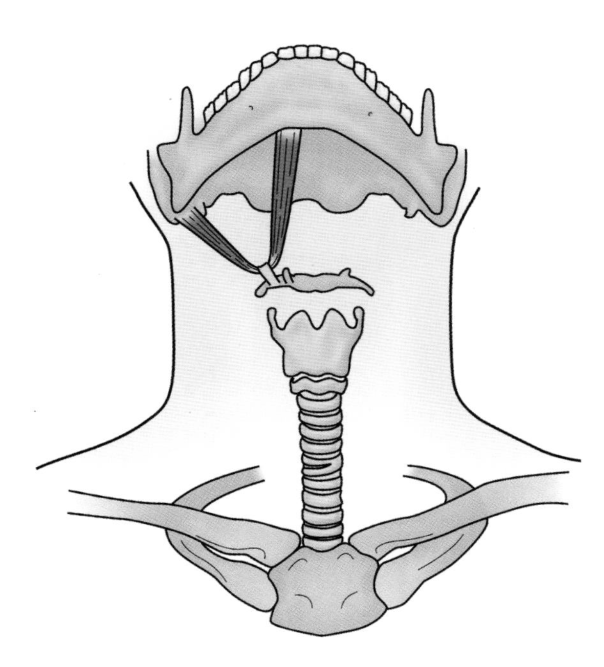

- *Concentric action:*
  - Elevates the hyoid and depresses the mandible at the TMJ (The posterior belly of this muscle is especially active in swallowing and chewing.)
- *Eccentric action:*
  - Restrains/controls (especially rapid movement) depression of the hyoid and elevation of the mandible
- *Isometric action:*
  - Stabilizes the hyoid bone
- *Origin, fixed end, proximal attachment, arises from:*
  - Posterior belly—mastoid notch of the temporal bone
  - Anterior belly—digastric fossa on the base of the mandible
- *Insertion, mobile end, distal attachment, attaches to:*
  - Body of the greater cornu of the hyoid bone by way of a fibrous sling of tissue
- *Innervation:*
  - Trigeminal (cranial nerve V) and facial (cranial nerve VII) nerves
- *Major synergists:*
  - Other suprahyoid muscles
- *Major antagonists:*
  - Infrahyoid muscles, temporalis, and masseter
- *Tender/trigger points:*
  - Belly of each division of the muscle
- *Common symptom/Common symptom/Referred pain pattern:*
  - Sternocleidomastoid area and bottom front teeth

Stylohyoid (STY-low-HY-oyd) (stylohyoideus)

Stylohyoid means "pen" and "U shaped."

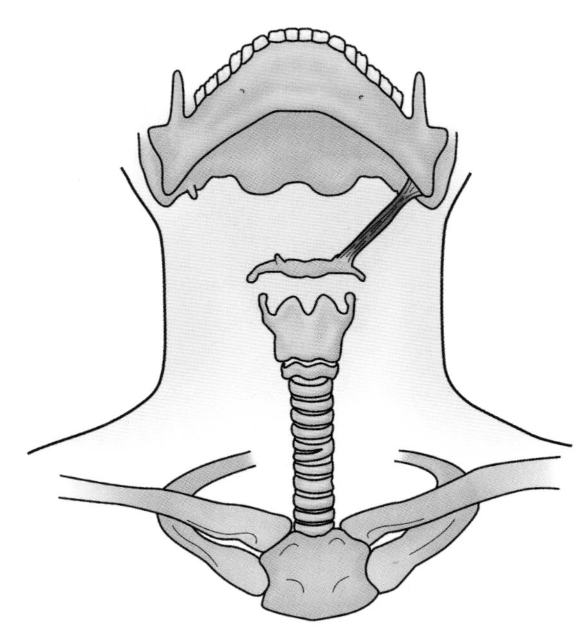

- *Concentric action:*
  - Elevates the hyoid (This muscle is effective at elevating the tongue.)
- *Eccentric action:*
  - Restrains/controls (especially rapid movement) depression of the hyoid
- *Isometric action:*
  - Stabilizes the hyoid bone
- *Origin, fixed end, proximal attachment, arises from:*
  - Posterior surface of the styloid process
- *Insertion, mobile end, distal attachment, attaches to:*
  - Body of the hyoid bone, at the junction with the greater cornu
- *Innervation:*
  - Facial nerve (cranial nerve VII, stylohyoid branch)
- *Major synergists:*
  - Other suprahyoid muscles
- *Major antagonists:*
  - Infrahyoid muscles, temporalis, and masseter
- *Tender/trigger points:*
  - Likely to form in the belly

Mylohyoid (MY-lo-HY-oyd) (mylohyoideus)

Mylohyoid means "molar" and "U shaped."

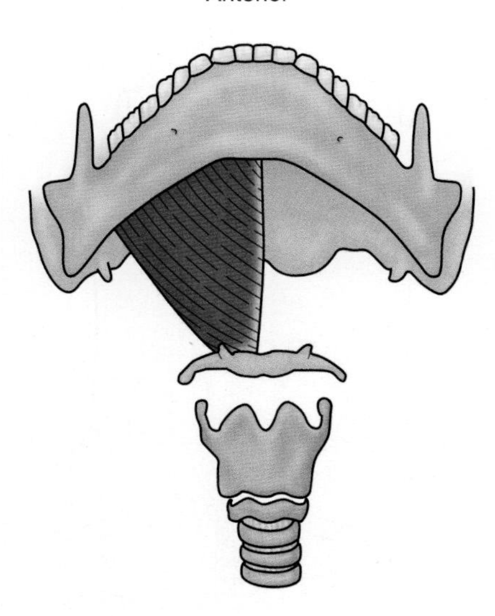

- *Concentric action:*
  - Elevates the hyoid and depresses the mandible at the TMJ (This muscle is important in elevating the floor of the mouth during the first stage of swallowing.)
- *Eccentric action:*
  - Restrains/controls (especially rapid movement) depression of the hyoid and elevation of the mandible
- *Isometric action:*
  - Stabilizes the hyoid bone
- *Origin, fixed end, proximal attachment, arises from:*
  - Mylohyoid line of the mandible
- *Insertion, mobile end, distal attachment, attaches to:*
  - Posterior fibers—anterior surface of the body of the hyoid bone near the inferior border
  - Middle and anterior fibers—median fibrous raphe stretching from the symphysis menti to the hyoid bone
- *Innervation:*
  - Mylohyoid branch of the inferior alveolar nerve of the trigeminal nerve (cranial nerve V)
- *Major synergists:*
  - Other suprahyoid muscles
- *Major antagonists:*
  - Infrahyoid muscles, temporalis, and masseter
- *Tender/trigger points:*
  - Likely to form in the belly

Geniohyoid (JEEN-ee-oh-HY-oyd) (geniohyoideus)

Geniohyoid means "chin" and "U shaped."

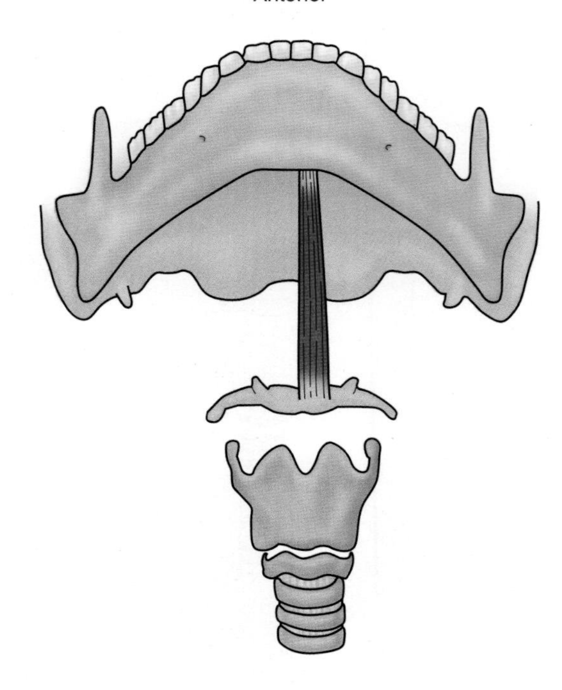

- *Concentric action:*
  - Elevates the hyoid and depresses the mandible at the TMJ (This muscle elevates the tongue and draws it forward.)
- *Eccentric action:*
  - Restrains/controls (especially rapid movement) depression of the hyoid and elevation of the mandible
- *Isometric action:*
  - Stabilizes the hyoid bone
- *Origin, fixed end, proximal attachment, arises from:*
  - Inferior mental spine on the posterior surface of the symphysis of the mandible
- *Insertion, mobile end, distal attachment, attaches to:*
  - Anterior surface of the body of the hyoid bone
- *Innervation:*
  - Hypoglossal nerve (cranial nerve XII)
- *Major synergists:*
  - Other suprahyoid muscles
- *Major antagonists:*
  - Infrahyoid muscles, temporalis, and masseter
- *Tender/trigger points:*
  - Likely to form in the belly

ACTIVITY 9.10

Draw and color the *muscles in the anterior triangle of the neck* in the spaces provided. For each muscle:

1. Label the origin and insertion attachment points: *O* for origin; *I* for insertion.
2. Place an X on the trigger points.
3. Palpate this muscle; identify the attachment points and the bellies of the muscles.
4. Move these muscles on yourself.

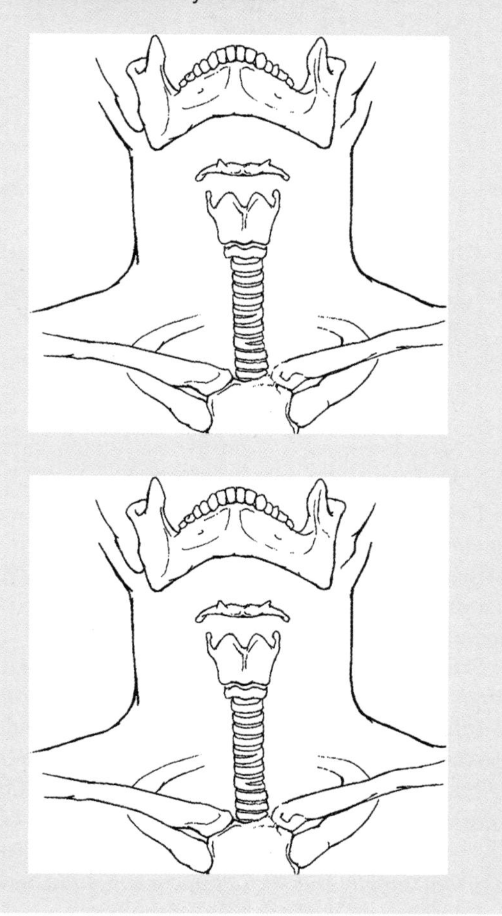

Infrahyoid Muscles

These muscles are located inferior to the hyoid bone. As a group, they depress the hyoid bone and influence swallowing and the production of sound.

Sternohyoid (STERN-oh-HY-oyd) (sternohyoideus)

Sternohyoid means "chest" and "U shaped."

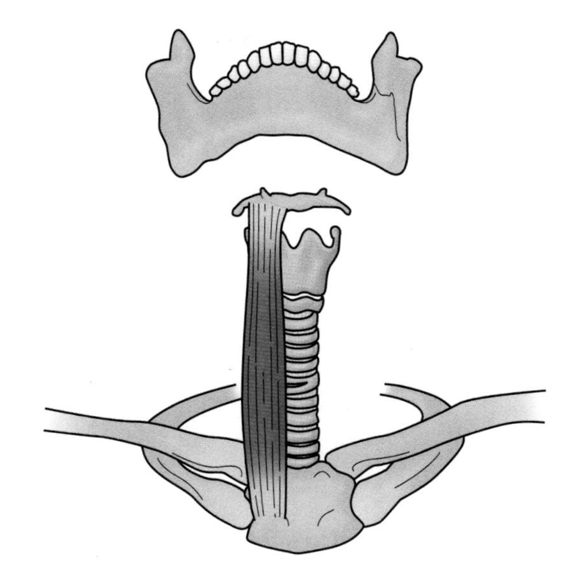

- *Concentric action:*
  - Depresses the hyoid (This muscle plays a part in speech and mastication.)
- *Eccentric action:*
  - Restrains/controls (especially rapid movement) elevation of the hyoid
- *Isometric action:*
  - Stabilizes the hyoid bone
- *Origin, fixed end, proximal attachment, arises from:*
  - Posterior surface of the medial end of the clavicle, posterior sternoclavicular ligament, and superior and posterior parts of the manubrium
- *Insertion, mobile end, distal attachment, attaches to:*
  - Inferior border of the body of the hyoid bone
- *Innervation:*
  - Branches from the ansa cervicalis of the cervical plexus
- *Major synergists:*
  - Thyrohyoid and omohyoid
- *Major antagonists:*
  - Suprahyoid muscles
- *Tender/trigger points:*
  - Likely to form in the belly

Sternothyroid (STERN-oh-THY-royd) (sternothyroideus)

Sternothyroid means "chest" and "shaped like a shield."

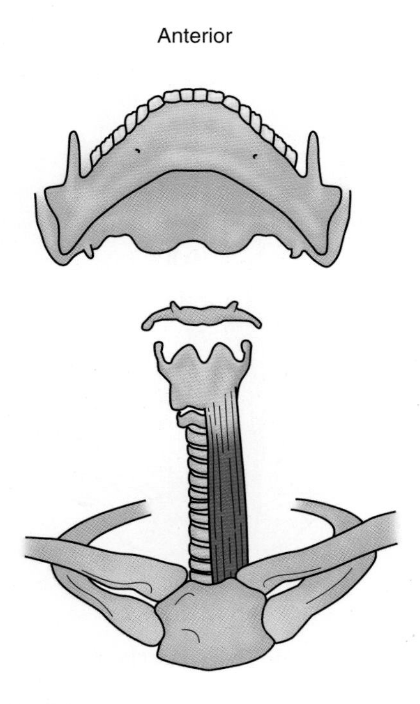

- *Concentric action:*
  - Depresses the thyroid cartilage
- *Eccentric action:*
  - Restrains/controls (especially rapid movement) elevation of the thyroid cartilage
- *Isometric action:*
  - Assists stabilization of the hyoid bone through its pull on the thyroid cartilage
- *Origin, fixed end, proximal attachment, arises from:*
  - Posterior surface of the manubrium and cartilage of the first rib
- *Insertion, mobile end, distal attachment, attaches to:*
  - Oblique line on the lamina of the thyroid cartilage
- *Innervation:*
  - Branches from the ansa cervicalis of the cervical plexus
- *Major synergists:*
  - Sternohyoid and omohyoid (if the thyroid cartilage is fixed to the hyoid bone)
- *Major antagonist:*
  - Thyrohyoid
- *Tender/trigger points:*
  - Likely to form in the belly

Omohyoid (OH-mo-HY-oyd) (omohyoideus)

Omohyoid means "shoulder" and "U shaped."

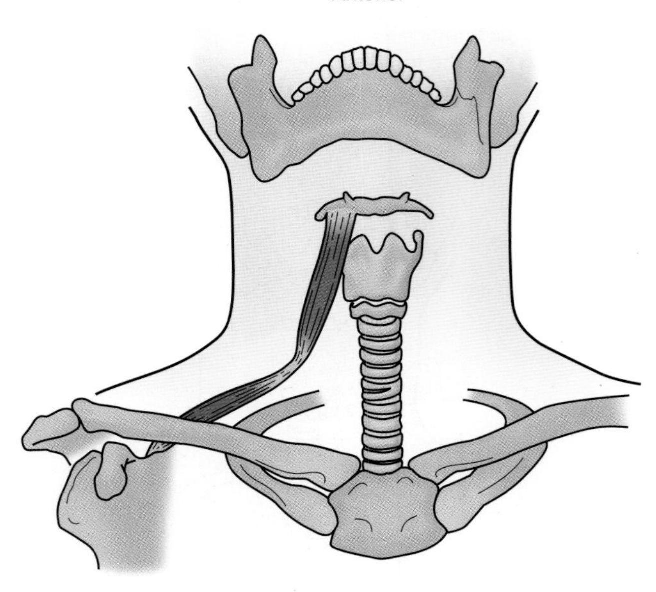

- *Concentric action:*
  - Depresses the hyoid
- *Eccentric action:*
  - Restrains/controls (especially rapid movement) elevation of the hyoid
- *Isometric action:*
  - Stabilizes the hyoid bone
- *Origin, fixed end, proximal attachment, arises from:*
  - Inferior belly—superior border of the scapula near the scapular notch and suprascapular ligament (ends at its central tendon attaching to the clavicle by a fibrous sling of tissue deep to the sternocleidomastoid)
  - Superior belly—from its central tendon at the clavicle
- *Insertion, mobile end, distal attachment, attaches to:*
  - Inferior border of the body of the hyoid bone
- *Innervation:*
  - Branches from the ansa cervicalis of the cervical plexus
- *Major synergists:*
  - Sternohyoid and thyrohyoid
- *Major antagonists:*
  - Suprahyoid muscles
- *Tender/trigger points:*
  - Likely to form in the belly

Thyrohyoid (THY-ro-HY-oyd) (thyrohyoideus)

Thyrohyoid means "shaped like a shield" and "U shaped."

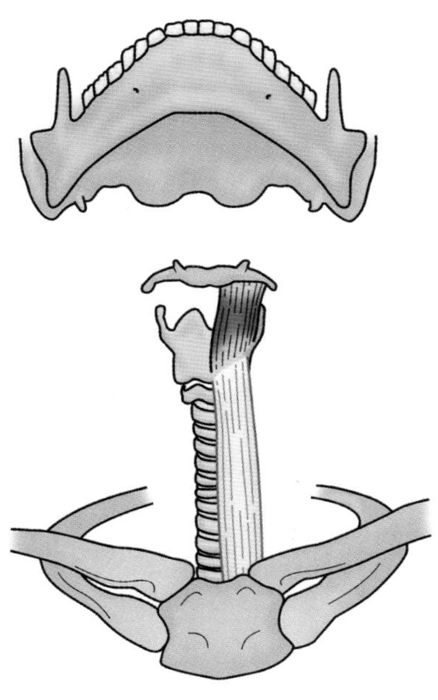

- *Concentric action:*
  - Depresses the hyoid and elevates the thyroid cartilage
- *Eccentric action:*
  - Restrains/controls (especially rapid movement) elevation of the hyoid and depression of the thyroid cartilage
- *Isometric action:*
  - Stabilizes the hyoid bone and the thyroid cartilage
- *Origin, fixed end, proximal attachment, arises from:*
  - Lamina of the thyroid cartilage at the oblique line
- *Insertion, mobile end, distal attachment, attaches to:*
  - Inferior border of the greater cornu and the body of the hyoid bone
- *Innervation:*
  - First cervical spinal nerve via the hypoglossal nerve (cranial nerve XII)
- *Major synergists:*
  - Infrahyoid muscles for depression of the hyoid and suprahyoid muscles for elevation of the thyroid cartilage (if the thyroid cartilage is fixed to the hyoid bone)
- *Major antagonists:*
  - Suprahyoid muscles for elevation of the hyoid and sternothyroid for depression of the thyroid cartilage
- *Tender/trigger points:*
  - Likely to form in the belly

ACTIVITY 9.11

Draw and color the *infrahyoid muscles* in the spaces provided. For each muscle:

1. Label the origin and insertion attachment points: *O* for origin; *I* for insertion.
2. Swallow to identify the hyoid bone and the action of these muscles.
3. Identify the attachment points and the bellies of the muscles.

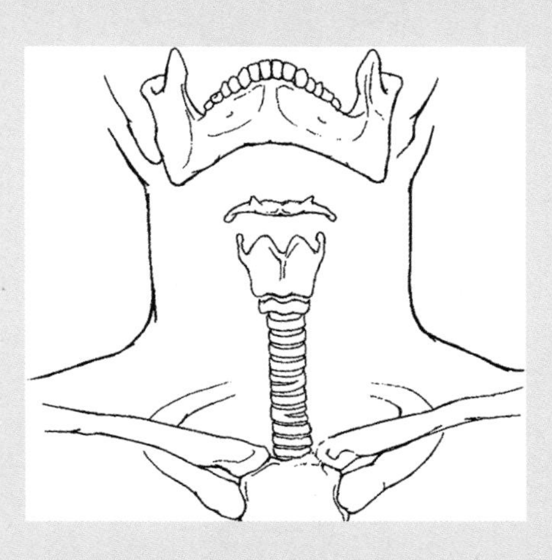

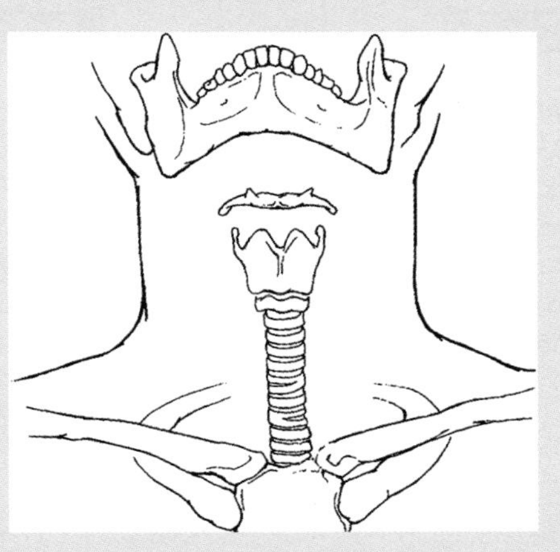

Longus colli (LONG-us KOAL-ee)

Longus colli means "long" and "belonging to the neck."

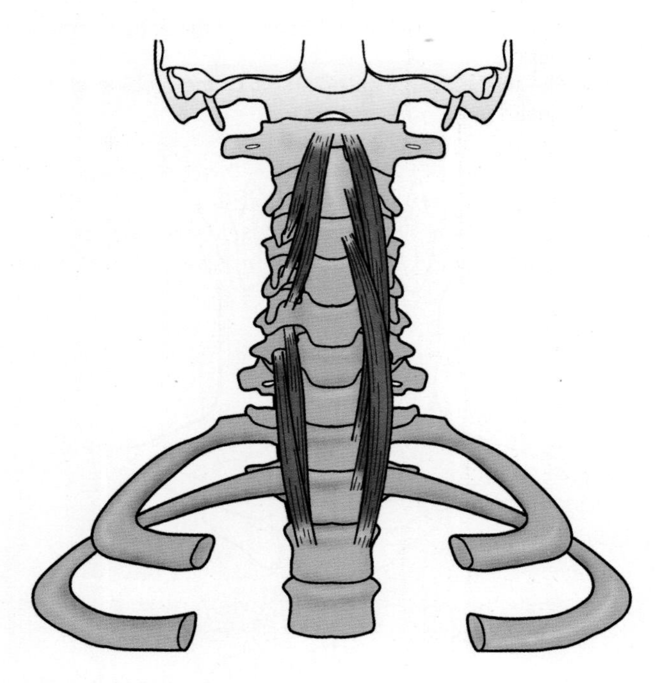

- *Concentric action:*
  - Flexion, lateral flexion, and contralateral rotation of the neck at the spinal joints
- *Eccentric action:*
  - Restrains/controls (especially rapid movement) extension, contralateral lateral flexion, and ipsilateral rotation of the neck
- *Isometric action:*
  - Stabilizes the cervical spine and can be compared with the psoas major and psoas minor in the lumbar region
- *Origin, fixed end, proximal attachment, arises from:*
  - Superior oblique portion—anterior tubercles of the transverse processes of the third, fourth, and fifth cervical vertebrae
  - Inferior oblique portion—anterior bodies of the first three thoracic vertebrae
  - Vertical portion—anterior bodies of the lower three cervical vertebrae and the upper three thoracic vertebrae
- *Insertion, mobile end, distal attachment, attaches to:*
  - Superior—anterior arch of the atlas
  - Inferior—anterior tubercles of the transverse processes of the fifth and sixth cervical vertebrae
  - Vertical—anterior bodies of the second, third, and fourth cervical vertebrae
- *Innervation:*
  - Ventral rami of the second through sixth cervical spinal nerves
- *Major synergists:*
  - Longus capitis, sternocleidomastoid, and scalene muscles
- *Major antagonists:*
  - Neck extensor group
- *Tender/trigger points:*
  - In the belly of the muscle (because of the presence of many vulnerable structures nearby, the practitioner must use caution when palpating this deep muscle)

The longus colli and longus capitis are important muscles to consider in any whiplash type of neck injury.

Longus capitis (LONG-us KAP-ih-tiss)

Longus capitis means "long" and "belonging to the head."

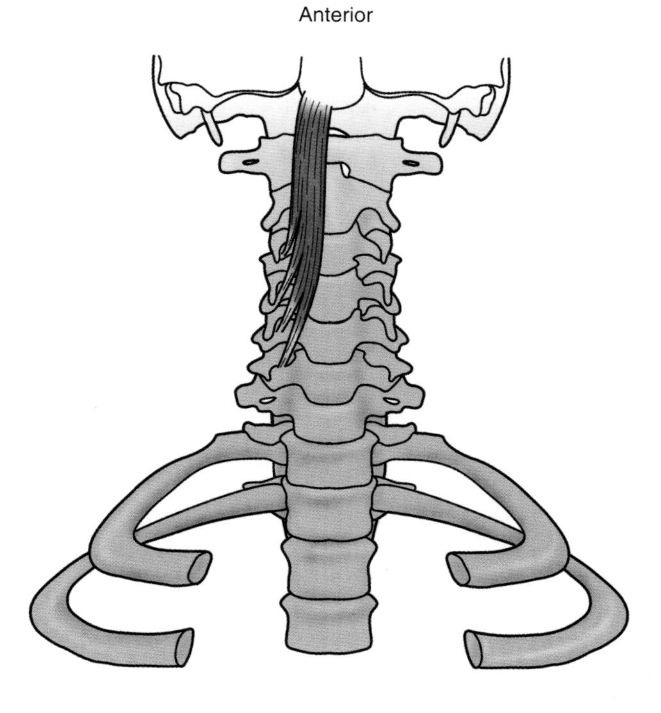

- *Concentric action:*
  - Flexion and lateral flexion of the head and the neck at the spinal joints
- *Eccentric action:*
  - Restrains/controls (especially rapid movement) extension and contralateral lateral flexion of the head and neck
- *Isometric action:*
  - Stabilizes the cervical spine
- *Origin, fixed end, proximal attachment, arises from:*
  - Anterior tubercles of the transverse processes of the third through sixth cervical vertebrae
- *Insertion, mobile end, distal attachment, attaches to:*
  - Inferior surface of the basilar part of the occipital bone just anterior to the foramen magnum
- *Innervation:*
  - Ventral rami of the first through third cervical spinal nerves
- *Major synergists:*
  - Longus colli, sternocleidomastoid, and scalene muscles
- *Major antagonists:*
  - Neck extensor group
- *Tender/trigger points:*
  - In the belly of the muscle (Because of the presence of many vulnerable structures nearby, the practitioner must use caution when palpating this deep muscle.)

ACTIVITY 9.12

Draw and color the muscles of the *deep anterior triangle of the neck* in the spaces provided. For each muscle:

1. Label the origin and insertion attachment points: *O* for origin; *I* for insertion.
2. Move these muscles on yourself.

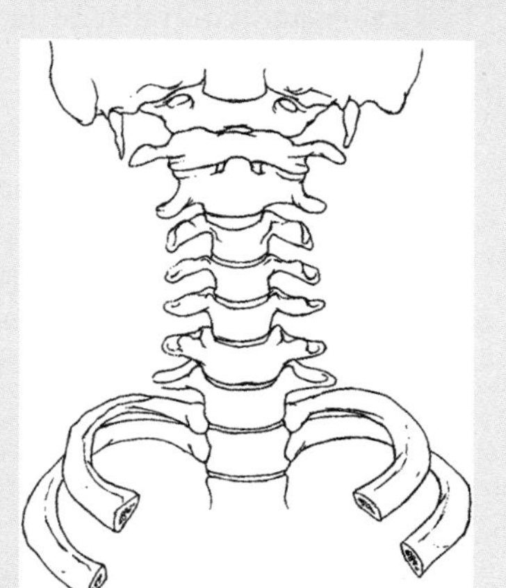

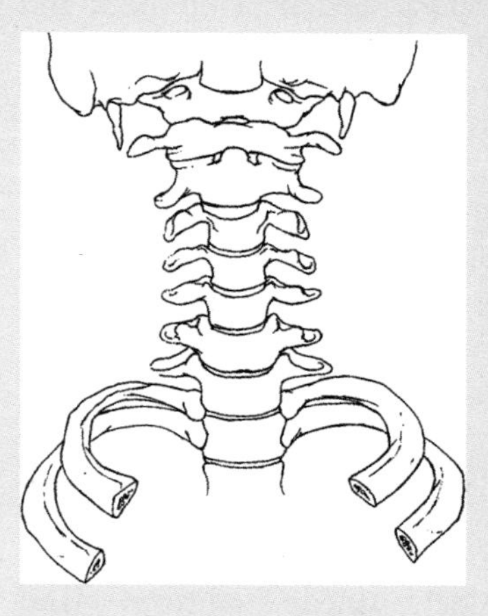

Scalene Group

Anterior scalene (scalenus anterior) (skay-LEE-nus)

Scalenus means "triangular with unequal sides;" *anterior* means "before" or "in front."

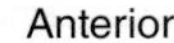

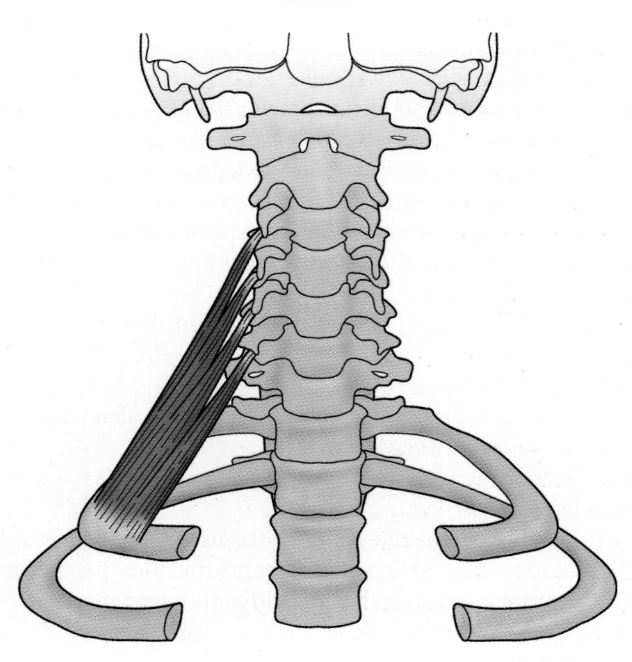

- *Concentric action:*
  - Flexion and lateral flexion of the neck at the spinal joints; elevation of the first rib at the sternocostal and costovertebral joints (thus functioning as an accessory muscle of respiration)
- *Eccentric action:*
  - Restrains/controls (especially rapid movement) extension and contralateral lateral flexion of the neck and depression of the first rib
- *Isometric action:*
  - Stabilizes the cervical spine
- *Origin, fixed end, proximal attachment, arises from:*
  - Anterior tubercles of the transverse processes of the third through sixth cervical vertebrae
- *Insertion, mobile end, distal attachment, attaches to:*
  - Scalene tubercle on the inner border of the first rib and superior surface of the first rib
- *Innervation:*
  - Ventral rami of the fourth through sixth cervical spinal nerves
- *Major synergists:*
  - Middle and posterior scalene muscles and sternocleidomastoid
- *Major antagonists:*
  - Neck extensors and lateral flexors on the opposite side of the neck
- *Tender/trigger points:*
  - Belly of the muscle near the rib attachment
- *Common symptom/Common symptom/Referred pain pattern:*
  - Pectoral region, rhomboid region, and the entire length of the arm into the hand

Middle scalene (scalenus medius) (skay-LEE-nus)

Scalenus means "triangular with unequal sides;" *medius* means "middle."

Anterior

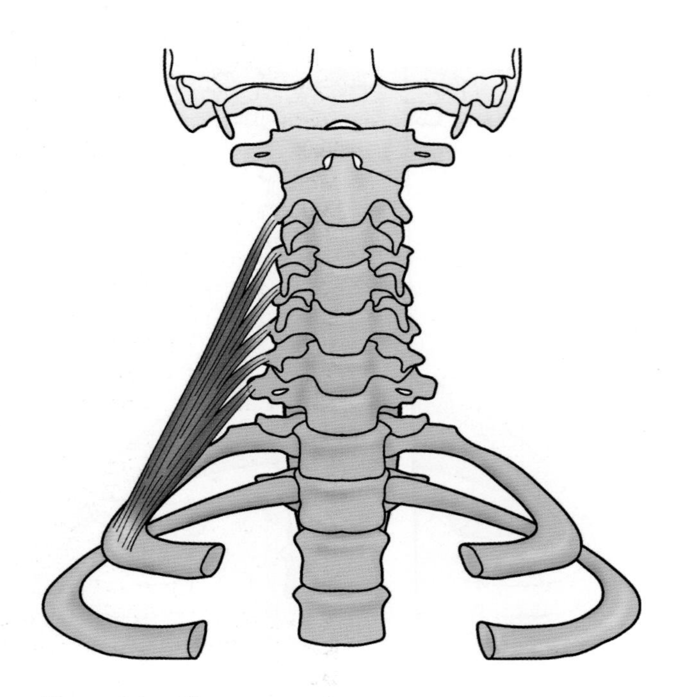

- *Concentric action:*
  - Flexion and lateral flexion of the neck at the spinal joints and elevation of the first rib at the sternocostal and costovertebral joints (thus functioning as an accessory muscle of respiration)
- *Eccentric action:*
  - Restrains/controls (especially rapid movement) extension and contralateral lateral flexion of the neck and depression of the first rib
- *Isometric action:*
  - Stabilizes the cervical spine
- *Origin, fixed end, proximal attachment, arises from:*
  - Posterior tubercles of the transverse processes of the second through seventh cervical vertebrae
- *Insertion, mobile end, distal attachment, attaches to:*
  - Superior surface of the first rib
- *Innervation:*
  - Ventral rami of the third through eighth cervical spinal nerves
- *Major synergists:*
  - Anterior and posterior scalene muscles and sternocleidomastoid
- *Major antagonists:*
  - Neck extensors and lateral flexors on the opposite side of the neck
- *Tender/trigger points:*
  - Belly of the muscle near the rib attachment
- *Common symptom/Common symptom/Referred pain pattern:*
  - Pectoral region, rhomboid region, and the entire length of the arm into the hand

Posterior scalene (scalenus posterior) (skay-LEE-nus)

Scalenus means "triangular with unequal sides;" *posterior* means "behind."

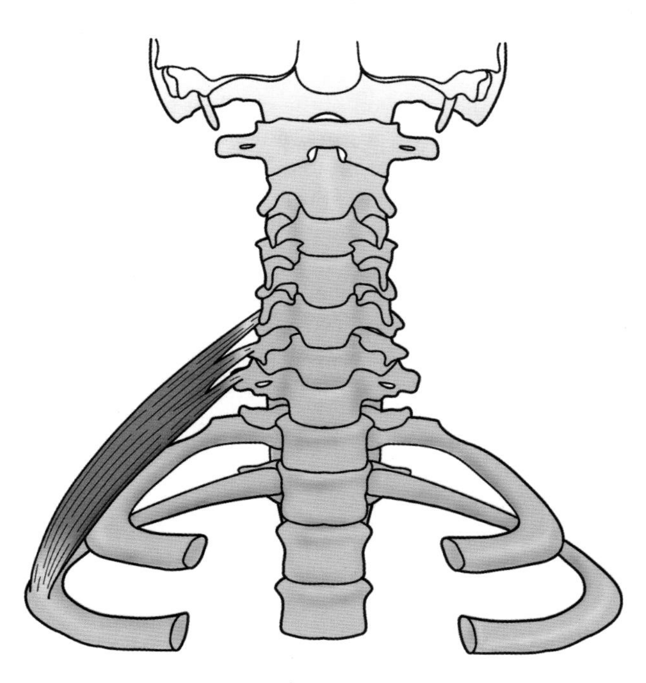

- *Concentric action:*
  - Lateral flexion of the neck at the spinal joints and elevation of the second rib at the sternocostal and costovertebral joints (thus functioning as an accessory muscle of respiration)
- *Eccentric action:*
  - Restrains/controls (especially rapid movement) contralateral lateral flexion of the neck and depression of the second rib
- *Isometric action:*
  - Stabilizes the cervical spine
- *Origin, fixed end, proximal attachment, arises from:*
  - Posterior tubercles of the transverse processes of the fifth through seventh cervical vertebrae
- *Insertion, mobile end, distal attachment, attaches to:*
  - Outer surface of the second rib
- *Innervation:*
  - Ventral rami of the sixth through eighth cervical spinal nerves
- *Major synergists:*
  - Anterior and middle scalene muscles and sternocleidomastoid
- *Major antagonists:*
  - Lateral flexors on the opposite side of the neck
- *Tender/trigger points:*
  - Belly of the muscle near the rib attachment
- *Common symptom/Common symptom/Referred pain pattern:*
  - Pectoral region, rhomboid region, and the entire length of the arm into the hand

ACTIVITY 9.13

Draw and color the *muscles of the scalene group* in the spaces provided. For each muscle:

1. Label the origin and insertion attachment points: *O* for origin; *I* for insertion.
2. Place an X on the trigger points.
3. Palpate this muscle; identify the attachment points and the bellies of the muscles.
4. Move these muscles on yourself.

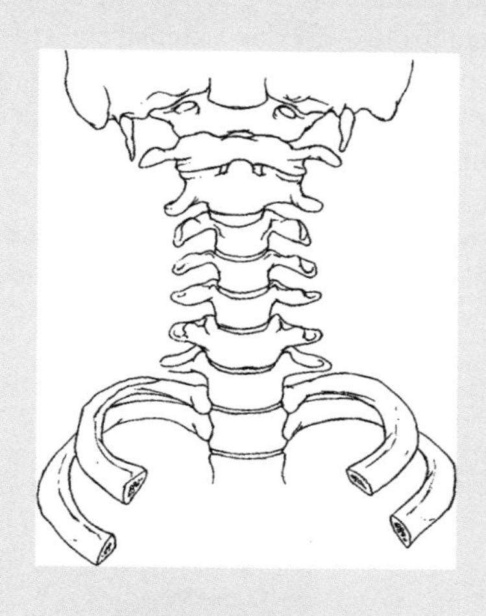

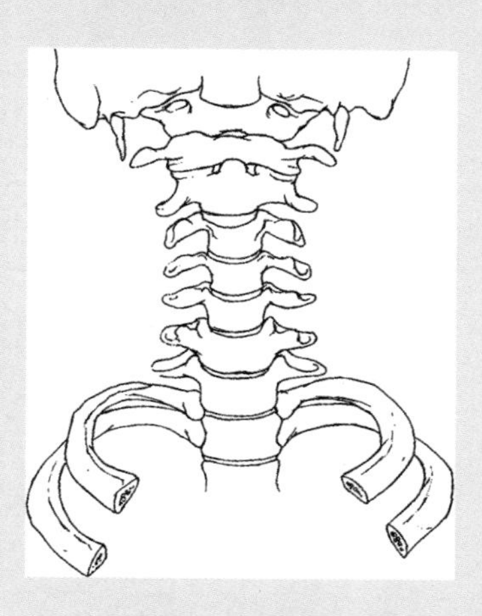

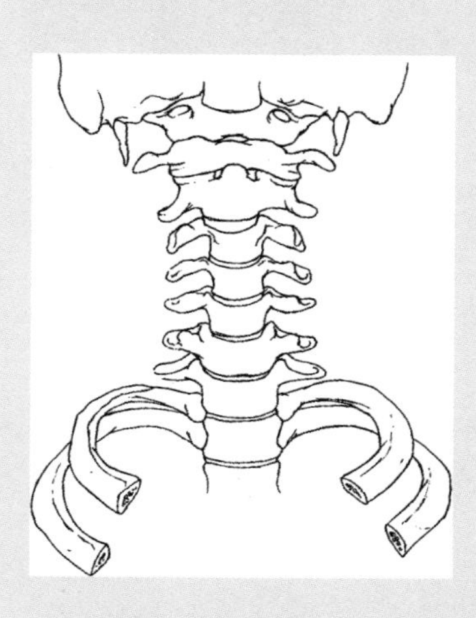

Deep Muscles of the Back and Posterior Neck

When concentrically contracted, the splenius muscles are responsible for neck and head extension, lateral flexion, and rotation. The deep, or intrinsic, back muscles associated with the vertebral column affect trunk movements. Isometrically, these muscles also play an important role in maintaining the normal curvature of the spine. The deep muscles of the back form a complex column that extends from the sacrum to the skull. Think of each of the individual deep back muscles as a string that, when pulled, causes one or more vertebrae to move on the vertebrae below. Because the attachments of the different muscle groups overlap extensively, entire regions of the vertebral column can move simultaneously and smoothly. Concentrically acting together, the deep back muscles can extend the trunk, neck, or head. Contraction of muscles on only one side causes extension, lateral flexion, and rotation of the trunk, neck, or head. Eccentric contraction restrains/controls (especially rapid movement) the opposite actions, primarily flexion, lateral flexion to the opposite side, and perhaps rotation.

The largest deep back muscle group is the erector spinae group. Assisting the long muscles of the back are a number of short muscles that extend from one vertebra to the next; these small intrinsic muscles act primarily as stabilizers for the spine. Postural deviation of any type—including forward head position or scoliosis, excessive kyphosis, and excessive lordosis or any rotational adaptation of the shoulder girdle and pelvic girdle—strains the deep postural muscles. These muscles are more involved in stabilization than mobility; therefore, when dysfunctional patterns exist, these muscles tend to shorten because of sustained isometric functioning. Massage affecting these muscles must be deep enough to access them without causing protective tensing (guarding) of the more superficial muscles. Massage is most effective when applied with a slow, sustained, broad-based compressive force that penetrates the superficial layers to affect the deep muscles (Fig. 9.17).

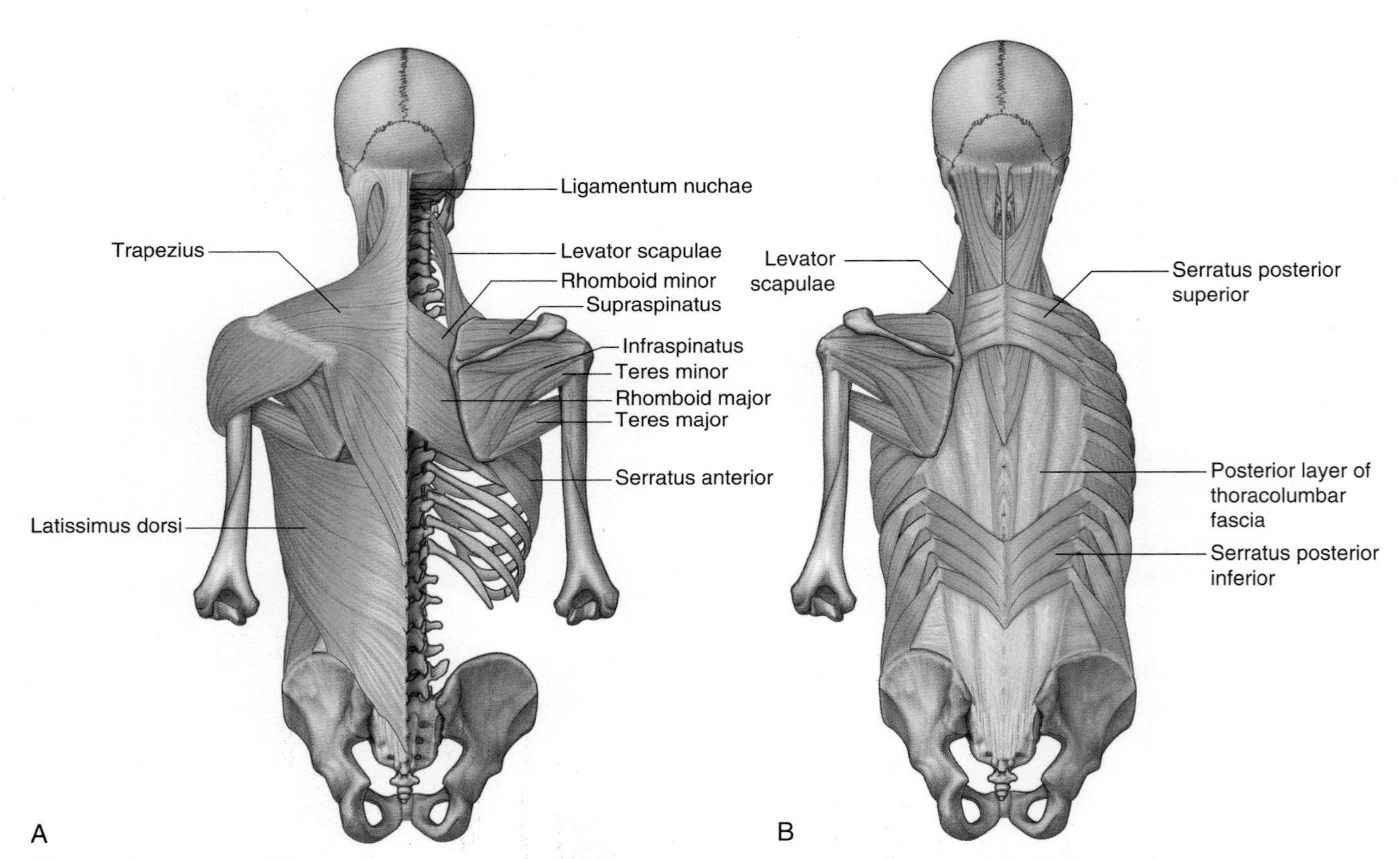

FIG. 9.17 (A) Superficial group of back muscles—the trapezius and latissimus dorsi, with the rhomboid major, rhomboid minor, and levator scapulae located deep to the trapezius in the superior part of the back. (B) Intermediate group of back muscles—serratus posterior muscles.

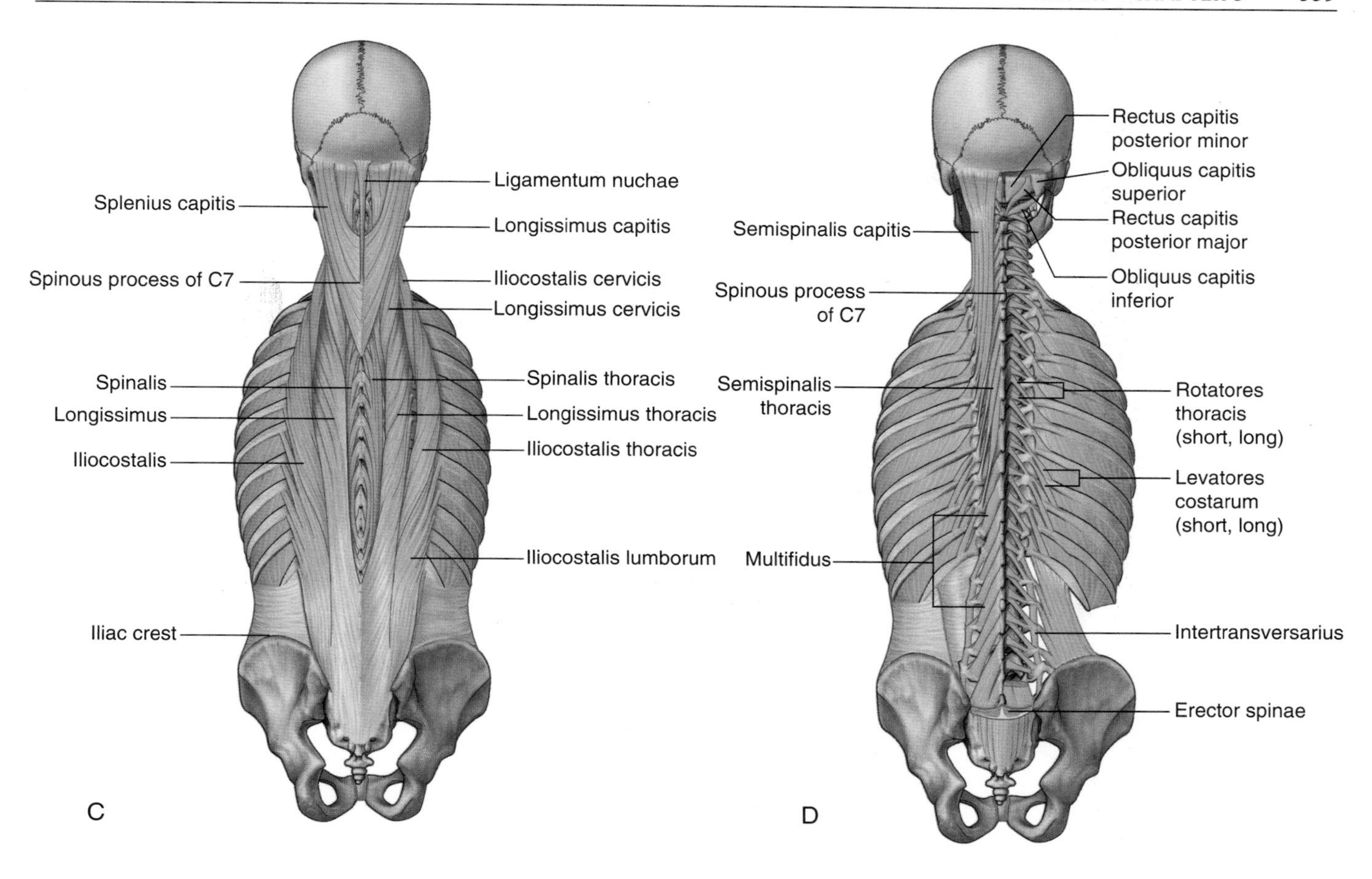

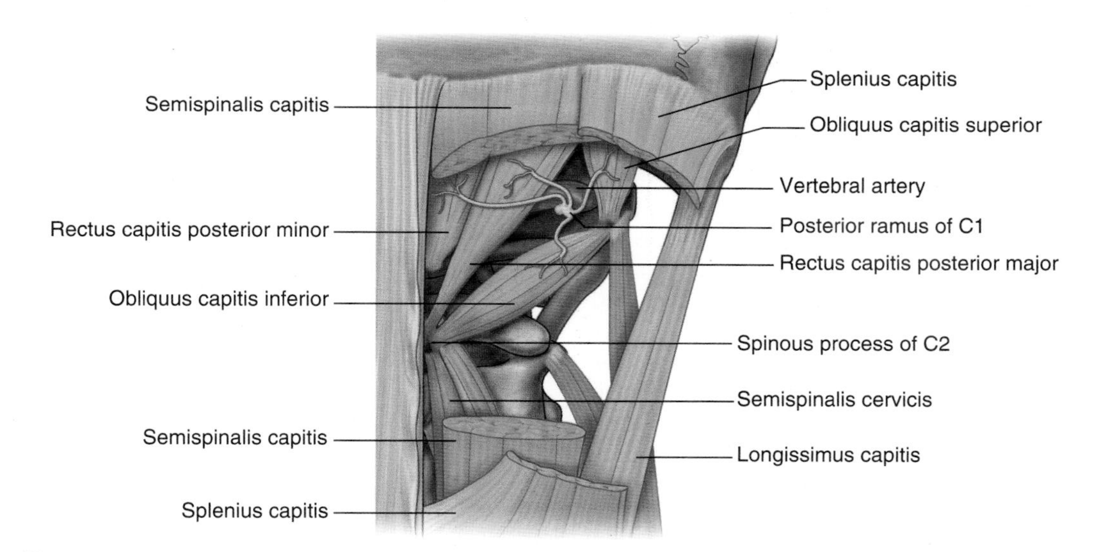

FIG. 9.17, cont'd (C) Deep group of back muscles—erector spinae muscles. (D) Deep group of back muscles—transversospinales and segmental muscles. (E) Deep group of back muscles—suboccipital muscles. This also shows the borders of the suboccipital triangle. (From Drake RL, Vogl W, Mitchell WM. *Gray's Anatomy for Students*. 2nd ed. Churchill Livingstone; 2010.)

Deep Posterior Cervical Muscles

Splenius capitis and splenius cervicis (SPLEEN-ee-us KAP-ih-tiss, SIR-vih-siss)

Splenius means "bandage," *capitis* means "head," and *cervicis* means "belonging to the neck."

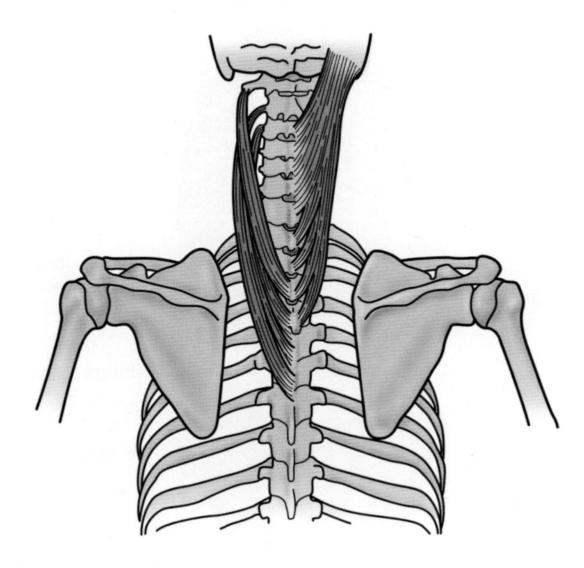

- *Concentric action:*
  - Extension, lateral flexion, and ipsilateral rotation of the head and the neck at the spinal joints
- *Eccentric action:*
  - Restrains/controls (especially rapid movement) flexion, contralateral lateral flexion, and contralateral rotation of the neck and the head
- *Isometric action:*
  - Stabilizes the cervical spine
- *Origin, fixed end, proximal attachment, arises from:*
  - Capitis—nuchal ligament and the spinous processes of the seventh cervical and first four thoracic vertebrae
  - Cervicis—spinous processes of the third through sixth thoracic vertebrae
- *Insertion, mobile end, distal attachment, attaches to:*
  - Capitis—lateral one-third of the superior nuchal line of the occipital bone deep to the attachment of the sternocleidomastoid and the mastoid process of the temporal bone
  - Cervicis—posterior tubercles of the transverse processes of the upper three cervical vertebrae
- *Innervation:*
  - Capitis—dorsal rami of the middle cervical spinal nerves
  - Cervicis—dorsal rami of the lower cervical spinal nerves
- *Major synergists:*
  - Posterior cervical extensors, opposite-sided upper trapezius, and opposite-sided sternocleidomastoid
- *Major antagonists:*
  - Anterior cervical flexors, same-sided upper trapezius, and same-sided sternocleidomastoid
- *Tender/trigger points:*
  - Belly of the muscles closer to the head
- *Referred pain patterns:*
  - To the top of the skull (the pain often feels as though it is inside the head), to the eye, and into the shoulder.

ACTIVITY 9.14

Draw and color the *deep posterior cervical muscles* in the spaces provided. For each muscle:

1. Label the origin and insertion attachment points: *O* for origin; *I* for insertion.
2. Place an X on the trigger points.
3. Palpate this muscle; identify the attachment points and the bellies of the muscles.
4. Move these muscles on yourself.

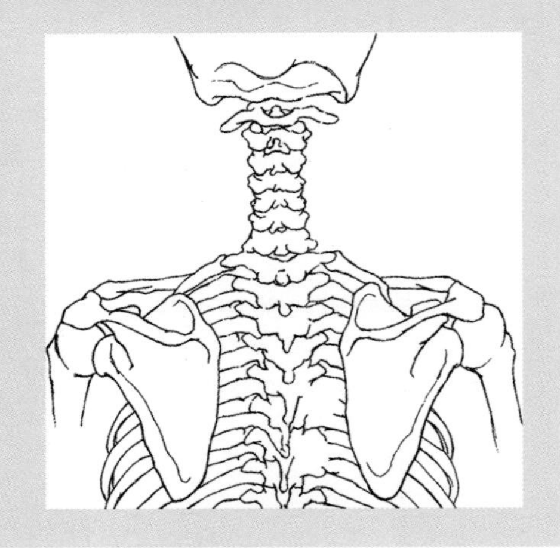

Vertebral Column Muscles, Erector Spinae Group

Also called the *sacrospinalis muscles*, the muscles in the erector spinae (ee-REK-tor SPIN-aye) group are the principal extensors of the spinal joints.

Iliocostalis lumborum, iliocostalis thoracis, and iliocostalis cervicis (ILL-ee-oh-kos-TAL-iss lum-BOR-um, thor-AH-siss, SIR-vih-siss)

Iliocostalis means "connecting the ilium" to the loins (lumborum), ribs (costa), chest (thoracis), and neck (cervicis).

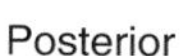

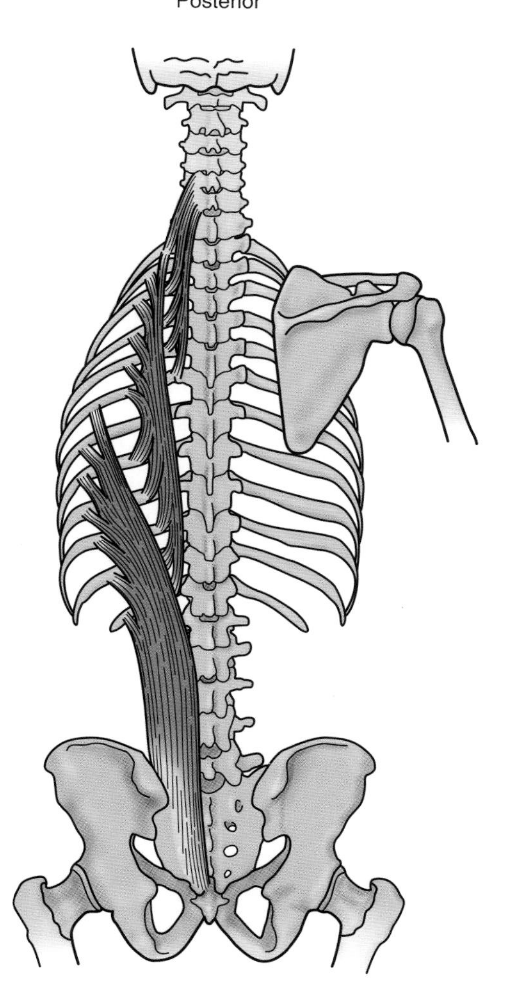

- *Concentric action:*
  - Extension, lateral flexion, and ipsilateral rotation of the trunk and neck at the spinal joints and anterior tilt of the pelvis at the lumbosacral joint
- *Eccentric action:*
  - Restrains/controls (especially rapid movement) flexion, contralateral lateral flexion, and contralateral rotation of the trunk and neck and allows posterior tilt of the pelvis
- *Isometric action:*
  - Stabilizes the spine and pelvis
- *Origin, fixed end, proximal attachment, arises from:*
  - Lumborum—medial iliac crest and medial and lateral sacral crests
  - Thoracis—lower six ribs medial to the tendons of the iliocostalis lumborum
  - Cervicis—angles of the third through sixth ribs
- *Insertion, mobile end, distal attachment, attaches to:*
  - Lumborum—inferior border at the angles of ribs 7 to 12
  - Thoracis—superior border at the angles of ribs 1 to 6 and transverse process of seventh cervical vertebra
  - Cervicis—posterior tubercles of the transverse processes of the fourth through sixth cervical vertebrae
- *Innervation:*
- Dorsal rami of the lower cervical, thoracic, and lumbar spinal nerves

Longissimus thoracis, longissimus cervicis, and longissimus capitis (lon-GISS-ih-mus thor-AH-siss, SIR-vih-siss, KAP-ih-tiss)

Longissimus means "the longest;" these muscles relate to the thorax, neck, and head, respectively.

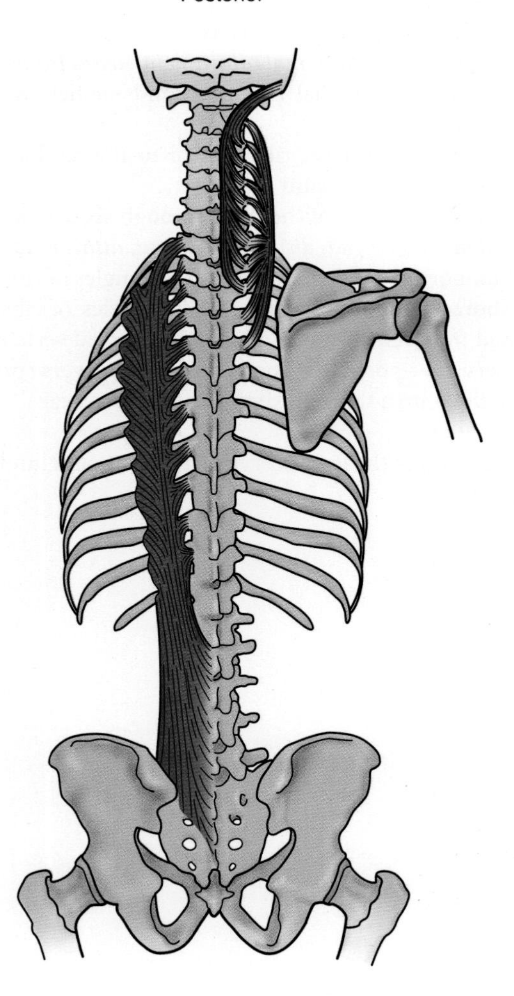

- *Concentric action:*
  - Extension, lateral flexion, and ipsilateral rotation of the trunk, neck, and head at the spinal joints and anterior tilt of the pelvis at the lumbosacral joint
- *Eccentric action:*
  - Restrains/controls (especially rapid movement) flexion, contralateral lateral flexion, and contralateral rotation of the trunk, neck, and head and allows posterior tilt of the pelvis
- *Isometric action:*
  - Stabilizes the spine and pelvis
- *Origin, fixed end, proximal attachment, arises from:*
  - Thoracis—transverse processes of the lumbar vertebrae, lumbocostal aponeurosis, and medial iliac crest and posterior sacrum
  - Cervicis—transverse processes of the upper five thoracic vertebrae
  - Capitis—transverse processes of the upper four or five thoracic vertebrae and articular processes of the lower three or four cervical vertebrae
- *Insertion, mobile end, distal attachment, attaches to:*
  - Thoracis—transverse processes of all thoracic vertebrae and lower 9 or 10 ribs
  - Cervicis—posterior tubercles of the transverse processes of the second through sixth cervical vertebrae
  - Capitis—mastoid process of the temporal bone
- *Innervation:*
  - Dorsal rami of the lower cervical, thoracic, and lumbar spinal nerves

Spinalis thoracis, spinalis cervicis, and spinalis capitis (spy-NAL-iss thor-AH-siss, SIR-vih-ciss, KAP-ih-tiss)

Spinalis means "related to the spine;" these muscles relate to the chest, neck, and head, respectively.

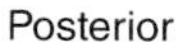

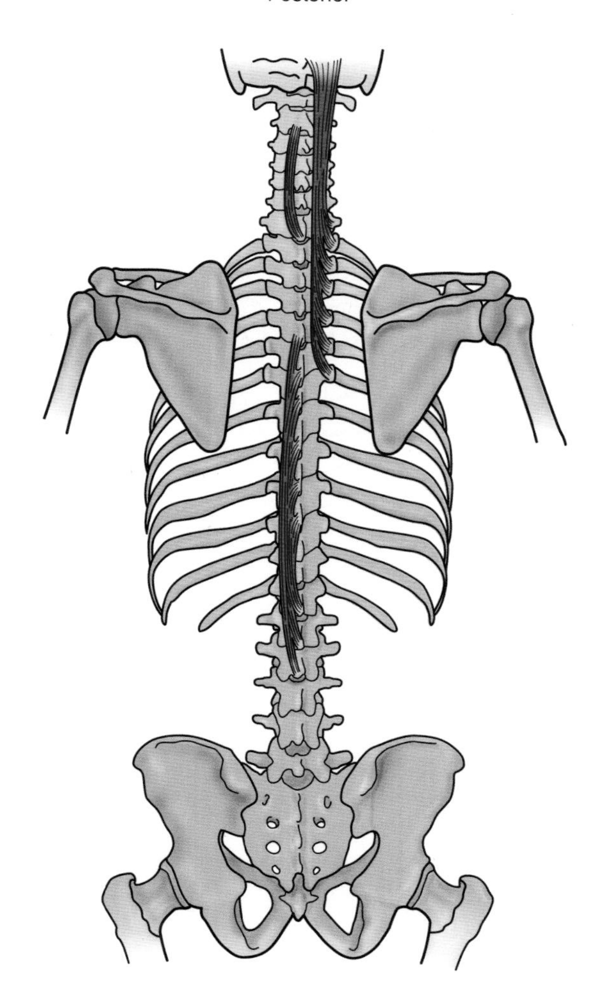

- *Concentric action:*
  - Extension, lateral flexion, and ipsilateral rotation of the trunk, neck, and head at the spinal joints
- *Eccentric action:*
  - Restrains/controls (especially rapid movement) flexion, contralateral lateral flexion, and contralateral rotation of the trunk, neck, and head
- *Isometric action:*
  - Stabilizes the spine
- *Origin, fixed end, proximal attachment, arises from:*
  - Thoracis—spinous processes of the first two lumbar and the last two thoracic vertebrae
  - Cervicis—spinous processes of the first and second thoracic and the seventh cervical vertebrae
  - Capitis—transverse processes of the upper seven thoracic and the seventh cervical vertebrae and articular processes of the fourth through sixth cervical vertebrae
- *Insertion, mobile end, distal attachment, attaches to:*
  - Thoracis—spinous processes of the fourth through eighth thoracic vertebrae
  - Cervicis—spinous processes of the second and third cervical vertebrae
  - Capitis—between the superior and inferior nuchal lines of the occipital bone
- *Innervation:*
  - Dorsal rami of the lower cervical, thoracic, and lumbar spinal nerves
  - Elements common to the erector spinae and transversospinalis group
- *Major antagonists:*
  - Flexors of the trunk (abdominal muscles)
- *Major synergists:*
  - Extension is assisted by the serratus posterior inferior and the quadratus lumborum; rotation is assisted by the abdominal obliques.
- *Tender/trigger points:*
  - The most common site for tender/trigger points is the superficial long-fibered, longitudinal muscles in the erector spinae group; tender/trigger points usually are found in the midscapular and lumbar regions.
- *Referred pain patterns:*
  - Scapular, lumbar, abdominal, and gluteal areas; also local area and adjacent spinal segment

ACTIVITY 9.15

Draw and color the *vertical muscles (erector spinae group)* in the spaces provided. For each muscle:

1. Label the origin and insertion attachment points: *O* for origin; *I* for insertion.
2. Place an X on the trigger points.
3. Palpate this muscle; identify the attachment points and the bellies of the muscles.
4. Move these muscles on yourself.

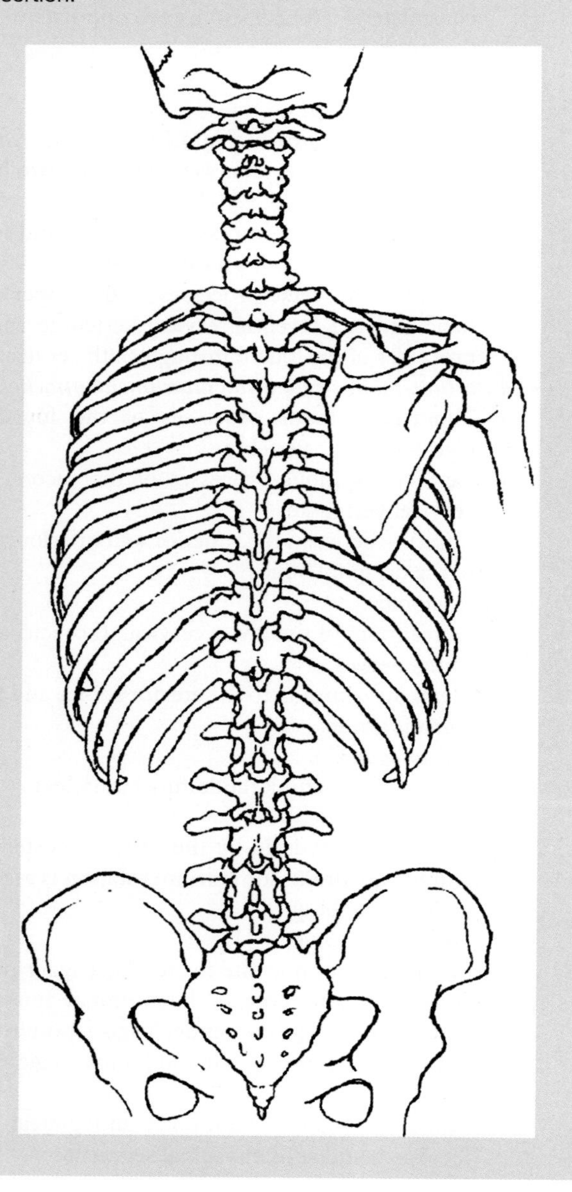

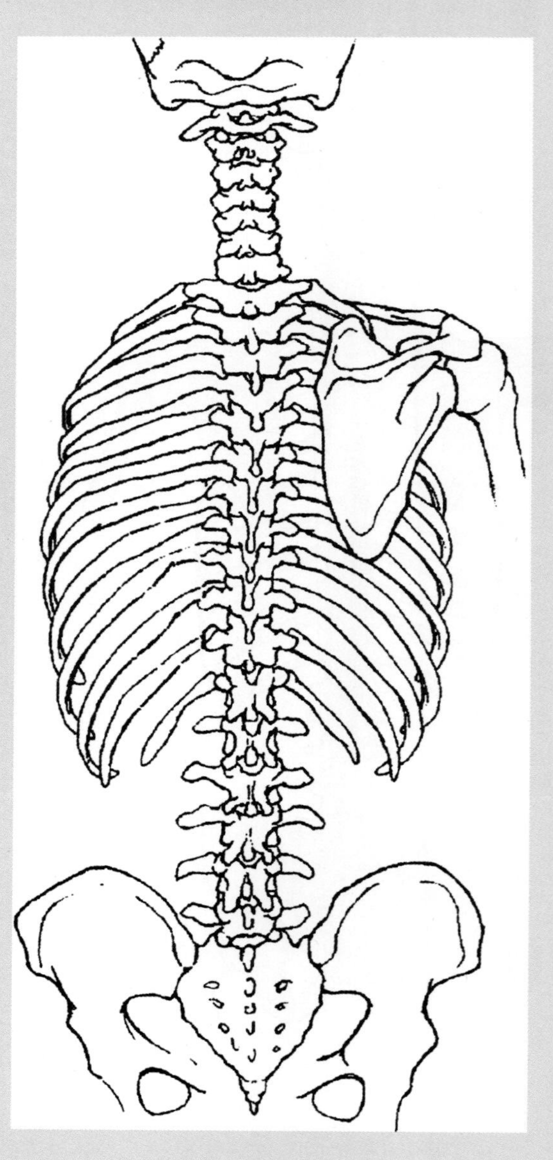

Transversospinales Group

The transversospinales group of muscles extends, laterally flexes, and contralaterally rotates the spinal joints and also functions to move and stabilize the pelvis.

> Semispinalis thoracis, semispinalis cervicis, and semispinalis capitis (sem-ee-spy-NAL-is thor-AH-siss, SIR-vih-siss, KAP-ih-tiss)

Semispinalis means "half" and "spine;" these muscles relate to the chest, neck, and head, respectively.

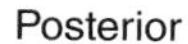

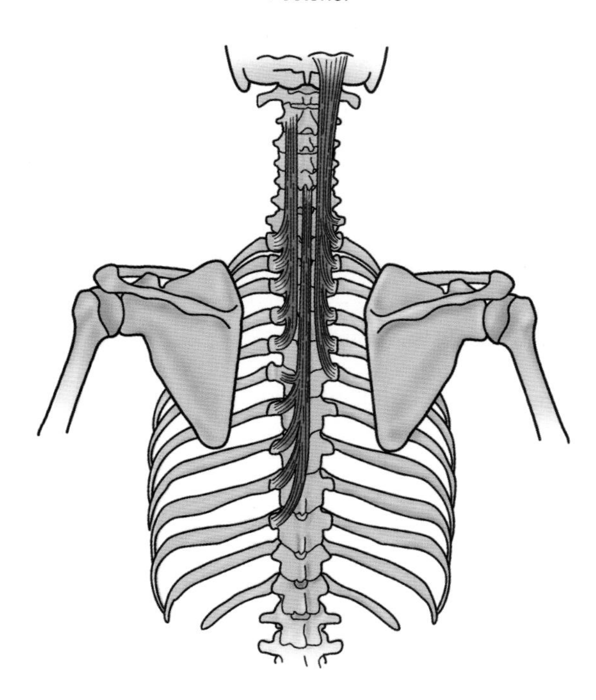

- *Concentric action:*
  - Extension and lateral flexion of the trunk, neck, and head at the spinal joints and contralateral rotation of the trunk and neck at the spinal joints
- *Eccentric action:*
  - Allows flexion and contralateral lateral flexion of the trunk, neck, and head and allows ipsilateral rotation of the trunk and neck
- *Isometric action:*
  - Stabilizes the spine
- *Origin, fixed end, proximal attachment, arises from:*
  - Thoracis—transverse processes of the last six thoracic vertebrae
  - Cervicis—transverse processes of the upper six thoracic and articular processes of the lower four cervical vertebrae
  - Capitis—transverse processes of the upper six thoracic vertebrae and the seventh cervical vertebrae; articular processes of the fourth through sixth cervical vertebrae
- *Insertion, mobile end, distal attachment, attaches to:*
  - Thoracis—spinous processes of the first four thoracic and the last two cervical vertebrae
  - Cervicis—spinous processes of the second through fifth cervical vertebrae
  - Capitis—between the superior and inferior nuchal lines of the occipital bone
- *Innervation:*
  - Thoracis—dorsal rami of the upper six thoracic spinal nerves
  - Cervicis—dorsal rami of the lower three cervical spinal nerves
  - Capitis—dorsal rami of the first six cervical spinal nerves
- *Major synergists:*
  - Multifidus and rotatores and extensors of the neck and head
- *Major antagonists:*
  - Flexors of the trunk (abdominal muscles)
- *Tender/trigger points:*
  - Belly of the muscles
- *Referred pain patterns:*
  - Local area

Multifidus (mul-tih-FYE-dus) (musculi multifidi)

Multifidus means "many split parts."

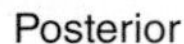

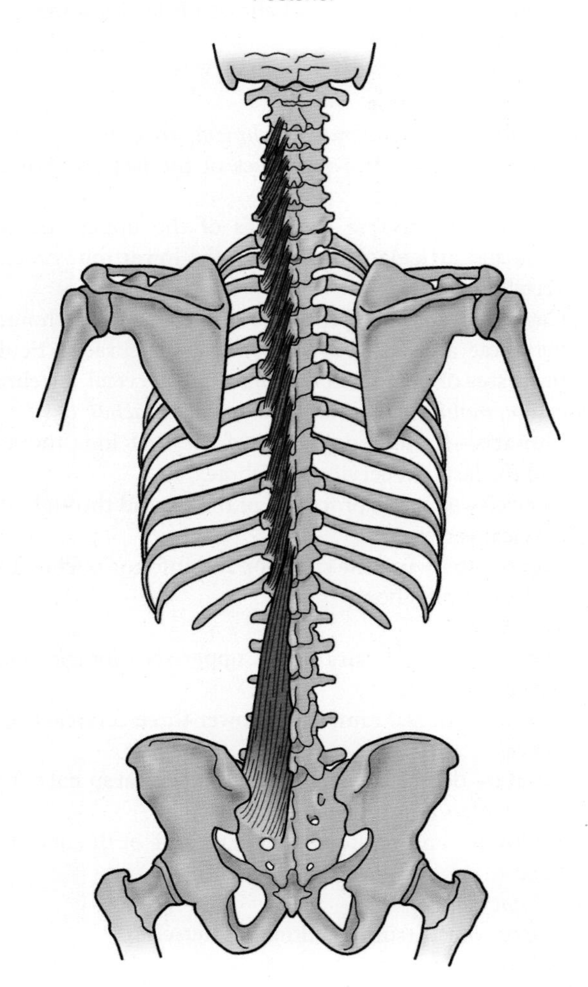

- *Concentric action:*
  - Contralateral rotation, lateral flexion, and extension of the trunk and neck at the spinal joints and anterior tilt and elevation of the pelvis at the lumbosacral joint
- *Eccentric action:*
  - Allows ipsilateral rotation, contralateral lateral flexion, and flexion of the trunk and neck and allows posterior tilt and depression of the pelvis
- *Isometric action:*
  - Stabilizes the spine and pelvis

  This muscle group provides proprioceptive input about posture and movement.
- *Origin, fixed end, proximal attachment, arises from:*
  - Articular processes of the last four cervical vertebrae, transverse processes of all thoracic vertebrae, mammillary processes of the lumbar vertebrae, posterior superior iliac spine, posterior sacroiliac ligaments, and posterior surface of the sacrum
- *Insertion, mobile end, distal attachment, attaches to:*
  - Spinous processes of the vertebrae two to four levels superior to the vertebrae of origin
- *Innervation:*
  - Dorsal rami of the spinal nerves
- *Major synergists:*
  - Semispinalis and rotatores
- *Major antagonists:*
  - Flexors of the trunk (abdominal muscles)
- *Tender/trigger points:*
  - Belly of the muscles
- *Referred pain patterns:*
  - Local area and sacroiliac joint

Rotatores (ro-TA-to-reez)

Rotatores means "one that rotates."

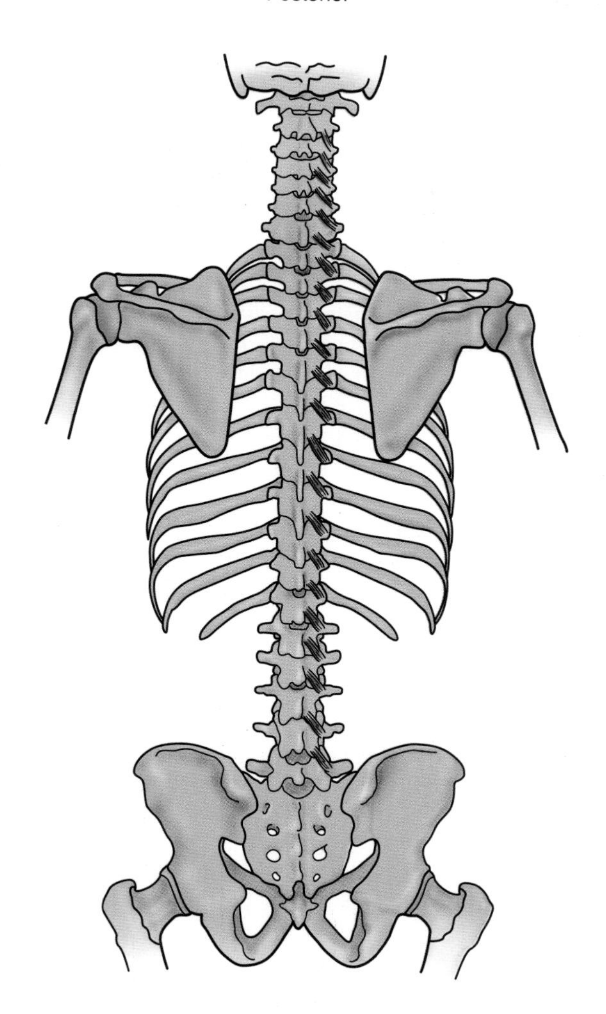

- *Concentric action:*
  - Contralateral rotation and extension of the trunk and neck at the spinal joints
- *Eccentric action:*
  - Restrains/controls (especially rapid movement) ipsilateral rotation and flexion of the trunk and neck
- *Isometric action:*
  - Stabilizes the vertebral column particularly on the transverse plane between each vertebra

  The rotatores are an important muscle group (with the multifidi) in providing proprioceptive posture information to the central nervous system.
- *Origin, fixed end, proximal attachment, arises from:*
  - Transverse process (inferiorly)
- *Insertion, mobile end, distal attachment, attaches to:*
  - Lamina one to two levels superior
- *Innervation:*
  - Dorsal rami of spinal nerves
- *Major synergists:*
  - Same-sided contralateral rotators of the trunk and neck and opposite-sided ipsilateral rotators of the trunk and neck
- *Major antagonists:*
  - Opposite-sided contralateral rotators of the trunk and neck and same-sided ipsilateral rotators of the trunk and neck
- *Tender/trigger points:*
  - Belly of the muscles
- *Referred pain patterns:*
  - Local area

Intertransversarii lumborum, intertransversarii thoracis, and intertransversarii cervicis (IN-ter-TRANS-ver-SAIR-ee-eye lum-BOR-um, thor-AH-siss, SIR-vih-siss)

Intertransversarii means "between or among the transverse processes of the vertebrae;" these muscles relate to the loins, thorax, and neck, respectively.

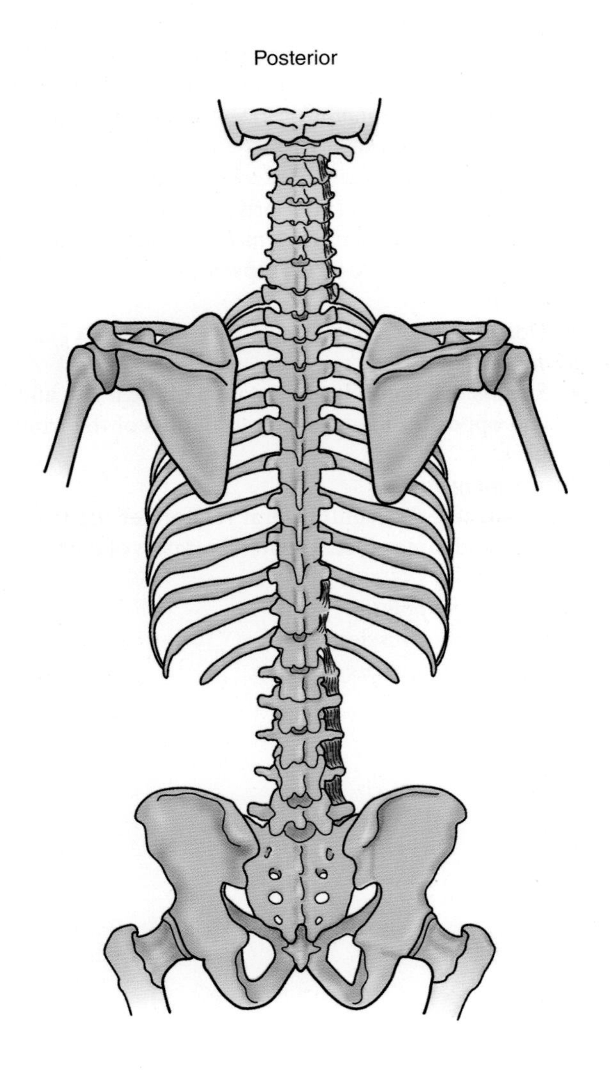

- *Concentric action:*
  - Lateral flexion of the trunk and neck at the spinal joints
- *Eccentric action:*
  - Restrains/controls (especially rapid movement) contralateral lateral flexion of the trunk and neck
- *Isometric action:*
  - Provides intersegmental stability of the spine in the frontal plane

  The intertransversarii muscles are active in proprioceptive input to the central nervous system.
- *Origin, fixed end, proximal attachment, arises from:*
  - Between transverse processes of the cervical, thoracic, and lumbar vertebrae (best developed in the cervical and lumbar regions)
- *Insertion, mobile end, distal attachment, attaches to:*
  - Between transverse processes of the cervical, thoracic, and lumbar vertebrae (best developed in the cervical and lumbar regions)
- *Innervation:*
  - Ventral and dorsal rami of the spinal nerves
- *Major synergists:*
  - Ipsilateral lateral flexors of the trunk and neck
- *Major antagonists:*
  - Contralateral lateral flexors of the trunk and neck
- *Tender/trigger points:*
  - Belly of the muscles
- *Referred pain patterns:*
  - Local area

Interspinales lumborum, interspinales thoracis, and interspinales cervicis (in-ter-spy-NAL-eez lum-BOR-um, thor-AH-siss, SIR-vih-siss)

Interspinales means "between or among the parts of the spine"; these muscles relate to the loins, chest, and neck, respectively.

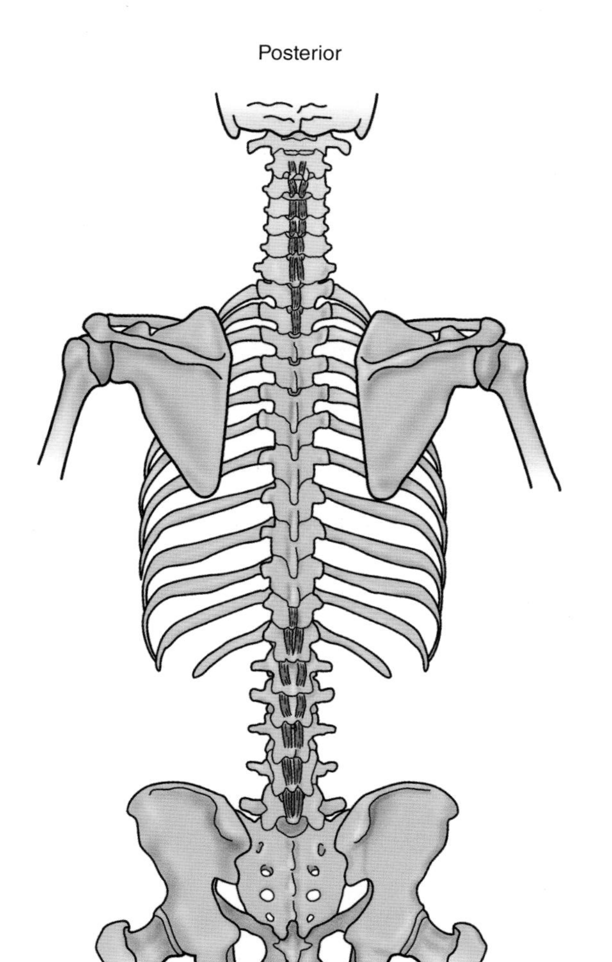

- *Concentric action:*
  - Extension of the trunk and neck at the spinal joints
- *Eccentric action:*
  - Restrains/controls (especially rapid movement) vertebral flexion
- *Isometric action:*
  - Provides intersegmental stability of the spine in the sagittal plane
  - Interspinales muscles provide proprioceptive input concerning spinal stabilization and neuromuscular control.
- *Insertion, mobile end, distal attachment, attaches to:*
  - Between the spinous processes of the vertebrae
- *Origin, fixed end, proximal attachment, arises from:*
  - Between the spinous processes of the vertebrae
- *Innervation:*
  - Dorsal rami of the spinal nerves
- *Major synergists:*
  - Extensors of the trunk and neck
- *Major antagonists:*
  - Flexors of the trunk and neck
- *Tender/trigger points:*
  - Belly of the muscle
- *Referred pain patterns:*
  - Local area

ACTIVITY 9.16

Draw and color the *transversospinales group* in the spaces provided. For each muscle:

1. Label the origin and insertion attachment points: *O* for origin; *I* for insertion.
2. Place an X on the trigger points.
3. Palpate this muscle; identify the attachment points and the bellies of the muscles.
4. Move these muscles on yourself.

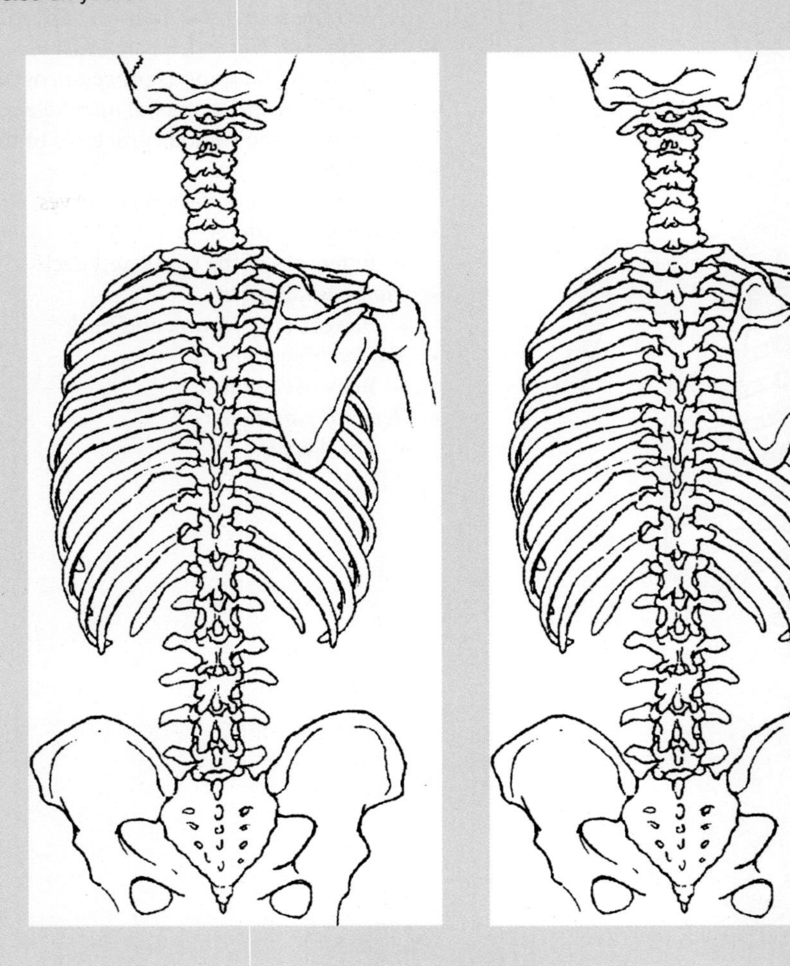

Suboccipital Muscles

As a group the suboccipital muscles extend and rotate the head at the atlantooccipital joint in small and precise movements. More often, these muscles isometrically function as stabilizers of the head. These muscles are also important postural muscles and are neurological reporting stations on balance and proprioceptive monitors of cervical spine and head position.

Rectus capitis posterior major (REK-tus KAP-ih-tiss)

Rectus means "straight," *capitis* means "belonging to the head," *posterior* means "behind," and *major* means "larger."

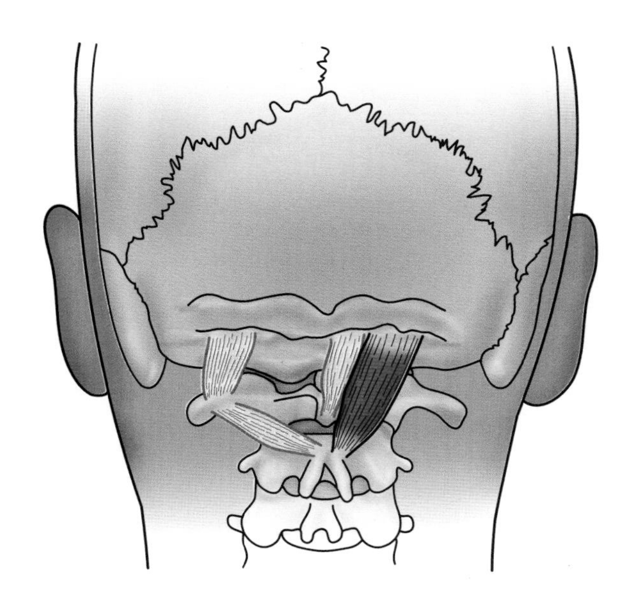

- *Concentric action:*
  - Extension, lateral flexion, and ipsilateral rotation of the head at the atlantooccipital joint
- *Eccentric action:*
  - Restrains/controls (especially rapid movement) flexion, contralateral lateral flexion, and contralateral rotation of the head
- *Isometric action:*
  - Stabilizes the upper cervical spine and head
- *Origin, fixed end, proximal attachment, arises from:*
  - Spinous process of the axis
- *Insertion, mobile end, distal attachment, attaches to:*
  - Lateral aspect of the inferior nuchal line of the occipital bone lateral to the rectus capitis posterior minor
- *Innervation:*
  - Dorsal ramus of the first cervical spinal nerve (the suboccipital nerve)
- *Major synergists:*
  - Semispinalis capitis, rectus capitis posterior minor, and the splenius capitis on the same side
- *Major antagonists:*
  - Rectus capitis anterior and the sternocleidomastoid on the same side
- *Tender/trigger points:*
  - Belly of the muscle, located with deep palpation at the base of the skull
- *Common symptom/Common symptom/Referred pain pattern:*
  - Around the ear on the same side, sensation of compressed junction of skull and neck, and bandlike headache

Rectus capitis posterior minor (REK-tus KAP-ih-tiss)

Rectus means "straight," *capitis* means "belonging to the head," *posterior* means "behind," and *minor* means "smaller."

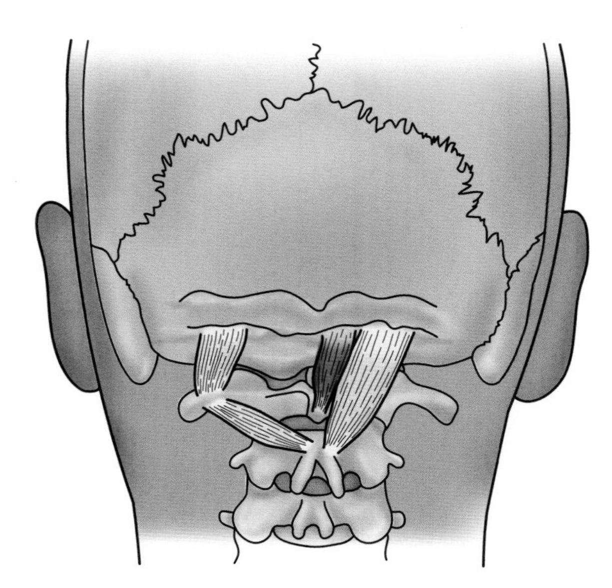

- *Concentric action:*
  - Extension of the head at the atlantooccipital joint (see Isometric Action)
- *Eccentric action:*
  - Restrains/controls (especially rapid movement) flexion of the head
- *Isometric action:*
  - Stabilizes the upper cervical spine and head

  Recent myographic studies indicate that this muscle does not act in extension beyond neutral position, but rather functions more importantly as a restraint to flexion and forward movement of the head; its proximal attachment weaves into the dura through the foramen magnum (DeStefano, 2011). This muscle actively provides proprioceptive input on positioning and posture to the central nervous system.
- *Origin, fixed end, proximal attachment, arises from:*
  - Posterior tubercle of the atlas
- *Insertion, mobile end, distal attachment, attaches to:*
  - Medial aspect of the inferior nuchal line of the occipital bone just superior to the foramen magnum
- *Innervation:*
  - Dorsal ramus of the first cervical spinal nerve (the suboccipital nerve)
- *Major synergists:*
  - Semispinalis capitis and rectus capitis posterior major
- *Major antagonists:*
  - Rectus capitis anterior and longus capitis on the opposite side
- *Tender/trigger points:*
  - Belly of the muscle, located with deep palpation at the base of the skull
- *Common symptom/Common symptom/Referred pain pattern:*
  - Around the ear on the same side, sensation of compressed junction of skull and neck, and bandlike headache

Oblique capitis superior (obliquus capitis superior) (oh-BLI-kwus KAP-ih-tiss)

Obliquus means "slanting," *capitis* means "head," and *superior* means "above" or "higher."

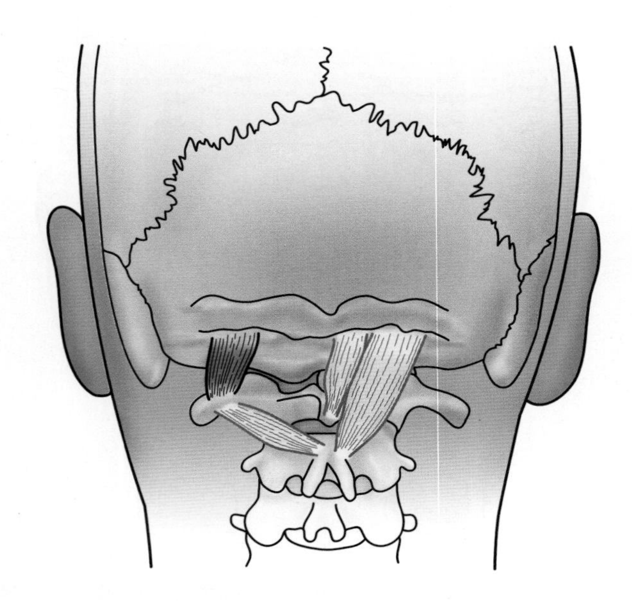

- *Concentric action:*
  - Extension and lateral flexion of the head at the atlanto-occipital joint
- *Eccentric action:*
  - Restrains/controls (especially rapid movement) flexion and contralateral lateral flexion of the head
- *Isometric action:*
  - Stabilizes the upper cervical spine and head
- *Origin, fixed end, proximal attachment, arises from:*
  - Superior surface of the transverse process of the atlas
- *Insertion, mobile end, distal attachment, attaches to:*
  - Between the superior and inferior nuchal lines of the occipital bone and lateral to the semispinalis capitis
- *Innervation:*
  - Dorsal ramus of the first cervical spinal nerve (the sub-occipital nerve)
- *Major synergists:*
  - Semispinalis capitis, rectus capitis posterior major, and rectus capitis posterior minor
- *Major antagonists:*
  - Rectus capitis anterior, sternocleidomastoid on the same side, and longus capitis on the opposite side
- *Tender/trigger points:*
  - Belly of the muscle, located with deep palpation at the base of the skull
- *Common symptom/Common symptom/Referred pain pattern:*
  - Around the ear on the same side, sensation of compressed junction of skull and neck, and bandlike headache

Oblique capitis inferior (obliquus capitis inferior) (oh-BLI-kwus KAP-ih-tiss)

Obliquus means "slanting," *capitis* means "head," and *inferior* means "lower" or "beneath."

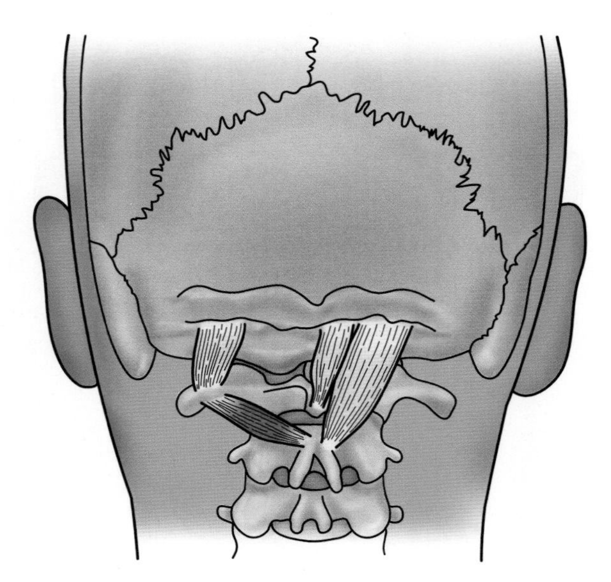

- *Concentric action*:
  - Ipsilateral rotation of the atlas at the atlantoaxial joint
- *Eccentric action:*
  - Restrains/controls (especially rapid movement) contralateral rotation of the atlas
- *Isometric action:*
  - Stabilizes the upper cervical spine
- *Origin, fixed end, proximal attachment, arises from:*
  - Superior part of the spinous process of the axis
- *Insertion, mobile end, distal attachment, attaches to:*
  - Inferior and posterior aspect of the transverse process of the atlas
- *Innervation:*
  - Dorsal ramus of the first cervical spinal nerve (the sub-occipital nerve)
- *Major synergists:*
  - Semispinalis capitis and the rectus capitis posterior major and rectus capitis posterior minor
- *Major antagonists:*
  - Rectus capitis anterior and rectus capitis lateralis on the opposite side
- *Tender/trigger points:*
  - Belly of the muscle, located with deep palpation at the base of the skull
- *Common symptom/Common symptom/Referred pain pattern:*
  - Around the ear on the same side, sensation of compressed junction of skull and neck, and bandlike headache

ACTIVITY 9.17

Draw and color the *suboccipital muscles* in the spaces provided. For each muscle:

1. Label the origin and insertion attachment points: *O* for origin; *I* for insertion.
2. Place an X on the trigger points.
3. Palpate this muscle; identify the attachment points and the bellies of the muscles.
4. Move these muscles on yourself.

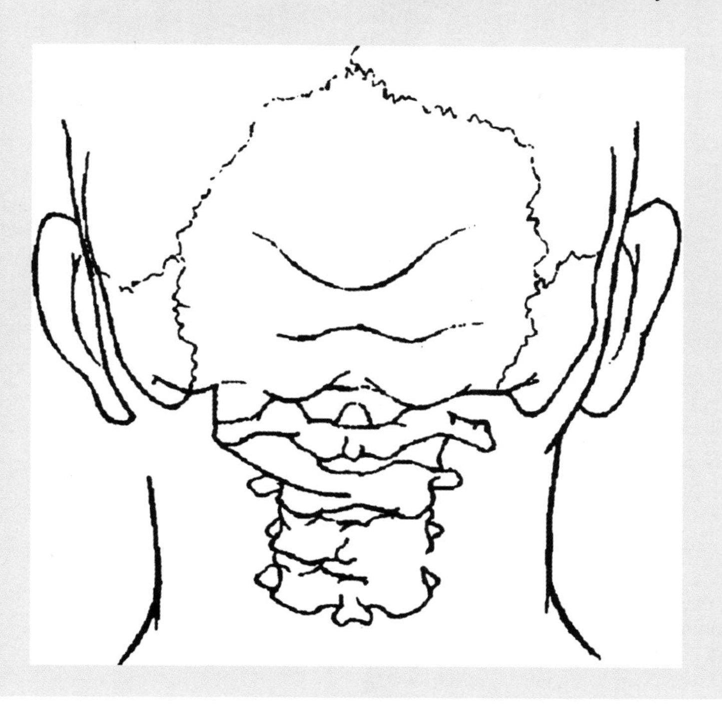

Muscles of the Torso

The primary function of the deep muscles of the thorax is to create movements necessary for breathing. Contraction of the diaphragm creates relaxed, quiet inspiration. Relaxed, quiet expiration requires no muscular contractions at all; rather, expiration is caused by the elastic recoil of the lungs themselves and the abdominal viscera that were stretched during inspiration. Forced inspiration and forced expiration result from the contraction of accessory muscles of respiration in addition to the diaphragm (Figs. 9.18 and 9.19).

Some anatomists have considered the abdominal and thorax muscle groups as one group. However, unlike the abdominal muscles, the thoracic muscles are short, extending between the ribs. When they contract, they elevate or depress the ribs. The external intercostal muscles (the most superficial layer) generally are accepted as elevating the ribs for inspiration, whereas the internal intercostal muscles (from the intermediate layer) depress the ribs for expiration. The transversus thoracis (the deepest layer) is also involved in depression of ribs.

The diaphragm is the most important muscle of inspiration and forms a muscular partition between the thoracic and abdominopelvic cavities. When relaxed, the diaphragm is dome shaped; but when it is contracted, its central dome moves inferiorly and flattens, increasing the volume of the thoracic cavity. The alternating contraction and relaxation of the diaphragm causes pressure changes in the abdominopelvic cavity that assists movement of lymph fluid as well as return of venous blood to the heart. We can contract the diaphragm to increase the intraabdominal pressure voluntarily to help evacuate urine or feces or to deliver a baby.

An increase in intraabdominal pressure also aids in lifting weight. When we take a deep breath to fixate our diaphragm, we can increase the abdominal pressure enough to support the spine while lifting a heavy weight. Fibers from the quadratus lumborum and psoas muscles weave into the diaphragm. With this direct relationship, we can see how low back function and breathing function are interrelated.

Forced breathing involves a number of other muscles that insert into the ribs. During forced inspiration, the scalene and sternocleidomastoid muscles may assist in lifting the ribs. Contraction of the abdominal wall muscles assists respiration. Massage in this area can positively influence effective breathing.

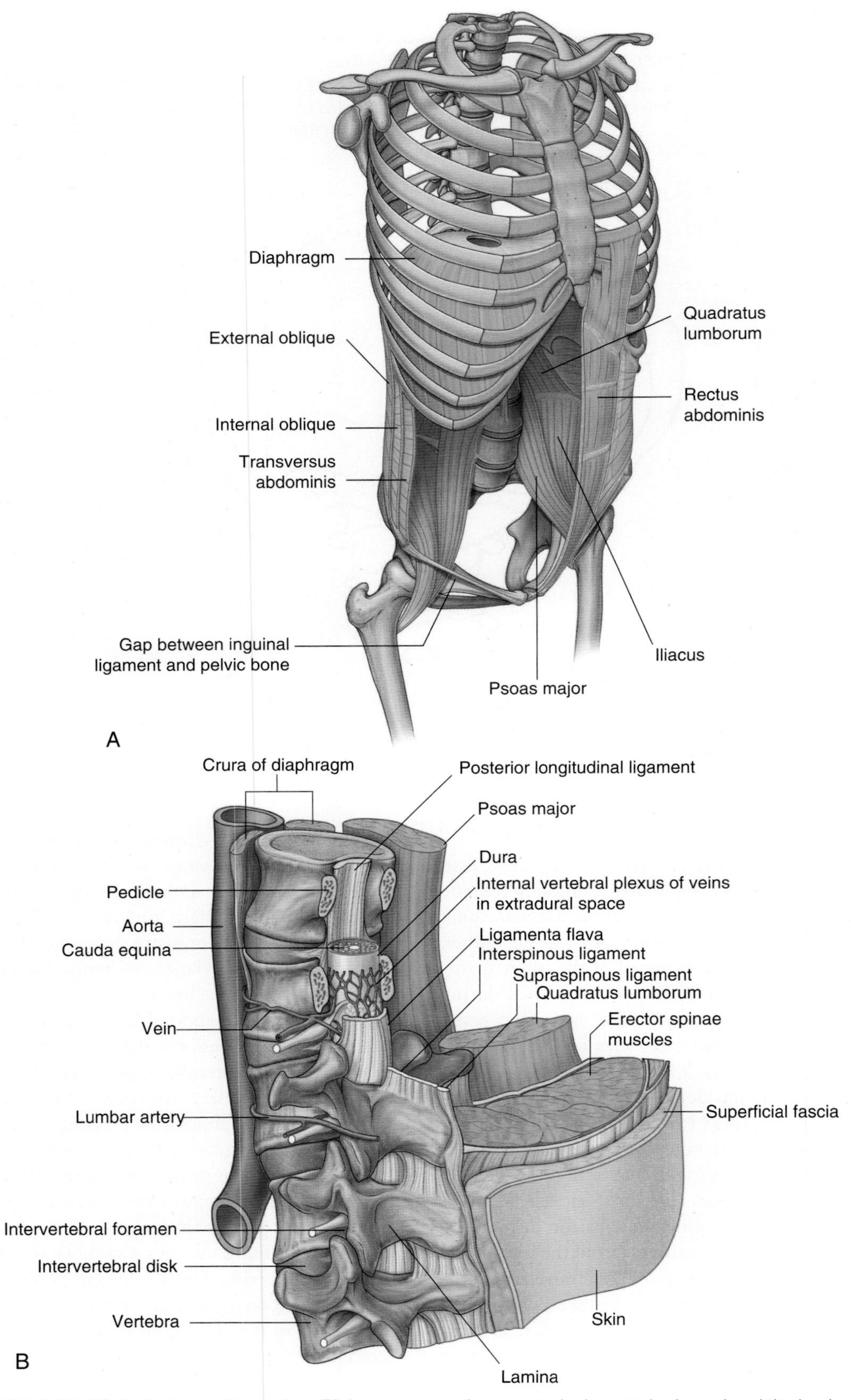

FIG. 9.18 (A) Abdominal wall muscles. (B) Arrangement of structures in the vertebral canal and the back.

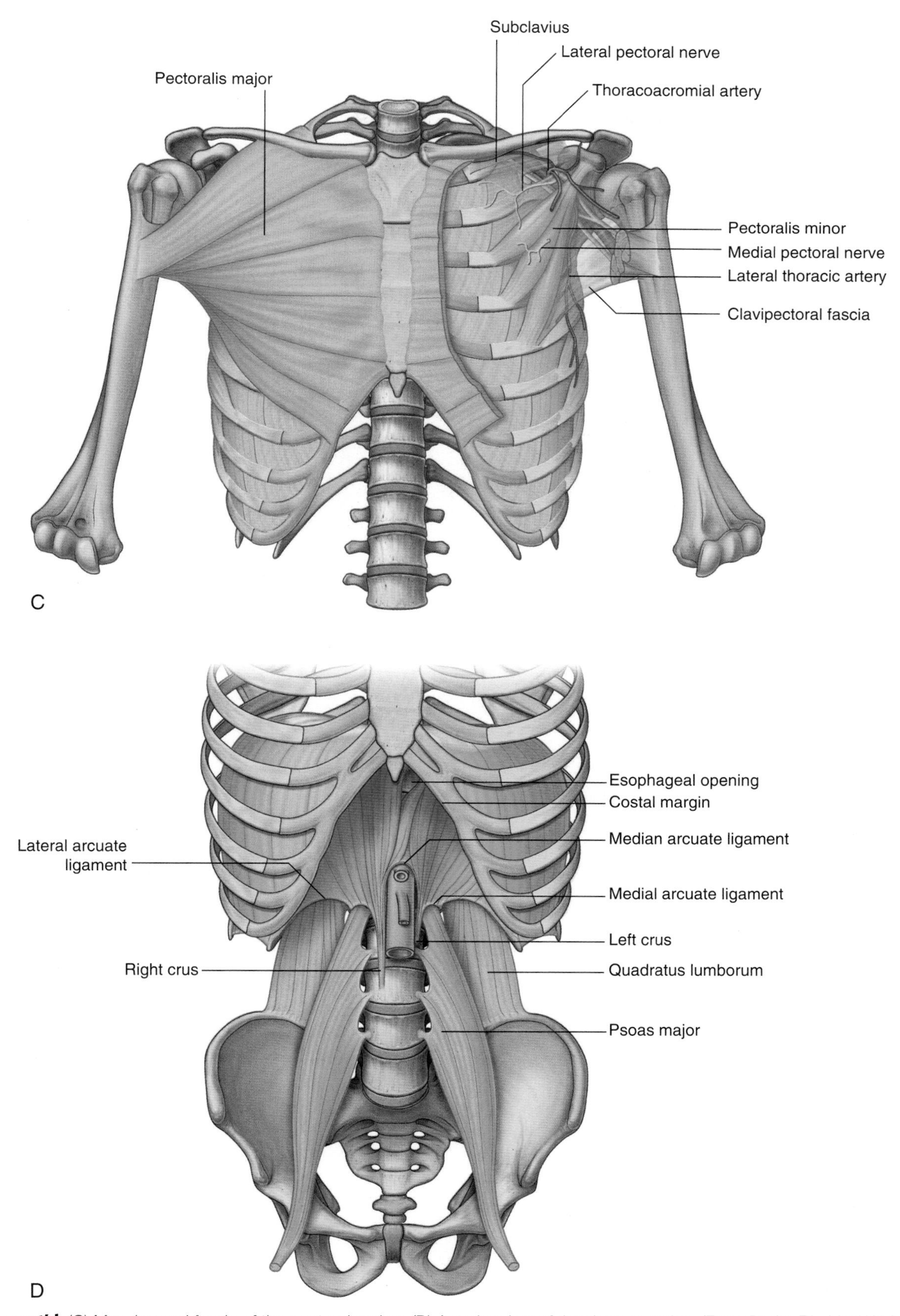

FIG. 9.18, cont'd (C) Muscles and fascia of the pectoral region. (D) Anterior view of the deep muscles. (From Drake RL, Vogl W, Mitchell WM. *Gray's Anatomy for Students*. 2nd ed. Churchill Livingstone; 2010.)

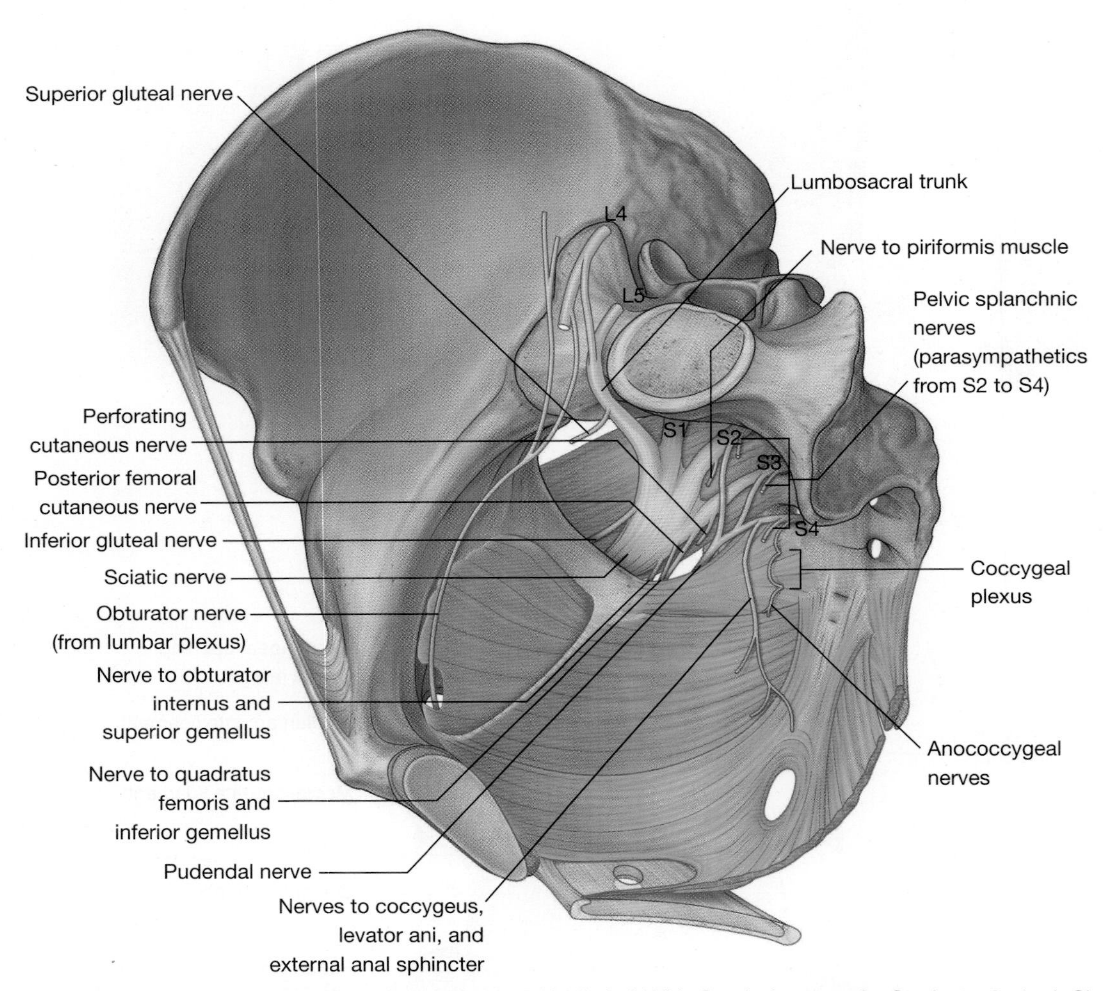

FIG. 9.19 Sacral and coccygeal plexuses. (From Drake RL, Vogl W, Mitchell WM. *Gray's Anatomy for Students*. 2nd ed. Churchill Livingstone; 2010.)

Muscles of the Thorax and Posterior Abdominal Wall

Serratus posterior superior (suhr-RATE-us)

Serratus means "saw shaped," *posterior* means "behind," and *superior* means "above."

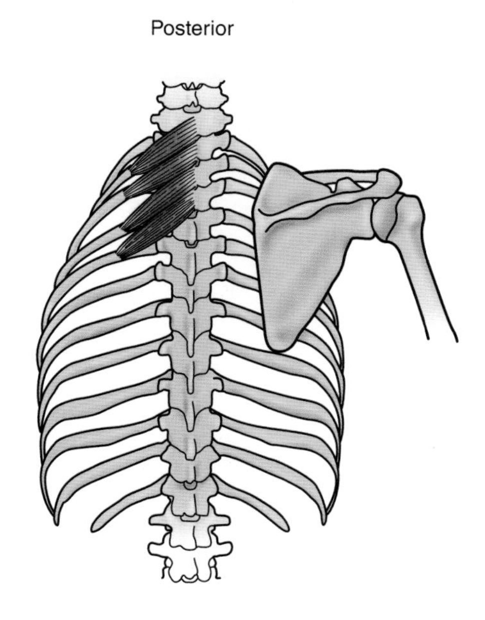

- *Concentric action:*
  - Elevates ribs 2 to 5 at the sternocostal and costovertebral joints during inspiration
- *Eccentric action:*
  - Restrains/controls (especially rapid movement) depression of ribs 2 to 5
- *Isometric action:*
  - Stabilizes the rib cage
- *Origin, fixed end, proximal attachment, arises from:*
  - Lower portion of the nuchal ligament and spinous processes of vertebrae C7–T3
- *Insertion, mobile end, distal attachment, attaches to:*
  - Superior borders and external surfaces of the second through fifth ribs, just lateral to their angles

  This muscle lies deep to the rhomboid muscles.
- *Innervation:*
  - Second through fifth intercostal nerves
- *Major synergists:*
  - Diaphragm and other muscles of inspiration
- *Major antagonists:*
  - Muscles of expiration, including the serratus posterior inferior
- *Tender/trigger points:*
  - Deep to the scapula near the insertion of the muscle on the ribs
- *Common symptom/Common symptom/Referred pain pattern:*
  - Deep to the superior portion of the scapula into the posterior deltoid, elbow, wrist, and ulnar portion of the hand

Serratus posterior inferior (suhr-RATE-us)

Serratus means "saw shaped," *posterior* means "behind," and *inferior* means "below."

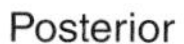

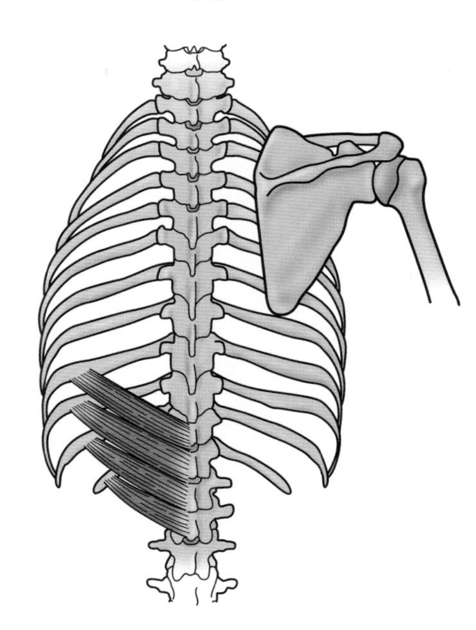

- *Concentric action:*
  - Depresses ribs 9 to 12 at the sternocostal and costovertebral joints during expiration
- *Eccentric action:*
  - Restrains/controls (especially rapid movement) elevation of ribs 9 to 12
- *Isometric action:*
  - Stabilizes the rib cage

  Some studies disagree that depression of ribs 9 to 12 for expiration is the function, finding no electromyographic activity of this muscle during respiration. Perhaps the serratus posterior inferior acts as a stabilizer during forced expirations such as coughing, which would be a concentric function.
- *Origin, fixed end, proximal attachment, arises from:*
  - Spines of T11, T12, and L1–L3; supraspinous ligament; and thoracolumbar fascia
- *Insertion, mobile end, distal attachment, attaches to:*
  - Inferior borders and outer surfaces of the lower four ribs (9–12) just lateral to the angles
- *Innervation:*
  - Subcostal nerve and intercostal nerves 9 to 11
- *Major synergists:*
  - Other muscles of expiration
- *Major antagonists:*
  - Diaphragm and serratus posterior superior
- *Tender/trigger points:*
  - Belly of the muscle near the eleventh rib
- *Common symptom/Common symptom/Referred pain pattern:*
  - Nagging ache in the area of the muscle

External intercostal muscles (in-ter-KOS-tal) (musculi intercostales externi)

Intercostal means "between or among the rib"; *external* means "on the outside."

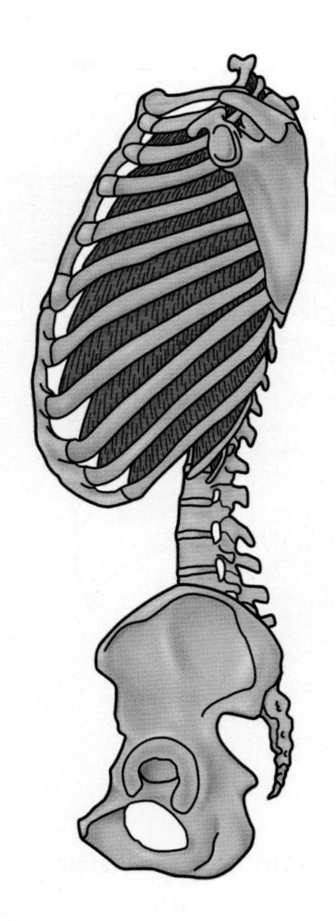

- *Concentric action:*
  - Elevates the ribs at the sternocostal and costovertebral joints, increasing the volume of the thoracic cavity for inspiration
  - The external intercostal muscles also may contribute to contralateral rotation of the trunk.
- *Eccentric action:*
  - Restrains/controls (especially rapid movement) depression of ribs
- *Isometric action:*
  - Stabilizes the rib cage
- *Origin, fixed end, proximal attachment, arises from:*
  - Eleven total—each arising from the inferior border of a rib
- *Insertion, mobile end, distal attachment, attaches to:*
  - Superior border of the inferior rib
- *Innervation:*
  - Adjacent intercostal nerves
- *Major synergists:*
  - Diaphragm and other muscles of inspiration
- *Major antagonists:*
  - Muscles of expiration
- *Tender/trigger points:*
  - The external intercostal muscles can develop trigger points, which can be located by palpating the muscles between the ribs.
- *Common symptom/Common symptom/Referred pain pattern:*
  - Spans the intercostal segment—especially noticeable with deep breathing or rotational movement

Internal intercostal muscles (in-ter-KOS-tal) (musculi intercostales interni)

Intercostal means "between or among the ribs"; *internal* means "on the inside."

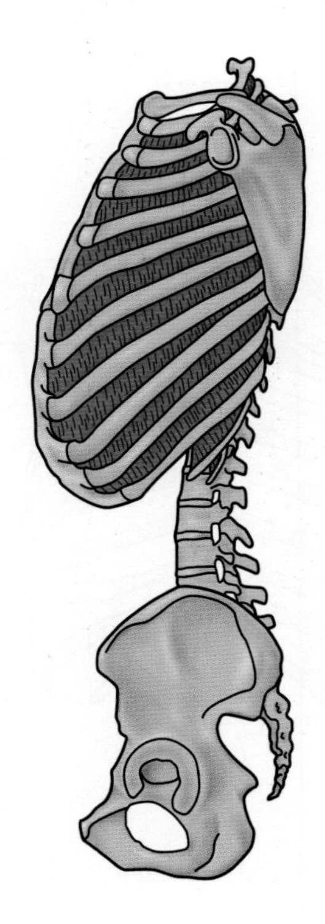

- *Concentric action:*
  - Depresses the ribs at the sternocostal and costovertebral joints, decreasing the volume of the thoracic cavity for expiration
  - The internal intercostal muscles also may contribute to ipsilateral rotation of the trunk.
- *Eccentric action:*
  - Restrains/controls (especially rapid movement) elevation of ribs
- *Isometric action:*
  - Stabilizes the rib cage
- *Origin, fixed end, proximal attachment, arises from:*
  - Eleven total, each arising from the ridge of the inner surface of a rib and corresponding costal cartilage
- *Insertion, mobile end, distal attachment, attaches to:*
  - Inferior border of the superior rib
- *Innervation:*
  - Adjacent intercostal nerves
- *Major synergists:*
  - Muscles of expiration
- *Major antagonists:*
  - Diaphragm and other muscles of inspiration
- *Tender/trigger points:*
  - The internal intercostal muscles can develop trigger points, which can be located by palpating the muscles between the ribs.
- *Common symptom/Common symptom/Referred pain pattern:*
  - Spans the intercostal segment, especially noticeable with deep breathing or rotational movement

Innermost intercostal muscles (in-ter-KOS-tal) (musculi intercostales intimi)

Intercostal means "between or among the ribs." The muscles of this small group attach to the internal aspects of two adjoining ribs. They are believed to act with the internal intercostal muscles.

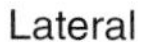

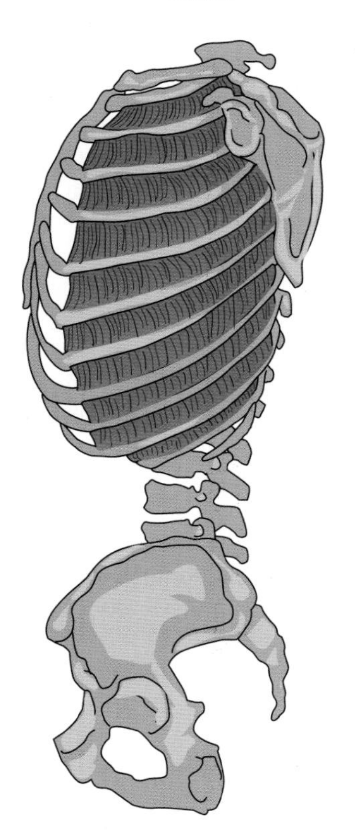

Transversus thoracis (trans-VER-sus thor-AH-siss)

Transversus means "lying crosswise"; and *thoracis* means "related to the chest."

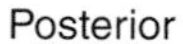

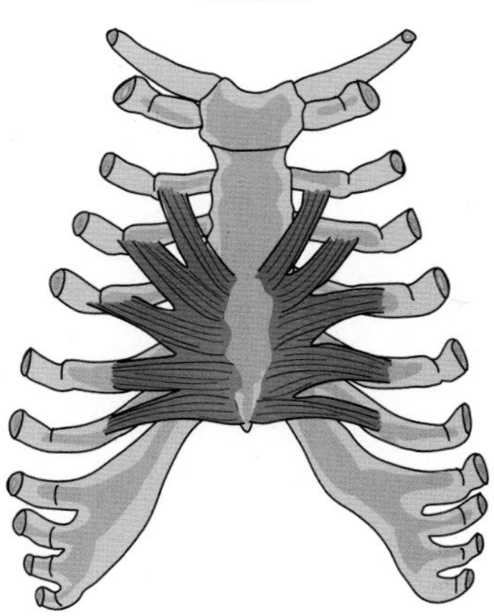

- *Concentric action:*
  - Depresses ribs 2 to 6 at the sternocostal and costovertebral joints
- *Eccentric action:*
  - Restrains/controls (especially rapid movement) elevation of ribs 2 to 6
- *Isometric action:*
  - Stabilizes the rib cage
- *Origin, fixed end, proximal attachment, arises from:*
  - Inner surface of the body of the sternum (caudal one-third), xiphoid process, and sternal ends of the costal cartilages of ribs 4 to 7
- *Insertion, mobile end, distal attachment, attaches to:*
  - Costal cartilages of the second through sixth ribs
- *Innervation:*
  - Adjacent intercostal nerves

  This muscle is on the inside of the rib cage.
- *Major synergists:*
  - Muscles of expiration
- *Major antagonists:*
  - Diaphragm and other muscles of inspiration
- *Tender/trigger points:*
  - Because of its location, this muscle is difficult to palpate for tender/trigger points.
- *Common symptom/Common symptom/Referred pain pattern:*
  - Spans the intercostal segment—especially noticeable with deep breathing or rotational movement

Diaphragm (DYE-ah-fram)

Diaphragm means "a partition or wall" (between the thoracic and abdominal cavities).

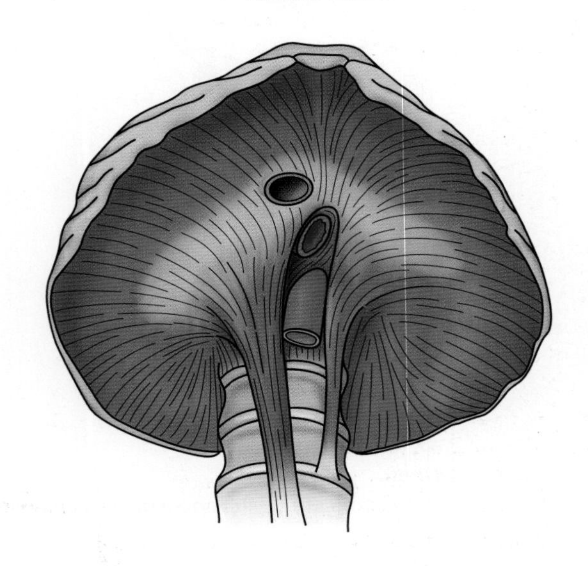

- *Concentric action:*
  - Inspiration (breathing in); diaphragmatic contractions increase the volume of the thoracic cavity
- *Eccentric action:*
  - Restrains/controls (especially rapid movement) expiration as the diaphragm relaxes (eccentrically contracts)
- *Isometric action:*
  - Stabilizes the thoracic and abdominopelvic cavities during breath holding and stabilizes the thoracic and lumbar spine
- *Origin, fixed end, proximal attachment, arises from:*
  - First three lumbar vertebrae, the lower six costal cartilages, and the inner surface of the xiphoid process
- *Insertion, mobile end, distal attachment, attaches to:*
  - Muscle fibers arch superiorly and inward to end in tendinous fibers, which form the central tendon; the central tendon is a large aponeurosis.

  The diaphragm is a broad, thin muscle that spans the thoracoabdominal cavity, separating the thorax from the abdomen. It can be visualized as plastic wrap around the edges of a bowl. The central tendon (the insertion) is not attached to any solid structure; rather, the middle of the plastic wrap becomes a thickened fascial structure. When the muscle component of the diaphragm contracts, it pulls and flattens the central tendon, which increases the volume of the thoracic cavity.
- *Innervation:*
  - Phrenic nerve (C3 to C5)
- *Major synergists:*
  - Accessory muscles of inspiration: external intercostal muscles, scalene muscles, and sternocleidomastoids
- *Major antagonists:*
  - Accessory muscles of expiration: internal intercostal muscles and anterior and anterolateral muscles of the abdominal wall. The elastic recoil of the soft tissues of the thoracic and abdominal cavities also provides an opposing force. The pelvic floor muscles may function as antagonists as well.

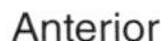

Quadratus lumborum (kwad-RATE-us lum-BOR-um)

Quadratus means "square shaped," and *lumborum* means "of the loins."

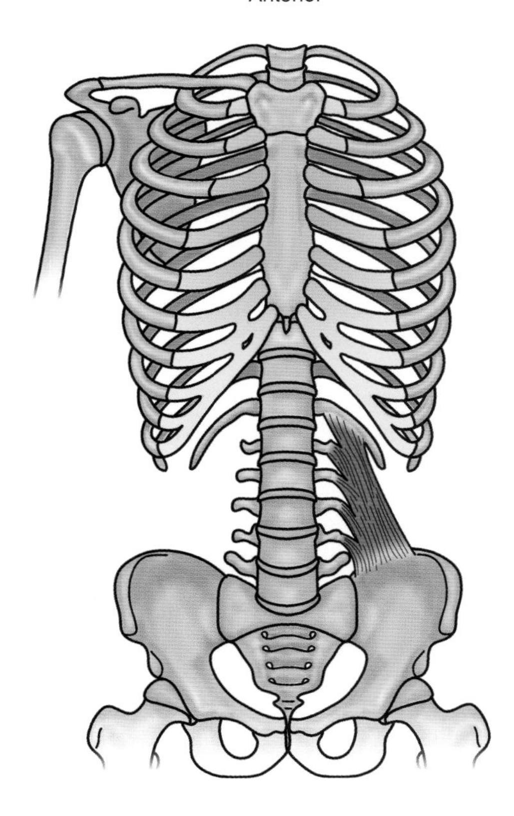

- *Concentric action:*
  - Elevation and anterior tilt of the pelvis at the lumbosacral joint, lateral flexion and extension of the trunk at the spinal joints, and depression of the twelfth rib at the costovertebral joints
- *Eccentric action:*
  - Allows depression and posterior tilt of the pelvis and allows contralateral lateral flexion and flexion of the trunk and elevation of the twelfth rib
- *Isometric action:*
  - Assists normal inspiration by stabilizing the twelfth rib against the pull of the diaphragm and also stabilizes the lumbar spine and pelvis
- *Origin, fixed end, proximal attachment, arises from:*
  - Iliolumbar ligament and posterior portion of the iliac crest
- *Insertion, mobile end, distal attachment, attaches to:*
  - Inferior border of the last rib and transverse processes of the first four lumbar vertebrae
- *Innervation:*
  - Ventral rami of the twelfth thoracic and upper three lumbar spinal nerves
- *Major synergists:*
  - Erector spinae group

  The quadratus lumborum also functions with the gluteus medius, tensor fascia lata, and adductors to stabilize the body in the frontal plane.
- *Major antagonists:*
  - Posterior fibers of gluteus medius and the anterior and contralateral anterolateral abdominal wall muscles
- *Tender/trigger points:*
  - Laterally near the rib or iliac attachment and medially near the iliac attachment at the transverse processes of the lumbar vertebra
- *Common symptom/Common symptom/Referred pain pattern:*
  - Gluteal and groin area, sacroiliac joint, and greater trochanter; these points are implicated in most low back pain. The dual function of lumbar stabilization (isometric function) and respiration (concentric function) can cause severe pain in the low back with a cough or sneeze if these trigger points are active. Low back pain often is related more to maintenance of posture than to trigger point activity; therefore finding corresponding pain patterns in the muscles that laterally flex the head and neck, such as the scalene muscles, is common.

Psoas major (SO-as)

Psoas means "of the loins"; *major* means "larger."

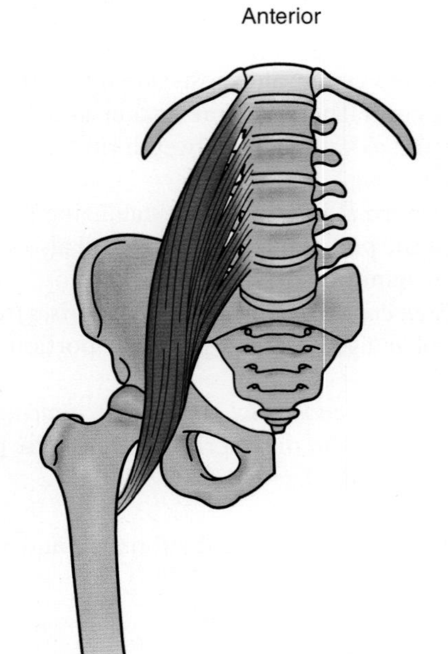

- *Concentric action:*
  - Flexion and lateral rotation of the thigh at the hip joint, flexion and lateral flexion of the trunk at the spinal joints, and anterior tilt of the pelvis at the hip joint
- *Eccentric action:*
  - Allows extension and medial rotation of the thigh and allows extension and contralateral lateral flexion of the trunk and posterior tilt of the pelvis
- *Isometric action:*
  - Stabilizes the lumbar spine and the lumbosacral and hip joints
- *Origin, fixed end, proximal attachment, arises from:*
  - Bodies and corresponding intervertebral disks of last thoracic and all lumbar vertebrae, anterior surface of transverse processes of all lumbar vertebrae, and tendinous arches extending across the sides of the bodies of the lumbar vertebrae
- *Insertion, mobile end, distal attachment, attaches to:*
  - Lesser trochanter of the femur
- *Innervation:*
  - Ventral rami of lumbar plexus nerves (L1–L3)
- *Major synergists:*
  - Iliacus, sartorius, rectus femoris, and anterior and anterolateral abdominal wall muscles
- *Major antagonists:*
  - Extensors of the thigh, extensors of the trunk, and posterior tilters of the pelvis
- *Tender/trigger points:*
  - Near both attachment points
- *Common symptom/Common symptom/Referred pain pattern:*
  - Entire lumbar area into the superior gluteal region and to the anterior thigh; may be associated with menstrual aching and can mimic appendicitis. Shortening of this muscle is a major cause of low back pain and often occurs during the isometric stabilization function. If tension or trigger point activity is located at the distal attachment, pain can mimic a groin pull. Because of postural reflexes, muscles that flex the head and neck are facilitated with psoas major activation. A common correlation exists between neck pain and stiffness to psoas major pain and low back stiffness. The massage therapist often must address both areas in sequence to be effective.

The psoas major and psoas minor are located on the anterior spine posterior to the abdominal muscles and viscera.

Psoas minor (SO-as)

Psoas means "of the loins"; *minor* means "smaller."

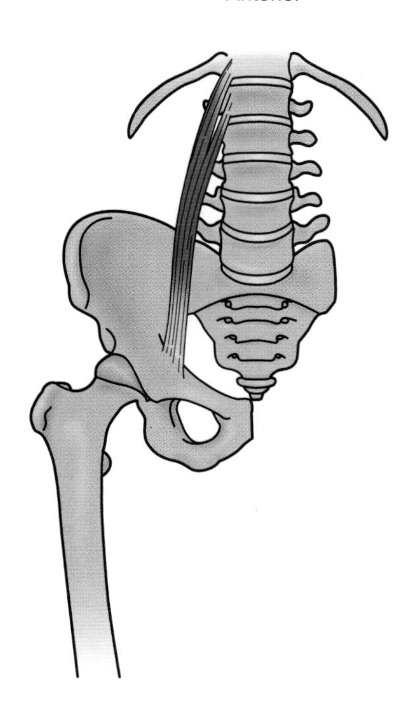

- *Concentric action:*
  - Flexion of the trunk at the spinal joints and posterior tilt of the pelvis at the lumbosacral joint
- *Eccentric action:*
  - Restrains/controls (especially rapid movement) extension of the trunk and anterior tilt of the pelvis

  This muscle is absent in approximately half of all human beings.
- *Origin, fixed end, proximal attachment, arises from:*
  - Sides of the bodies of the twelfth thoracic and first lumbar vertebrae and from the intervertebral disk between them
- *Insertion, mobile end, distal attachment, attaches to:*
  - Pectineal line of the pubis and the iliopectineal eminence of the ilium and pubis
- *Innervation:*
  - Branch from L1 spinal nerve

  The psoas major and psoas minor are located on the anterior spine posterior to the abdominal muscles and viscera.
- *Major synergists:*
  - Anterior and anterolateral abdominal wall muscles
- *Major antagonists:*
  - Erector spinae group
- *Tender/trigger points:*
  - Belly of the muscle
- *Common symptom/Common symptom/Referred pain pattern:*
  - Lumbar

Iliacus (ILL-ee-AK-us)

Iliacus means "of the hip."

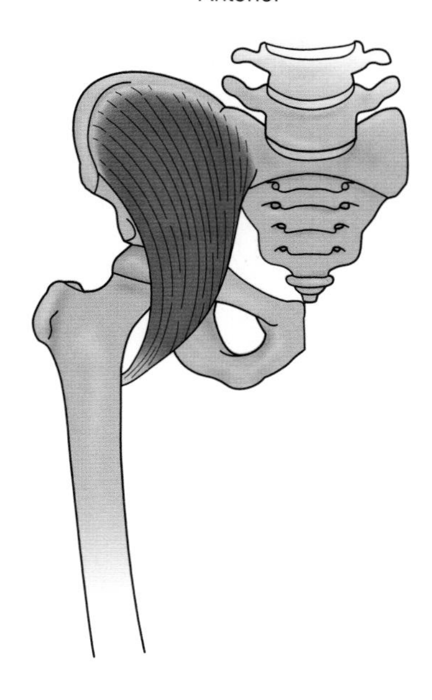

- *Concentric action:*
  - Flexion and lateral rotation of the thigh at the hip joint and anterior tilt of the pelvis at the lumbosacral joint
- *Eccentric action:*
  - Allows extension and medial rotation of the thigh and allows posterior tilt of the pelvis
- *Isometric action:*
  - Stabilizes the pelvis and the hip joint
- *Origin, fixed end, proximal attachment, arises from:*
  - Internal lip of the iliac crest; anterior sacroiliac, lumbosacral, and iliolumbar ligaments; superior two-thirds of the iliac fossa; and ala of the sacrum
- *Insertion, mobile end, distal attachment, attaches to:*
  - Lesser trochanter of the femur, into the posterior side of the psoas major tendon
- *Innervation:*
  - Femoral nerve (L2–L3)
- *Major synergist:*
  - Psoas major
- *Major antagonists:*
  - Gluteus maximus and hamstrings
- *Tender/trigger points:*
  - Inner border of the ilium posterior to the anterior superior iliac spine
- *Common symptom/Common symptom/Referred pain pattern:*
  - Hip and groin

ACTIVITY 9.18

Draw and color the *muscles of the thorax and posterior abdominal wall* in the spaces provided. For each muscle:

1. Label the origin and insertion attachment points: *O* for origin; *I* for insertion.
2. Place an X on the trigger points.
3. Palpate this muscle; identify the attachment points and the bellies of the muscles.
4. Move these muscles on yourself.

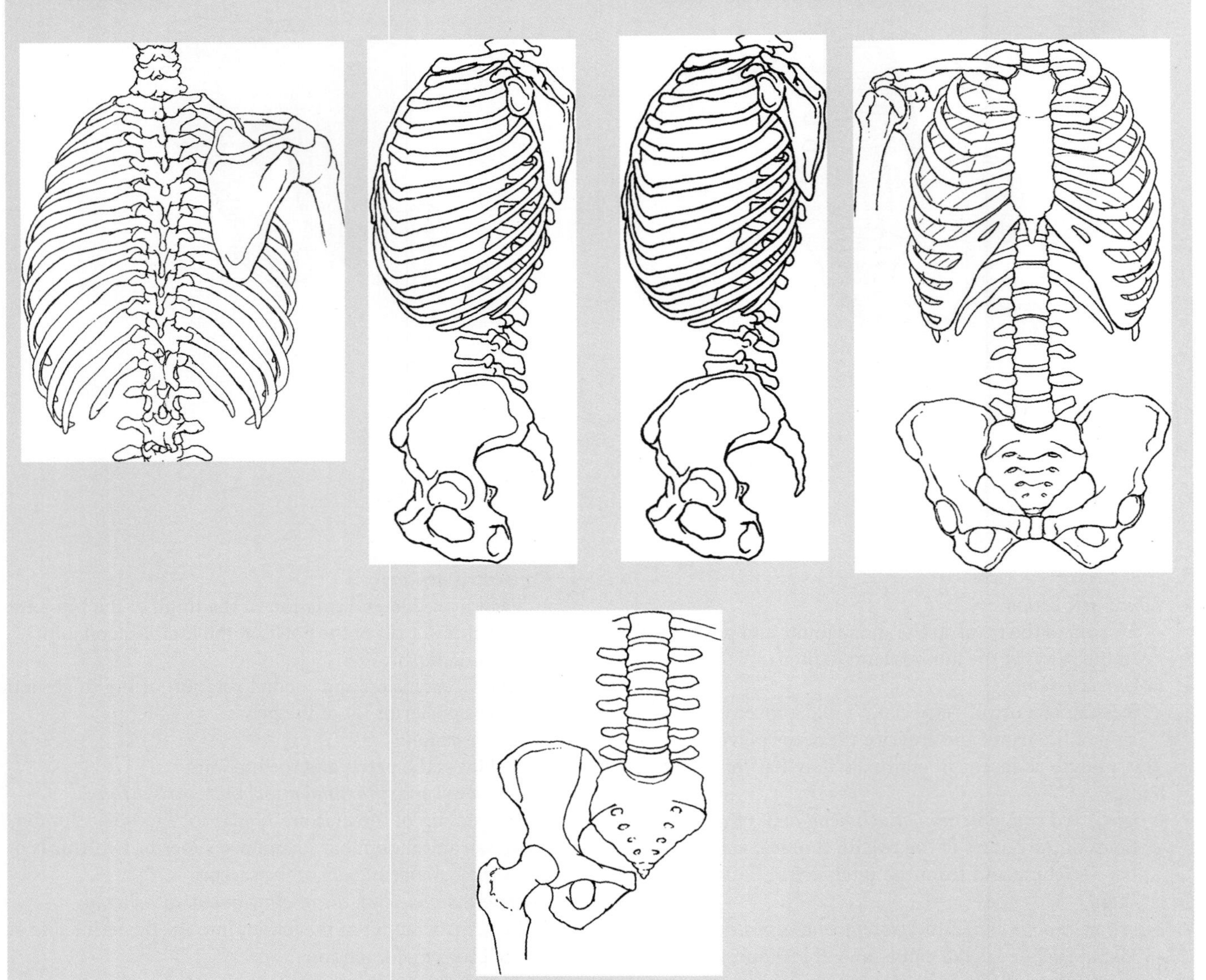

Muscles of the Anterior and Anterolateral Abdominal Wall

The abdominal muscles and extensive fascia form the anterior and anterolateral abdominal wall. The muscle fiber arrangement produces a crisscross fiber pattern similar to plywood, with vertical support provided by the rectus abdominis and the pyramidalis. These muscles attach directly or indirectly to a strong, fibrous cord in the midline of the abdomen called the *linea alba*, which is formed from the fusion of the two anterior abdominal aponeuroses. (Each abdominal aponeurosis is formed from the fusion of the aponeuroses of the external abdominal oblique and the transversus abdominis.) The linea alba extends from the xiphoid process to the symphysis pubis and contains the umbilicus.

As a group, these muscles act to compress the abdominal contents during expiration, urination, and defecation. They help maintain pressure on the curve of the low back, resisting excessive lumbar lordosis. Isometric stabilization is an important function of this group. Along with the deep muscles of the back, the abdominal muscles provide stability for the entire trunk of the body. The muscles also work with the adductors of the thighs at the hip joint to maintain upright posture. Massage application to this area is important because the muscles are involved in posture and breathing. The fascial aponeuroses may shorten, and the muscles are frequently weak and long. Methods to encourage normal muscle tone are effective. These exercises are usually called *core training*.

Rectus abdominis (REK-tus ab-DAHM-in-iss)

Rectus means "straight," and *abdominis* means "of the abdomen."

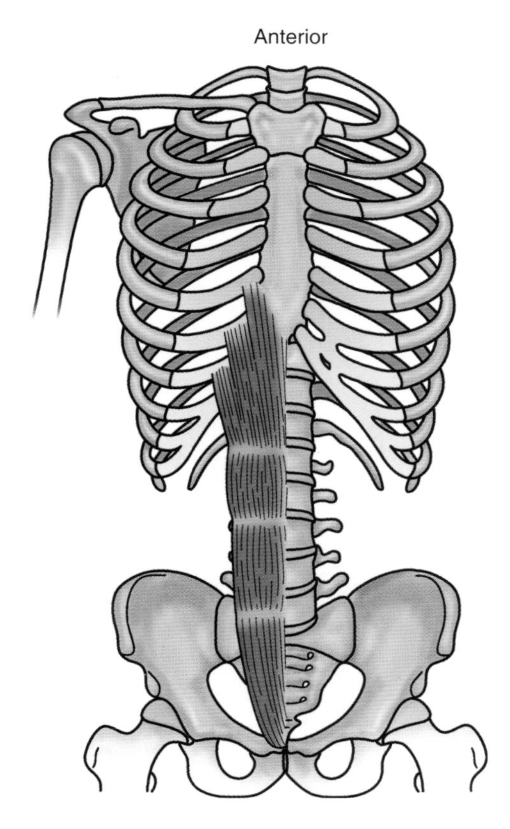

- *Concentric action:*
  - Flexion and lateral flexion of the trunk at the spinal joints, posterior tilt of the pelvis at the lumbosacral joint, and compression of the contents of the abdominal cavity (thereby supporting the abdominal viscera and assisting in forced expiration)
- *Eccentric action:*
  - Allows extension and contralateral lateral flexion of the trunk and allows anterior tilt of the pelvis
- *Origin, fixed end, proximal attachment, arises from:*
  - Pubis and the pubic symphysis
- *Insertion, mobile end, distal attachment, attaches to:*
  - Cartilages of the fifth, sixth, and seventh ribs and the xiphoid process of the sternum
- *Major synergists:*
  - External and internal abdominal obliques
- *Major antagonists:*
  - Extensors of the spine
- *Innervation:*
  - Anterior primary rami of the lower six intercostal nerves

External oblique (ex-TERN-al oh-BLEEK) (obliquus externus abdominis)

This muscle is located within the abdominal wall, superficial to the internal abdominal oblique; its fibers are slanted like pockets of a coat.

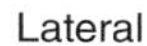

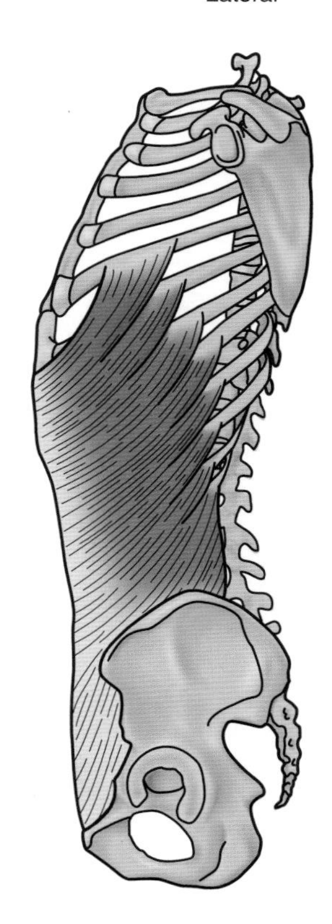

- *Concentric action:*
  - Flexion, lateral flexion, and contralateral rotation of the trunk at the spinal joints; posterior tilt of the pelvis at the lumbosacral joint; and compression of the contents of the abdominal cavity (thereby supporting the abdominal viscera and assisting in forced expiration)
- *Eccentric action:*
  - Allows extension, contralateral lateral flexion, and ipsilateral rotation of the trunk and allows anterior tilt of the pelvis
- *Origin, fixed end, proximal attachment, arises from:*
  - Outer lip of the iliac crest, pubic bone, and linea alba
- *Insertion, mobile end, distal attachment, attaches to:*
  - External surface of the lower eight ribs by interdigital slips
- *Innervation:*
  - Ventral rami of the lower six thoracic spinal nerves
- *Major synergists:*
  - Opposite-sided internal abdominal oblique and the rectus abdominis
- *Major antagonists:*
  - Extensors of the spine and opposite-sided external abdominal oblique

Internal oblique (in-TERN-al oh-BLEEK) (obliquus internus abdominis)

The internal oblique muscle is located within the anterolateral abdominal wall, deep to the external abdominal oblique and superficial to the transversus abdominis. The muscle is positioned at a slant.

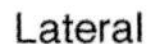

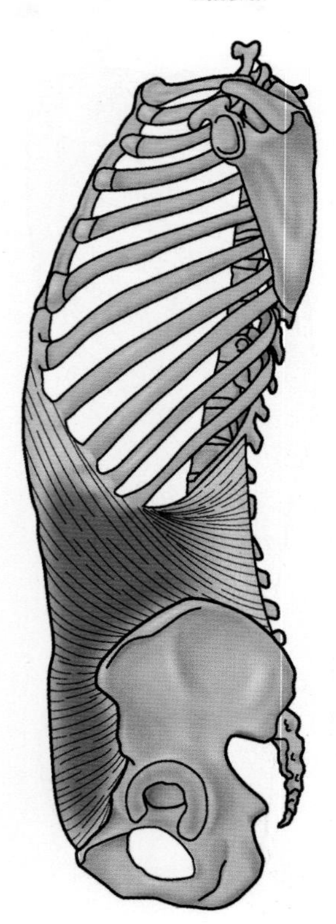

- *Concentric action:*
  - Flexion, lateral flexion, and ipsilateral rotation of the trunk at the spinal joints; posterior tilt of the pelvis at the lumbosacral joint; and compression of the contents of the abdominal cavity (thereby supporting the abdominal viscera and assisting in forced expiration)
- *Eccentric action:*
  - Allows extension, contralateral lateral flexion, and contralateral rotation of the trunk and allows anterior tilt of the pelvis
- *Origin, fixed end, proximal attachment, arises from:*
  - Inguinal ligament, iliac fascia, anterior two-thirds of the middle lip of the iliac crest, and lumbar fascia
- *Insertion, mobile end, distal attachment, attaches to:*
  - Upper fibers into cartilages of last three ribs; the remainder into the aponeurosis extending from the tenth costal cartilage to the pubic bone into the linea alba
- *Innervation:*
  - Ventral rami of the lower six thoracic and first lumbar spinal nerves
- *Major synergists:*
  - Opposite-sided external abdominal oblique and the rectus abdominis
- *Major antagonists:*
  - Extensors of the spine and opposite-sided internal abdominal oblique

Transversus abdominis (trans-VER-sus ab-DAHM-in-iss)

Transversus means "lying crosswise," and *abdominis* means "of the abdomen." The transversus abdominis is the innermost layer of the abdominal wall just superficial to the peritoneum.

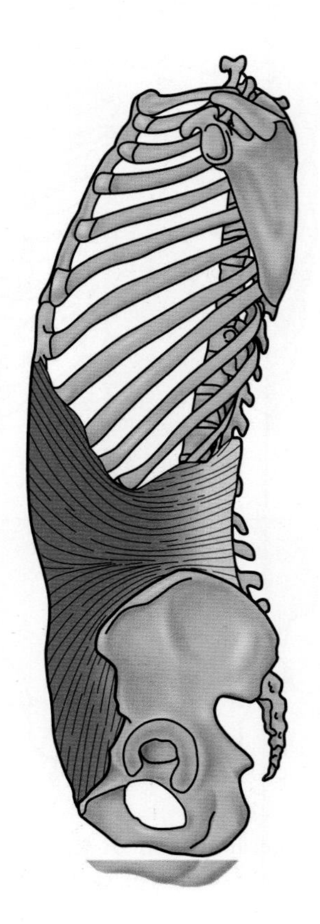

- *Concentric/isometric action:*
  - Compresses the contents of the abdomen, increasing intraabdominal pressure and thereby supporting the abdominal viscera and assisting in forced expiration
- *Origin, fixed end, proximal attachment, arises from:*
  - Inner surfaces of the cartilages of the last six ribs, anterior three fourths of the iliac crest, lateral one-third of the inguinal ligament, and thoracolumbar fascia
- *Insertion, mobile end, distal attachment, attaches to:*
  - Linea alba, abdominal aponeurosis, and pubis
- *Innervation:*
  - Ventral rami of the lower six thoracic and first lumbar spinal nerves
- *Major synergists:*
  - Rectus abdominis and external and internal abdominal obliques
- *Major antagonists:*
  - Not clearly defined

Pyramidalis (peer-AM-id-al-iss)

Pyramidalis means "pyramid shaped."

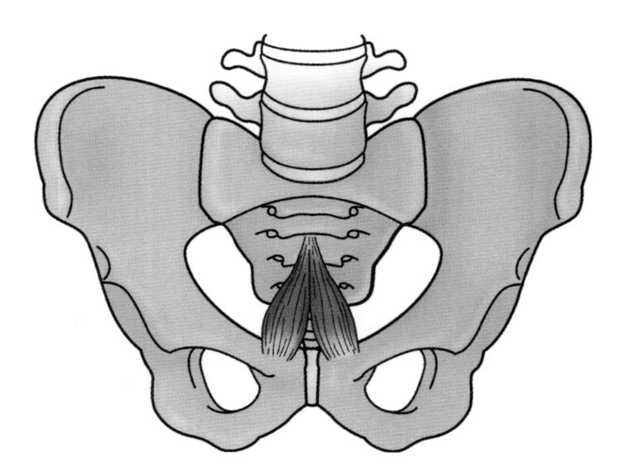

- *Action:*
  - Tenses the linea alba to compress the contents of the abdominal cavity (thereby supporting the abdominal viscera and assisting in forced expiration)
  - Although the pyramidalis is a striated muscle, it usually is not under voluntary control.
- *Origin, fixed end, proximal attachment, arises from:*
  - Ventral surface of the pubis and the pubic ligament
- *Insertion, mobile end, distal attachment, attaches to:*
  - Linea alba (between the pubis and the umbilicus)
- *Innervation:*
  - Subcostal nerve (ventral ramus of T12)

Cremaster (KREE-mast-er)

Cremaster means a "suspender."

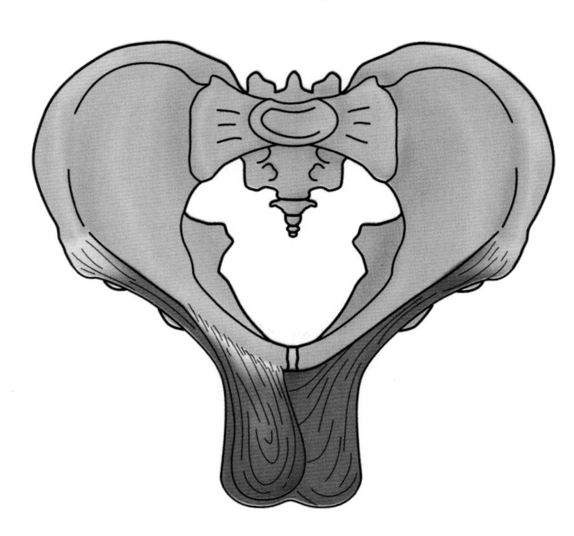

- *Action:*
  - Pulls the testes superiorly (to help regulate their temperature)
- *Origin, fixed end, proximal attachment, arises from:*
  - Lower edge of the internal oblique muscle and the middle aspect of the inguinal ligament
- *Insertion, mobile end, distal attachment, attaches to:*
  - Pubic tubercle and the crest of the pubis
- *Innervation:*
  - Genital branch of the genitofemoral nerve (L1–L2)
- *Synergists:*
  - Quadratus lumborum and diaphragm; rotation—lower serratus anterior and posterior, latissimus dorsi, iliocostalis
- *Antagonists:*
  - Flexion—paraspinal extensor group; rotation—contralateral muscles
- *Tender/trigger points:*
  - Located throughout the area but concentrated more in the external circle of the abdominal wall, rather than toward the middle near the umbilicus; the exceptions are points often found in the rectus abdominis just below the umbilicus on either side of the linea alba.
- *Common symptom/Common symptom/Referred pain pattern:*
  - Pain is likely to appear in the same quadrant and in the back; these tender/trigger points are capable of causing somatovisceral responses (e.g., vomiting, nausea, intestinal problems, diarrhea, bladder symptoms, pain).

ACTIVITY 9.19

Draw and color the *muscles of the anterior and anterolateral abdominal wall* in the spaces provided. For each muscle:

1. Label the origin and insertion attachment points: *O* for origin; *I* for insertion.
2. Place an X on the trigger points.
3. Palpate this muscle; identify the attachment points and the bellies of the muscles.
4. Move these muscles on yourself.

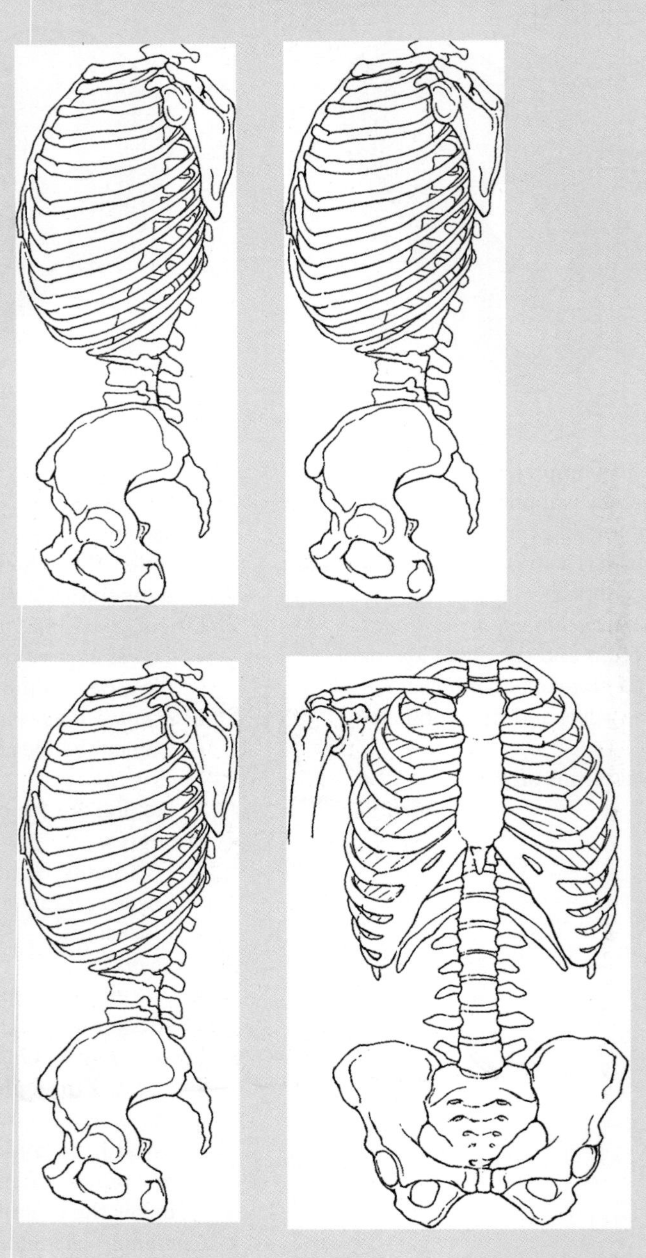

Pelvic and Perineal Muscles

The levator ani and the coccygeus muscles form the pelvic floor (also called the *pelvic diaphragm*) (see Fig. 9.19). These muscles close the inferior outlet of the pelvis; support and elevate the pelvic floor; and counterbalance increased intraabdominal pressure, which would expel the contents of the bladder, rectum, and uterus. The pelvic diaphragm has openings for the rectum, urethra, and vagina. The massage therapist usually does not massage this area with direct methods; however, attention to antagonistic and synergistic muscles that are accessed more easily is indicated. Isometric stabilization is a major function of these muscles.

Levator ani (le-VAY-tor AIN-eye)

Levator means "one that raises"; *ani* means "belonging to the anus or rectum."

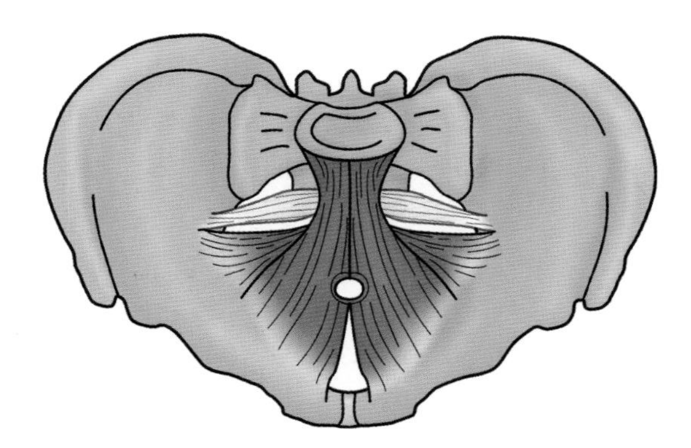

- *Action:*
  - Forms the floor of the pelvic cavity, constricts the lower end of the rectum and vagina, and supports and slightly raises the pelvic floor
- *Origin, fixed end, proximal attachment, arises from:*
  - Pelvic surfaces of the pubis, inner surface of the ischial spine, and the obturator fascia
- *Insertion, mobile end, distal attachment, attaches to:*
  - Last two segments of the coccyx, anococcygeal raphe uniting with fibers from the opposite side, and the sides of the rectum anterior into the perineal body
- *Innervation:*
  - Muscular branches of the perineal division of the pudendal nerve

Coccygeus (kok-SIH-jee-us)

Coccygeus means "related to the coccyx or tail bone."

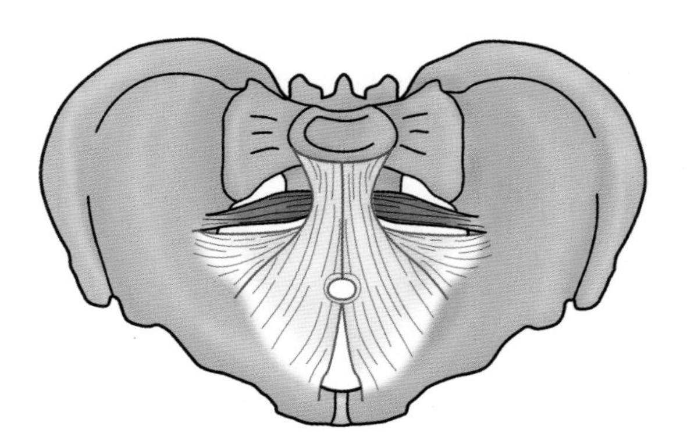

- *Action:*
  - Pulls forward and supports the coccyx; exerts rotary tension on the sacroiliac joint; and, with the levator ani and piriformis muscles, assists in closing the posterior part of the pelvic outlet and forms the supporting muscular diaphragm for the pelvic viscera
- *Origin, fixed end, proximal attachment, arises from:*
  - Pelvic surface of the spine of the ischium and the sacrospinous ligament
- *Insertion, mobile end, distal attachment, attaches to:*
  - Margin of the coccyx and the side of the fifth segment of the sacrum
- *Innervation:*
  - Branch of the fourth and fifth sacral nerves

External anal sphincter (sphincter ani externus) (SFINK-tur AIN-eye)

External means "on the outside," *sphincter* means "band," and *ani* means "related to the anus or rectum."

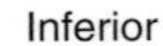

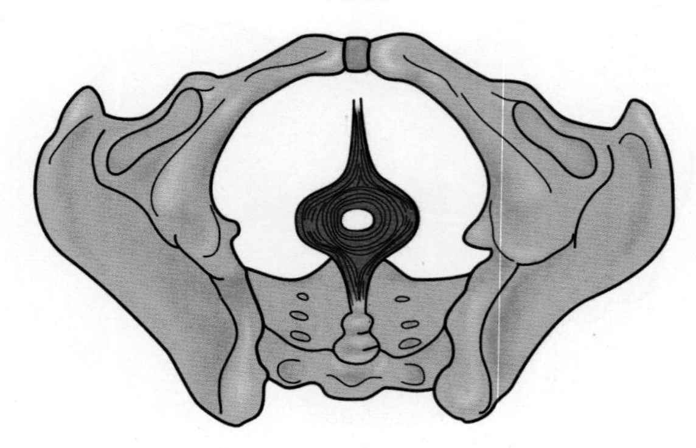

- *Action:*
  - Closes the anal orifice
- *Origin, fixed end, proximal attachment, arises from:*
  - Superficial fibers from the anococcygeal raphe; deeper fibers surround the anal canal
- *Insertion, mobile end, distal attachment, attaches to:*
  - Superficial fibers surround the anus, meeting posteriorly at the coccyx and anteriorly at the central point of the perineum
- *Innervation:*
  - Perineal branch of the fourth sacral nerve and the inferior rectal branch of the pudendal nerve

Deep transverse perineals (pair-i-NEE-als) (transversus perinei)

Transverse means "crossing" or "around"; *perineal* means "to empty or defecate."

Inferior

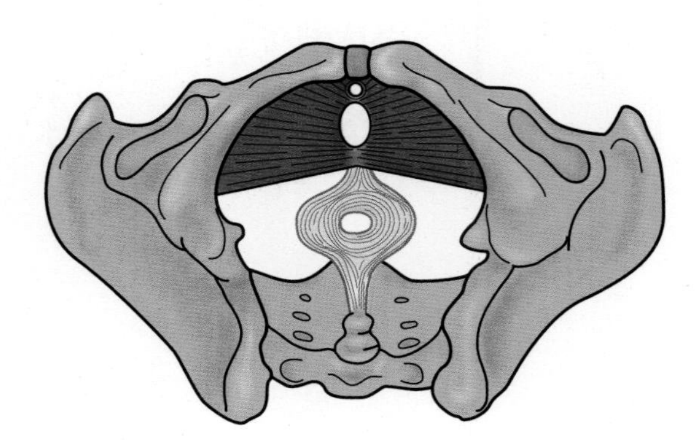

- *Action:*
  - Simultaneous contraction of both muscles helps to fix the perineal body.
- *Origin, fixed end, proximal attachment, arises from:*
  - Medial and anterior part of the ischial tuberosity
- *Insertion, mobile end, distal attachment, attaches to:*
  - Central tendinous point of the perineum
- *Innervation:*
  - Perineal branches of the pudendal nerve

Ischiocavernosus (ISS-she-oh-KAV-ern-oh-sus)

Ischiocavernosus means "hip" and "cavernlike."

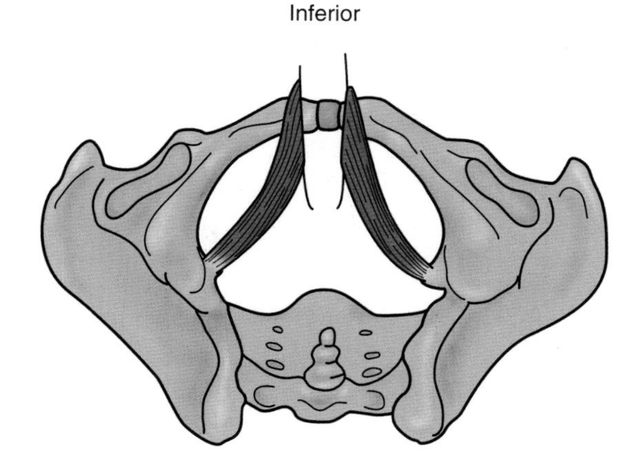

- *Action:*
  - Compresses the crus penis, which obstructs venous return and therefore is believed to play a part in maintaining erection of the penis or clitoris
- *Origin, fixed end, proximal attachment, arises from:*
  - Inner surface of the ischial tuberosity behind the crus penis or clitoris and the ramus of the ischium on both sides of the crus
- *Insertion, mobile end, distal attachment, attaches to:*
  - Aponeuroses on the sides and undersurface of the crus penis or clitoris
- *Innervation:*
- Perineal branch of the pudendal nerve (S2–S4)

Bulbospongiosus (BUL-bo-SPON-jee-oh-sus)

Bulbospongiosus means "bulb" and "spongy."

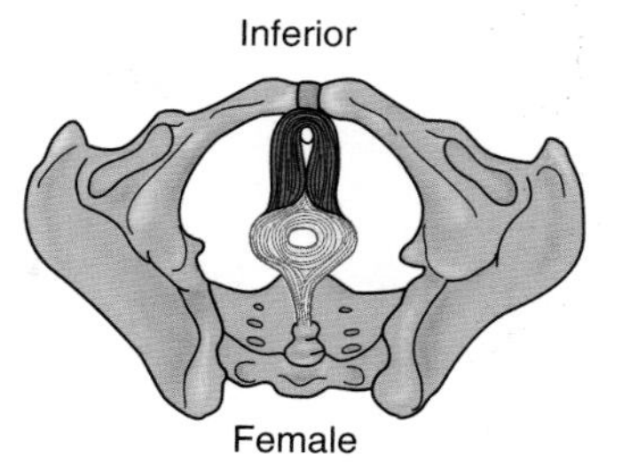

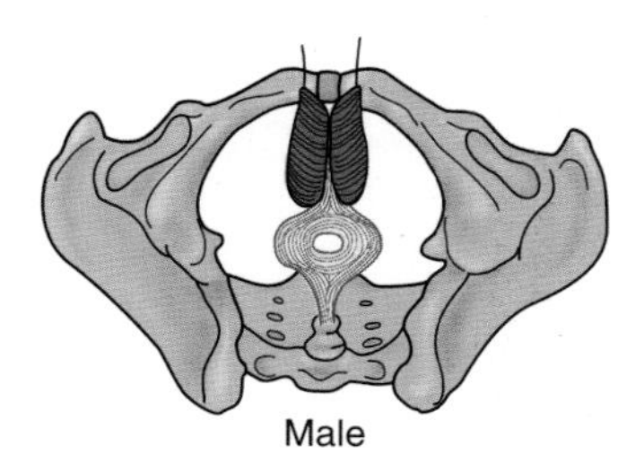

- *Action:*
  - Aids in emptying the urethra; the muscle is relaxed during the greater part of micturition, coming into action only at the end of the process, and can be used to assist urination; it constricts the orifice of the vagina and contributes to erection of the penis and clitoris.
- *Origin, fixed end, proximal attachment, arises from:*
  - Central tendinous point of the perineum, with fibers surrounding the vaginal orifice and vestibular bulbs (female)
- *Insertion, mobile end, distal attachment, attaches to:*
  - Lower surface of the perineal membrane, dorsal surface of the corpus spongiosum, deep fascia on the dorsum of the penis, and corpora cavernosa clitoris (female)
- *Innervation:*
  - Perineal branch of the pudendal nerve (S2–S4)

The following elements are common to the pelvic and perineal muscles:

Synergists:

All muscles are synergistic; the gluteus maximus supports the closure of the anus.

Antagonists:

No direct antagonist pattern to the pelvic floor has been identified in the literature; however, because the gluteus maximus is powerfully synergistic with these muscles, one could assume that antagonist patterns to the gluteus maximus, such as the psoas, would have an antagonistic influence on the pelvic floor muscles. The diaphragm muscle also may act as an antagonist to this muscle group.

Tender/trigger points:

Tender/trigger points do develop in these muscles. These tender/trigger points usually can be palpated internally, rectally, or vaginally.

Referred pain patterns:

To the pelvic floor itself and to the coccyx region

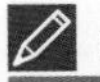

ACTIVITY 9.20

Draw and color the *pelvic and perineal muscles* in the spaces provided. For each muscle:

1. Label the origin and insertion attachment points: *O* for origin; *I* for insertion.
2. Move these muscles on yourself.

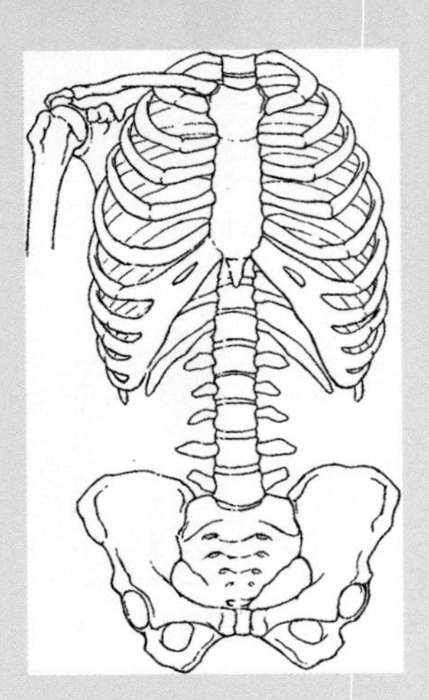

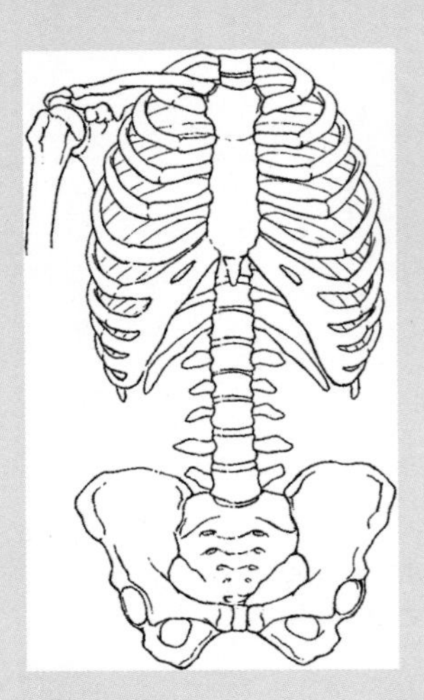

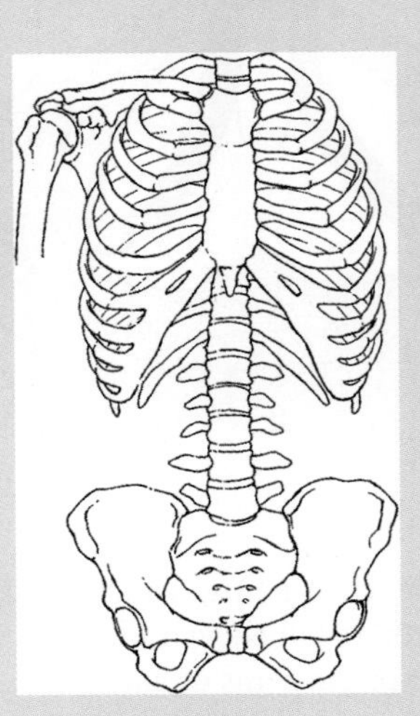

Muscles of Scapular Stabilization

The muscles of scapular stabilization hold the scapula to the rib cage (wall of the thorax) when acting isometrically and move the scapula during concentric and eccentric function (Fig. 9.20). The arrangement of the muscle attachments to the scapula requires cooperative concentric, eccentric, and isometric interaction to produce movement. Several muscles must act together to elevate or depress the scapula or to create other scapular movements at the scapulocostal joint.

The prime movers of scapular elevation at the scapulocostal joint (shrugging the shoulder) are the upper trapezius and the levator scapulae. The opposite rotational effects of the trapezius and levator scapulae on the scapula counterbalance each other.

Scapular depression at the scapulocostal joint results largely from gravitational pull, but when the scapula is depressed against resistance, the lower trapezius and serratus anterior are active. Serratus anterior activity creates the forward (pushing) movements of protraction (abduction) of the scapula at the scapulocostal joint on the chest wall. The trapezius and the rhomboid muscles provide retraction (adduction) of the scapula at the scapulocostal joint.

Although the serratus anterior and trapezius muscles are antagonists in the anterior/posterior movements of the scapula, they act together to create upward rotation of the scapula at the scapulocostal joint.

Clavicular movements accompany scapular movements. The clavicles rotate around their own axes as they move with scapular movements, giving stability and precision to these movements. Therapeutic massage methods easily address these more superficial muscles.

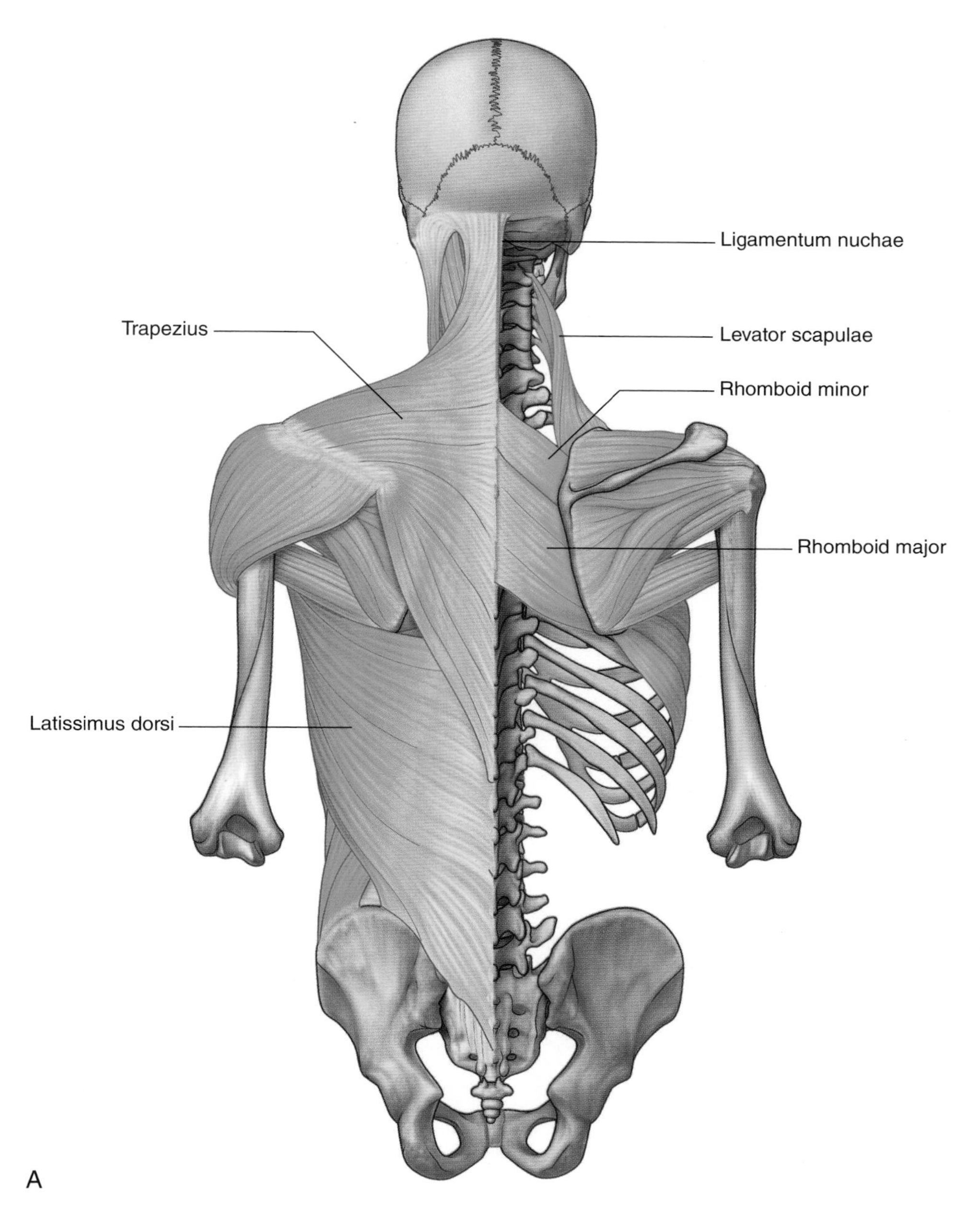

FIG. 9.20 Muscles of scapular stabilization: (A) surface and mid layer of muscles, (B) deep layer (From Drake RL, Vogl W, Mitchell WM. *Gray's Anatomy for Students*. 2nd ed. Churchill Livingstone; 2010.)

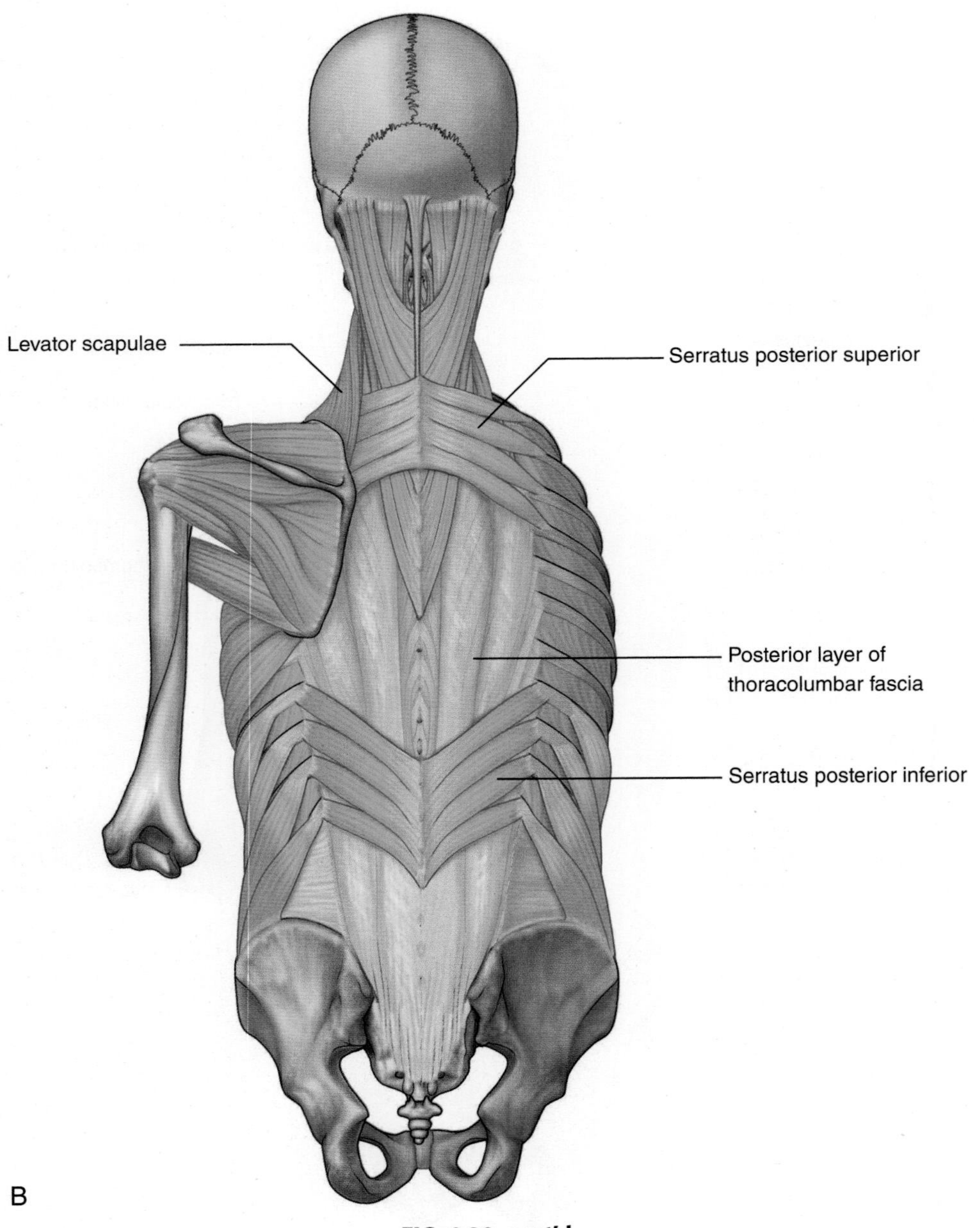

FIG. 9.20, cont'd

Trapezius (tra-PEE-zee-us)

Trapezius means "a figure with four unequal sides" (a trapezoid).

The trapezius usually is considered to consist of three functional parts: the upper trapezius, middle trapezius, and lower trapezius. Concentric, eccentric, and isometric contraction can occur simultaneously in different aspects of the muscle.

Posterior

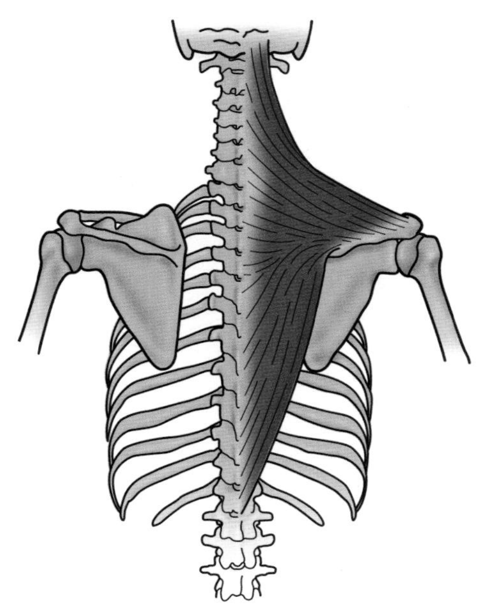

Concentric action:

Extension, lateral flexion, and contralateral rotation of the neck and head at the spinal joints (upper trapezius); elevation of the scapula at the scapulocostal joint (upper trapezius); retraction of the scapula at the scapulocostal joint (entire trapezius); depression of the scapula at the scapulocostal joint (lower trapezius); upward rotation of the scapula at the scapulocostal joint (upper and lower trapezius); and extension of the trunk at the spinal joints (middle and lower trapezius)

Many books divide the actions of the trapezius (and other muscles of the neck and trunk) into the actions created when the muscle contracts on one side (unilaterally) and when the right and left muscles contract (bilaterally). In this division, they often describe these actions in a manner that may be misleading. For example, they might state that the unilateral contraction of the upper trapezius causes lateral flexion and contralateral rotation of the neck at the spinal joints and that bilateral contraction of the upper trapezius muscles causes extension of the neck at the spinal joints. Although the bilateral trapezius contraction causes extension of the neck (and is pure extension because the opposite lateral flexions and opposite rotations cancel each other out), unilateral trapezius contraction also causes extension of the neck. This may not be immediately understood when actions are worded this way. No muscle can cause extension bilaterally if it cannot cause extension unilaterally.

What is valuable to take from this type of description is that when any muscle of the neck and trunk contracts bilaterally, its lateral flexion and rotation components always cancel each other out, and the resulting joint action is a pure sagittal plane movement—that is, flexion or extension. The other important thing to realize with all muscles of the neck and trunk is that the muscle on one side of the body always can be an antagonist to the same muscle on the other side of the body. For example, the right upper trapezius causes right lateral flexion of the neck, and the left upper trapezius causes left lateral flexion of the neck; hence they are antagonistic. Also, the right upper trapezius causes left rotation of the neck, and the left upper trapezius causes right rotation of the neck; hence they are antagonistic. Of course, regarding extension of the neck, because both sides can cause extension of the neck, they are synergistic. These principles are true and should be kept in mind for all muscles of the neck and trunk. As a rule, this text does not usually list the same muscle on the opposite side of the body in the synergist and antagonist sections.

Eccentric action:

Restrains/controls (especially rapid movement) flexion, contralateral lateral flexion, and ipsilateral rotation of the neck and head; depression, protraction (abduction), elevation, and downward rotation of the scapula; and flexion of the trunk

Isometric action:

Stabilizes the scapula and cervical spine

Origin, fixed end, proximal attachment, arises from:

Upper trapezius—external occipital protuberance; superior nuchal line, nuchal ligament; and spinous process of the seventh cervical vertebra

Middle trapezius—spinous processes of the first through fifth thoracic vertebrae

Lower trapezius—spinous processes of the sixth through twelfth thoracic vertebrae

Insertion, mobile end, distal attachment, attaches to:

Upper trapezius—lateral one-third of the clavicle and acromion process of the scapula

Middle trapezius—acromion process and spine of the scapula

Lower trapezius—root of the spine of the scapula

Innervation:

Spinal accessory nerve (cervical nerve XI) and ventral rami of third and fourth cervical spinal nerves

Major synergists:

Upper trapezius—semispinalis capitis, levator scapulae, serratus anterior, and sternocleidomastoid

Middle trapezius—rhomboid muscles and spinal extensors

Lower trapezius—serratus anterior, pectoralis minor, and spinal extensors

Major antagonists:

Upper trapezius—lower trapezius, rhomboid muscles, and flexors of the neck

Middle trapezius—pectoralis minor and serratus anterior

Lower trapezius—upper trapezius and levator scapulae

Tender/trigger points:

Upper trapezius near the acromion and clavicular attachments, middle trapezius near the spine of the scapula, and lower trapezius in the belly of the muscle

Referred pain patterns:

Neck posterior to the ear and to the temple, subscapular area, and acromial pain

Rhomboid major (ROM-boyd) (rhomboideus major)

Rhomboideus means "shaped like a rhombus" (a diamond shape); *major* means "larger."

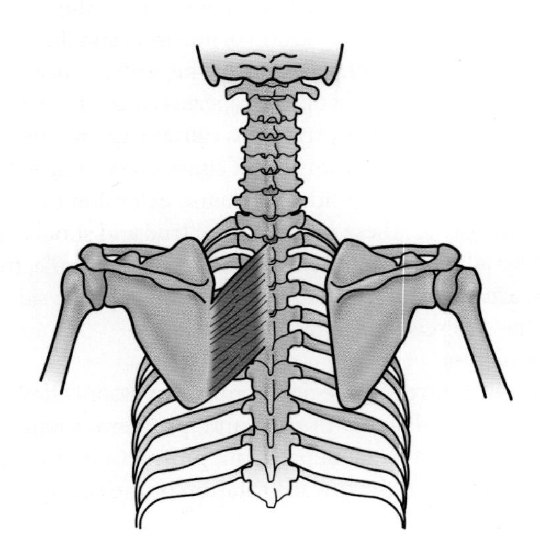

Concentric action:
Retraction (adduction), elevation, and downward rotation of the scapula at the scapulocostal joint
Eccentric action:
Restrains/controls (especially rapid movement) protraction (abduction), depression, and upward rotation of the scapula
Isometric action:
Stabilizes the scapula
Origin, fixed end, proximal attachment, arises from:
Spinous processes of the second through fifth thoracic vertebrae
Insertion, mobile end, distal attachment, attaches to:
Medial border of the scapula, between the spine and the inferior angle
Innervation:
Dorsal scapular nerve (C4–C5)
Major synergists:
Rhomboideus minor, trapezius, levator scapulae, and pectoralis minor
Major antagonists:
Serratus anterior, pectoralis minor, and trapezius
Tender/trigger points:
At the attachment point near the scapular border
Common symptom/Common symptom/Referred pain pattern:
Scapular region

Rhomboid minor (ROM-boyd) (rhomboideus minor)

Rhomboideus means "shaped like a rhombus" (a diamond shape); *minor* means "smaller."

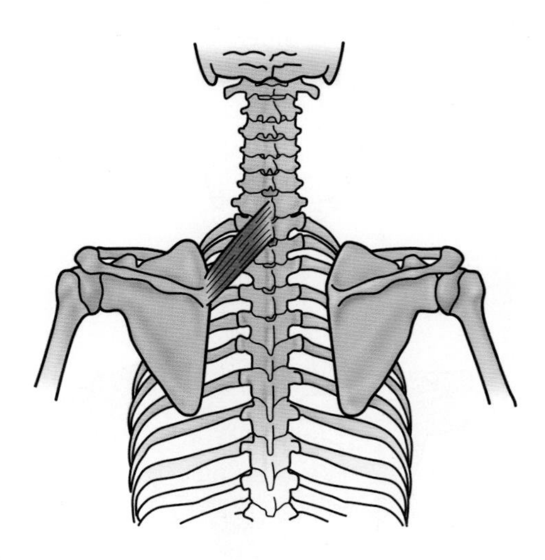

Concentric action:
Retraction (adduction), elevation, and downward rotation of the scapula at the scapulocostal joint
Eccentric action:
Restrains/controls (especially rapid movement) protraction, depression, and upward rotation of the scapula
Isometric action:
Stabilizes the scapula
Origin, fixed end, proximal attachment, arises from:
Ligamentum nuchae and spinous processes of the seventh cervical and first thoracic vertebrae
Insertion, mobile end, distal attachment, attaches to:
Medial border of the scapula at the root of the spine of the scapula
Innervation:
Dorsal scapular nerve (C4–C5)
Major synergists:
Rhomboideus major, trapezius, levator scapulae, and pectoralis minor
Major antagonists:
Serratus anterior, pectoralis minor, and trapezius
Tender/trigger points:
At the attachment point near the scapular border
Common symptom/Common symptom/Referred pain pattern:
Scapular region

Levator scapulae (le-VAY-tor SKAP-you-lee)

Levator scapulae means "to elevate the scapula."

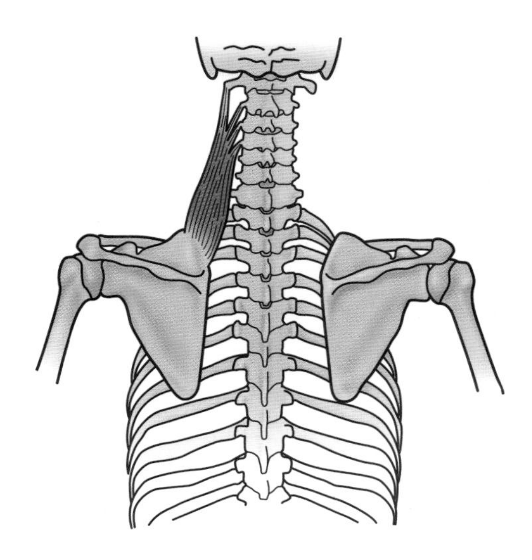

Concentric action:
Elevation and retraction (adduction) of the scapula at the scapulocostal joint and extension, lateral flexion, and ipsilateral rotation of the neck at the spinal joints
Eccentric action:
Allows depression and protraction (abduction) of the scapula and restrains/controls (especially rapid movement) flexion, contralateral lateral flexion, and contralateral rotation of the neck
Isometric action:
Stabilizes cervical/scapular function
Origin, fixed end, proximal attachment, arises from:
Transverse processes of the atlas and axis and the third and fourth cervical vertebrae
Insertion, mobile end, distal attachment, attaches to:
Medial border of the scapula between the superior angle and the root of the spine

The levator scapulae is a large muscle and has a rotation, or twist, which occurs in its design such that the attachments at the atlas and axis are from muscle fibers that attach to the inferior portion of the medial border of the scapula and the attachments at C4 are from fibers at the superior portion of the medial border.

Innervation:
Dorsal scapular nerve (C3–C5)
Major synergists:
Splenius cervicis and the upper trapezius
Major antagonists:
Serratus anterior and the sternocleidomastoid
Tender/trigger points:
Belly of the muscle just as it begins the twist in its fibers and at the attachment near the scapula
Referred pain patterns:
Angle of the neck at the trigger point and along the vertebral border of the scapula and stiff neck in rotation

Pectoralis minor (PEK-tor-al-iss)

Pectoralis means "related to the chest"; *minor* means "smaller."

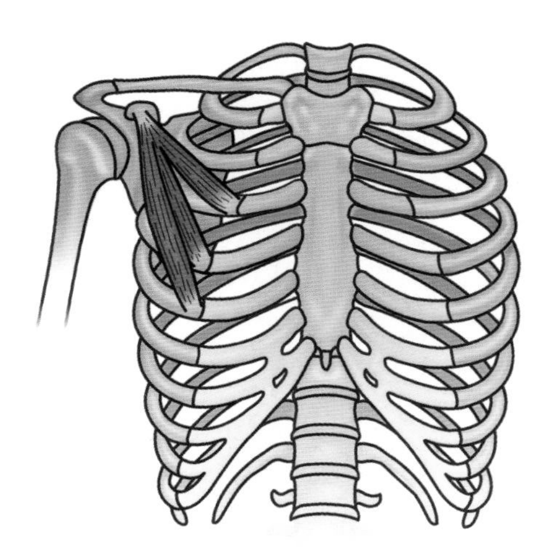

Concentric action:
Protraction (abduction), depression, and downward rotation of the scapula at the scapulocostal joint and elevation of ribs 3 to 5 at the sternocostal and costovertebral joints

This action assists in forced inspiration; therefore, the pectoralis minor is an accessory respiratory muscle.

Eccentric action:
Allows retraction (adduction), elevation, and upward rotation of the scapula and allows depression of ribs 3 to 5
Isometric action:
Stabilizes the scapula
Origin, fixed end, proximal attachment, arises from:
Third, fourth, and fifth ribs near the cartilage and the aponeurosis covering the intercostal muscles
Insertion, mobile end, distal attachment, attaches to:
Coracoid process of the scapula
Innervation:
Medial and lateral pectoral nerves (C5–T1)
Major synergists:
Serratus anterior, rhomboid muscles, and lower trapezius
Major antagonists:
Rhomboid muscles and upper trapezius
Tender/trigger points:
Near the attachment at the coracoid process and at the belly of the muscle
Common symptom/Common symptom/Referred pain pattern:
May mimic angina; front of the chest from the shoulder and down the ulnar side of the arm into the fingers

Serratus anterior (suhr-RATE-us)

Serratus means "sawlike"; *anterior* means "toward the front."

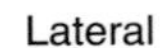

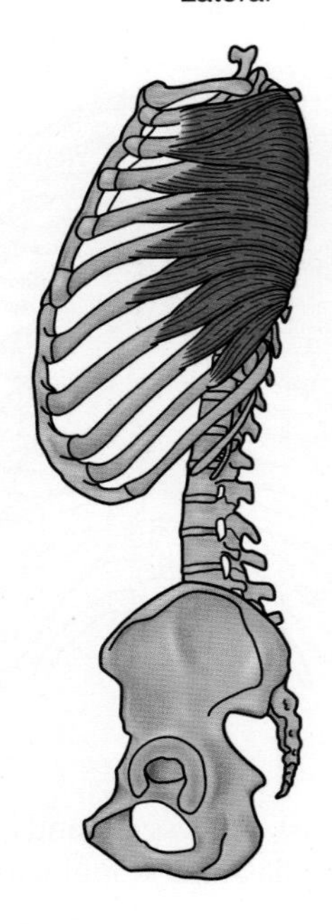

Concentric action:
Protraction (abduction) and upward rotation of the scapula at the scapulocostal joint and elevation of ribs 7 to 9 (assisting forced inspiration; therefore the serratus anterior is an accessory muscle of respiration)

Eccentric action:
Restrains/controls (especially rapid movement) retraction and downward rotation of the scapula

Isometric action:
Holds the medial border of the scapula firmly against the thorax, thereby preventing winging of the scapula

Origin, fixed end, proximal attachment, arises from:
External surfaces and superior borders of the upper eight or nine ribs

Insertion, mobile end, distal attachment, attaches to:
Costal surface of the medial border of the scapula
This muscle lies along the rib cage and is deep to the scapula.

Innervation:
Long thoracic nerve (C5–C7)

Major synergists:
Pectoralis minor and upper trapezius

Major antagonists:
Rhomboid muscles and middle trapezius

Tender/trigger points:
Along the midaxillary line near the ribs

Referred pain patterns:
Side and back of the chest and down the ulnar aspect of the arm into the hand
Injury may result in shortness of breath and pain during inhalation.

ACTIVITY 9.21

Draw and color the *muscles of scapular stabilization* in the spaces provided. For each muscle:

1. Label the origin and insertion attachment points: *O* for origin; *I* for insertion.
2. Place an X on the trigger points.
3. Palpate this muscle; identify the attachment points and the bellies of the muscles.
4. Move these muscles on yourself.

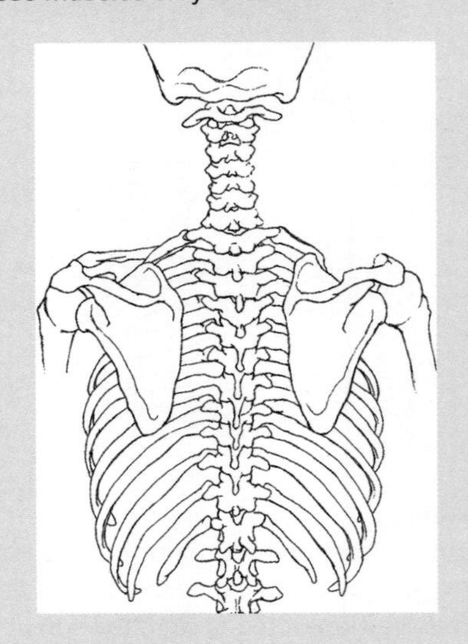

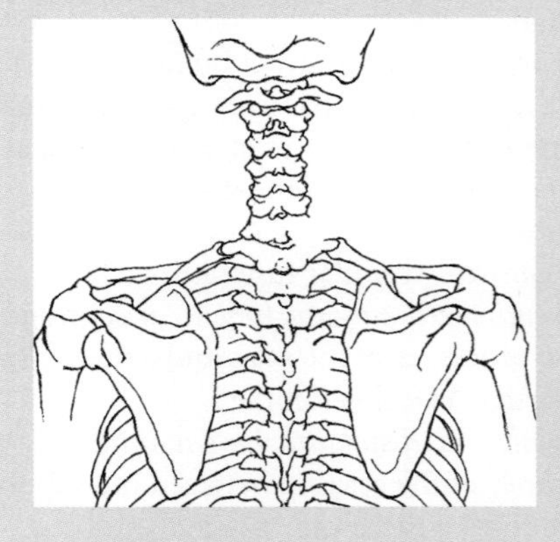

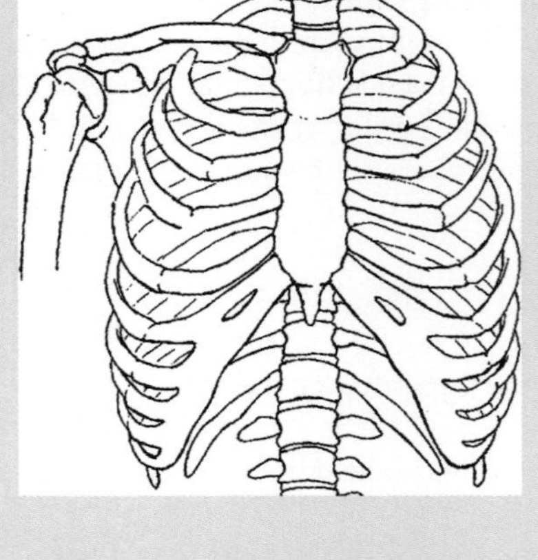

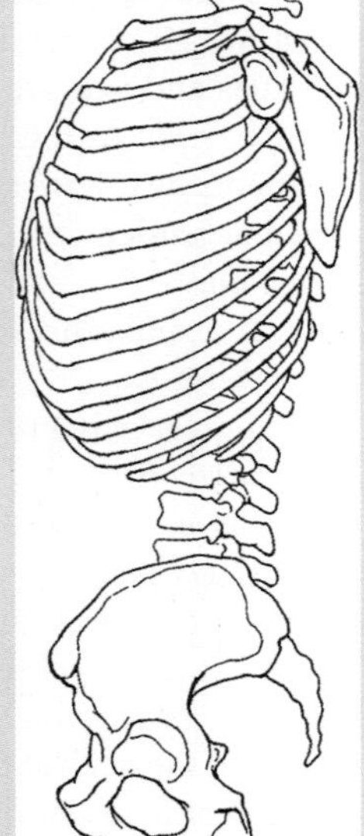

Muscles of the Musculotendinous (Rotator) Cuff

Nine muscles cross over the ball-and-socket joint of the shoulder to stabilize and move this joint (Fig. 9.21). Of these nine, the four "SITS" muscles are known as the rotator cuff muscles: the *s*upraspinatus, *i*nfraspinatus, *t*eres minor, and *s*ubscapularis. These muscles originate on the scapula, and their distal tendons blend into each other (and with the fibrous capsule of the shoulder joint). The main functions of these muscles are to hold the head of the humerus in the glenoid cavity and to reinforce the joint capsule; therefore they often sustain isometric contraction. The massage therapist can easily access all these muscles (except for the subscapularis). Because the subscapularis is located deep to the scapula, the best access position is supine with pressure applied through the axilla and toward the scapula. Caution must be taken not to press on the nerves and vessels in the area.

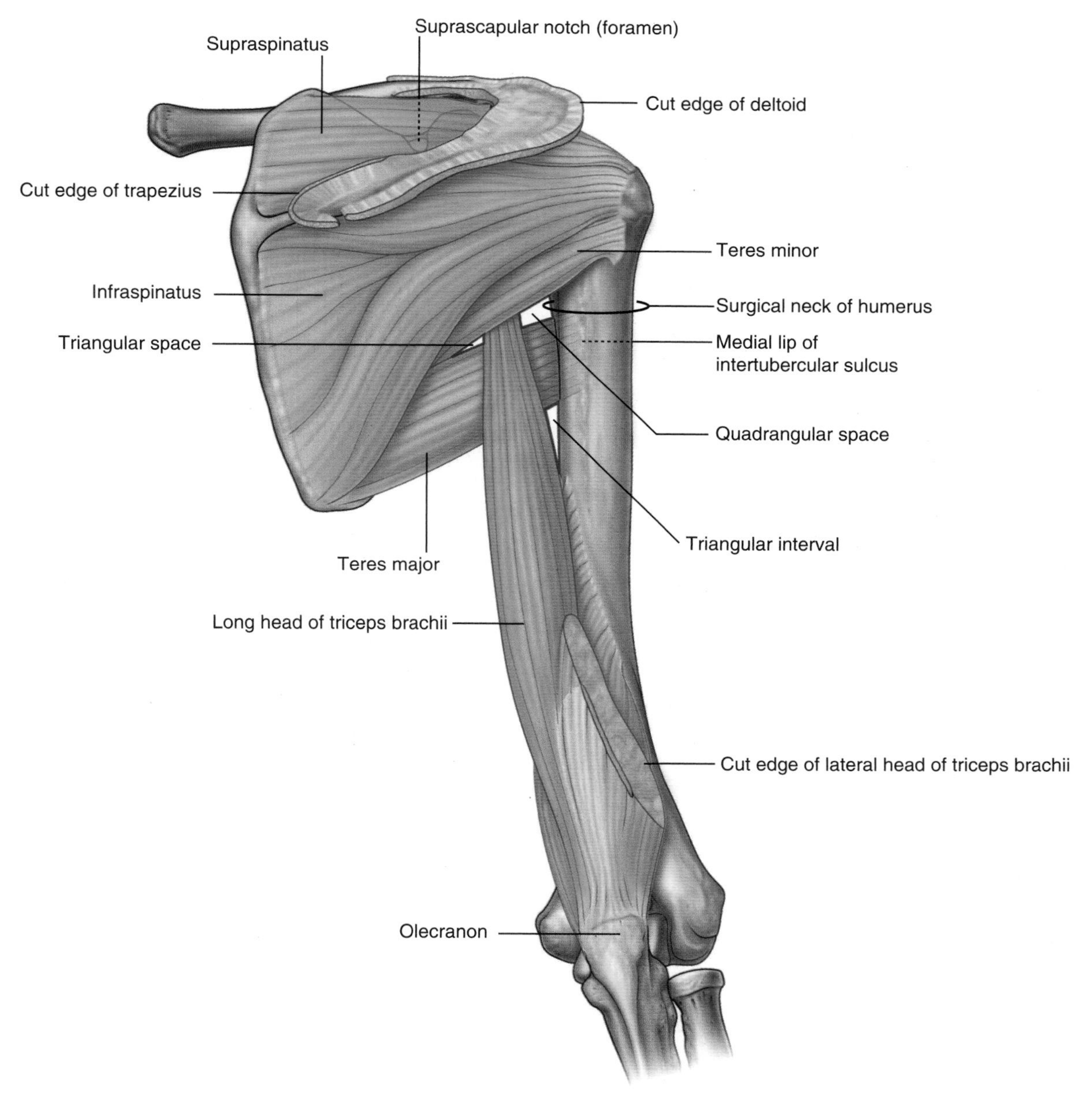

FIG. 9.21 Right posterior scapular region. (From Drake RL, Vogl W, Mitchell WM. *Gray's Anatomy for Students*. 2nd ed. Churchill Livingstone; 2010.)

Supraspinatus (SOO-prah-spy-NAH-tus)

Supraspinatus means "above the spine" (of the scapula).

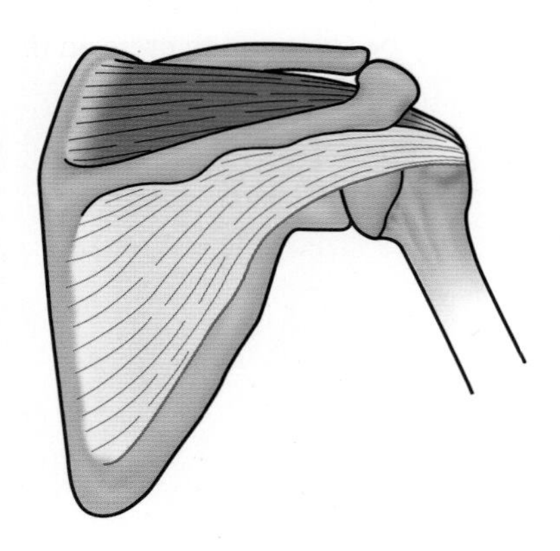

Concentric action:
Abduction of the arm at the shoulder joint
Eccentric action:
Restrains/controls (especially rapid movement) adduction of the arm
Isometric action:
Acts to stabilize the humeral head in the glenoid cavity during movements of the arm
Origin, fixed end, proximal attachment, arises from:
Medial two-thirds of the supraspinous fossa of the scapula
Insertion, mobile end, distal attachment, attaches to:
Superior facet of the greater tubercle of the humerus and the capsule of the shoulder joint
Innervation:
Suprascapular nerve (C5–C6)
Major synergist:
Deltoid

The rotator cuff muscles assist one another in stabilizing the head of the humerus in the glenoid fossa.

Major antagonists:
Latissimus dorsi, teres major, and pectoralis major
Tender/trigger points:
In the belly of the muscle and near the tendon at the humerus
Common symptom/Common symptom/Referred pain pattern:
Shoulder, deltoid, and down the arm to the elbow, often experienced as a dull ache

Infraspinatus (in-fra-spy-NAH-tus)

Infraspinatus means "below the spine" (of the scapula).

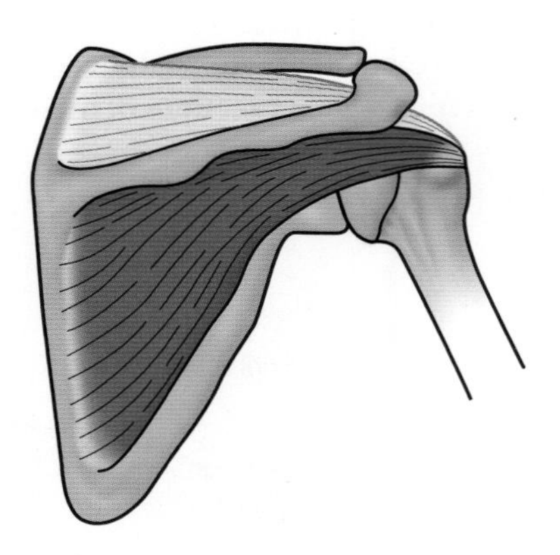

Concentric action:
Lateral rotation of the arm at the shoulder joint
Eccentric action:
Restrains/controls (especially rapid movement) medial rotation of the arm
Isometric action:
Acts to stabilize the humeral head in the glenoid cavity during movements of the arm
Origin, fixed end, proximal attachment, arises from:
Medial two-thirds of the infraspinous fossa
Insertion, mobile end, distal attachment, attaches to:
Middle facet of the greater tubercle of the humerus and the capsule of the shoulder joint
Innervation:
Suprascapular nerve (C5–C6)
Major synergists:
Teres minor and posterior deltoid

The rotator cuff muscles assist one another in stabilizing the head of the humerus in the glenoid fossa.

Major antagonists:
Subscapularis, pectoralis major, anterior deltoid, latissimus dorsi, and teres major
Tender/trigger points:
Belly of the muscle below the spine of the scapula and near the medial border of the scapula
Referred pain patterns:
Deep into the shoulder and deltoid area, down the arm, suboccipital area, and medial border of the scapula—which limits the ability to reach behind the back

Teres minor (TER-eez)

Teres means "smooth and round"; *minor* means "smaller."

Posterior

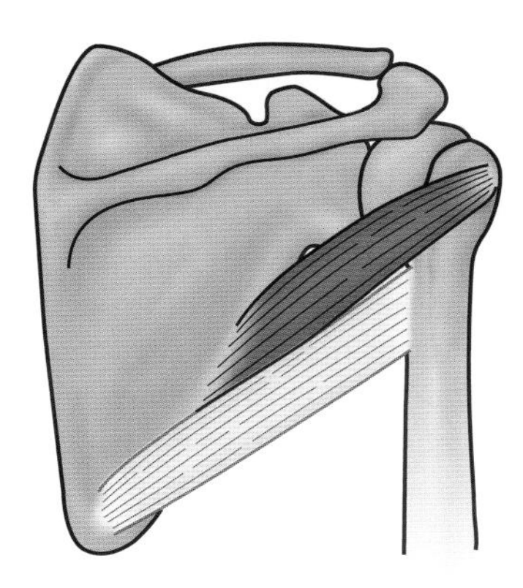

Concentric action:
Lateral rotation and adduction of the arm at the shoulder joint
Eccentric action:
Restrains/controls (especially rapid movement) medial rotation and abduction of the arm
Isometric action:
Acts to stabilize the humeral head in the glenoid cavity during movements of the arm
Origin, fixed end, proximal attachment, arises from:
Superior two-thirds, dorsal surface of the lateral border of the scapula
Insertion, mobile end, distal attachment, attaches to:
Inferior facet of the greater tubercle of the humerus and the capsule of the shoulder joint
Innervation:
Axillary nerve (C5–C6)
Major synergists:
Infraspinatus, posterior deltoid, and latissimus dorsi

The rotator cuff muscles assist one another in stabilizing the head of the humerus in the glenoid fossa.

Major antagonists:
Subscapularis, pectoralis major, anterior deltoid, and supraspinatus
Tender/trigger points:
Belly of the muscle closer to the attachment on the humerus
Common symptom/Common symptom/Referred pain pattern:
The posterior deltoid region often has limited range of motion for reaching behind the back, such as putting hands in the back pocket of pants.

Subscapularis (sub-SKAP-you-LAR-iss)

Subscapularis means "under (deep to) the shoulder blade."

This muscle often is implicated in "frozen shoulder" syndromes.

Anterior

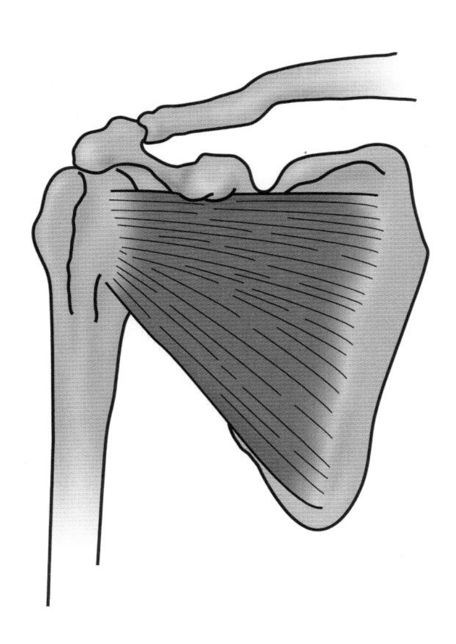

Concentric action:
Medial rotation of the arm at the shoulder joint
Eccentric action:
Restrains/controls (especially rapid movement) lateral rotation of the arm
Isometric action:
Acts to stabilize the humeral head in the glenoid cavity during movements of the arm
Origin, fixed end, proximal attachment, arises from:
Subscapular fossa of the scapula
Insertion, mobile end, distal attachment, attaches to:
Lesser tubercle of the humerus and the capsule of the shoulder joint
Innervation:
Upper and lower subscapular nerves (C5–C6)
Major synergists:
Pectoralis major, anterior deltoid, latissimus dorsi, and teres major

The rotator cuff muscles assist one another in stabilizing the head of the humerus in the glenoid fossa.

Major antagonists:
Infraspinatus, teres minor, and posterior deltoid
Tender/trigger points:
Access through the axilla near the attachment at the humerus and in the belly of the muscle
Common symptom/Common symptom/Referred pain pattern:
Posterior deltoid, scapular region, triceps area and into the wrist; often mistaken for bursitis because the pain often refers to insertion at the shoulder

ACTIVITY 9.22

Draw and color the *muscles of the rotator cuff* in the spaces provided. For each muscle:

1. Label the origin and insertion attachment points: *O* for origin; *I* for insertion.
2. Place an X on the trigger points.
3. Palpate this muscle; identify the attachment points and the bellies of the muscles.
4. Move these muscles on yourself.

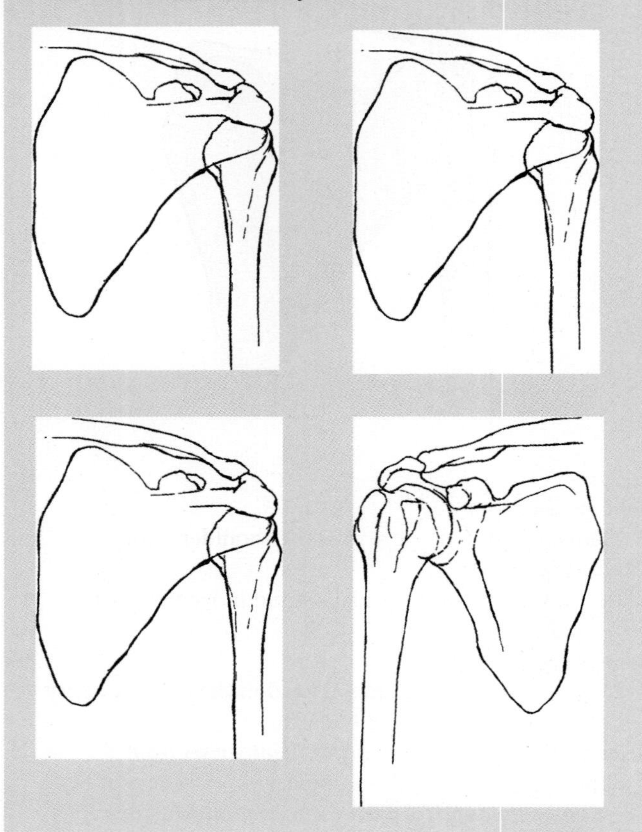

Muscles of the Shoulder Joint

In general, any muscle that crosses the shoulder joint anteriorly can flex the arm at the shoulder joint, and any muscle that crosses the shoulder joint posteriorly can extend the arm at the shoulder joint (Fig. 9.22). The deltoid is the prime mover of arm abduction at the shoulder joint but also is involved in flexion and extension of the arm at the shoulder joint. The main antagonists to abduction of the arm at the shoulder joint are the pectoralis major anteriorly and the latissimus dorsi posteriorly. Depending on the location and insertion points, the various muscles acting on the arm also provide lateral (external) and medial (internal) rotation of the arm at the shoulder joint. The interaction of these muscles is complex, and each muscle contributes to more than one movement.

Because these muscles are active during walking, all gait reflexes are involved with the shoulder muscles to promote the appropriate counterbalancing arm swing to the thigh swing. Facilitation occurs between muscles of the arms that flex and extend in conjunction with thigh muscles during contralateral gait patterns. The massage therapist often needs to consider the muscles of the shoulder joint with muscles of the hip joint and provide massage in a correlated pattern to be most effective. Although not listed with synergists, the shoulder joint flexors on one side work with hip joint flexors on the opposite side. Adductors and medial rotators of the arm at the shoulder joint on one side work with adductors and medial rotators of the thigh at the hip joint on the opposite side. The same pattern applies to lateral rotation. These muscles inhibit muscles on the same side of the body—that is, medial rotation of the arm at the shoulder joint and thigh at the hip joint on the right inhibit each other, as do the lateral rotators. Obviously, the same patterns occur on the left. Also, during normal gait, flexors and extensors of the arm at the shoulder joints interact. The flexors on the right work with extensors on the left and inhibit flexors on the left, and vice versa. The extensors on the right work with flexors on the left and inhibit the extensors on the left, and vice versa. Although this seems confusing, the patterns become apparent when observing gait. To understand this, the student should take a step—freeze—and then notice which muscles are interacting.

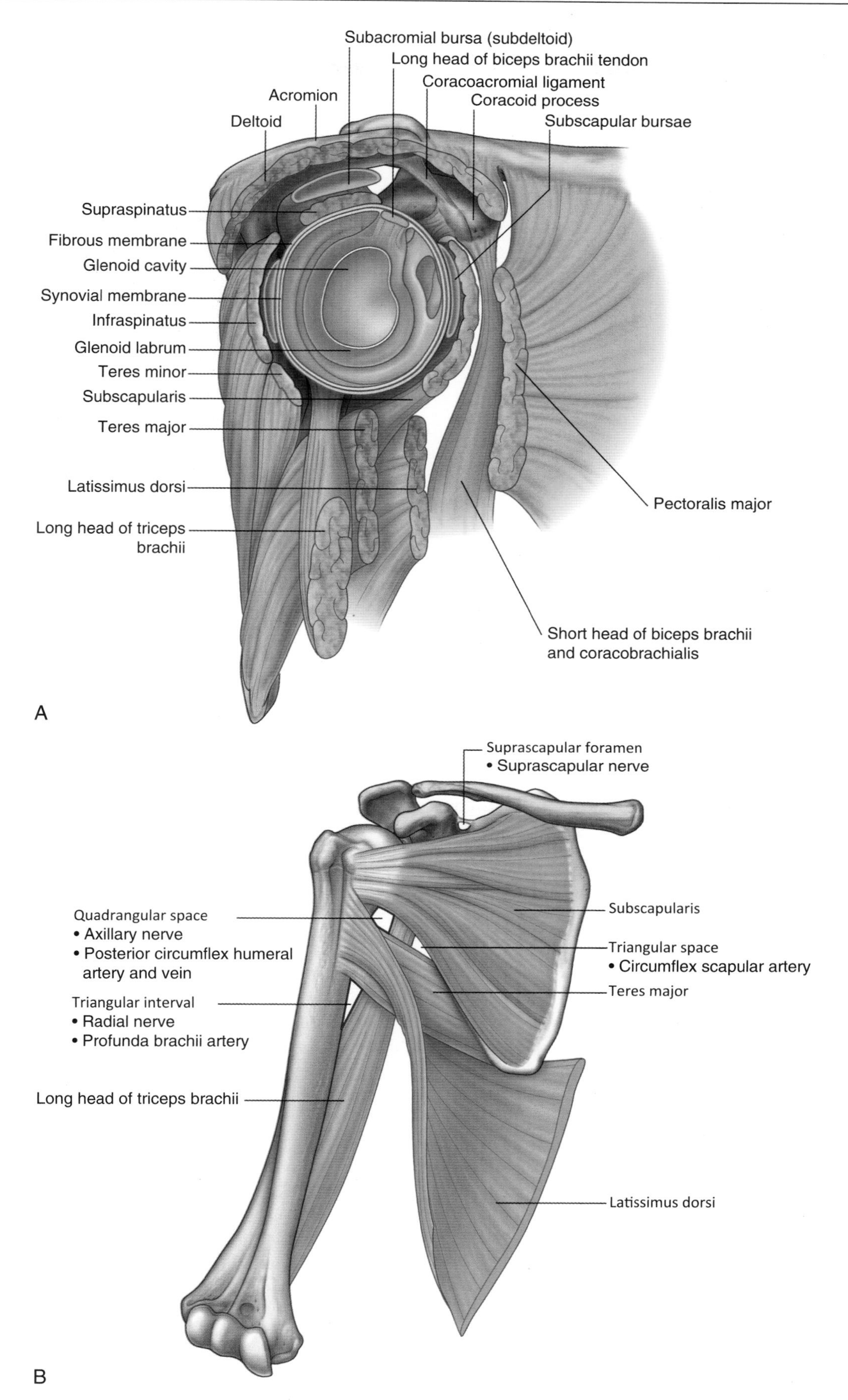

FIG. 9.22 (A) Lateral view of right glenohumeral joint and surrounding muscles with proximal end of humerus removed. (B) Posterior wall of the axilla. (From Drake RL, Vogl W, Mitchell WM. *Gray's Anatomy for Students*. 2nd ed. Churchill Livingstone; 2010.)

Deltoid (DEL-toyd) (deltoideus)

Deltoid means "triangular."

This muscle functions in three distinct patterns and can be thought of as three different muscles.

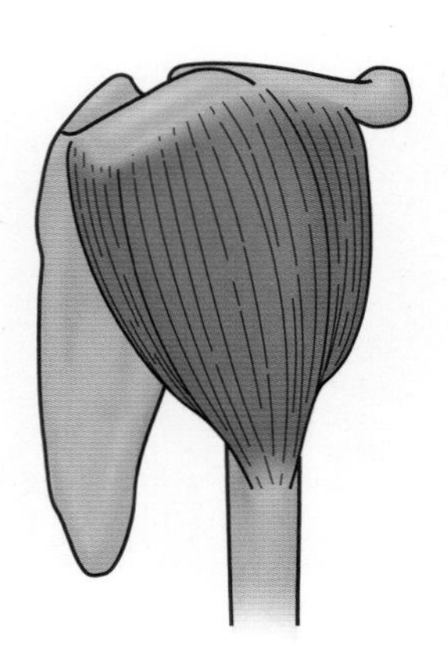

Concentric action:
- Anterior deltoid—flexion, medial rotation, and abduction of the arm at the shoulder joint
- Middle deltoid—abduction of the arm at the shoulder joint
- Posterior deltoid—extension, lateral rotation, and abduction of the arm at the shoulder joint

Eccentric action:
- The anterior deltoid muscle restrains/controls (especially rapid movement) extension, lateral rotation, and adduction of the arm. The middle deltoid muscle restrains/controls (especially rapid movement) adduction of the arm. The posterior deltoid muscle restrains/controls (especially rapid movement) flexion, medial rotation, and adduction of the arm.

Isometric action:
- Stabilizes glenohumeral joint during arm movement

Origin, fixed end, proximal attachment, arises from:
- Anterior deltoid—superior surface, lateral third of the clavicle
- Middle deltoid—lateral margin of the spine of the scapula and superior surface of the acromion
- Posterior deltoid—posterior border of the spine of the scapula

Insertion, mobile end, distal attachment, attaches to:
- Deltoid tuberosity of the humerus

Innervation:
- Axillary nerve (C5–C6)

Major synergists:
- Anterior deltoid—coracobrachialis, clavicular head of the pectoralis major, and biceps brachii
- Middle deltoid—supraspinatus
- Posterior deltoid—latissimus dorsi, teres major, and infraspinatus

Major antagonists:
- Pectoralis major and latissimus dorsi; the anterior and posterior deltoid muscles are antagonistic to each other.

Tender/trigger points:
- Anterior deltoid—near the clavicular attachment
- Posterior and middle deltoid—in the belly of the muscles

Common symptom/Common symptom/Referred pain pattern:
- Deltoid region and down the lateral side of the arm

Pectoralis major (PEK-tor-al-iss)

Pectoralis means "of the chest"; *major* means "larger."

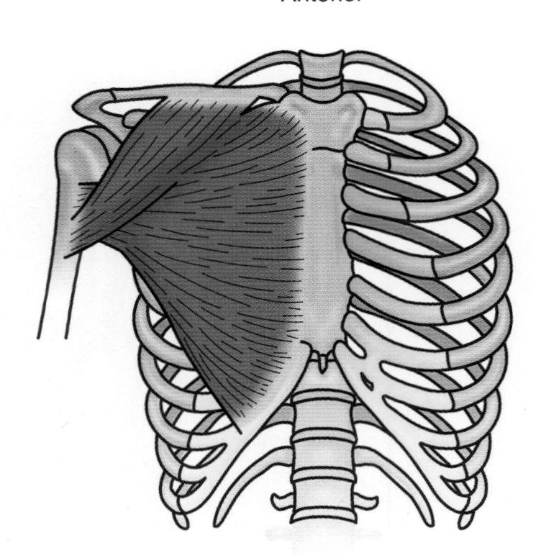

Concentric action:
- Entire muscle—adduction and medial rotation of the arm at the shoulder joint
- Clavicular head—flexion of the arm at the shoulder joint
- Sternocostal head—extension of the arm at the shoulder joint

Eccentric action:
- Restrains/controls (especially rapid movement) abduction and lateral rotation of the arm and also can restrain extension and flexion of the arm

Isometric action:
- Stabilizes the shoulder during overhead activity

Origin, fixed end, proximal attachment, arises from:
- Ventral surface of the sternum down to the seventh rib, medial half of the clavicle, cartilage of ribs 1 to 7, and aponeurosis of the external abdominal oblique muscle

Insertion, mobile end, distal attachment, attaches to:
- Lateral lip of the bicipital groove of the humerus

The attachment pattern for this muscle is complex and consists of several overlapping sheets of muscles in a fan arrangement with a spiraling distal attachment. The muscle is divided into clavicular, sternal, costal, and abdominal sections, each able to function independently.

Innervation:
- Medial and lateral pectoral nerves (C5–T1)

Major synergists:
- Clavicular head—anterior deltoid and coracobrachialis
- Sternocostal head—latissimus dorsi and teres major

Major antagonists:
- Clavicular head—latissimus dorsi and teres major
- Sternocostal head—anterior deltoid, supraspinatus, infraspinatus, and teres minor

Tender/trigger points:
- Belly of the muscle

Common symptom/Common symptom/Referred pain pattern:
- Chest and breast and down the ulnar aspect of the arm and forearm to the fourth and fifth fingers

Subclavius (sub-KLAVE-ee-us)

Subclavius means “below” and “little key” (referring to the clavicle).

This muscle often is considered with the clavicular portion of the pectoralis major.

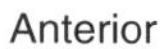

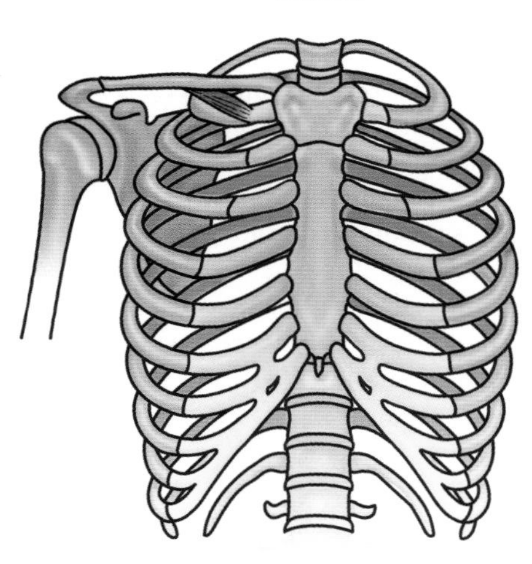

Concentric action:
Protraction and depression of the clavicle at the sternoclavicular joint

Eccentric action:
Restrains/controls (especially rapid movement) retraction and elevation of the clavicle at the sternoclavicular joint

Isometric action:
Stabilizes the clavicle

Origin, fixed end, proximal attachment, arises from:
Junction of the first rib and its costal cartilage

Insertion, mobile end, distal attachment, attaches to:
Inferior surface of the clavicle

Innervation:
Fifth and sixth cervical nerves (C5–C6)

Major synergists:
Deltoid muscle and pectoralis major

Major antagonists:
Sternocleidomastoid and upper trapezius

Tender/trigger points:
Belly of the muscle

Common symptom/Common symptom/Referred pain pattern:
Chest and breast region

Latissimus dorsi (la-TISS-ih-mus DOR-see)

Latissimus means "widest"; *dorsi* means "belonging to the back."

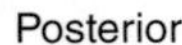

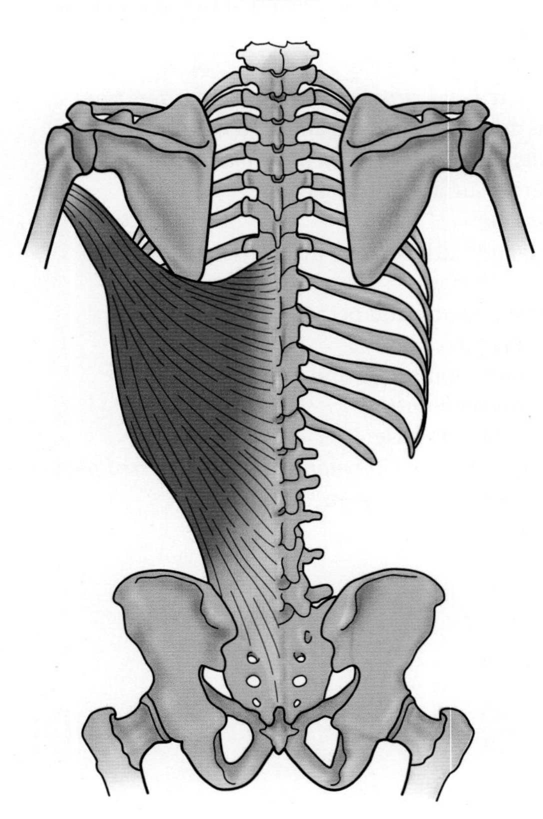

Concentric action:

Medial rotation, adduction, and extension of the arm at the shoulder joint; depression of the scapula at the scapulocostal joint; extension of the trunk at the spinal joints; and anterior tilt and elevation of the pelvis at the lumbosacral joint

Eccentric action:

Restrains/controls (especially rapid movement) lateral rotation, abduction, and flexion of the arm, elevation of the scapula, flexion of the trunk, and posterior tilt and depression of the pelvis

Isometric action:

Stabilizes the lumbar and pelvic area by maintaining tension on the thoracolumbar fascia

Origin, fixed end, proximal attachment, arises from:

Spinous processes of T7–L5, posterior one-third of the external lip of the iliac crest, posterior layer of the thoracolumbar fascia, and lower three or four ribs

Insertion, mobile end, distal attachment, attaches to:

Medial lip of the bicipital groove of the humerus just as the muscle begins to twist around the teres major

The latissimus dorsi is fan shaped and has a twist in its fibers such that the superior fibers attach more distally on the humerus and the inferior fibers attach more proximally on the humerus. Shortening in this muscle limits arm movement over the head and can cause the back of the lumbar area to feel tight.

Innervation:

Thoracodorsal nerve (C6–C8)

Major synergists:

Teres major, the long head of the triceps brachii, sternocostal head of the pectoralis major, subscapularis, and anterior deltoid muscle

Major antagonists:

Clavicular head of the pectoralis major, teres minor, infraspinatus, deltoid muscle, supraspinatus, levator scapulae, and rectus abdominis

Tender/trigger points:

Posterior axillary area and belly of the muscle near the rib attachments

Common symptom/Common symptom/Referred pain pattern:

Just below the scapula and into the ulnar side of the arm and anterior deltoid region and abdominal oblique area

Teres major (TER-eez)

Teres means "smooth and round"; *major* means "larger." This muscle may be fused with the latissimus dorsi.

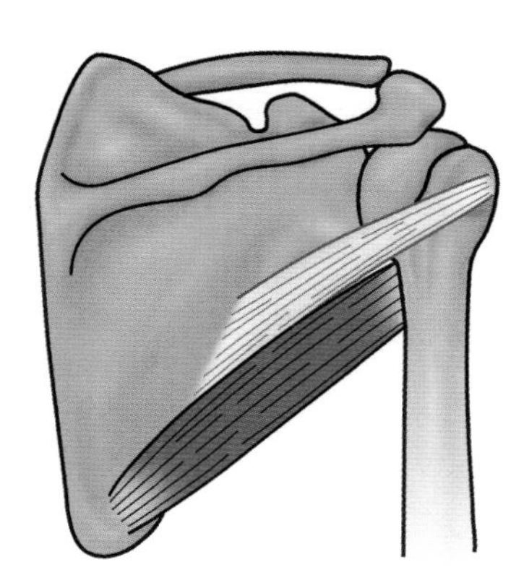

Concentric action:
Medial rotation, adduction, and extension of the arm at the shoulder joint and upward rotation of the scapula at the scapulocostal joint
Eccentric action:
Restrains/controls (especially rapid movement) lateral rotation, abduction, and flexion of the arm and restrains/controls (especially rapid movement) downward rotation of the scapula
Isometric action:
Stabilizes the glenohumeral joint
Origin, fixed end, proximal attachment, arises from:
Dorsal surfaces of inferior angle and lower third of lateral border of scapula
Insertion, mobile end, distal attachment, attaches to:
Medial lip of bicipital groove of the humerus
Innervation:
Lower subscapular nerve (C5–C7)
Major synergists:
Latissimus dorsi, subscapularis, and trapezius
Major antagonists:
Teres minor, infraspinatus, supraspinatus, anterior deltoid muscle, and pectoralis minor
Tender/trigger points:
Near the musculotendinous junction at both attachments and points at the attachments at the humerus; can be best reached through the axilla
Common symptom/Common symptom/Referred pain pattern:
Posterior deltoid region and down the dorsal portion of the arm

Coracobrachialis (KORE-a-koe-BRAY-kee-AL-iss)

Coracobrachialis means "crow's beak" and "of the arm."

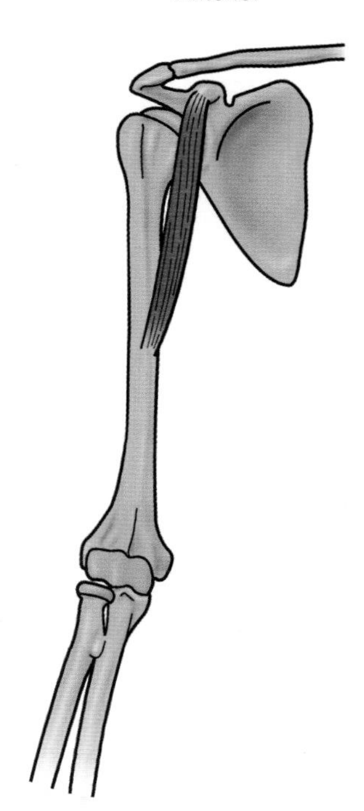

Concentric action:
Flexion and adduction of the arm at the shoulder joint
Eccentric action:
Restrains/controls (especially rapid movement) extension and abduction of the arm
Isometric action:
Stabilizes the shoulder and scapula
Origin, fixed end, proximal attachment, arises from:
Tip of the coracoid process of the scapula
Insertion, mobile end, distal attachment, attaches to:
Anteromedial surface of the middle of the shaft of the humerus, opposite the deltoid tuberosity
Innervation:
Musculocutaneous nerve (C5–C7)
Major synergists:
Pectoralis major and short head of biceps brachii
Major antagonist:
Posterior deltoid muscle
Tender/trigger points:
Near the musculotendinous junction and the coracoid attachment
Common symptom/Common symptom/Referred pain pattern:
Front of shoulder and posterior aspect of the arm down the triceps and posterior forearm into the posterior hand

ACTIVITY 9.23

Draw and color the *muscles of the shoulder joint* in the spaces provided. For each muscle:

1. Label the origin and insertion attachment points: *O* for origin; *I* for insertion.
2. Place an X on the trigger points.
3. Palpate this muscle; identify the attachment points and the bellies of the muscles.
4. Move these muscles on yourself.

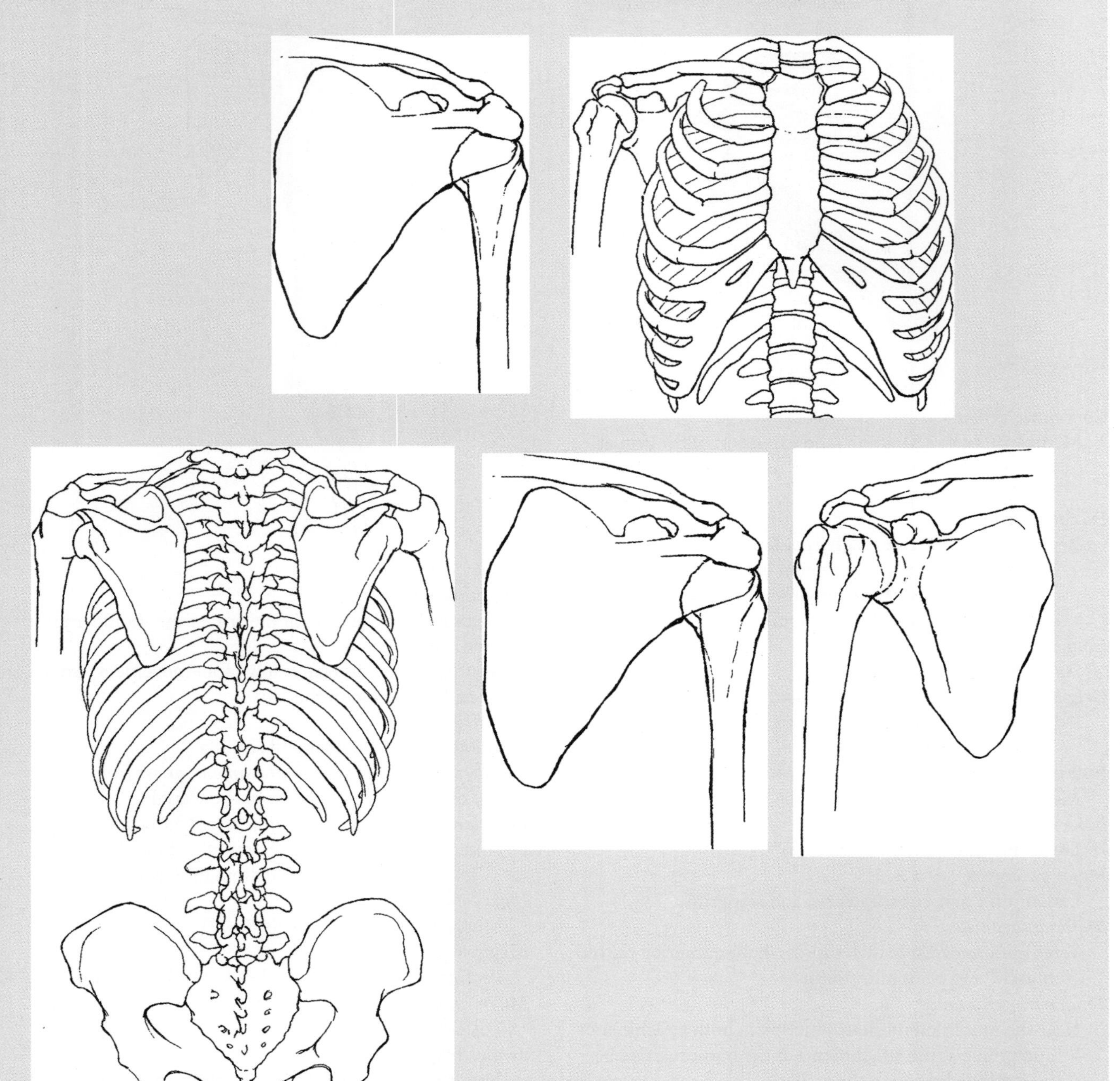

Muscles of the Elbow and Radioulnar Joints

The elbow is a hinge joint, and movements produced by the muscles at the elbow joint are limited entirely to flexion and extension of the forearm. Posterior arm muscles produce extension of the forearm at the elbow joint; anterior arm muscles produce flexion of the forearm at the elbow joint. The strongest elbow flexor is the brachialis. Reverse actions of flexion and extension of the arm at the elbow joint are also common. Pronation and supination take place at the radioulnar joints. Because of contralateral joint reflexes involved with gait, flexors of the forearm at the elbow joint work with flexors of the leg at the knee joint on the opposite side of the body, and extensors of the forearm at the elbow joint work with extensors of the leg at the knee joint on the opposite side of the body. Massage application is more effective when the massage therapist observes these interactions and considers the body-wide pattern. Dysfunction is common with static posture. Static position requires these muscles to hold contraction for prolonged periods. Examples are driving a car, holding a phone, computer work, and using hand tools. Repetitive-use activities, such as using a hammer or wrench, also strain this group of muscles (Fig. 9.23).

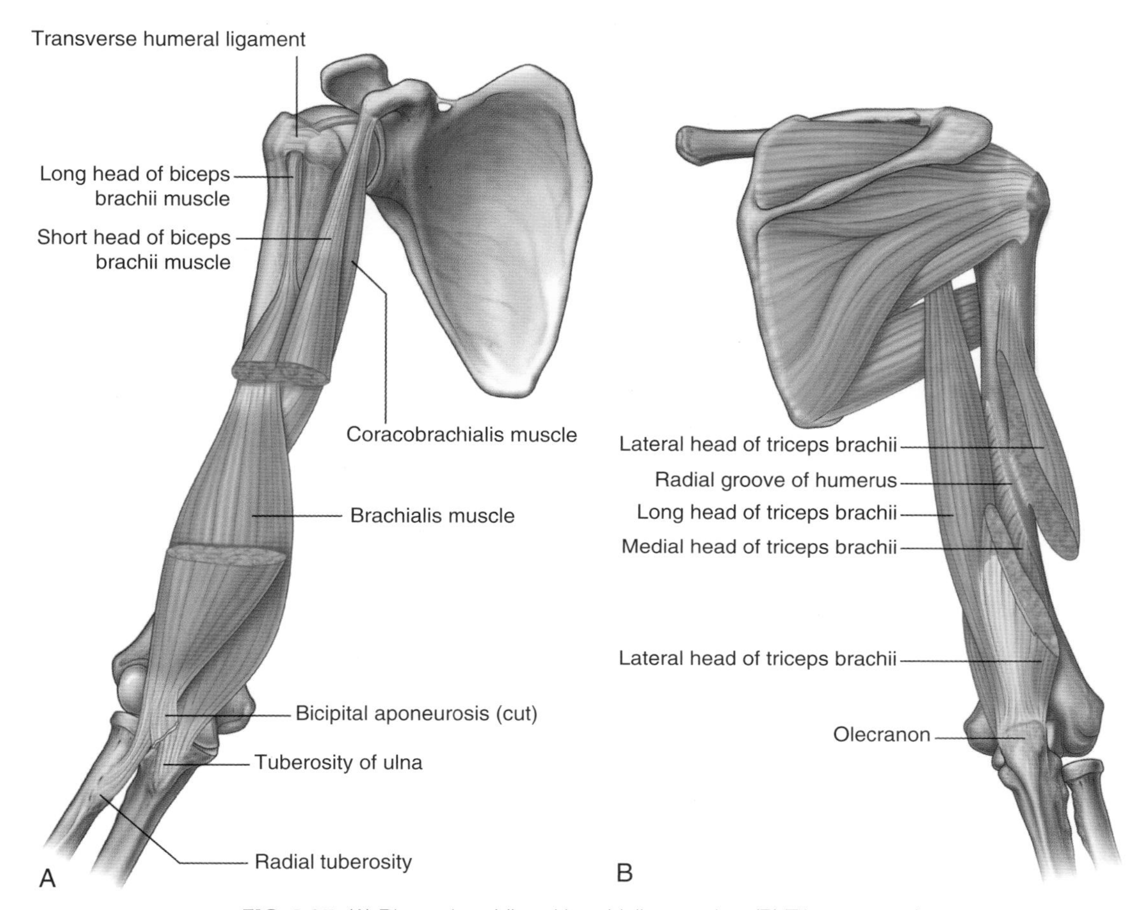

FIG. 9.23 (A) Biceps brachii and brachialis muscles. (B) Triceps muscle.

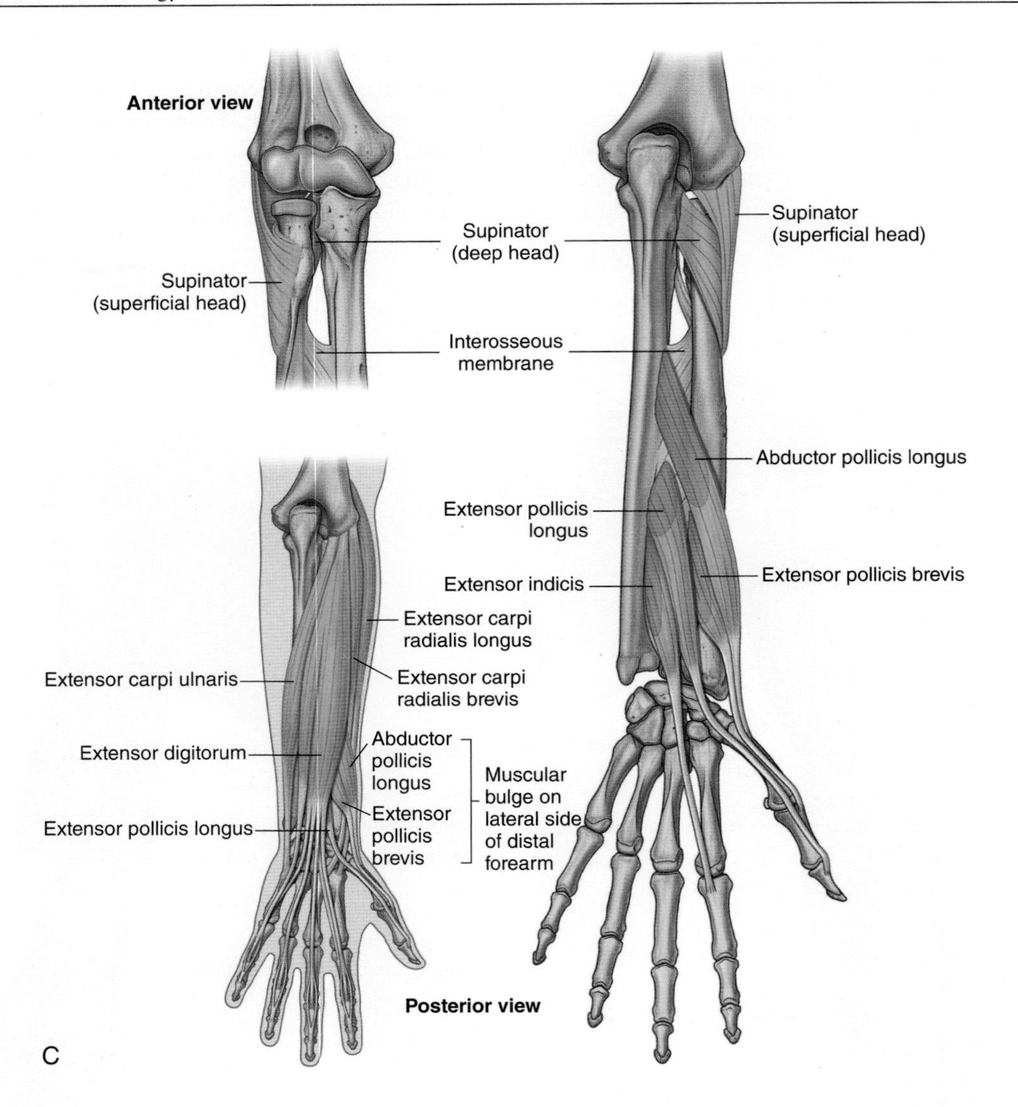

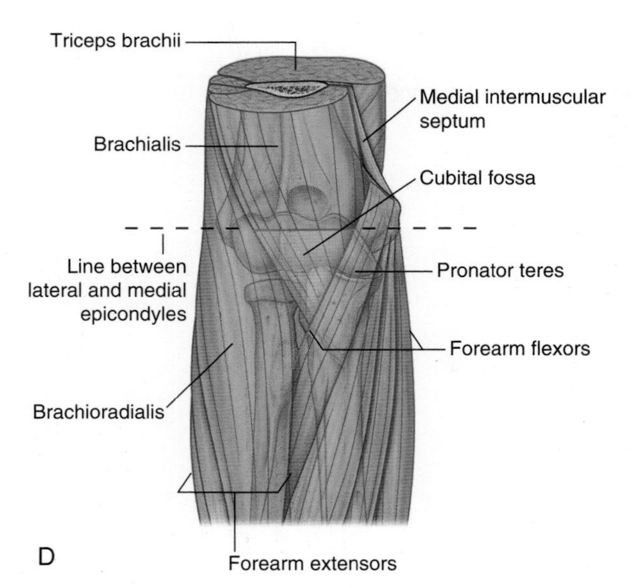

FIG. 9.23, cont'd (C) Deep layer of muscles in the posterior compartment of the forearm. (D) Cross section of the arm. (From Drake RL, Vogl W, Mitchell WM. *Gray's Anatomy for Students*. 2nd ed. Churchill Livingstone; 2010.)

Biceps brachii (BI-seps BRAY-kee-eye)

Biceps means "two heads"; *brachii* means "of the arm."

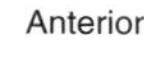

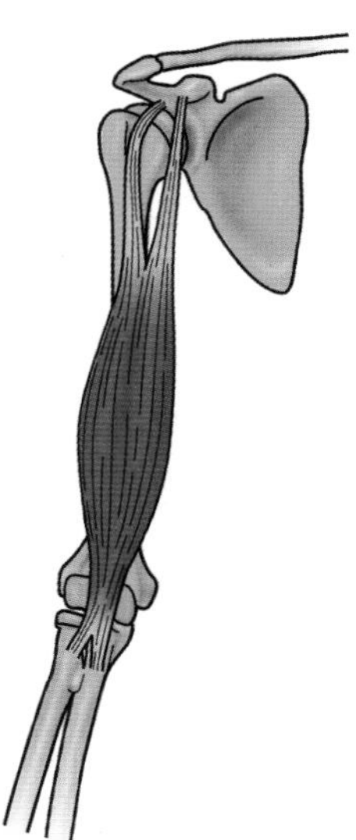

Concentric action:

Flexion of the forearm at the elbow joint, supination of the forearm at the radioulnar joints, and flexion of the arm at the shoulder joint

A common reverse action is flexion of the arm at the elbow joint, such as when doing a pull-up or chin-up.

Eccentric action:

Restrains/controls (especially rapid movement) extension and pronation of the forearm and extension of the arm

Isometric action:

Stabilizes the humerus at the shoulder and elbow joints during full extension and stabilizes the elbow joint when flexed and holding a weight

Origin, fixed end, proximal attachment, arises from:

Long head—supraglenoid tubercle of the scapula

Short head—tip of the coracoid process of the scapula

Insertion, mobile end, distal attachment, attaches to:

Tuberosity of the radius and aponeurosis of the proximal attachment (origin) of the wrist flexor muscles in the forearm

Innervation:

Musculocutaneous nerve (C5–C6)

Major synergists:

Brachialis, brachioradialis, supinator, and anterior deltoid muscle

Major antagonists:

Triceps brachii, pronator teres, pronator quadratus, and posterior deltoid muscle

Tender/trigger points:

In the belly of the long and short heads, closer to the elbow

Common symptom/Common symptom/Referred pain pattern:

Front of the shoulder at the anterior deltoid region and into the scapular region and also into the antecubital space (front of the elbow)

Brachialis (BRAY-kee-AL-iss)

Brachialis means "of the arm."

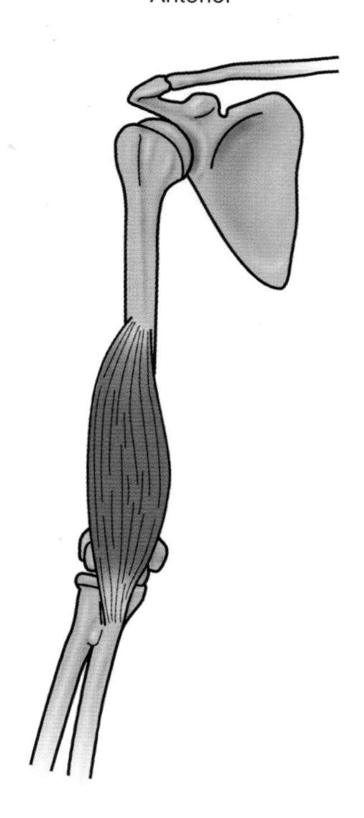

Concentric action:

Flexion of the forearm at the elbow joint

Eccentric action:

Restrains/controls (especially rapid movement) extension of the forearm

Isometric action:

Stabilizes the elbow joint

Origin, fixed end, proximal attachment, arises from:

Distal one half of the anterior surface of the humerus and the medial and lateral intermuscular septae

Insertion, mobile end, distal attachment, attaches to:

Coronoid process and tuberosity of the ulna

Innervation:

Musculocutaneous nerve (C5–C7)

Major synergists:

Biceps brachii and brachioradialis

Major antagonist:

Triceps brachii

Tender/trigger points:

Several locations in the belly of the muscle

Common symptom/Common symptom/Referred pain pattern:

Primarily to the thumb, with some pain in the anterior deltoid area and at the elbow

Brachioradialis (BRAY-kee-oh-RAY-dee-AL-iss)

Brachioradialis means "related to the arm" and "radius."

Anterior

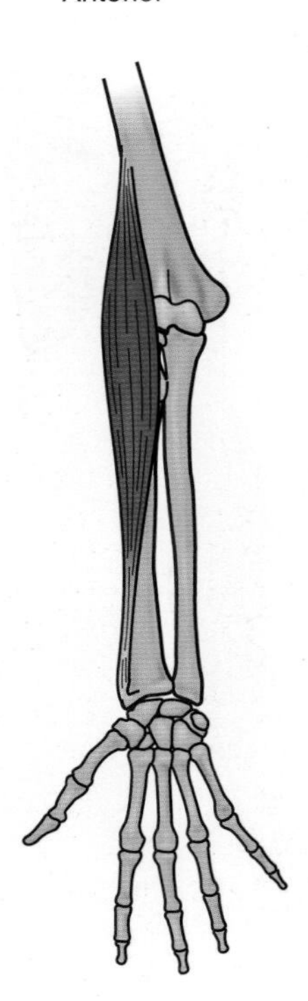

Concentric action:
Flexion of the forearm at the elbow joint; the brachioradialis also can assist in pronation and supination of the forearm at the radioulnar joints to midposition (halfway between full pronation and full supination)

Eccentric action:
Restrains/controls (especially rapid movement) extension of the forearm and can restrain pronation and supination of the forearm (beyond midposition)

Isometric action:
Stabilizes the elbow joint

Origin, fixed end, proximal attachment, arises from:
Proximal two-thirds of the lateral supracondylar ridge of the humerus and lateral intermuscular septum

Insertion, mobile end, distal attachment, attaches to:
Lateral side of the base of the styloid process of the radius

Innervation:
Radial nerve (C5–C6)

Major synergists:
Biceps brachii, brachialis, supinator, pronator teres, and pronator quadratus

Major antagonists:
Triceps brachii, supinator, pronator teres, and pronator quadratus

Tender/trigger points:
Belly of the muscle

Common symptom/Common symptom/Referred pain pattern:
Wrist and base of the thumb in the web space between the thumb and index finger and to the lateral epicondyle at the elbow

Pronator teres (PRO-nay-tor TER-eez)

Pronator means "one that causes pronation": *teres* means "round and smooth."

Anterior

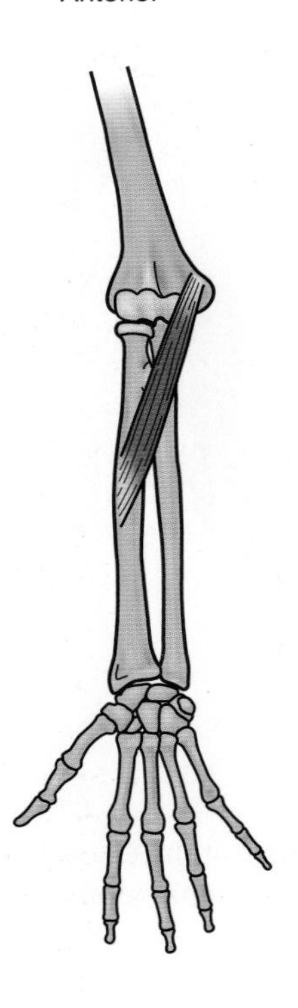

Concentric action:
Pronation of the forearm at the radioulnar joints and flexion of the forearm at the elbow joint

Eccentric action:
Restrains/controls (especially rapid movement) supination and extension of the forearm

Isometric action:
Stabilizes the elbow joint and the radioulnar joints

Origin, fixed end, proximal attachment, arises from:
Humeral head—medial epicondyle of the humerus, common flexor tendon, and deep antebrachial fascia
Ulnar head—medial side of the coronoid process of the ulna

Insertion, mobile end, distal attachment, attaches to:
Middle of lateral surface of radius

Innervation:
Median nerve (C6–C7)

Major synergists:
Pronator quadratus and all forearm flexors

Major antagonists:
Supinator, biceps brachii, and triceps brachii

Tender/trigger points:
Belly of the muscle near the elbow attachment

Common symptom/Common symptom/Referred pain pattern:
Radial side of the forearm into the wrist and thumb; may mimic carpal tunnel syndrome

Pronator quadratus (PRO-nay-tor kwad-RATE-us)

Pronator means "one that causes pronation"; *quadratus* means "square shaped."

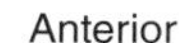

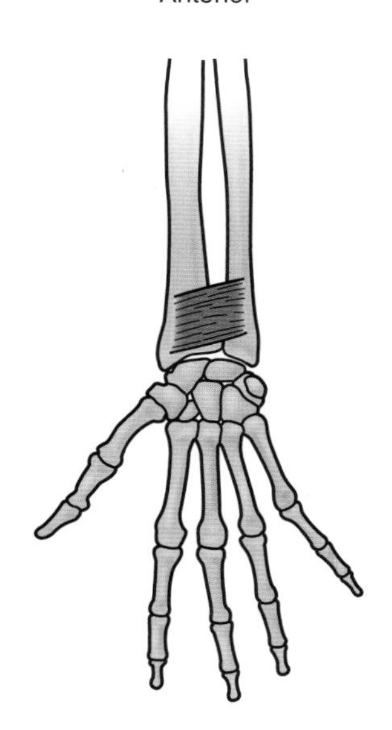

Concentric action:
Pronation of the forearm at the radioulnar joints
Eccentric action:
Restrains/controls (especially rapid movement) supination of the forearm
The pronator quadratus is the prime mover of pronation of the forearm.
Origin, fixed end, proximal attachment, arises from:
Medial side and anterior surface of the distal one-fourth of the ulna
Insertion, mobile end, distal attachment, attaches to:
Lateral side and anterior surface of the distal one-fourth of the radius
Innervation:
Anterior interosseous branch of the median nerve (C7–C8)
Major synergist:
Pronator teres
Major antagonists:
Supinator and biceps brachii
Tender/trigger points:
Belly of muscle
Common symptom/Common symptom/Referred pain pattern:
Local area

Triceps brachii (TRY-seps BRAY-kee-eye)

Triceps means "three heads"; *brachii* means "of the arm."

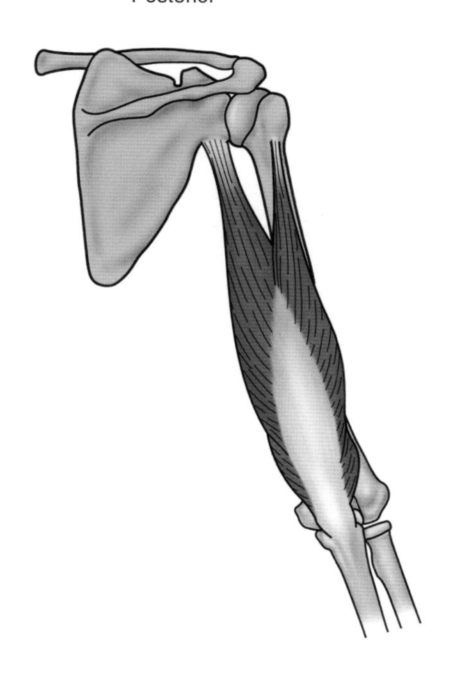

Concentric action:
Extension of the forearm at the elbow joint; in addition, the long head adducts and extends the arm at the shoulder joint
Eccentric action:
Restrains/controls (especially rapid movement) flexion of the forearm and abduction and flexion of the arm
Isometric action:
Stabilizes the elbow and shoulder joints
Origin, fixed end, proximal attachment, arises from:
Long head—infraglenoid tubercle of the scapula
Lateral head—lateral and posterior surfaces of the proximal one half of the shaft of the humerus and the lateral intermuscular septum
Medial (deep) head—distal half of the medial and posterior surfaces of the shaft of the humerus distal to the radial groove and the medial intermuscular septum
Insertion, mobile end, distal attachment, attaches to:
Posterior surface of the olecranon process of the ulna and antebrachial fascia
Innervation:
Radial nerve (C6–C8)
Major synergist:
Anconeus
Major antagonists:
Brachialis and biceps brachii
Tender/trigger points:
Belly of each head
Common symptom/Common symptom/Referred pain pattern:
Length of the posterior arm

Anconeus (an-KO-nee-us)

Anconeus means "elbow."

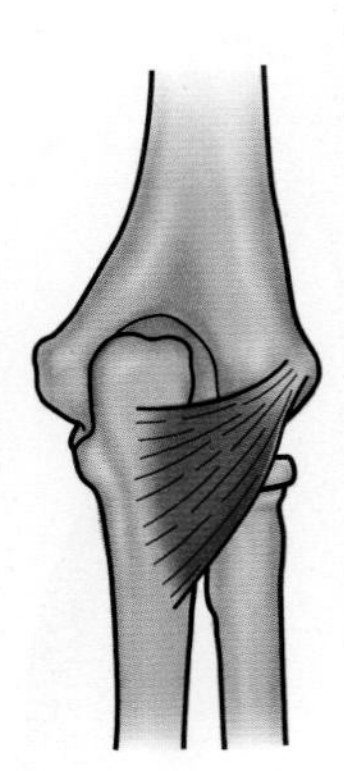

Concentric action:
Extension of the forearm at the elbow joint
Eccentric action:
Restrains/controls (especially rapid movement) flexion of the forearm
Isometric action:
Stabilizes the elbow joint
Origin, fixed end, proximal attachment, arises from:
Posterior surface of the lateral epicondyle of the humerus
Insertion, mobile end, distal attachment, attaches to:
Lateral side of the olecranon process and proximal one-fourth of the posterior surface of the shaft of the ulna
Innervation:
Radial nerve (C6–C8)
Major synergist:
Triceps brachii
Major antagonists:
Biceps brachii and brachialis
Tender/trigger points:
In the belly
Common symptom/Common symptom/Referred pain pattern:
Elbow at the lateral epicondyle

Supinator (SOOP-in-ATE-or)

Supinator means "one that causes supination."

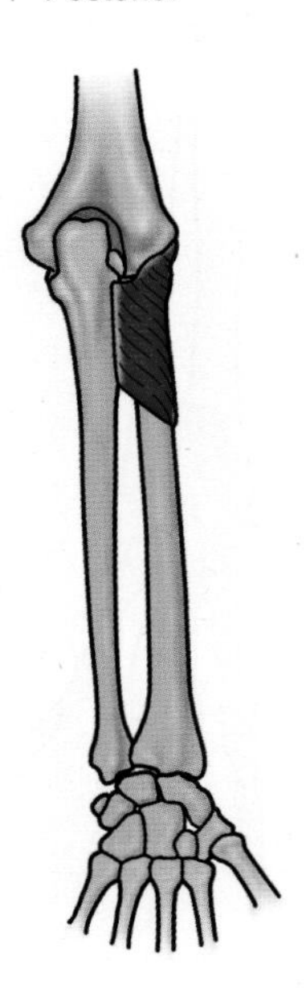

Concentric action:
Supination of the forearm at the radioulnar joints
Eccentric action:
Restrains/controls (especially rapid movement) pronation of the forearm
Isometric action:
Stabilizes the elbow and radioulnar joints
Origin, fixed end, proximal attachment, arises from:
Lateral epicondyle of the humerus, radial collateral ligament of the elbow joint, annular ligament of the radius, and supinator crest of the ulna
Insertion, mobile end, distal attachment, attaches to:
Lateral surface of the proximal one-third of the shaft of the radius, covering part of the anterior, medial, and posterior surfaces

The supinator is a large muscle that wraps around the bones of the forearm.

Innervation:
Deep branch of the radial nerve (C6–C7)
Major synergist:
Biceps brachii
Major antagonists:
Pronator teres and pronator quadratus
Tender/trigger points:
Near the radius in the antecubital space
Common symptom/Common symptom/Referred pain pattern:
Local area

ACTIVITY 9.24

Draw and color the *muscles of the elbow and radioulnar joints* in the spaces provided. For each muscle:

1. Label the origin and insertion attachment points: *O* for origin; *I* for insertion.
2. Place an X on the trigger points.
3. Palpate this muscle; identify the attachment points and the bellies of the muscles.
4. Move these muscles on yourself.

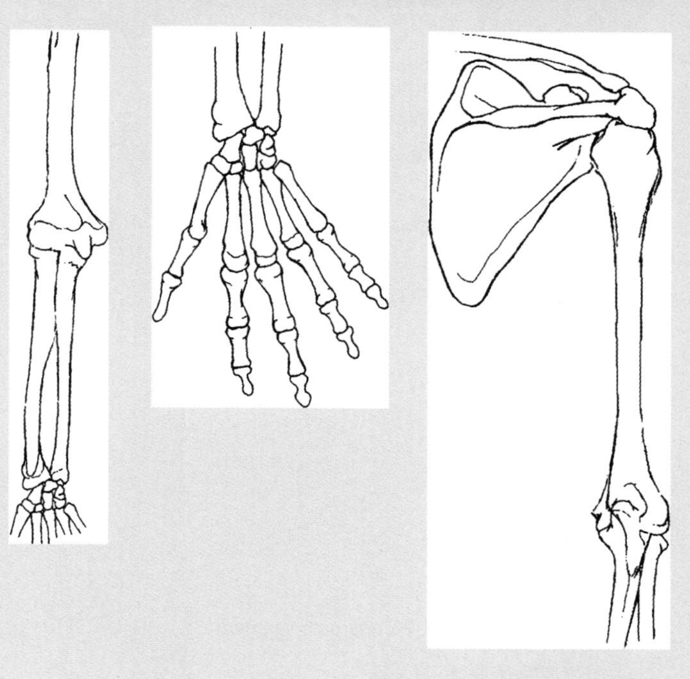

Muscles of the Wrist and Hand Joints

If all the muscles that move the hand actually were located in the hand, the hand would be too bulky to be functional. Instead, the bellies of these muscles are located closer to the elbow, tapering to long insertion tendons in the wrist and hand. Strong ligaments, called the *flexor* and *extensor retinacula*, secure the long, tendinous insertions, much like a bracelet at the wrist. Synovial tendon sheaths surround the tendons to assist their movements and reduce friction. Many of the forearm muscles attach on the humerus and cross the elbow and the wrist joints; however, their action on the elbow is usually insignificant. The forearm muscles are subdivided by fascial sheets into the anterior and posterior compartments, each having a superficial and a deep layer of muscles. Most muscles of the anterior compartment are wrist and finger flexors; the muscles of the posterior compartment are mainly wrist and finger extensors. These muscles have distinct layers, and massage application requires careful and gradual access to the deeper layers by penetrating through the superficial layers using a broad-based compressive force. A narrow-pointed contact with the tissue usually results in tensing and guarding by the superficial muscles (Fig. 9.24).

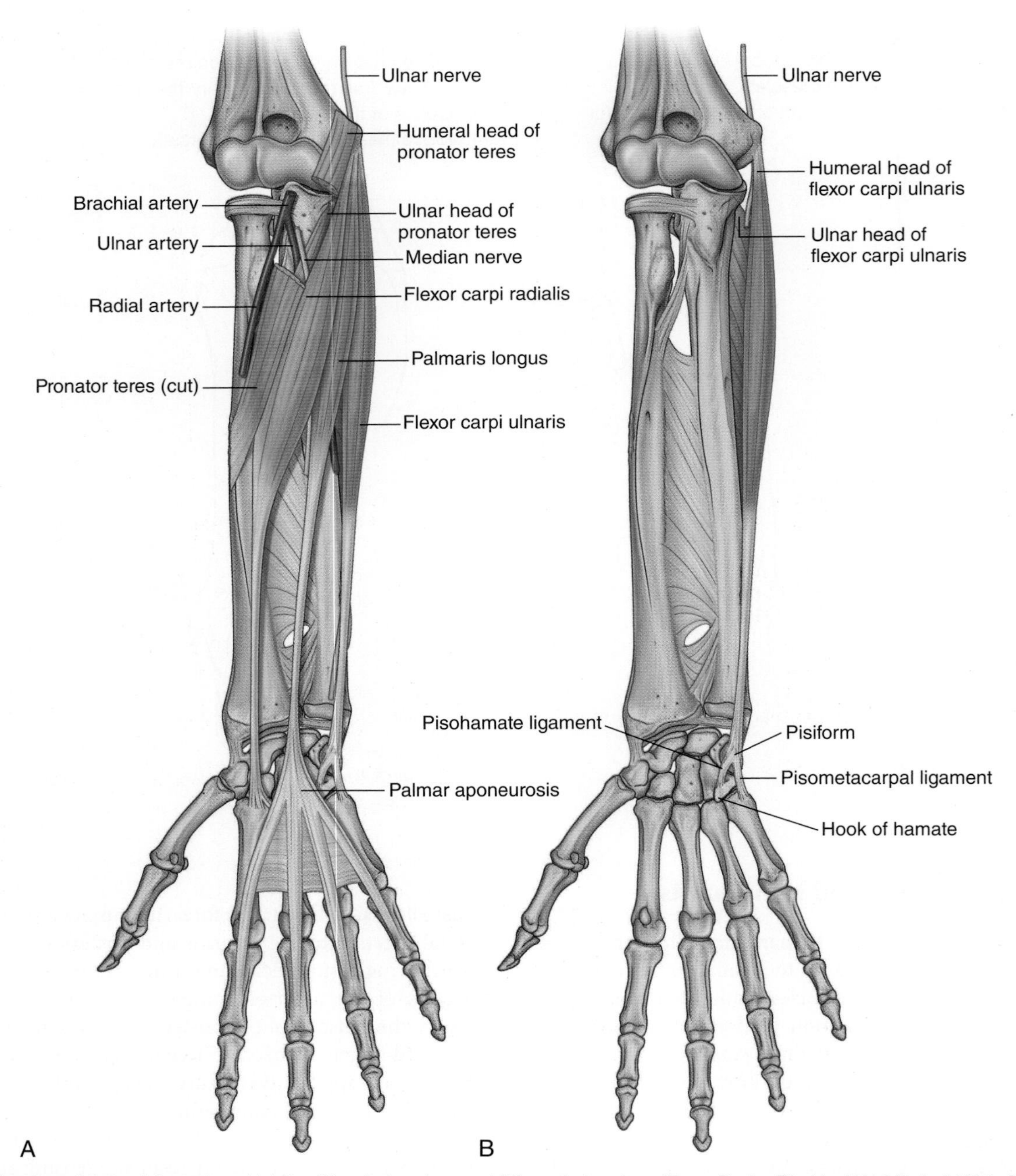

FIG. 9.24 Muscles of the wrist and hand joints: (A) anterior view and (B) posterior view. (From Drake RL, Vogl W, Mitchell WM. *Gray's Anatomy for Students*. 2nd ed. Churchill Livingstone; 2010.)

Anterior Flexor Group: Superficial Layer

Flexor carpi radialis (FLEKS-or KAR-pee RAY-dee-AL-iss)

Flexor means "to bend," *carpi* means "of the wrist," and *radialis* means "related to the radius."

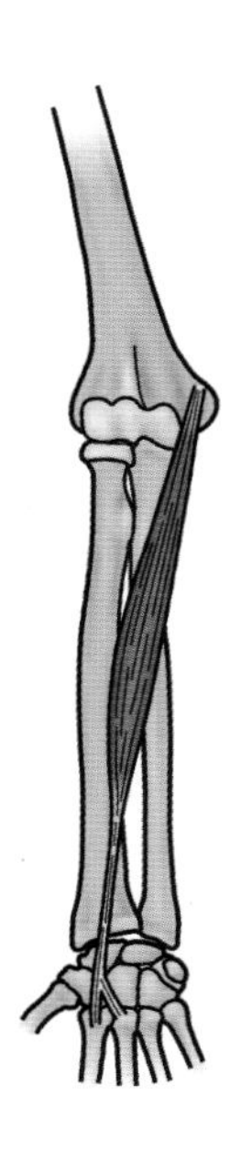

Concentric action:
Flexion and radial deviation (abduction) of the hand at the wrist joint, flexion of the forearm at the elbow joint, and pronation of the forearm at the radioulnar joints
Eccentric action:
Restrains/controls (especially rapid movement) extension and ulnar deviation (adduction) of the hand and extension and supination of the forearm
Isometric action:
Stabilizes the wrist
Origin, fixed end, proximal attachment, arises from:
Common flexor tendon from the medial epicondyle of the humerus and deep antebrachial fascia
Insertion, mobile end, distal attachment, attaches to:
Base of the second and third metacarpal bones
Innervation:
Median nerve (C6–C7)
Major synergists:
All flexors of the hand and the extensor carpi radialis longus and extensor carpi radialis brevis
Major antagonists:
All extensors of the hand and the flexor carpi ulnaris

Palmaris longus (pal-MAR-iss LONG-us)

Palmaris means "related to the palm"; *longus* means "long."

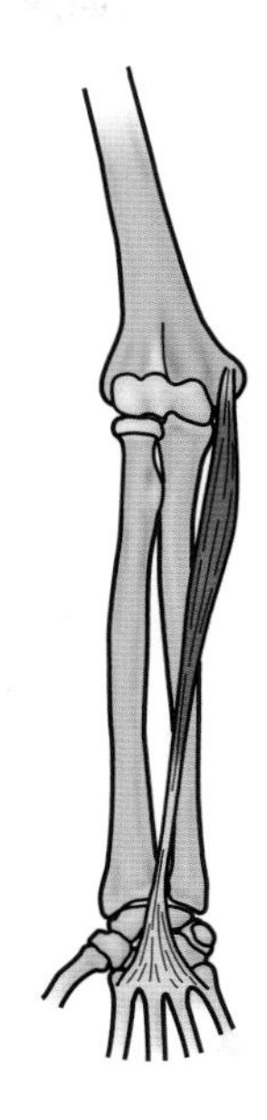

Concentric action:
Flexion of the hand at the wrist joint, flexion of the forearm at the elbow joint, and pronation of the forearm at the radioulnar joints
Eccentric action:
Restrains/controls (especially rapid movement) extension of the hand and extension and supination of the forearm
Isometric action:
Tenses the palmar fascia
Origin, fixed end, proximal attachment, arises from:
Common flexor tendon from the medial epicondyle of the humerus and deep antebrachial fascia
Insertion, mobile end, distal attachment, attaches to:
Flexor retinaculum and palmar aponeurosis
Innervation:
Median nerve (C7–C8)
Major synergists:
All flexors of the hand and the palmaris brevis
Major antagonists:
All extensors of the hand

The tendon of the palmaris longus is superficial to the antebrachial fascia of the wrist and is visible if one cups the hand and slightly flexes the wrist. This muscle is absent in about one-fourth of the population.

Flexor carpi ulnaris (FLEKS-or KAR-pee ul-NAR-iss)

Flexor means "to bend," *carpi* means "of the wrist," and *ulnaris* means "related to the ulna."

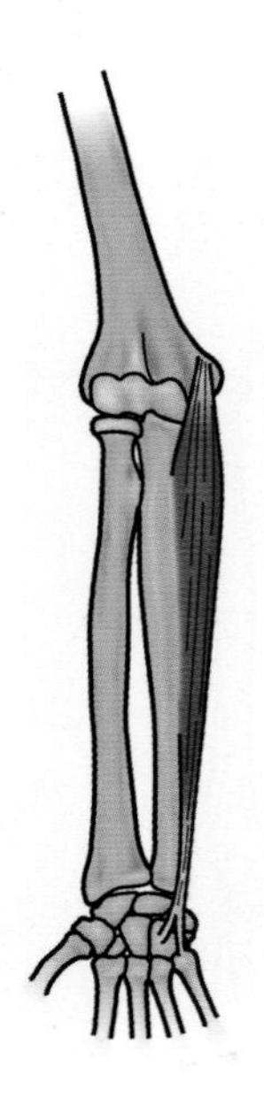

Concentric action:
Flexion and ulnar deviation (adduction) of the hand at the wrist joint and flexion of the forearm at the elbow joint

Eccentric action:
Restrains/controls (especially rapid movement) extension and radial deviation (abduction) of the hand and extension of the forearm

Isometric action:
Stabilizes the wrist

Origin, fixed end, proximal attachment, arises from:
Humeral head—common flexor tendon from the medial epicondyle of the humerus
Ulnar head—olecranon, proximal two-thirds of the posterior border of the ulna, and deep antebrachial fascia

Insertion, mobile end, distal attachment, attaches to:
Pisiform bone and, indirectly, by ligaments to the hamate and fifth metacarpal bones

Innervation:
Ulnar nerve (C7–C8)

Major synergists:
All flexors of the hand and the extensor carpi ulnaris

Major antagonists:
All extensors of the hand and the flexor carpi radialis

ACTIVITY 9.25

Draw and color the *muscles of the anterior flexor group: superficial layer* in the spaces provided. For each muscle:

1. Label the origin and insertion attachment points: *O* for origin; *I* for insertion.
2. Place an X on the trigger points.
3. Palpate this muscle; identify the attachment points and the bellies of the muscles.
4. Move these muscles on yourself.

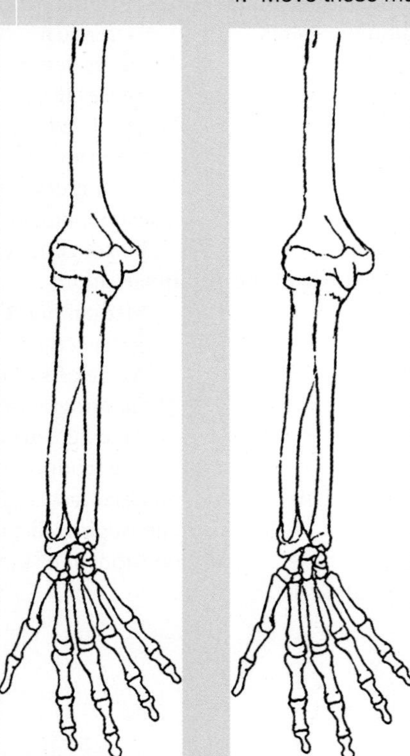

Anterior Flexor Group: Intermediate Layer

Flexor digitorum superficialis (FLEKS-or DIH-jih-TOR-um SOO-per-fish-ee-AL-us)

Flexor means "to bend," *digitorum* means "of the fingers or toes," and *superficialis* means "related to the top or surface."

Anterior

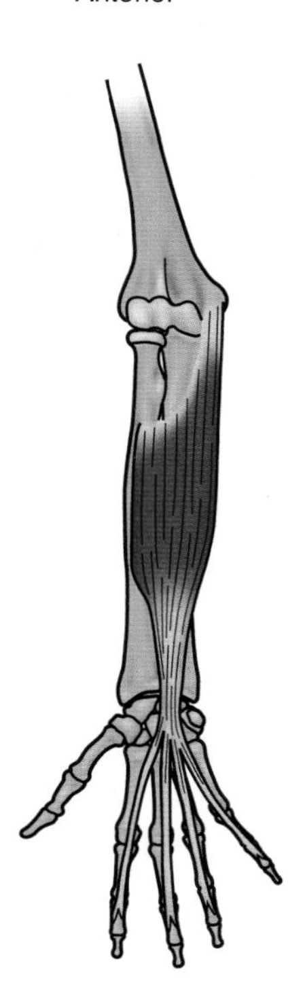

Concentric action:
Flexion of fingers 2 to 5 at the metacarpophalangeal and proximal interphalangeal joints and flexion of the hand at the wrist joint
Eccentric action:
Restrains/controls (especially rapid movement) finger extension and hand extension
Isometric action:
Stabilizes wrist and finger joints
Origin, fixed end, proximal attachment, arises from:
Humeral head—common flexor tendon from the medial epicondyle of the humerus, ulnar collateral ligament of the elbow joint, and deep antebrachial fascia
Ulnar head—medial side of the coronoid process of the ulna
Radial head—oblique line of the radius
Insertion, mobile end, distal attachment, attaches to:
Sides of the palmar surface of the middle phalanges of the second through fifth fingers
Innervation:
Median nerve (C7–T1)
Major synergist:
Flexor digitorum profundus
Major antagonist:
Extensor digitorum

ACTIVITY 9.26

Draw and color the *muscle of the anterior flexor group: intermediate layer* in the spaces provided:

1. Label the origin and insertion attachment points: *O* for origin; *I* for insertion.
2. Place an X on the trigger points.
3. Palpate this muscle; identify the attachment points and the belly of the muscle.
4. Move this muscle on yourself.

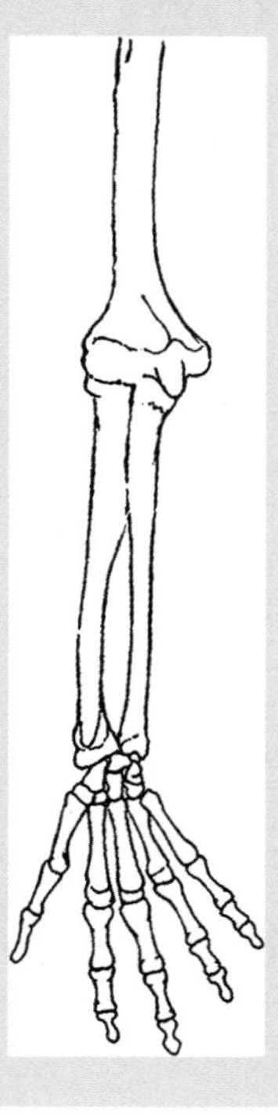

Anterior Flexor Group: Deep Layer

Flexor digitorum profundus (FLEKS-or DIH-jih-TOR-um pro-FUND-us)

Flexor means "to bend," *digitorum* means "related to the fingers or toes," and *profundus* means "deep."

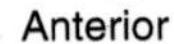

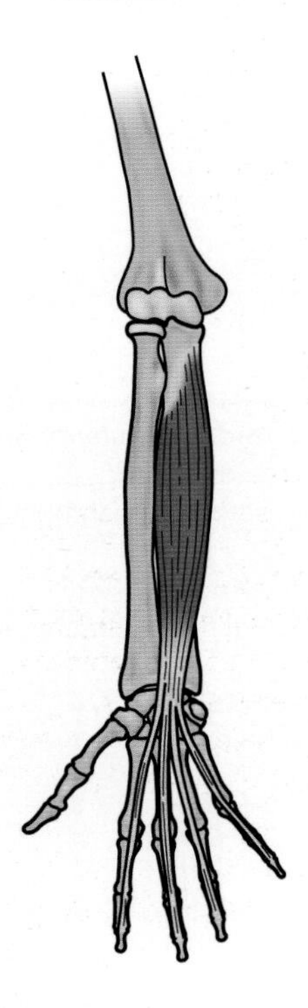

Concentric action:
Flexion of fingers 2 to 5 at the metacarpophalangeal, proximal, and distal interphalangeal joints and flexion of the hand at the wrist joint
Eccentric action:
Restrains/controls (especially rapid movement) extension of the fingers and extension of the hand
Isometric action:
Stabilizes wrist and finger joints
Origin, fixed end, proximal attachment, arises from:
Medial and anterior surfaces of the proximal half of the ulna, interosseous membrane, and deep antebrachial fascia
Insertion, mobile end, distal attachment, attaches to:
By four tendons into the distal phalanges of fingers 2 to 5 on the anterior surface
Innervation:
Ulnar nerve and interosseous branch of the median nerve (C7–T1)
Major synergist:
Flexor digitorum superficialis
Major antagonist:
Extensor digitorum

Flexor pollicis longus (FLEKS-or POLL-is-iss LONG-us)

Flexor means "to bend," *pollicis* means "of the thumb," and *longus* means "long."

Anterior

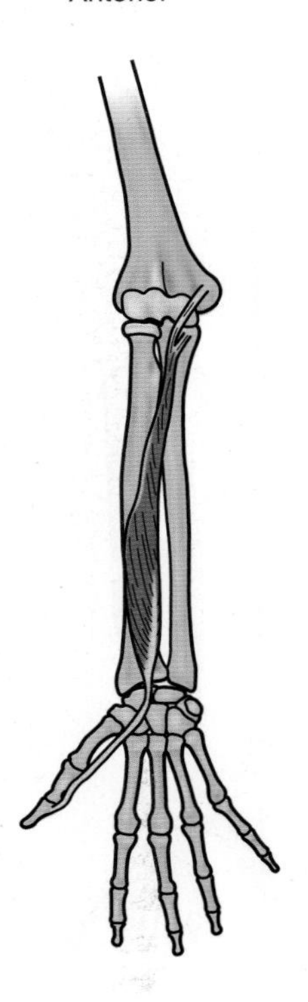

Concentric action:
Flexion of the thumb at the carpometacarpal, metacarpophalangeal, and interphalangeal joints
Eccentric action:
Restrains/controls (especially rapid movement) extension of the thumb
Isometric action:
Stabilizes the thumb
Origin, fixed end, proximal attachment, arises from:
Anterior surface of the radius medial epicondyle of the humerus, the coronoid process of the ulna, and interosseous membrane
Insertion, mobile end, distal attachment, attaches to:
Palmar surface of the base of the distal phalanx of the thumb
Innervation:
Anterior interosseous branch of the median nerve (C7–C8)
Major synergist:
Flexor pollicis brevis
Major antagonists:
Extensor pollicis longus and extensor pollicis brevis
Tender/trigger points
Elements common to the anterior flexion group:
Tender/trigger points:
In the belly
Common symptom/Common symptom/Referred pain pattern:
Into the wrist, associated fingers, or thumb and occasionally into the elbow

ACTIVITY 9.27

Draw and color the *muscles of the anterior flexor group: deep layer* in the spaces provided. For each muscle:

1. Label the origin and insertion attachment points: *O* for origin; *I* for insertion.
2. Place an X on the trigger points.
3. Palpate this muscle; identify the attachment points and the bellies of the muscles.
4. Move these muscles on yourself.

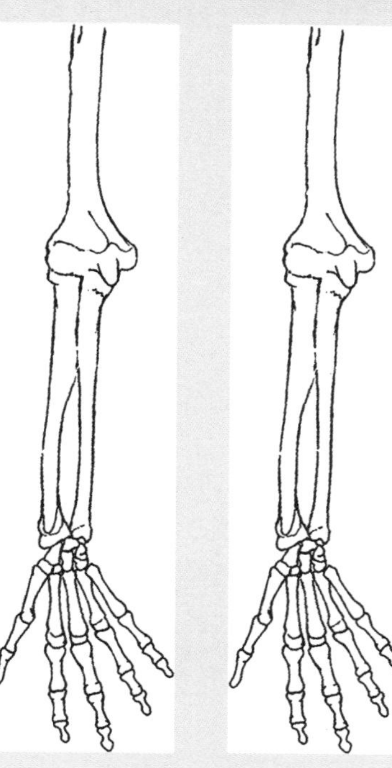

Posterior Extensor Group: Superficial Layer

Extensor carpi radialis longus (ex-STEN-sur KAR-pee RAY-dee-AL-iss LONG-us)

Extensor means "one that stretches," *carpi* means "related to the wrist," *radialis* means "related to the radius," and *longus* means "long."

Posterior

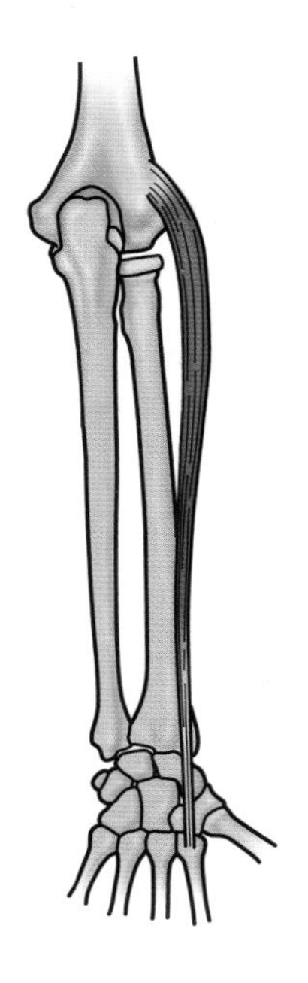

Concentric action:
Extension and radial deviation (abduction) of the hand at the wrist joint, flexion of the forearm at the elbow joint

Eccentric action:
Restrains/controls (especially rapid movement) flexion and ulnar deviation (adduction) of the hand, extension of the forearm, and pronation of the forearm at the radioulnar joint

Isometric action:
Stabilizes wrist and elbow joints

Origin, fixed end, proximal attachment, arises from:
Distal one-third of the lateral supracondylar ridge of the humerus and lateral intermuscular septum

Insertion, mobile end, distal attachment, attaches to:
Dorsal surface of the base of the second metacarpal bone on the radial side

Innervation:
Radial nerve (C5–C6)

Major synergists:
All extensors of the hand and the flexor carpi radialis

Major antagonists:
All flexors of the hand and the extensor carpi ulnaris

Extensor carpi radialis brevis (ex-STEN-sur KAR-pee RAY-dee-AL-iss BREV-iss)

Extensor means "one that stretches," *carpi* means "of the wrist," *radialis* means "related to the radius," and *brevis* means "short."

Posterior

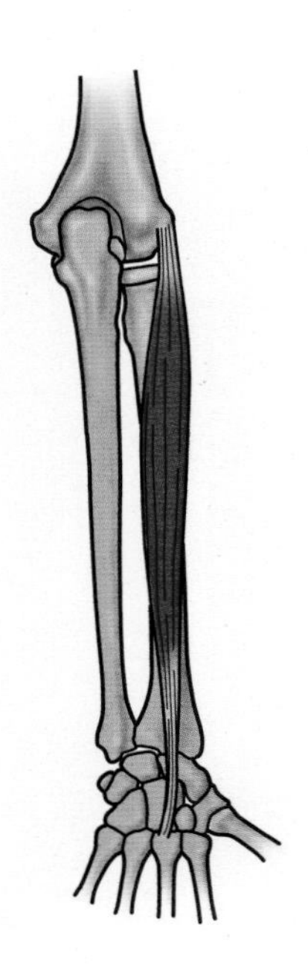

Concentric action:
Extension and radial deviation (abduction) of the hand at the wrist joint and flexion of the forearm at the elbow joint

Eccentric action:
Restrains/controls (especially rapid movement) flexion and ulnar deviation (adduction) of the hand and extension of the forearm

Isometric action:
Stabilizes the wrist joint

Origin, fixed end, proximal attachment, arises from:
Common extensor tendon from the lateral epicondyle of the humerus, radial collateral ligament of the elbow joint, and deep antebrachial fascia

Insertion, mobile end, distal attachment, attaches to:
Dorsal surface of the base of the third metacarpal bone

Innervation:
Posterior interosseous branch of the radial nerve (C7–C8)

Major synergists:
All extensors of the hand and the flexor carpi radialis

Major antagonists:
All flexors of the hand and the extensor carpi ulnaris

Extensor digitorum (ex-STEN-sur DIH-jih-TOR-um)

Extensor means "one that stretches"; *digitorum* means "of the fingers or toes."

Posterior

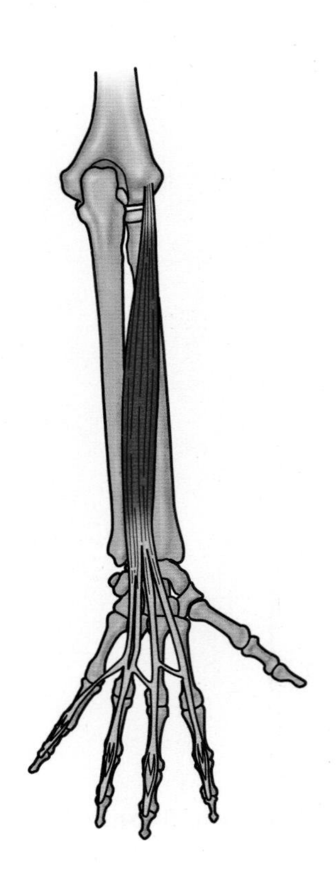

Concentric action:
Extension of fingers 2 to 5 at the metacarpophalangeal and proximal and distal interphalangeal joints and extension of the hand at the wrist joint

Eccentric action:
Restrains/controls (especially rapid movement) flexion of the fingers and flexion of the hand

Isometric action:
Stabilizes the finger and wrist joints

Origin, fixed end, proximal attachment, arises from:
Common extensor tendon from the lateral epicondyle of the humerus and intermuscular septa

Insertion, mobile end, distal attachment, attaches to:
By four tendons to the lateral and dorsal surface of the phalanges of the second through fifth digits

Innervation:
Posterior interosseous branch of the radial nerve (C7–C8)

Major synergists:
Extensor digiti minimi, extensor indicis, lumbrical muscles, palmar interossei, and dorsal interossei manus

Major antagonists:
Flexor digitorum superficialis and flexor digitorum profundus

The distal tendon of this muscle forms the dorsal digital expansion of fingers 2 to 5.

Extensor digiti minimi (ex-STEN-sur DIH-jih-tee MIN-ih-mee)

Extensor means "one that stretches," *digiti* means "of the fingers or toes," and *minimi* means "smallest."

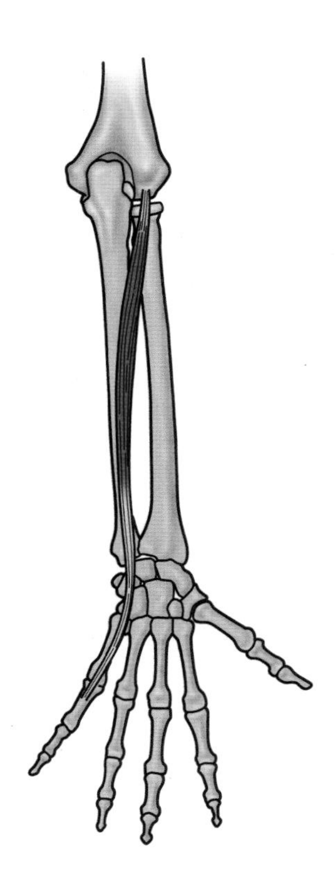

Concentric action:
Extension of the little finger at the metacarpophalangeal, proximal, and distal interphalangeal joints
Eccentric action:
Restrains/controls (especially rapid movement) flexion of the little finger
Isometric action:
Stabilizes the little finger
Origin, fixed end, proximal attachment, arises from:
Common extensor tendon from the lateral epicondyle of the humerus and intermuscular septa
Insertion, mobile end, distal attachment, attaches to:
Into the dorsal digital expansion of the little finger with the extensor digitorum tendon
Innervation:
Posterior interosseous branch of the radial nerve (C7–C8)
Major synergist:
Extensor digitorum
Major antagonists:
Flexor digitorum superficialis and flexor digitorum profundus

Extensor carpi ulnaris (ex-STEN-sur KAR-pee ul-NAR-iss)

Extensor means "one that stretches," *carpi* means "of the wrist," and *ulnaris* means "related to the ulna."

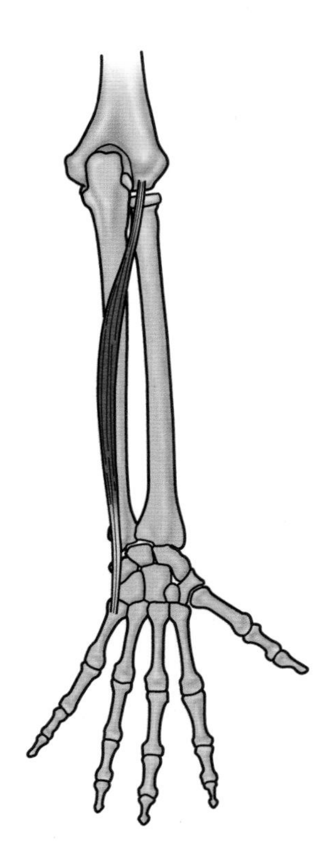

Concentric action:
Extension and ulnar deviation (adduction) of the hand at the wrist joint
Eccentric action:
Restrains/controls (especially rapid movement) flexion and radial deviation (abduction) of the hand
Isometric action:
Stabilizes the wrist joint
Origin, fixed end, proximal attachment, arises from:
Common extensor tendon from the lateral epicondyle of the humerus and the aponeurosis from the posterior border of the ulna
Insertion, mobile end, distal attachment, attaches to:
Posterior side of the base of the fifth metacarpal bone
Innervation:
Posterior interosseous branch of the radial nerve (C7–C8)
Major synergists:
All extensors of the hand and the flexor carpi ulnaris
Major antagonists:
All flexors of the hand and the extensor carpi radialis longus and extensor carpi radialis brevis

ACTIVITY 9.28

Draw and color the *muscles of the posterior extensor group: superficial layer* in the spaces provided. For each muscle:

1. Label the origin and insertion attachment points: *O* for origin; *I* for insertion.
2. Place an X on the trigger points.
3. Palpate this muscle; identify the attachment points and the bellies of the muscles.
4. Move these muscles on yourself.

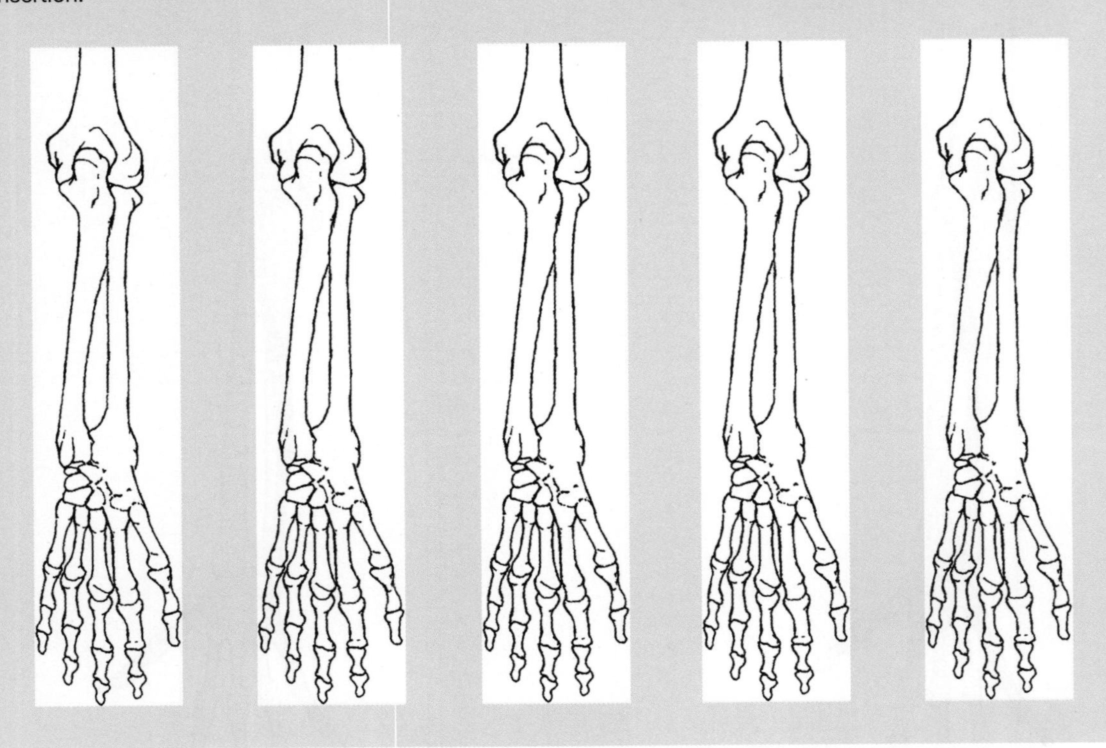

Posterior Extensor Group: Deep Layer

Extensor pollicis brevis (ex-STEN-sur POLL-is-iss BREV-iss)

Extensor means "one that stretches," *pollicis* means "of the thumb," and *brevis* means "short."

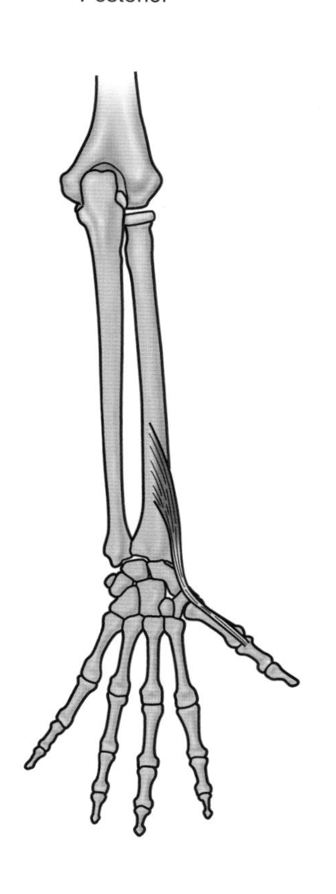

Concentric action:
Extension of the thumb at the carpometacarpal and metacarpophalangeal joints, abduction of the thumb at the carpometacarpal joint, radial deviation (abduction) of the hand at the wrist joint, and supination of the forearm at the radioulnar joints

Eccentric action:
Restrains/controls (especially rapid movement) flexion and adduction of the thumb, ulnar deviation (adduction) of the hand, and pronation of the forearm

Isometric action:
Stabilizes the thumb

Origin, fixed end, proximal attachment, arises from:
Posterior surface of the shaft of the radius distal to the origin of the abductor pollicis longus and the interosseous membrane

Insertion, mobile end, distal attachment, attaches to:
Base of the proximal phalanx of the thumb on the dorsal surface

Innervation:
Posterior interosseous branch of the radial nerve (C7–C8)

Major synergists:
Extensor pollicis longus, abductor pollicis longus, and abductor pollicis brevis

Major antagonists:
Flexor pollicis longus, flexor pollicis brevis, and adductor pollicis

Abductor pollicis longus (ab-DUCK-tur POLL-is-iss LONG-us)

Abductor means "one that leads away," *pollicis* means "of the thumb," and *longus* means "long."

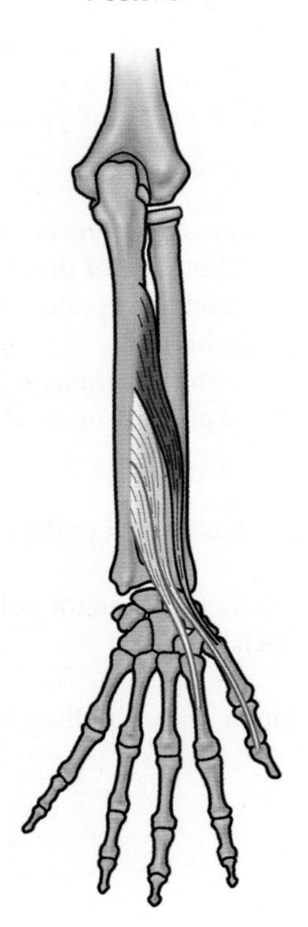

Concentric action:
Abduction and extension of the thumb at the carpometacarpal joint, radial deviation (abduction) and flexion of the hand at the wrist joint, and supination of the forearm at the radioulnar joints
Eccentric action:
Restrains/controls (especially rapid movement) adduction and flexion of the thumb, ulnar deviation (adduction) and extension of the hand, and pronation of the forearm
Isometric action:
Stabilizes the thumb and the wrist joint
Origin, fixed end, proximal attachment, arises from:
Posterior surface of the shaft of the ulna distal to the origin of the supinator, interosseous membrane, and posterior surface of the middle one-third of the shaft of the radius
Insertion, mobile end, distal attachment, attaches to:
Base of the first metacarpal bone of the thumb on the lateral side
Innervation:
Posterior interosseous branch of the radial nerve (C7–C8)
Major synergists:
Abductor pollicis brevis, extensor pollicis longus, and extensor pollicis brevis
Major antagonists:
Adductor pollicis, flexor pollicis longus, and flexor pollicis brevis

Extensor pollicis longus (ex-STEN-sur POLL-is-iss LONG-us)

Extensor means "one that stretches," *pollicis* means "of the thumb," and *longus* means "long."

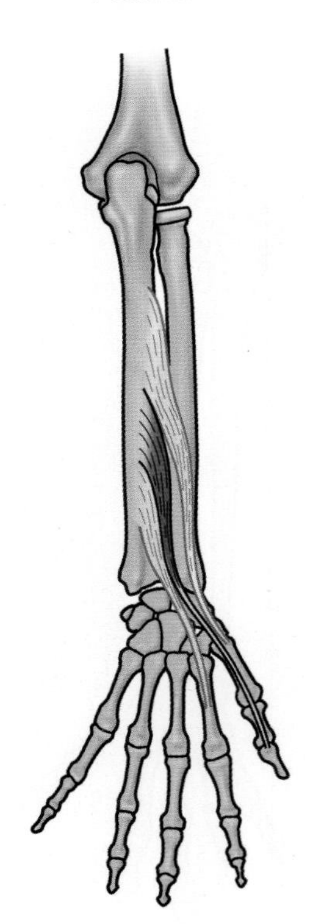

Concentric action:
Extension of the thumb at the carpometacarpal, metacarpophalangeal, and interphalangeal joints; radial deviation (abduction) of the hand at the wrist joint; and supination of the forearm at the radioulnar joints
Eccentric action:
Restrains/controls (especially rapid movement) flexion of the thumb, ulnar deviation (adduction) of the hand, and pronation of the forearm
Isometric action:
Stabilizes the thumb and the wrist joint
Origin, fixed end, proximal attachment, arises from:
Middle one-third of the posterior surface of the ulna distal to the origin of the abductor pollicis longus and the interosseous membrane
Insertion, mobile end, distal attachment, attaches to:
Dorsal surface of the base of the distal phalanx of the thumb
Innervation:
Posterior interosseous branch of the radial nerve (C7–C8)
Major synergist:
Extensor pollicis brevis
Major antagonists:
Flexor pollicis longus and flexor pollicis brevis

Extensor indicis (ex-STEN-sur IN-dih-siss)

Extensor means "one that stretches"; *indicis* means "of the index finger."

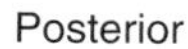
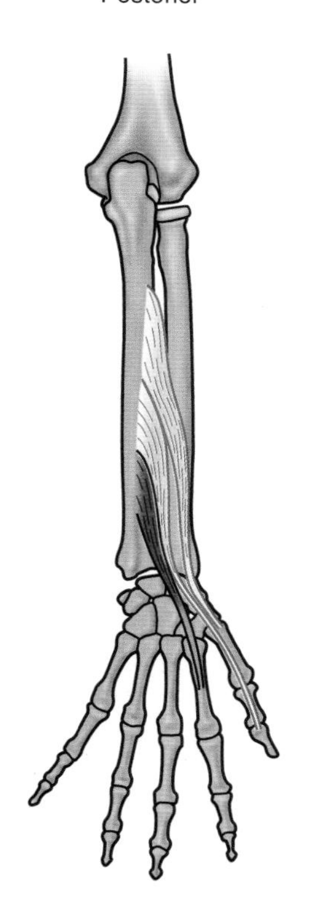

Concentric action:
Extension of the index finger at the metacarpophalangeal, proximal, and distal interphalangeal joints; adduction of the index finger at the metacarpophalangeal joint; and supination of the forearm at the radioulnar joints

Eccentric action:
Restrains/controls (especially rapid movement) flexion and abduction of the index finger and pronation of the forearm

Isometric action:
Stabilizes the index finger

Origin, fixed end, proximal attachment, arises from:
Posterior surface of the ulna and the interosseous membrane

Insertion, mobile end, distal attachment, attaches to:
Into the dorsal digital expansion of the index finger with the extensor digitorum tendon

Innervation:
Posterior interosseous branch of the radial nerve (C7–C8)

Major synergist:
Extensor digitorum

Major antagonists:
Flexor digitorum superficialis and flexor digitorum profundus

Elements common to the posterior extensor group muscles:

Major synergists:
For extension, all extensors are synergistic with each other; for radial deviation of the hand, the extensor carpi radialis muscles are synergistic with the flexor carpi radialis; for ulnar deviation, the extensor and flexor carpi ulnaris muscles are synergistic.

Major antagonists:
The flexor group; the ulnar deviation and radial deviation groups are antagonistic to each other

Tender/trigger points:
Belly of each muscle, located nearer the elbow

Common symptom/Common symptom/Referred pain pattern:
From the lateral epicondyle at the elbow down the dorsum of the forearm to various parts of the hand, especially to the web of the thumb

ACTIVITY 9.29

Draw and color the *muscles of the posterior extensor group: deep layer* in the spaces provided. For each muscle:

1. Label the origin and insertion attachment points: *O* for origin; *I* for insertion.
2. Place an X on the trigger points.
3. Palpate this muscle; identify the attachment points and the bellies of the muscles.
4. Move these muscles on yourself.

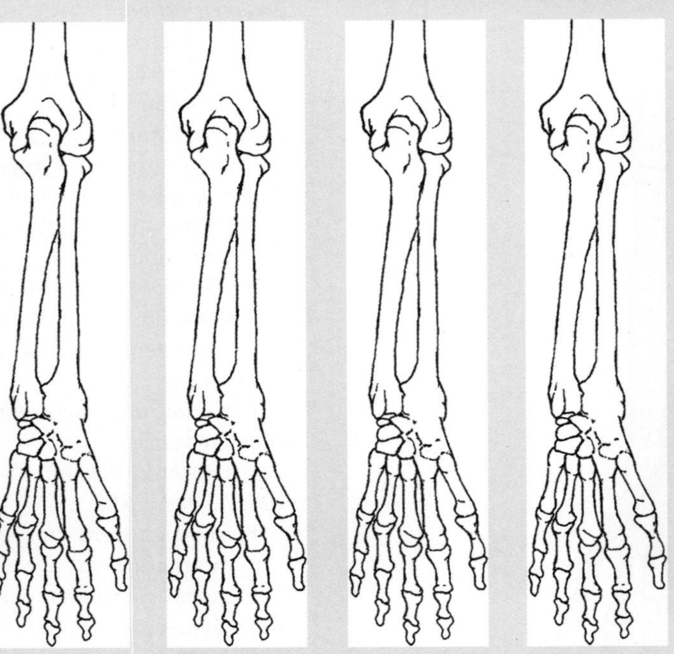

Intrinsic Muscles of the Hand

Intrinsic muscles of the hand are small muscles that are located wholly within the hand (i.e., they originate and insert within the hand). The complex and intricate nature of these muscles allows for an almost limitless variety of fine hand movements. The delicacy of the muscles and the interactive pattern of their layout are unique to the human hand (Fig. 9.25).

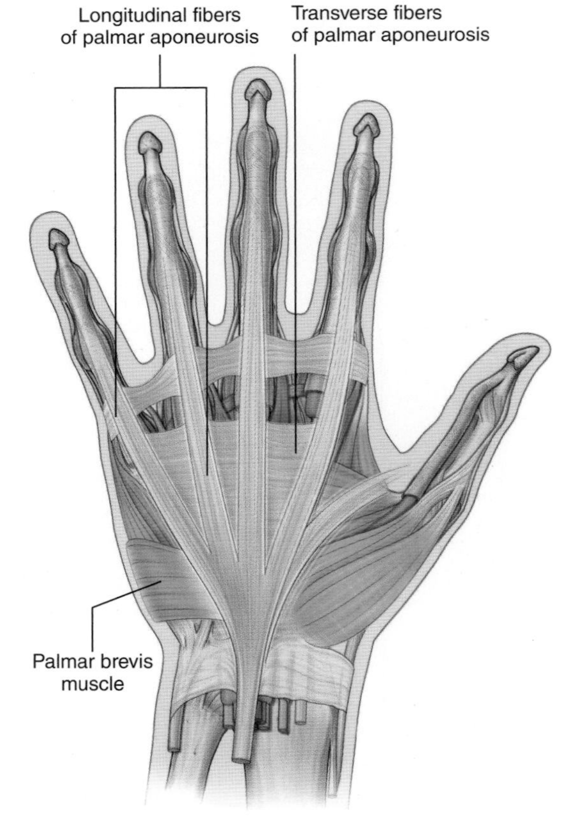

FIG. 9.25 Palmar aponeurosis. (From Drake RL, Vogl W, Mitchell WM. *Gray's Anatomy for Students*. 2nd ed. Churchill Livingstone; 2010.)

Thenar Eminence Muscles

Opponens pollicis (oh-PONE-ens POLL-is-iss)

Opponens means "opposing"; *pollicis* means "of the thumb."

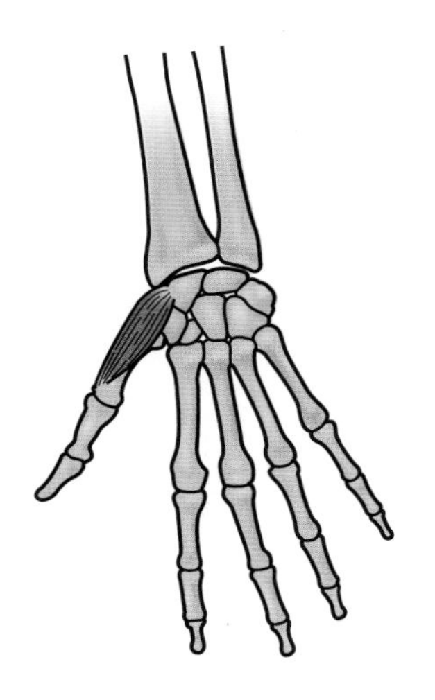

Concentric action:
Opposition of the thumb at the carpometacarpal joint (opposition is the movement in which the thumb pad comes to meet the finger pad of any other finger; opposition of the thumb is usually considered to be a combination of abduction, flexion, and medial rotation of the thumb at the carpometacarpal joint)

Eccentric action:
Restrains/controls (especially rapid movement) reposition of the thumb

Isometric action:
Stabilizes the thumb

Origin, fixed end, proximal attachment, arises from:
Flexor retinaculum and trapezium bone

Insertion, mobile end, distal attachment, attaches to:
Anterior surface on the radial side of the first metacarpal bone

Innervation:
Median and ulnar nerves (C8 to T1)

Major synergists:
Flexor pollicis brevis and abductor pollicis brevis

Major antagonists:
Extensor pollicis longus, extensor pollicis brevis, and adductor pollicis

Tender/trigger points:
In the belly of the muscle

Common symptom/Common symptom/Referred pain pattern:
Into the thumb and the wrist

Abductor pollicis brevis (ab-DUCK-tur POLL-is-iss BREV-iss)

Abductor means "one that leads away," *pollicis* means "of the thumb," and *brevis* means "short."

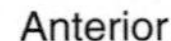

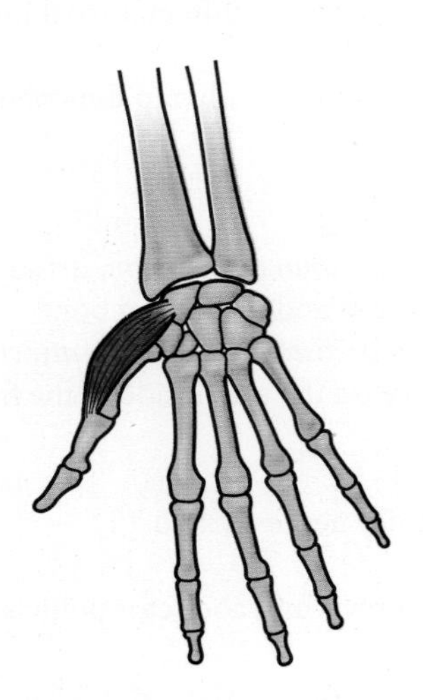

Concentric action:
Abduction of the thumb at the metacarpophalangeal joint

Eccentric action:
Restrains/controls (especially rapid movement) adduction of the thumb

Isometric action:
Stabilizes the thumb

Origin, fixed end, proximal attachment, arises from:
Flexor retinaculum, tubercle of the trapezium bone, and tubercle of the scaphoid bone

Insertion, mobile end, distal attachment, attaches to:
Radial side of the base of the proximal phalanx of the thumb and dorsal digital expansion

Innervation:
Median nerve (C8–T1)

Major synergist:
Abductor pollicis longus

Major antagonist:
Adductor pollicis

Tender/trigger points:
In the belly of the muscle

Common symptom/Common symptom/Referred pain pattern:
Into the thumb and the wrist

Flexor pollicis brevis (FLEKS-or POLL-is-iss BREV-iss)

Flexor means "one that bends," *pollicis* means "of the thumb," and *brevis* means "short."

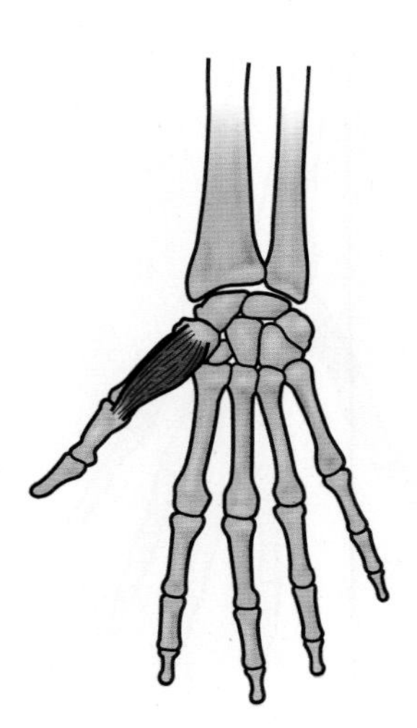

Concentric action:
Flexion of the thumb at the carpometacarpal and metacarpophalangeal joints

Eccentric action:
Restrains/controls (especially rapid movement) extension of the thumb

Isometric action:
Stabilizes the thumb

Origin, fixed end, proximal attachment, arises from:
Superficial head—flexor retinaculum and trapezium bone
Deep head—trapezoid and capitate bones

Insertion, mobile end, distal attachment, attaches to:
Radial side of the base of the proximal phalanx of the thumb and dorsal digital expansion

Innervation:
Median and ulnar nerves (C8 to T1)

Major synergist:
Flexor pollicis longus

Major antagonists:
Extensor pollicis longus and extensor pollicis brevis

Tender/trigger points:
In the belly of the muscle

Common symptom/Common symptom/Referred pain pattern:
Into the thumb and the wrist

ACTIVITY 9.30

Draw and color the *thenar eminence muscles* in the spaces provided. For each muscle:

1. Label the origin and insertion attachment points: *O* for origin; *I* for insertion.
2. Place an X on the trigger points.
3. Palpate this muscle; identify the attachment points and the bellies of the muscles.
4. Move these muscles on yourself.

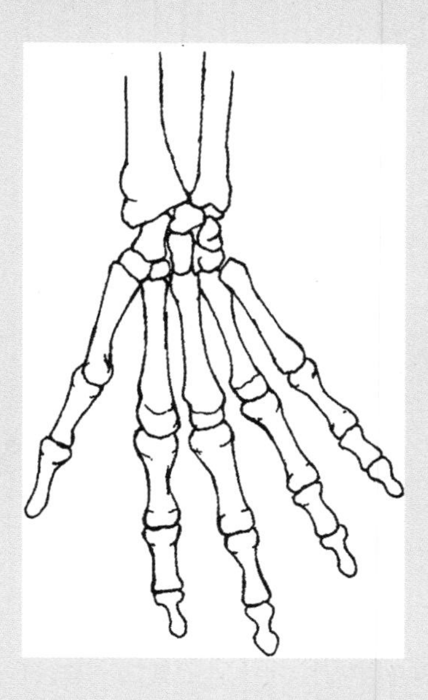

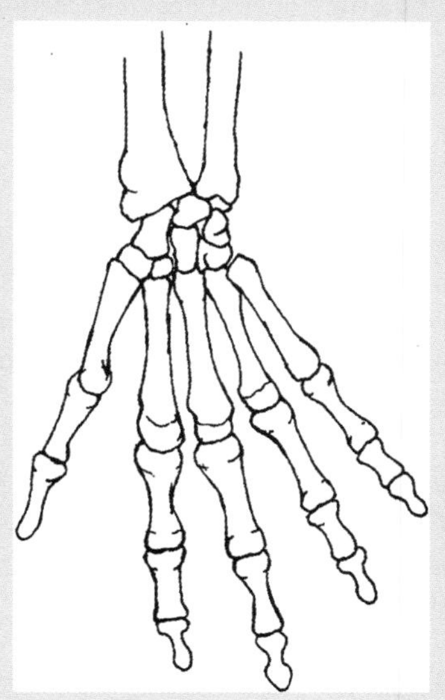

Hypothenar Muscles

Opponens digiti minimi (oh-PONE-ens DIH-jih-tee MIN-ih-mee)

Opponens means "opposing," *digiti* means "of the fingers or toes," and *minimi* means "smallest."

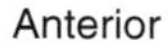

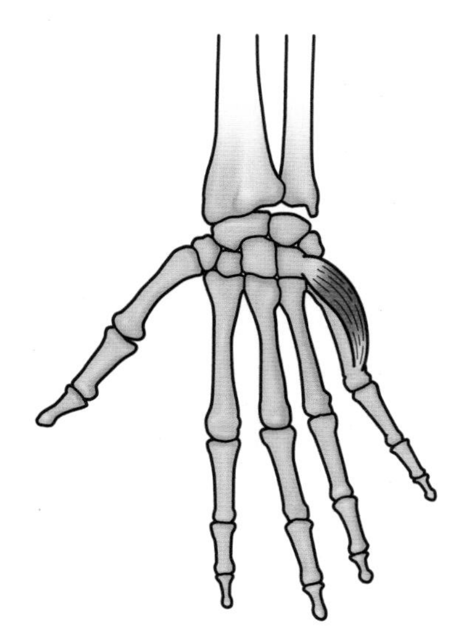

Concentric action:
Opposition of the little finger at the carpometacarpal joint
Opposition is the movement in which the finger pad of the little finger comes to meet the finger pad of the thumb. Opposition of the little finger is actually a combination of flexion, adduction, and lateral rotation of the little finger at the carpometacarpal joint.

Eccentric action:
Restrains/controls (especially rapid movement) reposition of the little finger

Isometric action:
Stabilizes the little finger

Origin, fixed end, proximal attachment, arises from:
Flexor retinaculum and the hook of the hamate bone

Insertion, mobile end, distal attachment, attaches to:
Entire length of the fifth metacarpal bone on the ulnar side

Innervation:
The ulnar nerve (C8–T1)

Major synergists:
Flexor digitorum superficialis, flexor digitorum profundus, and palmar interossei (No. 3)

Major antagonists:
Extensor digitorum, extensor digiti minimi, and abductor digiti minimi manus

Tender/trigger points:
In the belly of the muscle

Common symptom/Common symptom/Referred pain pattern:
Into the little finger and wrist

Abductor digiti minimi manus (ab-DUCK-tur DIH-jih-tee MIN-ih-mee MAN-us)

Abductor means "one that leads away," *digiti* means "of the fingers or toes," *minimi* means "smallest," and *manus* means "of the hand."

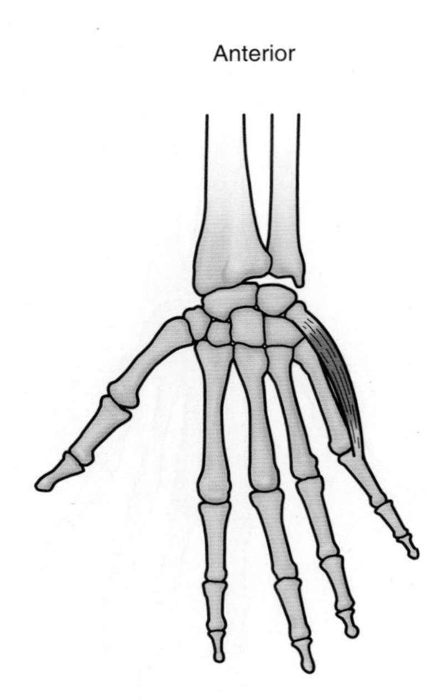

Concentric action:
Abduction of the little finger at the metacarpophalangeal joint
Eccentric action:
Restrains/controls (especially rapid movement) adduction of the little finger
Isometric action:
Stabilizes the little finger
Origin, fixed end, proximal attachment, arises from:
Tendon of the flexor carpi ulnaris and the pisiform bone
Insertion, mobile end, distal attachment, attaches to:
Base of the proximal phalanx of the little finger on the ulnar side and dorsal digital expansion
Innervation:
Ulnar nerve (C8–T1)
Major synergists:
No major synergists
Major antagonists:
Palmar interossei (No. 3)
Tender/trigger points:
In the belly of the muscle
Common symptom/Common symptom/Referred pain pattern:
Into the little finger and wrist

Flexor digiti minimi manus (FLEKS-or DIH-jih-tee MIN-ih-mee MAN-us)

Flexor means "one that bends," *digiti* means "of the fingers or toes," *minimi* means "smallest," and *manus* means "of the hand."

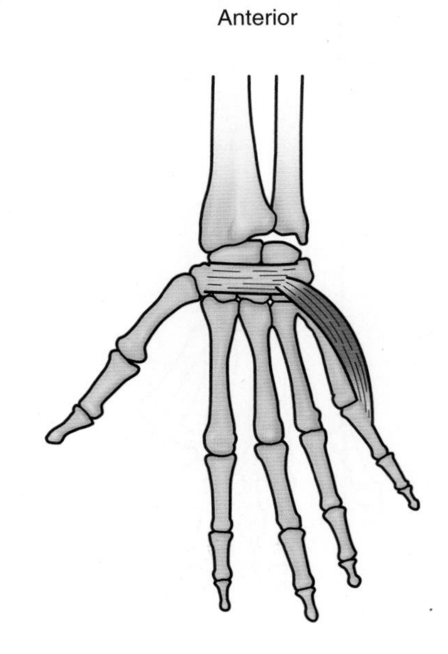

Concentric action:
Flexion of the little finger at the metacarpophalangeal joint
Eccentric action:
Restrains/controls (especially rapid movement) extension of the little finger
Isometric action:
Stabilizes the little finger
Origin, fixed end, proximal attachment, arises from:
Hook of the hamate bone and flexor retinaculum
Insertion, mobile end, distal attachment, attaches to:
Base of the proximal phalanx of the little finger on the ulnar side
Innervation:
Ulnar nerve (C8–T1)
Major synergists:
Flexor digitorum superficialis and flexor digitorum profundus
Major antagonists:
Extensor digitorum and extensor digiti minimi
Tender/trigger points:
In the belly of the muscle
Common symptom/Common symptom/Referred pain pattern:
Into the little finger and wrist

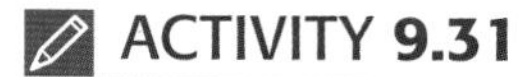

ACTIVITY 9.31

Draw and color the *hypothenar muscles* in the spaces provided. For each muscle:

1. Label the origin and insertion attachment points: *O* for origin; *I* for insertion.
2. Place an X on the trigger points.
3. Palpate this muscle; identify the attachment points and the bellies of the muscles.
4. Move these muscles on yourself.

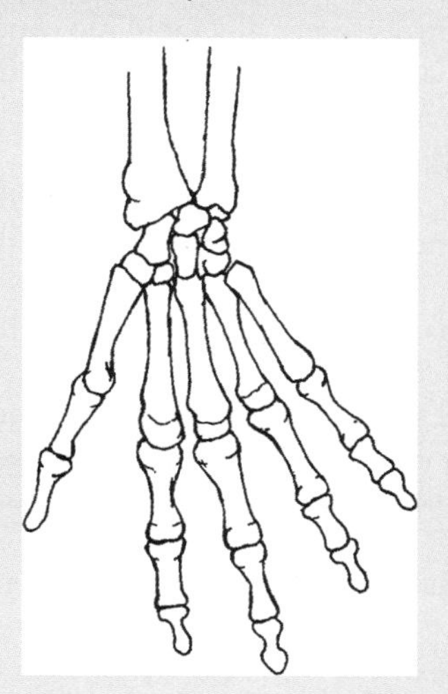

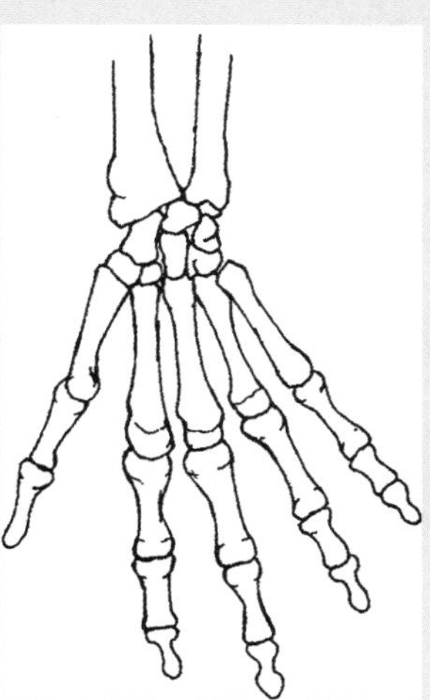

Central Compartment Muscles

Adductor pollicis (ad-DUCK-tur POLL-is-iss)

Adductor means "one that leads toward"; *pollicis* means "of the thumb."

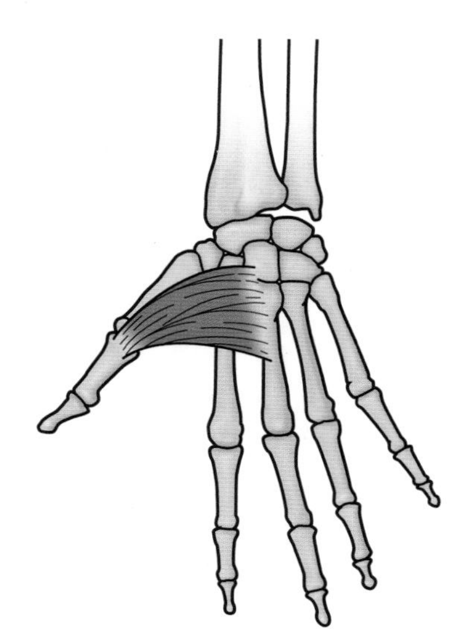

Concentric action:
Adduction of the thumb at the carpometacarpal joint

Eccentric action:
Restrains/controls (especially rapid movement) abduction of the thumb

Isometric action:
Stabilizes the thumb

Origin, fixed end, proximal attachment, arises from:
Oblique head—trapezium, trapezoid, and capitate bones and the base of the second and third metacarpal bones
Transverse head—palmar surface of the third metacarpal

Insertion, mobile end, distal attachment, attaches to:
Ulnar side of the base of the proximal phalanx of the thumb

Innervation:
Ulnar nerve (C8–T1)

Major synergists:
There are no major synergists.

Major antagonists:
Abductor pollicis longus and abductor pollicis brevis

Tender/trigger points:
In the belly of the muscle

Common symptom/Common symptom/Referred pain pattern:
Into the associated finger; commonly associated with Heberden nodes, which develop on the dorsolateral or dorsomedial aspect of the terminal phalanx at its joint

Palmar interossei (PAL-mar INT-er-OSS-ee-eye)

Interossei means "between the bones"; *palmar* means "of the palm."

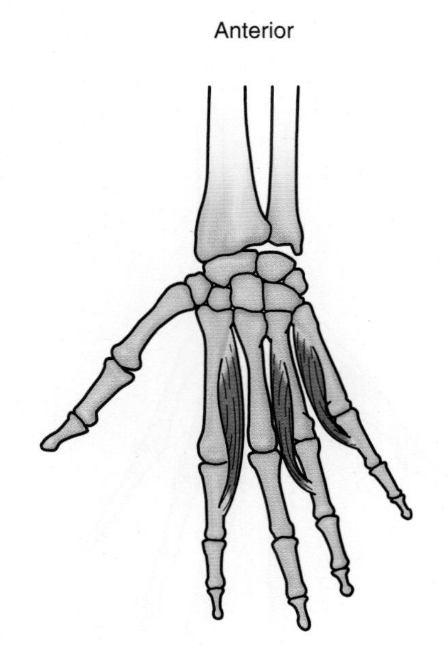

Concentric action:
Adduction of the index, ring, and little fingers (2, 4, and 5) at the metacarpophalangeal joints (adduction of a finger is a movement toward an imaginary line drawn through the middle of the middle finger); flexion of fingers 2, 4, and 5 at the metacarpophalangeal joints; and extension of fingers 2, 4, and 5 at the proximal and distal interphalangeal joints

Eccentric action:
Restrains/controls (especially rapid movement) abduction, extension, and flexion of fingers 2, 4, and 5

Isometric action:
Stabilizes fingers 2, 4, and 5

Origin, fixed end, proximal attachment, arises from:
First—ulnar side of the base of the second metacarpal bone
Second—radial side of the base of the fourth metacarpal bone
Third—radial side of the base of the fifth metacarpal bone

Insertion, mobile end, distal attachment, attaches to:
First—ulnar side of the proximal phalanx of the index finger
Second—radial side of the proximal phalanx of the ring finger
Third—radial side of the proximal phalanx of the little finger

Innervation:
Ulnar nerve (C8–T1)

Major synergists:
Lumbricals manus

Major antagonists:
Dorsal interossei

Tender/trigger points:
In the belly of the muscle

Common symptom/Common symptom/Referred pain pattern:
Into the associated finger; commonly associated with Heberden nodes, which develop on the dorsolateral or dorsomedial aspect of the terminal phalanx at its joint

Dorsal interossei dorsales manus (DOR-sal INT-er-OSS-ee-eye MAN-us)

Interossei means "between the bones," *dorsales* means "related to the back," and *manus* means "of the hand."

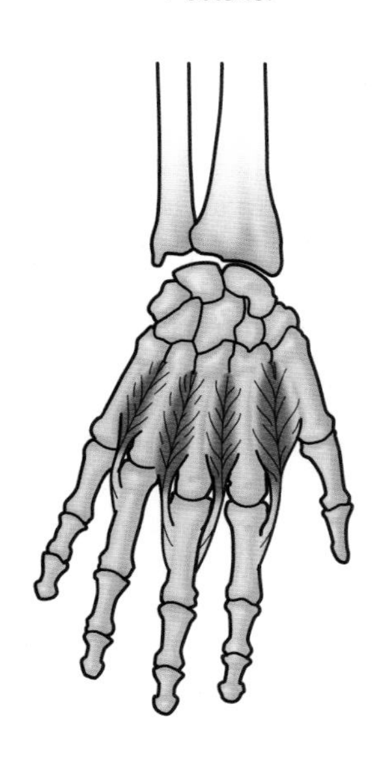

Concentric action:
Abduction of the index, middle, and ring fingers (fingers 2 to 4) at the metacarpophalangeal joints (abduction of a finger is a movement away from an imaginary line drawn through the middle of the middle finger); flexion of fingers 2 to 4 at the metacarpophalangeal joints; and extension of fingers 2 to 4 at the proximal and distal interphalangeal joints

Eccentric action:
Restrains/controls (especially rapid movement) adduction, extension, and flexion of fingers 2 to 4

Isometric action:
Stabilizes fingers 2 to 4

Origin, fixed end, proximal attachment, arises from:
First—adjacent sides of the first and second metacarpal bones
Second—adjacent sides of the second and third metacarpal bones
Third—adjacent sides of the third and fourth metacarpal bones
Fourth—adjacent sides of the fourth and fifth metacarpal bones

Insertion, mobile end, distal attachment, attaches to:
First—radial side of the proximal phalanx of the index finger
Second—radial side of the proximal phalanx of the middle finger
Third—ulnar side of the proximal phalanx of the middle finger
Fourth—ulnar side of the proximal phalanx of the ring finger

Innervation:
Ulnar nerve (C8–T1)

Major synergists:
Lumbricals manus

Major antagonists:
Palmar interossei

Tender/trigger points:
In the belly of the muscle

Common symptom/Common symptom/Referred pain pattern:
Into the associated finger; commonly associated with Heberden nodes, which develop on the dorsolateral or dorsomedial aspect of the terminal phalanx at its joint

Lumbricals manus (LUM-brih-kals MAN-us)

Lumbricals means "earthworms"; *manus* means "of the hand."

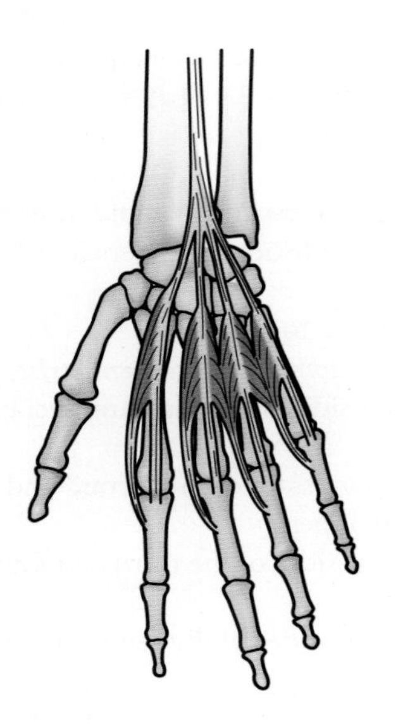

Concentric action:
Extension of the index, middle, ring, and little fingers at the interphalangeal joints and flexion of the index, middle, ring, and little fingers at the metacarpophalangeal joints

Origin, fixed end, proximal attachment, arises from:
First and second—radial surface of the flexor digitorum profundus tendons of the index and middle fingers, respectively
Third—adjacent sides of the flexor digitorum profundus tendons of the middle and ring fingers
Fourth—adjacent sides of the flexor digitorum profundus tendons of the ring and little fingers

Insertion, mobile end, distal attachment, attaches to:
Into the radial border of the dorsal digital expansion on the dorsal aspect of the digits

Innervation:
Median and ulnar nerves (C8 to T1)

Major synergists:
Palmar interossei and dorsal interossei manus, flexor digitorum superficialis, flexor digitorum profundus, and extensor digitorum

Major antagonists:
Flexor digitorum superficialis, flexor digitorum profundus, extensor digitorum

Tender/trigger points:
In the belly of the muscle

Common symptom/Common symptom/Referred pain pattern:
Into the associated finger; commonly associated with Heberden nodes, which develop on the dorsolateral or dorsomedial aspect of the terminal phalanx at its joint

ACTIVITY 9.32

Draw and color the *central compartment muscles* in the spaces provided. For each muscle:

1. Label the origin and insertion attachment points: *O* for origin; *I* for insertion.
2. Place an X on the trigger points.
3. Palpate this muscle; identify the attachment points and the bellies of the muscles.
4. Move these muscles on yourself.

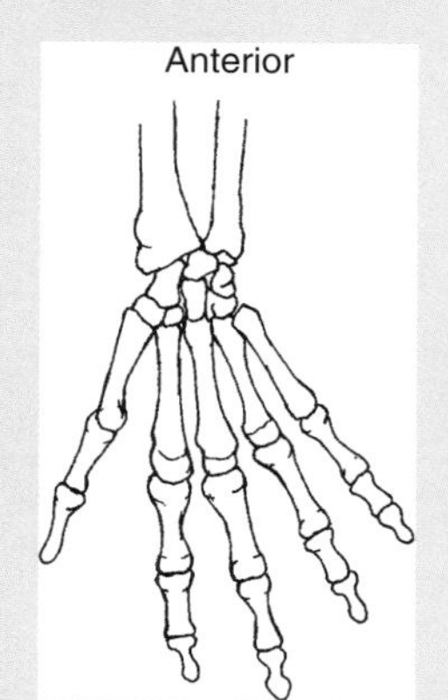

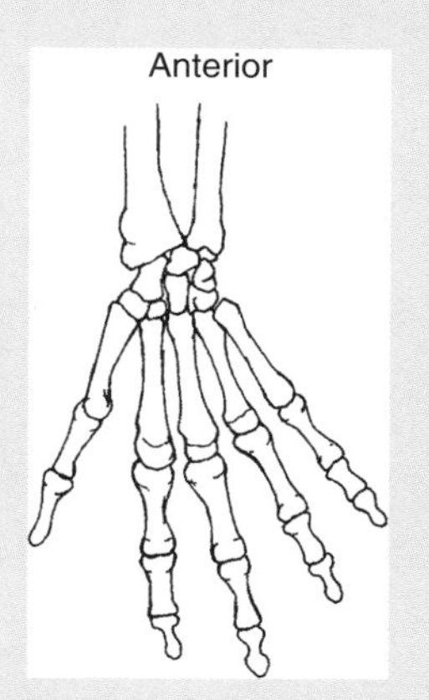

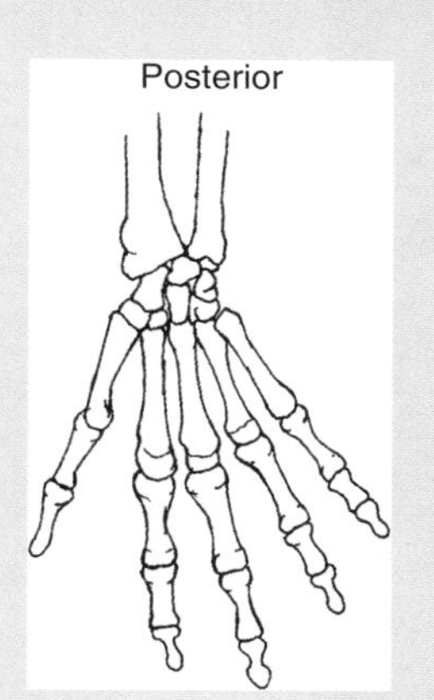

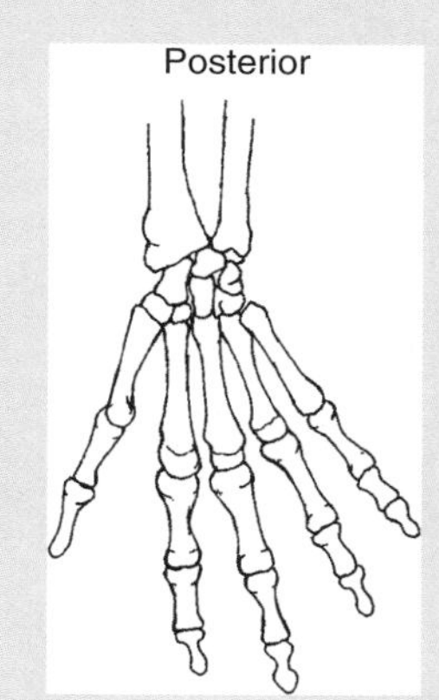

Muscles of the Gluteal Region

The muscles of the gluteal region are some of the most powerful muscles of the body. The more superficial muscles, especially the large gluteus maximus, extend the thigh during forceful extension. The gluteus maximus also stabilizes the iliotibial band and thoracolumbar fascia. The gluteus medius and gluteus minimus are especially strong at abduction and medial (internal) rotation of the thigh. The deep lateral (external) rotators of the thigh at the hip joint are six small, deep muscles of the gluteal region that oppose medial rotation. As a group, the gluteal muscles are related to shoulder extensors and flexors and arm medial and lateral rotators because of gait (walking) reflex patterns to promote the appropriate counterbalancing arm swing. Facilitation between muscles of the arms that flex and extend along with thigh muscles in contralateral patterns occurs.

The massage therapist usually needs to consider the muscles of the shoulder joint with muscles of the hip joint and apply massage in a correlated pattern. Although not listed with synergists and antagonists, the flexors of the thigh at the hip joint work with flexors of the arm at the shoulder joint on the opposite side (i.e., right with left and left with right). These muscles also display inhibitory patterns with each other. For example, right extensors of the thigh at the hip joint are inhibitory to left flexors of the arm at the shoulder joint. On the same side (right arm with right thigh, left arm with left thigh), flexors and extensors work with each other. Adductors and medial rotators of the shoulder joint work with adductors and medial rotators of the hip joint on the opposite side. This same concept is true for abductors and lateral rotators. Conversely, same-side adductors of the shoulder and hip are inhibitory to each other, as are same-side abductors and lateral rotators. Although these patterns may seem confusing, the connection becomes apparent if you take a step and analyze the patterns of the muscles that are working together (Fig. 9.26).

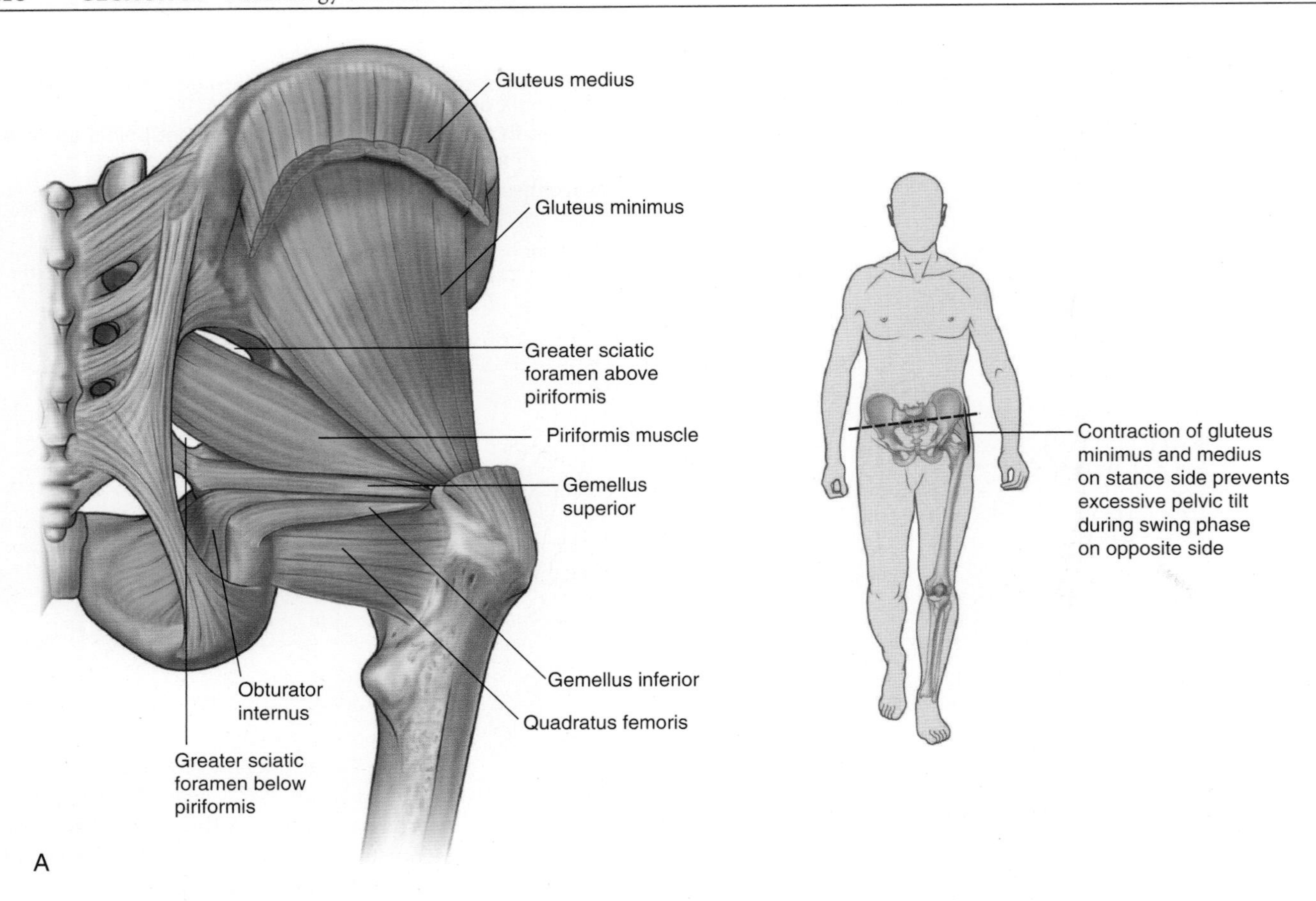

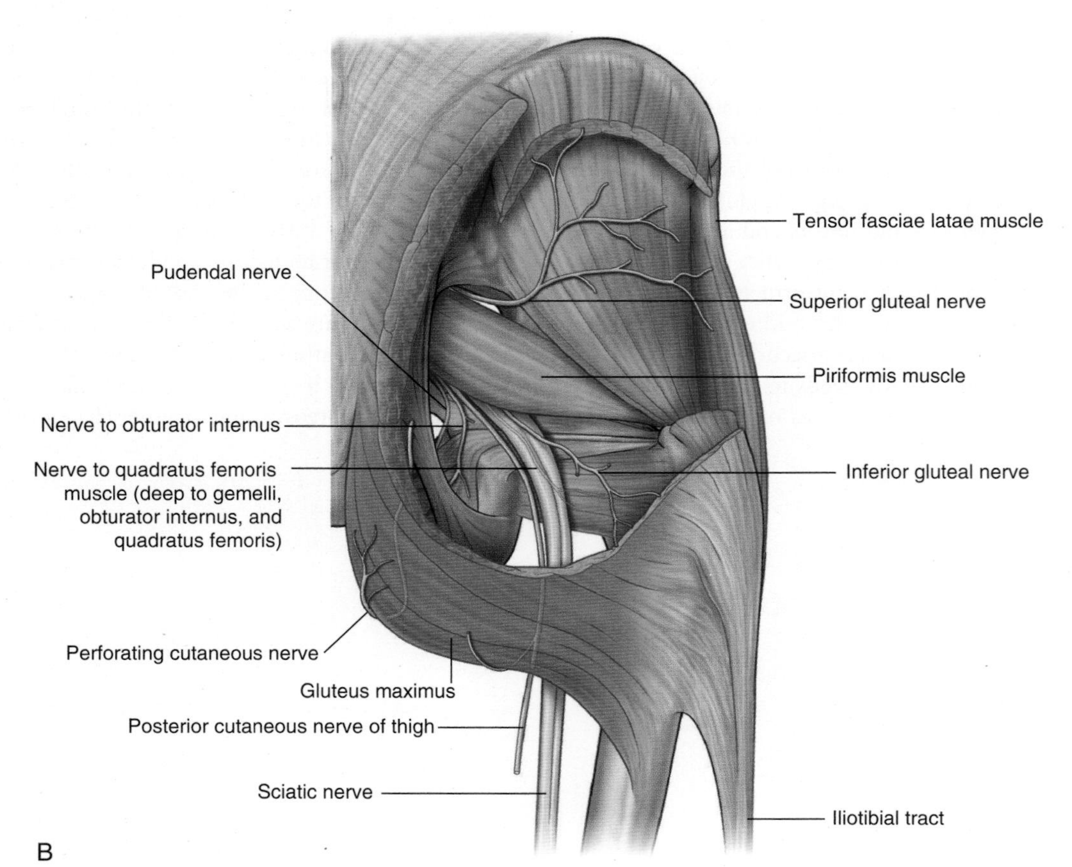

FIG. 9.26 (A) Deep muscles in the gluteal region. (B) Nerves of the gluteal region, posterior view. (From Drake RL, Vogl W, Mitchell WM. *Gray's Anatomy for Students*. 2nd ed. Churchill Livingstone; 2010.)

Gluteus maximus (GLUE-tee-us MAX-uh-mus)

Gluteus means "buttocks"; *maximus* means "greatest or largest."

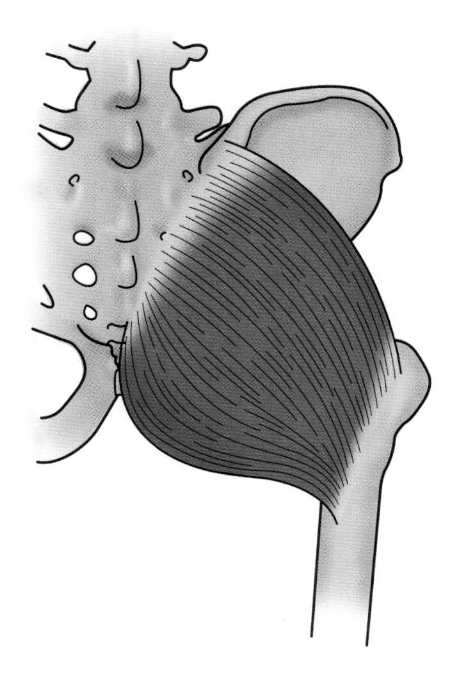

Concentric action:

Extends and laterally rotates the thigh at the hip joint—the upper fibers abduct the thigh at the hip joint, and the lower fibers adduct the thigh at the hip joint—and provides posterior tilt of the pelvis at the hip joint

The gluteus maximus is active primarily during strenuous activity, such as running, jumping, and climbing stairs.

Eccentric action:

Restrains/controls (especially rapid movement) flexion and medial rotation of the thigh and anterior tilt of the pelvis

The upper fibers restrain adduction of the thigh, and the lower fibers restrain abduction of the thigh.

Isometric action:

These muscles are important postural muscles that help maintain the upright posture, stabilize the pelvis, and provide tension to the iliotibial band to keep the fascial band taut.

Origin, fixed end, proximal attachment, arises from:

Posterior gluteal line of the ilium, dorsal surface of the lower aspect of the sacrum and the side of the coccyx, sacrotuberous ligament and gluteal aponeurosis, and aponeurosis of the erector spinae

Insertion, mobile end, distal attachment, attaches to:

Iliotibial band of the fascia lata and gluteal tuberosity of the femur

Innervation:

Inferior gluteal nerve (L5–S2)

Major synergists:

Hamstring muscles and piriformis

Major antagonists:

Iliopsoas, tensor fasciae latae, and gluteus medius (anterior fibers)

Tender/trigger points:

Three main areas—near the sacrum at the musculotendinous junction midway down from the iliac crest, near the ischial tuberosity, and in the belly of the muscle closer to the lower fibers

Common symptom/Common symptom/Referred pain pattern:

Regionally into the gluteal area, especially to the ischial tuberosity, the tip of the greater trochanter, and the sacrum

A shortened and tight gluteus maximus can be responsible for tightness of the iliotibial band and thoracolumbar fascia. These superficial muscles are thick and require firm massage application to be effective. The smaller, deeper muscle layers have to be accessed by pressure that penetrates through the gluteus maximus. Positioning the client so that this muscle is in a passive contraction by propping the client such that the attachments of the muscle are closer together is helpful. If no active contraction is taking place, the area becomes softer and it is easier for compressive forces of massage to reach the underlying muscle layers.

Gluteus medius (GLUE-tee-us MEED-ee-us)

Gluteus means "buttocks"; *medius* means "middle."

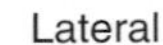

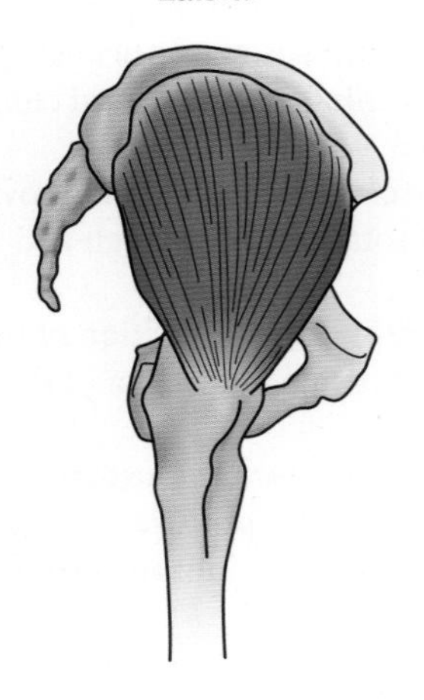

Concentric action:
- Abducts the thigh at the hip joint
- Anterior fibers medially rotate and flex the thigh at the hip joint and allow anterior tilt of the pelvis at the hip joint; posterior fibers laterally rotate and extend the thigh at the hip joint and allow posterior tilt of the pelvis at the hip joint.

Eccentric action:
- Restrains/controls (especially rapid movement) adduction of the thigh
- The anterior fibers restrain extension and lateral rotation of the thigh and posterior tilt of the pelvis; the posterior fibers restrain flexion and medial rotation of the thigh and anterior tilt of the pelvis.

Isometric action:
- Stabilizes the pelvis (especially when a person is standing on one foot)

Origin, fixed end, proximal attachment, arises from:
- External surface of the ilium inferior to the iliac crest, between the anterior and posterior gluteal lines, and the gluteal aponeurosis

Insertion, mobile end, distal attachment, attaches to:
- Lateral surface of the greater trochanter of the femur

Innervation:
- Superior gluteal nerve (L4–S1)

Major synergists:
- Gluteus minimus, tensor fasciae latae, and piriformis

Major antagonists:
- The adductors of the thigh

Tender/trigger points:
- Along the musculotendinous junction at the iliac crest

Common symptom/Common symptom/Referred pain pattern:
- Low back, posterior crest of the ilium to the sacrum, and to the posterior and lateral areas of the buttock into the upper thigh

Gluteus minimus (GLUE-tee-us MIN-ih-mus)

Gluteus means "buttocks"; *minimus* means "smallest."

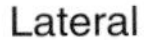

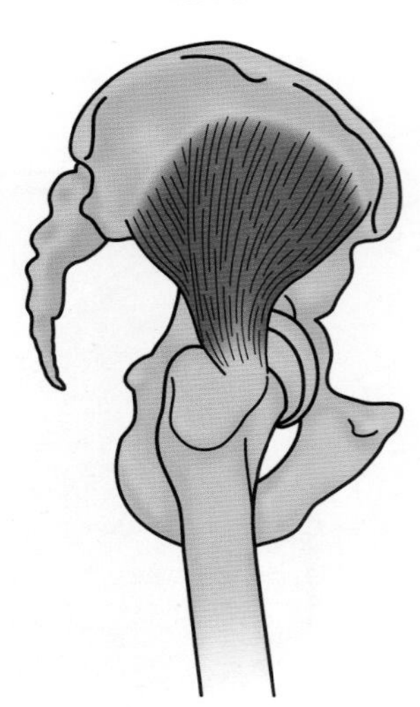

Concentric action:
- Abducts the thigh at the hip joint, medially rotates and flexes the thigh at the hip joint, and allows anterior tilt of the pelvis at the hip joint

Eccentric action:
- Restrains/controls (especially rapid movement) adduction of the thigh
- The anterior fibers restrain extension and lateral rotation of the thigh and posterior tilt of the pelvis.

Isometric action:
- Stabilizes the pelvis (especially when a person is standing on one foot)

Origin, fixed end, proximal attachment, arises from:
- External surface of the ilium inferior to the iliac crest, between the anterior and inferior gluteal lines

Insertion, mobile end, distal attachment, attaches to:
- Anterior border of the greater trochanter of the femur

Innervation:
- Superior gluteal nerve (L4–S1)

Major synergist:
- Gluteus medius

Major antagonists:
- Adductors of the thigh

Tender/trigger points:
- Belly of the muscle

Common symptom/Common symptom/Referred pain pattern:
- Lower lateral buttock and down the lateral to posterior aspect of the thigh, knee, and leg to the ankle

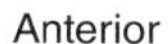

Tensor fasciae latae (TEN-sore FAH-she-e LAT-e)

Tensor means "one that stretches," *fasciae* means "bands or bandages," and *latae* means "wide."

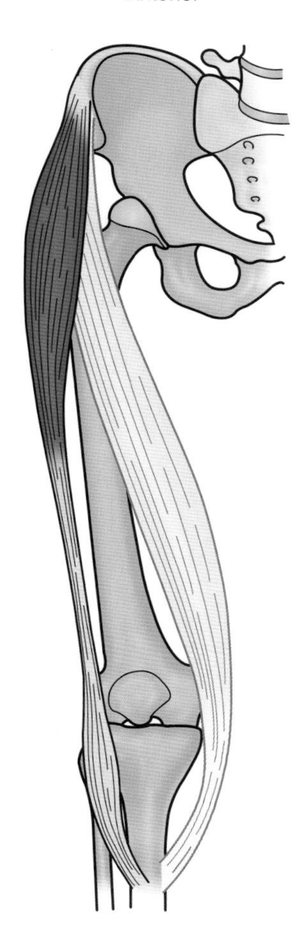

Concentric action:
Flexion, medial rotation, and abduction of the thigh at the hip joint; anterior tilt of the pelvis at the hip joint; and extension of the leg at the knee joint

Eccentric action:
Restrains/controls (especially rapid movement) extension, lateral rotation, and adduction of the thigh and allows posterior tilt of the pelvis and flexion of the leg

Isometric action:
Tenses the iliotibial band, counterbalancing the backward pull of the gluteus maximus on the iliotibial band, and stabilizes the pelvis and the knee

Origin, fixed end, proximal attachment, arises from:
Anterior aspect of the outer lip of the iliac crest and outer surface of the anterior superior iliac spine

Insertion, mobile end, distal attachment, attaches to:
Iliotibial band, one-third of the way down the thigh

Innervation:
Superior gluteal nerve (L4–S1)

Major synergists:
Gluteus medius (anterior fibers) and iliopsoas

Major antagonists:
Gluteus medius (posterior fibers), adductors of the thigh group, gluteus maximus, and hamstrings

Tender/trigger points:
In the belly of the muscle and near the distal attachment

Common symptom/Common symptom/Referred pain pattern:
Localized in the hip and down the lateral side of the thigh to the knee

ACTIVITY 9.33

Draw and color the *gluteal muscles* and tensor fasciae latae in the spaces provided. For each muscle:

1. Label the origin and insertion attachment points: *O* for origin; *I* for insertion.
2. Place an X on the trigger points.
3. Palpate this muscle; identify the attachment points and the bellies of the muscles.
4. Move these muscles on yourself.

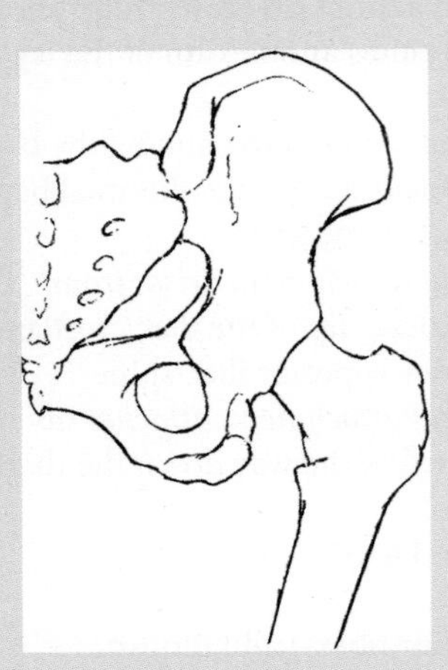

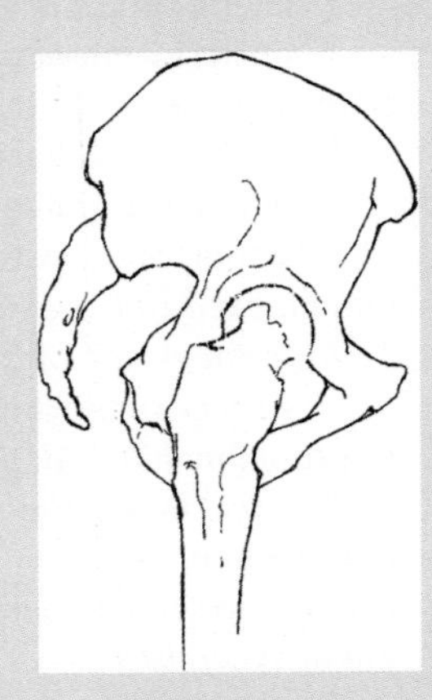

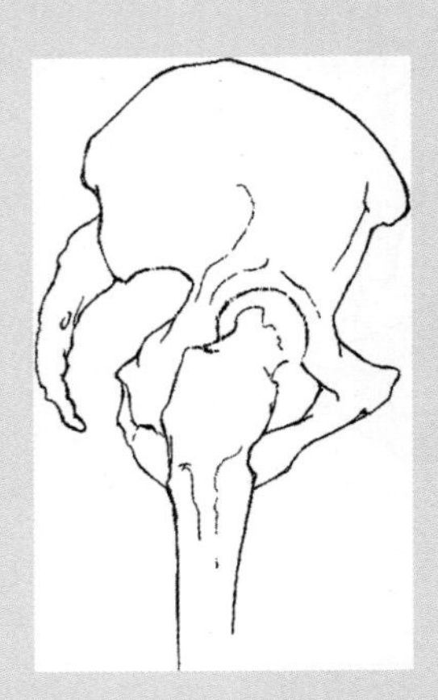

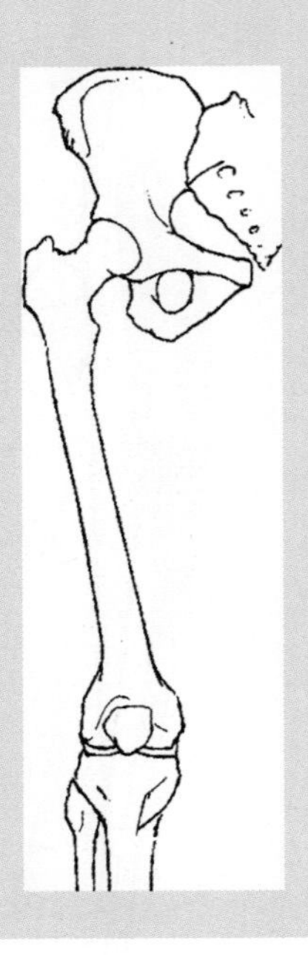

Deep Lateral Rotators of the Thigh at the Hip Joint

Piriformis (PEER-ih-FOR-miss)

Piriformis means "pear shaped."

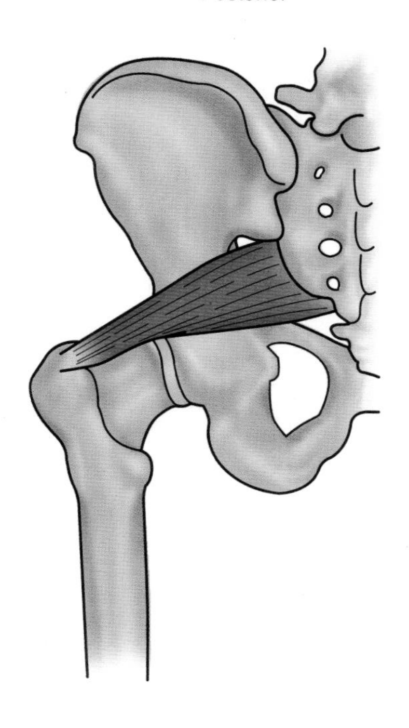

Concentric action:
Lateral rotation of the thigh at the hip joint and abduction and medial rotation of the thigh at the hip joint if the thigh is first in a position of flexion at the hip joint

Eccentric action:
Restrains/controls (especially rapid movement) medial rotation of the thigh and also may restrain adduction and lateral rotation of the thigh (if the thigh is in a position of flexion)

Isometric action:
Stabilizes the hip joint

Origin, fixed end, proximal attachment, arises from:
Anterior surface of the sacrum between the first through fourth sacral foramina and the pelvic surface of the sacrotuberous ligament

Insertion, mobile end, distal attachment, attaches to:
Superior border of the greater trochanter of the femur

Innervation:
Lumbosacral plexus (L5–S2)

Major synergists:
All deep lateral rotators of the thigh at the hip joint are synergistic with one another; posterior fibers of the gluteus medius are also major synergists.

Major antagonists:
Anterior fibers of the gluteus medius, gluteus minimus, and the tensor fasciae latae

Tender/trigger points:
The main tender/trigger points in the piriformis muscle are near the attachments. The belly may have tender/trigger points as well. Tension in this muscle can cause entrapment of the sciatic nerve, which normally passes inferior to the piriformis but in some individuals passes through the muscle, predisposing the person to symptoms of sciatica.

Common symptom/Common symptom/Referred pain pattern:
Sacroiliac region, entire buttock, and down the posterior thigh to just proximal to the knee

Obturator internus (OB-tur-ATE-or in-TER-nus)

Obturator means "one that covers an opening"; *internus* means "interior."

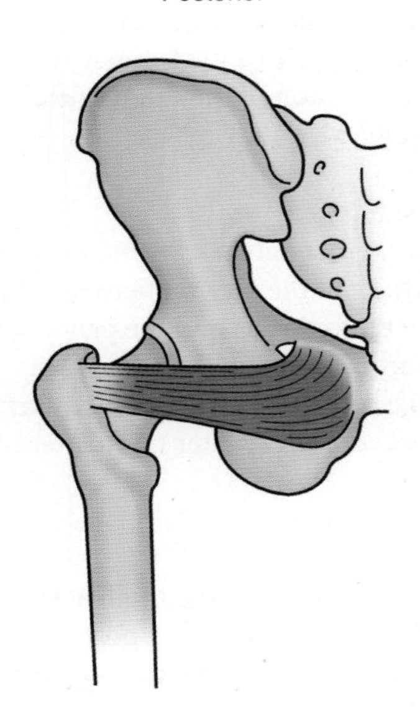

Concentric action:
Lateral rotation of the thigh at the hip joint and abduction of the thigh at the hip joint if the thigh is first in a position of flexion at the hip joint

Eccentric action:
Restrains/controls (especially rapid movement) medial rotation of the thigh and also may restrain adduction of the thigh (if the thigh is in a position of flexion)

Isometric action:
Stabilizes the hip joint

Origin, fixed end, proximal attachment, arises from:
Internal surface of the obturator membrane and the margins of the obturator foramen (on the ilium, ischium, and pubis)

Insertion, mobile end, distal attachment, attaches to:
Medial surface of the greater trochanter of the femur

Innervation:
Nerve to obturator internus from the lumbosacral plexus (L5–S1)

Major synergists:
All deep lateral rotators of the thigh at the hip joint are synergistic with one another; posterior fibers of the gluteus medius are also major synergists.

Major antagonists:
Anterior fibers of the gluteus medius, gluteus minimus, and the tensor fasciae latae

Tender/trigger points:
The belly of the muscle

Common symptom/Common symptom/Referred pain pattern:
Sacroiliac region, entire buttock, and down the posterior thigh to just proximal to the knee joint

Obturator externus (OB-tur-ATE-or ex-STIR-nus)

Obturator means "one that covers an opening"; *externus* means "exterior."

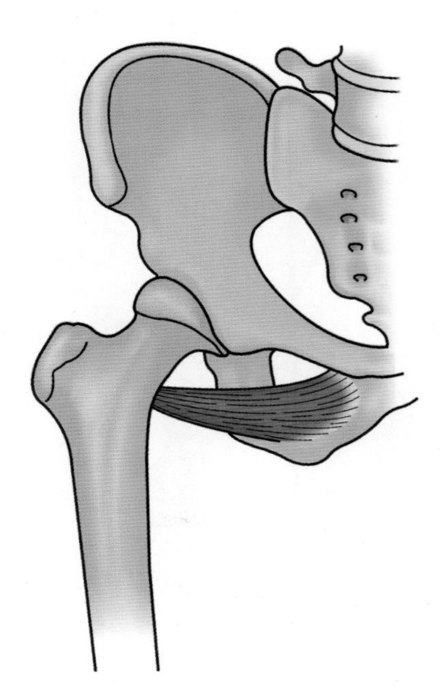

Concentric action:
Lateral rotation of the thigh at the hip joint

Eccentric action:
Restrains/controls (especially rapid movement) medial rotation of the thigh

Isometric action:
Stabilizes the hip joint

Origin, fixed end, proximal attachment, arises from:
External surface of the obturator membrane and the margins of the obturator foramen (on the ischium and pubis)

Insertion, mobile end, distal attachment, attaches to:
Trochanteric fossa of the femur

Innervation:
Obturator nerve (L3–L4)

Major synergists:
All deep lateral rotators of the thigh at the hip joint are synergistic with one another; posterior fibers of the gluteus medius are also major synergists.

Major antagonists:
Anterior fibers of the gluteus medius, gluteus minimus, and the tensor fasciae latae

Tender/trigger points:
The belly of the muscle

Common symptom/Common symptom/Referred pain pattern:
Sacroiliac region, entire buttock, and down the posterior thigh to just proximal to the knee joint

Gemellus superior (JEM-ell-us)

Gemellus means "twin"; *superior* means "above."

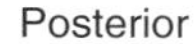

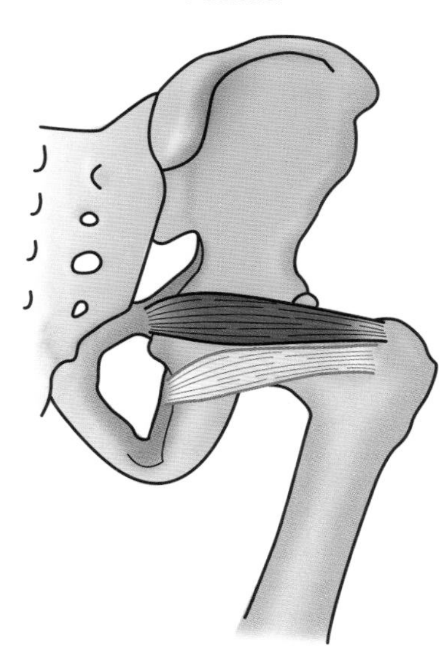

Concentric action:
Lateral rotation of the thigh at the hip joint and abduction of the thigh at the hip joint if the thigh is first in a position of flexion at the hip joint

Eccentric action:
Restrains/controls (especially rapid movement) medial rotation of the thigh and also may restrain adduction of the thigh (if the thigh is in a position of flexion)

Isometric action:
Stabilizes the hip joint

Origin, fixed end, proximal attachment, arises from:
Dorsal surface of the ischial spine

Insertion, mobile end, distal attachment, attaches to:
Medial surface of the greater trochanter of the femur

Innervation:
Nerve to obturator internus (L5–S1)

Major synergists:
All deep lateral rotators of the thigh at the hip joint are synergistic with one another; posterior fibers of the gluteus medius are also synergistic.

Major antagonists:
Anterior fibers of the gluteus medius, gluteus minimus, and the tensor fasciae latae

Tender/trigger points:
The belly of the muscle

Common symptom/Common symptom/Referred pain pattern:
Sacroiliac region, entire buttock, and down the posterior thigh to just proximal to the knee joint

Gemellus inferior (JEM-ell-us)

Gemellus means "twin"; *inferior* means "below."

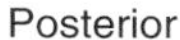

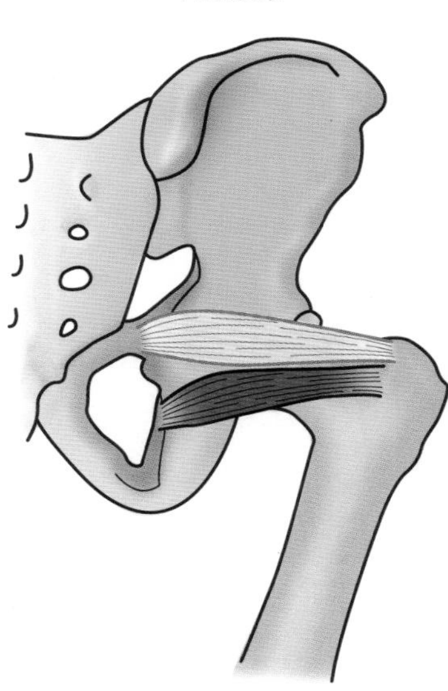

Concentric action:
Lateral rotation of the thigh at the hip joint and abduction of the thigh at the hip joint if the thigh is first in a position of flexion at the hip joint

Eccentric action:
Restrains/controls (especially rapid movement) medial rotation of the thigh and also may restrain adduction of the thigh (if the thigh is in a position of flexion)

Isometric action:
Stabilizes the hip joint

Origin, fixed end, proximal attachment, arises from:
Upper part of the ischial tuberosity

Insertion, mobile end, distal attachment, attaches to:
Medial surface of the greater trochanter

Innervation:
Lumbosacral plexus

Major synergists:
All deep lateral rotators of the thigh at the hip joint are synergistic with one another; posterior fibers of the gluteus medius are synergistic.

Major antagonists:
Anterior fibers of the gluteus medius, gluteus minimus, and the tensor fasciae latae

Tender/trigger points:
The belly of the muscle

Common symptom/Common symptom/Referred pain pattern:
Sacroiliac region, entire buttock, and down the posterior thigh to just proximal to the knee joint

Quadratus femoris (kwad-RATE-us FEM-or-iss)

Quadratus means "square shaped"; *femoris* means "related to the thigh."

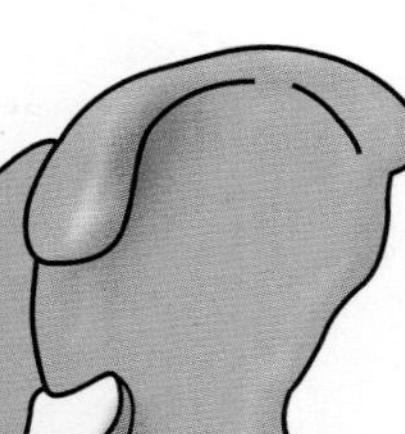

Concentric action:
Lateral rotation and adduction of the thigh at the hip joint (if the thigh is in a position of flexion)

Eccentric action:
Restrains/controls (especially rapid movement) medial rotation of the thigh and also may restrain abduction of the thigh

Isometric action:
Stabilizes the hip joint

Origin, fixed end, proximal attachment, arises from:
Lateral border of the ischial tuberosity

Insertion, mobile end, distal attachment, attaches to:
Small tubercle on the upper part of the intertrochanteric crest of the femur

Innervation:
Nerve to quadratus femoris from the lumbosacral plexus (L5 and S1)

Major synergists:
All deep lateral rotators of the thigh at the hip joint are synergistic with one another; posterior fibers of the gluteus medius are also synergistic.

Major antagonists:
Anterior fibers of the gluteus medius, gluteus minimus, and the tensor fasciae latae

Tender/trigger points:
The belly of the muscle

Common symptom/Common symptom/Referred pain pattern:
Sacroiliac region, entire buttock, and down the posterior thigh to just proximal to the knee joint

ACTIVITY 9.34

Draw and color the *deep lateral rotators of the thigh at the hip joint* in the spaces provided. For each muscle:

1. Label the origin and insertion attachment points: *O* for origin; *I* for insertion.
2. Place an X on the trigger points.
3. Palpate this muscle; identify the attachment points and the bellies of the muscles.
4. Move these muscles on yourself.

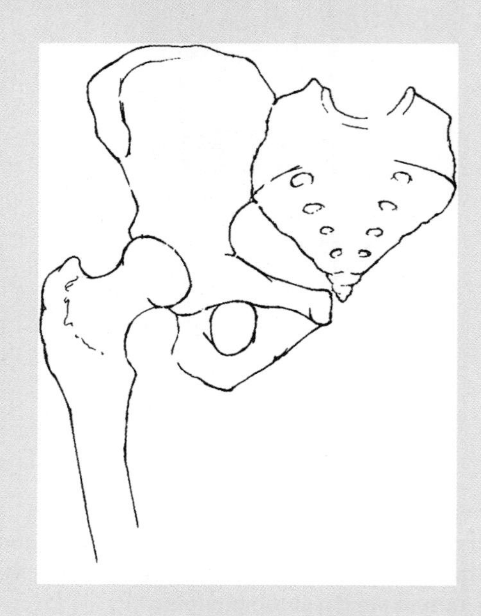

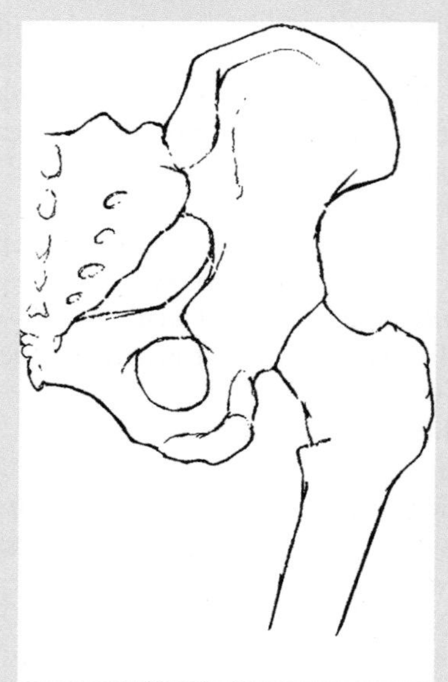

Muscles of the Posterior Thigh

The hamstring muscle group crosses two joints—the hip and the knee. These muscles posteriorly tilt the pelvis at the hip joint, extend the thigh at the hip joint, and flex the leg at the knee joint. The muscles of the massive hamstring group are the main extensors of the thigh. Because these muscles are active during walking, all gait reflexes are involved with the shoulder muscles to promote the appropriate counterbalancing arm swing. Facilitation between muscles of the arms that flex and extend occur along with thigh muscles in contralateral patterns. The massage therapist usually needs to consider the muscles of the shoulder joint with muscles of the hip and massage in a correlated pattern. Although not listed with synergists and antagonists, the flexors of the arm at the shoulder joint work with the flexors of the thigh at the hip joint on the opposite side (i.e., right with left and left with right). This concept is also true for the extensors of the arm and thigh. These muscles show patterns of inhibition as well; for example, right-side extensors of the thigh at the hip joint inhibit right-side extensors of the arm at the shoulder joint. Adductors and medial rotators of the arm at the shoulder joint work with adductors and medial rotators of the thigh at the hip joint on the opposite side. This concept holds true for abductors and lateral rotators as well. Of course, these muscles also exhibit inhibitory patterns.

These muscles are thick, and massage application must address the muscles adequately but not painfully compress them against the underlying bone. The side-lying position naturally moves these muscles away from the bone making it most suitable for applying compressive force during massage. These muscles tend to adhere together. Although this may be a compensation pattern for repetitive movement in extension of the thigh at the hip joint or flexion of the leg at the knee joint, adhesion can reduce and interfere with range of motion of the associated joints (Fig. 9.27).

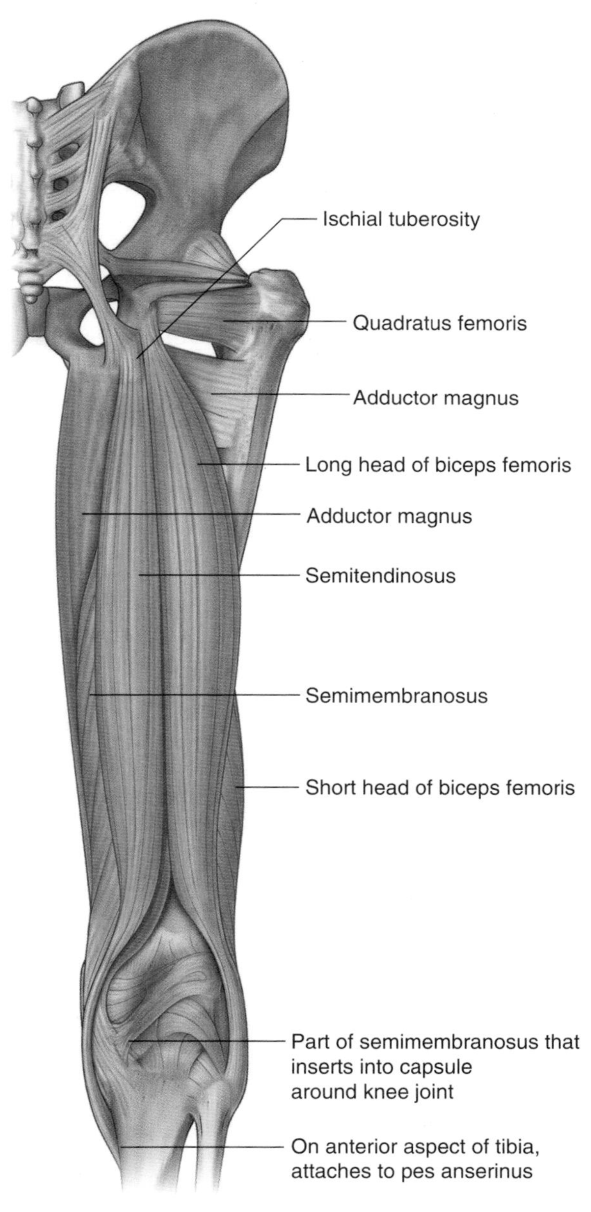

FIG. 9.27 Muscles of the posterior compartment of the thigh, posterior view. (From Drake RL, Vogl W, Mitchell WM. *Gray's Anatomy for Students*. 2nd ed. Churchill Livingstone; 2010.)

Biceps femoris (BI-seps FEM-or-iss)

Biceps means "two headed"; *femoris* means "related to the thigh."

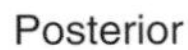

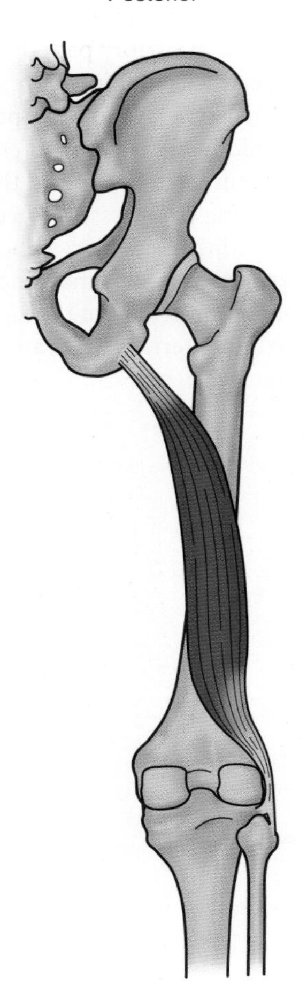

Concentric action:
Entire muscle—flexion and lateral rotation of the leg at the knee joint (The knee joint must be semiflexed for lateral rotation to occur.)
Long head—extension of the thigh at the hip joint and posterior tilt of the pelvis at the hip joint

Eccentric action:
Restrains/controls (especially rapid movement) extension and medial rotation of the leg and restrains/controls (especially rapid movement) flexion of the thigh and anterior tilt of the pelvis

Isometric action:
Stabilizes the hip and knee joints

Origin, fixed end, proximal attachment, arises from:
Long head—posterior part of the ischial tuberosity and the sacrotuberous ligament
Short head—lateral lip of the linea aspera, lateral intermuscular septum, and proximal two-thirds of the supracondylar line

Insertion, mobile end, distal attachment, attaches to:
Lateral side of the fibular head, lateral condyle of the tibia, and deep fascia on the lateral aspect of the leg

Innervation:
Tibial and common fibular portions of the sciatic nerve (L5–S2)

Major synergists:
Semitendinosus, semimembranosus, and gluteus maximus

Major antagonists:
Quadriceps femoris group, iliopsoas, and tensor fasciae latae

Tender/trigger points:
Several areas in the belly of the muscle and at the musculotendinous junction near the knee joint

Common symptom/Common symptom/Referred pain pattern:
Ischial tuberosity, back of the knee, and the entire posterior thigh and leg to midcalf

Semitendinosus (SEM-ee-TEN-din-oh-sus)

Semitendinosus means "half tendon."

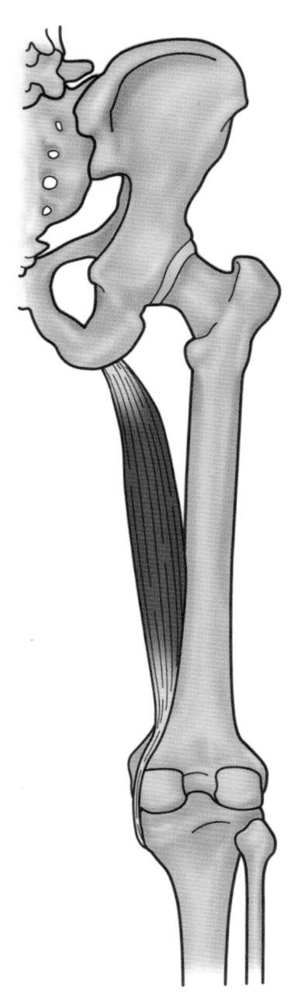

Concentric action:
Flexion and medial rotation of the leg at the knee joint (the knee joint must be semiflexed for medial rotation to occur), extension of the thigh at the hip joint, and posterior tilt of the pelvis at the hip joint

Eccentric action:
Restrains/controls (especially rapid movement) extension and lateral rotation of the leg and allows flexion of the thigh and anterior tilt of the pelvis

Isometric action:
Stabilizes the knee and hip joints

Origin, fixed end, proximal attachment, arises from:
Distal part of the medial aspect of the ischial tuberosity

Insertion, mobile end, distal attachment, attaches to:
Proximal anteromedial tibia at the pes anserinus tendon and deep fascia of the leg

Innervation:
Tibial portion of the sciatic nerve (L5–S2)

Major synergists:
Semimembranosus, biceps femoris, and gluteus maximus

Major antagonists:
Quadriceps femoris group, iliopsoas, and tensor fasciae latae

Tender/trigger points:
Several areas in the belly of the muscle and at the musculotendinous junction near the knee joint

Common symptom/Common symptom/Referred pain pattern:
Ischial tuberosity, back of the knee, and the entire posterior thigh and leg to midcalf

Semimembranosus (SEM-ee-MEM-bran-oh-sus)

Semimembranosus means "half membrane."

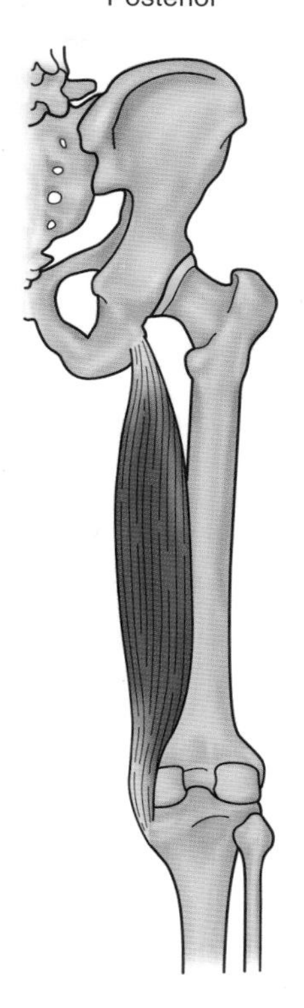

Concentric action:
Flexion and medial rotation of the leg at the knee joint (the knee joint must be semiflexed for medial rotation to occur), extension of the thigh at the hip joint, and posterior tilt of the pelvis at the hip joint. The semimembranosus also serves to move the medial meniscus posteriorly during knee flexion.

Eccentric action:
Restrains/controls (especially rapid movement) extension and lateral rotation of the leg and allows flexion of the thigh and anterior tilt of the pelvis

Isometric action:
Stabilizes the knee and hip joints

Origin, fixed end, proximal attachment, arises from:
Upper lateral aspect of the ischial tuberosity

Insertion, mobile end, distal attachment, attaches to:
Posteromedial surface of the medial condyle of the tibia; attaches to the medial meniscus

Innervation:
Tibial portion of the sciatic nerve (L5–S2)

Major synergists:
Semitendinosus, biceps femoris, and gluteus maximus

Major antagonists:
Quadriceps femoris group, iliopsoas, and tensor fasciae latae

Tender/trigger points:
Several areas in the belly of the muscle and at the musculotendinous junction near the knee joint

Common symptom/Common symptom/Referred pain pattern:
Ischial tuberosity, back of the knee, and the entire posterior thigh and leg to midcalf

ACTIVITY 9.35

Draw and color the *muscles of the posterior thigh* in the spaces provided. For each muscle:

1. Label the origin and insertion attachment points: *O* for origin; *I* for insertion.
2. Place an X on the trigger points.
3. Palpate this muscle; identify the attachment points and the bellies of the muscles.
4. Move these muscles on yourself.

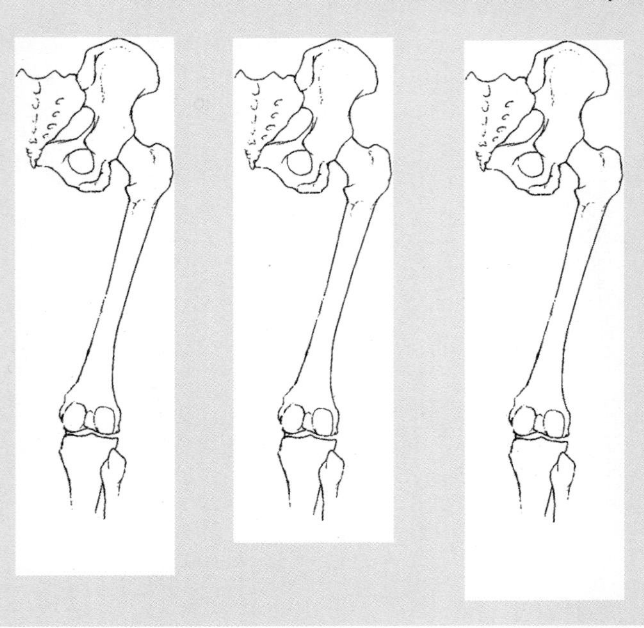

Muscles of the Medial Thigh

The medial thigh muscles, called the *adductor group of the thigh*, adduct the thigh at the hip joint. Interaction between abduction and adduction of the thighs (co-contraction) keeps the weight of the body balanced over the weight-bearing lower extremity when a person is walking (when standing on one foot). Because of gait reflexes, these muscles work with adductors of the arm at the shoulder joint and inhibit abductors of the arm at the shoulder joint on the opposite side. These muscles also work with the abdominal muscles to support the trunk and pelvis in an upright position.

This muscle group is massive, and the massage therapist can manage it most easily with the client in the side-lying position with the top lower extremity bent and flexed forward to expose the adductor muscles of the bottom thigh (Fig. 9.28).

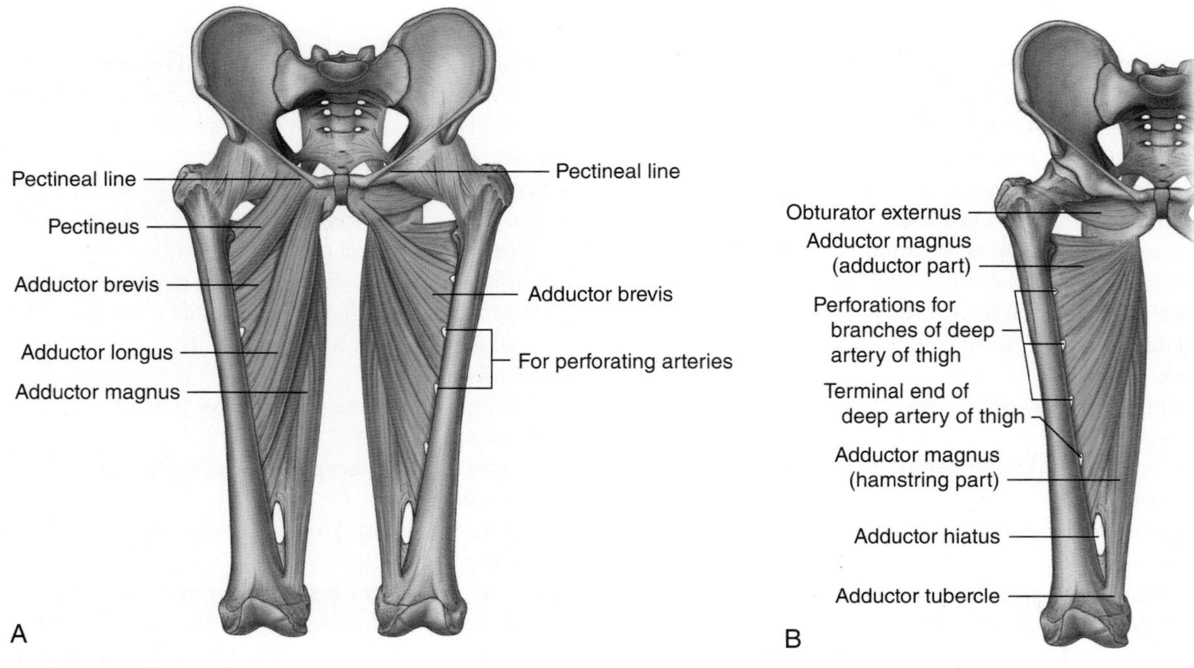

FIG. 9.28 A, Pectineus, adductor longus, and adductor brevis muscles, anterior view. **B**, Adductor magnus and obturator externus muscles, anterior view. (From Drake RL, Vogl W, Mitchell WM. *Gray's Anatomy for Students*. 2nd ed. Churchill Livingstone; 2010.)

Gracilis (gra-SIL-iss)

Gracilis means "slender."

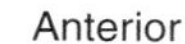

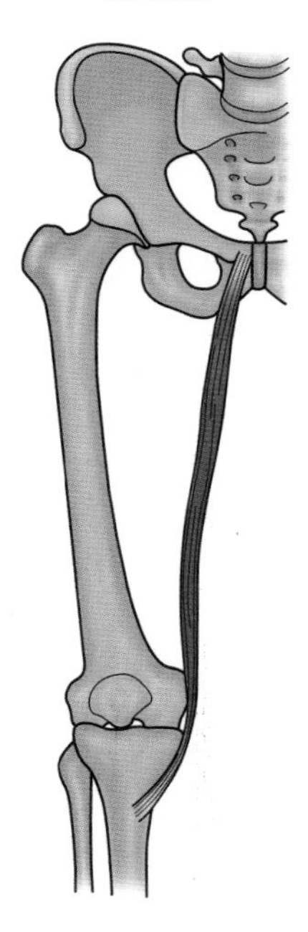

Concentric action:
Adduction and flexion of the thigh at the hip joint, anterior tilt of the pelvis at the hip joint, and flexion and medial rotation of the leg at the knee joint

The knee joint must be semiflexed for medial rotation to occur.

Eccentric action:
Restrains/controls (especially rapid movement) abduction and extension of the thigh and allows posterior tilt of the pelvis and extension and lateral rotation of the leg

Isometric action:
Stabilizes the pelvis at the hip joint and assists in controlling and stabilizing the valgus angulation of the knee joint

Origin, fixed end, proximal attachment, arises from:
Inferior half of the symphysis pubis and inferior ramus of the pubic bone

Insertion, mobile end, distal attachment, attaches to:
Proximal anteromedial tibia at the pes anserinus tendon

Innervation:
Obturator nerve (L2–L3)

Major synergists:
The adductor group of the thigh is synergistic, as are the iliopsoas and sartorius.

Major antagonists:
Gluteus medius and gluteus minimus, tensor fasciae latae, and hamstrings

Tender/trigger points:
Within the belly of each muscle and near the ischial tuberosity attachment

Common symptom/Common symptom/Referred pain pattern:
Deep in the groin, into the medial thigh and downward to the knee and leg; may mimic hamstring tension

Adductor magnus (ad-DUCK-tur MAG-nus)

Adductor means "to lead toward"; *magnus* means "great."

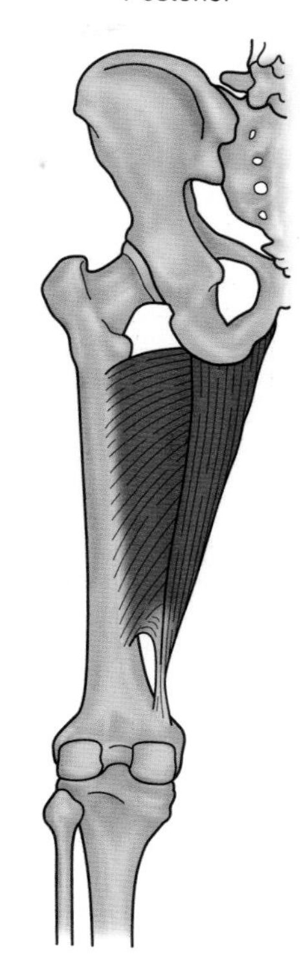

Concentric action:
Adduction and extension of the thigh at the hip joint and posterior tilt of the pelvis at the hip joint

Eccentric action:
Restrains/controls (especially rapid movement) abduction and flexion of the thigh and anterior tilt of the pelvis

Isometric action:
Stabilizes the pelvis at the hip joint

Origin, fixed end, proximal attachment, arises from:
Inferior ramus of the pubis and the ramus of the ischium (anterior fibers); posterior fibers attach to the ischial tuberosity

Insertion, mobile end, distal attachment, attaches to:
Gluteal tuberosity, linea aspera, medial supracondylar line, and adductor tubercle of the femur

Innervation:
Obturator and tibial division of sciatic nerves (L2 to L4)

Major synergists:
The adductor group of the thigh is synergistic, as are the hamstrings.

Major antagonists:
Gluteus medius and gluteus minimus, tensor fasciae latae, and iliopsoas

Tender/trigger points:
Within the belly of each muscle and near the ischial tuberosity attachment

Common symptom/Common symptom/Referred pain pattern:
Deep in the groin, into the medial thigh and downward to the knee and leg; may mimic hamstring tension

Adductor longus (ad-DUCK-tur LONG-us)

Adductor means "to lead toward"; *longus* means "long."

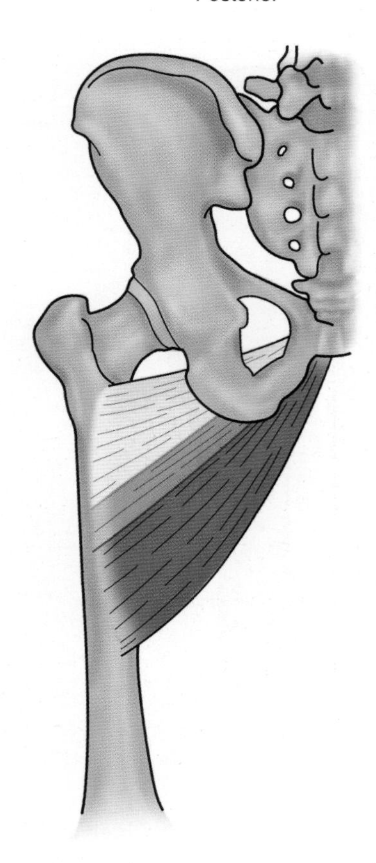

Concentric action:
Adduction and flexion of the thigh at the hip joint and anterior tilt of the pelvis at the hip joint
Eccentric action:
Restrains/controls (especially rapid movement) abduction and extension of the thigh and posterior tilt of the pelvis
Isometric action:
Stabilizes the pelvis at the hip joint
Origin, fixed end, proximal attachment, arises from:
Anterior pubis between the crest and symphysis
Insertion, mobile end, distal attachment, attaches to:
Middle one-third of the medial lip of the linea aspera of the femur
Innervation:
Obturator nerve (L2–L4)
Major synergists:
The adductor group of the thigh is synergistic, as is the iliopsoas.
Major antagonists:
Gluteus medius and gluteus minimus, tensor fasciae latae, and hamstrings
Tender/trigger points:
Within the belly of each muscle and near the ischial tuberosity attachment
Common symptom/Common symptom/Referred pain pattern:
Deep in the groin, into the medial thigh and downward to the knee and leg; may mimic hamstring tension

Adductor brevis (ad-DUCK-tur BREV-us)

Adductor means "to lead toward;" *brevis* means "short."

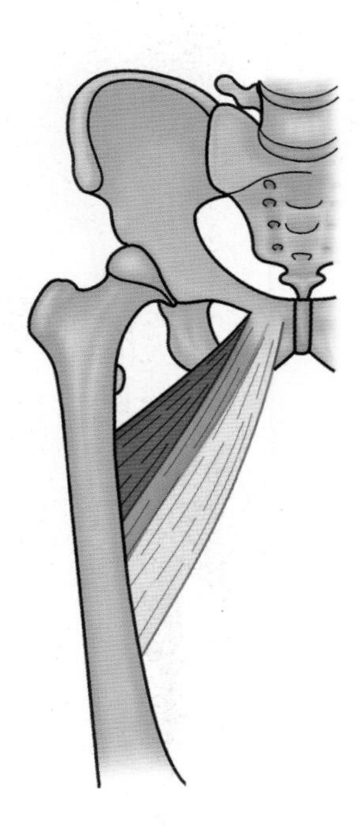

Concentric action:
Adduction and flexion of the thigh at the hip joint and anterior tilt of the pelvis at the hip joint
Eccentric action:
Restrains/controls (especially rapid movement) abduction and extension of the thigh and posterior tilt of the pelvis
Isometric action:
Stabilizes the pelvis at the hip joint
Origin, fixed end, proximal attachment, arises from:
Outer surface of the inferior ramus of the pubis between the gracilis and the obturator externus
Insertion, mobile end, distal attachment, attaches to:
Linea aspera of the femur
Innervation:
Obturator nerve (L2–L3)
Major synergists:
The adductor group of the thigh group is synergistic, as is the iliopsoas.
Major antagonists:
Gluteus medius and gluteus minimus, tensor fasciae latae, and hamstrings
Tender/trigger points:
Within the belly of each muscle and near the ischial tuberosity attachment
Common symptom/Common symptom/Referred pain pattern:
Deep in the groin, into the medial thigh and downward to the knee and leg; may mimic hamstring tension

Pectineus (PEK-tih-NEE-us)

Pectineus means "related to the pubic bone."

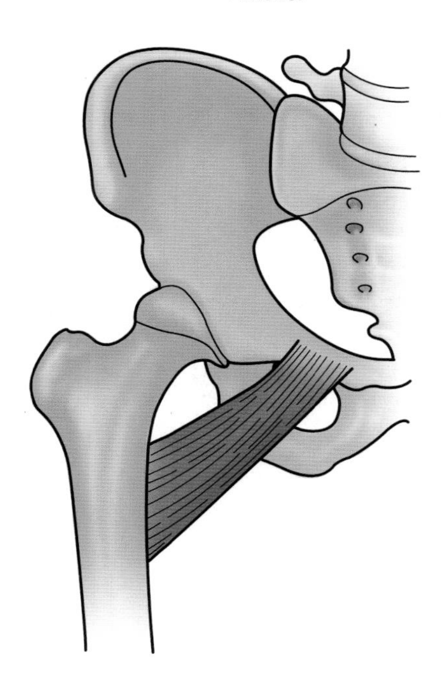

Concentric action:
Adduction and flexion of the thigh at the hip joint and anterior tilt of the pelvis at the hip joint

Eccentric action:
Restrains/controls (especially rapid movement) abduction and extension of the thigh and posterior tilt of the pelvis

Isometric action:
Stabilizes the pelvis at the hip joint

Origin, fixed end, proximal attachment, arises from:
Pectineal line of the pubis (on the superior ramus of the pubis)

Insertion, mobile end, distal attachment, attaches to:
Pectineal line of the femur (line extending from the lesser trochanter of the femur to the linea aspera)

Innervation:
Femoral nerve (L2–L3)

Major synergists:
The adductor group of the thigh is synergistic, as is the iliopsoas.

Major antagonists:
Gluteus medius and gluteus minimus, tensor fasciae latae, and hamstrings

Tender/trigger points:
Within the belly of each muscle and near the ischial tuberosity attachment

Common symptom/Common symptom/Referred pain pattern:
Deep in the groin, into the medial thigh and downward to the knee and leg; may mimic hamstring tension

ACTIVITY 9.36

Draw and color the *muscles of the medial thigh* in the spaces provided. For each muscle:

1. Label the origin and insertion attachment points: *O* for origin; *I* for insertion.
2. Place an X on the trigger points.
3. Palpate this muscle; identify the attachment points and the bellies of the muscles.
4. Move these muscles on yourself.

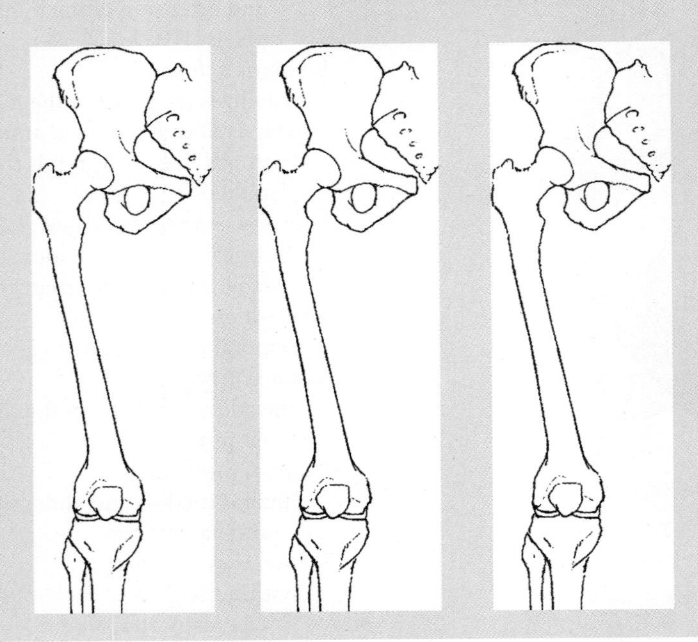

Muscles of the Anterior Thigh

The majority of the musculature of the anterior thigh is composed of the muscles of the quadriceps femoris group; the main action of this group is to extend the leg at the knee joint. The quadriceps femoris and hamstring muscle groups obviously are antagonistic, yet together they ensure the stability of the knee joint. The vastus lateralis and vastus medialis of the quadriceps femoris group also function together for proper tracking of the patella. The rectus femoris of the quadriceps femoris group is the only one that also crosses the hip joint. Because the rectus femoris crosses the hip joint anteriorly, it can flex the thigh at the hip joint. Another muscle of the anterior thigh is the sartorius, which also flexes the thigh at the hip joint and flexes the leg at the knee joint. The rectus femoris and sartorius fall into gait patterns and reflexes with flexors and extensors of the arm at the shoulder joint. The remaining quadriceps femoris muscles work with muscles that flex and extend the forearm at the elbow joint; these patterns are synergistic on opposite sides and antagonistic on the same side. Muscles of the anterior thigh can adhere to each other, particularly the rectus femoris to the underlying vastus intermedius. Should this happen, the rectus femoris will not have the necessary functional range during flexion of the thigh at the hip joint and extension of the leg at the knee joint. Adhesion compromises range of motion, and pain occurs, usually in the knee.

A major function of the quadriceps femoris group is to move the thigh into extension at the knee; this is sometimes called a *reverse action* because the proximal attachment moves in this situation and the distal attachment stays fixed. Examples would be standing up from a seated position or coming up into a straight-leg position from a squat. This action requires moving the upper body and the thigh. Therefore the quadriceps femoris group is large and strong (Fig. 9.29).

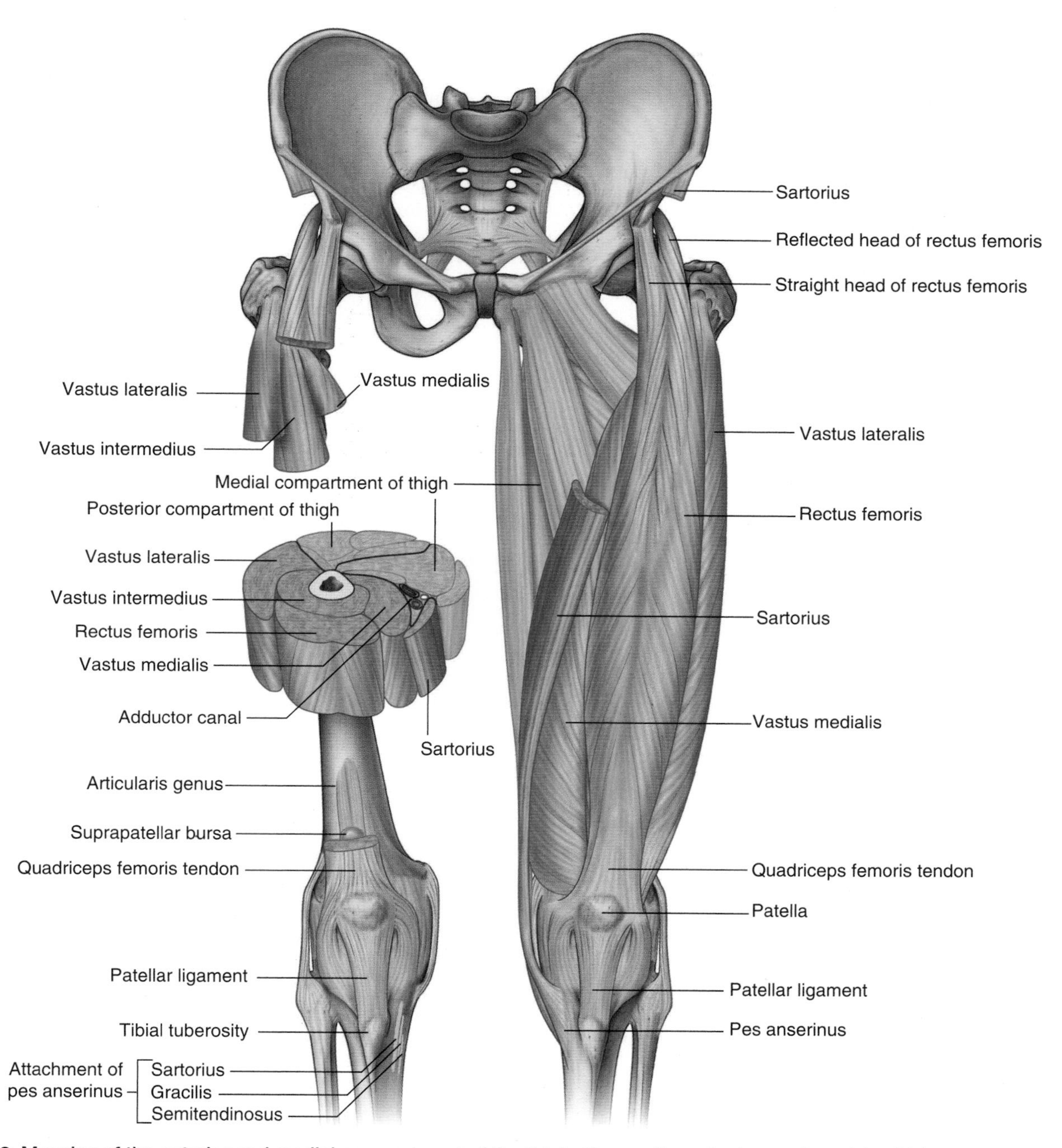

FIG. 9.29 Muscles of the anterior and medial compartment of the thigh. Composite and cutaway view of the thigh.

Sartorius (sar-TOR-ee-us)

Sartorius means "tailor."

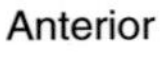

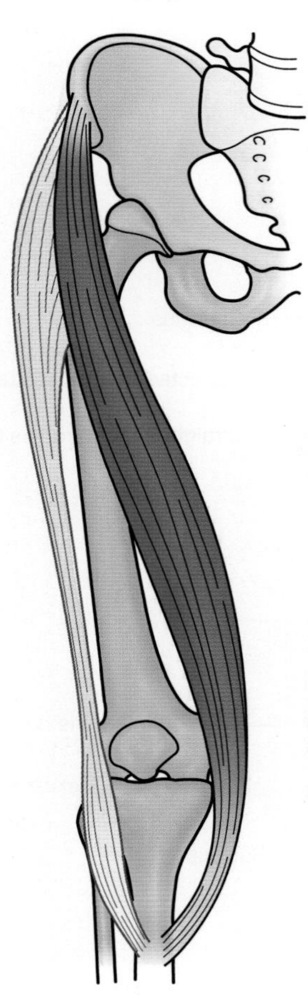

Concentric action:
Flexion, lateral rotation, and abduction of the thigh at the hip joint; flexion and medial rotation of the leg at the knee joint (The knee joint must be semiflexed for medial rotation to occur.); and anterior tilt of the pelvis at the hip joint

Eccentric action:
Restrains/controls (especially rapid movement) extension, medial rotation, and adduction of the thigh and allows extension and lateral rotation of the leg and posterior tilt of the pelvis

Isometric action:
Stabilizes the knee and hip joints

Origin, fixed end, proximal attachment, arises from:
Anterior superior iliac spine

Insertion, mobile end, distal attachment, attaches to:
Proximal anteromedial tibia at the pes anserinus tendon

Innervation:
Femoral nerve (L2–L3)

Major synergists:
Iliopsoas, rectus femoris, lateral rotator group of the thigh, and gluteus medius

Major antagonists:
Hamstrings, tensor fasciae latae, adductor group of the thigh, and quadriceps femoris group

Tender/trigger points:
Three or four areas along the belly of the muscle

Common symptom/Common symptom/Referred pain pattern:
Entire anterior thigh, with concentration at the knee

Rectus femoris (REK-tus FEM-or-iss)

The first muscle of the quadriceps femoris group, *rectus* means "straight" or "upright"; *femoris* means "related to the thigh." *Quadriceps* means "four headed."

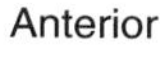

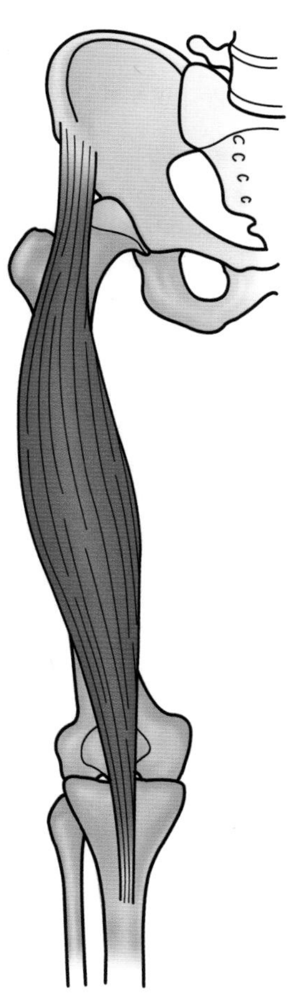

Concentric action:
Extension of the leg at the knee joint, flexion of the thigh at the hip joint, and anterior tilt of the pelvis at the hip joint

Eccentric action:
Restrains/controls (especially rapid movement) flexion of the leg and allows extension of the thigh and posterior tilt of the pelvis

Isometric action:
Stabilizes the knee and hip joints

Origin, fixed end, proximal attachment, arises from:
Anterior inferior iliac spine; groove above the rim of the acetabulum

Insertion, mobile end, distal attachment, attaches to:
Tibial tuberosity, by way of the patella and patellar ligament

Innervation:
Femoral nerve (L2–L4)

Major synergists:
All quadriceps femoris muscles are synergistic, as are the iliopsoas and sartorius.

Major antagonists:
Hamstrings and gluteus maximus

Tender/trigger points:
Near the attachment at the pelvis

Common symptom/Common symptom/Referred pain pattern:
Entire anterior thigh, with concentration at the knee

Vastus lateralis (VAS-tus LAT-ter-al-us)

The second muscle of the quadriceps femoris group, *vastus* means "vast" or "large"; *lateralis* means "related to the side." *Quadriceps* means "four headed."

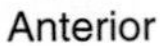

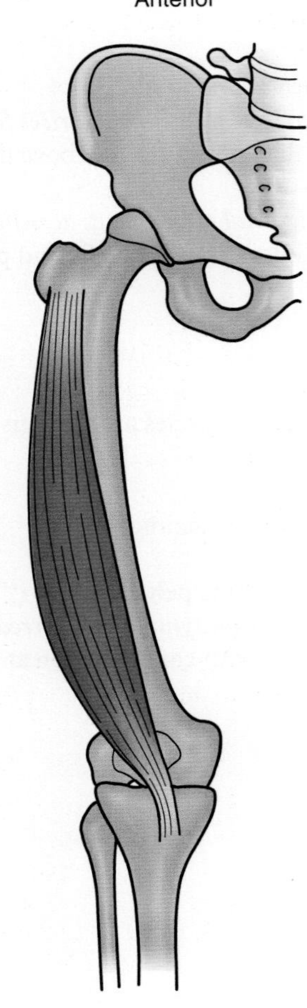

Concentric action:
Extension of the leg at the knee joint
The vastus lateralis also exerts a lateral pull on the patella.
Eccentric action:
Restrains/controls (especially rapid movement) flexion of the leg at the knee joint
The vastus lateralis also restrains/controls the medial pull on the patella by the vastus medialis.
Isometric action:
Stabilizes the patella and the knee joint (and the iliotibial band)
Origin, fixed end, proximal attachment, arises from:
Linea aspera, anterior aspect of the greater trochanter, gluteal tuberosity, and lateral intermuscular septum
Insertion, mobile end, distal attachment, attaches to:
Tibial tuberosity, by way of the patella and patellar ligament
Innervation:
Femoral nerve (L2–L4)
Major synergists:
All quadriceps femoris muscles are synergistic.
Major antagonists:
Hamstrings
Tender/trigger points:
Several locations at each attachment and in the belly of the muscle
Common symptom/Common symptom/Referred pain pattern:
Entire anterior thigh, with concentration at the knee
A tight vastus lateralis, not the iliotibial band, is usually responsible for shortening and pain in the lateral thigh.

Vastus medialis (VAS-tus MEE-dee-al-us)

The third muscle of the quadriceps femoris group, *vastus* means "vast" or "large"; *medialis* means "related to the middle." *Quadriceps* means "four headed."

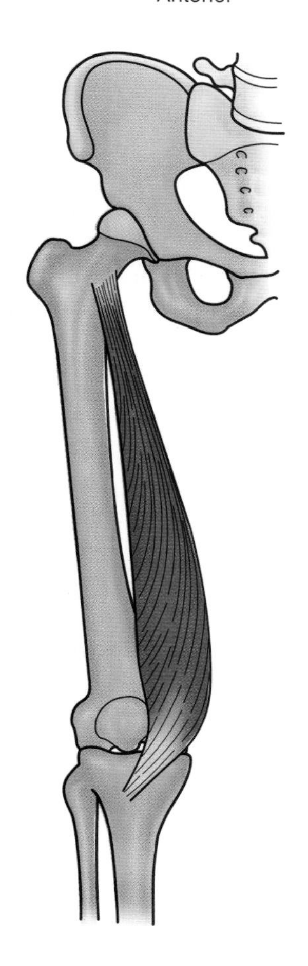

Concentric action:
Extension of the leg at the knee joint
The vastus medialis also exerts a medial pull on the patella.

Eccentric action:
Restrains/controls (especially rapid movement) flexion of the leg at the knee joint
The vastus medialis also restrains/controls the lateral pull on the patella by the vastus lateralis.

Isometric action:
Stabilizes the patella and the knee joint

Origin, fixed end, proximal attachment, arises from:
Linea aspera, intertrochanteric line, medial supracondylar line, and medial intermuscular septum

Insertion, mobile end, distal attachment, attaches to:
Tibial tuberosity, by way of the patella and patellar ligament

The lower fibers of the vastus medialis often are called the *vastus medialis oblique* (VMO); the upper fibers often are called the *vastus medialis longus* (VML).

Innervation:
Femoral nerve (L2–L4)

Major synergists:
All quadriceps femoris muscles are synergistic.

Major antagonists:
Hamstrings

Tender/trigger points:
In the belly of the muscle, near the attachment just above the knee, and in the oblique portion (VMO)

Common symptom/Common symptom/Referred pain pattern:
Entire anterior thigh, with concentration at the knee

Vastus intermedius (VAS-tus in-ter-MEE-dee-us)

The fourth muscle of the quadriceps femoris group, *vastus* means "vast" or "large"; *intermedius* means "among the middle." *Quadriceps* means "four headed."

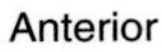

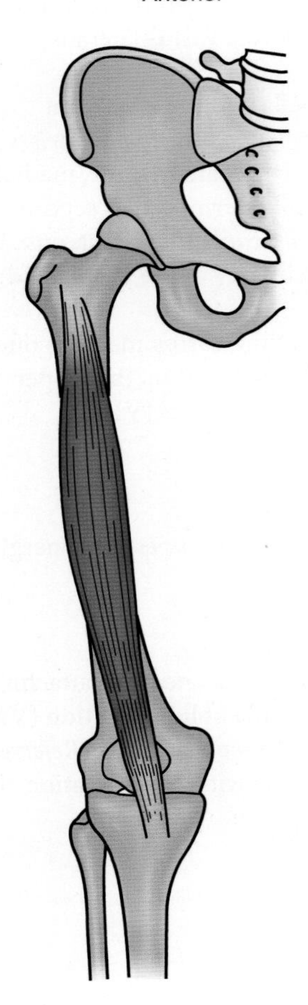

Concentric action:
Extension of the leg at the knee joint
Eccentric action:
Restrains/controls (especially rapid movement) flexion of the leg
Isometric action:
Stabilizes the patella and the knee joint
Origin, fixed end, proximal attachment, arises from:
Linea aspera, anterior and lateral surfaces of the proximal two-thirds of the shaft of the femur, and intermuscular septum
Insertion, mobile end, distal attachment, attaches to:
Tibial tuberosity, by way of the patella and patellar ligament

A portion of the vastus intermedius can be considered a separate muscle called the *articularis genus*, which is responsible for lifting the joint capsule of the knee during extension so that it is not pinched between the patella and femur.

Innervation:
Femoral nerve (L2–L4)
Major synergists:
All quadriceps femoris muscles are synergistic.
Major antagonists:
Hamstrings
Tender/trigger points:
Near the proximal attachment at the musculotendinous junction
Common symptom/Common symptom/Referred pain pattern:
Entire anterior thigh, with concentration at the knee

ACTIVITY 9.37

Draw and color the *muscles of the medial and anterior thigh* in the spaces provided. For each muscle:

1. Label the origin and insertion attachment points: *O* for origin; *I* for insertion.
2. Place an X on the trigger points.
3. Palpate this muscle; identify the attachment points and the bellies of the muscles.
4. Move these muscles on yourself.

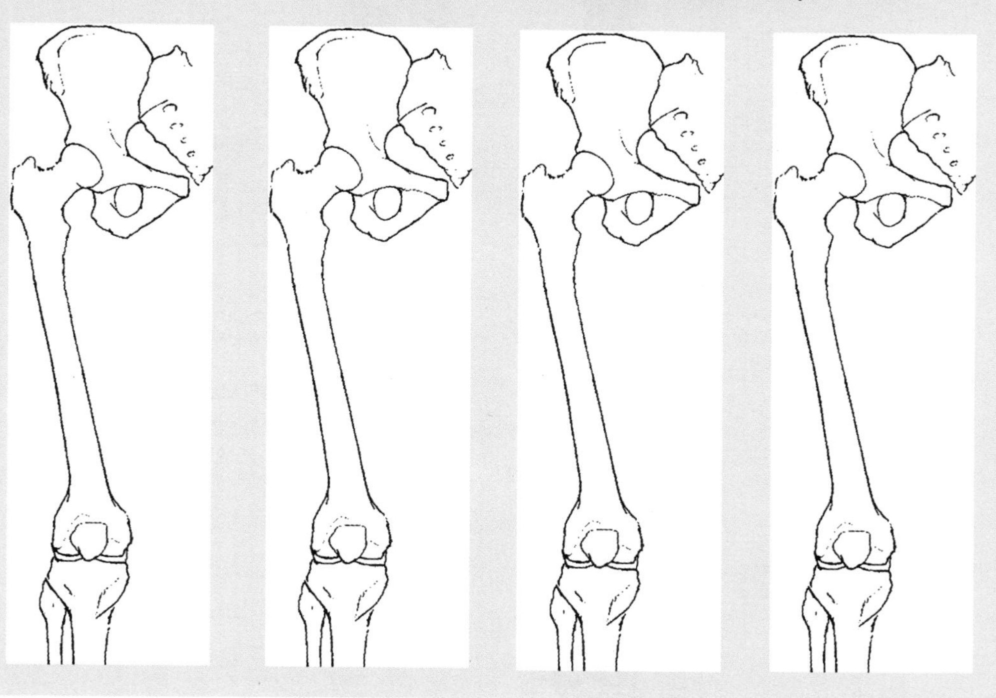

Muscles of the Anterior and Lateral Leg

The muscles of the leg are primarily important for their actions at the foot (Fig. 9.30). These muscles produce dorsiflexion and plantar flexion movements of the foot at the ankle joint and inversion and eversion movements of the foot at the tarsal (subtalar) joints. Many of these muscles also flex and extend the toes at the metatarsophalangeal and interphalangeal joints. The muscles of the anterior leg primarily provide dorsiflexion of the foot at the ankle joint and extension of the toes at the metatarsophalangeal and interphalangeal joints. The muscles of the posterior leg primarily provide plantar flexion of the foot at the ankle joint and flexion of the toes at the metatarsophalangeal and interphalangeal joints. Dorsiflexion of the foot is important in preventing the toes from dragging during walking; plantar flexion of the foot is important for pushing off during walking. The lateral leg muscles evert the foot at the tarsal (subtalar) joints and provide plantar flexion of the foot at the ankle joint.

The deep fascia of the leg is continuous with the iliotibial band, which expands and ensheaths the thigh and binds the leg muscles together. This construction helps prevent excessive swelling of the muscles during exercise. This same fascial sheath supports a pumping action that aids the circulation of blood and lymph, particularly venous return flow. The fascia divides the leg muscles into the anterior, lateral, and posterior compartments, each with its own nerve and blood supply. The leg fascia thickens at the ankles to form the retinacula, which secure the muscle tendons in place as they cross the ankles into the feet. Because of this extensive fascial structure, massage is effective when applied in a slow, sustained manner with a drag that addresses the viscous quality of the tissue. Although most of these muscles primarily produce movements of the foot, any muscle that crosses the knee joint is involved in the function and dysfunction of the knee joint. Because the hip, knee, and ankle joints function as a complex unit and closed kinematic chain when standing, all muscles affecting these joints interact with one another.

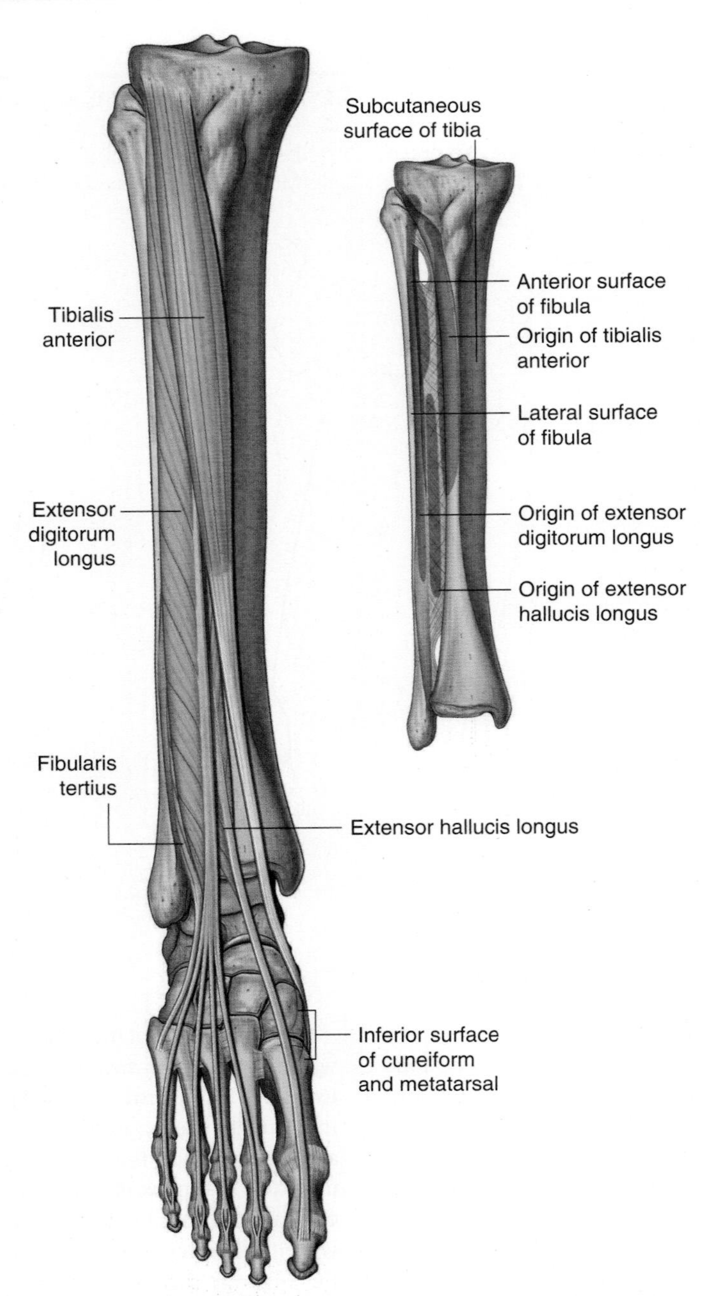

FIG. 9.30 Muscles of the anterior compartment of the leg. (From Drake RL, Vogl W, Mitchell WM. *Gray's Anatomy for Students*. 2nd ed. Churchill Livingstone; 2010.)

Anterior Muscles

Tibialis anterior (TIB-ee-AL-iss)

Tibialis means "related to the shin bone"; *anterior* means "before" or "in front."

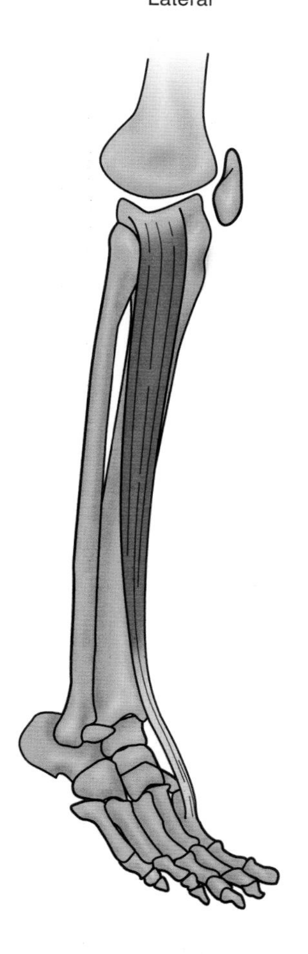

Concentric action:
Dorsiflexion of the foot at the ankle joint and inversion of the foot at the tarsal joints

Eccentric action:
Restrains/controls (especially rapid movement) plantar flexion and eversion of the foot

Isometric action:
Stabilizes the ankle joint

Origin, fixed end, proximal attachment, arises from:
Lateral condyle and proximal two-thirds of the anterior surface of the tibia, interosseous membrane, deep fascia, and lateral intermuscular septum

Insertion, mobile end, distal attachment, attaches to:
At the foot on the medial plantar surface of the medial cuneiform bone and base of the first metatarsal bone

Innervation:
Deep fibular nerve (L4–L5)

Major synergists:
Extensor digitorum longus, extensor hallucis longus, and tibialis posterior

Major antagonists:
Gastrocnemius, soleus, and fibularis muscles

Tender/trigger points:
In the belly of the muscle

Common symptom/Common symptom/Referred pain pattern:
Down the leg to the ankle and into the toes

Extensor digitorum longus (ex-STEN-sur DIH-jih-TOR-um LONG-us)

Extensor means "one that stretches," *digitorum* means "of the fingers and toes," and *longus* means "long."

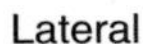

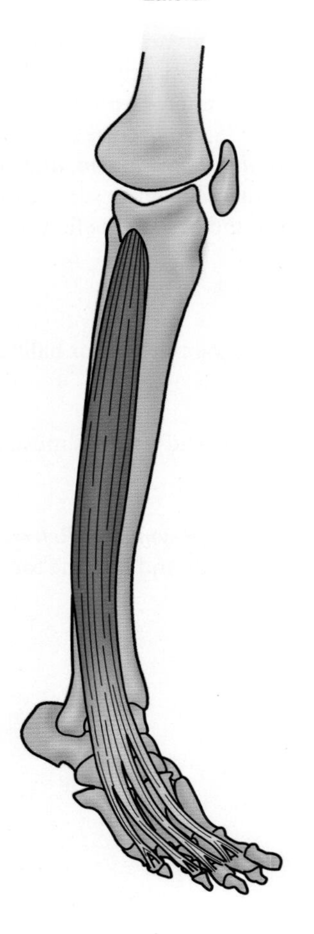

Concentric action:
Extension of toes 2 to 5 at the metatarsophalangeal and interphalangeal joints, dorsiflexion of the foot at the ankle joint, and eversion of the foot at the tarsal joints

Eccentric action:
Restrains/controls (especially rapid movement) flexion of the toes and allows plantar flexion and inversion of the foot

Isometric action:
Stabilizes joints of the ankle and foot

Origin, fixed end, proximal attachment, arises from:
Lateral condyle of the tibia, proximal two-thirds of the anterior surface of the shaft of the fibula, interosseous membrane, deep fascia, and intermuscular septa

Insertion, mobile end, distal attachment, attaches to:
By four tendons to the second through fifth digits; each tendon divides into an intermediate slip, which attaches to the base of the middle phalanx, and two lateral slips, which attach to the base of the distal phalanx.

The distal tendons of the extensor digitorum longus create the dorsal digital expansion of toes 2 to 5.

Innervation:
Deep fibular nerve (L5–S1)

Major synergists:
Extensor digitorum brevis, tibialis anterior, and fibularis muscles

Major antagonists:
Flexor digitorum longus, flexor digitorum brevis, tibialis anterior, and tibialis posterior

Tender/trigger points:
In the belly of the muscle

Common symptom/Common symptom/Referred pain pattern:
Down the leg to the ankle and into the toes

Extensor hallucis longus (ex-STEN-sur HAL-uh-siss LONG-us)

Extensor means "one that stretches," *hallucis* means "related to the big toe," and *longus* means "long."

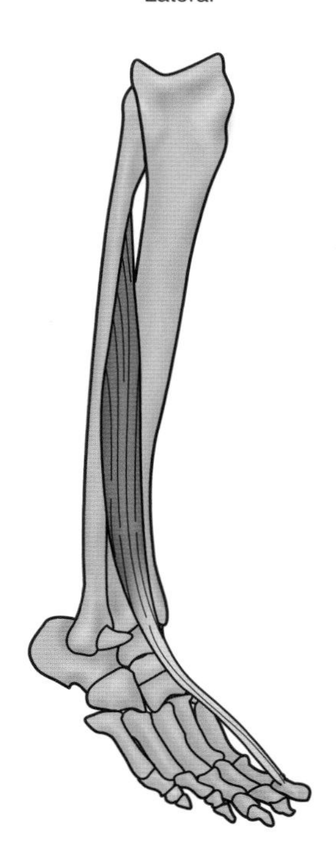

Concentric action:
Extension of the big toe at the metatarsophalangeal and interphalangeal joints, dorsiflexion of the foot at the ankle joint, and inversion of the foot at the tarsal joints

Eccentric action:
Restrains/controls (especially rapid movement) flexion of the great toe and allows plantar flexion and eversion of the foot

Isometric action:
Stabilizes the great toe and assists in stabilizing the ankle

Origin, fixed end, proximal attachment, arises from:
Middle third of the anterior surface of the fibula and adjacent interosseous membrane

Insertion, mobile end, distal attachment, attaches to:
Base of the distal phalanx of the great toe

Innervation:
Deep fibular nerve (L5–S1)

Major synergists:
The tibialis anterior, digitorum longus, peroneus tertius, and extensor hallucis longus are synergistic for dorsiflexion.

Major antagonists:
Eversion and inversion—tibialis anterior, digitorum longus
Dorsiflexion—gastrocnemius, soleus, peroneus longus and peroneus brevis, flexors of the toes, tibialis posterior

Tender/trigger points:
In the belly of each muscle

Common symptom/Common symptom/Referred pain pattern:
Down the leg to the ankle and into the toes

Fibularis (peroneus) tertius (fib-you-LAR-iss TER-she-us)

Fibularis means "related to the pin or fibula"; *tertius* means "the third."

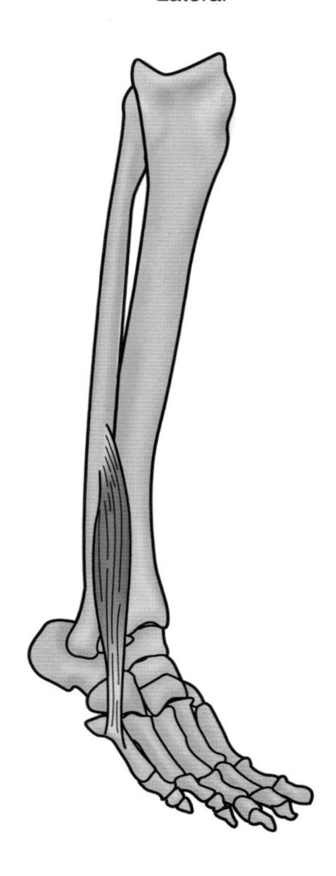

Concentric action:
Dorsiflexion of the foot at the ankle joint and eversion of the foot at the tarsal joints

Eccentric action:
Restrains/controls (especially rapid movement) plantar flexion and inversion of the foot

Isometric action:
Assists in stabilizing the ankle joint

Origin, fixed end, proximal attachment, arises from:
Distal one-third of the anterior surface of the fibula, interosseous membrane, and intermuscular septum

Insertion, mobile end, distal attachment, attaches to:
Dorsal surface of the base of the fifth metatarsal bone

Innervation:
Deep fibular nerve (L5–S1)

Major synergists:
Extensor hallucis brevis and tibialis anterior

Major antagonists:
Flexor hallucis longus, flexor hallucis brevis, and fibularis muscles

Tender/trigger points:
In the belly of the muscle

Common symptom/Common symptom/Referred pain pattern:
Down the leg to the ankle and into the toes

ACTIVITY 9.38

Draw and color the *anterior leg muscles* in the spaces provided. For each muscle:

1. Label the origin and insertion attachment points: *O* for origin; *I* for insertion.
2. Place an X on the trigger points.
3. Palpate this muscle; identify the attachment points and the bellies of the muscles.
4. Move these muscles on yourself.

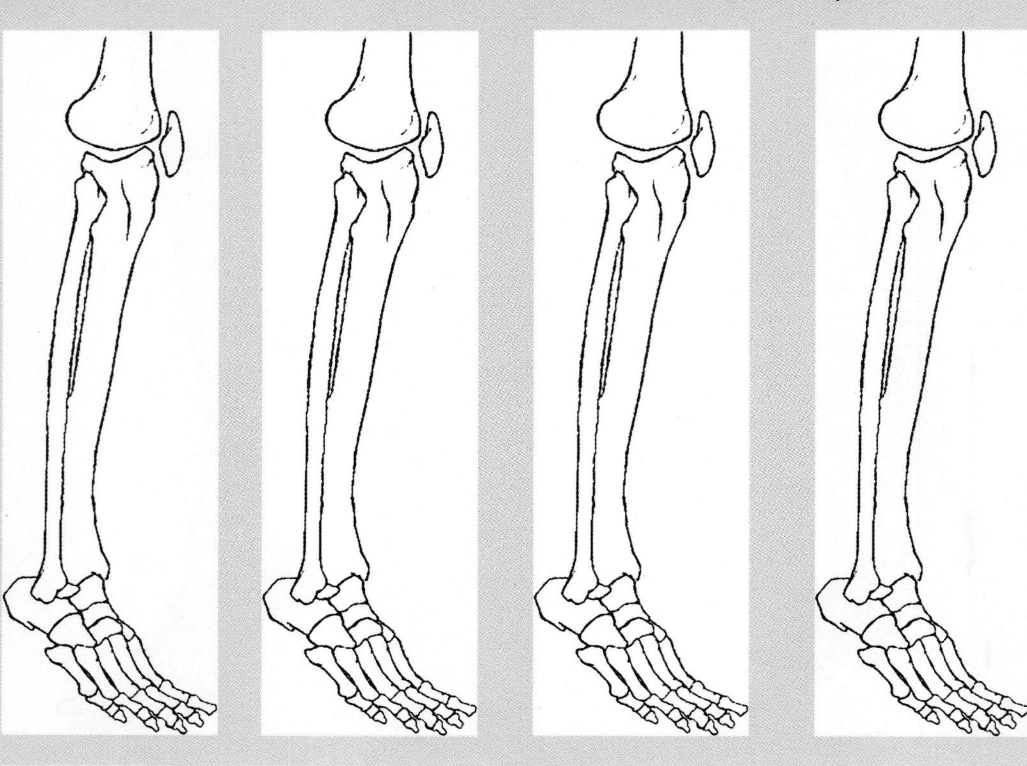

Lateral Muscles

Fibularis (peroneus) longus (fib-you-LAR-iss LONG-us)

Fibularis means "related to the pin or fibula"; *longus* means "long."

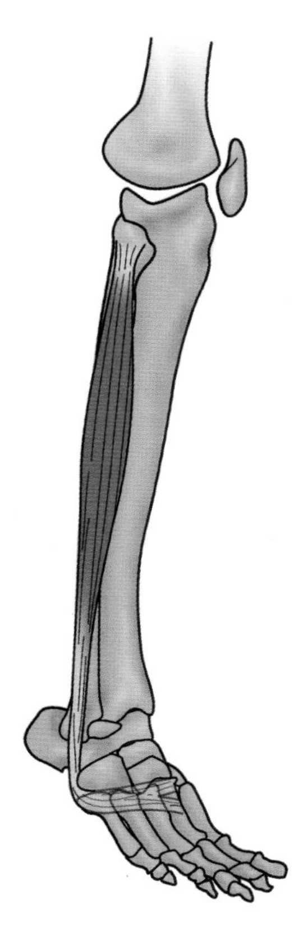

Concentric action:
Eversion of the foot at the tarsal joints and plantar flexion of the foot at the ankle joint

Eccentric action:
Restrains/controls (especially rapid movement) inversion and dorsiflexion of the foot

Isometric action:
Stabilizes the ankle joint

Origin, fixed end, proximal attachment, arises from:
Lateral condyle of the tibia, head and proximal half of the lateral surface of the fibula, intermuscular septa, and adjacent deep fascia

Insertion, mobile end, distal attachment, attaches to:
Lateral side of the base of the first metatarsal bone and the medial cuneiform bone

Innervation:
Superficial fibular nerve (L5–S1)

Major synergist:
Fibularis brevis

Major antagonist:
Tibialis anterior

Tender/trigger points:
Located at the origin and insertion near the musculotendinous junction

Common symptom/Common symptom/Referred pain pattern:
To the lateral malleolus and the heel

Fibularis (peroneus) brevis (fib-you-LAR-iss BREV-iss)

Fibularis means "related to the pin or fibula"; *brevis* means "smaller."

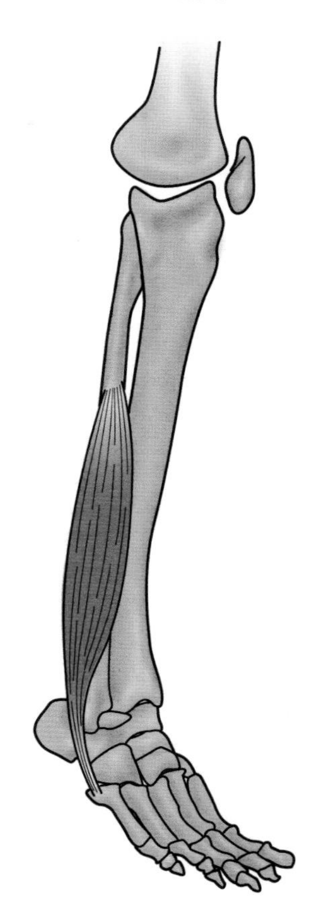

Concentric action:
Eversion of the foot at the tarsal joints and plantar flexion of the foot at the ankle joint

Eccentric action:
Restrains/controls (especially rapid movement) inversion and dorsiflexion of the foot

Isometric action:
Stabilizes the ankle joint

Origin, fixed end, proximal attachment, arises from:
Distal half of the lateral surface of the fibula and adjacent intermuscular septum

Insertion, mobile end, distal attachment, attaches to:
Tuberosity at the base of the fifth metatarsal bone on the lateral side

Innervation:
Superficial fibular nerve (L5–S1)

Major synergist:
Fibularis longus

Major antagonist:
Tibialis anterior

Tender/trigger points:
Located at the origin and insertion near the musculotendinous junction

Common symptom/Common symptom/Referred pain pattern:
To the lateral malleolus and the heel

ACTIVITY 9.39

Draw and color the *lateral leg muscles* in the spaces provided. For each muscle:

1. Label the origin and insertion attachment points: *O* for origin; *I* for insertion.
2. Place an X on the trigger points.
3. Palpate this muscle; identify the attachment points and the bellies of the muscles.
4. Move these muscles on yourself.

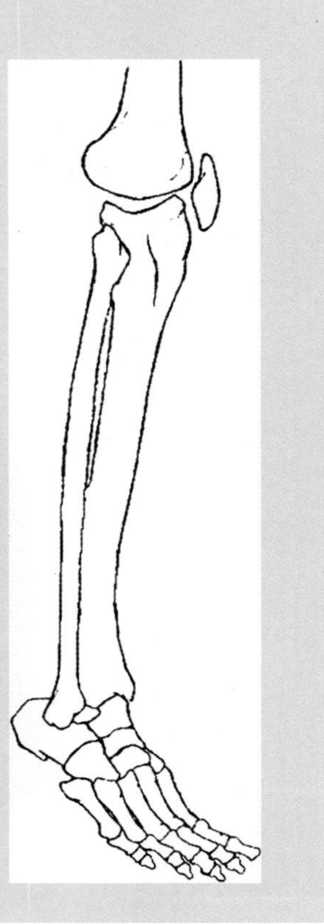

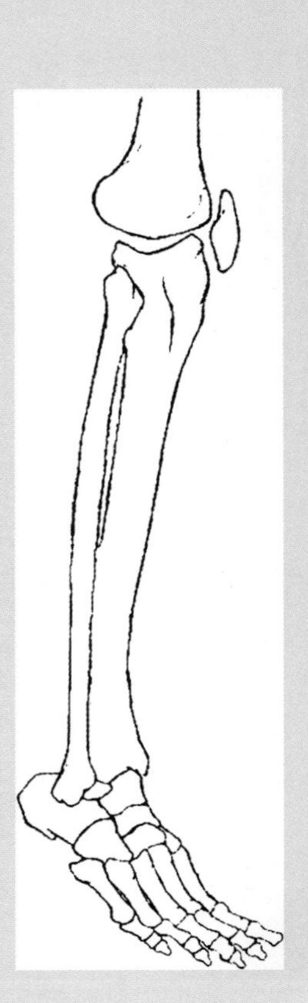

Muscles of the Posterior Leg

The majority of the posterior leg muscles provide plantar flexion of the foot at the ankle joint and invert the foot at the tarsal joints; many of them also flex the toes at the metatarsophalangeal and interphalangeal joints (Fig. 9.31). Plantar flexion lifts the entire weight of the body to allow a person to stand on tiptoe and provides the necessary forward thrust for walking and running. Plantar flexion is a powerful movement. The popliteus muscle, which crosses the knee, is important in unlocking the extended knee (by medial rotation of the leg at the knee joint) in preparation for flexion of the leg at the knee joint. Because they cross the knee joint posteriorly, the gastrocnemius and plantaris muscles assist with flexion of the leg at the knee joint. The gastrocnemius and soleus can become adhered together, which interferes with the function of the gastrocnemius, often causing knee pain, stiffness, and ankle restriction.

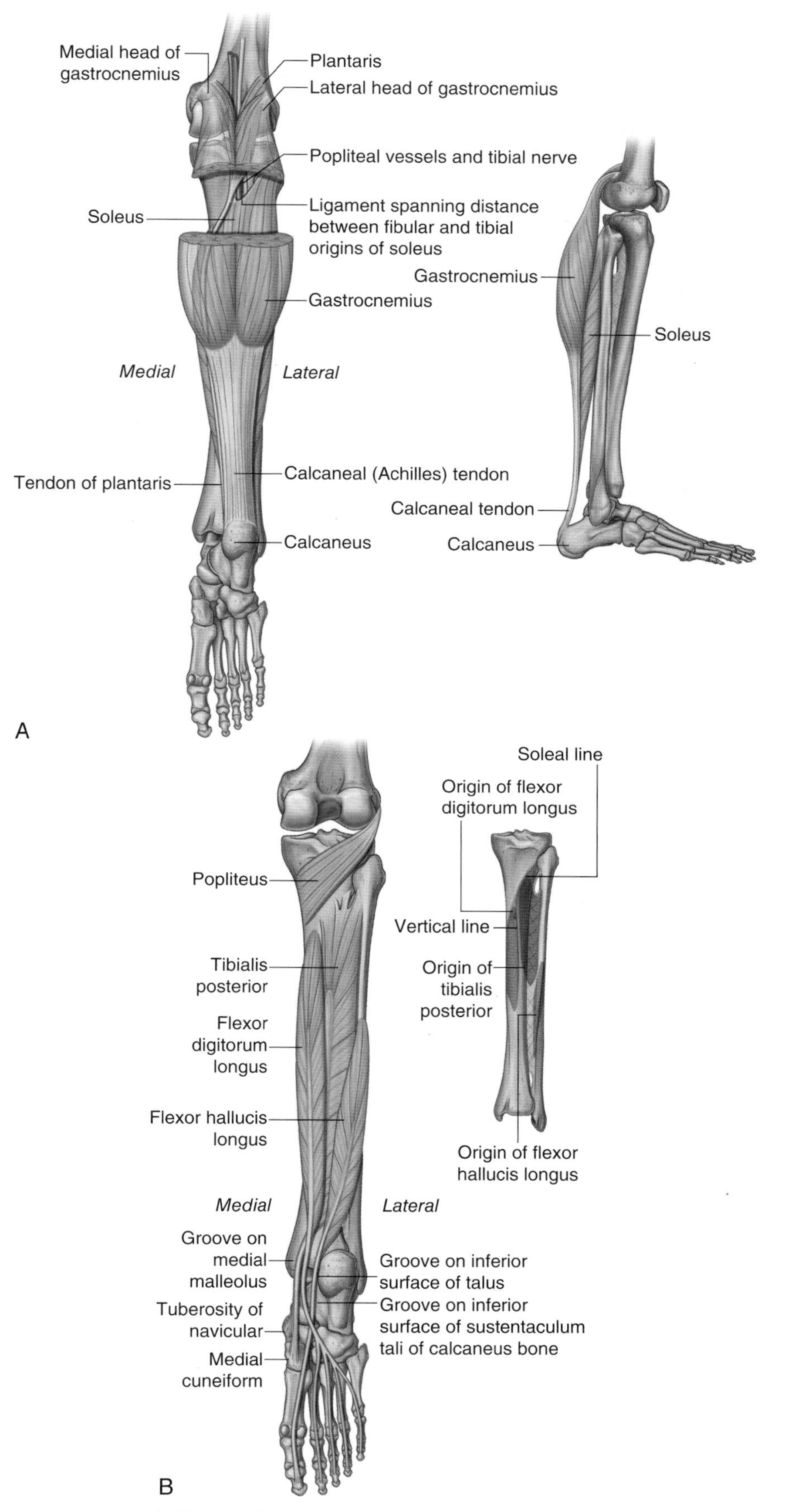

FIG. 9.31 (A) Superficial group of muscles in the posterior compartment of the leg, posterior view. (B) Deep group of muscles in the posterior compartment of the leg. (From Drake RL, Vogl W, Mitchell WM. *Gray's Anatomy for Students*. 2nd ed. Churchill Livingstone; 2010.)

Gastrocnemius (GAS-trok-NEEM-ee-us)

Gastrocnemius means "belly" and "leg."

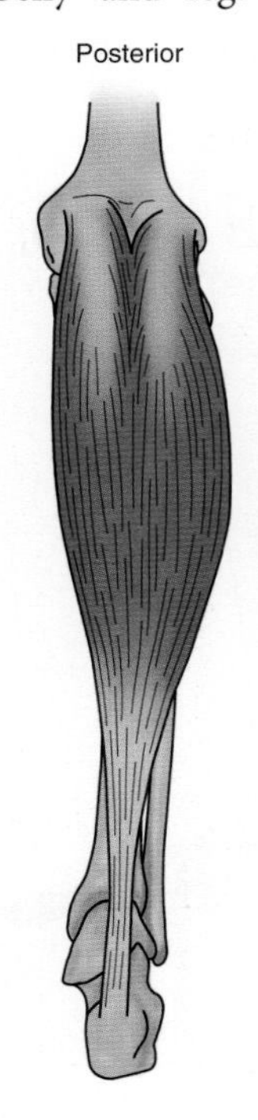

Concentric action:
Plantar flexion of the foot at the ankle joint, inversion of the foot at the tarsal joints, and flexion of the leg at the knee joint

Eccentric action:
Allows dorsiflexion and eversion of the foot and allows extension of the leg

Isometric action:
Stabilizes the knee and ankle joints and is involved in maintaining balance in static standing

Origin, fixed end, proximal attachment, arises from:
Medial head—proximal posterior part of the medial condyle of the femur and capsule of the knee joint
Lateral head—distal part of the lateral supracondylar line and lateral condyle of the femur and capsule of the knee joint

Insertion, mobile end, distal attachment, attaches to:
Calcaneus (with the soleus) by way of the calcaneal (Achilles) tendon

Innervation:
Tibial nerve (S1–S2)

Major synergists:
Soleus and hamstring muscles

Major antagonists:
Tibialis anterior, extensor digitorum longus, extensor hallucis longus, and quadriceps femoris muscles

Tender/trigger points:
In the belly of the muscle and at the attachment near the knee in each head of this muscle

Common symptom/Common symptom/Referred pain pattern:
Down the posterior leg to the heel and the sole of the foot into the plantar surface of the toes; can be a factor in knee pain and restricted mobility of the knee and ankle

Soleus (SOL-ee-us)

Soleus means "sandal" or "sole of the foot."

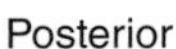

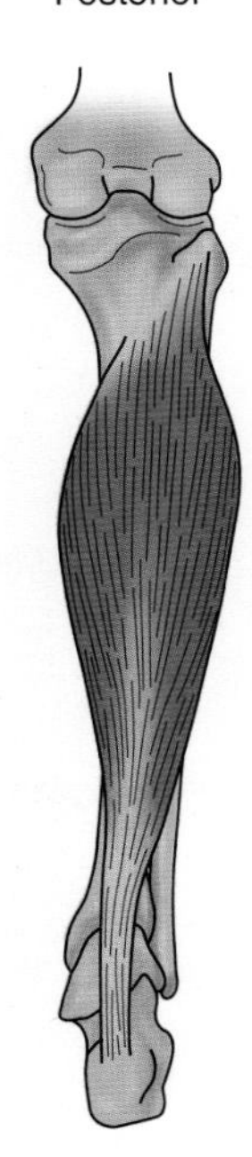

Concentric action:
Plantar flexion of the foot at the ankle joint and inversion of the foot at the tarsal joints

Eccentric action:
Restrains/controls (especially rapid movement) dorsiflexion and eversion of the foot

Isometric action:
Stabilizes the ankle joint
Because of its thick, large venous sinuses, tough fascial covering, and vein structure, the soleus is an effective musculovenous pump that functions as a "second heart," especially during strenuous running and jumping activities.

Origin, fixed end, proximal attachment, arises from:
Posterior surface of the head and proximal one-third of the posterior surface of the fibula, soleal line of the tibia, and fibrous band between the tibia and the fibula

Insertion, mobile end, distal attachment, attaches to:
Calcaneus (with the gastrocnemius) via the calcaneal (Achilles) tendon

Innervation:
Tibial nerve (S1–S2)

Major synergist:
Gastrocnemius

Major antagonists:
Tibialis anterior, extensor digitorum longus, and extensor hallucis longus

Tender/trigger points:
Near the proximal and distal attachments

Common symptom/Common symptom/Referred pain pattern:
Down the posterior leg to the heel and the sole of the foot into the plantar surface of the toes; can be a factor in knee pain and restricted mobility of the knee and ankle

Plantaris (plan-TAR-iss)

Plantaris means "the sole of the foot."

Posterior

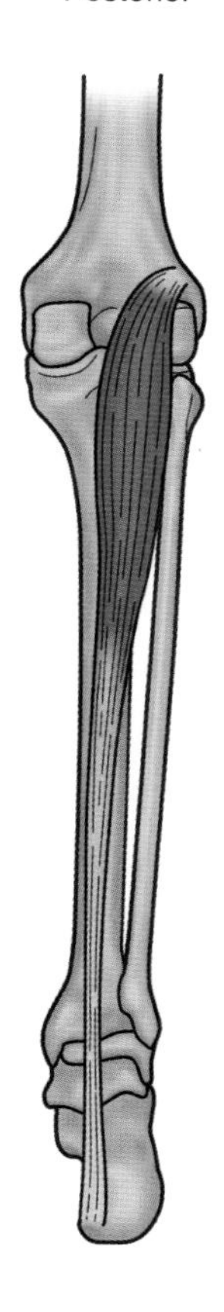

Concentric action:
Plantar flexion of the foot at the ankle joint and flexion of the leg at the knee joint
Eccentric action:
Restrains/controls (especially rapid movement) dorsiflexion of the foot and extension of the leg
Isometric action:
Stabilizes the ankle and knee joints
Origin, fixed end, proximal attachment, arises from:
Distal part of the lateral supracondylar line of the femur and oblique popliteal ligament
Insertion, mobile end, distal attachment, attaches to:
Posterior medial part of the calcaneus with the calcaneal tendon
Innervation:
Tibial nerve (S1–S2)
Major synergists:
Gastrocnemius and soleus
Major antagonists:
Tibialis anterior and quadriceps femoris group
Tender/trigger points:
In the belly of the muscle at the back of the knee joint
Common symptom/Common symptom/Referred pain pattern:
Down the posterior leg to the heel and the sole of the foot into the plantar surface of the toes; can be a factor in knee pain and restricted mobility of the knee and ankle

Flexor hallucis longus (FLEKS-or HAL-uh-siss LONG-us)

Flexor means "to bend," *hallucis* means "related to the big toe," and *longus* means "long."

Posterior/Inferior

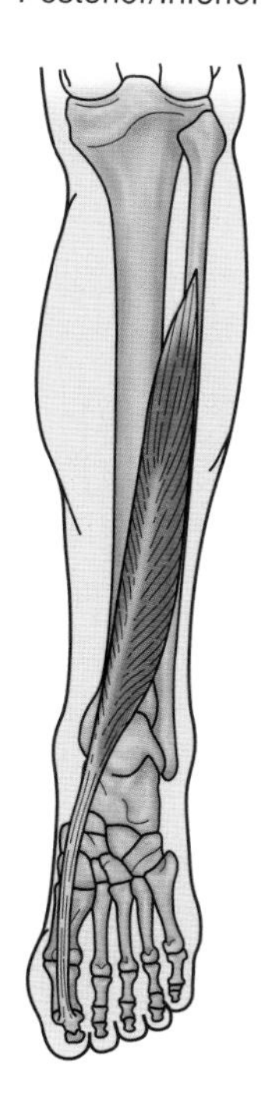

Concentric action:
Flexion of the big toe at the metatarsophalangeal and interphalangeal joints, plantar flexion of the foot at the ankle joint, inversion of the foot at the tarsal joints
Eccentric action:
Restrains/controls (especially rapid movement) extension of the big toe and dorsiflexion and eversion of the foot
Isometric action:
Stabilizes the big toe, ankle, and foot
Origin, fixed end, proximal attachment, arises from:
Distal two-thirds of the posterior surface of the fibula, interosseous membrane, and adjacent intermuscular septum and fascia
Insertion, mobile end, distal attachment, attaches to:
Plantar aspect of the base of the distal phalanx of the big toe (sole of foot)
Innervation:
Tibial nerve (L5–S2)
Major synergist:
Flexor hallucis brevis
Major antagonists:
Extensor hallucis longus and extensor hallucis brevis
Tender/trigger points:
In the belly of the muscle
Common symptom/Common symptom/Referred pain pattern:
Down the posterior leg to the heel and the sole of the foot into the plantar surface of the toes; can be a factor in knee pain and restricted mobility of the knee and ankle

Flexor digitorum longus (FLEKS-or DIH-jih-TOR-um LONG-us)

Flexor means "to bend," *digitorum* means "related to the fingers or toes," and *longus* means "long."

Posterior/Inferior

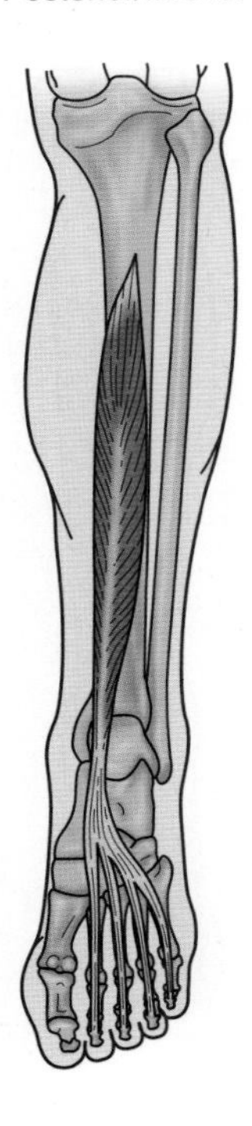

Concentric action:
Flexion of toes 2 to 5 at the metatarsophalangeal and interphalangeal joints, plantar flexion of the foot at the ankle joint, and inversion of the foot at the tarsal joints
Eccentric action:
Allows extension of the toes and allows dorsiflexion and eversion of the foot
Isometric action:
Stabilizes the ankle joint and the toes
Origin, fixed end, proximal attachment, arises from:
Middle one-third of the posterior surface of the shaft of the tibia and the fascia covering the tibialis posterior
Insertion, mobile end, distal attachment, attaches to:
Bases of the distal phalanges of the second through fifth digits (sole of foot)
Innervation:
Tibial nerve (L5–S2)
Major synergist:
Flexor digitorum brevis
Major antagonists:
Extensor digitorum longus and extensor digitorum brevis
Tender/trigger points:
In the belly of the muscle
Common symptom/Common symptom/Referred pain pattern:
Down the posterior leg to the heel and the sole of the foot into the plantar surface of the toes; can be a factor in knee pain and restricted mobility of the knee and ankle

Tibialis posterior (TIB-ee-AL-iss)

Tibialis means "related to the shin bone"; *posterior* means "coming after" or "behind."

Posterior/Inferior

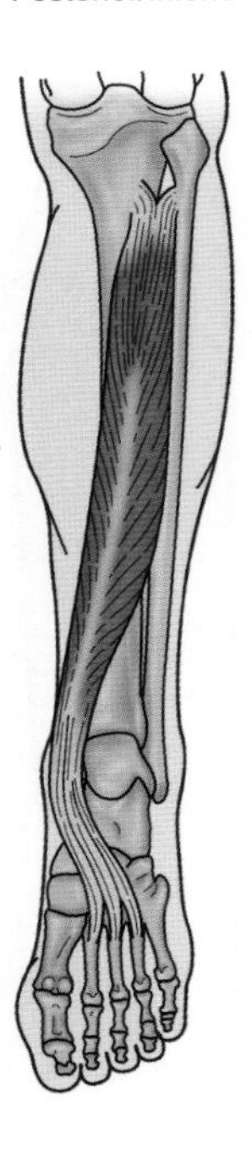

Concentric action:
Plantar flexion of the foot at the ankle joint and inversion of the foot at the tarsal joints
Eccentric action:
Restrains/controls (especially rapid movement) dorsiflexion and eversion of the foot
Isometric action:
Stabilizes the ankle joint
Origin, fixed end, proximal attachment, arises from:
Proximal two-thirds of the posterior surface of the tibia, fibula, and the interosseous membrane and intermuscular septa
Insertion, mobile end, distal attachment, attaches to:
Tuberosity of the navicular bone, calcaneus, three cuneiform bones and the cuboid bone, and bases of the second through fourth metatarsal bones (sole of foot)
Innervation:
Tibial nerve (L4–L5)
Major synergists:
Tibialis anterior, flexor digitorum longus, and flexor hallucis longus
Major antagonists:
Fibularis longus, fibularis brevis, and tibialis anterior
Tender/trigger points:
Belly of the muscle near the knee joint
Common symptom/Common symptom/Referred pain pattern:
Down the posterior leg to the heel and the sole of the foot into the plantar surface of the toes; can be a factor in knee pain and restricted mobility of the knee and ankle

Popliteus (pop-LIT-ee-us)

Popliteus means "hollow of the knee."

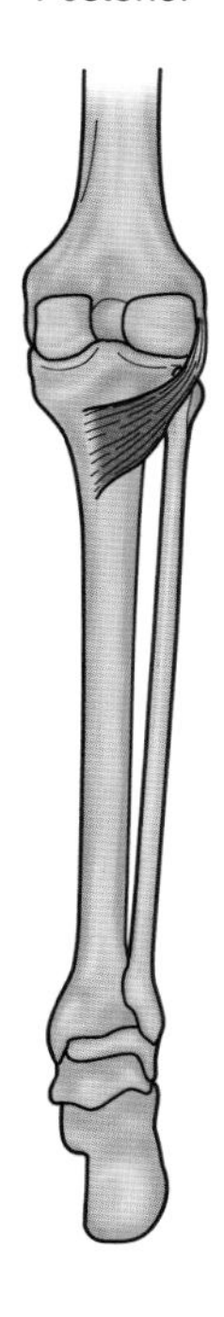

Concentric action:

With the proximal attachment (origin) fixed, medial rotation and flexion of the leg at the knee joint. The medial rotation of the knee joint is considered to be important for flexing the fully extended knee. The reverse action of lateral rotation of the thigh at the knee joint is also important for beginning flexion of the thigh at the knee joint in a weight-bearing lower extremity. The popliteus also moves the lateral meniscus posteriorly during knee flexion.

Eccentric action:

Restrains/controls (especially rapid movement) lateral rotation and extension of the leg

Isometric action:

Stabilizes the knee joint

Origin, fixed end, proximal attachment, arises from:

Lateral surface of the lateral condyle of the femur, oblique popliteal ligament, and lateral meniscus of the knee

Insertion, mobile end, distal attachment, attaches to:

Triangular area above the soleal line on the posterior and medial surfaces of the tibia, as well as the fascia covering its surface

Innervation:

Tibial nerve (L4–S1)

Major synergists:

Semitendinosus, semimembranosus, sartorius, and gracilis

Major antagonists:

Biceps femoris and the quadriceps femoris group

Tender/trigger points:

Belly of the muscle

Common symptom/Common symptom/Referred pain pattern:

To the back of the knee

ACTIVITY 9.40

Draw and color the *posterior leg muscles* in the spaces provided. For each muscle:

1. Label the origin and insertion attachment points: *O* for origin; *I* for insertion.
2. Place an X on the trigger points.
3. Palpate this muscle; identify the attachment points and the bellies of the muscles.
4. Move these muscles on yourself.

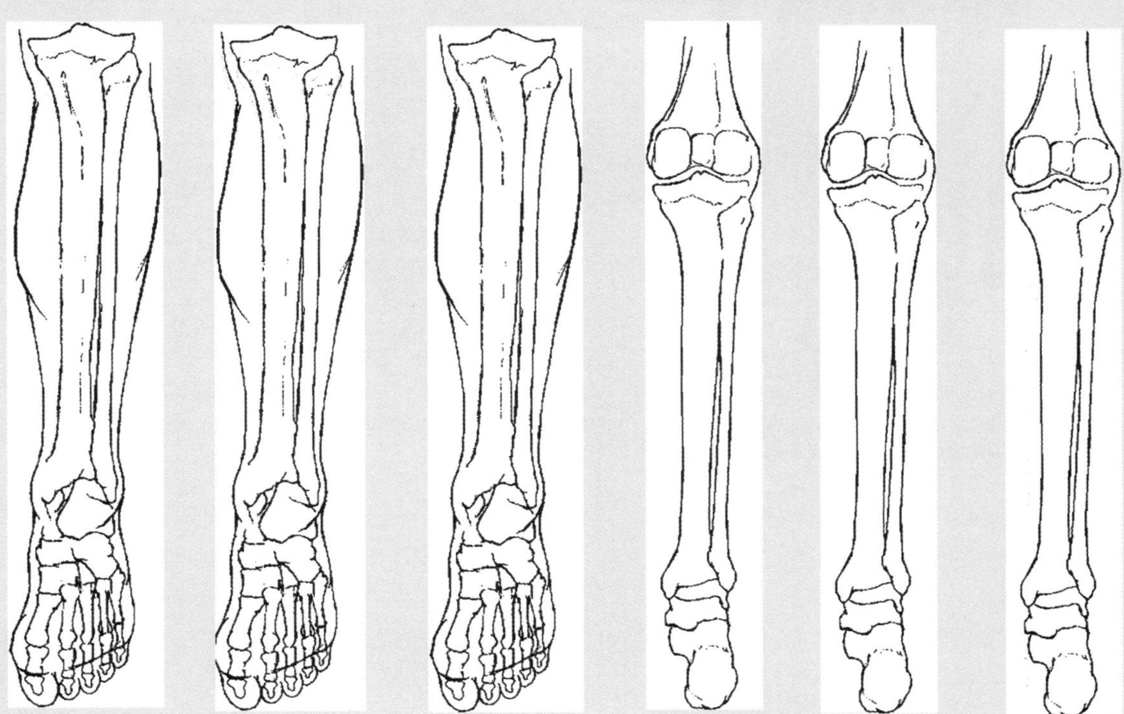

Intrinsic Muscles of the Foot

Intrinsic muscles of the foot are small muscles located entirely within the foot (i.e., they originate and insert within the foot). The muscles of the sole of the foot work concentrically and eccentrically to help flex, extend, abduct, and adduct the toes; they also work isometrically with the tendons of the leg muscles to support the arches of the foot. These muscles are numerous, their arrangement is complex, and their actions are interdependent. Although only the classic concentric mover functions of these muscles are listed, note that the primary function of these muscles is stabilization and proprioceptive feedback on foot position (Fig. 9.32).

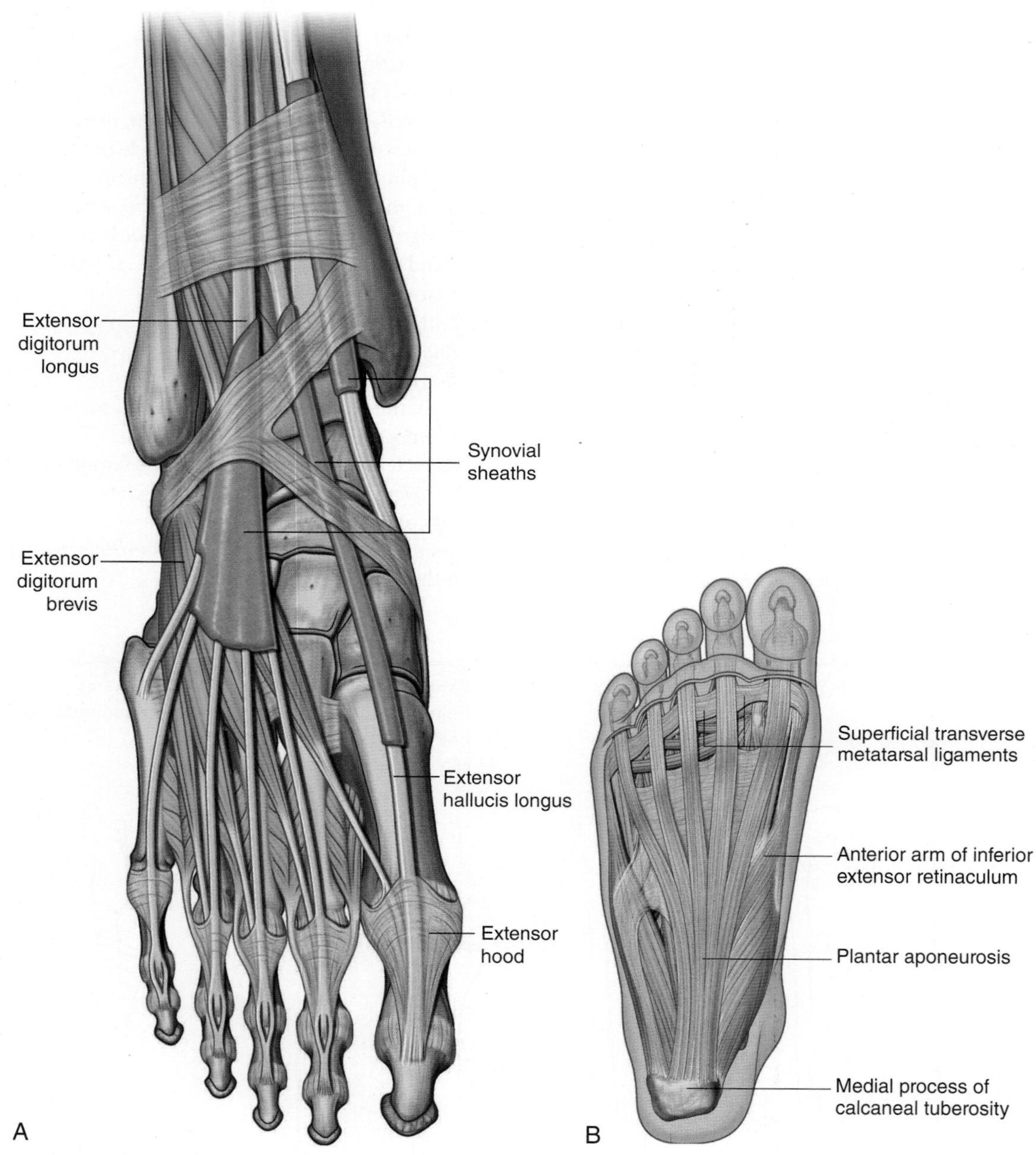

FIG. 9.32 (A) Extensor digitorum brevis and dorsal interossei pedis muscles. (B) Plantar aponeurosis. (From Drake RL, Vogl W, Mitchell WM. *Gray's Anatomy for Students*. 2nd ed. Churchill Livingstone; 2010.)

Dorsal Aspect

Extensor digitorum brevis (ex-STEN-sur DIH-jih-TOR-um BREV-us)

Extensor means "to stretch," *digitorum* means "related to the fingers or toes," and *brevis* means "short."

The most medial portion of the extensor digitorum brevis inserts into the dorsal surface of the base of the proximal phalanx of the big toe and sometimes is called the *extensor hallucis brevis muscle.*

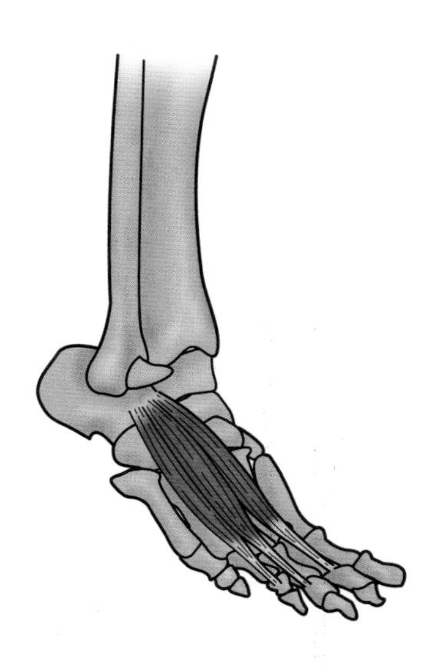

Concentric action:
Extension of the big toe at the metatarsophalangeal joint and extension of toes 2 to 4 at the metatarsophalangeal and interphalangeal joints

Eccentric action:
Restrains/controls (especially rapid movement) flexion of the big toe and flexion of toes 2 to 4

Origin, fixed end, proximal attachment, arises from:
Dorsal surface of the calcaneus, lateral talocalcaneal ligament, and inferior extensor retinaculum

Insertion, mobile end, distal attachment, attaches to:
First tendon into the dorsal surface of the base of the proximal phalanx of the great toe and lateral sides of the tendons of the extensor digitorum longus (dorsal digital expansion) to the second, third, and fourth toes

Innervation:
Deep fibular nerve (L5–S1)

Major synergists:
Extensor digitorum longus and extensor hallucis longus

Major antagonists:
Flexor digitorum longus, flexor hallucis longus, and flexor digitorum brevis

Tender/trigger points:
The belly of the muscle

Common symptom/Common symptom/Referred pain pattern:
The entire foot, with areas concentrated at the large toe, the ball of the foot, and the heel

ACTIVITY 9.41

Draw and color the *muscle of the dorsal aspect of the foot* in the space provided:

1. Label the origin and insertion attachment points: *O* for origin; *I* for insertion.
2. Place an X on the trigger points.
3. Palpate this muscle; identify the attachment points and the bellies of the muscles.
4. Move muscle on yourself.

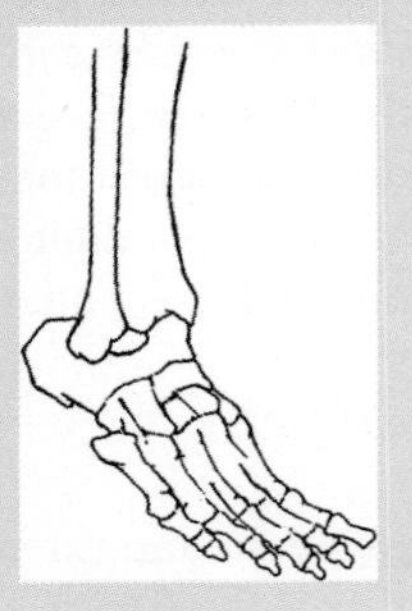

Plantar Aspect: Superficial Layer

Abductor hallucis (ab-DUCK-tur HAL-uh-siss)

Abductor means "to lead away from"; *hallucis* means "big toe."

Inferior/plantar surface

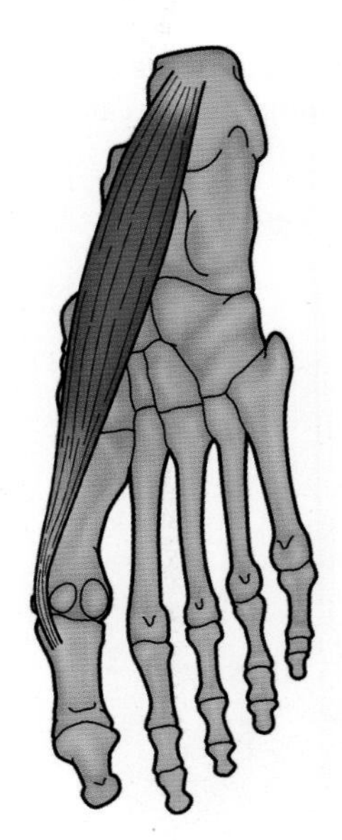

Concentric action:
Abduction and flexion of the big toe at the metatarsophalangeal joint

Eccentric action:
Restrains/controls (especially rapid movement) adduction and extension of the big toe

Origin, fixed end, proximal attachment, arises from:
Medial process of the calcaneal tuberosity, flexor retinaculum, plantar aponeurosis, and adjacent intermuscular septum

Insertion, mobile end, distal attachment, attaches to:
Medial side of the base of the proximal phalanx of the great toe

Innervation:
Medial plantar nerve (S1–S2)

Major synergist:
Flexor hallucis brevis

Major antagonist:
Adductor hallucis

Tender/trigger points:
The belly of the muscle

Common symptom/Common symptom/Referred pain pattern:
The entire foot, with areas concentrated at the large toe, the ball of the foot, and the heel

Flexor digitorum brevis (FLEKS-or DIH-jih-TOR-um BREV-iss)

Flexor means "to bend," *digitorum* means "related to fingers or toes," and *brevis* means "short."

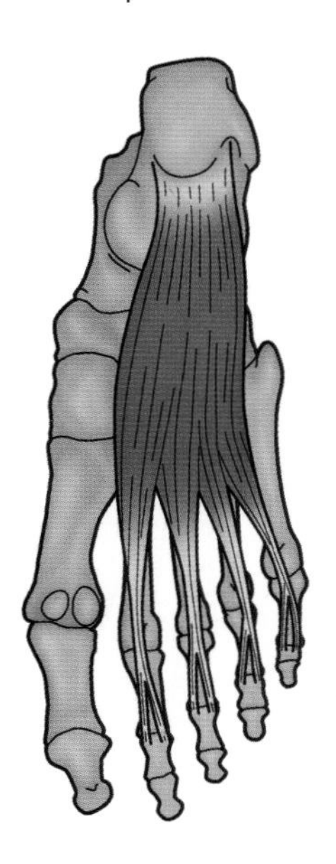

Concentric action:
Flexion of toes 2 to 5 at the metatarsophalangeal and proximal interphalangeal joints
Eccentric action:
Restrains/controls (especially rapid movement) extension of toes 2 to 5
Origin, fixed end, proximal attachment, arises from:
Medial process of the calcaneal tuberosity, plantar aponeurosis, and adjacent intermuscular septa
Insertion, mobile end, distal attachment, attaches to:
Medial and lateral sides of the middle phalanges of the second through fifth toes
Innervation:
Medial plantar nerve (S1 and S2)
Major synergists:
Flexor digitorum longus and quadratus plantae
Major antagonists:
Extensor digitorum longus and extensor digitorum brevis
Tender/trigger points:
The belly of the muscle
Common symptom/Common symptom/Referred pain pattern:
The entire foot, with areas concentrated at the large toe, the ball of the foot, and the heel

Abductor digiti minimi pedis (ab-DUCK-tur DIH-jih-tee MIN-ih-mee PEE-dis)

Abductor means "to lead away from," *digiti* means "related to the fingers or toes," *minimi* means "smallest," and *pedis* means "of the foot."

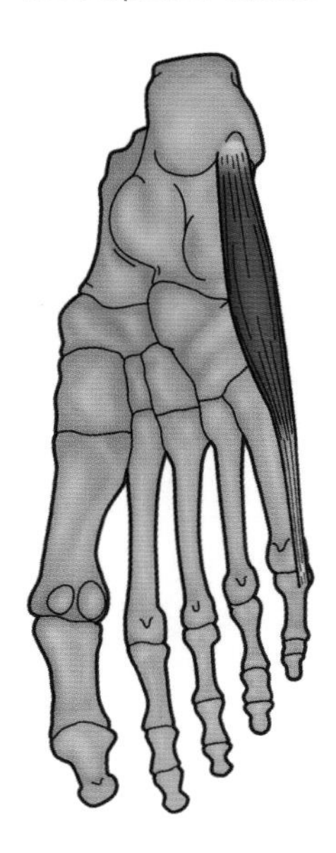

Concentric action:
Abduction and flexion of the fifth toe at the metatarsophalangeal joint
Eccentric action:
Restrains/controls (especially rapid movement) adduction and extension of the fifth toe
Origin, fixed end, proximal attachment, arises from:
Lateral process of the calcaneal tuberosity, plantar aponeurosis, and intermuscular septum
Insertion, mobile end, distal attachment, attaches to:
Lateral side of the base of the proximal phalanx of the fifth toe
Innervation:
Lateral plantar nerve (S2–S3)
Major synergist:
Flexor digitorum brevis
Major antagonist:
Plantar interosseous (No. 3)
Tender/trigger points:
The belly of the muscle
Common symptom/Common symptom/Referred pain pattern:
The entire foot, with areas concentrated at the large toe, the ball of the foot, and the heel

ACTIVITY 9.42

Draw and color the *muscles of the plantar aspect (superficial layer) of the foot* in the spaces provided. For each muscle:

1. Label the origin and insertion attachment points: *O* for origin; *I* for insertion.
2. Place an X on the trigger points.
3. Palpate this muscle; identify the attachment points and the bellies of the muscles.
4. Move these muscles on yourself.

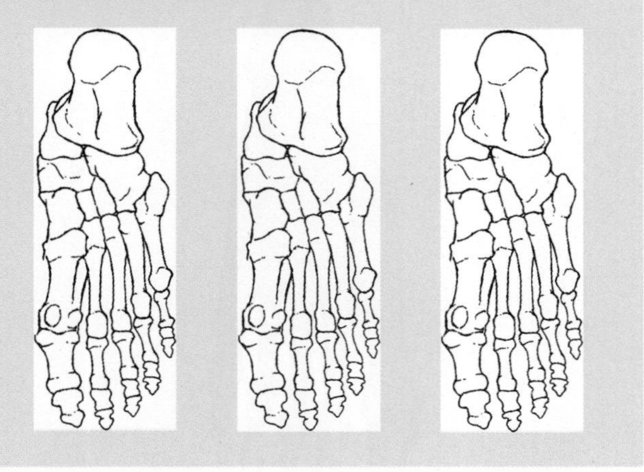

Plantar Aspect: Second Layer

Quadratus plantae (kwad-RATE-us PLAN-tie)

Quadratus means "square shaped"; *plantae* means "for the sole of the foot."

Inferior/Plantar surface

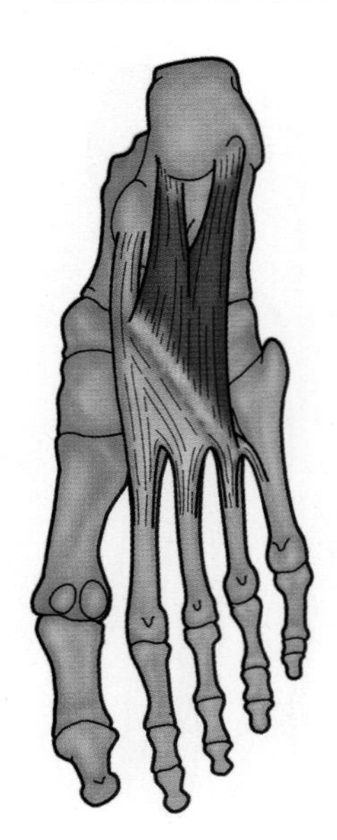

Concentric action:
Flexion of toes 2 to 5 at the metatarsophalangeal and interphalangeal joints
The quadratus plantae acts to modify the line of pull of the flexor digitorum longus.

Eccentric action:
Restrains/controls (especially rapid movement) extension of toes 2 to 5

Origin, fixed end, proximal attachment, arises from:
Medial head—medial surface of the calcaneus and medial border of the long plantar ligament
Lateral head—lateral inferior surface of the calcaneus, lateral border of the plantar surface of the calcaneus, and lateral border of the long plantar ligament

Insertion, mobile end, distal attachment, attaches to:
Lateral margin of the flexor digitorum longus tendon

Innervation:
Lateral plantar nerve (S2–S3)

Major synergists:
Flexor digitorum longus and flexor digitorum brevis

Major antagonists:
Extensor digitorum longus and extensor digitorum brevis

Tender/trigger points:
The belly of the muscle

Common symptom/Common symptom/Referred pain pattern:
The entire foot, with areas concentrated at the large toe, the ball of the foot, and the heel

Lumbricals pedis (LUM-brih-kals PEE-dis)

Lumbricals means "earthworms"; *pedis* means "of the foot."

Inferior/Plantar surface

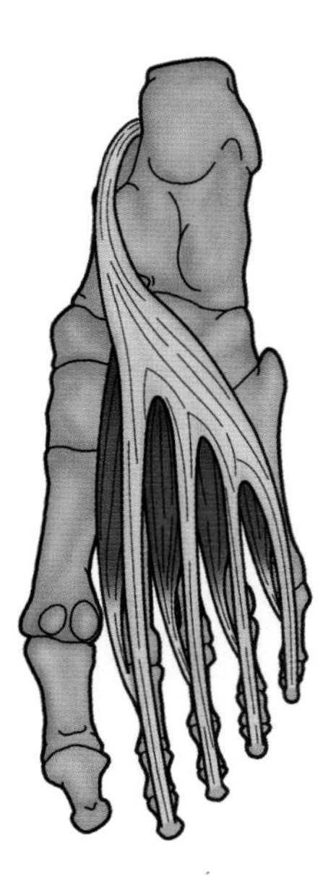

Concentric action:
Flexion of toes 2 to 5 at the metatarsophalangeal joints and extension of toes 2 to 5 at the proximal and distal interphalangeal joints

Eccentric action:
Restrains/controls (especially rapid movement) extension and flexion of toes 2 to 5

Origin, fixed end, proximal attachment, arises from:
First—From the medial side of the first flexor digitorum longus tendon
Second—From adjacent sides of the first and second flexor digitorum longus tendons
Third—From adjacent sides of the second and third flexor digitorum longus tendons
Fourth—From adjacent sides of the third and fourth flexor digitorum longus tendons

Insertion, mobile end, distal attachment, attaches to:
Distal tendons of the extensor digitorum longus (dorsal digital expansion) into the base of the middle and distal phalanges of the second through fifth toes

Innervation:
Medial and lateral plantar nerves (S1–S3)

Major synergists:
Flexor digitorum longus and extensor digitorum longus

Major antagonists:
Flexor digitorum longus and extensor digitorum longus

Tender/trigger points:
The belly of the muscle

Common symptom/Common symptom/Referred pain pattern:
The entire foot, with areas concentrated at the large toe, the ball of the foot, and the heel

ACTIVITY 9.43

Draw and color the *muscles of the plantar aspect (second layer) of the foot* in the spaces provided. For each muscle:

1. Label the origin and insertion attachment points: *O* for origin; *I* for insertion.
2. Place an X on the trigger points.
3. Palpate this muscle; identify the attachment points and the bellies of the muscles.
4. Move these muscles on yourself.

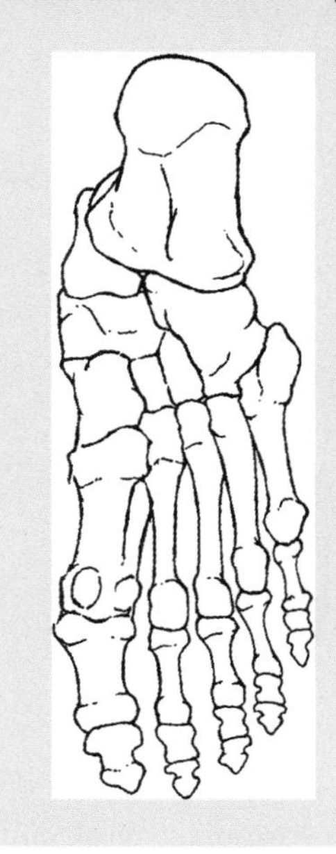

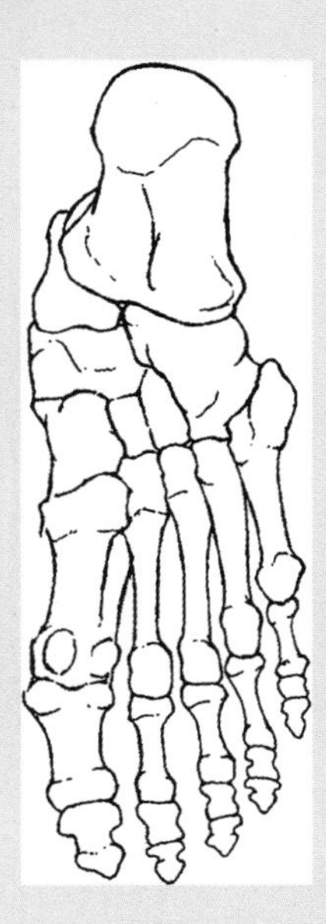

Plantar Aspect: Third Layer

Flexor hallucis brevis (FLEKS-or HAL-uh-siss BREV-us)

Flexor means "to bend," *hallucis* means "big toe," and *brevis* means "short."

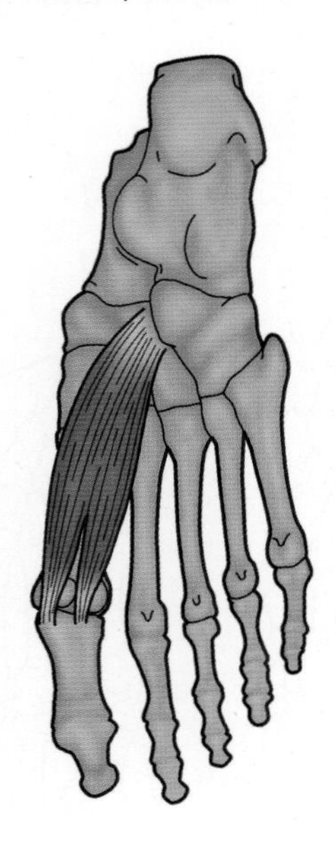

Concentric action:
Flexion of the big toe at the metatarsophalangeal joint
Eccentric action:
Restrains/controls (especially rapid movement) extension of the big toe
Origin, fixed end, proximal attachment, arises from:
Medial aspect of the plantar surface of the cuboid bone, lateral cuneiform bone, and from the tendon of the tibialis posterior
Insertion, mobile end, distal attachment, attaches to:
Medial and lateral sides of the base of the proximal phalanx of the great toe
Innervation:
Medial plantar nerve (S1–S2)
Major synergist:
Flexor hallucis longus
Major antagonists:
Extensor hallucis longus and extensor digitorum brevis (medial part)
Tender/trigger points:
The belly of the muscle
Common symptom/Common symptom/Referred pain pattern:
The entire foot, with areas concentrated at the large toe, the ball of the foot, and the heel

Adductor hallucis (ad-DUCK-tur HAL-uh-siss)

Adductor means "to lead toward"; *hallucis* means "big toe."

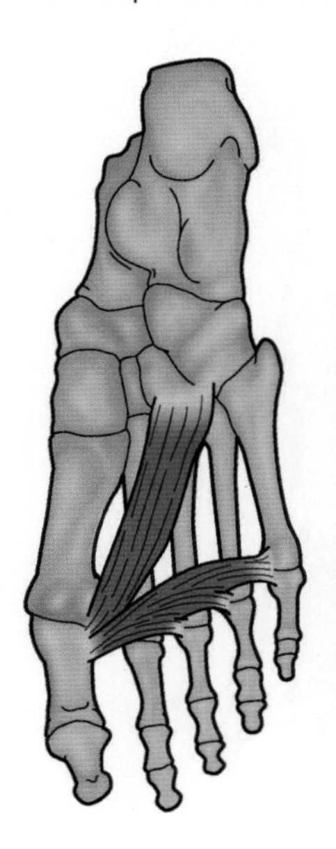

Concentric action:
Adduction and flexion of the big toe at the metatarsophalangeal joint
Eccentric action:
Restrains/controls abduction and extension of the big toe
Origin, fixed end, proximal attachment, arises from:
Oblique head—bases of the second, third, and fourth metatarsal bones and sheath of the tendon of the fibularis longus
Transverse head—plantar metatarsophalangeal ligaments of the third, fourth, and fifth digits and deep transverse metatarsal ligament of the sole
Insertion, mobile end, distal attachment, attaches to:
Lateral side of the base of the proximal phalanx of the big toe
Innervation:
Lateral plantar nerve (S2–S3)
Major synergists:
Flexor hallucis longus and flexor hallucis brevis
Major antagonist:
Abductor hallucis
Tender/trigger points:
The belly of the muscle
Common symptom/Common symptom/Referred pain pattern:
The entire foot with areas concentrated at the large toe, the ball of the foot, and the heel

Flexor digiti minimi pedis (FLEKS-or DIH-jih-tee MIN-ih-mee PEE-dis)

Flexor means "to bend," *digiti* means "related to the fingers and toes," *minimi* means "smallest," and *pedis* means "of the foot."

Occasionally, some of the deeper fibers of the flexor digiti minimi pedis reach the lateral part of the distal half of the fifth metatarsal bone; this sometimes is described as a distinct muscle, the opponens digiti minimi pedis.

Inferior/plantar surface

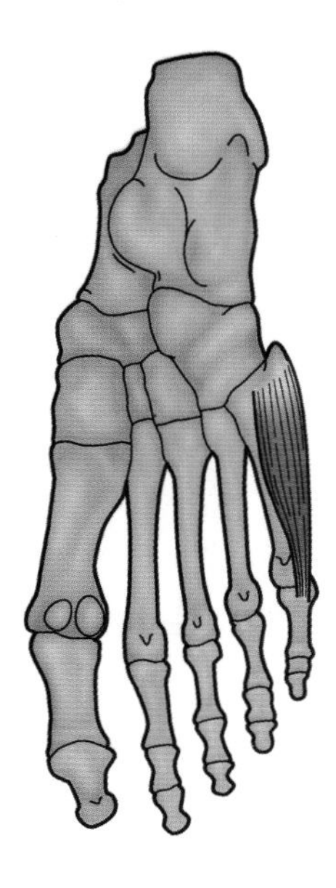

Concentric action:
Flexion of the little toe at the metatarsophalangeal joint
Eccentric action:
Restrains/controls extension of the little toe
Origin, fixed end, proximal attachment, arises from:
Medial part of the plantar surface of the base of the fifth metatarsal bone and sheath of the fibularis longus
Insertion, mobile end, distal attachment, attaches to:
Plantar surface of the base of the proximal phalanx of the little toe
Innervation:
Lateral plantar nerve (S2–S3)
Major synergists:
Flexor digitorum longus and flexor digitorum brevis
Major antagonist:
Extensor digitorum longus
Tender/trigger points:
The belly of the muscle
Common symptom/Common symptom/Referred pain pattern:
The entire foot, with areas concentrated at the large toe, the ball of the foot, and the heel

ACTIVITY **9.44**

Draw and color the *muscles of the plantar aspect (third layer) of the foot* in the spaces provided. For each muscle:

1. Label the origin and insertion attachment points: *O* for origin; *I* for insertion.
2. Place an X on the trigger points.
3. Palpate this muscle; identify the attachment points and the bellies of the muscles.
4. Move these muscles on yourself.

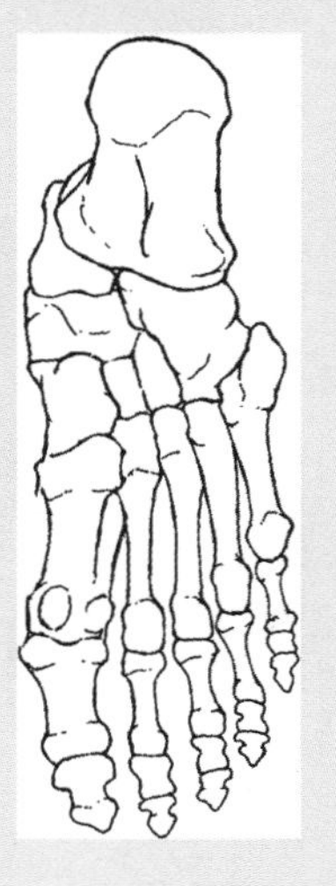

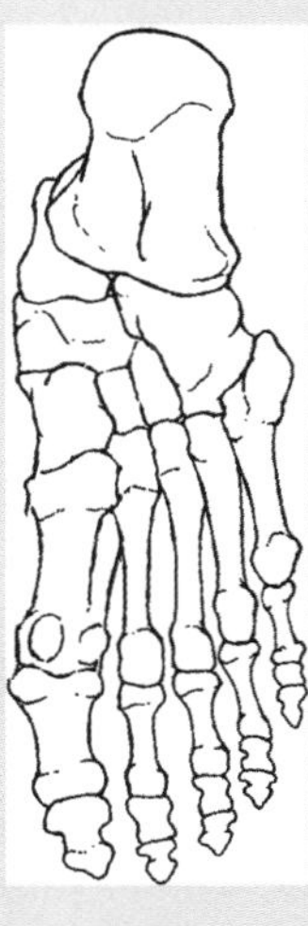

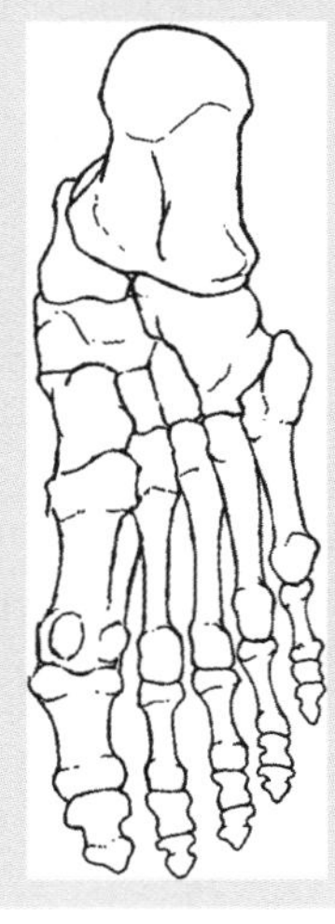

Plantar Aspect: Fourth Layer

Plantar interossei (plan-TAR INT-er-OSS-ee-eye)

Plantar means "sole of the foot"; *interossei* means "between the bones."

Inferior/plantar surface

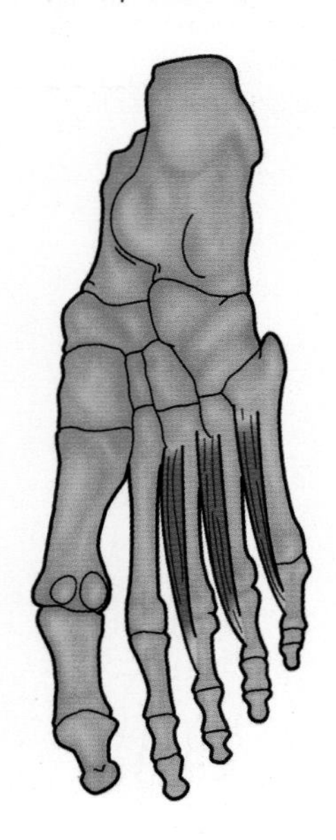

Concentric action:
Adduction of toes 3 to 5 at the metatarsophalangeal joints (adduction of a toe is a movement toward an imaginary line drawn through the middle of the second toe), flexion of toes 3 to 5 at the metatarsophalangeal joints, and extension of toes 3 to 5 at the proximal and distal interphalangeal joints

Eccentric action:
Restrains/controls (especially rapid movement) abduction, extension, and flexion of toes 3 to 5

Origin, fixed end, proximal attachment, arises from:
Three plantar interossei arise from the base and medial sides of the shafts of the third, fourth, and fifth metatarsals.

Insertion, mobile end, distal attachment, attaches to:
Medial sides of the bases of the proximal phalanges of the same toes and the dorsal digital expansion

Innervation:
Lateral plantar nerve (S2–S3)

Major synergist:
Lumbricals pedis

Major antagonist:
Dorsal interossei pedis

Tender/trigger points:
The belly of the muscle

Common symptom/Common symptom/Referred pain pattern:
The entire foot, with areas concentrated at the large toe, the ball of the foot, and the heel

Dorsal interossei pedis (DOOR-sul INT-er-OSS-ee-eye PEE-dis)

Dorsal means "on or near the back," *interossei* means "between the bones," and *pedis* means "of the foot."

Inferior/plantar surface

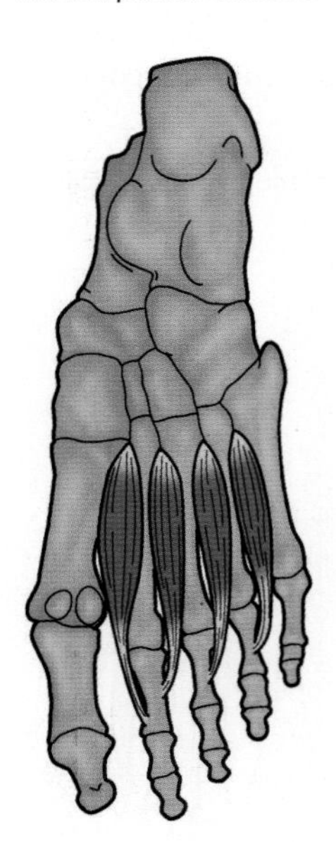

Concentric action:
Abduction of toes 2 to 4 at the metatarsophalangeal joints (abduction of a toe is a movement away from an imaginary line drawn through the middle of the second toe), flexion of toes 2 to 4 at the metatarsophalangeal joints, and extension of toes 2 to 4 at the proximal and distal interphalangeal joints

Eccentric action:
Restrains/controls (especially rapid movement) adduction, extension, and flexion of toes 2 to 4.

Origin, fixed end, proximal attachment, arises from:
Each arises by way of two heads from adjacent sides of the metatarsal bones between which they are placed.

Insertion, mobile end, distal attachment, attaches to:
Bases of the proximal phalanges of toes 2 to 4 and distal tendons of the extensor digitorum longus (dorsal digital expansion)

Innervation:
Lateral plantar nerve (S2–S3)

Major synergist:
Lumbricals pedis

Major antagonist:
Plantar interossei

Tender/trigger points:
Belly of the muscle

Common symptom/Common symptom/Referred pain pattern:
The entire foot, with areas concentrated at the large toe, the ball of the foot, and the heel

ACTIVITY 9.45

Draw and color the *muscles of the plantar aspect (fourth layer) of the foot* in the spaces provided. For each muscle:

1. Label the origin and insertion attachment points: *O* for origin; *I* for insertion.
2. Place an X on the trigger points.
3. Palpate this muscle; identify the attachment points and the bellies of the muscles.
4. Move these muscles on yourself.

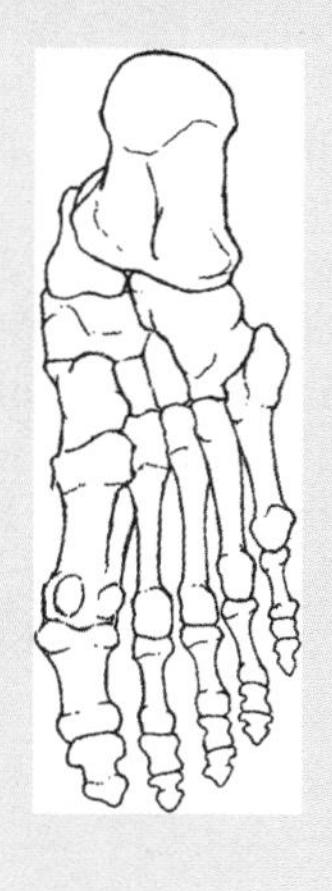

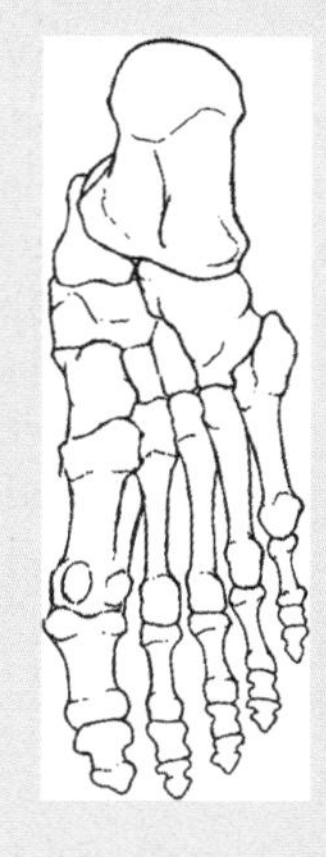

Section Summary

Explain the three types of muscle actions.

Concentric: muscle shortens, accelerating motion, functioning as the prime mover/agonist. Eccentric: muscle lengthens, decelerating motion, typically functioning as the antagonist. Isometric: muscle contracts but produces no motion, functioning as the stabilizer (fixator)/neutralizer.

Describe how muscles are named.

Muscles are named based on their location, function, shape, fiber direction, number of heads/divisions, attachment points, and size.

Apply knowledge of the muscular system to therapeutic massage application.

Massage application first addresses superficial layers of muscle, then deeper layers. Superficial muscles tend to be large prime movers. Deeper muscles tend to be small stabilizers. Muscle dysfunction of one muscle can/may cause dysfunction of related synergists and/or antagonists. Shape and fiber direction of muscle correlates with its function. Massage best affects muscle tissue when multiple mechanical force loads are applied, such as tension (gliding) parallel to fiber direction (with the grain), bending/torsion (kneading) perpendicular to the fiber direction (against the grain). Muscle actions and attachment locations inform the direction of active and passive joint movement and application of muscle energy techniques. Trigger points often correlate with symptomatic referred pain.

PATHOLOGICAL CONDITIONS

SECTION OBJECTIVES

Chapter objective covered in this section:

13. Identify common pathology related to muscles and explain indications and contraindications for massage.

After completing this section, the student will be able to:

- Describe categories of medications used to treat pathological conditions of muscles.
- Explain massage adaptation related to pathological conditions of muscles.

Mechanisms of Disease

Whenever the myofascial system is stressed, a fairly predictable sequence of events occurs:

1. Causal factors can lead to increased muscle tension and retention of metabolic wastes. Causal factors include congenital factors or predisposition, overuse, misuse, abuse, and disuse of the body, postural stress, chronic stressful emotional states, and so forth.
2. Increased tension leads to localized ischemia and edema.
3. Pain results.
4. Pain increases tension or spasm, which increases pain.
5. Inflammation or chronic irritation may result.
6. Neurological reporting stations in tense tissue bombard the central nervous system with information, which leads to hyperactivity.
7. Macrophages and fibroblasts are activated.
8. Connective tissue fiber production increases, with increasing shortening of fascia.
9. Because fascia is continuous throughout the body, any distortions in one area could create distortions elsewhere, affecting structures supported by or attached to the fascia, including the nerves, muscles, lymph, and blood vessels.
10. Changes occur in the muscular tissues, leading to chronic tension related to tone and stiffness, which leads to densification and ultimately fibrotic changes. Increased tension in a muscle causes inhibition of the antagonist muscles and facilitation in the synergists.
11. Chain reactions in myotatic units occur. Typically, muscles used for posture become shortened, and muscles used for motion tend to weaken. This effect alters gait reflexes, and synergists can become dominant, causing muscle firing patterns to be altered.
12. Sustained increases in muscle tension cause ischemia in tendinous areas, and areas of periosteal pain develop.
13. Abnormal biomechanics and body-wide compensatory patterns develop. Torsion patterns at the shoulder and pelvic girdle are common. Gait patterns are compromised.
14. Joint restriction or imbalance or both develop, and fascial shortening, stiffening, and immobility increase.

15. Localized tender/trigger points develop or worsen.
16. Generalized fatigue develops as a result of wasted energy used to maintain unproductive compensation patterns as well as interrupted sleep patterns.
17. Sympathetic arousal is heightened, perpetuating dysfunctional patterns.
18. Immune response is altered, increasing susceptibility to disease.

Massage Intervention

Muscle dysfunction in the concentric action often results in short, tense muscles that do not relax and lengthen eccentrically when necessary. Tender/trigger points often set up in the muscle belly. Concentric contraction dysfunction is an important place to begin treatment by using methods to inhibit and lengthen the muscle. Ideally after lengthening, muscles will respond to strengthening procedures.

Muscle dysfunction in the eccentric action phase often results in tense but elongated and strained muscles that are not concentrically shortening, so they attempt recruitment of synergists to function. Tender/trigger points often set up near the attachments. Massage therapy application should avoid specifically addressing eccentric tight patterns with methods that would relax and elongate the muscle further.

Isometric muscle dysfunction usually results in agonist and antagonist patterns interacting simultaneously to stabilize a joint dysfunction. This dysfunction is usually caused by joint laxity, guarding of an injury, or overuse. If this continues for a time, fibrosis is common, as well as reduced ability for concentric and eccentric function. Mobility and coordination decrease because stabilizing function is prioritized over mobility.

Intervention should focus on reversing nonproductive patterns and supporting resourceful compensation patterns that develop in response to chronic problems. The goal is to calm the nervous system and support connective tissue pliability and layer sliding. Connective tissue responds to methods that affect the viscoelastic and colloid properties. Muscle shortening patterns related to the nervous system respond to compression and drag that stimulates proprioceptors. Muscle energy methods systematically use contraction and relaxation of muscles, combined with lengthening to restore normal resting length of the muscles. Tender/trigger points respond to methods that reduce nervous system hyperactivity, such as muscle energy methods and compression. Calming of sympathetic arousal is also necessary.

Medications

Pathological conditions of the muscles are treated with antiinfectives, antiinflammatories, and muscle relaxants. Pain is treated with analgesics. Infections are treated with antibiotics, antivirals, and antifungal and antiparasitic medications. Steroidal and nonsteroidal antiinflammatory medications ease inflammation. Muscle relaxants soothe spasm and hypertonic muscles. Low doses of antidepressants sometimes assist the client with sleep restoration and support of other restorative processes.

These drugs may be prescription or over-the-counter medications. Any form of medication or herbal remedy may have effects on the client that need to be taken into consideration when developing a treatment plan. Consideration must also be given to the interaction between massage and the effects of medication. Many medications used to treat muscle dysfunction determine the intensity of pressure and the duration and amount of stretch one can apply to the tissues.

Any time infection is present and is being treated with medication the system already is stressed. Therapeutic methods support the healing process by promoting general relaxation but are to be performed gently so as not to place additional demand on the system. When clients use antiinflammatory drugs, the practitioner should avoid methods that produce inflammation. Muscle relaxants interfere with the normal feedback systems of stretch and tension receptors. Because these medications interrupt this protective mechanism, the massage therapist must take care with any type of lengthening or stretching methods. Because analgesics interfere with the normal pain response, feedback from the client may be inaccurate. It is necessary to adjust intensity and duration.

Specific Disorders

Conditions

Muscle Pain: Local and Systemic

The medical term for muscle pain is *myalgia*. Local muscle pain affects an area of the body and is usually related to tension, stress, overuse, and minor injuries. Examples of local pain are:

- Contusion
- Sprains and strains
- Muscle cramp
- Repetitive strain injury
- Overexertion

Other causes are:

- Claudication-related pain caused by too little blood flow, usually during exercise.
- Chronic exertional compartment syndrome. During exercise, increased blood flow causes muscles to expand. If the fascia that binds the muscle fibers in a compartment doesn't also expand, pressure builds up in the compartment, cutting off some of the muscle's blood supply.

INDICATIONS/CONTRAINDICATIONS for Therapeutic Massage

Caution should be taken with muscle pain in general. Myalgia is often a symptom of an underlying condition. Referral for diagnosis is indicated, especially if there is no logical explanation for the discomfort.

Caution for local pain is important because this type of pain is often related to injury. Avoid the area or use a palliative-type massage application. Various strategies are used to treat both local and systemic myalgia, including massage and other forms of soft tissue work, biofeedback, relaxation training, exercise, and flexibility methods. Systemic muscle pain responds to whole-body therapy, which not only addresses the immediate areas but also relaxes the entire body.

Systemic muscle pain is pain throughout the whole body. It is more often the result of an infection or illness or a side effect of a medication. A number of conditions can be associated with generalized aching perceived to be muscle pain. Examples include:

- Chronic fatigue syndrome
- Myofascial pain syndrome
- A variety of autoimmune conditions
- Hypothyroidism
- Viral illness (influenza-like illness)
- Lyme disease

Stress-Induced Muscle Tension and Headache

Stress-induced muscle tension can result in myalgia, or muscle pain. The contracted muscles exert pressure on the nerves and blood vessels in the area, causing the pain. The stress-induced headache is a dull, persistent ache with feelings of tightness around the head, temples, forehead, and occipital area. It is often accompanied by stiffness in the neck and back. The headache may be less intense in the morning and worsen as the day goes on.

INDICATIONS/CONTRAINDICATIONS for Therapeutic Massage

Various strategies are used to treat stress-induced muscle tension headaches, including massage and other forms of soft tissue work, biofeedback, relaxation training, exercise, and flexibility methods. Headaches respond best to whole-body therapy, which not only addresses the immediate areas but also relaxes the entire body.

Cramps/Spasms

Cramps are painful muscle spasms or involuntary twitches. Cramps involve the whole muscle; spasms involve individual motor units within a muscle. Cramps often result from mild myositis or fibromyositis, but they can be a symptom of any irritation or of an electrolyte imbalance. Clonic spasms alternate contraction and relaxation in the muscle. Tonic spasms, or tetany, are sustained muscle contractions usually caused by disorders of the central nervous system.

INDICATIONS/CONTRAINDICATIONS for Therapeutic Massage

Cramps and spasms may seem benign, but they can be symptomatic of more severe underlying conditions. If there does not seem to be a logical reason for the cramps or spasms or if the cramps or spasms occur frequently, the practitioner should refer the client for a diagnosis. Simple cramps or spasms can be managed by firmly pushing the belly of the muscle together and or applying firm compression into the cramping tissue.

Fibromyalgia

Fibromyalgia is a syndrome with symptoms of widespread pain or aching, persistent fatigue, generalized morning stiffness, nonrestorative sleep, and multiple tender points. These symptoms often are found with headaches, irritable bladder, dysmenorrhea, cold sensitivity, Raynaud phenomenon, restless legs, atypical patterns of numbness and tingling, and complaints of weakness. The onset usually is gradual, often following prolonged exposure to damp cold, a bacterial or viral infection, or prolonged physical or emotional stress. Chronic fatigue syndrome also may be present.

A neurochemical imbalance, central nervous system hypersensitivity, and a disrupted sleep pattern, coupled with the dysfunction of myofascial repair mechanisms, seem to be contributing factors. Treatment protocols aim at sleep restoration and a gradual rebuilding of the myofascial system. Diet and lifestyle changes, moderate exercise, and various forms of complementary therapies and mind/body approaches are beneficial. If necessary, low doses of antidepressants often can help restore sleep patterns.

INDICATIONS/CONTRAINDICATIONS for Therapeutic Massage

General constitutional approaches seem to work best to aid in symptomatic pain reduction and restoration of the sleep pattern. The practitioner should avoid any form of therapy that causes therapeutic inflammation, including intense exercise and stretching programs, until healing mechanisms in the body are functioning. Exercise programs should be gentle and slow. If tender points have been injected with antiinflammatory medications, anesthetics, or other substances, the massage therapist should not massage over the area.

Contracture

Contracture is the chronic shortening of a muscle, especially the connective tissue component. Volkmann ischemic contracture occurs in the upper or lower extremity when the blood supply is cut off and can be caused by tight casts, tourniquets, fractures, dislocations, or vascular spasms. The ischemia can lead to fibrosis and can result in the contracture of the muscles, tendons, and fascia.

INDICATIONS/CONTRAINDICATIONS for Therapeutic Massage

Gentle, slow intervention using connective tissue methods and stretching may improve stiffening within contractures. Applying soft tissue and movement methods may prevent or slow the development of a contracture. The reason for the contracture must be taken into consideration when developing a treatment plan for managing this condition.

Dupuytren Contracture

The first sign of Dupuytren contracture is a thickened plaque overlying the tendon of the ring finger and occasionally the little finger at the level of the distal palmar crease. The skin in this area puckers, and a thickened, fibrotic cord develops between the palm and the finger. Flexion contracture of the fingers may increase gradually.

INDICATIONS/CONTRAINDICATIONS for Therapeutic Massage

Treatment is contraindicated regionally if methods increase symptoms.

Torticollis

Torticollis, or wry neck, involves a spasm or shortening of one of the sternocleidomastoid muscles. The condition may be congenital, acute, or chronic. Congenital torticollis can be caused by the fetal position or by a birth injury; acute torticollis is associated with cold or flu symptoms; chronic torticollis results from emotional stress, trauma, or infection.

INDICATIONS/CONTRAINDICATIONS for Therapeutic Massage

Management of torticollis with massage therapy involves relaxing the neck, lengthening the contracted muscles, and improving range of motion. Avoiding pressure on the vessels under the sternocleidomastoid muscle is important.

Anterior Compartment Syndrome

The anterior compartment of the leg is surrounded by a tough fascial sheath containing the tibialis anterior, the extensor digitorum longus, the extensor hallucis longus, and the fibularis tertius, as well as nerves and blood vessels. Any condition that increases pressure in this compartment interferes with blood flow and compresses the nerves. The affected person usually has a tight feeling in the calf and pain, numbness, and tingling. Overuse, repetitive stress, and accelerated growth of the muscles are common causal factors.

INDICATIONS/CONTRAINDICATIONS for Therapeutic Massage

Treatment is contraindicated regionally unless supervised by the diagnosing or treating healthcare provider. Massage methods may soften the connective tissue sheath, relieving some of the pressure, but they also could aggravate the inflammatory process.

Flaccidity and Spasticity

A muscle with decreased tone is flaccid; a muscle with excessive tone is spastic. Flaccid or spastic muscles often are associated with motor neuron disorders. The reason for the change in tone determines the appropriateness of massage or movement therapy. These conditions differ from general muscle tension or weakness in that the dysfunction has a physical cause rather than a functional one.

INDICATIONS/CONTRAINDICATIONS for Therapeutic Massage

Massage therapy is indicated for both general relaxation and pain management. However, if these conditions result from a nervous system dysfunction, it is unlikely that massage will alter the specific condition. Caution is necessary because normal feedback mechanisms are altered and the client is unable to provide accurate feedback. Increased spasticity can be a result of massage; therefore, it is necessary to carefully monitor the result of massage. Flaccid muscles offer little resistance to compressive force, and the tissues may be injured if pressure is excessive.

Injuries

Muscle Strain

Injury to skeletal muscles caused by overexertion or trauma can result in muscle strain. Muscle strains involve overstretching or tearing of muscle fibers and associated connective tissue. Although the inflammation may subside in a few hours or days, repair of damaged muscle fibers usually takes weeks, and some damaged muscle cells may be replaced by fibrous tissue, forming scars.

INDICATIONS/CONTRAINDICATIONS for Therapeutic Massage

Direct work over the area of injury is contraindicated regionally until all signs of inflammation have dissipated. Gentle range of motion exercises can support healing. Do not stretch the area in the acute healing phase. Methods to manage distortion in posture resulting from compensation in the rest of the body are helpful.

Contusion

Compressive trauma to the muscles may cause a muscle bruise, or contusion, that involves local internal bleeding and inflammation. Severe trauma to a skeletal muscle may cause a crush injury that damages the affected muscle tissue and releases the muscle fiber contents into the bloodstream. This situation can be life-threatening because the reddish muscle pigment myoglobin can accumulate in the blood and cause kidney failure.

INDICATIONS/CONTRAINDICATIONS for Therapeutic Massage

Direct work over the area of injury is contraindicated regionally until all signs of inflammation have dissipated.

Whiplash

Whiplash is an injury to the soft tissues of the neck caused by sudden hyperextension or flexion (or both) of the neck. The most common cause is an automobile accident resulting in pain, swelling, stiffness, and spasm in the shoulders and neck. In extension injuries, the muscles most likely to be injured are the sternocleidomastoid, scalene muscles, infrahyoid muscles, suprahyoid muscles, levator scapulae, longus colli, suboccipital muscles, and rhomboid muscles. In flexion injuries the muscles most likely to be injured are the trapezius, splenius capitis, and semispinalis capitis. A side injury affects the sternocleidomastoid, suboccipital muscles, levator scapulae, splenius capitis, and splenius cervicis. Vestibular system damage to the inner ear may result in dizziness, nausea, vomiting, headache, and gait problems.

INDICATIONS/CONTRAINDICATIONS for Therapeutic Massage

Direct intervention during the acute phase is contraindicated unless closely supervised by a physician or other qualified healthcare professional. Massage is a valuable part of rehabilitation in the subacute phase and can help restore function if the condition is chronic. Extension injury is more severe and requires careful intervention.

Rotator Cuff Tear

Repeated impingement, overuse, or other conditions may weaken the rotator cuff and eventually cause partial or complete tears. The condition is more common after age 40. Prior injury may increase the likelihood of a tear. Symptoms include weakness, atrophy of the supraspinatus and infraspinatus muscles, pain, and tenderness. A complete tear of the supraspinatus tendon severely impairs active abduction at the glenohumeral joint. An attempt to abduct the arm instead produces a characteristic shoulder shrug.

INDICATIONS/CONTRAINDICATIONS for Therapeutic Massage

Work on acute myofascial tears is contraindicated. However, massage therapy may be indicated in the rehabilitative process and as part of a supervised treatment protocol. Compensatory patterns can be managed or improved with massage.

Rhabdomyolysis

Rhabdomyolysis is the breakdown of muscle tissue that leads to the release of the protein myoglobin into the bloodstream. Myoglobin breaks down into substances that can damage kidney cells. Rhabdomyolysis may be caused by injury or any other condition that damages skeletal muscle, including crush injury, heatstroke, extensive burns, blocked blood vessels, seizure, and intense exercise/exertional rhabdomyolysis.

There are multiple potential causes of rhabdomyolysis, which can be organized into three categories:

- Traumatic or muscle compression
- Nontraumatic exertional
- Nontraumatic nor exertional

Common symptoms are:

- Brown or cola/tea-colored urine
- Muscle pain and weakness
- Nausea and vomiting

INDICATIONS/CONTRAINDICATIONS for Therapeutic Massage

This condition can range from mild to severe. The more severe manifestation of rhabdomyolysis is a medical emergency. Mild manifestation can be mistaken for other conditions. Causes of rhabdomyolysis are additive, meaning that overexertion, combined with heat exhaustion and reduced fluid intake or excessive sweating, can combine to create a more serious condition. Extreme and excessive heavy pressure when used in massage can create a type of localized crush injury. This obviously needs to be avoided. However, if a person with mild rhabdomyolysis, regardless of causal factors, receives this type of massage application, it is plausible that the results of the massage can add to the severity. Caution is needed when working with people who have risk factors for the condition. Be especially cautious with those who may have a mild or moderate case of exertional rhabdomyolysis that is mistaken for delayed onset muscle soreness.

Myopathies

Muscular Dystrophy

The term *muscular dystrophy* encompasses a group of disorders characterized by atrophy of skeletal muscles with no malfunction of the nervous system. The muscle protein dystrophin declines or is lacking. Some forms of muscular dystrophy can be fatal.

The most common form of muscular dystrophy is Duchenne muscular dystrophy (DMD), also called *pseudohypertrophy* (meaning "false muscle growth") because the atrophy of muscle is masked by excessive replacement of muscle by fat and fibrous tissue. DMD usually begins with mild leg muscle weakness that progresses rapidly to include the shoulder muscles.

The first signs of DMD become apparent at about 3 years of age, and the child usually is affected severely within 5 to 10 years. Death from respiratory or cardiac muscle weakness often occurs by 21 years of age.

Many pathophysiologists believe that DMD is caused by a missing fragment in the X chromosome, although other factors may be involved. Because girls have two X chromosomes and boys only one, genetic diseases involving X chromosome abnormalities are more likely to occur in boys. This is true because girls with one affected X chromosome may not exhibit an X-linked disease if the other X chromosome is normal.

Some less devastating forms of muscular dystrophy are fascioscapulohumeral dystrophy, which affects the fascia and shoulder girdle muscles, and limb-girdle dystrophy, which affects the pelvic and shoulder girdle muscles.

INDICATIONS/CONTRAINDICATIONS for Therapeutic Massage

Careful intervention may slow the atrophy. Passive and active joint movement methods not only directly affect the muscles and joints but also aid in the circulation and elimination processes. Abdominal massage may help with constipation. Methods that cause any inflammation should not be used.

Myositis Ossificans

Myositis ossificans involves an inflammatory process that stimulates the formation of osseous tissue in the fascial components of muscles. The disease may occur with no apparent cause or may occur after a fracture or contusion. The onset of muscle pain is gradual.

INDICATIONS/CONTRAINDICATIONS for Therapeutic Massage

Treatment is contraindicated regionally in myositis ossificans.

Muscle Infections

Several bacteria, viruses, and parasites may infect muscle tissue, often producing local or widespread myositis (muscle inflammation). Trichinosis, which is caused by a parasite, is an example of such an infection. The muscle pain and stiffness that sometimes accompany influenza is another example of myositis. Poliomyelitis is a viral infection of the nerves that control skeletal muscle movement. Polio is usually asymptomatic in populations where there is poor sanitation. It enters the body by way of a fecal-oral route and usually passes through the body without causing disease; but in a small number of cases, it enters the central nervous system and causes the "polio" symptoms we recognize. Poliomyelitis often causes paralysis that may progress to death. Virtually eliminated in the United States through an effective vaccine, polio nonetheless still affects millions around the world who have not been vaccinated.

More common is the occurrence of postpolio syndrome in people who had polio years ago. The symptoms are weakness, fatigue, intolerance to cold, and general aching pain.

INDICATIONS/CONTRAINDICATIONS for Therapeutic Massage

For postpolio syndrome, general constitutional approaches seem to work best to aid in overall pain reduction and restoration of the sleep pattern. Any form of therapy that causes therapeutic inflammation, including intense exercise and stretching programs, should not be used.

Acquired Metabolic and Toxic Myopathies

Acquired metabolic myopathies often result from disorders of the endocrine system. Nutritional and vitamin deficiency, especially protein deficiency and lack of vitamins C, D, and E, may lead to myopathy.

Toxic myopathies are related to certain drugs and chemicals. Corticosteroid therapy may cause steroid-induced muscle weakness. An excessive alcohol intake can result in breakdown of striated muscles, which can affect skeletal and other muscles.

INDICATIONS/CONTRAINDICATIONS for Therapeutic Massage

Treatment for these types of myopathies usually is not contraindicated, as long as the therapeutic approaches are general and focus on supporting body restoration and the healing processes. Regional avoidance of steroid injection sites is indicated. The massage therapist must take care in toxic conditions not to tax an already overloaded system. A general therapeutic approach over a longer period is indicated.

Section Summary

- Describe categories of medications used to treat pathological conditions of muscles.
  Analgesics treat pain. Antibiotic/antiviral/antifungal/antiparasitic medications treat infections. Steroidal/nonsteroidal antiinflammatory medications treat inflammation. Muscle relaxants soothe spasm and hypertonic muscles.
- Explain massage adaptation related to pathological conditions of muscles.
  Intervention should focus on reversing nonproductive patterns and supporting resourceful compensation patterns that develop in response to chronic problems. Caution is required to avoid overstressing a system that is already stressed. Interactions of medications and massage must be considered. The massage therapist should always carefully research and study indications and contraindications when working with pathological conditions.

SUMMARY

Just as muscles are able to function concentrically, eccentrically, and isometrically, massage professionals play various roles. You, the massage professional, are the one who provides the massage application, educates the client in wellness strategies, supports other professions in multidisciplinary teams, and maintains stability in scope of practice and ethical boundaries in the professional relationship. Much like muscles, your job requires a specific action, depending on the demands, and usually is an ever-changing dynamic process. Competency is measured by how you are able to take information and use it in a multidimensional way and in functional units. This chapter presented functional patterns of muscle interaction. This information is used functionally in massage practice in multiple ways as well. Understanding the location and various actions of muscles and their relationship to the rest of the body influences skilled assessment, clinical reasoning, decision making regarding appropriate methods to achieve outcomes for the session, charting and other forms of written documentation, and interaction with other health professionals.

This chapter has taken an in-depth look at the muscular system, including the complex fascial network. We have explored individual muscles and mapped the interdependent nature of muscular action in the synergist and antagonist pattern of each muscle. We have discussed the progression of pathological conditions in muscle dysfunction, along with the indications and contraindications for massage for specific muscle-related dysfunctions.

We explore the larger picture of dynamic movement in the next chapter, in which we see all the parts—bones, joints, and muscles—as a functioning unit that is more than the sum of its parts.

Visit the Evolve website: https://evolve.elsevier.com/Fritz/essential/

CRITICAL THINKING/CLINICAL REASONING

Each chapter will feature a critical thinking and clinical reasoning application of the content related to massage therapy practice. A client scenario will be presented with recommendations for additional research often using MedlinePlus or PubMed. Relevant questions based on the chapter content outline are provided to guide discussion. There are no specific current answers to the questions. However, responses should be supportive of evidence-informed practices and based on biological plausibility if sufficient research is not available. The author's decision-making process related to the scenario and questions is on the Evolve site. Compare and contrast your thoughts and discussion to that of the author and determine where you agree or disagree.

Scenario

Sabina is a 36-year-old computer programmer. She experiences frequent tension headaches and neck and shoulder pain. She stretches throughout the day and does yoga three times a week. Her worst habit is drinking a lot of coffee even though she knows it makes her jittery. She has not been getting to sleep until after midnight.

Lately she has not been able to stretch out the tension, so she wants to start receiving massage weekly. During the intake assessment she indicates that she was in a minor car accident 2 months ago and was very sore for a couple of days. She did not go to the doctor. When asked when her symptoms increased, she said about a month ago.

- What are the major myofascial structures in the areas where Sabina is experiencing symptoms?
- What are the major common attachment points for the muscle structures in these areas?
- How are Sabina's headache, coffee intake, occupation, and breathing interrelated?
- How might a suspected whiplash injury influence the function of the tissues in the target area?
- How might regular yoga practice influence Sabina's condition?
- The muscles in the target area are primarily two shapes—cylindrical with vertical fiber arrangement and triangular with diagonal fiber arrangement. What does this suggest about function in the area?
- Observational assessment identifies that Sabina has a slightly anteriorly rotated shoulder with a change in scapular position. The pectoralis minor is palpated as tender. What is the major synergist with attachments on the ribs? What are the antagonists and what is their likely status? Which antagonist would most likely be involved with the tension headache?
- During conversation Sabina discloses that her low back and hips are also stiff. Is there a logical connection between the target area and these symptoms?
- What would be the most conservative but beneficial massage care plan?

The Evolve website provides support for review of the chapter content and chapter quizzes to help you prepare for the MBLEx or other massage therapy certification or licensing exams. End of chapter questions for discussion and review answer key and rationales and author's response to critical thinking and clinical reasoning scenarios.

MULTIPLE CHOICE QUESTIONS FOR REVIEW AND DISCUSSION

The answers, with rationales, can be found on the Evolve site.

These questions are used for review and discussion. It is as important to understand why wrong answers are wrong as it is to know why the correct answer is correct. The answers to the questions, with rationales and explanations about why the correct answer is correct and why wrong answers are wrong, can be found on the Evolve site. Guidance also is provided on how questions are developed and how the textbook content can be presented in a multiple-choice question format. At the end of the question section here in the textbook, you will find an exercise that asks you to write more questions. Use the various questions in the chapter as examples. This is one of the best study strategies for test-taking.

It is important to understand that the actual licensing exam you take may not contain any of the specific questions found in this textbook or in the review material and practice tests on the Evolve site. Therefore, just because you can answer any of these questions correctly does not mean you will pass the licensing exam. The questions are content and style examples to help you prepare—this is why understanding why wrong answers are wrong is just as important as identifying the correct answer. Also, make sure you understand all the terminology used in the questions and possible answers in the review and discussion questions. Look up words you do not understand.

1. If the concentric function of a muscle is extension and lateral flexion, then which of the following is the eccentric function of that same muscle?
   a. Stabilizes the adjacent joint
   b. Elevation and rotation of the area
   c. Restrains flexion and controls extension
   d. Assists extension and lateral flexion
2. If the concentric function of a muscle is to extend and laterally rotate the thigh at the hip joint, which of the following would be synergist and antagonist muscles?
   a. Hamstrings and iliopsoas
   b. Quadratus femoris and fibularis
   c. Popliteus and plantaris
   d. Quadratus lumborum and transverse abdominis oblique
3. What relationship do the tibialis anterior and the extensor digitorum longus have?
   a. They are located in the thigh.
   b. Both muscles are synergists to each other.
   c. The muscles are concentric eccentric antagonists.
   d. Both muscles function at the knee.
4. If the attachment of a muscle is located closer to the torso and would be listed as fixed end in an attachment description, which of the following would be correct?
   a. Distal insertion
   b. Distal origin
   c. Proximal origin
   d. To insertion
5. A client complains of fatigue and muscle soreness after attempting to push a car that was stuck. Which of the following best describes this action?

   a. No movement was produced, so static force was generated.
   b. Dynamic force was used because the car did not move.
   c. Static force produced movement and energy expenditure.
   d. Because the car did not move, little energy was expended.
6. During assessment, the massage professional realizes that a client is excessively flexible. Which muscle functions would seem to be impaired?
   a. Produce movement
   b. Generate heat
   c. Maintain posture
   d. Stabilize joints
7. A client was a sprinter in high school track and was effective during short and quick runs. Now 10 years later the client is complaining of lacking the endurance to run 5 miles as part of a fitness program. The client is in good physical condition with no apparent reason for the difficulties. Which of the following offers the most plausible explanation for the client's condition?
   a. The person has an abundance of slow twitch fibers in relationship to fast twitch fibers.
   b. The person has an increased ability to manage oxygen debt.
   c. The person's legs have a genetic tendency toward a makeup of more white anaerobic fibers.
   d. The person has increased slow twitch fibers in the postural muscles.
8. A client is complaining of tender areas in the postural muscles along the spine. Assessment indicates a series of trigger points in these muscles. The massage professional must determine how much compressive force to apply to the trigger points and how long to hold the contraction. Which of the following will affect this decision?
   a. These muscles contain more slow twitch red fibers that are fatigue resistant.
   b. These muscles are prone to oxygen debt.
   c. These muscles have an abundance of fast twitch and intermediate fibers.
   d. These muscles require a maximal stimulus to respond to treatment.
9. A client is complaining of pain when straightening the elbow. Palpation of the triceps at the musculotendinous junction indicates more tenderness at the distal attachment when the muscle is activated. What is the most likely reason for this?
   a. The distal attachment is the fixed attachment and would be more tender during movement.
   b. The distal attachment is the is the origin and is straining at the intermuscular septa.
   c. The belly of the muscle located at the distal attachment is highly innervated.
   d. The distal attachment is the more movable attachment, so it would produce more tenderness upon motion.
10. A client is experiencing a limitation in range of motion of the hip into abduction. Assessment indicates shortening and tension in the adductor group of muscles. Which of the following is the most likely source of the limited range of motion?
    a. Agonists
    b. Synergists
    c. Antagonists
    d. Fixators
11. A client lifted a box that was unexpectedly heavy. Now the client is experiencing residual weakness in the biceps and brachialis muscles and tension in the triceps muscle group. Which of the following reflexes best explains this situation?
    a. Stretch reflex
    b. Tendon reflex
    c. Withdrawal reflex
    d. Crossed extensor reflex
12. A client's job requires them to perform the same repetitive lift and hand squeeze task. They have been doing this job for 8 months. In the beginning, their arms were sore and a bit swollen but that went away. In the past 3 months the pain and tension in the arms have returned and have begun to increase. Which of the following best describes the client's current condition?
    a. Chain reaction in myotatic units has occurred.
    b. Pain increases tension or spasm, which increases pain.
    c. Joint restriction and fascial shortening decrease mobility.
    d. Generalized fatigue has developed from an interrupted sleep pattern.
13. Which of the following conditions is most likely to benefit directly from a nonspecific general massage session?
    a. Contusion
    b. Anterior compartment syndrome
    c. Muscle tension headache
    d. Spasticity
14. Two clients describe accidents in which the muscles of their upper thigh were cut and now healed. Client A has a mobile scar with near normal function. Client B has tissue rigidity and reduced movement. What is the most plausible explanation?
    a. Client A limited exercise and kept the area tightly wrapped during the healing process.
    b. Client B had more satellite cell activity during healing, causing increased scar tissue.
    c. Client A exercised during healing to stimulate satellite cells.
    d. Client B experienced increased circulation and reduced adhesions.
15. A client has been working on a project that required gripping a hammer for an extended period. Now the client is complaining of weakness when attempting to extend the wrist. Which of the following is the most likely explanation?
    a. The flexor muscle group of the hand and wrist increased tone levels, resulting in inhibition of the extensor group of muscles in the forearm.

b. The flexor digitorum superficialis and profundus are weak from fatigue, so the wrist extensors have been facilitated.
c. The deep layer of the posterior wrist extensor group is antagonistic to the superficial layer of this same muscle group, resulting in weakness in the wrist extensors.
d. The flexor carpi ulnaris and the extensor carpi ulnaris are in spasm, resulting in inhibition of the abductor pollicis longus.

16. A client with fibromyalgia has been referred by the physician for massage. A treatment plan has been requested for approval before treatment begins. Which of the following would be the best approach?
 a. General massage with active assisted joint movement and stretching
 b. General massage with friction methods to active tender points
 c. Localized massage to the feet and ischemic compression to active trigger points
 d. General massage to support restorative sleep and symptomatic pain management
17. Which of the following medications likely would be prescribed for tendinitis?
 a. Antibiotic
 b. Muscle relaxant
 c. Anticoagulant
 d. Antiinflammatory
18. A client is taking an over-the-counter analgesic. What concern would the massage professional have while providing massage?
 a. Feedback mechanisms for pain will be altered.
 b. Blood pressure may fall dangerously low.
 c. The infection may be spread.
 d. Inflammation may be increased.
19. Which of the following conditions presents regional contraindications for massage?
 a. Post-polio syndrome
 b. Myositis ossificans
 c. Muscular dystrophy
 d. Myasthenia gravis
20. If the major function of a muscle is to stabilize, then which of the following muscle functions is involved?
 a. Isometric
 b. Concentric
 c. Eccentric
 d. Kinetic

CHAPTER

10 Biomechanics Basics

https://evolve.elsevier.com/Fritz/essential/

CHAPTER OBJECTIVES

After completing this chapter, the learner will be able to:

1. Explain the basic principles of biomechanics.
2. Implement biomechanical principles in massage therapy body mechanics and ergonomics.
3. Explain and assess the function of the kinetic chain.
4. List principles of a massage intervention plan based on efficient biomechanical movement.
5. Assess biomechanical function using individual joint assessment.
6. Assess biomechanical functions for regions of the body.
7. Identify and describe the three main biomechanical dysfunctional patterns and the associated indications and contraindications for massage.

CHAPTER OUTLINE

KEY TERMS

acceleration: The rate of change in velocity.
balance: The ability to control equilibrium.
biomechanics: The science concerned with the internal and external forces acting on the human body and the effects produced by these forces.
center of gravity: An imaginary midpoint or center of the weight of a body or object, where the body or object could balance on a point.
effort: The force applied to overcome resistance.
equilibrium: The result when all forces acting on an object are equal.
force: Push or pull on an object in an attempt to affect motion or shape.
gait: The rhythmic and alternating motions of the legs, trunk, and arms, resulting in the propulsion of the body.
gait cycle: Begins when the heel of one foot strikes the floor and continues until the same heel strikes the floor again. The cycle is subdivided into the stance phase and swing phase.
inertia: (in-NUR-shuh) The property of matter by which it remains at rest or in uniform motion in the same straight line unless acted upon by some external force.
kinesiology: (ki-nee-see-OL-o-jee) The study of movement that combines the fields of anatomy, physiology, physics, and geometry and relates them to human movement.
kinetic chain: An integrated functional unit. The kinetic chain is made up of the myofascial system (muscle, ligament, tendon, and fascia), the articular (joint) system, and the nervous system. Each of these systems works interdependently to allow structural and functional efficiency in all three planes of motion: sagittal, frontal, and transverse.
lever: (LE-ver) A solid mass, such as a crowbar or a person's arm, that rotates around a fixed point called the fulcrum. The rotation is produced by a force applied to a lever at some distance from the fulcrum.
resistance: The opposition to force.
stability: The resistance to change in the acceleration of the body or the resistance to the disturbance of the equilibrium of the body.
vector: The direction of the force.

Chapter 10 is the final chapter in the kinesiology and biomechanics section of this textbook. Chapters 7 to 9 targeted the anatomy and physiology of the bones, joints, and muscles, providing the foundation for learning about kinesiology and biomechanics. This chapter is about kinesiology and

LEARNING HOW TO LEARN

There is a difference between learning the names of parts and what parts can do and learning the ways various parts work together to create a combined outcome. Think of a bike. It has multiple parts. One of the parts is a wheel. The wheel is part of the bike, but the wheel is not the bike. Okay—a little weird, but consider a movement, such as walking. Walking requires bones, joints, muscles, and at least the nervous system and circulatory system, if not the rest. So muscles are part of walking, but walking is a lot more than muscles.

This chapter is not specifically about parts. You learned the parts in previous chapters. This chapter is about understanding the relationships of those parts. You will need to remember the names of the parts (e.g., bones, joints, and muscles), or you will be confused. If you do not remember the meaning of a word, you will have to look it up. The best way to study this chapter is to make up examples. The chapter presents lots of examples, but the examples that you make up are even better.

The information in this chapter is also about doing. For example, pressure is the amount of force on a specific area. During massage application, the method called *compression* generates compressive stress. The amount of pressure used during the massage depends on variations in the compressive load applied to the body.

Now do something: Get a balloon, blow it up, and then watch and feel what happens when you press on it.

Have fun!

biomechanics. These four chapters combine to create an understanding of why, how, and what happens when we move. The foundation laid in this chapter prepares the massage therapist to provide massage therapy related to the outcome of functional mobility. There is a focus on the practical integration of assessment and interventions that can be incorporated into the massage session when mobility is the focus.

Recall that kinesiology is:

1. The science dealing with the interrelationship of anatomy and the physiology of the body with respect to movement
2. The study of movement that blends anatomy, physiology, physics, and geometry and relates them to human movement

Kinesiology is the study of body movement. It involves a lot of anatomy and physiology. **Biomechanics**, the study of the mechanical processes of human movement, is an aspect of the larger field of kinesiology. Kinesiology includes the biomechanics of motion combined with the neural and cardiovascular elements of movement. Biomechanics is the study of the effects of movement on the body. It involves a lot of math and measurement, more accurately called detailed force equations and/or objective measurements. Within the field of biomechanics, the specific focus is on mechanical movement. This includes the articulation of joints and the participation of tendons and muscles in the coordination of physical activity. What occurs because of the mechanical forces applied to the body during massage requires an understanding of biomechanics. A functional understanding of biomechanics is important both for the person receiving the massage and for the practitioner, so that they can use leverage and good posture to reduce harmful forces on both their bodies. You need to understand biomechanics before you are able to perform physical assessment and develop care and treatment plans for clients with goals related to posture and movement. People with an interest in biomechanics may also be interested in the development of ergonomic systems to protect people at work and play by reducing the risk of injury. Biomechanics in relation to massage involves how we stand, move, push, pull, and do massage. Ergonomics involves the height and width of the massage table, size of the room, type of tools used, clothing and shoes, temperature, how long we work, and so on (Box 10.1).

Biomechanics is often referred to as the link between structure and function. *Kinematics* is defined as the study of motion without regard to the forces that cause that motion. *Kinetics* is the study of motion under the action of forces.

BIOMECHANICS

SECTION OBJECTIVES

Chapter objective covered in this section:

1. Explain the basic principles of biomechanics.
2. Implement biomechanical principles in massage therapy.

After completing this section, the learner will be able to:

- Define biomechanics.
- Explain the lever and fulcrum and the application of force.
- Describe the center of gravity of the body, balance, equilibrium, and stability.
- Identify common postural deviations.
- Explain gait.

Biomechanics is the science concerned with the internal and external forces acting on the human body and the effects produced by these forces. Movement is a fundamental characteristic of human behavior and is accomplished by the contraction of skeletal muscles acting within a system of levers and pulleys formed by bones, tendons, and ligaments that network into the unified tensegrity system of the body.

Because a variety of forces may act on the human body, the massage therapist must have a basic understanding of biomechanical principles. Understanding these principles helps us in assessing and observing the body and in clinical reasoning methods used to develop treatment plans.

An understanding of biomechanics includes the following:

- Application of the mechanical principles in the study of living organisms.
- The science of movement of a living body, including how muscles, bones, tendons, and ligaments work together to produce movement.
- The study of mechanical principles and actions applied to living bodies. This may involve looking at the static (nonmoving) or dynamic (moving) systems associated with various activities.
- The application of mechanical principles (e.g., engineering) to human movement.

It is important to distinguish between two types of motion:

- Linear (or translational) motion: Movement in a particular direction (e.g., walking down a sidewalk)

Box 10.1 Biomechanics Related to Body Mechanics and Ergonomics

Biomechanical principles have direct application to therapeutic massage application. Body mechanics refers to the way we move our bodies. How efficiently the massage therapist uses their body will influence their career success. All forces should be applied in the direction of the intended motion. During massage, when we point our feet toward the direction of the stroke, we are applying this principle.

A total force is the sum of the forces of each body segment contributing to the act if the forces are applied in a single direction and proper sequence with timing. This principle is important to massage-related body mechanics. When we stack the joints and are stable and lean forward from the ankles, we can apply more force with less effort. We want the force produced to move into the client's tissues, not be dissipated. That is why we need to maintain the joints in a stable position. This is especially true of the elbow. If you let your elbow bend when using your hand to apply the force, most of it is lost (absorbed). This is not a problem when we use our forearm for massage so long as the shoulder remains stable.

If one or both feet are not in the proper alignment, the energy that creates the force will be wasted. We should have our weight distributed to the back foot with a concentration toward the heel.

Maintain a stable asymmetrical stance. The feet should be shoulder width apart with one foot forward. Avoid having the legs too close together or far apart.

Stand up. Avoid bending or excessive lunge position. Especially avoid bending/reaching and twisting. The height of

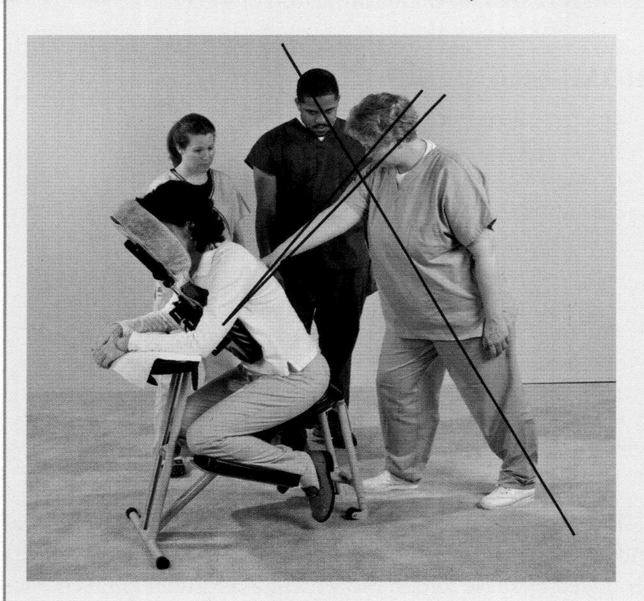

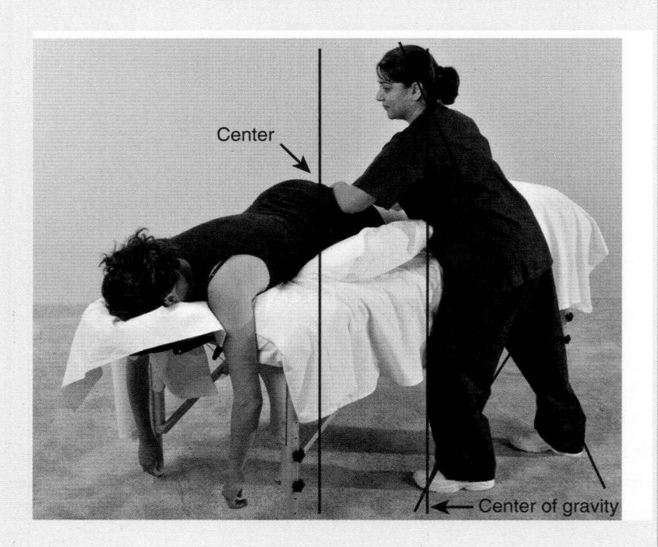

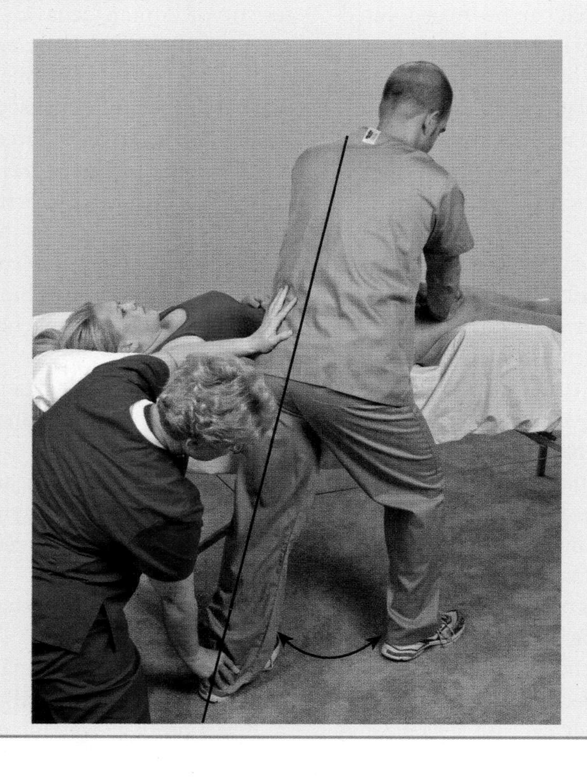

Continued

Box 10.1 Biomechanics Related to Body Mechanics and Ergonomics—cont'd

the massage table generally is measured by the practitioner's hip height.

Push instead of pull. Lean forward to push when possible. When you push an object, you use the muscles in your legs. When pulling, there is a tendency to use the back muscles to yank and pull. It is easier to keep your back straight while pushing.

Ergonomics is an applied science concerned with designing and arranging things people use so that the people and things interact most efficiently and safely. It is also called human engineering. Ergonomics is based on the principle that the job should be adapted to fit the person, rather than forcing the person to fit the job. It focuses design and function of the work environment. Ergonomics includes restructuring or changing workplace conditions to make the job easier and reducing stressors that cause cumulative trauma disorders and repetitive motion injuries. For massage therapy practice, ergonomics involves the massage table's height and width, the size of the massage area, the space around the massage table, temperature and ventilation, uniforms, shoes, access to equipment, scheduling, and rest breaks.

- Rotational motion: Movement about an axis that results in rotation (e.g., a ballet dancer's toe spin)

Force

Because biomechanics is the science concerned with the internal and external forces acting on the human body and the effects produced by these forces, we need to understand the properties of force. Throughout the textbook, mechanical forces have been described and discussed.

Force causes change. Forces push or pull on an object in an attempt to affect motion or shape. The human body moves because of internal forces, such as muscle contraction, and external forces, such as being pulled by a dog on a leash. Therapeutic massage purposefully applies external forces to trigger a change in the homeostatic mechanisms of the body. Forces generated by massage load soft tissue and create tension, torsion, bend, shear, and compression stress and strain.

The term *stress*, when related to biomechanics, describes force applied to a certain area of an object that will not move, so instead the applied force causes deformation (a change in shape). *Strain* is the response of the object to an applied stress. When a material is loaded with a force, it produces stress, which then causes a material to deform, which is the strain (Box 10.2).

Technically, force is the product of mass multiplied by acceleration. A **vector** is the direction of the force. The magnitude of a vector is the result of the vertical and horizontal components of an applied force. Most massage application involves applying a force down (vertical) into the tissue and then pushing forward or pulling back (horizontal). The magnitude of a massage application involves how much pressure is pressed down into the tissue, combined with how much force is applied to push tissue away or pull tissue toward our hands during massage application. For example, a light pressure application on the skin combined with a slight push forward has less magnitude compared to more pressure down into muscle tissue combined with a push forward. Mass is the amount of matter or material substance that forms or comprises a body. For our purposes, weight and mass are the same. The weight multiplied by the speed or **acceleration** determines the amount of force. A feather floating softly down to touch our arm exerts less force than a bowling ball thrown down an alley.

The following elements influence or are related to force and massage application:

- *Pressure:* Pressure is the amount of force on a specific area. During massage application, the method called *compression* generates a compressive load. The amount of pressure used during the massage depends on variations in the compressive load and size of the surface area where the load is applied to the body. For example, if the compressive load is applied to a large area of the body using the forearm, the load is the same, but the experience of pressure will be less than if the same load is applied to a small area of the body using the point of the elbow. The small contact area from the point of the elbow increases the experience of the pressure. This is because the load is spread over different surface areas. However, tissue injury is more likely with a load applied to a small area than the same load applied to a large area. If the area where the force is applied is smaller, then the pressure on a surface would be greater, increasing the strain on the tissue.
- *Inertia:* **Inertia** is the property of matter by which it remains at rest or in uniform motion in the same straight line unless acted upon by some external force. Because force is required to change inertia, any activity that is conducted at a steady pace in a consistent direction conserves energy. Any irregularly paced or multidirectional activity costs energy. A movement example is handball, which is more fatiguing than dancing. To support the body mechanics of the massage therapist, massage methods should be applied using a steady pace in a consistent direction. For example, massage strokes are typically slow, even, and rhythmic. The body mechanics of leaning on tissue with your body weight is essentially the inertia of falling forward.
- *Acceleration:* Acceleration is the rate of change in velocity, which is the speed of something in a specific direction. To begin to move the body and attain speed generally requires a strong muscular force. Weight (mass) coupled with the influence of gravity affects speed and acceleration during physical movements. Accelerating a 200-pound adult takes more muscle force than accelerating a 50-pound child. Acceleration occurs in the same direction as the force that caused it. The change in acceleration is directly proportional to the force causing it and inversely proportional to the mass of the body. This means that a large force provides

Box 10.2 Force, Stress, Strain, and Application

Types of Biomechanical Stress

Compression stress: Acts to shorten or flatten body tissues
Tension stress: Acts to lengthen/elongate body tissues
Shear stress: Causes one tissue to slide over another
Terms for tissue behavior when stress is applied:

- *Elastic:* Deforms under stress but returns to its original size and shape when the stress is released. There is no permanent deformation. An example is a rubber band.
- *Viscous:* Deforms steadily under stress. An example is modeling clay.
- *Viscoelastic:* Combines elastic and viscous behavior. An example is yeast bread dough.
- *Brittle:* Deforms by fracturing. An example is a potato chip or corn chip.
- *Ductile:* Deforms without breaking and results in permanent deformation. An example is bending a piece of wire.
- *Plastic:* Does not deform until a threshold stress has been exceeded. An example is stretching plastic wrap.

We never actually see the stress. We only see the results of stress as it deforms tissue (i.e., changes shape). This is the strain on the tissue. *Strain* is defined as the amount of deformation a tissue experiences compared to its original size and shape. Too much strain on tissue causes injury.

- *Longitudinal or linear strain:* Strain that changes the length without changing direction. Can be either compressional or tensional. Compressional linear strain that shortens the tissue. Tension longitudinal strain that lengthens the tissue.
- *Shear strain:* Strain that changes the angles of an object. Shear strain causes lines to rotate.

Massage Examples

1. Soft tissue is viscoelastic.
   Massage application: Gliding with moderate pressure
   Results in: Tissue loaded with combined compressive stress and tension stress
   Creates: Longitudinal tensional strain
   Outcome: Temporarily elongates tissue
2. Soft tissue is viscoelastic.
   Massage application: Kneading with moderate drag
   Results in: Tissue loaded with combined compressive stress, tension stress, and shear stress
   Creates: Shear strain
   Outcome: Temporarily elongates, lifting and sliding of tissue layers
3. Soft tissue is viscoelastic.
   Massage application: Compression
   Results in: Tissue loaded with compressive stress
   Creates: Compressional linear strain
   Outcome: Temporarily elongates tissue under the point of pressure application and shortening of tissue surrounding the point of pressure application

Injury Examples

1. Soft tissue is viscoelastic.
   Action causing injury: Being hit by a ball
   Results in: Tissue loaded with compressive stress
   Creates: Compressional linear strain
   Outcome: Contusion/bruise
2. Bone is brittle.
   Action causing injury: Falling down stairs
   Results in: Tissue loaded with combined compressive stress, tension stress, and shear stress
   Creates: Longitudinal tensional, compressional, and shear strain
   Outcome: Broken bone
3. Ligaments are plastic.
   Action causing injury: Landing wrong after a jump
   Results in: Tissue loaded with combined compressive stress, tension stress, and shear stress
   Creates: Longitudinal tensional, compressional, and shear strain
   Outcome: Sprained ankle and knee

a greater degree of acceleration than a small force. Given the same amount of force, more acceleration occurs on a light body than on a heavy one. The concept of acceleration would suggest that more muscle effort is required by the massage therapist each time a new massage stroke begins.

- *Speed:* Speed is a variable of massage application. Typically, the speed of a massage method is slow; however, some methods (e.g., percussion [tapotement]) are fast. Massage methods that are applied at a fast speed require the most effort.
- *Resistance:* **Resistance** opposes force. Newton's law of reaction says that for every action, there is an opposite and equal reaction. As we place force on the floor by walking on it, the floor provides equal resistance back in the opposite direction to the soles of our feet. Walking on a wood floor is easier than walking on a sandy beach because of the difference in the reaction of the two surfaces. The wood floor resists the weight and pushes back, making walking easier, whereas the sand dissipates the force and requires more effort with each step. The massage client's body tissues provide resistance to the force created by the massage stroke. The surface of the body—especially with the application of a lubricant—offers little resistance to the massage application. However, more resistance is experienced when the pressure increases to access deeper tissues. Also, some individuals have denser tissue and therefore offer more resistance to the mechanical forces created by massage.
- *Effort:* **Effort** is the force applied to overcome resistance. It takes more effort by the massage therapist to work on tissues that are dense and thick. It also takes effort to hold surface tissues at their binding endpoints, such as when performing certain myofascial release methods. It takes less effort to work on the surface tissues of the body, especially when a lubricant is used that increases the slipperiness of the skin.

Levers and Fulcrums

Levers can be used to increase the force with the same amount of effort. Think of a crowbar, which most of us have used to lift

Practical Application

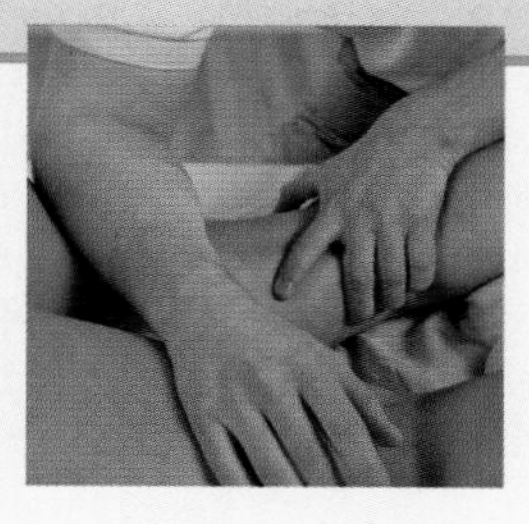

Because massage therapy is the application of mechanical forces, it is helpful to relate the elements that influence force to massage.

When applying pressure to a client, especially during a gliding application, it is always more efficient to go uphill than downhill. Whenever a force vector is applied at an angle, the force can be broken down into its horizontal and vertical components. When applying force to a client going uphill, both the horizontal and vertical components of the force go into the client's tissue. However, when applying a force downhill, only the vertical component of the force goes into the client's tissue; the horizontal component goes out into space away from the body, like pushing into the air, and is wasted (Fig. 10.1).

or move an object. Levers help a given effort move a heavier load or move a load farther than could otherwise be done. A lever is a rigid bar or mass that rotates around a fixed point, called the *axis of rotation*, or *fulcrum*. Rotation is produced by applying force to a lever at some distance from the fulcrum. A force applied to a lever reduces the effort needed to overcome resistance.

In the body, joints are the fulcrums and bones are the levers. Muscle contraction provides the effort and applies it at the muscle attachment points on a bone. The load that is moved includes the bone, the overlying tissues, and anything else one tries to move with that particular lever, such as a book bag. Forces, when working on a joint that is a fulcrum in the body, cause a rotational effect. This is known as a *moment* or *torque*. The body may be considered a series of interconnected levers. For example, in the forearm, the radius and ulna act as a lever, with the elbow joint as the fulcrum.

Torque can be considered the rotational equivalent of force. Because nearly all joint motions occur about an axis of rotation, the internal and external forces acting at a joint are expressed as a torque. The interaction of internal and external forces ultimately controls our movement and posture. As described earlier, internal forces usually arise from muscular activation, whereas external forces arise from gravity or other external sources. These competing forces interact through a system of bony levers, with the pivot point, or fulcrum, located at the axis of rotation of our joints. Through these systems of levers, the internal and external forces are converted to internal and external torques, ultimately causing movement—or rotation—of the joints. The amount of torque generated across a joint depends on two things: (1) the amount of force exerted and (2) the distance between the force and the axis of rotation. This distance, called the *moment arm*, is the length between the axis of rotation and the perpendicular intersection of the

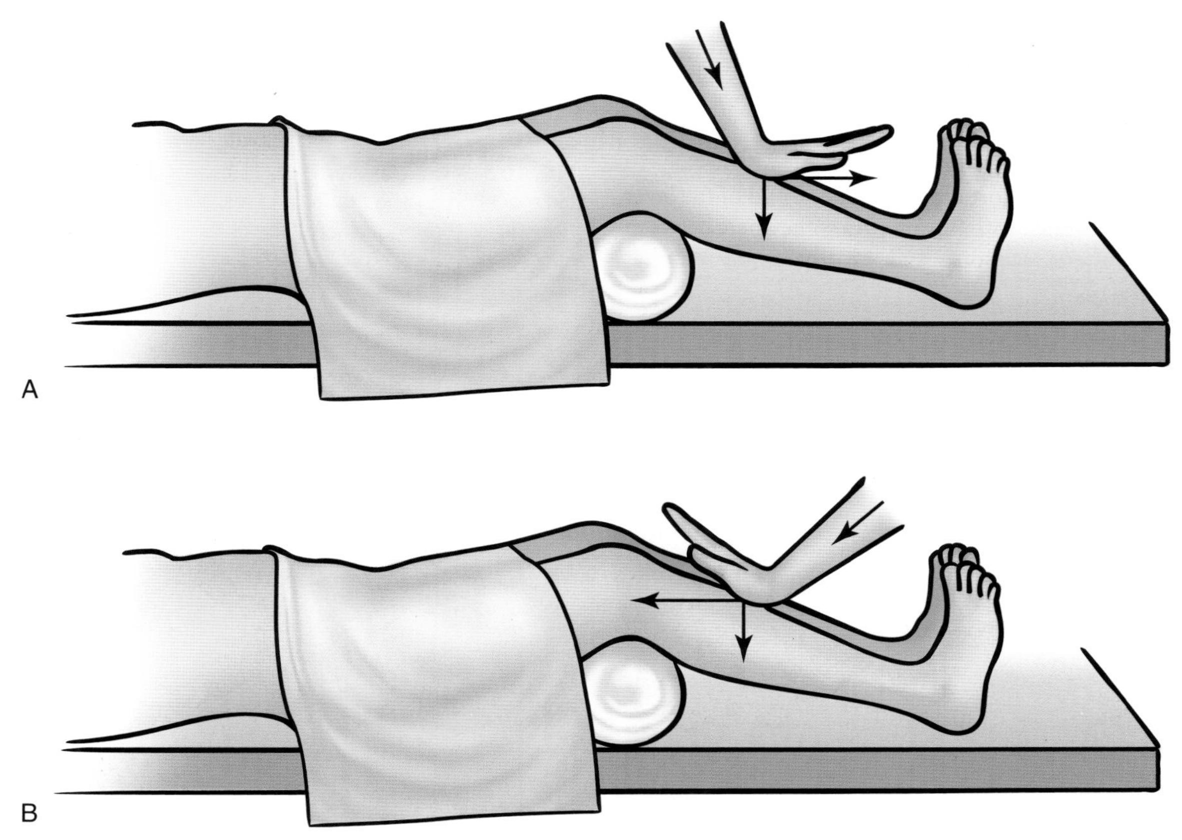

FIG. 10.1 (A) When a force is applied downhill, only the vertical component of the force goes into the client's tissue; the horizontal component goes out into space, like pushing into the air, and is wasted. (B) When applying a force to a client going uphill, both the horizontal and vertical components of the force go into the client's tissue.

MENTORING TIP

This information may seem somewhat abstract. To gain clarity explore YouTube videos. Use search terms such as *mechanical force, applied force, force versus pressure, simple machines, and levers*. Many of the terms used in the textbook can be used as search terms. It is often really helpful to watch videos made for elementary school-age kids. As the textbook author, I must make complex concepts as basic as possible and relevant to the practice of massage therapy. When I need to better understand something, I explore online learning sites for kids and websites for kids. When working to understand kinesiology and biomechanics, a video clip is worth a hundred words.

force. The product of a force and its moment arm is equal to the torque (or rotational force) generated about an axis of rotation.

Mechanical Advantage and Disadvantage

Mechanical advantage means that less effort is required to move an object, and *mechanical disadvantage* requires more effort to move the same object (Fig. 10.2).

Regardless of the type, all levers follow the same basic principles:

- Lever systems that operate at a mechanical advantage are slower, more stable, and used where strength is a priority.
- In lever systems that operate at a mechanical disadvantage, force is lost but speed is gained.

There are three types of levers: first class, second class, and third class.

First-Class Levers

In first-class levers, the effort is applied at one end of the lever and the load at the other, with the fulcrum somewhere between them. Teeter-totters, scissors, and crowbars are familiar examples of first-class levers. The use of a first-class lever occurs when you lift your head from looking down at the floor to looking straight ahead. Some first-class levers in the body operate at a mechanical advantage when the effort is farther from the joint than the load and is less than the load to be moved. Other muscles operate at a mechanical disadvantage when the effort is closer to the joint and greater than the load to be moved (Fig. 10.3).

Second-Class Levers

In second-class levers, the effort is applied at the end of the lever and the fulcrum is located at the other end, with the load at some intermediate point between them. A wheelbarrow is an example of this type of lever. Second-class levers are uncommon in the body, and the best example of their use is standing on your toes. Joints forming the ball of the foot act together as the fulcrum. The load is the entire body weight. The calf muscles inserted into the calcaneus exert the effort, pulling the heel upward. All second-class levers in the body work at a mechanical advantage because the muscle distal attachment is

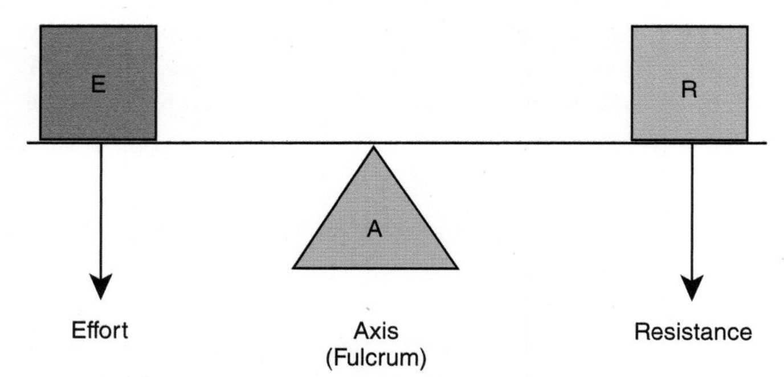

FIG. 10.3 A first-class lever has its axis of motion (*A*) between the force of effort (*E*) and the force of resistance (*R*). Modified from Roberts SL, Falkenburg SA. *Biomechanics: Problem Solving for Functional Activity*. Mosby; 1992.

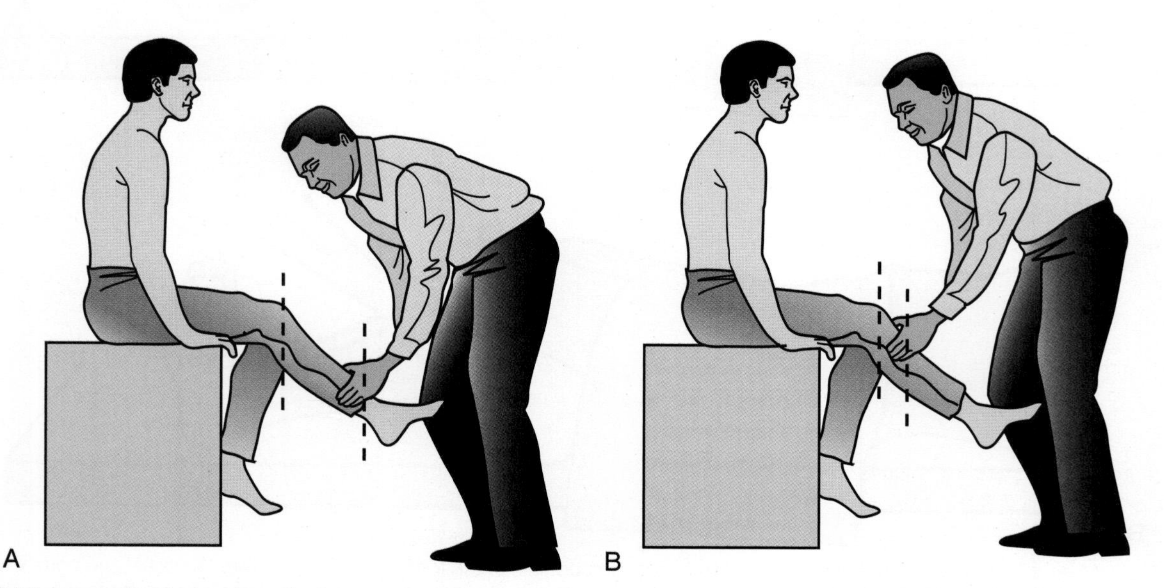

FIG. 10.2 (A) Force applied farther from the joint results in mechanical advantage. (B) Force applied near the joint results in a mechanical disadvantage.

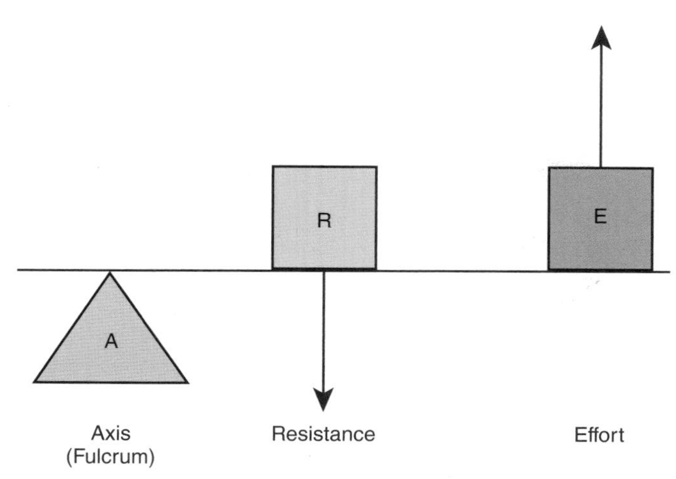

FIG. 10.4 In a second-class lever, the force of resistance (*R*) lies between the axis of movement (*A*) and the force of effort (*E*). (Modified from Roberts SL, Falkenburg SA. *Biomechanics: Problem Solving for Functional Activity*. Mosby; 1992.)

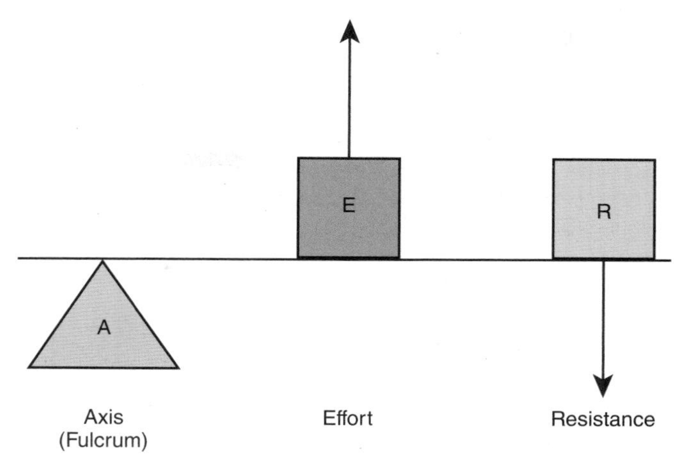

FIG. 10.5 With a third-class lever, the force of effort (*E*) lies between the axis (*A*) and the force of resistance (*R*). (Modified from Roberts SL, Falkenburg SA. *Biomechanics: Problem Solving for Functional Activity*. Mosby; 1992.)

always farther from the fulcrum than the load to be moved. Second-class levers are levers of strength, with speed and range of motion sacrificed (Fig. 10.4).

Third-Class Levers

With third-class levers, the effort is applied at a point between the load and the fulcrum. These levers operate with greater speed and are always at a mechanical disadvantage. Tweezers or forceps provide this type of leverage. Most of the body operates with a third-class lever system that permits a muscle to be inserted close to a joint, allowing rapid extensive movement with little shortening of the muscle. As an example, the biceps muscle of the arm provides the effort, the fulcrum is the elbow, and the force is exerted on the proximal radius. The load to be lifted is the distal forearm and anything carried in the hand or over the forearm (Fig. 10.5).

Balance, Equilibrium, and Stability

Balance is the ability to control equilibrium. The two types of balance are static (or still) and dynamic (or moving).

Equilibrium means that all forces acting on an object are equal. Equilibrium may be static or dynamic. A body at rest or completely motionless is in static equilibrium. Dynamic equilibrium occurs when all of the applied and internal forces acting on the moving body are in balance, resulting in movement with no change in speed or direction. For us to control equilibrium to achieve balance, we need to maximize stability.

Stability is the resistance to change in the acceleration of the body or the resistance to the disturbance of the equilibrium of the body. Determining the center of gravity of the body and changing it appropriately may enhance stability.

In biomechanical terms, the concept of center refers to the center of gravity, the midpoint or center, of the weight of a body or object. The **center of gravity** is the point at which all the mass, or weight, of the body, is balanced equally or distributed equally in all directions. The anatomical center of gravity can be calculated if the body is at rest; however, the anatomical center of gravity changes constantly as the body moves. The position of the center of gravity depends on the arrangement of the body segments and changes with every movement. Any loss of biomechanical stability, such as with a missing limb or altered posture, alters not only the total body weight distribution but also the center of gravity.

Functions of the nervous system contribute to balance. The semicircular canals of the inner ear, vision, touch, pressure, and proprioceptive sense provide balance information. The body is in a constant dynamic state of adjustment to maintain balance, reflecting dynamic homeostasis.

Balance Principles

- A person is balanced when the center of gravity falls within the base of support.
- A person is balanced in direct proportion to the size of the base of support. The larger the base of support, the more balance.
- A person is balanced depending on the weight, or mass. The greater the weight, the more balance.
- A person's balance depends on the height of the center of gravity. The lower the center of gravity, the more balance.
- A person's balance depends on where the center of gravity is in relation to the base of support. If the center of gravity is near the edge of the base, less balance is present. However, in anticipation of an oncoming force, a person may improve stability by placing the center of gravity closer to the side of the base of support expected to receive the force.
- In anticipation of an oncoming force, a person may increase stability by enlarging the size of the base of support in the direction of the anticipated force.
- A person may enhance equilibrium by increasing the friction between the body and the surface it contacts.
- Rotation around an axis is easier to balance. A bike that is moving is easier to balance than a stationary bike.

Practical Application

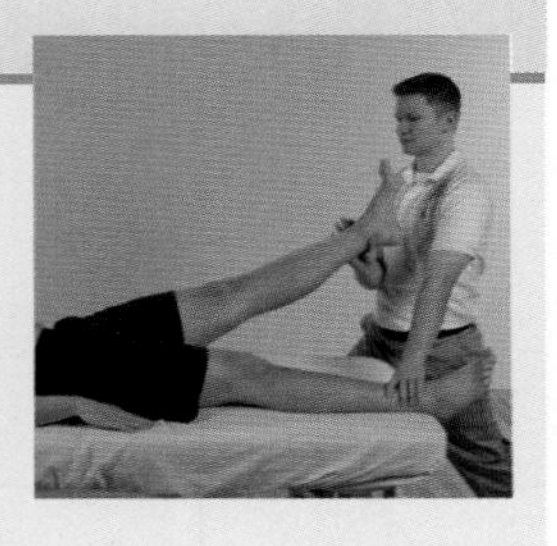

Muscles can function in multiple ways to meet various tasks, such as maintaining balance. Most daily activities require the coordination of complex neuromuscular interactions. Sometimes muscles are required to function for prolonged periods without fatiguing, and at other times muscles must provide maximal effort for only a few seconds. Muscles have three major actions: isometric, concentric, and eccentric. Muscles must be able to shorten and lengthen to provide a range of motion at joints, yet they must generate enough power to move a load at each end of the range. Muscles must be able to hold a static position to provide stability. The nervous system accomplishes the fine control of muscle contraction over a wide range of lengths, tensions, speeds, and loads.

When giving a massage, we have to assess for these functions. Massage application depends on accurate functional assessment. We can observe a muscle contract through its range of motion. When muscles move a joint, its ability to stabilize is decreased, and vice versa. Muscles that span a long distance, such as the biceps brachii of the arm, are most efficient in supplying movement through a longer range of motion. Other muscles are more effective at stabilizing the joint than moving it. The supraspinatus of the shoulder joint is a good example; its line of pull is mostly vertical and close to the axis of the shoulder joint. Therefore, the supraspinatus has a short range of motion, which makes this muscle more effective at stabilizing than moving the shoulder joint. Opposing muscle groups generate parallel forces to provide stability; this is achieved through cocontraction. As presented in Chapter 9 and expanded upon in this chapter, muscle/fascial units coordinated by the nervous system work together to support stability and mobility. The more integrated movement is understood, the more beneficial the massage.

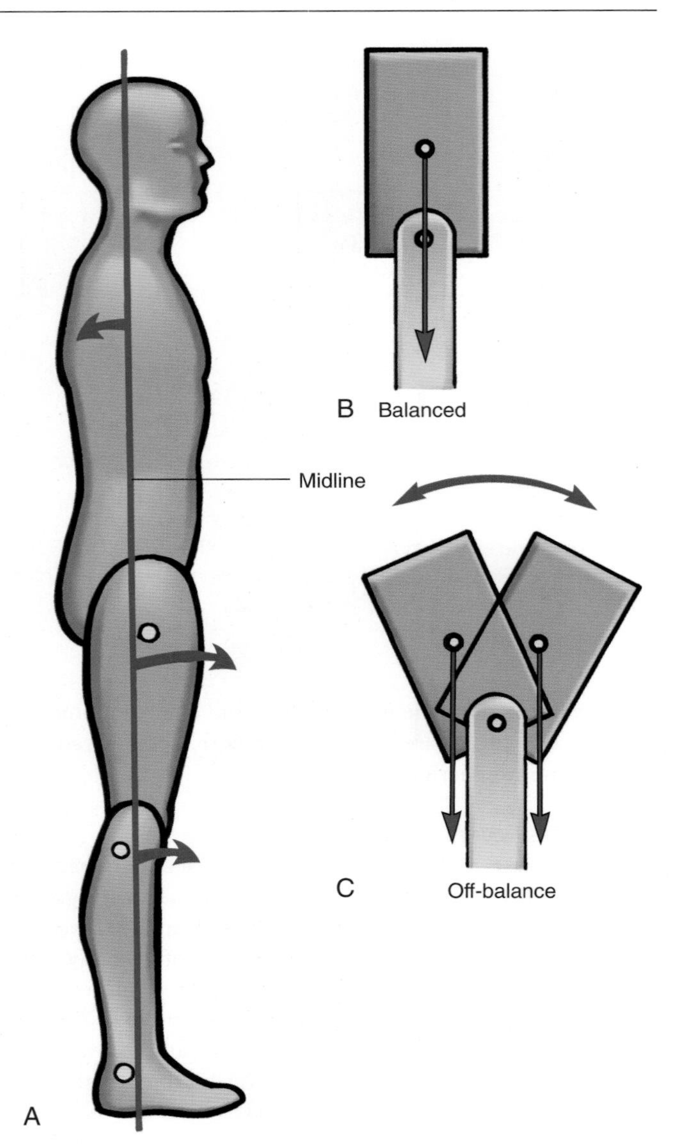

FIG. 10.6 (A) In normal, relaxed standing, the leg and trunk tend to rotate slightly off the midline of the body but maintain a counterbalancing force. Balance is achieved in (B) but not (C). Whenever the trunk moves off this midline balance point, the body must compensate. (From Fritz S. *Mosby's Fundamentals of Therapeutic Massage*. 4th ed. Mosby/Elsevier; 2009.)

Posture

The postural muscles help us to maintain our upright position in gravity. This is quite a task because the center of gravity constantly changes with each movement. When we lie down, we relieve the postural muscles of this task.

Efficient posture is important because it reduces the amount of stress placed on ligaments, muscles, and tendons, improves function, and decreases the amount of muscle energy needed to keep the body upright (Fig. 10.6). There are many postural variations. The concept of an ideal posture has not stood up to research evaluation. It is possible to have multiple deviations away from the ideal and remain functional. However, a level of symmetry is considered efficient. Observation and palpation of symmetry in relation to the interrelated moving parts of the body are a helpful assessment approach.

Recall from Chapter 7 that the vertebral column is a column of block-shaped bones stacked in counterbalancing anterior-posterior curves. At birth, the entire vertebral column is concave anteriorly and called the *primary curve*. As the child grows, anteriorly convex curves of the cervical and lumbar regions develop. These curves are maintained during rest and activity and function as shock absorbers. The thoracic and sacral curves counter the cervical and lumbar curves. The thoracic and sacral curves are concave anteriorly and convex posteriorly. Conversely, the lumbar and cervical curves are convex anteriorly and concave posteriorly. Any change of these vertebral curves, such as an increase or decrease, results in poor posture. For example, a sway back is an increased lumbar curve, or *hyperlordosis*, whereas a flat back is a decreased thoracic curve. Any lateral curvature of the spine is a pathological condition called *scoliosis*.

The pelvis should be in a neutral position, defined as:

- The anterior superior iliac spine and posterior superior iliac spine are level with each other in a transverse plane.
- The anterior superior interior spine is in the same vertical plane as the symphysis pubis.

When the pelvis is in a neutral position, the lumbar curve has the optimal amount of curvature. When the pelvis is tilted anteriorly, the amount of lumbar curvature increases, causing lordosis. When the pelvis is tilted posteriorly, the amount of curve decreases, causing a flat back.

When weight is distributed evenly on both legs, the pelvis should remain level from side to side, with the anterior superior iliac spine and anterior superior interior spine at the same level. During the normal walking gait, the pelvis dips from side to side as weight shifts from stance to swing phase. This lateral pelvic tilt is controlled by the hip abductors, mainly the gluteus medius and gluteus minimus, and the trunk lateral flexors, primarily the erector spinae and quadratus lumborum.

In the upright position, posture depends primarily on muscle contractions and fascial support to remain upright in gravity. The muscles most involved are called *antigravity muscles*. The antigravity muscles are primarily the hip and knee extensors and the trunk and neck extensors. Other muscles maintaining the upright position are the trunk and neck flexors and lateral flexors, hip abductors and adductors, and ankle pronators (everters) and supinators (inverters). If all of these muscles were to relax, the body would collapse.

The ankle plantar flexors and dorsiflexors are also antigravity muscles and are important in controlling postural sway. Postural sway is the anterior-posterior motion of the upright body caused by motion occurring primarily at the ankles. This sway results from the constant displacement and correction of the center of gravity within the base of support.

A person's posture can be assessed most accurately using a plumb line suspended from the ceiling or a posture grid placed behind the person as a point of reference (Fig. 10.7). A plumb line is a string or cord with a weight attached to the lower end. Because the string is weighted, it makes a perfectly straight vertical line in gravity. It is important to remember that we are all slightly asymmetrical. When comparing an individual's body against a postural grid, it is not realistic to expect that someone's posture will line up perfectly, nor is it a realistic massage outcome goal to expect to shift posture to perfect symmetry. The grid helps identify exaggerated areas of postural asymmetry that may be problematic.

Lateral View

In the standing position and viewed from the lateral position, the plumb line should be aligned so that it passes slightly in front of the lateral malleolus. For ideal posture, the body segments should be aligned so that the plumb line passes through the listed landmarks as follows:

Head	Through the ear lobe
Shoulder	Through the tip of the acromion process
Thoracic spine	Anterior to the vertebral bodies
Lumbar spine	Through the vertebral bodies
Pelvis	Level
Hip	Through the greater trochanter (slightly posterior to the hip joint axis)
Knee	Slightly posterior to the patella (slightly anterior to the knee joint axis) with the knees in extension
Ankle	Slightly anterior to the lateral malleolus with the ankle joint in a neutral position between dorsiflexion and plantar flexion

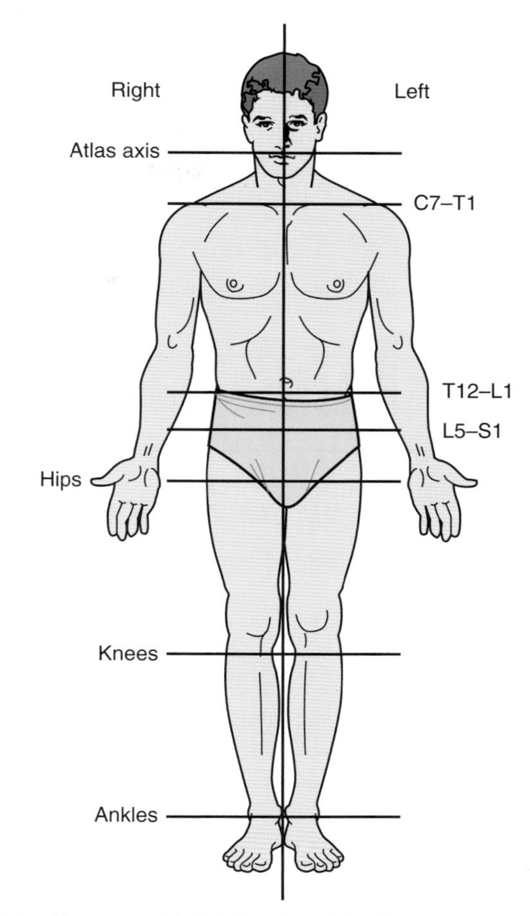

FIG. 10.7 Posture grid. Gridlines help identify symmetry or deviations in symmetry. As shown in the figure, no one is perfectly symmetrical. It is the degree of variation and the limitation in function that determines the degree of dysfunction.

Anterior View

In the standing position and viewed from the anterior position, the plumb line should be aligned to pass through the midsagittal plane of the body, thus dividing the body into two halves. The body segments should be aligned as follows:

Head	Extended and level, not flexed or hyperextended
Shoulders	Level and not elevated or depressed
Sternum	Centered in the midline
Hips	Level with the anterior superior iliac and anterior superior interior spines in the same plane
Legs	Slightly apart
Knees	Level and not bowed or knock-kneed
Ankles	Normal arch in feet
Feet	Slight toeing outward

Posterior View

In the standing position and viewed from the posterior position, the plumb line should be aligned to pass through the midsagittal plane of the body, dividing the body into two halves. The body segments should be aligned as follows:

Head	Extended, not flexed or hyperextended
Shoulders	Level and not elevated or depressed
Spinous processes	Centered in the midline
Hips	Level with posterior superior iliac spine and in the same plane with anterior superior iliac spine
Legs	Slightly apart
Knees	Level and not bowed or knock-kneed
Ankles	Calcaneus should be straight

Postural Stabilization

Stabilization of the body during normal movement occurs in soft tissues between movement segments. For example, the muscles located between the base of the skull and the top of the shoulders or the muscles located between the last thoracic vertebrae and the top of the hips are considered segments. These patterns balance each other to provide postural stability in a diagonal counterbalancing function. Compensation and dysfunction can occur as well. For example, if the right hip is elevated because of muscles tensing in the back, typically there is a compensation tension pattern in the anterior muscles on the left between vertebrae C7 and T12. Another example is pain in the quadriceps on the left that shows a compensation pattern in the calf on the right and the tissue between the hips and S1 on the right posterior. Tension also may develop in the tissues on the top of the left foot.

The body must be balanced in three dimensions against the forces of gravity to provide stability in the upright position and for locomotion. Balanced daily against the forces of gravity, the body reacts to pain, injury, and other stimuli through complex compensations involving many polysynaptic reflex arcs. Some compensation patterns are resourceful, such as when the body is required to adapt to a trauma or repetitive use pattern. Massage applications should support these changes. Some compensation patterns become pathological or maladaptive and increase strain in the system. Therapeutic massage can assist in reversing some of these nonproductive patterns. Any form of compensation can yield a confusing combination of signs and symptoms. Symptoms may range from complaints of left scapular pain after a right quadriceps injury to complaints of pain on the front left side of the neck after an injury to the right calf. Signs, such as decreased movement of extremities, splinting, and lack of bilateral symmetry, also may be observable.

Sitting, Standing, and Bending

Squatting down to pick up an object is more efficient than bending over at the hip joint and then lifting. Bending over puts an enormous strain on the back. Half the body weight is being moved in addition to the weight of the object being lifted. When squatting down and then moving from a squat to a standing position, keep weight distributed over the entire bottom of the foot, particularly the heels. The tendency is to bear weight on the ball of the foot and toes. This position causes instability in the ankle and knee.

When in the seated position, moving to a standing position begins by leaning forward at the hips and leading with the head. The momentum carries the body forward into a semisquat. The leg muscles then lift the body into a standing position (Fig. 10.8).

Walking/Gait

Locomotion, or walking, is the act of moving from one place to another. Gait is the means of achieving this action. Despite years of scientific study, we still do not know exactly why we stand upright and walk. The question remains as to how much of locomotion is innate and how much is learned. Human beings certainly are driven to walk. Most authorities agree that the urge and the "hardwiring" for bipedal (two-legged)

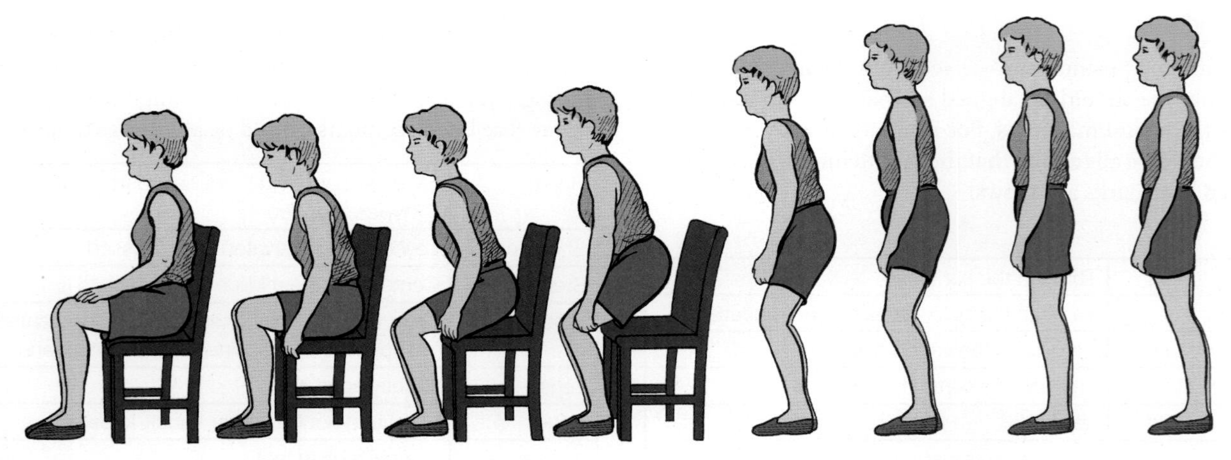

FIG. 10.8 Sit-to-stand viewed laterally. (Modified from Gillen G, Burkhardt A. *Stroke Rehabilitation: A Function-Based Approach*. 3rd ed. Mosby/Elsevier; 2011.)

locomotion are with us from birth, and the coordination of all the components necessary to accomplish the task is learned.

Controlling bipedal locomotion is not an easy task. Reflexive coordination by the central nervous system is an essential part of the walking pattern. The central nervous system coordinates muscles to generate the locomotion pattern through the following actions:

- Producing the effort necessary to move the body
- Adapting changes in the center of gravity
- Coordinating the movements and projected movements of the limbs
- Adapting to changing conditions and joint positions
- Coordinating visual, auditory, vestibular, and peripheral afferent information

Understanding reflex patterns is an important part of understanding how we walk. Because most reflex actions involve a great many reflex arcs, local stimulation of a small number of receptors leads to a large number of outgoing impulses to muscles and glands. The result is a widespread and generalized reflex response. Most reflexes are polysynaptic, using many sensory neurons, interneurons, and motor neurons. Breaking down these complex functional patterns is often confusing (Whittle, 2007; Sahrmann, 2002). We can simplify this process for understanding gait.

Walking is an activity in which a person moves their body into and out of balance with each step. When standing and while walking, our center of gravity is located in our pelvis at the upper sacral region anterior to the second sacral vertebra. Our head is balanced on top of the spine, and the center of gravity for the head is in front of the ear by the cheek.

Watching toddlers as they start to walk reveals that from the beginning, walking is counterbalanced by the activity of the arms, hands, head, and pelvis. This counterbalancing action becomes important in understanding the complex system of reflex control of gait patterns.

Normal Adult Walking Cycle

Simply stated, we walk around on two legs composed of three segments each: the thigh, lower leg, and foot. On top of our legs are the trunk, head, and arms. The whole arm unit is used as a counterbalance and for momentum and moves opposite the leg movement. This pattern is linked by the contralateral reflex arc mechanism (Fig. 10.9). A practice protocol for gait assessment can be found at the end of the chapter.

When we walk, peripheral receptors in our joints and muscles detect changes in muscle length and force, joint position, and weight-bearing status of the limbs. Righting reflexes involving the eyes and ears, together with tonic neck reflexes, maintain an upward, level, and forward head position, whereas ocular/pelvic reflexes balance the head and pelvis position. Sensory receptors on the soles of the feet relay postural information about weight distribution (Viseux, 2020). Mechanoreceptors, the pressure receptors in the sole of the foot, are involved in postural control (Yamashita et al., 2024). The relationship between the movement of the legs when walking and the independent use of the arm/hand complex depends on the task and environment.

Flexion and extension of the hip joints cause some rotation in the lumbar spine, and to keep the head facing forward and the eyes level, the thorax and cervical spine rotate in the opposite direction. Reciprocal movements of the upper and lower limbs occur with the right upper limb flexing at the shoulder joint simultaneously with flexion at the left hip joint. Normally, the shoulder joint starts to flex or extend slightly before the same movement occurs in the elbow joint. These movements again serve to keep the head and trunk oriented and to counterbalance the body weight in gravity.

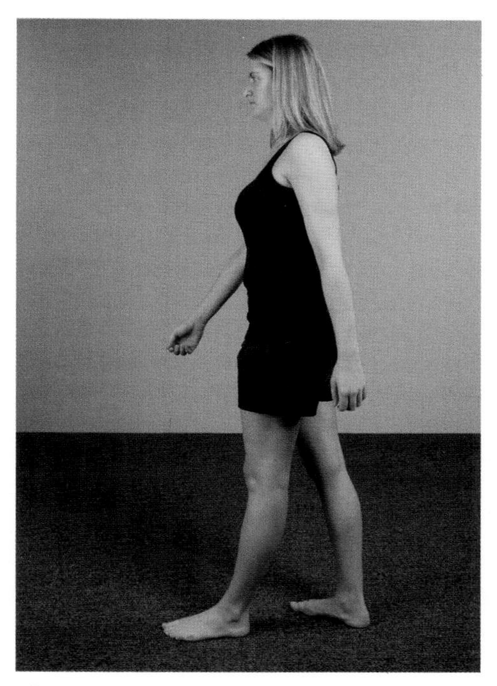

FIG. 10.9 Counterbalance is shown as the arm moves opposite the leg. (From Fuhr A. *The Activator Method*. 2nd ed. Mosby/Elsevier; 2008.)

Gait Cycle

Gait is defined as the rhythmic and alternating movement of the legs along with the trunk and the arms, which results in the propulsion of the body mass. Gait is an automatic function coordinated by innate and learned reflexes. Muscles certainly work together to create movement, but an interesting note is that in large portions of the gait cycle, little or no muscle activity occurs in most of the muscle groups, pointing to the energy-efficient nature of walking.

A **gait cycle** is the period during which a complete sequence of events takes place; it begins when the heel of one foot strikes the floor. The gait cycle is subdivided into the stance phase and the swing phase. The stance phase occurs when the limb under consideration is in contact with the floor. During walking, a period always occurs when both feet are in contact with the floor; this is called a double stance. The swing phase occurs when the foot is not in contact with the floor.

In the average walking pattern, the stance phase takes about 60% of the gait cycle, and the swing phase about 40%. As the speed of walking, or cadence, increases, the length of time in the stance phase decreases. Double-stance time increases with slow walking.

The components of the stance phase are heel strike, foot flat, midstance, heel-off, and toe-off (Fig. 10.10). The components of the swing phase are acceleration, midswing, deceleration, and arm swing (Fig. 10.11).

Heel strike = Initial contact
Hip 25° Flexion Hip extensors eccentric
Knee 0° Quadriceps concentric
Ankle 0° Tibials concentric
A
Foot Flat = Loading Response
Hip 26° Flexion Hip extensors eccentric and hip abductors isometric
Knee 15° Flexion Quadriceps eccentric
Ankle 10° Plantar flexion Pretibials eccentric
B
Midstance = Midstance
• The body (center of gravity) reaches its highest point in the gait cycle
Hip 0° Hip abductors isometric
Knee 0° Quadriceps concentric initially, then no muscle activity
Ankle 0° Plantar flexors (calf) eccentric
C
Toe-Off = Preswing
Hip 0° Adductor longus
Knee 40° Knee flexion No muscle activity
Ankle 20° Plantar flexion Plantar flexors concentric initially, then no muscle activity
D
Heel-Off = Terminal Stance
Hip 20° Hip hyperextension No muscle activity
Knee 0° No muscle activity
Ankle 10° Dorsiflexion Plantar flexors (calf) eccentric
E

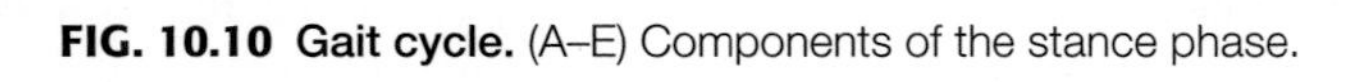

FIG. 10.10 Gait cycle. (A–E) Components of the stance phase.

Section Summary

- Define biomechanics.
  - The science of internal and external forces acting on the human body and the effects produced by these forces.
- Explain the lever and the fulcrum and the application of force.
  - A lever is a rigid mass that rotates around a fixed point called the *fulcrum (axis of rotation)*. Force applied to a lever reduces the effort needed to overcome resistance. In the body, joints are fulcrums and bones are levers.
- Describe the center of gravity of the body and also balance, equilibrium, and stability.

Practical Application

The massage therapist often can trace dysfunctional patterns through these basic reflex principles. For example, a client complains of a stiff left shoulder and cannot remember how the pain began but can remember walking around an amusement park with a blister on the right heel. This dysfunctional pattern may result from a change in gait, developed from an alteration in the reciprocal counterbalancing pattern, which eventually led to shoulder pain. The shoulder difficulty may be relieved by addressing neuromuscular tension patterns in the right leg and hip. Many such patterns could develop in different clients. By paying attention to the reflex pattern operating in the body and understanding the gait cycle and the kinetic chain, the massage therapist can manage this type of soft-tissue dysfunction more effectively.

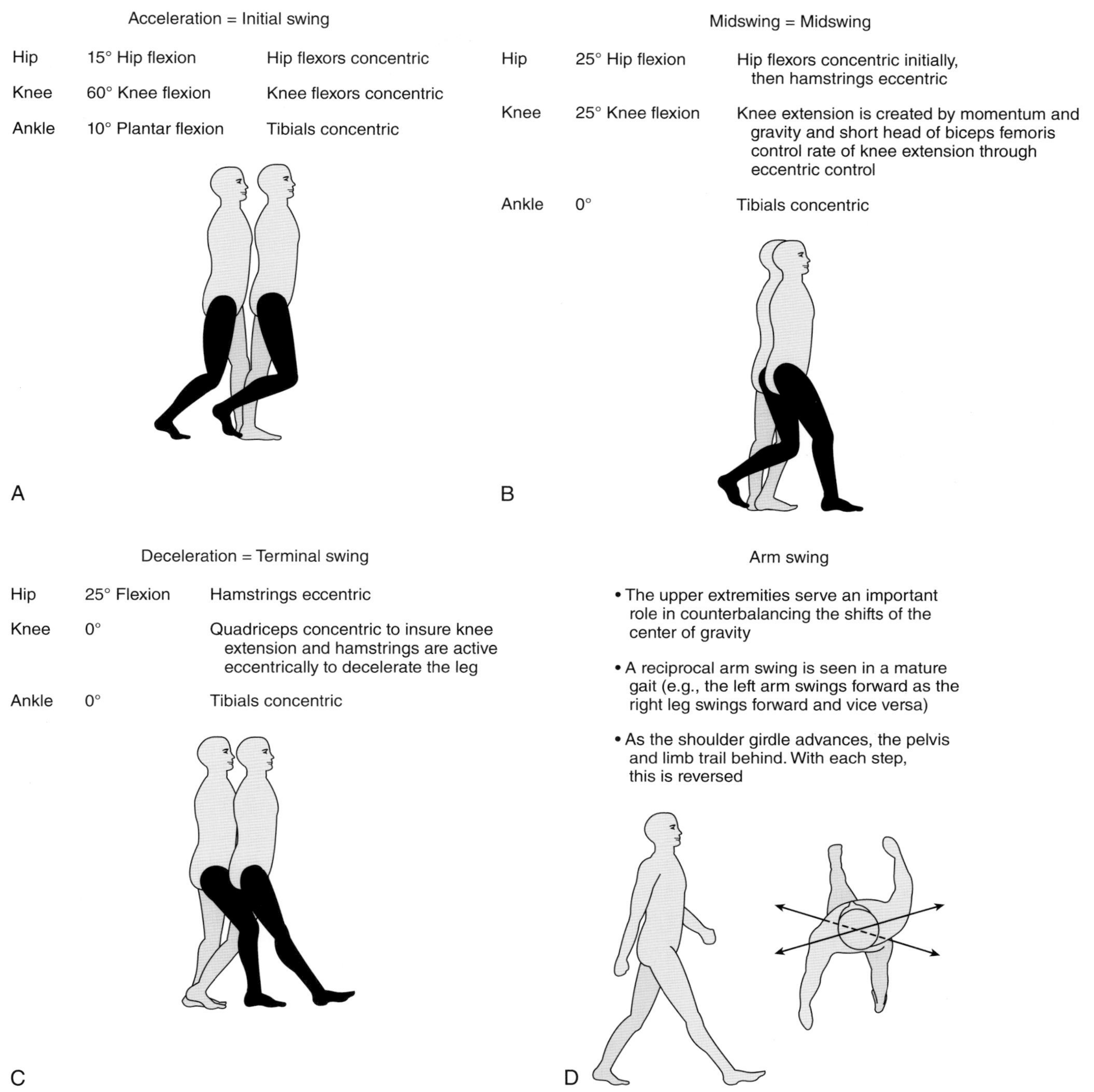

Acceleration = Initial swing

Hip	15° Hip flexion	Hip flexors concentric
Knee	60° Knee flexion	Knee flexors concentric
Ankle	10° Plantar flexion	Tibials concentric

A

Midswing = Midswing

Hip	25° Hip flexion	Hip flexors concentric initially, then hamstrings eccentric
Knee	25° Knee flexion	Knee extension is created by momentum and gravity and short head of biceps femoris control rate of knee extension through eccentric control
Ankle	0°	Tibials concentric

B

Deceleration = Terminal swing

Hip	25° Flexion	Hamstrings eccentric
Knee	0°	Quadriceps concentric to insure knee extension and hamstrings are active eccentrically to decelerate the leg
Ankle	0°	Tibials concentric

C

Arm swing

- The upper extremities serve an important role in counterbalancing the shifts of the center of gravity
- A reciprocal arm swing is seen in a mature gait (e.g., the left arm swings forward as the right leg swings forward and vice versa)
- As the shoulder girdle advances, the pelvis and limb trail behind. With each step, this is reversed

D

FIG. 10.11 Gait cycle. (A–D) Components of the swing phase.

- The center of gravity is the point where all the mass, or weight, of the body, is balanced/distributed in all directions. While standing/walking, the anatomical center of gravity is located in the pelvis/upper sacral region, which can be calculated if the body is at rest but changes constantly as the body moves. Balance is the ability to control equilibrium statically or dynamically. Equilibrium means all static or dynamic forces acting on an object are equal. Stability is the resistance to disruption of equilibrium.
- Identify common postural deviations.
  - Increased lumbar curve, or lordosis, correlates with anterior tilt of the pelvis. A decreased thoracic curve, or flat back, correlates with the posterior tilt of the pelvis. Lateral curvature of the spine, called *scoliosis*, correlates with elevation/depression of the pelvis.
- Explain gait.
  - Gait is the rhythmic and alternating movement of the legs along with the trunk and arms, resulting in the propulsion of the body. Many innate and learned reflexes coordinate this action. A gait cycle is a period during which a complete sequence of events takes place, subdivided into the stance phase (heel strike, foot flat, midstance, heel-off, toe-off), and swing phase (acceleration, midswing, deceleration, arm swing).

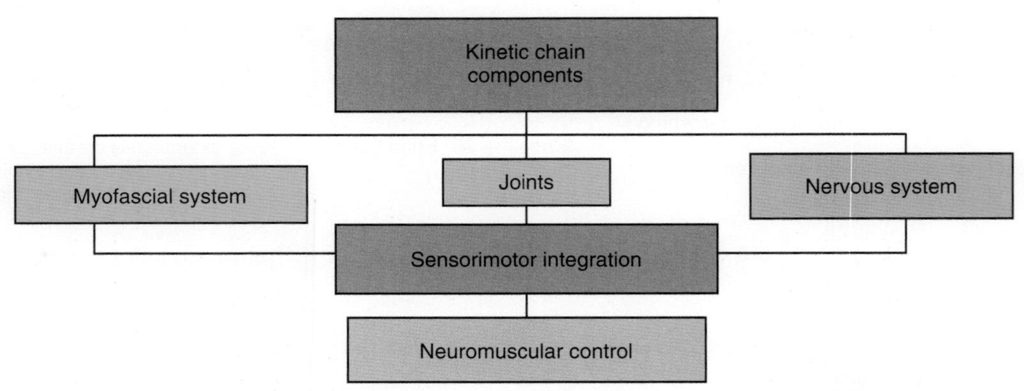

FIG. 10.12 Kinetic chain components.

KINETIC CHAIN

SECTION OBJECTIVES

Chapter objective covered in this section:

3. Explain and assess the function of the kinetic chain.

After completing this section, the learner will be able to:

- Define kinetic chain.
- Explain the function of muscular inner and outer units.
- Describe and assess muscle synergies organized as muscle firing patterns/activation sequences.

The **kinetic chain** is an integrated functional unit (Fig. 10.12). The kinetic chain is different from previously described open and closed kinematic chains, which refer to single or multiple linked joint functions. The kinetic chain network systems of the body involve human movement. Kinetic means force(s), and chain means connected or linked together. Specifically, the kinetic chain is made up of the myofascial system (muscle, ligament, tendon, and fascia), the articular (joint) system, and the nervous system. Each of these systems works interdependently to allow structural and functional efficiency in all three planes of motion: sagittal, frontal, and transverse. If one or more of the systems do not work efficiently, compensations and adaptations occur in the remaining systems, leading to stress in the body and eventually resulting in the development of dysfunctional patterns.

For example, if you change the position of one joint either by faulty movement patterns or posture, this will affect the position and forces on all other joints and the associated soft tissue. Recall the three main functions of the nervous system:

- Sensory function: Senses changes in either external or internal environmental
- Integrative function: Combines and interprets the information gathered from all the senses to plan a response to restore homeostasis
- Motor function: Directs the neuromuscular system to produce the response based on the integrative plan

The result of the integration of the kinetic chain is effective and efficient functional movement.

All functional movement patterns involve acceleration provided by concentric muscle action, stabilization provided by isometric muscle action, and deceleration provided by eccentric action. All three actions occur at every joint in the kinetic chain and all three planes of motion with each movement pattern. Muscles also must react proprioceptively to gravity, momentum, external forces, and forces created by other functioning muscles.

This kinetic chain model considers the body as a linked system of interdependent segments involving the entire neuromuscular connective tissue articular system linking each segment to the next (Adeel et al., 2024). The parts of the body act as a system of chain links so that the energy or force generated by one part of the body can be transferred successively to the next link. The optimum coordination (timing) of these body segments and their movements allow for the efficient transfer of energy and power up through the body, moving from one body segment to the next. Each movement in the sequence builds upon the previous motion.

Biomechanical principles are used to analyze the movement of the body. Dysfunction in the kinetic chain is often caused by muscle imbalances that allow for faulty movement patterns at a joint or joints somewhere along the chain. A common dysfunction is a change in the length-tension relationship of muscle structures.

The concept of the *length-tension relationship* describes how much force a muscle can generate when stimulated to contract. Resting length is often the ideal length of a muscle and the length at which it can generate the most active force. Contraction of muscles begins at a cellular level with actin and myosin. It is the pulling of the actions by myosin heads toward each other, creating cross bridges, that exerts the force. When the resting length of a muscle is considered too short, there is too much overlap between the actin and myosin. You learned in Chapter 9 that muscle contraction occurs as actin filaments slide over one another, and muscular contraction is halted by the butting of myosin filaments against the Z-discs. In a short muscle fiber the actin has already moved together and therefore, when stimulated to contract, cannot exert a significant pulling force. If the muscle structure is too long, the actin filaments become pulled away from the myosin filaments and from each other. Very few cross-bridges can form. Less tension is produced. When the filaments are pulled too far from one another, they no longer interact and cross-bridges fail to form. No contraction results. This principle demonstrates the length-tension relationship. The central nervous system maintains muscle tone so that muscles are contracted partially to maintain resting muscle length near the optimum—not too short, not too long, but just right. The natural resting length of our skeletal muscles maximizes the ability of the muscle to contract when stimulated.

Length-tension relationships are important because if muscle lengths are altered as a result of postural distortion or joint dysfunction, they will not be able to produce an efficient movement pattern. Faulty length-tension relationships are also responsible for most common postural problems. Connective tissue binding, joint injury, degeneration, or neurological and balance problems are also causes of dysfunction. Regardless of where the problem begins, eventually the entire chain is affected. Massage therapy techniques can be used to support joint and soft tissue mobility and neuromuscular function.

Muscles function cooperatively in integrated groups to provide neuromuscular control during movements and can be divided into two main groups (each with multiple names, depending on the resource): the inner unit (stabilizers/postural muscles/local) and the outer unit (movers/phasic muscles/global). This classification type was described by Professor Anders Bergmark during the 1980s (Bergmark, 1989; Fig. 10.13).

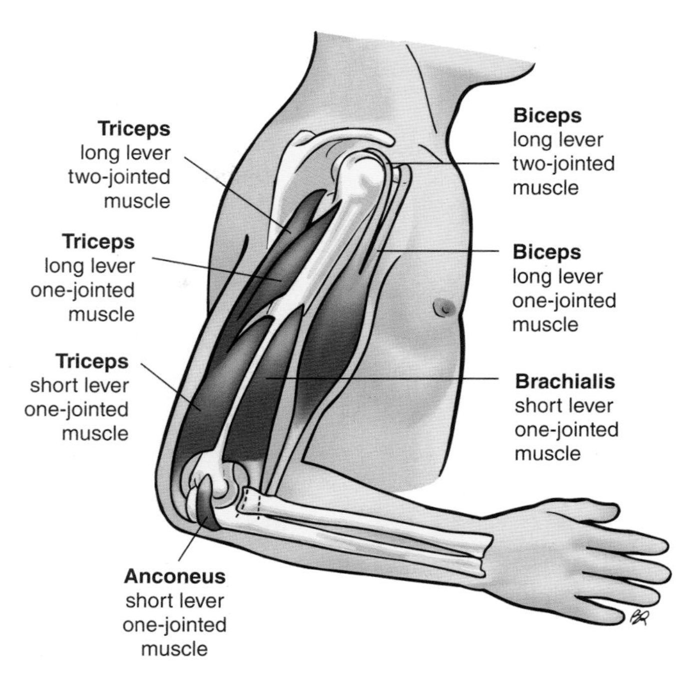

FIG. 10.13 The inner unit primarily consists of intrinsic muscles that function at only one joint and are involved predominantly in joint support or stabilization. The outer unit muscles typically cross two or more joints and are predominantly responsible for movement and typically consist of more superficial and extrinsic muscles that attach from the limbs and shoulder and pelvic girdles to the trunk (core).

Inner Unit/Local

The inner unit primarily consists of intrinsic muscles that function at only one joint and are involved predominantly in joint support or stabilization. Joint support systems consist of muscles that are not movement specific but that provide stability to allow the movement of a joint. Joint support systems also have a broad spectrum of attachments to the joint capsule that make them ideal for increasing joint stability. This group provides stability to the core and peripheral joints. These muscles tend to be inhibited in response to altered movement, which reduces the ability to respond to stimuli appropriately; this typically results in a loss of proper strength (weakness).

The postural/core/stabilization portion of the inner unit of the kinetic chain consists of the lumbo-pelvic-hip complex, thoracic spine, and cervical spine and operates as an integrated functional unit to stabilize the kinetic chain dynamically during functional movements of the limbs and head.

The joint support system of the core consists of muscles that have their proximal attachment to the spine. The peripheral joints in the shoulders, pelvic girdle, and limbs also contain inner units of muscles. An example of a peripheral joint support system is the rotator cuff for the glenohumeral joint that provides dynamic stabilization for the humeral head in the glenoid fossa during movement. Some examples of muscles that are primarily stabilizers are:

- Deep cervical flexors
- Rotator cuff
- Rhomboids
- Mid and lower trapezius
- Transversus abdominis
- Multifidus
- Diaphragm
- Muscles of the pelvic floor
- Gluteus medius and minimus
- External rotators of the hip
- Vastus medialis obliquus

Outer Unit/Global

The outer unit muscles are predominantly responsible for movement and typically consist of more superficial and extrinsic muscles that attach from the limbs and shoulder and pelvic girdles to the trunk (core) (Fig. 10.14). The outer unit muscles are usually larger than the inner unit and are associated with the movement of the trunk and limbs. Global muscles have greater biomechanical advantages to manipulate the movement of one or more joints. These muscles tend to become tight as a result of a decrease in the resting length of a muscle, as well as short and the common occurrence of a heightened neurological state.

The major global muscles include:

- Sternocleidomastoid
- Upper trapezius
- Levator scapulae
- Pectoralis major
- Deltoid
- Latissimus dorsi
- Rectus abdominis
- External obliques
- Erector spinae
- Gluteus maximus
- Hamstrings
- Rectus femoris
- Iliopsoas
- Adductors
- Gastrocnemius/soleus

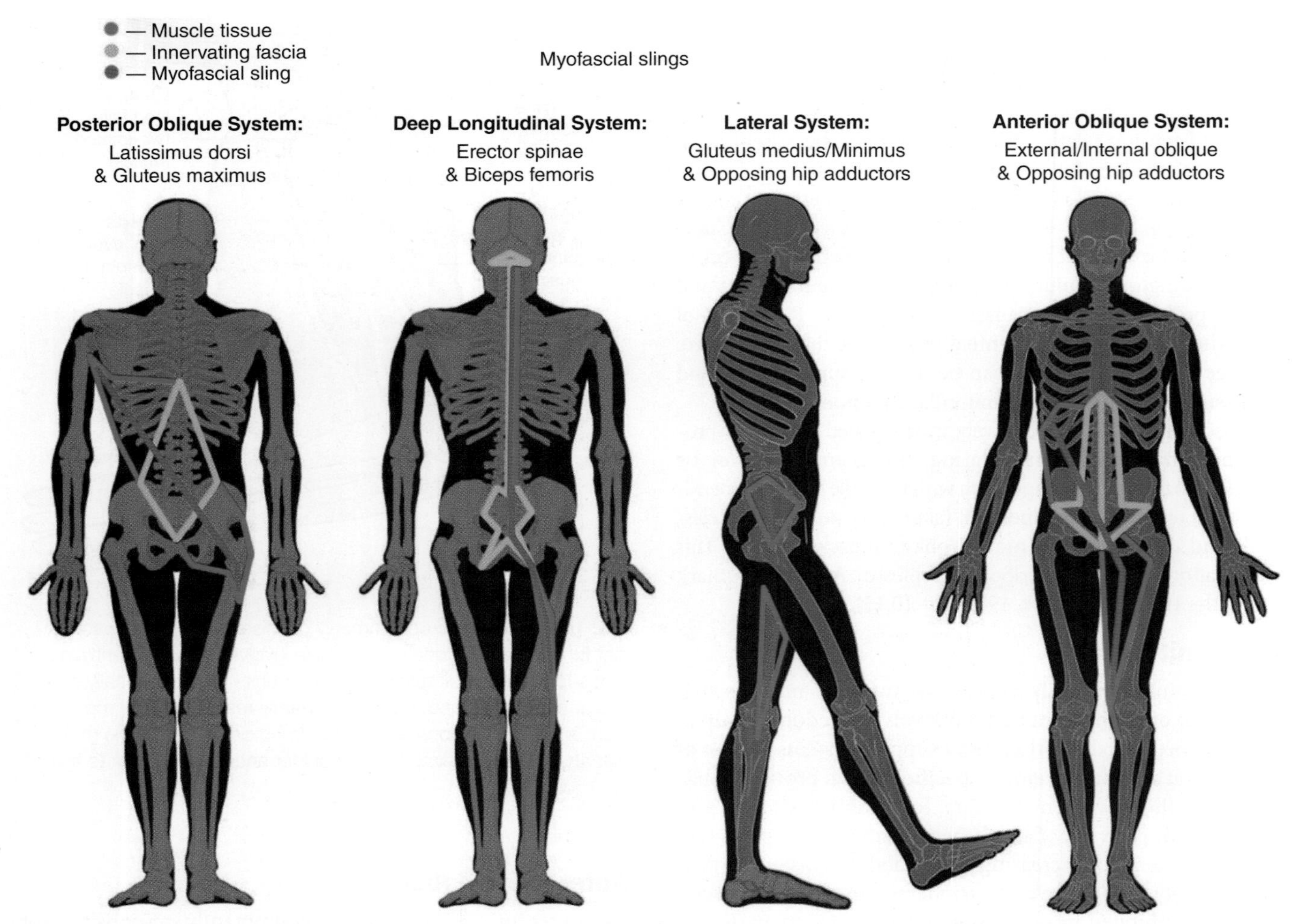

FIG. 10.14 Slings (also referred to as chains) are a functional component of the musculoskeletal system. Slings help to transfer force through the trunk and facilitate rotational movements, supporting movement and stability.

Transverse Diaphragms: Focus of Intervention

The transverse diaphragms are layers of connective tissues and fascia that run transversely through the body. These layers are perpendicular to the common myofascial planes, which run longitudinally through the body. Transverse diaphragms occur in what is known as transitional zones (anatomically known as junctions), where the function of the spinal column changes. There are four major diaphragms in the body: the cranial base, thoracic inlet/outlet, respiratory diaphragm, and pelvic floor. They occur at the junctions where the regions of the vertebrae change function and where spinal rotation more easily occurs (Standen, 2017).

- Craniocervical—the cranial base. This is the site of the tonic neck reflexes, which influence postural muscular tone throughout the trunk.
- Cervicothoracic—the thoracic inlet (clinically the thoracic outlet). This is also where the brachial plexus passes.
- Thoracolumbar—the respiratory diaphragm (or thoracic diaphragm in anatomy). This diaphragm separates the thoracic cavity (heart, lungs, and ribs) from the abdominal cavity and performs an important function in respiration. Contraction and relaxation of this diaphragm provide the function for breathing and it also produces alternating intrathoracic and intraabdominal pressure gradients, which provide the pumping mechanism for venous and lymphatic circulation.

The pelvic diaphragm, spanning anteriorly to posteriorly from the pubis to the coccyx, comprises the levator ani and the ischiococcygeus. Its openings include the anal canal and urethra, and the vagina in females (Zink and Lawson, 1979).

Muscle/Motor Synergy Relationships: Muscle Firing Patterns/Activation Sequences

Muscle synergies, also known as motor synergies, are thought to be patterns of coordinated muscle activation by the central nervous system (CNS) (Zhao et al., 2023). Although the exact mechanisms of coordinated motor control remain largely unknown, a conceptual framework for understanding the neural basis of muscle synergies is helpful for the massage therapist. The idea of "working together" describes how the nervous system functionally groups muscles in a task-specific way streamlining movement control (O'Reilly and Delis, 2024). Muscles rarely work in isolation; the concept of muscle/motor synergies facilitates movement by allowing muscles and joints to operate as a cohesive unit. Joint motion is caused by muscles pulling on bones. Because muscles are recruited as synergies, multiple muscles will transmit force onto their respective bones, creating movement at the joints. For example, during the simple act of shoulder extension, the latissimus dorsi, teres major, and posterior deltoid all work together as a cohesive unit to perform the movement pattern. The central nervous system recruits the appropriate muscles in specific firing patterns to generate the appropriate muscle functions of acceleration, deceleration, or stability. The term *activation sequence* is now beginning to be used in place of firing patterns to describe this interactive function of muscles. Firing patterns that become abnormal, with the synergist becoming dominant, compromise efficient movement and strain the joint position. Although speed factors in strength and is required for action, it also influences the firing patterns. The general firing pattern sequence is (1) prime movers, (2) stabilizers, and (3) synergists. It is also possible that the stabilizers contract first to position the bone ends of the joint (sometimes called centrate). Regardless, if the stabilizer also has to move the area (acceleration) or control movement (deceleration), it typically becomes short and tight. If the synergist fires before the prime mover, the movement is awkward and labored.

If one muscle is tight and short, reciprocal inhibition occurs; that is, a tight muscle causes decreased nervous stimulation to its functional antagonist, causing it to reduce activity. For example, tight, short psoas reduces the function of the gluteus maximus. The activation and force production of the prime mover (gluteus maximus) decreases, leading to compensation and substitution by the synergists (hamstrings) and stabilizers (erector spinae), creating an altered firing pattern.

The most common activation sequence dysfunction is synergistic dominance, in which a synergist compensates for a prime mover to produce the movement. For example, if a client has a weak gluteus medius, synergists (tensor fasciae latae, adductor complex, and quadratus lumborum) become dominant to compensate for the weakness. This alters normal joint alignment, which further alters the normal length-tension relationships of the muscles around the joint. Massage therapy intervention can be used to normalize activation sequences by inhibiting the dominate synergists by applying inhibitory pressure in the belly of the muscles and activating the prime movers by having the client contract the muscle group.

There are other ways to classify functional movement groups or muscle synergies., including the following:

- The erector spinae, thoracolumbar fascia, sacrotuberous ligament, and biceps femoris assist in stabilizing the sacroiliac joint. Dysfunction in these structures can lead to sacroiliac joint pain. Often called the *deep longitudinal subsystem*, this function group helps to stabilize the body in the sagittal plane and provides force transmission through muscle chains longitudinally from the foot and ankle to the trunk and back down.
- The superficial erector spinae, psoas, deep erector spinae, transverse abdominis, abdominal obliques, diaphragm, lumbar multifidus, and muscles of the pelvic floor provide intersegmental stabilization of the trunk during functional movement. Also called the *intrinsic stabilization subsystem*, dysfunction in any of these structures can lead to sacroiliac joint instability and low back pain.
- The internal oblique, external oblique, adductor group, external rotator hip group, contralateral gluteus maximus and latissimus dorsi, anterior and posterior tibialis, soleus and gastrocnemius, and fibularis group create a stabilizing force for sacroiliac joint function, aid in the stability and rotation of the pelvis, and contribute to leg swing. Combined these muscles are called the *oblique subsystem*, consisting of an anterior and posterior portion. This functional group functions primarily in the transverse plane. The oblique subsystem integrates activities involving the trunk and the upper and lower extremities, especially during walking. When we walk our pelvis must rotate in the transverse plane to create a swinging motion for the legs, as does the shoulder girdle in the opposite direction to allow arm swing. Dysfunction in this group often leads to sacroiliac joint dysfunction and rotational strain in the lumbar spine, pelvic area, and knee, which can also affect the ankle. The weakening of the gluteus maximus or latissimus dorsi (or both) also may lead to increased tension in the hamstrings and therefore cause recurring hamstring strains.
- The gluteus medius, tensor fasciae latae, adductor group, and quadratus lumborum are responsible for pelvic-femoral stability. Also called the *lateral subsystem*, this functional group provides frontal plane stabilization of the lumbo-pelvic hip complex transfer of force between lower and upper extremities. During single-leg functional movements (e.g., walking, lunges, or stair climbing), the ipsilateral gluteus medius, tensor fasciae latae, and adductors combine with the contralateral quadratus lumborum to control the pelvis and femur. Dysfunction can create instability and strain during walking, running, and jumping activities.

Anatomy Slings: Another Way to Describe the Same Concepts

Anatomy slings were first described in the 1990s by Dr. Andry Vleeming, researcher and professor of anatomy. Functional myofascial chains and muscle synergy relationships can also be thought of as slings. The term "myofascial" relates to the various structures involved within a sling. Anatomy slings consist of muscles, fascia, and ligaments all working together to create stability and mobility (Vleeming et al., 1993). By now, it is obvious that nothing in our body functions independently. In biomechanics, it is necessary to understand that any mechanical load is distributed through a continuous network of fascia, ligaments, and muscles supporting the entire skeleton and producing movement (Vleeming et al., 2012; Schuenke et al., 2012).

Whether called myofascial chains, kinetic chain relationships, or anatomical slings, these functional units allow mechanical forces to be transmitted, creating stability and mobility. These same interrelationships are considered force couple relationships. A *force couple* can be defined as two or more muscles generating forces in different directions, resulting in a turning movement. Force couples can also create stability when equal and opposing rotations create a canceling movement. All muscles that work together to provide stability and mobility can be seen in a force couple relationship. Dr. Vleming organized force couples as myofascial slings. This approach is similar to the previous discussion about kinetic chain relationships.

Anterior Oblique System

(1) External oblique, (2) contralateral internal oblique, (3) contralateral adductors: Functions to create force closure, increasing stability of the pubic symphysis and sacroliac joint.

Posterior Oblique System

(1) Latissimus dorsi, (2) thoracolumbar fascia, (3) contralateral gluteus maximus: Functions to create force closure of the sacroiliac joint and transfers mechanical forces through the pelvic girdle during rotational activities and gait.

Deep Longitudinal System

(1) Erector spinae, (2) sacrotuberous ligament and multifidus, (3) biceps femoris, (4) peroneus longus, (5) anterior tibialis: Functions to use the thoracolumbar fascia and erector spinae muscles to transmit kinetic energy above the pelvis, while using the biceps femoris to communicate between the pelvis and the lower extremity.

Lateral System

(1) Gluteus medius and minimus, (2) contralateral adductors, (3) contralateral quadratus lumborum: Functions to provide frontal plane stability of the pelvic girdle during standing and walking.

As a massage practitioner it is important to understand that the body moves in coordinate units organized by the system. The various models previously described can help with the critical thinking process during assessment. By having the client produce a functional movement, such as standing on one foot, and observing how they complete the task can indicate the quality of movement and suggest a focus for massage intervention. Understanding that "everything is connected" supports the value of an intelligent purposeful whole-body approach to therapeutic massage practice.

Section Summary

- Define a kinetic chain.
  - A kinetic chain is the linked interdependent segments of the myofascial system (muscle, tendon, ligament, fascia), articular system (joints), and nervous system, which work together to produce structured, efficient motion. The dysfunction of one system creates added stress (compensation/adaptation) in the remaining systems.
- Explain the function of muscular inner and outer units.
  - Inner units (stabilizers/postural muscles/local) primarily consist of intrinsic muscles that function at only one joint and are involved predominantly in joint support/stabilization. Outer units (movers/phasic muscles/global) primarily consist of superficial/extrinsic muscles that attach the limbs and shoulder/pelvic girdles to the trunk and are predominantly responsible for movement.
- Describe and assess muscle/motor synergies organized as muscle firing patterns/activation sequences.
  - Muscle firing patterns/activation sequences are typically (1) prime movers, (2) stabilizers, and (3) synergists. The most common dysfunction is synergistic dominance, meaning synergists compensate for prime mover inhibition. *Simplified* firing pattern/activation sequences: Trunk flexion: (1) obliques. (2) rectus abdominis. Hip extension: (1) gluteus maximus, (2) proximal hamstrings, (3) contralateral lumbar erector spinae. Hip abduction: (1) gluteus medius, (2) tensor fasciae latae, (3) quadratus lumborum. Knee flexion: (1) distal hamstrings, (2) gastrocnemius. Knee extension: (1) vastus medialis, (2) vastus lateralis, (3) rectus femoris. Shoulder abduction: (1) supraspinatus, (2) middle deltoid.

ASSESSMENT BASED ON BIOMECHANICS

SECTION OBJECTIVES

Chapter objectives covered in this section:

4. List principles of a massage intervention plan based on efficient biomechanical movement.
5. Assess biomechanical function using individual joint assessment.
6. Assess biomechanical functions for regions of the body.

After completing this section, the learner will be able to:

- Describe two types of information assessed using movement patterns.
- Give an example of resistance and stabilization application during assessment.
- Give an example of clinical reasoning applied to individual joint assessment.
- Assess individual joint range of motion.
- Assess the body by region.

The clinical reasoning process is essential when assessing for biomechanical function and developing intervention, or treatment, plans. This section provides specific assessment protocols for the body. Refer to Chapter 3 for a review of the clinical reasoning process.

Intervention plans should work toward the client's goals. Optimally intervention should result in positive change related to the client's perception and ability to perform daily activities. For example, a plan based on the client's goal to achieve more effective shoulder movement could be: "Client indicates that more effective shoulder movement could result in improved golf performance and the reduction of shoulder stiffness after the game. Improved shoulder movement would be encouraged with the use of weekly therapeutic massage and daily yoga practice."

A plan based on efficient biomechanical movement would focus on reestablishing or supporting effective movement patterns based on these principles:

- Biomechanically efficient movement is smooth, bilaterally symmetrical, and coordinated, with an easy, effortless use of the body. Noticeable variations from this standard should be noted during the assessment.
- Each jointed area has a movement pattern. Movement involves bones; joints; ligaments; capsular components and design; tendons; muscle shapes and fiber types; interlinked fascial networks; nerve distribution; and myotatic units of prime movers, antagonists, synergists, fixators, and kinetic chain interactions.
- Reflexes, including positional and righting reflexes of vision and the inner ear, have body-wide influence—as does circulatory distribution.
- General systemic balance and nutritional influences affect biomechanical movement.
- Assessment should also identify areas of resourceful and successful compensation. These compensation patterns occur when the body has been required to adapt to some sort of trauma or repetitive use pattern. Permanent adaptive changes, although not as efficient as optimal functioning, are the best pattern the body can develop in response to an irreversible change in the system. Resourceful compensation should be supported, not eliminated.
- An efficient movement pattern is assessed as all parts functioning in a well-orchestrated manner. Causal factors in a dysfunction can be from any one or a combination of these elements. A multidisciplinary diagnosis is often necessary to

identify the interconnected pattern of the pathological condition.

Individual Joint Assessment

The following sections explore movement assessments for individual jointed areas by applying a force to load the muscles to determine the response in the jointed area.

Remember that each joint movement pattern is part of an interconnected aspect of the kinetic chain and the tensegrity nature of the design of the body. Posture and movement dysfunction should be identified in an individual joint pattern and then addressed in broader terms of kinetic chain interactions, muscle tension-length relationships, and the effects of stress and strain on the entire system.

Assessing a movement pattern gives two types of information:

- Step 1: When a jointed area moves into flexion and the joint angle decreases, the prime mover and synergists concentrically shorten, antagonists eccentrically lengthen, and the fixators isometrically stabilize. Body-wide stabilization patterns also come into play to assist in allowing the motion. During the assessment, apply resistance to load the prime mover groups and synergists to check for the neurological function of strength and, to a lesser degree, endurance as the contraction is held for a time.
- Step 2: At the same time, the antagonist pattern of the tissues that are lengthened when positioned as in step 1 can be assessed for increased tension patterns or connective tissue shortening. Dysfunction shows itself in a limited range of motion by restricting the movement pattern.

Therefore, when placing a jointed area into flexion, assess the extensors for increased tension or shortening. When the jointed area moves into extension, the opposite becomes the case. The same holds for adduction and abduction, internal and external rotation, and plantar and dorsal flexion, for example.

Resistance (pressure against) applied to the muscles is focused at the end of the lever system for mechanical advantage. For example, when assessing the function of the shoulder, focus resistance at the distal end of the humerus, not at the wrist. When assessing the extension of the hip, place resistance at the end of the femur. When assessing flexion of the knee, place resistance at the distal end of the tibia. The therapist applies resistance slowly, smoothly, and firmly at an appropriate intensity determined by the size of the muscle mass.

Stabilization is essential to assess movement patterns accurately. Allow only the area being assessed to move. Movement in any other part of the body needs to be stabilized. The massage therapist usually applies a stabilizing force. As one hand applies resistance, the other provides stabilization. Sometimes the client can provide the stabilization. Some modalities use straps to provide stabilization. The easiest way to identify the area to be stabilized is to move the area to be assessed through the range of motion. At the end of the range, some other part of the body will begin to move; this is the area of stabilization. Return the body to a neutral position, provide the appropriate stabilization to the area identified, and begin the assessment procedure.

Range of motion of a joint is measured in degrees. A full circle is 360 degrees. A flat horizontal line is 180 degrees. Two perpendicular lines (as in the shape of a capital L) create a 90-degree angle. Various ranges of motion are possible. For example, when the range of motion of a joint allows 0 to 90 degrees of flexion, anything less is hypomobile and anything more is hypermobile. A great degree of variability exists among individuals as to the actual normal range of motion; the degrees provided are general guidelines (Fig. 10.15). Range of motion is measured from the anatomical position. Regardless of whether the client is standing, supine, or side-lying, anatomical position is considered 0 degrees of motion.

In actual professional practice, the therapist picks and chooses which assessments to perform according to the client's goals and intervention processes. The activities that follow in the chapter are arranged to represent (agonist/antagonist) myotonic units (e.g., trunk extension/flexion and hip adduction/abduction).

During assessments, muscles should be able to hold against appropriate resistance without strain or pain from the pressure and without recruiting or using other muscles. Apply appropriate resistance slowly and steadily and with just enough force for the muscles to respond to the stimulus. Large muscle groups require more force than small ones. The position should be easy to assume and comfortable to maintain for a short duration—10 to 30 seconds. Contraindications to this type of assessment include joint and disk dysfunction, acute pain, recent trauma, and inflammation.

The results of the assessment are analyzed using the clinical reasoning process to identify the appropriate function of each area or dysfunction (discussed later in the Pathological Conditions section of the chapter).

General Guidelines to Assist the Clinical Reasoning Process

- If an area is hypomobile, consider tension or shortening in the antagonist pattern as a possible cause.
- If an area is hypermobile, consider instability of the joint structure or muscle weakness in the fixation pattern or problems with antagonist/agonist cocontraction function.
- If an area cannot hold against resistance, consider weakness from reciprocal inhibition of the muscles of the prime movers/agonist due to synergistic dominance and/or tension in the antagonist pattern as possible causes. Motor nerve problems could also be a cause.
- If pain occurs on passive movement, consider joint capsular dysfunction and nerve entrapment syndromes as possible causes.
- If pain occurs during active movement, consider muscle and fascial involvement as a possible cause.
- Always consider body-wide reflexive patterns, as discussed in the Postural Stabilization section, as possible causes.
- The ability to resist the applied force should be the same or similar bilaterally.
- The client should be able to assume opposite movement patterns easily.
- Bilateral asymmetry, pain, weakness, inability to assume the isolation position or to move into the opposite position, or fatigue or a heavy sensation may indicate dysfunction.
- Intervention or referral depends on the severity of the condition (stages 1, 2, or 3) and whether the dysfunction is related to the joints, neuromuscular system, or myofascial tissues.

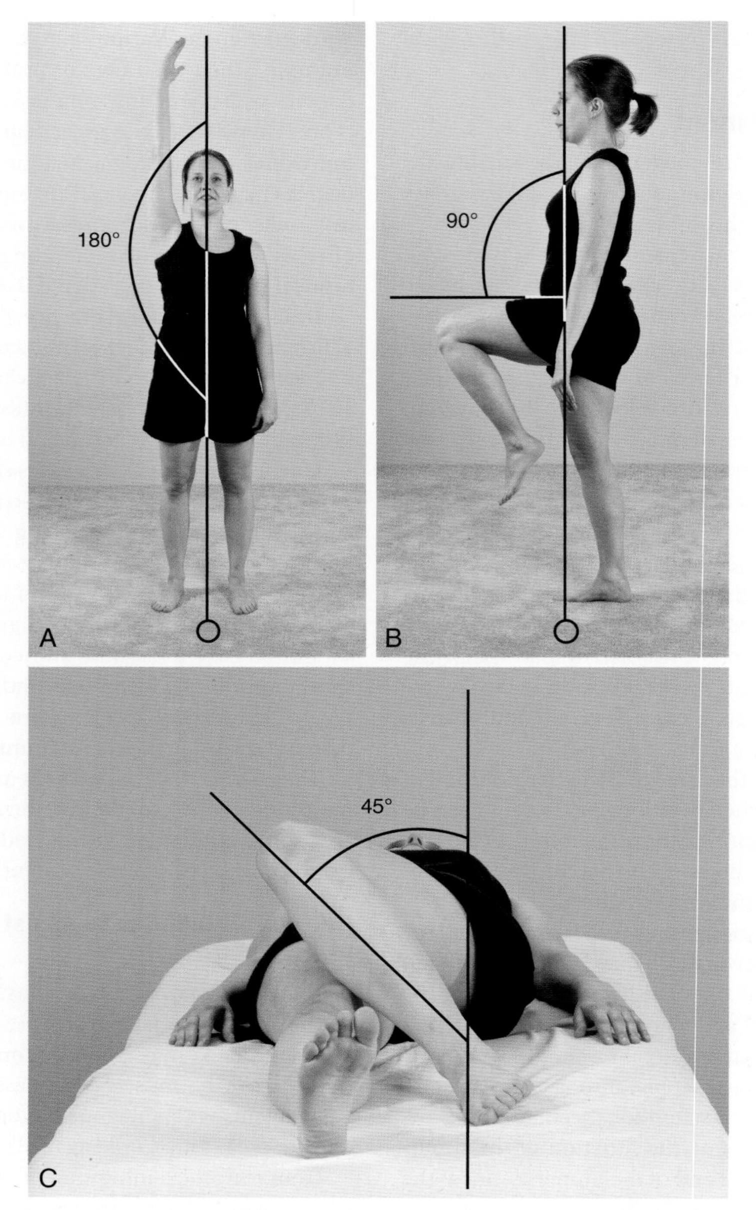

FIG. 10.15 (A–C) Examples of how to measure degrees of range of motion.

Biomechanics by Region

This part of the chapter describes the kinesiology and biomechanics of the body in a regional format. Each region is discussed, and then activities are provided to help you integrate the information. Assessment activities teach you how to muscle test and assess for range of motion. For each jointed region, the following information is provided:

- Name of the movement
- Muscles involved
- Range of motion
- Position of client
- Isolation and assessment

The activities are organized so that those movements within the same plane are adjacent. For example: Trunk flexion/trunk extension, and shoulder adduction/abduction. This means that the muscles involved in the movements would be agonist/antagonist pairs.

- The muscles that produce trunk flexion would have the trunk exterior muscles as the antagonist. The shoulder adductors would be the antagonist for the shoulder abductors.

This is important because a decrease in the range of motion of a joint is often due to shortening in the antagonist muscles.

- If the shoulder cannot abduct to the indicated range of motion, it may be that the shoulder adductors are short.

These activities are excellent for helping you provide results for clients. In addition to aiding in assessment, each of the positions can be a starting point for various types of massage applications, including active and passive joint movement and stretching.

If you are not sure about a specific muscle listed, return to Chapter 9 and review. If you are not clear on how the specific joint is designed, return to Chapters 7 and 8 for review.

The information in this section consolidates the content you learned in Chapters 7–9. In these chapters, you learned about individual parts of the anatomy and physiology. However, none of the individual structures can operate individually. Bones, joints, and muscles all work together under the direction of the nervous system. In this section, you will learn how all the bones, joints, muscles, and associated connective tissue function together.

Head/Neck Region

The neck connects to the head in the thorax and contains the C1 to C7 cervical vertebrae, spinal cord, 32 muscles, ligaments, pharynx, larynx, trachea, thyroid gland, esophagus, lymph glands, hyoid bone, blood vessels, and spinal nerves.

The cervical vertebrae allow the head and neck to be moved into flexion, extension, lateral flexion, and rotation. Combinations of these movements are also possible. The small bodies and thick disks of the cervical vertebrae tend to increase mobility. Side bending is somewhat restricted by the rectangular shape of the vertebral bodies. The atlas and axis (C1 and C2) form a pivot joint that allows the head and C1 to rotate almost 90 degrees, such as in a "no" motion. The short spinous processes of C3 to C6 allow for good extension of the head and neck.

Intervertebral disks make up approximately 25% of the height of the cervical spine. The ligaments connecting the occiput to the atlas are dense and broad. These ligaments protect the entrance of the spinal cord through the foramen magnum into the skull. The atlantoaxial (C1 and C2) joint almost totally depends on the ligamentous structure. The cervical spine from C2 to C7 is reinforced by anterior and posterior longitudinal ligaments. These ligaments limit the amount of flexion and extension.

The body moves and is balanced at certain points throughout our form. Two of these movement segments fall within the head/neck area: one at the atlas and skull and one at C6 to C7. (The other locations are T12/L1, L4/L5/S1, acetabulum/hips, knees, and ankles, as previously described.)

All muscles that act on the head attach to the skull. Those that are anterior to the frontal plane midline are termed *capital flexors*. Those muscles that lie behind the frontal plane midline are termed *capital extensors*. Their center of motion is in the atlantooccipital or atlantoaxial joints.

Practical Application

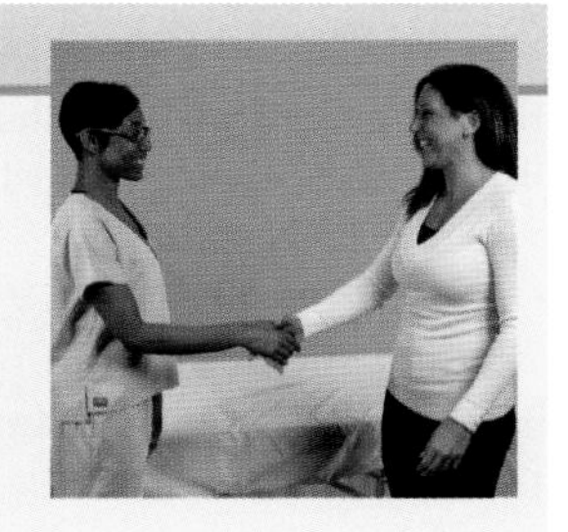

Massage clients expect results from the massage. They tell us during assessment, "It hurts when I do this." Then they move their head or arm or bend over and twist or bend and straighten their knee or ankle. Each of those movements can be found in the activities in the following sections. When a client performs a joint movement, look through the figures in the various activities to find the one that matches. For example, if a client shows you that it hurts to bend and straighten her elbow, go to the section on the elbow and to the corresponding activity to find the pertinent information.

Muscles that act on the cervical spine are attached to the skull and the cervical and thoracic vertebrae, sternum, clavicle, ribs, and scapula. Most movement occurs at C6 to C7.

The muscles of the erector spinae group are considered stabilizers of the spinal column. The deep muscles extend, rotate, laterally flex, and stabilize the cervical region. All the muscles serve to maintain the correct position of the head and spine while we are moving (e.g., walking, sitting). These muscles are adapted physiologically to work in a relay manner so that they do not fatigue under normal conditions.

The sternocleidomastoid is primarily responsible for flexion and rotation of the head and neck. Extension, particularly extension and rotation, involves the splenius muscles together with the erector spinae and the upper trapezius muscles. The neck extensors, trapezius, scalenes, sternocleidomastoid, and levator scapulae are considered major postural muscles in the body. The responsibility of these muscles is taxing even when the body has good posture and no pathological condition is present. Many muscles of the neck are called on to assist in breathing if incorrect breathing patterns exist.

Trunk and Thorax Region

The biomechanics of the trunk and thorax are unique because the vertebral column is composed of 24 intricate and complex articulating vertebrae and 31 pairs of spinal nerves. Vertebral motion is greatest where the articulating surfaces and disks are large.

Spinal or Vertebral Movements

Movement depends on a finely integrated system of muscles that are deep (composed of numerous small bundles that attach from vertebra to vertebra) or superficial (arranged in large, broad sheets).

The name given to the region of movement often precedes the descriptions of spinal or vertebral movements. For example, flexion of the trunk at the lumbar spine is known as *lumbar flexion*, and extension of the neck often is referred to as *cervical extension*. The movement of the head between the cranium and the first cervical vertebra is called *capital movement*. Movements occurring among the other cervical vertebrae are called *cervical movements*. These motions usually occur together.

The five spinal movements are:

- *Spinal flexion:* Spinal flexion is the anterior movement of the spine in the sagittal plane. In the cervical region, the head moves toward the chest. In the thoracic and lumbar regions, the thorax moves toward the pelvis.
- *Spinal extension:* Spinal extension is the posterior movement of the spine in the sagittal plane to return from flexion. In the cervical region, the head moves away from the chest. The thorax moves away from the pelvis.
- *Lateral flexion (side bending):* Lateral flexion in the frontal plane occurs in the cervical region when the head moves laterally toward the shoulder. In the thoracic and lumbar regions, the thorax moves laterally toward the pelvis. Movement can be to the left or right.
- *Reduction:* Reduction is the return movement from lateral flexion to neutral.
- *Spinal rotation (left or right):* Spinal rotation in the transverse plane is the rotary or twisting movement of the spine.

In the cervical region, the chin rotates from neutral toward the shoulder. In the thoracic and lumbar regions, the thorax rotates to one side.

As explained previously, each pair of vertebrae constitutes a vertebral motion segment, the basic movable unit of the back. Except for the atlantoaxial joint formed by the first two cervical vertebrae, little movement is possible between any two vertebrae. The amount of movement varies, depending on the shape of the vertebrae, the thickness of the intervertebral disk (thicker disks providing greater mobility), and any rib articulations. However, the cumulative effect of the movements from several adjacent vertebrae allows for substantial movements within a given area. Most of the spinal column movement occurs in the cervical and lumbar regions. Of course, some thoracic movement occurs, but it is slight compared with that of the neck and lower back.

Rotation screws the superior vertebra down into the adjacent vertebra, compressing the disk. Prime mover muscles contract while the contralateral muscles lengthen. Ligament structures are twisted.

In flexion, the anterior muscles contract, the posterior muscles lengthen, the superior vertebra tilts toward the front, and the disks are compressed anteriorly and expand posteriorly while the nucleus moves slightly to the back. The superior articular facets slide forward on the inferior ones. The posterior ligaments are stretched, and the anterior ligaments slacken.

In extension, just the opposite occurs. The posterior muscles contract and the anterior muscles lengthen. The superior vertebra tilts toward the back. The disk is compressed posteriorly and expands anteriorly, and the nucleus moves slightly to the front. The articular facets are pressed together. The anterior ligaments are stretched, and the posterior ligaments slacken. Lateral flexion follows the same pattern (Fig. 10.16).

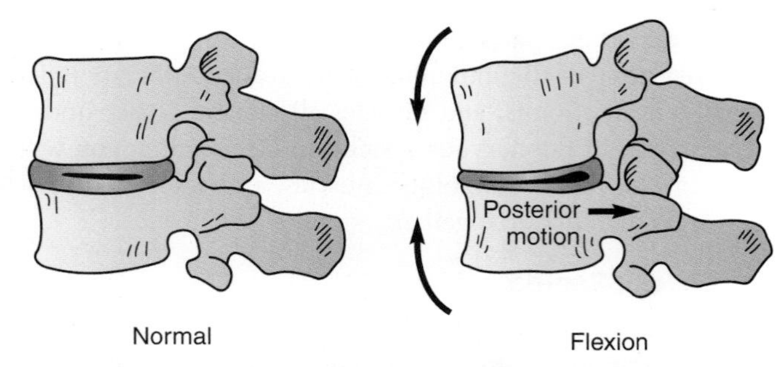

FIG. 10.16 Movement of the spine from a position of extension into flexion causes the nucleus to move in a posterior direction. (Adapted from Shankman GA. *Fundamental Orthopedic Management for the Physical Therapist Assistant*. 3rd ed. Mosby/Elsevier; 2011.)

Thoracic Vertebral Column Region

The thoracic vertebrae are structured to articulate with the ribs, with stability as the main function of this outer unit region. This area does not move extensively, but small movements at the facet joints are ongoing with the breathing process.

A few large extrinsic muscles and numerous small intrinsic muscles are found in this area. *Extrinsic muscles* are defined as muscles that link a limb to the trunk of the body. *Intrinsic muscles* are muscles that are entirely within the body part or segment (inner unit). The largest muscle is the erector spinae (sacrospinalis), which extends on each side of the spinal column from the pelvic region to the cranium.

The erector spinae muscles function best when the pelvis is held up in front, thus pulling them down slightly in the back.

As the spine is held straight and the ribs are raised, the chest raises and consequently makes the abdominal muscles more effective in holding the pelvis up in front and flattening the abdominal wall.

Lumbar Vertebral Column Region

The five lumbar vertebrae are the most massive of the spinal column. These vertebrae carry a large share of the upper body weight, balancing the torso on the sacrum. The combined unit of the vertebrae and disks in the upright position forms the lumbar spinal curve. The lumbar vertebral disks are strong, short, and thick. The ligaments provide stability in all directions. This is the most frequently injured area of the back.

The lumbar vertebral group has less mobility than the cervical region but more than the thoracic region. Because of the absence of ribs and the shape of the spinous processes, the lumbar spine is freer in flexion and extension. Rotation, however, is limited by the amount of tension created in the surrounding ligaments and annulus fibrosis of the disks.

Motions of the lumbar spine include flexion, extension, lateral flexion, and rotation. More motion takes place at L5/S1 (the lumbosacral junction) than at L1/L2.

The angle formed between L5 and S1 is called the *lumbosacral angle*. This angle is approximately 41 degrees in the normal individual. This is typically a neutral position in that no erector spinae force needs to be exerted as a counterbalance. When special conditions exist (e.g., obesity, pregnancy, abdominal muscle weakness, wearing of high heels, foot pronation, and poor posture), this angle increases undesirably, which can lead to lumbar pain and dysfunction (Fig. 10.17).

Abdominal muscles initiate flexion, whereas the erector spinae resists flexion. Intrinsic muscles of the back provide extension, whereas the abdominal muscles (mainly the rectus abdominis) resist. Lateral bending occurs with spinal rotation. Ipsilateral structures tend to relax, whereas contralateral structures resist. Lumbosacral rotation takes place with a variety of complex tension and relaxation patterns. Rotation is limited by the straight, posteriorly oriented spinous processes (Activity 10.1).

Abdominal Region

Abdominal muscles do not extend from bone to bone but attach into tendinous bands and aponeurosis (fascia) around the rectus abdominis area. The abdominal muscles are the rectus abdominis, external oblique, internal oblique, and transversus abdominis.

The rectus abdominis muscle controls the tilt of the pelvis and the consequent curvature of the lower spine. Holding the pelvis up in front makes the erector spinae muscle more effective as an extensor of the spine and makes the hip flexors (e.g., the iliopsoas) more effective.

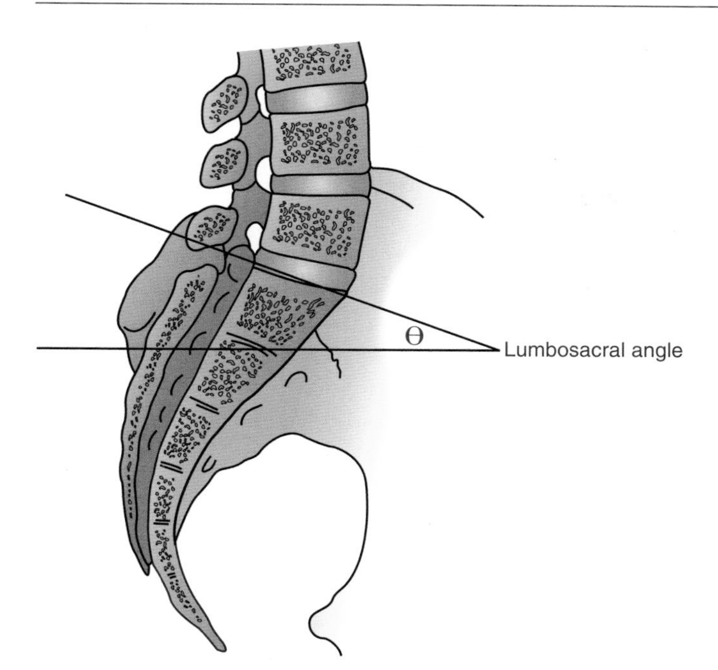

FIG. 10.17 The lumbosacral angle. (Modified from Malone TR, McPoil T, Nitz AJ. *Orthopedic and Sports Physical Therapy*. 3rd ed. Mosby; 1997.)

The internal oblique muscles run diagonally in the direction opposite that of the external oblique muscles. The left internal oblique muscle causes rotation to the left, and the right internal oblique muscle causes rotation to the right. In rotary movements, the internal oblique muscle and the opposite-side external oblique muscle always work together.

The transversus abdominis is the chief muscle of forced expiration. The transversus abdominis and the external oblique and internal oblique muscles are effective in helping to hold the abdomen flat.

Thoracic Region

As discussed in Chapter 7, the skeletal foundation of the thorax is formed by 12 pairs of ribs, the manubrium, the body of the sternum, and the xiphoid process. Breathing is a major function of the thorax. Breathing involves inspiration, or inhaling, and expiration, or exhaling. The primary muscles of inspiration are the diaphragm and the external intercostal muscles.

During quiet respiration, the diaphragm may act alone, or a slight rhythmic activity may occur in the scalenus anterior and scalenus medius and the intercostal muscles. In deep inspiration, the action of the primary muscles increases, and the sternocleidomastoid and scalenes assist in raising the ribs. Forced inspiration involves any muscles that stabilize or elevate the shoulder girdle to elevate the ribs directly or indirectly.

Expiration is primarily passive as relaxation of the prime movers and the weight of gravity pulls the rib cage down. The primary muscles of expiration are the internal intercostal muscles. Forced expiration involves muscles that force the rib cage down (quadratus lumborum) or compress the abdominal cavity (oblique and transverse abdominal muscles), forcing the diaphragm upward.

There are two different types of breathing patterns: diaphragmatic and thoracic. Diaphragmatic, or abdominal, breathing is the natural way to breathe and occurs in infants and sleeping adults. Inhalation deep into the lungs occurs by the contraction of the diaphragm, flattening its dome shape and resulting in negative pressure in the lungs, which fill with air to equalize the pressure. The diaphragm then relaxes, expelling the air by its upward movement. Diaphragmatic breathing is even and relaxed.

Thoracic, or chest, breathing is common in persons with anxiety or other emotional distress. Anxious persons may experience breath holding, hyperventilation syndrome, constricted breathing, shortness of breath, or fear of fainting. Thoracic breathing occurs in persons who wear restrictive clothing, actively hold in their abdominal muscles, or lead sedentary or stressful lives. Chest breathing is often shallow, irregular, and rapid. On inhalation, the chest expands and the shoulders rise to take in air. Dysfunctional patterns can develop if the accessory muscles of respiration (scalenes, sternocleidomastoid, serratus posterior superior, levator scapulae, rhomboid muscles, abdominal muscles, and quadratus lumborum) are used constantly for regular breathing when forced inhalation and expiration are not required.

Shoulder Region

The complicated framework of the shoulder not only is extremely mobile but also provides a secure and stable immovable point for specific actions, such as lifting, thrusting, shoving, and pushing heavy objects. This region consists of the shoulder girdle and the shoulder, or glenohumeral joint.

Shoulder Girdle Region

The shoulder girdle is made up of the scapula and clavicle (which generally move as a unit) and associated soft tissues. The clavicle has two synovial gliding joints. The sternoclavicular joint is medial, and the acromioclavicular joint is lateral. When analyzing scapulothoracic movements, realize that the scapula moves on the rib cage, because the joint motion occurs at the sternoclavicular joint and, to a lesser extent, at the acromioclavicular joint.

The movements of the sternoclavicular joint include elevation, depression, rotation, protraction, and retraction. For full abduction to occur, the clavicle must rotate 50 degrees posteriorly. Movement at the joint occurs indirectly as a result of scapular movement. The characteristics of the joint are influenced indirectly by the movement of the glenohumeral joint. Although no direct muscular attachments cross this joint, several muscles have an indirect influence on the movement, especially the pectoralis major, subclavius, sternocleidomastoid, sternothyroid and sternohyoid, scalenus medius and scalenus posterior, and upper trapezius.

The acromioclavicular joint contributes little to scapular movement because its joint surfaces do not allow much angular movement. A rotary and hingelike motion takes place at this joint, chiefly with elevation of the arm above 90 degrees. The S shape of the clavicle provides extra motion during the elevation of the arm.

ACTIVITY 10.1

In this activity, you will be working with a partner to assess individual movement patterns, normal function, and possible dysfunction in each other. First, one of you should isolate the specified movement patterns on each side of your partner, one side at a time, and assess for normal function by applying a gentle pressure opposite to the action of the isolation position. The body should be stabilized so that only the isolated area is moving. In some instances, the ability to assume the position and maintain it indicates normal function. Muscles should be able to hold against gravity or the applied pressure without strain or pain. The position itself should be easy to assume and comfortable to maintain for a short duration—10 to 30 seconds. The bilateral movement patterns should be the same. The opposite movement pattern also should be easily performed.

Dysfunction may be indicated by bilateral asymmetry, pain, weakness, fatigue, a heavy sensation (binding), and inability to assume the isolation position or move into the opposite position. Intervention or referral depends on the severity of the condition and whether the dysfunction is neuromuscular, myofascial, or joint related.

Note: Do not perform these assessments if contraindications exist. Contraindications to this type of assessment include joint and disk dysfunction, acute pain, recent trauma, and inflammation.

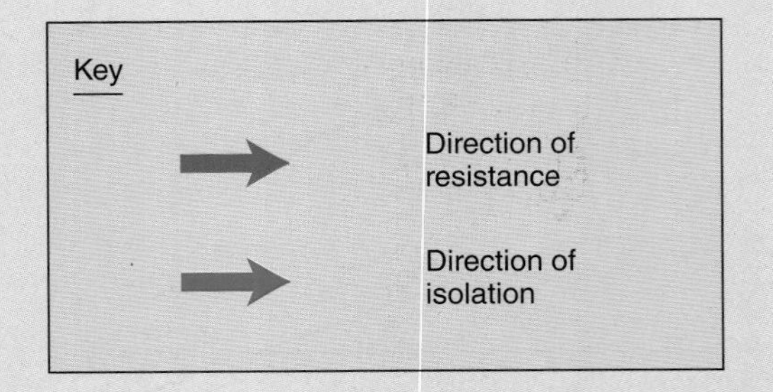

ACTIVITY 10.1—cont'd

Trunk Extension

Assesses for strength and endurance in the isolation position and tension or shortening in the flexion pattern

Muscles Involved

Erector spinae (sacrospinalis) group: Iliocostalis, longissimus, and spinalis
Splenius cervicis and splenius capitis
Semispinalis
Multifidus

Range of Motion

Thoracic spine: No range of motion
Lumbar spine: 0 to 25 degrees

Position of Client

Prone, with hands clasped behind head; client may hold hands behind back.

Isolation and Assessment

The client extends the lumbar spine until the head and chest are raised from the table. The ability to perform tests indicates normal function. No resistance is required.

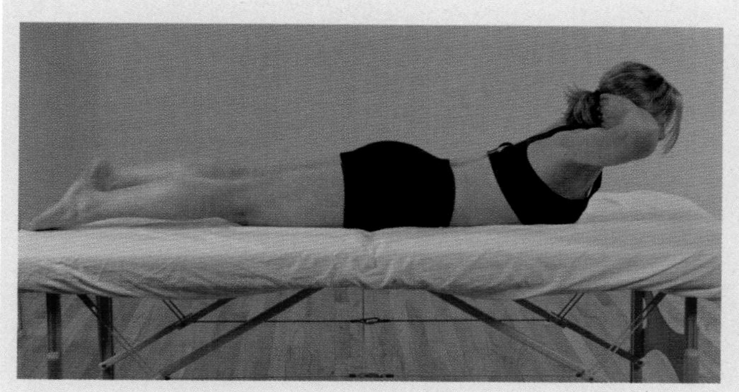

Trunk extension

Trunk Flexion

Assesses for strength and endurance in the isolation position and tension or shortening in the extension pattern

Muscles Involved

Rectus abdominis
Internal and external obliques
Psoas major and psoas minor

Range of Motion

0 to 50 degrees (beyond 50 degrees, any additional flexion comes from pelvic rotation)

Position of the Client

Supine, with hands clasped behind the head or crossed in front and placed on shoulders, knees bent, feet flat

Note: Client is not to lift head with hands.

Isolation and Assessment

Client tucks chin to chest and brings shoulders toward thighs. The ability to clear scapulae from the table indicates good function. No resistance is required.

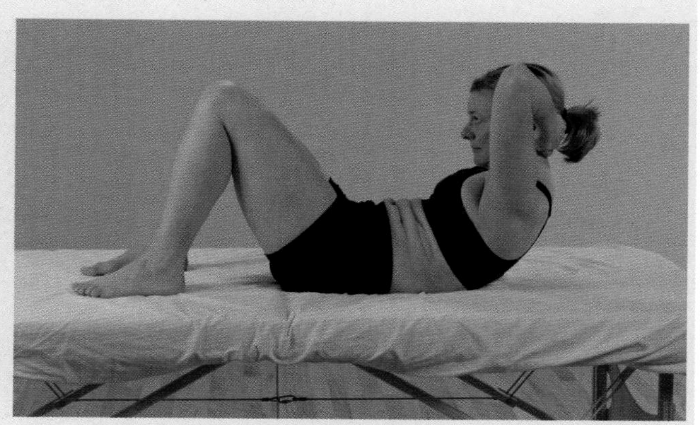

Trunk flexion

Continued

ACTIVITY 10.1—cont'd

Trunk Rotation

Assesses for strength and endurance in the isolation position and tension or shortening in the contralateral pattern

Muscles Involved

External obliques
Internal obliques
Latissimus dorsi
Rectus abdominis
Deep back muscles (unilateral test)

Range of Motion

0 to 45 degrees

Position of Client

Supine, with knees bent and feet flat, hands clasped across the chest or held beside ears

NOTE: Client is not to lift head with hands.

Isolation and Assessment

Client slowly flexes and rotates trunk to one side. After returning to the supine position, movement is repeated on the opposite side. The ability to clear scapulae from the table indicates good function.

Right shoulder to left knee tests the right external obliques and left internal obliques. Left shoulder to right knee tests the left external obliques and right internal obliques.

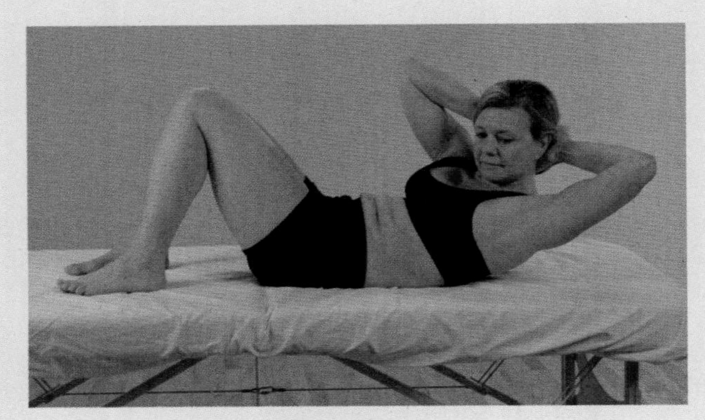

Trunk rotation

Elevation of the Pelvis (More Correctly Known as Lateral Tilt)

Assesses for strength and endurance in the isolation position and tension or shortening in the contralateral pattern

Muscles Involved

Quadratus lumborum
Latissimus dorsi
Internal abdominal obliques
Iliocostalis lumborum

Range of Motion

Not applicable

Position of Client

Prone with hip and lumbar spine in extension, hip slightly abducted, feet off the end of table; the client grasps the edges of the table to provide stabilization during resistance.

Isolation and Assessment

Client brings iliac crest toward ribs on one side while examiner applies resistance to lower leg to pull hip down.

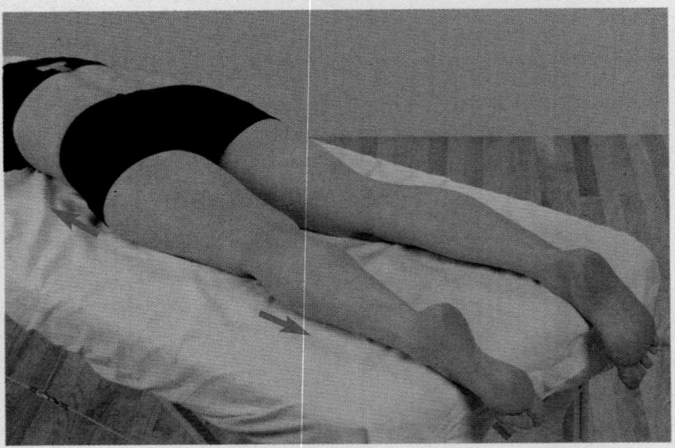

Elevation of the pelvis, lateral tilt

ACTIVITY 10.1—cont'd

Capital Extension

Assesses for strength and endurance in the isolation position and tension or shortening in the flexion pattern

Muscles Involved

Rectus capitis posterior major
Rectus capitis posterior minor
Longissimus capitis
Obliquus capitis superior
Obliquus capitis inferior
Splenius capitis
Semispinalis capitis

Range of Motion

0 to 25 degrees

Position of Client

Prone with the head off the end of the table, arms at the sides

NOTE: Do not do this test if the client has cervical disk problems.

Isolation and Assessment

Client lifts chin away from the chest as if beginning to nod "yes." The cervical spine is not extended. The examiner applies resistance to the back of the head.

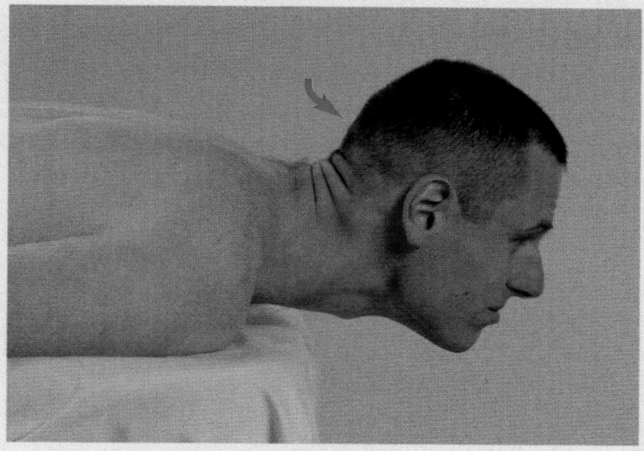

Capital extension

Capital Flexion

Assesses for strength and endurance in the isolation position and tension or shortening in the extension pattern

Muscles Involved

Rectus longus
Capitis anterior

Range of Motion

0 to 10 or 15 degrees

Position of Client

Supine

NOTE: Do not do this test if the client has cervical disk problems.

Isolation and Assessment

Client tucks chin into the neck as if nodding "yes." Head remains on the table. No motion should occur at the cervical spine. No resistance is required.

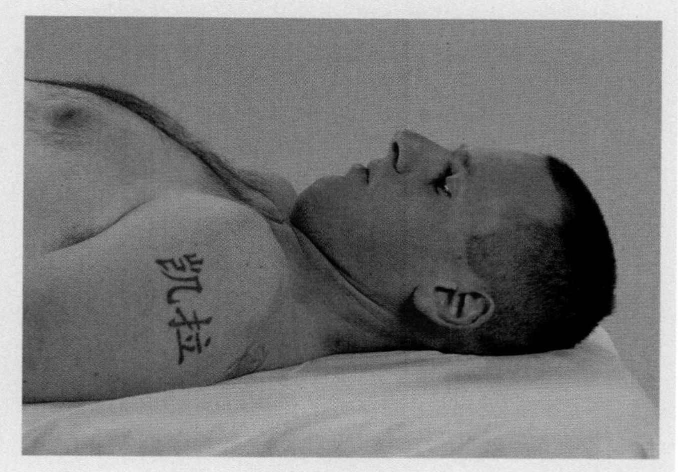

Capital flexion

Continued

ACTIVITY 10.1—cont'd

Cervical Extension
Assesses for strength and endurance in the isolation position and tension or shortening in the flexion pattern

Muscles Involved
Longissimus cervicis
Semispinalis cervicis
Iliocostalis cervicis
Splenius capitis and splenius cervicis

Range of Motion
0 to 25 degrees

Position of Client
Prone, with the head off the end of the table, arms along the sides

Note: Do not do this test if client has cervical disk problems.

Isolation and Assessment
Client extends neck by lifting head toward the ceiling. No resistance is required. The ability to hold the head up against gravity indicates normal function.

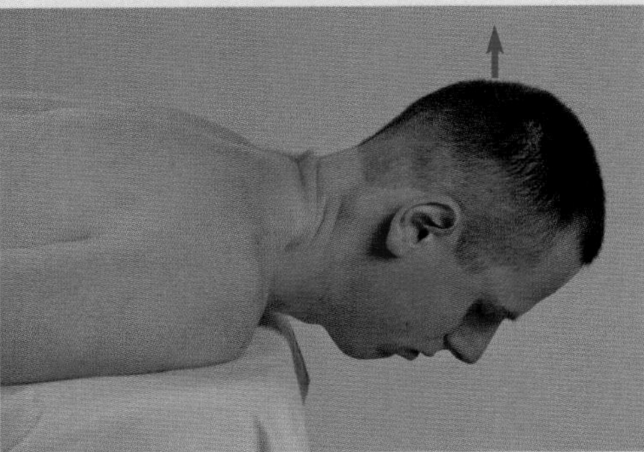
Cervical extension

Cervical Flexion
Assesses for strength and endurance in the isolation position and tension or shortening in the extension pattern

Muscles Involved
Scalenus anterior, scalenus medius, and scalenus posterior
Sternocleidomastoid
Longus colli

Range of Motion
0 to 35 or 45 degrees

Note: Women usually have greater cervical lordosis than men, so they likely could have a greater arc of motion.

Position of Client
Supine, with arms at the sides and head supported on the table

Note: Do not do this test if client has cervical disk problems.

Isolation and Assessment
Client lifts head off the table and tucks chin. This is a weak muscle group, so no resistance is required.

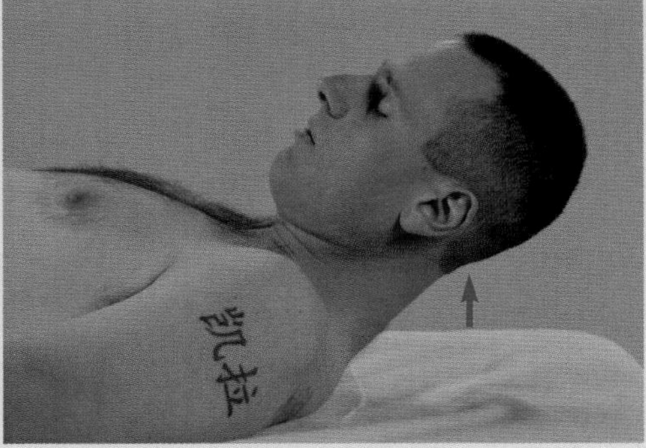

Cervical flexion

Cervical Rotation
Assesses for strength and endurance in the isolation position and tension or shortening in the contralateral pattern

Muscles Involved
Sternocleidomastoid
Rectus capitis posterior major
Obliquus capitis inferior
Longissimus capitis

Range of Motion
0 to 45 or 55 degrees
Two separate actions will be tested.

Position of Client
Supine
Begin with the head supported on the table and turn to one side.

Isolation and Assessment
Client lifts head off the table without any additional rotation, returns to the start position, and repeats on the other side. No resistance is required.

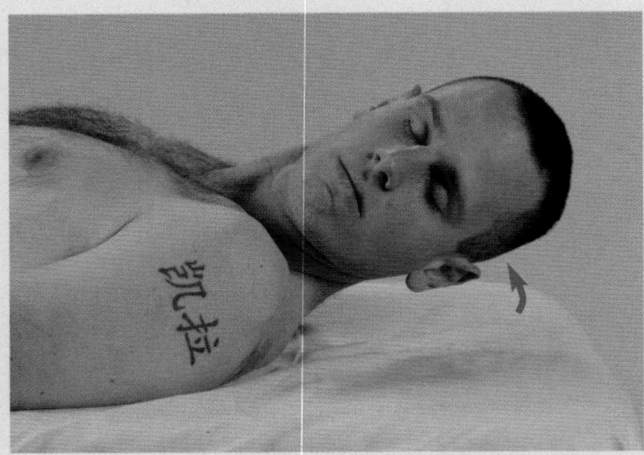

Cervical rotation 1

Position of Client
Supine, with cervical spine in neutral flexion and extension
Begin with the head supported on the table and turned to one side.

Isolation and Assessment
Client rotates the head to neutral (nose facing the ceiling) against resistance. Make sure the client does not lift the head off the table. Repeat on the opposite side.

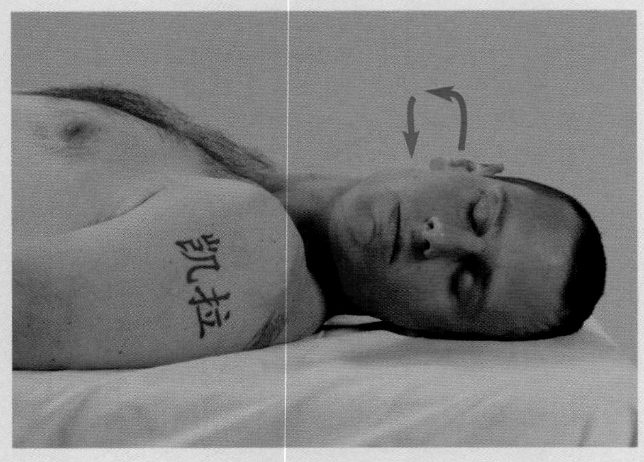

Cervical rotation 2

The scapulae rotate at the acromioclavicular joint at the beginning of the scapular movement. Of the approximately 60 degrees that scapular movement contributes to the elevation of the arm, about 30 degrees occurs at the sternoclavicular joint and the remaining 30 degrees occurs from the combined effects of clavicular rotation, which causes the clavicular joint surfaces to face upward, and the acromioclavicular movement that occurs at the acromioclavicular joint.

The acromioclavicular joint allows the widening and narrowing of the angle between the clavicle and the scapula (from above). Narrowing occurs during protraction; widening occurs during retraction. The joint also allows for rotation of the scapula upward when the inferior angle moves away from the midline, and it allows for rotation of the scapula downward when the inferior angle moves toward the midline. The acromioclavicular joint also allows rotation of the scapula in such a way that the inferior angle swings anteriorly and posteriorly. Although no muscles directly cause movements of the acromioclavicular joint, the deltoid, upper trapezius, and subclavius muscles indirectly affect it.

The subacromial space is located between the top of the arm bone (humerus) and a bony prominence on the shoulder blade (acromion). The coracoacromial ligament completes the arch. It contains the belly and tendon of the supraspinatus muscle, as well as the long head of the biceps. Conditions range from subacromial bursitis to rotator cuff tendinopathy, and full-thickness rotator cuff tears. The bursa allows the rotator cuff tendons to glide freely when you move your arm.

Glenohumeral Joint

The shoulder, or glenohumeral joint, includes the scapula, humerus, and associated soft tissues. The only attachment of the shoulder joint to the axial skeleton is the clavicle at the sternoclavicular joint.

The glenohumeral joint is a ball-and-socket joint and is the articulation between the glenoid fossa of the scapula and the head of the humerus. Movements of the shoulder joint are many and varied. This mobile joint allows adduction, abduction, flexion, extension, hyperextension, horizontal adduction and abduction, and lateral and medial rotation of the humerus in all planes: sagittal, frontal, and transverse.

Movement of the humerus without scapular movement is unusual. Much of the movement of the scapula is related to movement at the glenohumeral joint. Flexion and abduction of the humerus elevates and abducts the scapula with upward rotation. Adduction and extension of the humerus results in depression, rotation downward, and adduction of the scapula. The scapula is abducted with humeral internal rotation and horizontal adduction. Scapular adduction accompanies external rotation and horizontal abduction of the humerus.

Because the shoulder joint has such a wide range of motion in so many different planes, it also has a certain amount of laxity, which often results in instability, such as rotator cuff impingement and dislocations. Often the price of mobility is instability. The concept that the more mobile a joint is, the less stable it is, and that the more stable it is, the less mobile it is, applies generally throughout the body but especially in the shoulder joint.

An important, protective fibro-osseous arch over the glenohumeral arch is formed by the coracoacromial ligament, together with the acromion (or the lateral end of the clavicle articulating directly with the acromion and indirectly with the coracoid process through the coracoclavicular ligaments) and coracoid process. This arch forms a secondary restraining socket for the humeral head, preventing superior dislocation or displacement.

At the brim of the glenoid fossa is a fibrocartilaginous ring called the *glenoid labrum* that adds stability and substance to this shallow and mobile articulation.

The glenoid labrum merges with several ligaments and tendons to form the joint capsule of the glenohumeral joint. Tendons that connect at this joint are from the muscles of the subscapularis, infraspinatus, teres minor, and supraspinatus, also known as *SITS*, or rotator cuff muscles, because they contribute to the rotation of the humerus. In reality, numerous muscles and tendons intersect the glenohumeral joint, and because of their attachment points, they contribute to the stability of the joint through their tension lines of pull. The deltoid forms a hood over the small muscles that closely surround the joint and acts as a shock absorber to protect the joint from impact.

The deep fascia covering the deltoid, known as the *deltoid aponeurosis*, is a fibrous layer that covers the outer surface of the muscle. The deep fascia is thick and strong behind, where it is continuous with the infraspinatus fascia and thinner over the rest of the muscle. In front, the deltoid aponeurosis is continuous with the fascia covering the pectoralis major. Above, the deltoid aponeurosis is attached to the clavicle, the acromion, and the spine of the scapula; below, it is continuous with the deep fascia of the arm. This extensive fascial network provides dynamic stability.

Scapulothoracic Junction

The scapulothoracic junction meets the criteria of a joint in that it allows the scapula to glide over the ribs and is separated by muscle, fascia, and bursae. The junction is not a true synovial joint because it does not have regular synovial features and its movement depends totally on the sternoclavicular and acromioclavicular joints. Even though scapular movement occurs as a result of motion at the sternoclavicular and acromioclavicular joints, the scapula can be described as having a total range of 25 degrees of abduction-adduction, 60 degrees of upward-downward rotation, and 55 degrees of elevation-depression. A large subscapular bursal sheet and fat pad enhance the gliding of this junction.

In analyzing shoulder girdle movements, focusing on a specific bony landmark, such as the inferior angle (posteriorly), glenoid fossa (laterally), and acromion process (anteriorly), often is helpful. All the following movements have their pivotal point where the clavicle joins the sternum at the sternoclavicular joint. Movements of the shoulder girdle can be described as movements of the scapula.

Movements of the Scapula

The following movements involve the scapula:

- *Abduction (protraction):* Movement of the scapula laterally away from the spinal column

- *Adduction (retraction):* Movement of the scapula medially toward the spinal column
- *Upward rotation:* Turning the glenoid fossa upward and moving the inferior angle superiorly and laterally away from the spinal column
- *Downward rotation:* Returning the inferior angle medially and inferiorly toward the spinal column and the glenoid fossa to its normal position
- *Elevation:* Upward or superior movement, as in shrugging the shoulders
- *Depression:* Downward or inferior movement, as in returning to normal position

Movements of the Glenohumeral Joint

The glenohumeral joint allows the following movements:

- *Abduction:* Lateral movement of the humerus out to the side and away from the body
- *Adduction:* Movement of the humerus medially toward the body from abduction
- *Flexion:* Movement of the humerus anteriorly
- *Extension:* Movement of the humerus posteriorly
- *Horizontal adduction (flexion):* Movement of the humerus in a horizontal or transverse plane toward and across the chest
- *Horizontal abduction (extension):* Movement of the humerus in a horizontal or transverse plane away from the chest
- *External rotation:* Movement of the humerus laterally around its long axis away from the midline
- *Internal rotation:* Movement of the humerus medially around its long axis toward the midline
- The shoulder joint and shoulder girdle work together in carrying out upper extremity activities. Table 10.1 shows a pairing of shoulder girdle and shoulder joint movements.

Table 10.1 Shoulder Joint

Shoulder Joint	Shoulder Girdle
Abduction	Upward rotation
Adduction	Downward rotation
Flexion	Elevation, upward rotation, protraction
Extension	Depression, downward rotation, retraction
Internal rotation	Abduction (protraction)
External rotation	Adduction (retraction)
Horizontal abduction	Adduction (retraction)
Horizontal adduction	Abduction (protraction)

Shoulder Girdle Muscles

Five muscles are involved primarily in the shoulder girdle: trapezius, levator scapulae, rhomboid muscles, serratus anterior, and pectoralis minor. Grouping the muscles of the shoulder girdle separately from the shoulder joint is helpful to avoid confusion. All five shoulder girdle muscles have their proximal attachment on the axial skeleton, with their distal attachment located on the scapula or clavicle. Shoulder girdle muscles do not attach to the humerus, nor do they cause actions of the shoulder joint. The shoulder girdle muscles are essential in providing dynamic stability of the scapula so that it can serve as a base of support for shoulder joint activities. The trapezius and serratus anterior muscles upwardly rotate and are important stabilizers. The lower fibers of the trapezius muscle stabilize each scapula to prevent unwanted protraction caused by the serratus anterior and pectoralis minor.

The trapezius muscle fixates the scapula for deltoid action by preventing the glenoid fossa from being pulled down when the arms lift objects. The muscle is used strenuously when lifting with the hands, as in picking up a heavy wheelbarrow. The trapezius must prevent the scapula from being pulled downward, such as when an object is held overhead or a person is carrying an object that is resting on the tip of the shoulder.

Shrugging the shoulder calls the levator scapulae muscle into play, along with the upper trapezius muscle.

The rhomboids fix the scapula in adduction/retraction when the muscles of the shoulder joint adduct or extend the arm. The trapezius and rhomboid muscles work together to produce adduction, with slight elevation of the scapula. To prevent this elevation, the latissimus dorsi muscle is called into play. The serratus anterior muscle acts in movements drawing the scapula forward with slight upward rotation and works along with the pectoralis major muscle in actions such as throwing a baseball. A winged scapula condition indicates a definite weakness of the serratus anterior.

The pectoralis minor muscle is used, along with the serratus anterior muscle, in true abduction (protraction) without rotation. When true abduction of the scapula is necessary, the serratus anterior draws the scapula forward with a slight upward rotation and the pectoralis minor pulls forward with a slight downward rotation. The two pulling together give true abduction. These muscles work together in most movements of pushing with the hands.

Most of the scapular action involves force couples. A force couple occurs when two or more muscles pull in different directions to accomplish the same action (Fig. 10.18). During assessment and massage application all structures involved in force couples must be addressed.

Glenohumeral Joint Muscles

Muscles of the glenohumeral joint contribute to more than one action when the humerus is in a sequence of movement. The muscles involved in flexion of the shoulder and glenohumeral joint cross the joint anteriorly. The primary flexors are the pectoralis major, anterior deltoid, and coracobrachialis. Synergists to flexion are the biceps brachii.

In an extension of the glenohumeral joint, when movement meets no resistance, gravity is the prime mover, with the flexor muscles eccentrically contracting to control the action of extension. When resistance occurs, the posterior muscles of the glenohumeral joint go to work, specifically the teres major, latissimus dorsi, and sternocostal pectoralis. Synergists for extension are the posterior deltoid, particularly when the humerus is rotated externally, and the triceps brachii (long head) when the elbow is flexed or fully extended.

Two primary movers are involved in the abduction of the glenohumeral joint: the middle deltoid and supraspinatus. Both muscles intersect the shoulder superior to the glenohumeral joint. The supraspinatus begins the movement of abduction for approximately the first 15 to 30 degrees. The middle deltoid is

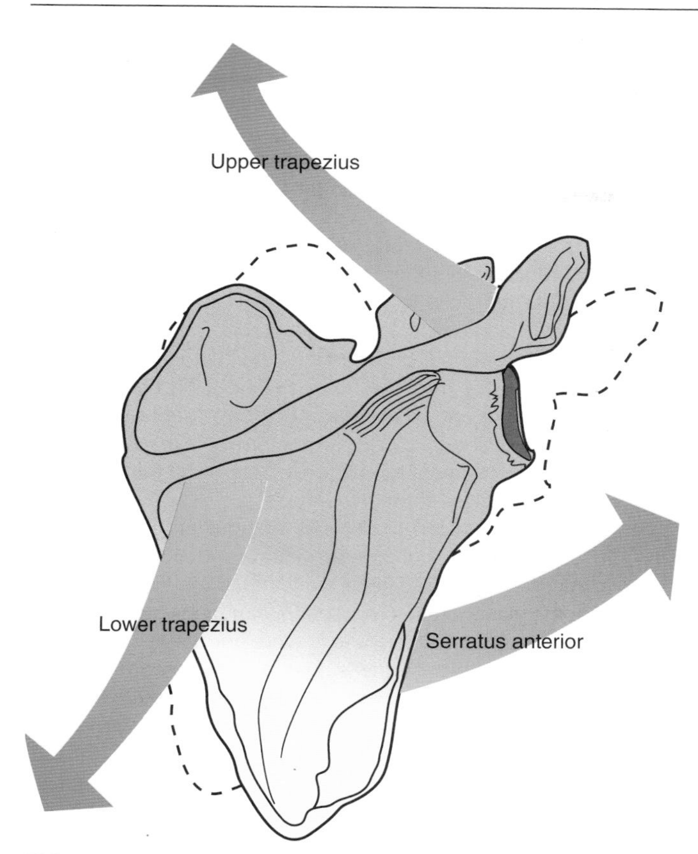

FIG. 10.18 The upper trapezius, lower trapezius, and serratus anterior pull in three different directions to achieve one type of motion—upward rotation of the scapula. This is called a *force couple*.

active up to 90 degrees. Past 90 degrees, the scapula needs to rotate to achieve up to 180 degrees of abduction. To counteract superior dislocation, the infraspinatus, subscapularis, and teres major shorten to control the action of the middle deltoid.

Adduction of the glenohumeral joint is another movement in which, if no resistance occurs, gravity is the prime mover, with the abductors as the antagonists controlling the speed of the motion. With resistance, the principal adductors are the latissimus dorsi, teres major, and pectoralis major sternal, all positioned inferior to the glenohumeral joint. The synergists are the biceps (short head) and triceps (long head).

Medial rotation of the humerus results from the subscapularis and teres major as the prime movers. Both attach to the anterior aspect of the humerus. Synergists to medial rotation are the pectoralis major, anterior deltoid, latissimus dorsi, and biceps brachii (short head).

Muscles attaching to the posterior aspect of the humerus generate the lateral rotation, specifically the infraspinatus and teres minor.

Horizontal adduction results from the actions of anterior muscles, which include the anterior deltoid, pectoralis major, and coracobrachialis.

Horizontal abduction is affected by the middle and posterior deltoid, infraspinatus, and teres minor, muscles located on the posterior aspect of the joint. The synergists to horizontal abduction are the teres major and latissimus dorsi (Activity 10.2).

A modified force couple functions at the glenohumeral joint because the two forces involved are not opposite to one another. Instead, the deltoid produces a superior force, while the subscapularis and infraspinatus/teres minor produce a compressive and inferior force. The combined compressive forces of the subscapularis and infraspinatus/teres minor pull the head of the humerus into the glenoid fossa, counteracting the superior shear force of the deltoid muscle.

Elbow Region

The elbow is considered a stable joint with firm osseous support and is composed of three articulations: the humeroulnar joint, humeroradial joint, and radioulnar joint. The elbow is a uniaxial hinge joint that moves in only one plane along a single axis. The action of the elbow is flexion/extension. The elbow is capable of moving from 0 degrees of extension to approximately 145 to 150 degrees of flexion.

After the elbow flexes beyond 20 degrees, its bony stability is somewhat unlocked, allowing for more side-to-side laxity. In flexion, the stability of the elbow depends on the lateral or radial collateral ligament, with most of the work done by the medial or ulnar collateral ligament.

The radioulnar joint is classified as a trochoid or pivot-type joint. The radial head rotates around its location at the proximal ulna. This rotary movement is accompanied by the distal radius rotating around the distal ulna. The radial head is maintained in its joint by the annular ligament. The radioulnar joint can supinate approximately 80 to 90 degrees from the neutral position. Pronation varies from 70 to 90 degrees.

Practically any movement of the upper extremity involves the elbow and radioulnar joints. Often these joints are grouped because of their close anatomic relationship. The radioulnar joint motion may be attributed incorrectly to the wrist joint because it appears to occur there. However, with close inspection, the elbow joint and its movements may be distinguished clearly from those of the radioulnar joints, just as the radioulnar movements may be distinguished from those of the wrist.

When the arm is in an anatomically extended position, the longitudinal axes of the upper arm and forearm form a valgus angle at the elbow joint known as the *carrying angle*; this angle approximates 5 degrees in males and between 10 and 15 degrees in females. Anatomically, the carrying angle is designed to fit closely into the waist depressions immediately superior to the iliac crest. The carrying angles should be bilaterally symmetric.

The olecranon fossa of the humerus, which receives the olecranon of the ulna during extension, is filled with fat and covered by a portion of the triceps muscle and aponeurosis.

The cubital fossa is defined by the brachioradialis laterally and the pronator teres medially, with the biceps tendon, brachial artery, and median and musculocutaneous nerves passing through this area. The biceps tendon is a taut, long structure that is medial to the brachioradialis muscle, and the pulse of the brachial artery can be palpated medial to the biceps tendon.

Movements of the Elbow

The elbow allows the following movements

- *Flexion:* Movement of the forearm to the shoulder by bending the elbow to decrease its angle

ACTIVITY 10.2

In this activity, you will be working with a partner to assess individual movement patterns, normal function, and possible dysfunction in each other. First, one of you should isolate the specified movement patterns on each side of your partner, one side at a time, and assess for normal function by applying a gentle pressure opposite the action of the isolation position. The body should be stabilized so that only the isolated area is moving. In some instances, the ability to assume the position and maintain it indicates normal function. Muscles should be able to hold against gravity or the applied pressure without strain or pain. The position itself should be easy to assume and comfortable to maintain for a short duration—10 to 30 seconds. The bilateral movement patterns should be the same. The opposite movement pattern also should be able to be done easily.

Dysfunction may be indicated by bilateral asymmetry, pain, weakness, fatigue, a heavy sensation (binding), and the inability to assume the isolation position or move into the opposite position. Intervention or referral depends on the severity of the condition and whether the dysfunction is neuromuscular, myofascial, or joint related.

Note: Do not perform these assessments if contraindications exist. Contraindications to this type of assessment include joint and disk dysfunction, acute pain, recent trauma, and inflammation.

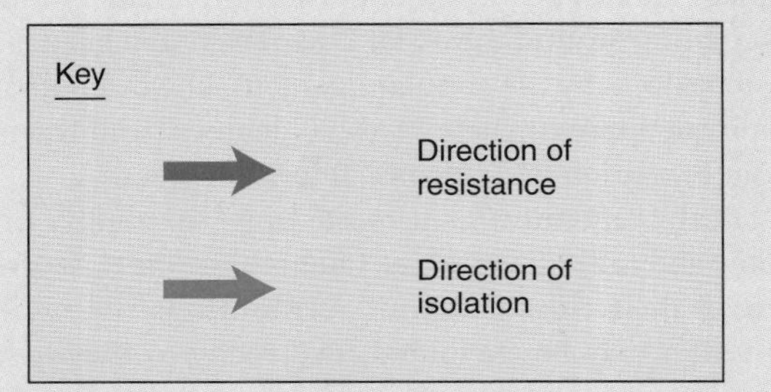

Before starting scapular motion assessments, do a visual assessment of your partner to check for variations in position and symmetry. Asymmetry often shows as one shoulder or scapula that is higher, especially in those who carry briefcases, purses, or babies on one side.

Working with your partner, determine the position of the scapulae at rest and whether the two sides are symmetric. The normal scapula lies close to the rib cage with the vertebral border nearly parallel and 1 to 3 inches lateral to the spinous processes. The inferior angle is tucked in. If the inferior angle of the scapula is tilted away from the rib cage, check for tightness of the pectoralis minor and weakness of the lower trapezius.

The most prominent abnormal posture of the scapula is "winging," in which the vertebral border tilts away from the rib cage, a sign of serratus anterior weakness.

Within the total arc of 180 degrees of shoulder forward flexion, 120 degrees is glenohumeral motion and 60 degrees is scapular motion. Because these movements are not isolated, saying that the glenohumeral and scapular motions coexist after 60 degrees and up to 150 degrees is more correct.

Passively raise your partner's test arm in forward flexion completely above his or her head to determine scapular mobility. The scapula should start to rotate at about 60 degrees, although considerable individual variation exists.

Check that the scapula remains in its rest position at ranges of shoulder flexion less than 60 degrees, with some variation among individuals. If the scapula moves as the glenohumeral joint moves below 60 degrees (i.e., within this range, they move as a unit), limited glenohumeral motion is evident, but the scapula may move through a complete or even excessive range.

From greater than 60 degrees to about 150 or 160 degrees in active and passive motion, the scapula moves in concert with the humerus.

ACTIVITY 10.2—cont'd

Scapular Abduction (Protraction)

Assesses for strength and endurance in the isolation position and tension or shortening in the scapular adduction pattern

Muscles Involved

Serratus anterior
Pectoralis minor

Range of Motion

0 to 15 degrees

Position of Client

Seated, with legs over the end or side of the table, and hands at the sides on top of the table

Isolation and Assessment

Client flexes the straight arm to approximately 130 degrees and reaches forward to protract the scapula. The examiner palpates the medial border of the scapula and applies resistance to the arm.

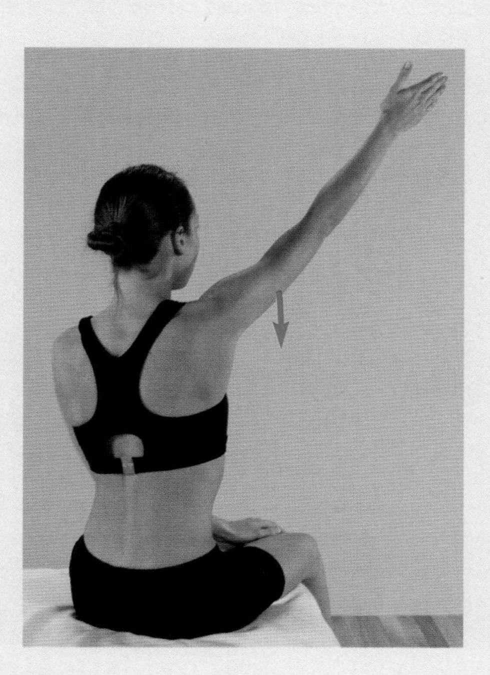

Scapular Adduction (Retraction)

Assesses for strength and endurance in the isolation position and tension or shortening in the scapular abduction pattern

Muscles Involved

Trapezius (middle fibers)
Rhomboideus major and rhomboideus minor
Latissimus dorsi

Range of Motion

0 to 20 degrees

Position of Client

Seated with legs over the edge of the table
Shoulder abducted to 90 degrees and externally rotated
Elbow flexed to a right angle and held at shoulder level

Isolation and Assessment

Client horizontally abducts the arm to adduct the scapula while the examiner applies resistance to the posterior arm above the elbow to push the arm into horizontal adduction.

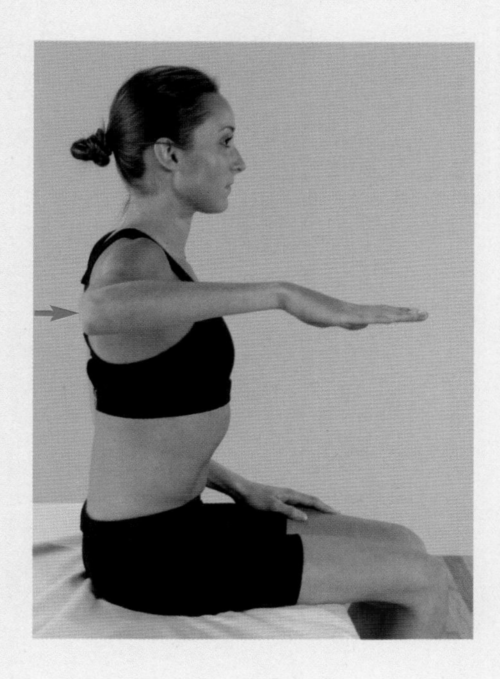

Continued

ACTIVITY 10.2—cont'd

Scapular Elevation

Assesses for strength and endurance in the isolation position and tension or shortening in the scapular depression pattern

Muscles Involved

Trapezius (upper fibers)
Levator scapulae
Rhomboideus major and rhomboideus minor

Range of Motion

0 to 40 degrees

Position of Client

Seated, with legs over the side of the table and arms relaxed

Isolation and Assessment

Client lifts shoulders toward ears, as in shrugging, while examiner applies resistance to push the shoulders down.

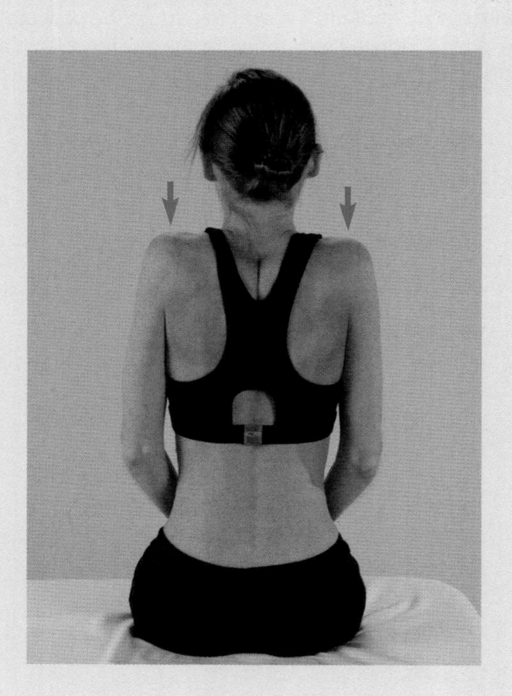

Scapular Upward Rotation With Abduction

Assesses for strength and endurance in the isolation position and tension or shortening in the scapular downward rotation pattern

Muscles Involved

Upper and lower trapezius
Anterior serratus
Pectoralis minor

Range of Motion

Reliable values are not available.

Position of Client

Seated, with legs over the side of the table, arms resting at the sides

Isolation and Assessment

Client flexes shoulder forward to 120 degrees with no rotation or horizontal movement while examiner applies resistance to arm just above the elbow to push it down.

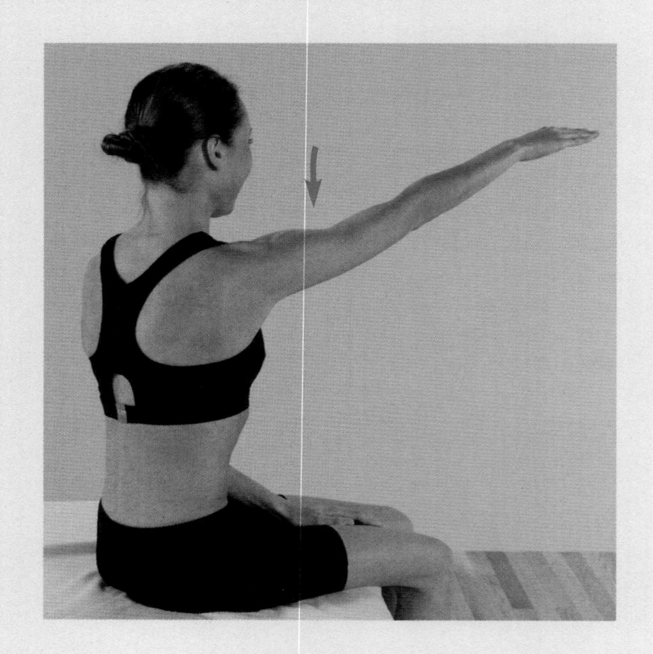

ACTIVITY 10.2—cont'd

Scapular Depression With Adduction and Downward Rotation

Assesses for strength and endurance in the isolation position and tension or shortening in the scapular elevation and upward rotation pattern

Muscles Involved

Lower trapezius
Lower anterior serratus
Levator scapula
Rhomboideus major and rhomboideus minor
Latissimus dorsi

Range of Motion

Reliable values are not available.

Position of Client

Prone
Head may be turned to either side for comfort.
Internally rotate shoulder, flex elbow, and adduct arm across back.
Hand rests on the lower back near the waist.

Isolation and Assessment

Client further adducts the arm by attempting to touch the opposite side. Examiner applies resistance to the medial side of the upper arm to pull it away from the body.

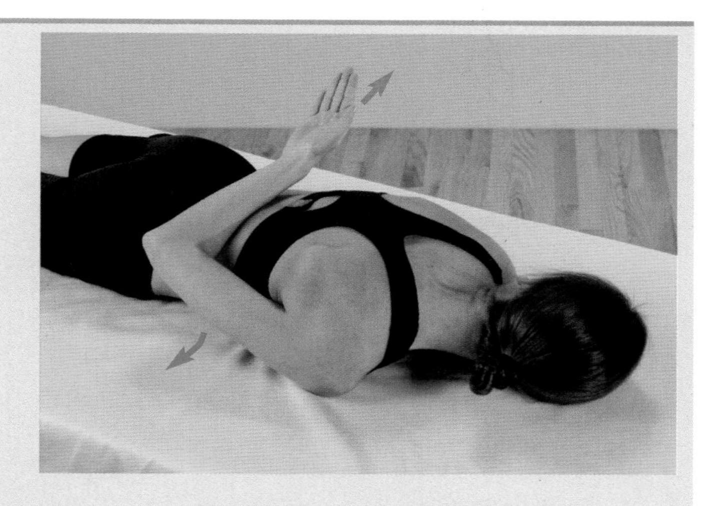

Continued

ACTIVITY 10.2—cont'd

Shoulder Flexion

Assesses for strength and endurance in the isolation position and tension or shortening in the shoulder extension and adduction pattern

Muscles Involved

Deltoid (anterior and middle)
Supraspinatus
Pectoralis major (upper)
Coracobrachialis
Biceps brachii
Subscapularis

Range of Motion

0 to 180 degrees (including scapular movement)

Position of Client

Seated with knees bent off the table, arms at sides, elbows slightly flexed, and forearm pronated

Isolation and Assessment

Client flexes shoulder to 90 degrees without rotation or horizontal movement while examiner applies resistance to upper arm above elbow to push arm down.

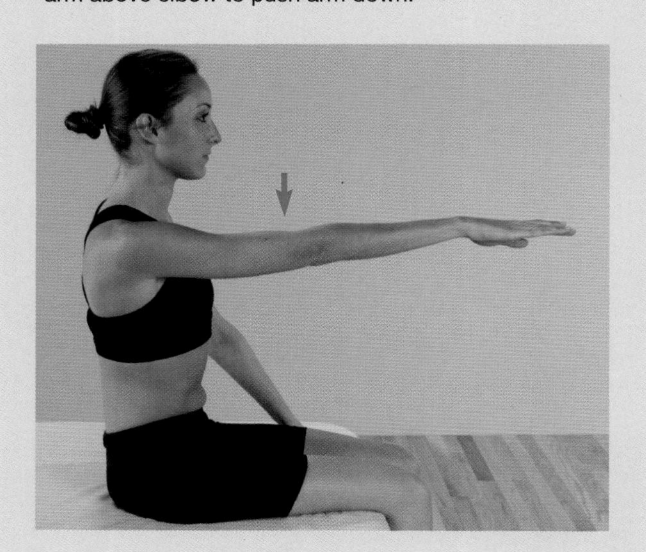

Shoulder Extension

Assesses for strength and endurance in the isolation position and tension or shortening in the shoulder flexion pattern

Muscles Involved

Latissimus dorsi
Deltoid (posterior)
Teres major
Triceps brachii (long head)

Range of Motion

0 to 45 degrees

Position of Client

Prone, with arms at sides and shoulder internally rotated (palm up)
Elbow remains extended throughout isolation

Isolation and Assessment

Client lifts arm off the table and holds while examiner applies resistance to the posterior arm above elbow to push it down.

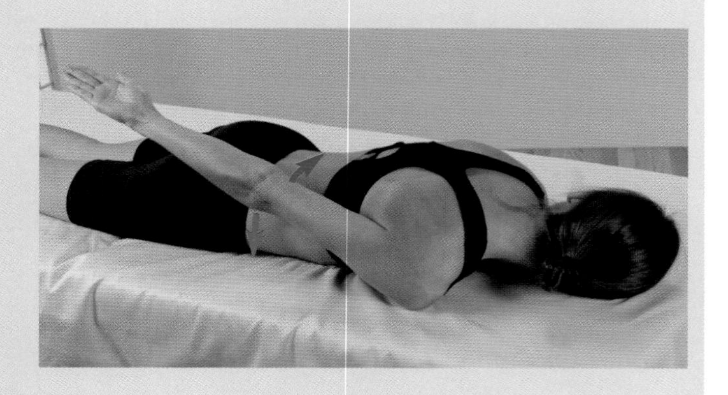

ACTIVITY 10.2—cont'd

Shoulder Horizontal Abduction

Assesses for strength and endurance in the isolation position and tension or shortening in the shoulder horizontal adduction pattern

Muscles Involved

Deltoid (posterior fibers)
Infraspinatus
Teres minor

Range of Motion

0 to 90 degrees (beginning at 90 degrees flexion)

Position of Client

Prone with shoulder abducted to 90 degrees, elbow flexed, upper arm supported on table, and forearm off the edge of the table.

Isolation and Assessment

Client horizontally (posteriorly) abducts shoulder (lifts elbow toward the ceiling) while examiner applies resistance to the posterior arm above elbow to push the arm down.

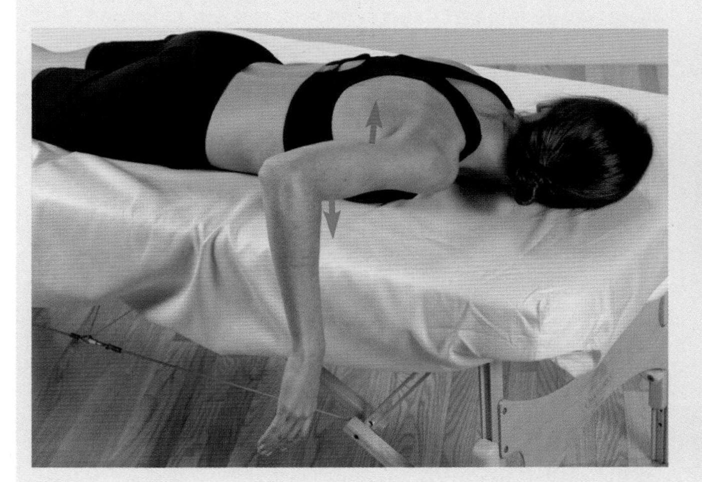

Shoulder Horizontal Adduction

Assesses for strength and endurance in the isolation position and tension or shortening in the shoulder horizontal abduction pattern

Muscles Involved

Pectoralis major
Deltoid (anterior fibers)

Range of Motion

0 to 40 degrees when starting from a position of 90 degrees of forward flexion

Position of Client

Supine

Shoulder abducted to 90 degrees, upper arm supported on a table, and elbow flexed to 90 degrees

Isolation and Assessment

Client horizontally adducts arm to move it across the chest while examiner applies resistance to the medial side of the upper arm above the elbow to push it down.

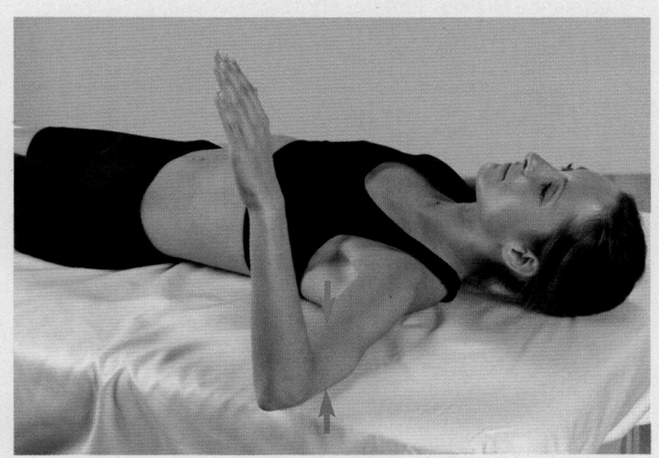

Continued

ACTIVITY 10.2—cont'd

Shoulder External or Lateral Rotation

Assesses for strength and endurance in the isolation position and tension or shortening in the shoulder internal or medial rotation pattern

Muscles Involved

Infraspinatus
Teres minor
Deltoid (posterior)

Range of Motion

0 to 90 degrees

Position of Client

Prone, with head turned toward the test side

Shoulder is abducted to 90 degrees with upper arm fully supported on a table, elbow flexed, and forearm hanging over the edge of the table

Isolation and Assessment

Client moves forearm upward toward the level of the table, keeping an upper arm on the table, while examiner applies resistance to distal forearm above the wrist to push it down.

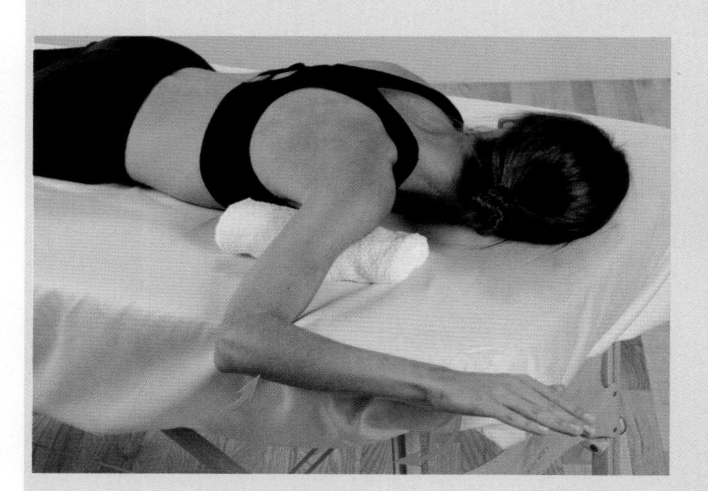

Shoulder Internal or Medial Rotation

Assesses for strength and endurance in the isolation position and tension or shortening in the shoulder external or lateral rotation pattern

Muscles Involved

Subscapularis
Pectoralis major
Latissimus dorsi
Teres major
Deltoid (anterior)

Range of Motion

0 to 80 degrees

Position of Client

Prone with shoulder abducted to 90 degrees, upper arm supported on a table, elbow flexed, and forearm hanging over the edge of the table.

Examiner stabilizes upper arm

Isolation and Assessment

Client moves forearm through internal rotation (backward and upward) while examiner applies resistance to forearm above the wrist to push it down.

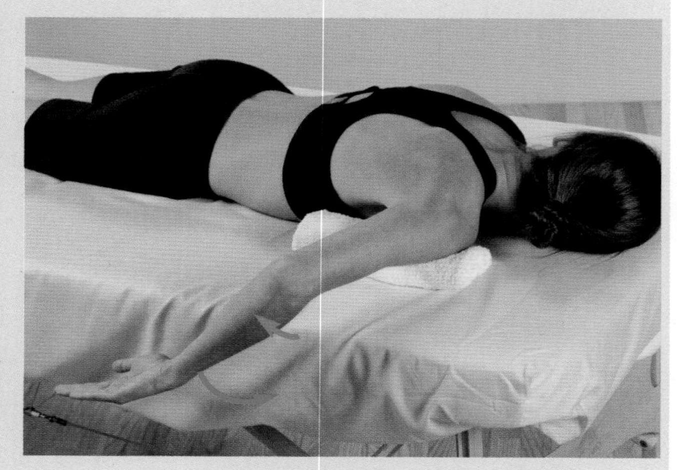

- *Extension:* Movement of the forearm away from the shoulder by straightening the elbow to increase its angle
- *Pronation:* Internal rotary movement of the radius on the ulna that results in the hand moving from the palm-up to the palm-down position
- *Supination:* External rotary movement of the radius on the ulna that results in the hand moving from the palm-down to the palm-up position

Elbow Muscles

The elbow flexors are the biceps brachii, brachialis, and brachioradialis. The triceps brachii is the primary elbow extensor, assisted by the anconeus. The pronator group consists of the pronator teres, pronator quadratus, and brachioradialis. The brachioradialis also assists with supination, which is controlled mainly by the supinator muscle and the biceps brachii.

Wrist and Hand Region

The joints of the wrist, hand, and fingers often are taken for granted, even though the fine motor characteristics of this area are essential in skilled activities requiring precise functioning of the wrist and hand. Anatomically and structurally, the human wrist and hand have highly developed, complex mechanisms capable of a variety of movements. The amazing diversity of motion results from the arrangement of the 29 bones, more than 25 joints, and more than 30 muscles (of which 15 are intrinsic muscles with proximal attachment and distal attachment found inside the hand). This complexity may be simplified by relating the functional anatomy to the major actions of the joints: flexion, extension, abduction, and adduction of the wrist and hand.

Wrist motion occurs primarily between the distal radius and the proximal carpal row, consisting of the scaphoid, lunate, and triquetrum. The joint allows 70 to 90 degrees of flexion and 65 to 85 degrees of extension. The wrist can abduct 15 to 25 degrees and adduct 25 to 40 degrees.

Each finger has three joints. In these joints 0 to 40 degrees of extension and 85 to 100 degrees of flexion are possible. The proximal interphalangeal joint, classified as a hinge joint, can move from full extension to 90 to 120 degrees of flexion. The distal interphalangeal joints, also classified as hinge joints, can flex 80 to 90 degrees from full extension.

The thumb has only two joints. The metacarpophalangeal joint moves from full extension into 40 to 90 degrees of flexion. The interphalangeal joint can flex 80 to 90 degrees. The carpometacarpal joint of the thumb is a unique saddle-type joint having 50 to 70 degrees of abduction and can flex approximately 15 to 45 degrees and extend 0 to 20 degrees. Numerous ligaments support and provide static stability to many joints of the wrist and hand.

Movements of the Wrist and Hand

The following are movements of the wrist and hand:

- *Flexion:* Moving the palm or the phalanges toward the anterior or volar aspect of the forearm
- *Extension:* Moving the back of the hand or the phalanges toward the posterior or dorsal aspect of the forearm
- *Abduction (radial flexion or deviation):* Movement of the thumb side of the hand toward the lateral aspect or radial side of the forearm
- *Adduction (ulnar flexion or deviation):* Movement of the little-finger side of the hand toward the medial aspect or ulnar side of the forearm
- *Opposition:* Movement of the thumb across the palmar aspect to oppose any or all of the phalanges

Muscles of the Wrist and Hand

The extrinsic muscles of the wrist and hand may be grouped according to function and location. The wrist flexor-pronator muscle group includes the pronator teres, flexor carpi radialis, flexor carpi ulnaris, and palmaris longus.

All the wrist flexors generally have their proximal attachments on the anteromedial aspect of the proximal forearm and medial epicondyle of the humerus, whereas their distal attachments are on the anterior aspect of the wrist and hand.

The wrist extensors include the extensor carpi radialis longus, extensor carpi radialis brevis, and extensor carpi ulnaris muscles. The wrist extensors generally have their proximal attachments on the posterolateral aspect of the proximal forearm and lateral humeral epicondyle, and their distal attachments are located on the posterior aspect of the hand and wrist.

The wrist abductors include the flexor carpi radialis, extensor carpi radialis longus, extensor carpi radialis brevis, abductor pollicis longus, extensor pollicis longus, and extensor pollicis brevis. These muscles generally cross the wrist joint anterolaterally and posterolaterally to insert on the radial side of the hand. The flexor carpi ulnaris and extensor carpi ulnaris adduct the wrist and cross the wrist joint anteromedially and posteromedially to insert on the ulnar side of the hand.

Nine other muscles function primarily to move the phalanges but also are involved in wrist joint actions because they originate on the forearm and cross the wrist. These muscles are generally weaker in their actions on the wrist. The flexor digitorum superficialis and flexor digitorum profundus are finger flexors, and they also assist in wrist flexion along with the flexor pollicis longus, which is a thumb flexor. The extensor digitorum, extensor indicis, and extensor digiti minimi are finger extensors and also assist in wrist extension, along with the extensor pollicis longus and extensor pollicis brevis, which extend the thumb. The abductor pollicis longus abducts the thumb and assists in wrist abduction.

Intrinsic hand muscles have their proximal attachment and distal attachment within the hand. They are primarily responsible for fine and precise movements of the fingers and thumb. Those acting on the thumb, located in the thenar eminence, include the opponens pollicis, abductor pollicis brevis, and flexor pollicis brevis. Those acting on the little finger are the opponens digiti minimi, abductor digiti minimi, and flexor digiti minimi brevis. These muscles are located in the hypothenar eminence. Acting with the thenar muscles, they function in opposition, allowing effective grasping movements.

The lumbricales flex the metacarpophalangeal joint and extend the interphalangeal joints. The dorsal and palmar interossei muscles are involved with the adduction and abduction of the fingers. The adductor pollicis and abductor pollicis muscles adduct and abduct the thumb. With these actions, the hand can hold and manipulate small objects, such as a pencil (Activity 10.3).

ACTIVITY 10.3

In this activity, you will be working with a partner to assess individual movement patterns, normal function, and possible dysfunction in each other. First, one of you should isolate the specified movement patterns on each side of your partner, one side at a time, and assess for normal function by applying gentle pressure opposite to the action of the isolation position. The body should be stabilized so that only the isolated area is moving. In some instances, the ability to assume the position and maintain it indicates normal function. Muscles should be able to hold against gravity or the applied pressure without strain or pain. The position itself should be easy to assume and comfortable to maintain for a short duration—10 to 30 seconds. The bilateral movement patterns should be the same. The opposite movement pattern also should be able to be done easily.

Dysfunction may be indicated by bilateral asymmetry, pain, weakness, fatigue, a heavy sensation (binding), and inability to assume the isolation position or move into the opposite position. Intervention or referral depends on the severity of the condition and whether the dysfunction is neuromuscular, myofascial, or joint related.

Note: Do not perform these assessments if contraindications exist. Contraindications to this type of assessment include joint and disk dysfunction, acute pain, recent trauma, and inflammation.

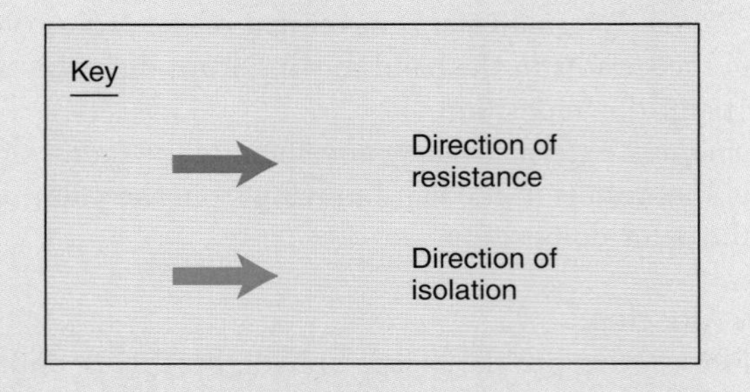

ACTIVITY 10.3—cont'd

Elbow Flexion

Assesses for strength and endurance in the isolation position and tension or shortening in the elbow extension pattern

Muscles Involved

Biceps brachii (short head)
Brachialis
Brachioradialis
Pronator teres

Range of Motion

0 to 150 degrees

Position of Client

Seated, with arms at sides

Three separate muscles can be isolated depending on the position of the forearm:

- Biceps brachii: Forearm in supination
- Brachialis: Forearm in pronation
- Brachioradialis: Forearm in mid-position between pronation and supination

Client's forearm is flexed to 90 degrees, and the examiner stabilizes it at the elbow

Isolation and Assessment (All Three Forearm Positions)

Client flexes elbow through a range of motion while examiner applies resistance to the distal forearm.

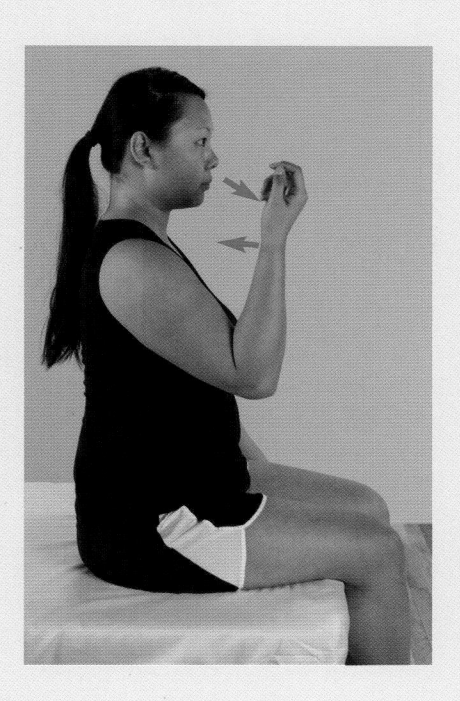

Elbow Extension

Assesses for strength and endurance in the isolation position and tension or shortening in the elbow flexion pattern

Muscles Involved

Triceps brachii
Anconeus

Range of Motion

No range of motion

Position of Client

Standing or seated with arm to be tested able to extend without touching the table

Forearm is flexed, and the examiner stabilizes it at the elbow

Isolation and Assessment

Client extends elbow to end of available range without extending shoulder. Examiner applies resistance at the wrist to prevent the action.

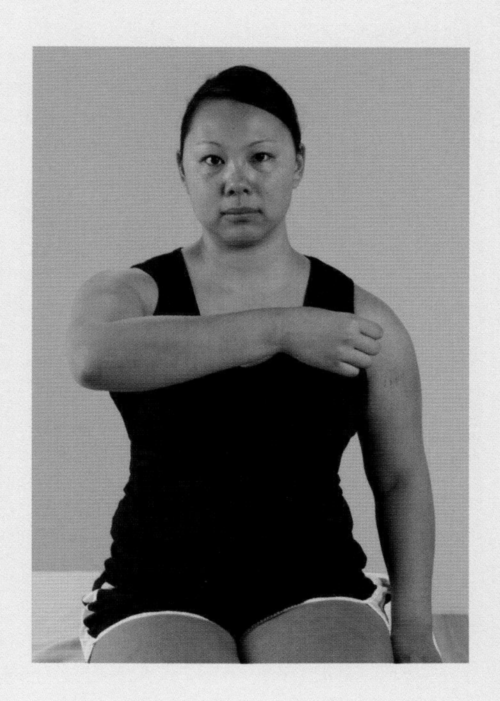

Continued

ACTIVITY 10.3—cont'd

Forearm Supination

Assesses for strength and endurance in the isolation position and tension or shortening in the pronation pattern

Muscles Involved

Supinator

Biceps brachii

Range of Motion

0 to 90 degrees

Position of Client

Seated, arm at side and elbow flexed to 90 degrees, and forearm in neutral or mid-position

Examiner stabilizes at the elbow with one hand and grasps the forearm above the wrist with the other hand

Isolation and Assessment

Client supinates the forearm until the palm faces the ceiling while the examiner resists the motion.

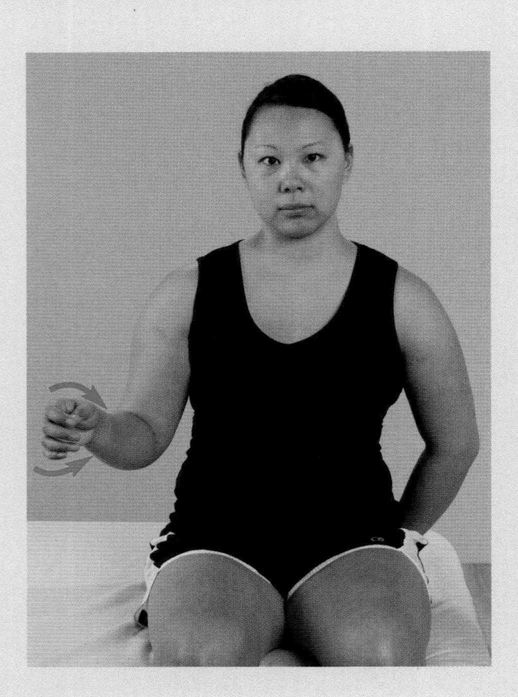

Forearm Pronation

Assesses for strength and endurance in the isolation position and tension or shortening in the supination pattern

Muscles Involved

Pronator teres

Pronator quadratus

Flexor carpi radialis

Range of Motion

0 to 80 degrees

Position of Client

Seated, with the arm at the side and elbow flexed to 90 degrees, and forearm in the neutral position

Examiner stabilizes at the elbow with one hand and grasps the forearm at wrist with the other hand

Isolation and Assessment

Client pronates the forearm until the palm faces downward while the examiner resists the motion.

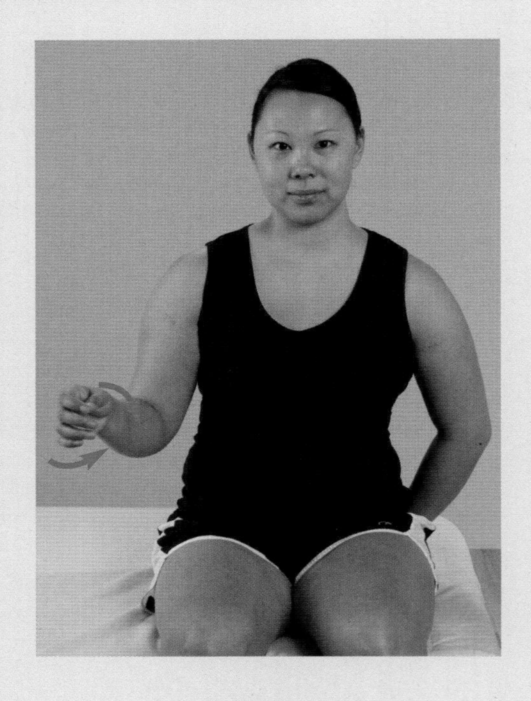

ACTIVITY 10.3—cont'd

Wrist Flexion

Assesses for strength and endurance in the isolation position and tension or shortening in the extension pattern

Muscles Involved

Flexor carpi radialis
Flexor carpi ulnaris
Palmaris longus
Abductor pollicis longus
Flexor digitorum superficialis
Flexor pollicis longus
Flexor digitorum profundus

Range of Motion

0 to 80 degrees

Position of Client

Seated with elbow flexed if needed and the forearm supinated while supported on its dorsal surface on a table
Wrist position is neutral

Isolation and Assessment

Client flexes the wrist while the examiner resists action. Make sure the client's thumbs and fingers are relaxed.

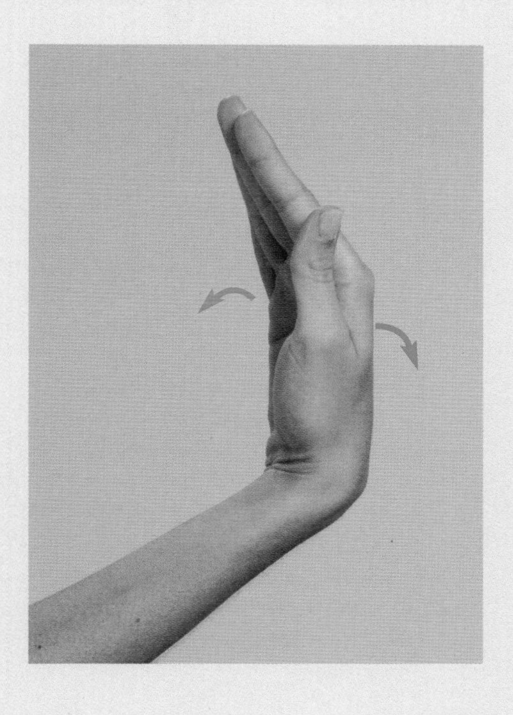

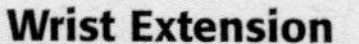

Wrist Extension

Assesses for strength and endurance in the isolation position and tension or shortening in the flexion pattern

Muscles Involved

Extensor carpi radialis longus
Extensor carpi radialis brevis
Extensor carpi ulnaris
Extensor digitorum
Extensor digiti minimi
Extensor indicis
Extensor pollicis longus

Range of Motion

0 to 85 degrees

Position of Client

Seated, with the elbow flexed as needed, and forearm pronated while arm is supported on the table

Isolation and Assessment

Client hyperextends wrist while examiner resists action. Client's thumb and fingers stay relaxed.

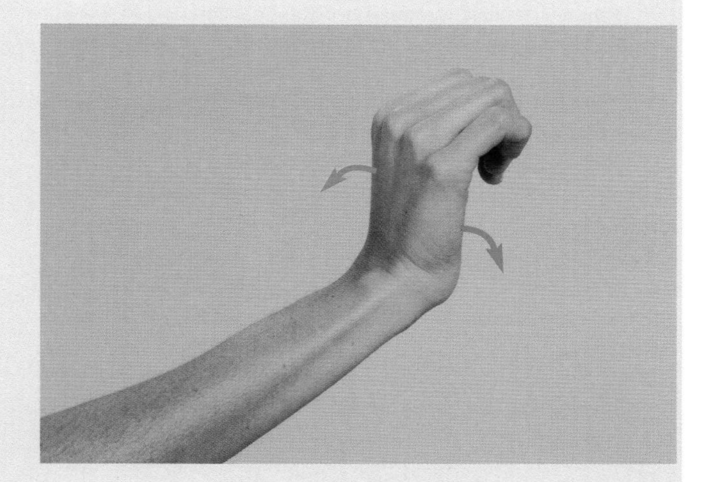

Continued

ACTIVITY 10.3—cont'd

Finger Flexion

Assesses for strength and endurance in the isolation position and tension or shortening in the finger extension pattern

Muscles Involved

Lumbricales
Dorsal interossei
Palmar interossei
Flexor digitorum superficialis
Flexor digitorum profundus

Range of Motion

0 to 100 degrees

Position of Client

Seated, with elbow flexed and forearm supinated and supported on a table
Wrist is maintained in the neutral position
Begin with metacarpophalangeal joints fully extended and interphalangeal joints flexed
Each finger is to be isolated separately

Isolation and Assessment

Client flexes the metacarpophalangeal joint (bends knuckles) and extends the interphalangeal (finger) joints while the examiner resists metacarpophalangeal flexion. Make sure the client does not flex the interphalangeal joint.

Finger Extension

Assesses for strength and endurance in the isolation position and tension or shortening in the finger flexion pattern

Muscles Involved

Extensor digitorum
Extensor indicis
Extensor digiti minimi

Range of Motion

0 to 15 degrees

Position of Client

Seated, with forearm in pronation and supported on a table and wrist in neutral

Isolation and Assessment

No resistance is required. Ability to perform isolation indicates normal function
Extensor digitorum: Client extends metacarpophalangeal joints (all fingers simultaneously), allowing the interphalangeal joints to be in slight flexion
Extensor indicis: Client extends the metacarpophalangeal joint of the index finger
Extensor digiti minimi: Client extends the joint of the fifth digit

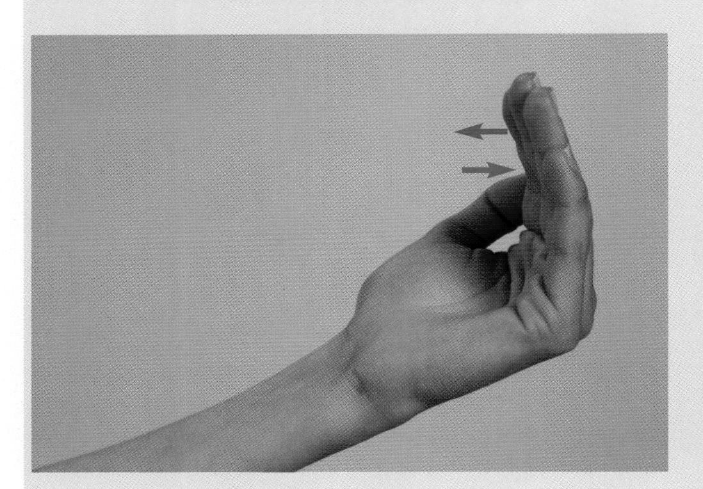

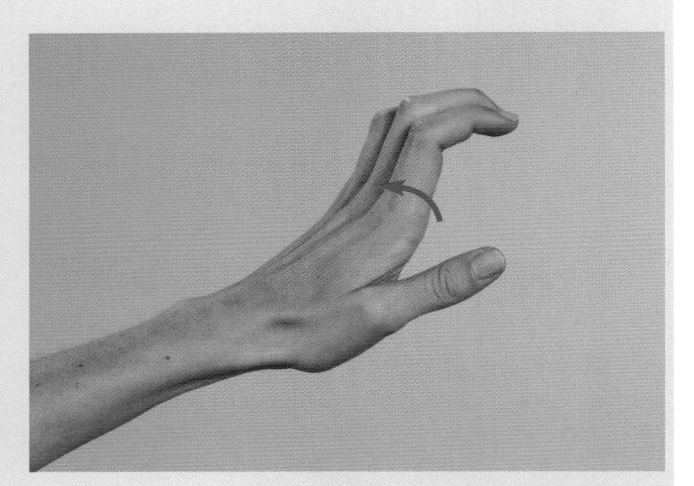

ACTIVITY 10.3—cont'd

Finger Abduction

Assesses for strength and endurance in the isolation position and tension or shortening in the finger adduction pattern

Muscles Involved

Dorsal interossei

Abductor digiti minimi

Range of Motion

0 to 20 degrees

Position of Client

Seated, with the forearm pronated and supported and wrist in the neutral position

Fingers are abducted (separated), and metacarpophalangeal joints remain neutral

Isolation and Assessment

Each finger is isolated separately against resistance given near the distal end of the finger to push it together with other fingers.

Dorsal interossei:

- Abduction of ring finger toward little finger (includes abductor digiti minimi)
- Abduction of the middle finger toward the ring finger
- Abduction of the middle finger toward the index finger
- Abduction of the index finger toward the thumb

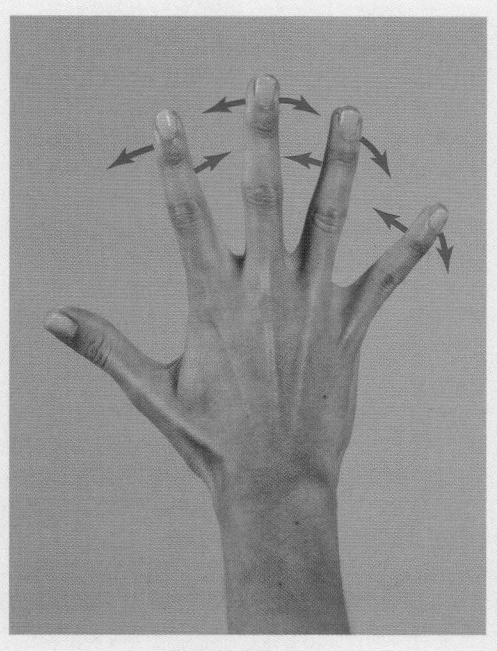

Finger abduction

Finger Adduction

Assesses for strength and endurance in the isolation position and tension or shortening in the finger abduction pattern

Muscles Involved

Palmar interossei

Range of Motion

0 to 20 degrees

Position of Client

Seated, with elbow flexed, forearm pronated and supported, wrist in neutral, and fingers extended and adducted (together)

Metacarpophalangeal joints are neutral

Isolation and Assessment

Fingers are tested separately; middle finger is not tested because it has no palmar interossei muscle. Examiner applies resistance near the distal end of the finger to pull it away from other fingers. Adduction of the little finger is toward the ring finger. Adduction of the ring finger is toward the middle finger. Adduction of the index finger is toward the middle finger. Adduction of the thumb is toward the index finger.

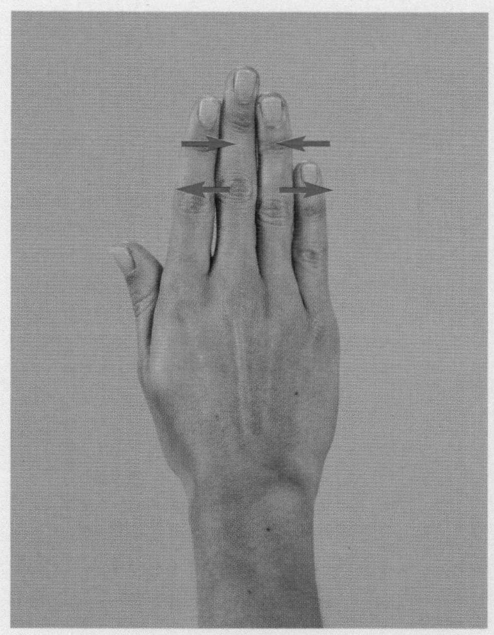

Finger adduction

Continued

ACTIVITY 10.3—cont'd

Thumb Adduction, Flexion, and Medial Rotation

Assesses for strength and endurance in the isolation position and tension or shortening in the thumb extension pattern

Thumb extensors are extrinsic muscles.

The thumb has 0 to 20 degrees of extension.

Muscles Involved

Flexor pollicis brevis
Flexor pollicis longus
Adductor pollicis

Range of Motion

Metacarpophalangeal flexion: 0 to 50 degrees
Interphalangeal flexion: 0 to 80 degrees
Adduction: 0 to 70 degrees

Position of Client

Seated, with the forearm supinated and supported and wrist in the neutral position

Carpometacarpal joint and interphalangeal joints are neutral

Thumb is in adduction

Isolation and Assessment

Client flexes the metacarpophalangeal joint of the thumb to slide thumb across palm while examiner applies resistance to pull the thumb back between carpometacarpal and interphalangeal joints. Interphalangeal joint does not flex.

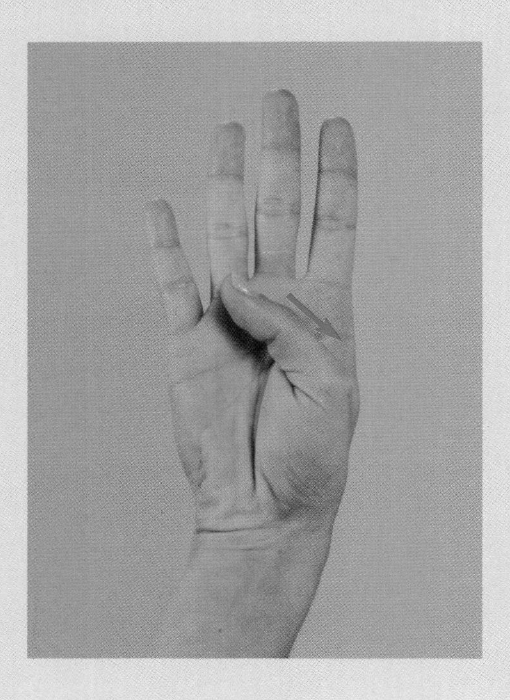

Thumb Opposition

Assesses for strength and endurance in the isolation position and tension or shortening in the thumb opposition pattern

Muscles Involved

Opponens pollicis
Opponens digiti minimi

Range of Motion

0 to 70 degrees

Position of Client

Seated, with forearm supinated and supported, wrist in neutral position, and thumb in palmar abduction

Opponens pollicis: Apply resistance for the opponens pollicis at the head of the first metacarpal in the direction of lateral rotation, extension, and adduction

Isolation and Assessment

Client medially rotates and flexes thumb toward little finger while little finger flexes and rotates toward thumb such that pads of digits touch (not tips of digits).

The examiner applies resistance on the palmar surface of the thumb and fifth metacarpal to bring them apart.

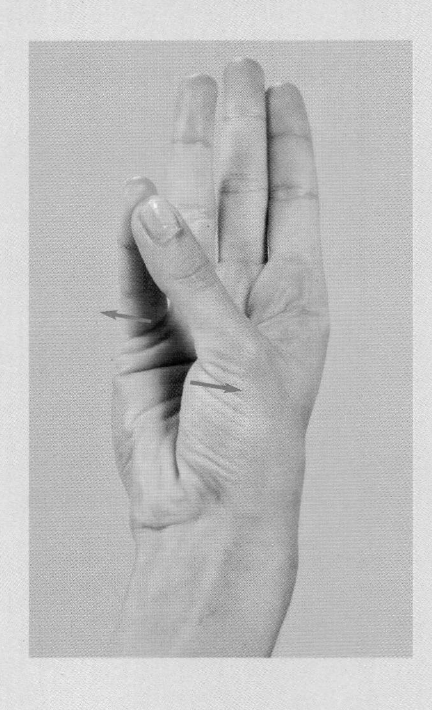

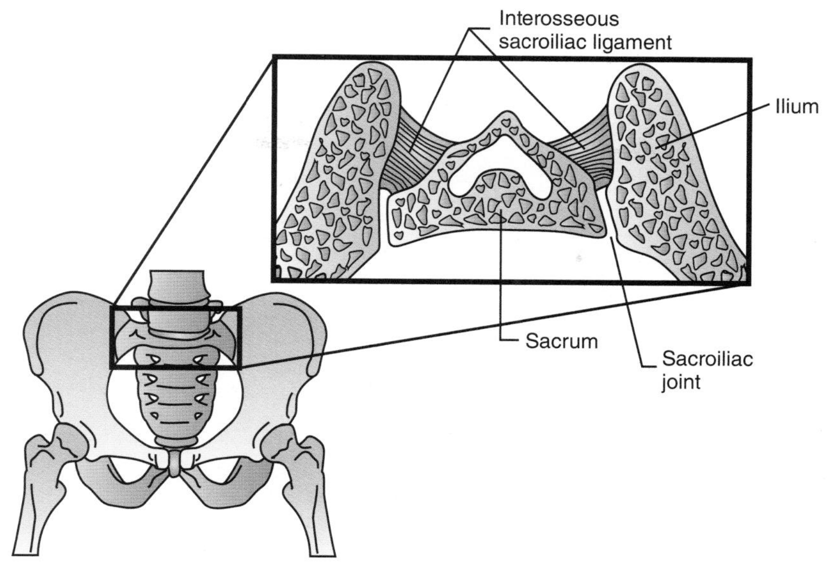

FIG. 10.19 Cross section of the sacroiliac joints.

Pelvic Girdle and Hip Joint Region

The pelvis consists of three bones and three joints. The bones are the two fused coxal bones (made up of the ilium, ischium, and pubis) and the sacrum. The three joints are the two sacroiliac articulations and the symphysis pubis.

Motion in the Pelvic Girdle

The pelvic girdle functions as one unit, with all three bones moving at all three joints. The lower extremities, the vertebral column, and the trunk influence the pelvic girdle. The unit moves around a vertical axis. In a movement to the left, the symphysis turns left of the midline, the right coxal turns forward, the left coxal turns backward, and the sacrum turns a little to the left. The reverse happens when rotating to the right.

The pelvic girdle moves back and forth within three planes for a total of six different movements. Analyzing the pelvic girdle activity to determine the exact location of the movement is important to prevent confusion.

All pelvic girdle rotation results from motion at the right hip, left hip, or lumbar spine. Although movement does not have to occur in all three of these areas, it must occur in at least one area for the pelvis to rotate in any direction. Even though the sacroiliac joints are synovial joints, they permit little movement and even fuse in many persons later in life. This general reduction of motion is related to degenerative changes, such as osteoarthritis (Fig. 10.19).

Four groups of ligaments form the main bond that keeps the ilium and sacrum in approximation. Stability of the sacroiliac joints is crucial because they maintain support for a large portion of the body weight. More movement (and therefore less stability) is present in the sacroiliac joints of females, who have smaller and flatter surfaces involving only the first two sacral vertebrae, than in men, who have longer, more concave surfaces involving the first three sacral vertebrae.

When weight shifts from one leg to the other while standing, the symphysis may show an upward/downward motion of 2 mm. During pregnancy, the symphysis may separate 5 to 9 mm.

During normal walking, motions involve the entire pelvic girdle and both hip joints. When the pelvic girdle rotates forward, hip flexion occurs; when it rotates backward, hip extension occurs. The symphysis pubis serves as the axis for the rotation. Jogging and running result in a faster and greater range of these movements.

Muscular attachments to the pelvic girdle are extensive, but no muscles directly influence the sacroiliac joint. Indirect actions come from the abdominal muscles, which are inserted on the superior aspect of the pelvic girdle and are joined by the quadratus lumborum.

Six groups of hip and thigh muscles are attached to the pelvic girdle and lower extremities. These hip muscles highly influence the movement of the two coxal bones within the pelvic girdle. Anterior to the sacroiliac joint are two important muscles, the psoas and piriformis.

The psoas crosses over the anterior aspect of the sacroiliac joint and goes from the lumbar region to insert into the lesser trochanter of the femur. The right and left piriformis muscles originate from the anterior surface of the sacrum, pass through the sciatic notch, and insert into the greater trochanter of the femur. Muscle imbalance in any of these groups can affect pelvic function adversely.

The pelvic girdle is thought to be of importance within the craniosacral system. Theory indicates that the sacrum has mobility between the two coxals as part of the craniosacral rhythm. Any changes or alterations in the biomechanical function of the pelvic girdle can influence the craniosacral mechanism negatively; the reverse is also true.

Because the pelvis is the supporting base of the spine, dysfunctions in its joints have a significant effect on the lumbar spine. Sacroiliac pain is usually a dull ache in the bones above the buttock on one side. Because the nerves in that region are not specific, pain caused by the sacroiliac joint can be felt in the groin, back of the thigh, and lower abdomen.

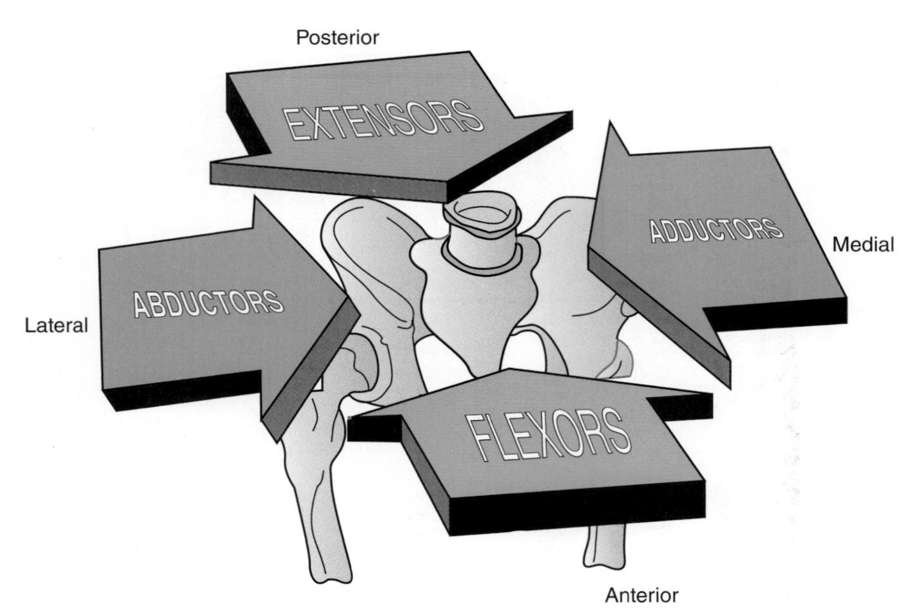

FIG. 10.20 Position and function of the hip to support multiaxial joint function.

One of the most common dysfunctions occurs when leaning forward to lift some heavy object instead of going into the bent-knee position. If the abdominal muscles are strong and support the anterior pelvis, stabilizing the trunk to maintain a more or less constant balance between the trunk and the pelvis, no dysfunction happens. But if the abdominal muscles and the sacrotuberous ligaments are weak, dysfunction and pain could occur.

Hip Joint

Except for the glenohumeral joint, the hip joint is one of the most mobile joints of the body, largely because of its multiaxial arrangement. Unlike the glenohumeral joint, the bony architecture of the hip joint provides a great deal of stability, resulting in few hip joint dislocations. An extremely strong and dense ligamentous capsule reinforces the joint, especially the anterior portion (Fig. 10.20).

Because of individual differences, some disagreement exists regarding the exact range of each movement in the hip joint, but the ranges are generally 0 to 130 degrees of flexion, 0 to 30 degrees of extension, 0 to 35 degrees of abduction, 0 to 30 degrees of adduction, 0 to 45 degrees of internal rotation, and 0 to 50 degrees of external rotation.

Movements of the Pelvis and Hip Joints

Anterior and posterior pelvic rotations occur in the sagittal plane, whereas right and left lateral rotation occurs in the frontal plane. Right transverse (clockwise) rotation and left transverse (counterclockwise) rotation occur in the horizontal or transverse plane of motion. The movements are as follows:

- *Anterior pelvic rotation:* Anterior movement of the upper pelvis; the iliac crest tilts forward in a sagittal plane.
- *Posterior pelvic rotation:* Posterior movement of the upper pelvis; the iliac crest tilts backward in a sagittal plane (Fig. 10.21).
- *Left lateral pelvic rotation (tilt):* In the frontal plane the left pelvis moves superiorly in relation to the right pelvis; the left pelvis rotates upward or the right pelvis rotates downward.
- *Right lateral pelvic rotation (tilt):* In the frontal plane the right pelvis moves superiorly in relation to the left pelvis; the right pelvis rotates upward, or the left pelvis rotates downward (Fig. 10.22).
- *Left transverse pelvic rotation:* In a transverse (horizontal) plane of motion, the pelvis rotates to the left of the body; the right iliac crest moves anteriorly in relation to the left iliac crest, which moves posteriorly.
- *Right transverse pelvic rotation:* In a transverse (horizontal) plane of motion, the pelvis rotates to the right of the body; the left iliac crest moves anteriorly in relation to the right iliac crest, which moves posteriorly (Fig. 10.23).
- *Hip flexion:* Movement of the femur straight anteriorly toward the pelvis.
- *Hip extension:* Movement of the femur straight posteriorly away from the pelvis.
- *Hip abduction:* Movement of the femur laterally to the side away from the midline.
- *Hip adduction:* Movement of the femur medially toward the midline.
- *Hip external rotation:* Rotary movement of the femur laterally around its longitudinal axis away from the midline.
- *Hip internal rotation:* Rotary movement of the femur medially around its longitudinal axis toward the midline.

The lumbar spine, hip joint, and pelvic girdle work together in carrying out lower extremity activities.

Table 10.2 shows a comparison of pelvic girdle, lumbar spine, and hip joint movements.

Muscles of the Hip Joint

At the hip joint are six two-joint muscles that have one action at the hip and another at the knee. The muscles usually involved in hip and pelvic girdle motions depend largely on the direction of the movement and the position of the body in relation to the

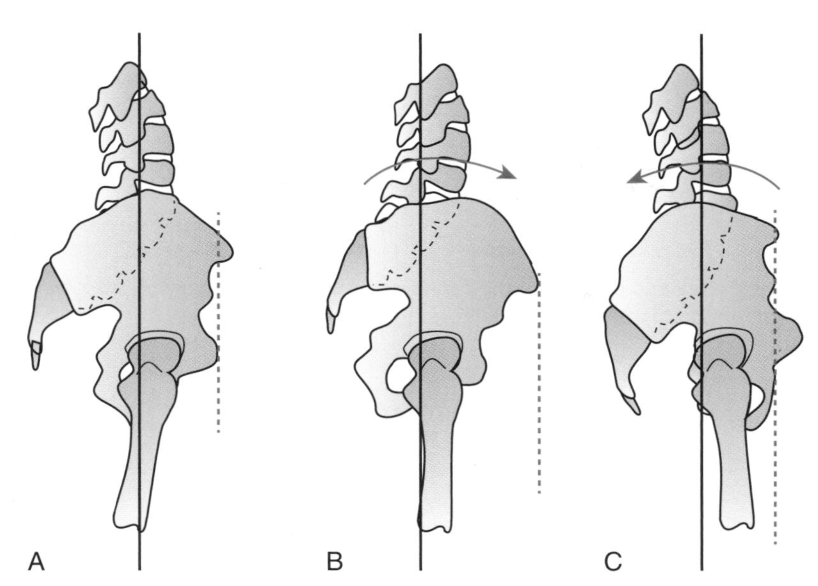

FIG. 10.21 Sagittal plane pelvic movement. (A) In the neutral position, the anterior superior iliac spine and the pubic symphysis are in the same vertical plane. (B) Anterior rotation. Pelvis tilts forward, moving the anterior superior iliac spine anterior to the pubic symphysis. (C) Posterior rotation. Pelvis tilts backward, moving the anterior superior iliac spine posterior to the pubic symphysis.

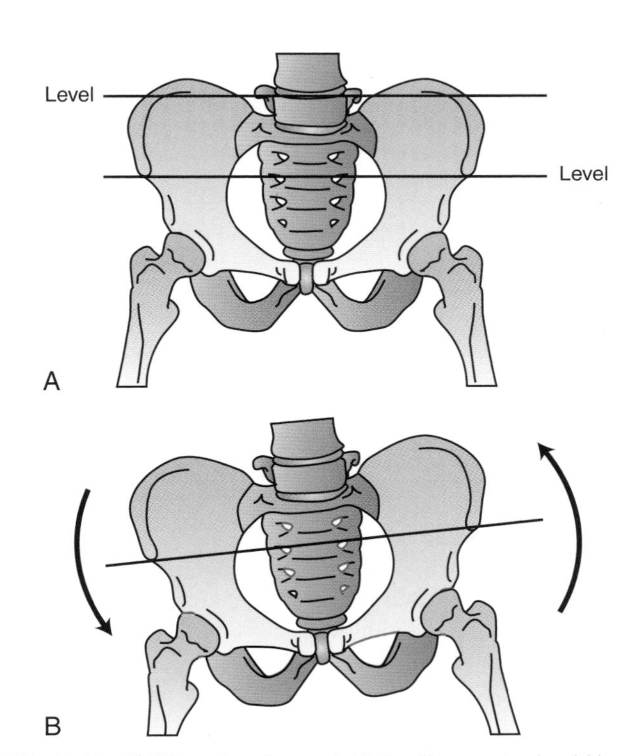

FIG. 10.22 (A) When standing upright, the iliac crests should be level in the frontal plane, and the anterior superior iliac spines on the left and right should be level. (B) Frontal plane pelvic movement tilt.

earth and its gravitational forces. In addition, note that the body part that moves the most is the part least stabilized. For example, when a person is standing on both feet and contracting the hip flexors, the trunk and pelvis flex anteriorly; however, when the person is lying supine and contracting the hip flexors, the thighs move forward into flexion on the stable pelvis. In another example, the hip flexor muscles are used in moving the legs toward the trunk, but the extensor muscles are used eccentrically when the pelvis and trunk move downward slowly on the femur and concentrically when the trunk is raised on the femur, such as when rising to the standing position.

In the downward phase of the knee-bend exercise, the movement at the hips and knees is flexion. The muscles involved primarily are the hip and knee extensors in eccentric contraction to control the trunk.

The iliopsoas muscle provides stabilization and powerful actions such as raising the legs from a supine position on the floor. The proximal attachment in the lower back tends to move the lower back anteriorly or, in the supine position, pulls the lower back up as it raises the legs. For this reason, lower back problems are common with this activity because leg raising is primarily hip flexion, not abdominal action. Strong abdominal muscles prevent lower back strain by pulling up on the front of the pelvis and thus flattening the back.

The sartorius, a two-joint muscle, is effective as a hip or knee flexor and is weak when both actions occur at the same time. When the knees are extended, the sartorius becomes a more effective hip flexor.

The rectus femoris muscle pulls from the anterior inferior iliac spine of the ilium to rotate the pelvis anteriorly. Only the abdominal muscles, particularly the rectus abdominis, can prevent this from occurring. In older adults, the pelvis may be tilted forward permanently. The relaxed abdominal wall does not hold the pelvis up, and therefore an increased lumbar curve results. The rectus femoris muscle is a powerful extensor of the knee when the hip is extended but is weak when the hip is flexed.

The pectineus muscles tend to rotate the pelvis anteriorly. The abdominal muscles pulling up on the pelvis in front counteract this tilting.

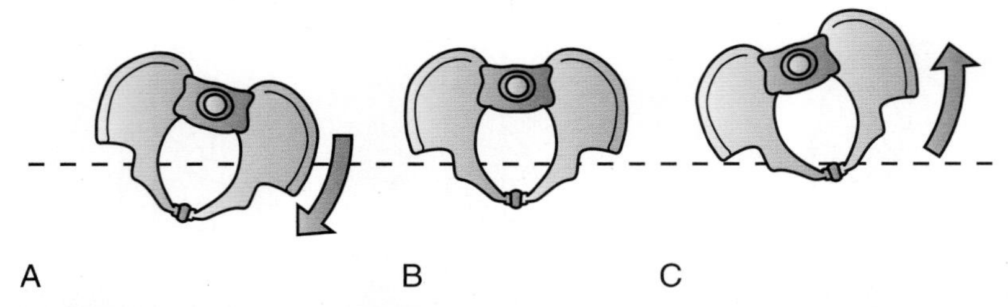

FIG. 10.23 A superior view of the transverse rotation of the pelvis in the transverse plane: (A) left forward rotation, (B) neutral position of the pelvis, and (C) left backward rotation of the pelvis.

Table 10.2 Pelvic Girdle, Lumbar Spine, and Hip Joint Movements

Pelvic Rotations	Lumbar Spine Motion	Right Hip Motion	Left Hip Motion
Anterior rotation	Extension	Flexion	Flexion
Posterior rotation	Flexion	Extension	Extension
Right lateral rotation	Right lateral flexion	Adduction	Abduction
Left lateral rotation	Left lateral flexion	Abduction	Adduction
Right transverse rotation	Left lateral rotation	Internal rotation	External rotation
Left transverse rotation	Right lateral rotation	External rotation	Internal rotation

The tensor fasciae latae muscle is used when flexion and internal rotation take place. This muscle also aids in preventing external rotation of the femur as it is flexed by other flexor muscles.

Typical action of the gluteus medius and gluteus minimus muscles occurs in walking. As the weight of the body shifts to one leg, these muscles prevent the opposite hip from sagging. Weakness in the gluteus medius and gluteus minimus can result in what is known as the *Trendelenburg gait*. With this weakness, the individual's opposite hip sags on weight bearing because the hip abductors cannot maintain proper alignment. As the body ages, the gluteus medius and gluteus minimus muscles tend to lose their effectiveness. Walking loses its easy spring and becomes more labored.

The gluteus maximus muscle comes into action when movement between the pelvis and the femur approaches and goes beyond 15 degrees of extension. As a result, the gluteus maximus is not used extensively in ordinary walking but is important in the extension of the thigh with external rotation and stabilization between the lumbar dorsal fascia and iliotibial band.

The six deep lateral rotator muscles—piriformis, gemellus superior, gemellus inferior, obturator externus, obturator internus, and quadratus femoris—provide powerful movements of external rotation of the femur. Standing on one leg and forcefully turning the body away from that leg is accomplished by contraction of these muscles.

The hamstrings (semitendinosus, semimembranosus, and biceps femoris), together with the gluteus maximus muscle, act in the extension of the thigh when the knees are straight. These muscles are used in ordinary walking as extensors of the hip and allow the gluteus maximus to stabilize the movement. When the trunk is bent forward with the knees straight, the hamstring muscles have a powerful pull on the rear pelvis and tilt it down in the back. If the knees are flexed when this movement takes place, the gluteus maximus chiefly does the work.

The adductor brevis, adductor longus, adductor magnus, and gracilis provide powerful movement of the thighs toward each other and are important postural muscles (Activity 10.4).

Knee Region

The knee joint is the largest and most complex joint in the body and is primarily a hinge joint. The combined functions of weight bearing and locomotion place considerable stress and strain on the knee joint. The ligaments provide static stability to the knee joint, and contractions of the quadriceps and hamstrings produce dynamic stability.

The knee includes the articulation of the femur and tibia and the patella, which covers it anteriorly. The knee acts as part of a closed kinematic chain with the lumbar spine, hip, and ankle. Weight-bearing forces normally bisect the knee even though it has a slight valgus angulation. A slight hyperextension of both knees when standing is normal (more in females). The extension ends when the capsule and ligaments twist and draw tight, locking the joint in its close-packed position. The range of motion of the knee is 5 to 10 degrees of hyperextension, 135 to 150 degrees of flexion with soft tissue of the calf and thigh limiting flexion, and 10 degrees of internal or external tibial rotation. With the knee flexed 30 degrees or more, approximately 30 degrees of internal rotation and 45 degrees of external rotation can occur. The external rotation of the tibia toward the end of the extension and internal rotation during the beginning of flexion are automatic because of the shape of the articulating bones.

The quadriceps pull the patella in line with the femur. The patellar tendon pulls the patella in line with the tibia. The quadriceps (Q) angle is the angle formed by these two pulls. The tension from the quadriceps and patellar tendon plus the anterior projection of the lateral femoral condyle and the deep patellar groove in the femur hold the patella in place during

ACTIVITY 10.4

In this activity, you will be working with a partner to assess individual movement patterns, normal function, and possible dysfunction in each other. First, one of you should isolate the specified movement patterns on each side of your partner, one side at a time, and assess for normal function by applying gentle pressure opposite to the action of the isolation position. The body should be stabilized so that only the isolated area is moving. In some instances, the ability to assume the position and maintain it indicates normal function. Muscles should be able to hold against gravity or the applied pressure without strain or pain. The position itself should be easy to assume and comfortable to maintain for a short duration—10 to 30 seconds. The bilateral movement patterns should be the same. The opposite movement pattern also should be able to be done easily. Dysfunction may be indicated by bilateral asymmetry, pain, weakness, fatigue, a heavy sensation (binding), and the inability to assume the isolation position or move into the opposite position.

Intervention or referral depends on the severity of the condition and whether the dysfunction is neuromuscular, myofascial, or joint related.

Note: Do not perform these assessments if contraindications exist. Contraindications to this type of assessment include joint and disk dysfunction, acute pain, recent trauma, and inflammation.

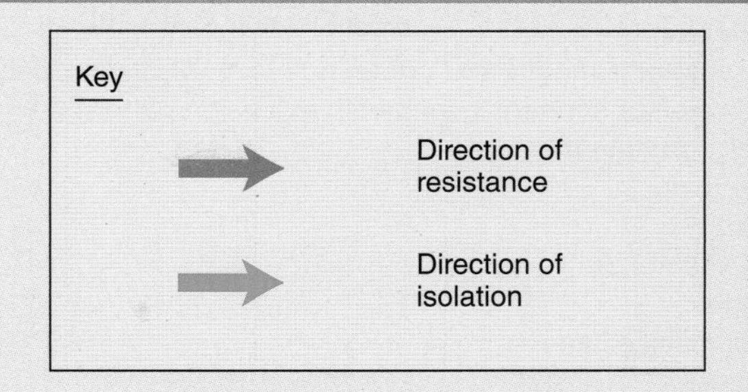

ACTIVITY 10.4—cont'd

Hip Flexion

Assesses for strength and endurance in the isolation position and tension or shortening in the hip extension pattern

Muscles Involved

Psoas major
Iliacus
Rectus femoris
Sartorius
Tensor fasciae latae
Pectineus
Adductor brevis
Adductor longus
Adductor magnus

Range of Motion

0 to 130 degrees

Position of Client

Seated, knees bent with thighs fully supported on the table and feet hanging over the edge

Client may use arms for stability

Isolation and Assessment

Client flexes hip through full range while examiner applies resistance on anterior thigh above the knee to push the leg down.

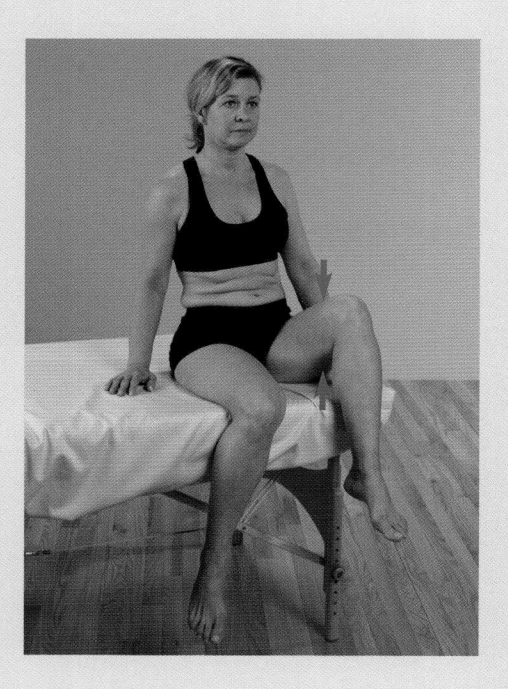

Hip Extension

Assesses for strength and endurance in the isolation position and tension or shortening in the hip flexion pattern

Muscles Involved

Gluteus maximus
Semitendinosus
Semimembranosus
Biceps femoris (long head)

Range of Motion

0 to 30 degrees

Position of Client

Prone, with arms overhead or abducted to hold sides of table

Place pillows under hips to help flex hips for start position

Isolation and Assessment

Client extends the hip through the entire available range of motion while the knee is extended. The entire leg should clear the table. Examiner applies resistance to the posterior thigh above the knee to push the leg down.

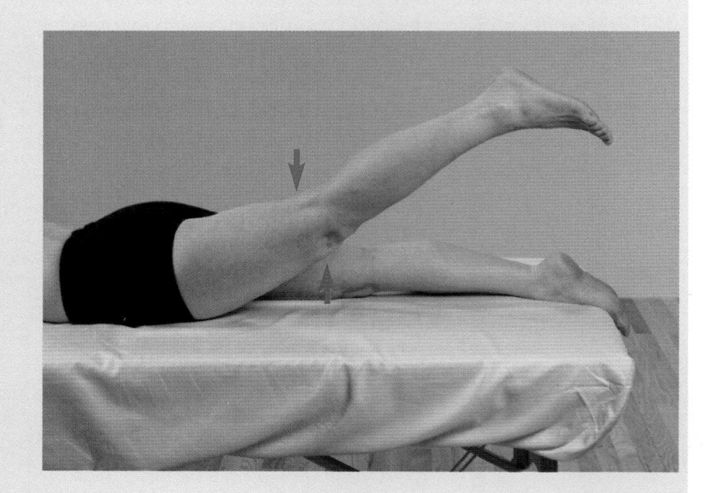

 ACTIVITY **10.4—cont'd**

Hip Abduction

Assesses for strength and endurance in the isolation position and tension or shortening in the hip adduction pattern

Muscles Involved

Gluteus medius
Gluteus minimus
Tensor fasciae latae
Gluteus maximus (upper fibers)

Range of Motion

0 to 35 degrees

Position of Client

Side-lying on the nontest side, hip and knee flexed for stability
Hip is slightly extended on the leg to be tested

Isolation and Assessment

Client abducts the hip through the range of motion leading with heel to prevent flexing or rotating the hip. Examiner applies resistance to the lateral aspect of the thigh above the knee to push the leg down.

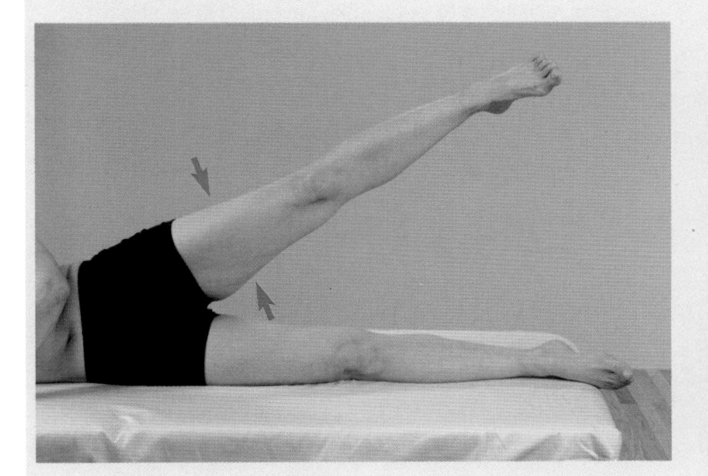

Hip Adduction

Assesses for strength and endurance in the isolation position and tension or shortening in the hip abduction pattern

Muscles Involved

Adductor magnus
Adductor brevis
Adductor longus
Pectineus
Gracilis

Range of Motion

0 to 15 to 30 degrees

Position of Client

Side-lying on the test side with the uppermost limb in 25 degrees of abduction, supported by the examiner
The therapist cradles the leg with the forearm; the hand supports the limb on the medial surface of the leg

Isolation and Assessment

Client adducts the hip until the lower limb contacts the upper one. No resistance is required.

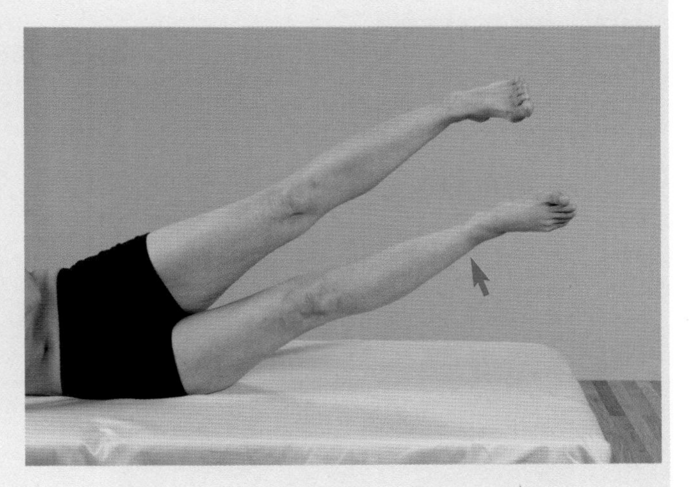

Continued

ACTIVITY 10.4—cont'd

Hip External or Lateral Rotation

Assesses for strength and endurance in the isolation position and tension or shortening in the hip internal or medial rotation pattern

Muscles Involved

Obturator externus
Obturator internus
Quadratus femoris
Piriformis
Gemellus superior
Gemellus inferior
Gluteus maximus
Sartorius

Range of Motion

0 to 45 degrees

Position of Client

Seated, with hips flexed but not rotated
Patella in line with the anterior superior interior spine
Examiner stabilizes the outer thigh above the knee
Trunk is supported by placing hands at the sides

Isolation and Assessment

Client externally rotates the hip by bringing the sole toward the opposite calf while the examiner applies resistance to the inner ankle. It is important to avoid knee stress with resistance.

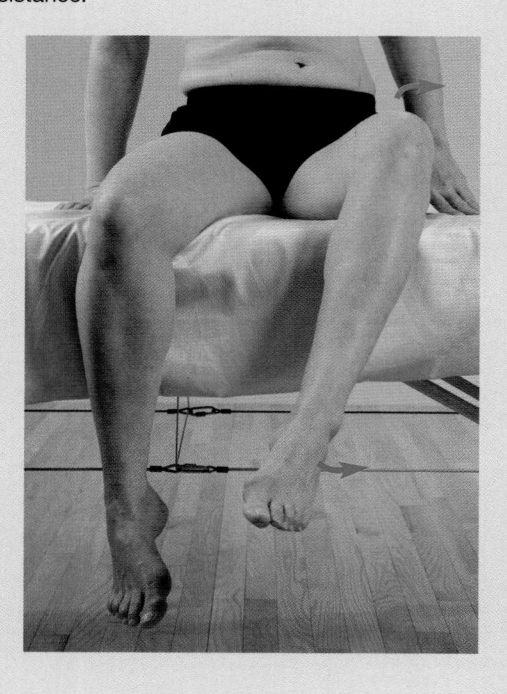

Hip Internal or Medial Rotation

Assesses for strength and endurance in the isolation position and tension or shortening in the lateral or external hip rotation pattern

Muscles Involved

Gluteus minimus
Gluteus medius
Tensor fasciae latae

Range of Motion

0 to 50 degrees

Position of Client

Seated, with hips flexed, patella in line with the anterior superior iliac spine
Arms at the sides to support the trunk
Examiner stabilizes the medial thigh just above the knee

Isolation and Assessment

Client internally rotates hip, turning sole of foot to the side and bringing the knee toward the opposite leg while examiner applies resistance to outer ankle, avoiding knee strain.

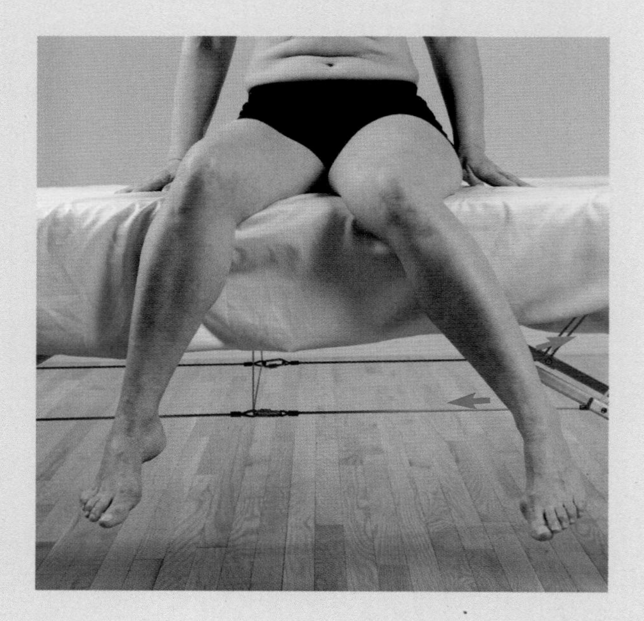

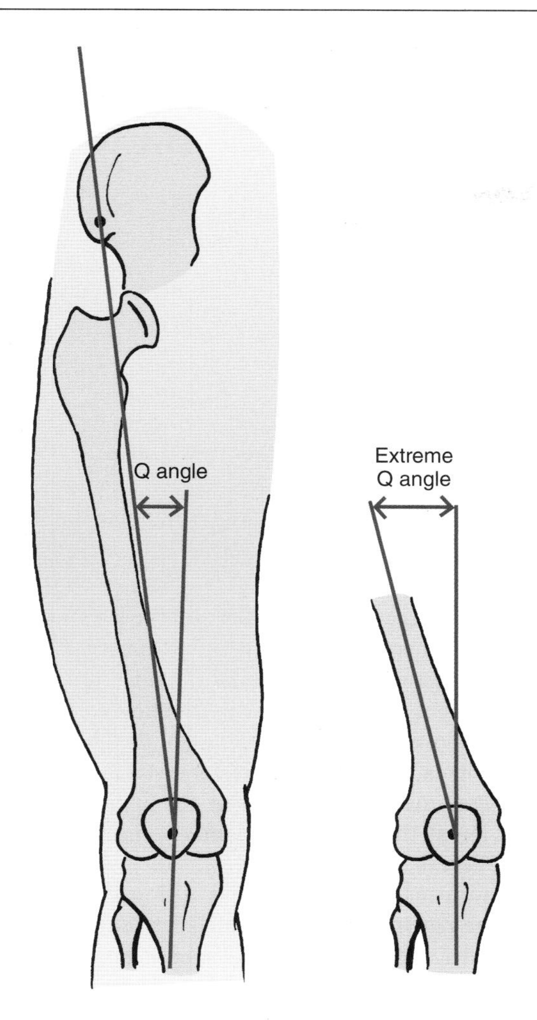

FIG. 10.24 The quadriceps angle (*Q angle*) is measured from the anterior superior iliac spine through the axis of the patella and distally to the distal attachment of the patellar tendon on the tibial tuberosity. (Modified from Shankman GA. *Fundamental Orthopedic Management for the Physical Therapist Assistant*. 3rd ed. Mosby/Elsevier; 2011.)

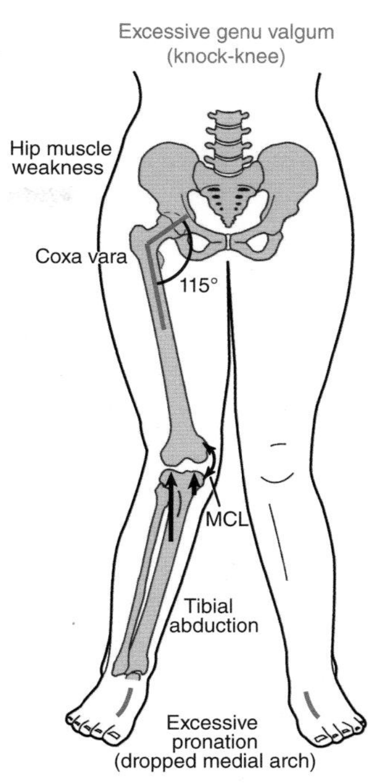

FIG. 10.25 Excessive valgus angulation. *MCL*, Medial collateral ligament. (From Neumann DA. *Kinesiology of the Musculoskeletal System: Foundations for Rehabilitation*. 2nd ed. Mosby/Elsevier; 2010.)

flexion. As the muscle contracts, the patella moves out of the groove and lateral, and the Q angle decreases. The lateral femoral condyle and the contraction of the vastus medialis muscle (oblique pattern) help prevent lateral dislocation of the patella. This is particularly important for a female because their broader pelvis causes a greater Q angle and a stronger lateral pull (Fig. 10.24).

The superior tibiofemoral joint aids the knee in supporting one-sixth of the body weight. The joint glides anteriorly during knee flexion and rotates with ankle dorsiflexion. Joint dysfunctions (such as hypomobility) can lead to lateral knee, leg, or ankle pain.

Other Major Knee Components

Two cartilaginous menisci partially fill the space between the articulating surfaces of the tibia and femur. Both menisci are thicker on the periphery than in the center margin. They move with the tibia during flexion or extension and with the femur in rotation. Menisci improve weight distribution by increasing the contact area between the two long bones. They act as shock absorbers by spreading the stress over the articulating surfaces, reducing friction and cartilage wear. They are part of the locking mechanism of the knee, which prevents hyperextension by directing the movement of the articulating condyles.

The medial (tibial) collateral ligament is a strong, broad, triangular strap that attaches to the medial epicondyle of the femur. The ligament helps prevent anterior tibial displacement on the femur. The lateral collateral ligament is shorter and more rounded than the medial collateral ligament and is located between the biceps femoris tendon externally and the popliteus tendon internally. The lateral collateral ligament does not attach to the lateral meniscus. Its fibers are tight, especially during knee extension, tibial adduction, and lateral rotation. The lateral collateral ligament helps protect the lateral aspect of the knee from varus stress. Excessive varus (bowlegs) and valgus (knock-knees) are two of the more common deformities of the knee joint (Fig. 10.25).

The medial collateral ligament and lateral collateral ligament twist in relationship with each other to protect the knee externally from excessive tibial rotation and extension. The cruciate ligaments are the main rotary stabilizers and cross each other within the knee capsule. These ligaments are vital in maintaining the anterior, posterior, and rotary stability of the knee joint. They aid the rolling and gliding movements of the tibia on the femur and are rotary guides for the screw-home, or locking, mechanism of the knee.

The screw-home mechanism occurs with rotary movement of the knee (Fig. 10.26). This rotary motion results not from

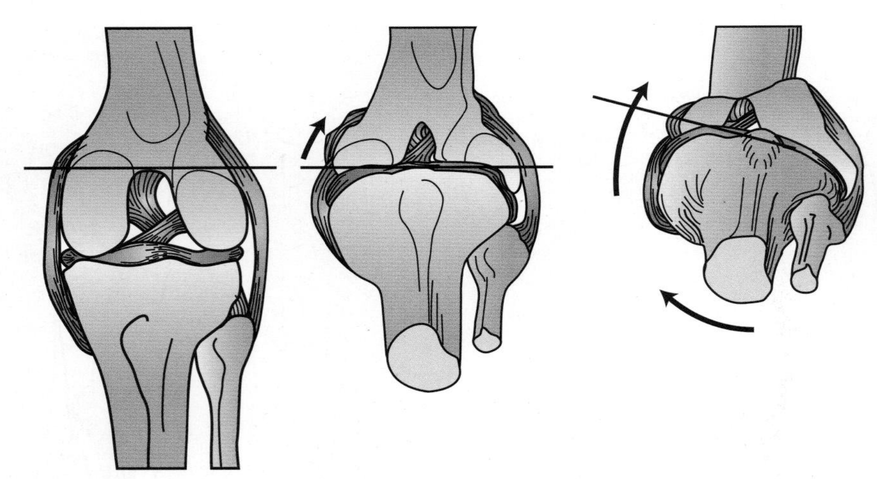

FIG. 10.26 The screw-home motion of the knee. In the non-weight-bearing position, the tibia laterally rotates on the femur as the knee moves into the last few degrees of extension.

muscle action, but instead from joint and menisci structure. The articular surface of the medial femoral condyle is longer than that of the lateral condyle. In addition, the C shape of the medial meniscus allows the medial tibial condyle to rotate around the femoral condyle. The lateral meniscus is shaped like an O, holds the lateral tibial condyle more securely against the femoral condyle, and does not allow motion. As a result of these structural features, the medial condyle of the tibia rotates on the femur during the last 15 degrees of knee extension in an external direction in the non-weight-bearing position. In the weight-bearing position, the femur medially rotates on the tibia when the knee is extended fully. This action locks the knee into extension, which allows us to stand without using muscle action but instead being supported by the ligaments at the hip. This saves energy and allows us to stand for extended periods without fatigue. The popliteus muscle unlocks the knee to begin flexion.

The knee joint is well supplied with synovial fluid from a synovial cavity that lies under the patella and between the surfaces of the tibia and the femur. Commonly, this synovial cavity is called the *capsule* of the knee. More than 10 bursae are located in the knee, some of which are connected to the synovial cavity. Bursae are located where they can absorb shock or prevent friction.

Movements of the Knee

Flexion and extension of the knee occur in the sagittal plane, whereas internal and external rotation occurs in the horizontal plane:

- *Flexion:* Bending or decreasing the angle of the knee, characterized by the heel moving toward the buttocks
- *Extension:* Straightening or increasing the angle of the knee
- *External rotation:* Rotary motion of the lower leg laterally away from the midline
- *Internal rotation:* Rotary motion of the lower leg medially toward the midline

Muscles of the Knee

The muscles that flex and medially rotate the knee are the hamstrings, sartorius, gracilis, gastrocnemius, and popliteus. The popliteus muscle is the only flexor of the leg found only at the knee. All other flexors are two-joint muscles. Two-joint muscles are most effective when the proximal attachment or distal attachment is fixed by the contraction of the muscles that prevent movement in the direction of the pull.

The popliteus provides posterolateral stability to the knee and assists the medial hamstrings in the internal rotation of the lower leg at the knee. The plantaris and gastrocnemius assist with flexion.

The quadriceps extends the knee. All quadriceps muscles attach to the patella and by the patellar tendon to the tibial tuberosity. All these muscles are superficial and palpable except the vastus intermedius, which is under the rectus femoris. The quadriceps muscles generally are designed to be 25% to 33% stronger than the hamstring muscle group (knee flexors). Proper tracking of the patella is provided by the relationship between the vastus medialis (primarily oblique portion) and vastus lateralis.

The tensor fasciae latae assists with flexion and extension. The semimembranosus and semitendinosus (medial hamstrings) muscles are assisted by the popliteus to rotate the knee internally, whereas the biceps femoris (lateral hamstrings) is responsible for external knee rotation. The pes anserinus is the tendinous expansion of the sartorius, gracilis, and semitendinosus muscles at the medial border of the tibial tuberosity.

Ankle and Foot Region

The ankle joint is made up of the talus, distal tibia, and distal fibula. The ankle joint allows approximately 50 degrees of plantar flexion and 15 to 20 degrees of dorsiflexion. A greater range of dorsiflexion is possible when the knee is flexed, which reduces the tension of the biarticular gastrocnemius muscle.

Inversion and eversion, although commonly thought to be ankle joint movements, technically occur in the subtalar and transverse tarsal joints. These joints combine to allow approximately 20 to 30 degrees of inversion and 5 to 25 degrees of eversion. Minimal movement occurs within the remainder of the intertarsal and tarsometatarsal arthrodial joints.

The structural complexity of the foot is demonstrated by its 26 bones, 19 large muscles, many small (intrinsic) muscles,

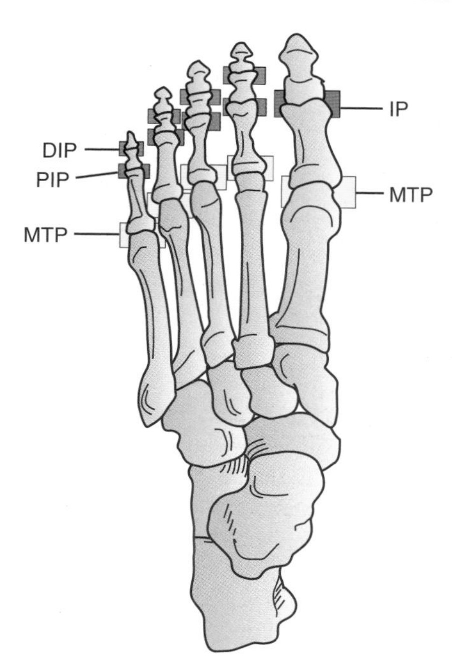

FIG. 10.27 Joints of the phalanges of the foot. *DIP*, Distal interphalangeal; *IP*, interphalangeal; *MTP*, metatarsophalangeal; *PIP*, proximal interphalangeal.

and more than 100 ligaments. The bones of the foot connect with the upper bony structure of the upper body through the fibula and tibia. Body weight is transferred from the tibia to the talus and calcaneus.

Support and propulsion are the two functions of the foot. Proper functioning and adequate development of the muscles of the foot and the practice of proper foot mechanics are essential for everyone. In our modern society, foot trouble is one of the most common ailments. Poor foot mechanics begun in early life invariably led to foot discomfort in later years.

The metatarsophalangeal joint of the great toe flexes 45 degrees and extends 70 degrees, whereas the interphalangeal joint can flex from 0 degree of full extension to 90 degrees of flexion. The metatarsophalangeal joints of the four lesser toes allow approximately 40 degrees of flexion and 40 degrees of extension. The metatarsophalangeal joints also adduct minimally. The proximal interphalangeal joints in the lesser toes flex from 0 degree of extension to 35 degrees of flexion. The distal interphalangeal joints flex 60 degrees and extend 30 degrees. Much variation exists from joint to joint and person to person in all of these joints (Fig. 10.27).

Ligaments in the foot and the ankle have the difficult task of maintaining the position of the arches in the foot. The foot has three longitudinal arches: the medial, lateral, and transverse. Individual long arches vary from high, medium, and low, but a low arch is not necessarily a weak arch.

The medial longitudinal arch is located on the medial side of the foot and extends from the calcaneus to the talus, the navicular, the three cuneiform bones, and the proximal ends of the three medial metatarsals. The lateral longitudinal arch is located on the lateral side of the foot and extends from the calcaneus to the cuboid bone and proximal ends of the fourth and fifth metatarsals. The transverse arch extends across the

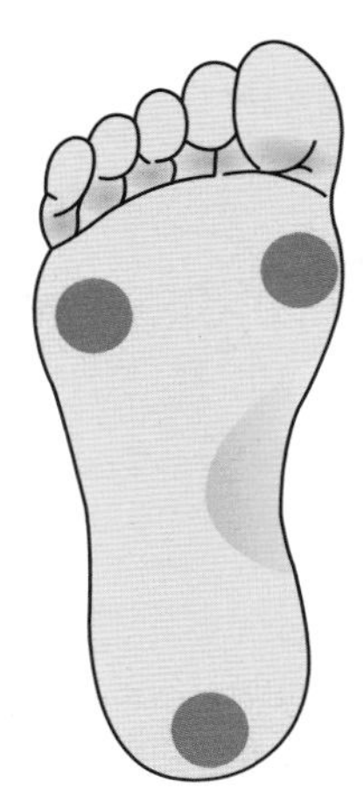

FIG. 10.28 The main weight-bearing surfaces of the foot.

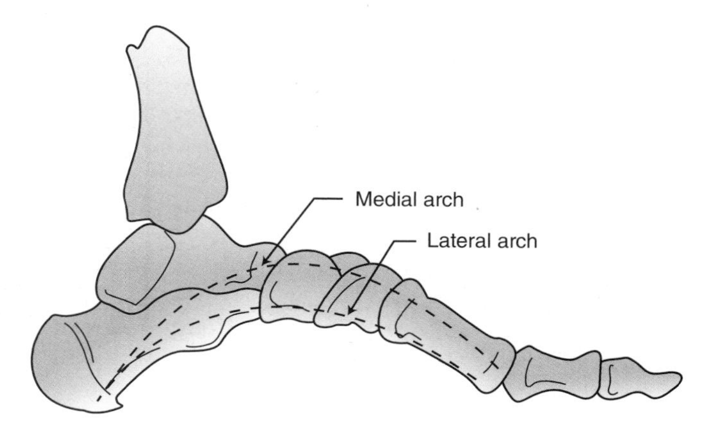

FIG. 10.29 Longitudinal arches of the foot.

foot from one metatarsal bone to the other. A vast network of fascia in the sole of the foot supports the arches. Plantar fascia with the muscles provides the spring to the arch structure (Figs. 10.28 and 10.29).

Movements of the Ankle and Foot

The following are movements of the ankle and foot (Fig. 10.30):

- *Dorsiflexion:* Movement of the top of the ankle and foot toward the anterior tibial bone, accomplished by the flexor muscles of the ankle
- *Plantar flexion:* Movement of the ankle and foot away from the tibia, accomplished by the extensor muscles of the ankle
- *Eversion (pronation):* Turning the ankle and foot outward, away from the midline, with weight on the medial edge of the foot
- *Inversion (supination):* Turning the ankle and foot inward, toward the midline, with weight on the lateral edge of the foot
- *Toe flexion:* Movement of the toes toward the plantar surface of the foot
- *Toe extension:* Movement of the toes away from the plantar surface of the foot

Muscles of the Ankle and Foot

The large number of muscles in the ankle and foot may be grouped according to location and function. In general, the

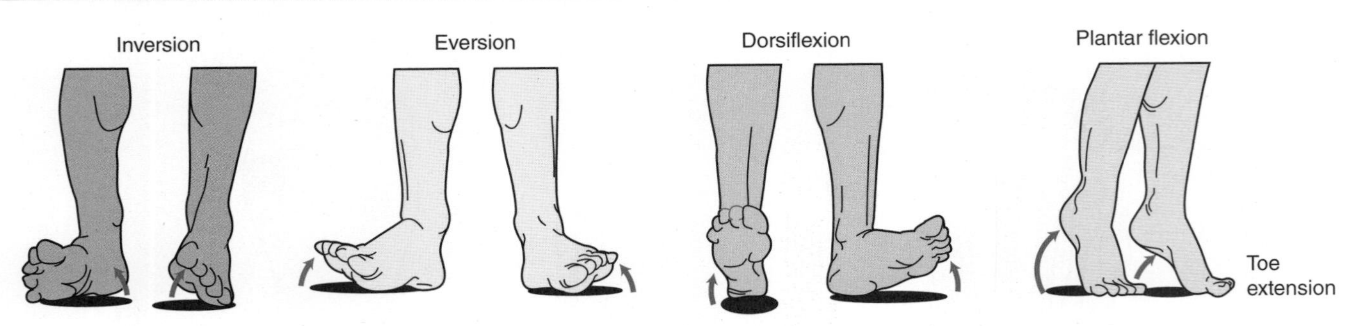

FIG. 10.30 Quick tests for foot and ankle range of motion.

muscles located on the anterior of the ankle and foot are the dorsal flexors. Those to the posterior are plantar flexors. Muscles that are everters are located more to the lateral side, and the invertors are located medially. The muscular strength patterns are not balanced. Plantar flexion is dominant over dorsiflexion, and inversion dominates eversion.

The gastrocnemius muscle is more effective as a knee flexor if the foot is elevated and more effective as a plantar flexor of the foot if the knee is held in extension. You can observe this when someone sits too close to the wheel when driving a car. When the knees are bent, the muscle becomes an ineffective plantar flexor, and the person finds it difficult to depress the brakes.

The soleus muscle is one of the most important plantar flexors of the ankle. This is especially true when the knee is flexed. When the knee is slightly flexed, the effect of the gastrocnemius is reduced, thereby placing more work on the soleus.

The tibialis posterior muscle pulls down from the underside and contracts to invert and plantar flex the foot. Use of the tibialis posterior in plantar flexion and inversion gives support to the longitudinal arch of the foot.

Passing down the back of the lower leg under the medial malleolus and then forward, the flexor digitorum longus muscle draws the four lesser toes down into flexion toward the heel as it plantar flexes the ankle. This muscle is important in helping other foot muscles maintain the longitudinal arch.

Pulling from the underside of the great toe, the flexor hallucis muscle may work independently of the flexor digitorum longus muscle or with it.

The fibularis longus muscle passes behind and beneath the lateral malleolus and under the foot from the outside to the inner surface. Because of its line of pull, the peroneus longus is a strong everter and assists in plantar flexion.

When the fibularis longus muscle is used effectively with the other ankle flexors, it helps support the transverse arch as it flexes.

The fibularis brevis muscle passes down behind and under the lateral malleolus to pull on the base of the fifth metatarsal. The fibularis brevis is a primary everter of the foot and assists in plantar flexion. In addition, the fibularis brevis aids in maintaining the longitudinal arch as it depresses the foot.

The tibialis anterior muscle holds up the inner margin of the foot. However, as it contracts, the tibialis anterior muscle dorsiflexes the ankle and is an antagonist to the plantar flexors of the ankle. The tibialis anterior is forced to contract strongly when a person ice skates or walks on the outside of the foot, and the muscle strongly supports the long arch in inversion.

Strength is necessary for the extensor digitorum longus muscle to maintain the balance between the plantar and the dorsal flexors. The strength of the ankle is evident when the gastrocnemius, soleus, tibialis posterior, fibularis longus, fibularis brevis, digitorum longus, flexor digitorum brevis, and flexor hallucis longus muscles are all used effectively in walking.

Intrinsic Muscles of the Foot

The intrinsic muscles of the foot have their proximal attachment and distal attachment on the bones within the foot. Four layers of these muscles are found on the plantar surface of the foot. These muscles are involved with dorsiflexion and plantar flexion of the toes:

- *First layer (most superficial):* Adductor hallucis, flexor digitorum brevis, and abductor digiti quinti pedis
- *Second layer:* Quadratus plantae and lumbricales (four)
- *Third layer:* Flexor hallucis brevis, flexor digiti quinti brevis pedis, and adductor hallucis
- *Fourth layer (deepest):* Interossei (seven) (Activity 10.5)

Section Summary

- Describe two types of information assessed using movement patterns.
  - The capacity for prime movers/synergists to concentrically shorten and the capacity for antagonists to eccentrically lengthen.
- Give an example of resistance and stabilization application during assessment.
  - Stabilization is used to ensure only the assessed area moves (applied near the moving joint). Resistance is applied at the distal end of the lever system of the area being assessed. Example: shoulder flexion—stabilization is focused on the scapula (to assure that only the glenohumeral joint moves)—resistance is focused at the distal end of the humerus (not at the wrist).
- Give an example of clinical reasoning applied to individual joint assessment.
  - If pain occurs during passive joint movement, joint capsular dysfunction and/or nerve entrapment may be causal. If pain occurs during active joint movement, muscle/fascial dysfunction may be causal. Thus, if pain occurs during active joint movement but *not* during passive joint movement, it is more likely muscle/fascial dysfunction is causal than joint capsular dysfunction.
- Assess individual joint range of motion.
  - See Fig. 10.15.

ACTIVITY 10.5

In this activity, you will be working with a partner to assess individual movement patterns, normal function, and possible dysfunction in each other. First, one of you should isolate the specified movement patterns on each side of your partner, one side at a time, and assess for normal function by applying gentle pressure opposite to the action of the isolation position. The body should be stabilized so that only the isolated area is moving. In some instances, the ability to assume the position and maintain it indicates normal function. Muscles should be able to hold against gravity or the applied pressure without strain or pain. The position itself should be easy to assume and comfortable to maintain for a short duration—10 to 30 seconds. The bilateral movement patterns should be the same. The opposite movement pattern also should be able to be done easily.

Dysfunction may be indicated by bilateral asymmetry, pain, weakness, fatigue, a heavy sensation (binding), and the inability to assume the isolation position or move into the opposite position. Intervention or referral depends on the severity of the condition and whether the dysfunction is neuromuscular, myofascial, or joint related.

Note: Do not perform these assessments if contraindications exist. Contraindications to this type of assessment include joint and disk dysfunction, acute pain, recent trauma, and inflammation.

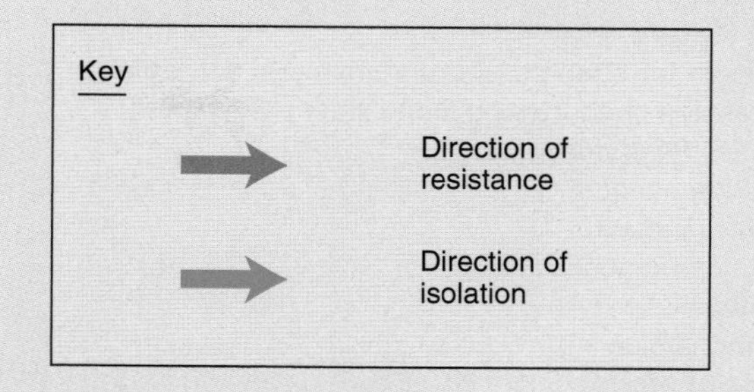

ACTIVITY 10.5—cont'd

Knee Flexion

Assesses for strength and endurance in the isolation position and tension or shortening in the extension pattern

Muscles Involved

Biceps femoris
Semitendinosus
Semimembranosus
Popliteus
Gastrocnemius

Range of Motion

0 to 150 degrees

Position of Client

Prone, with limbs straight and toes hanging over the edge of the table

Examiner applies light to moderate counterpressure to hamstrings

Isolation and Assessment

Client flexes knee through the full range, keeping thigh in contact with the table. Examiner applies resistance gradually to the posterior leg proximal to the ankle joint after the knee reaches 45 degrees to straighten the leg.

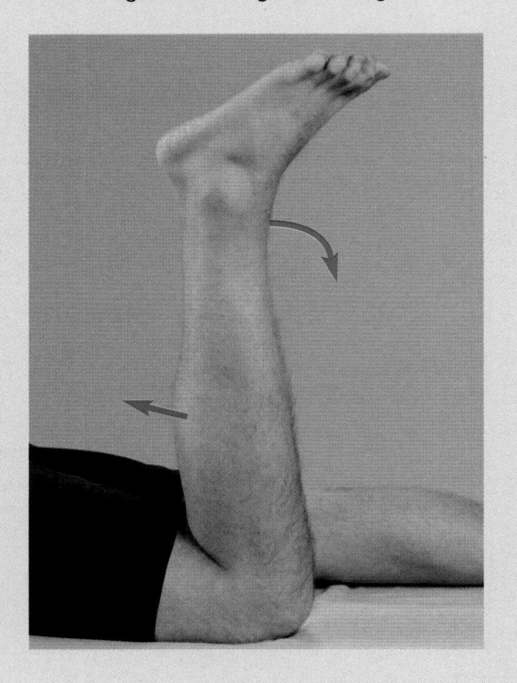

Knee Extension

Assesses for strength and endurance in the isolation position and tension or shortening in the flexion pattern

Muscles Involved

Rectus femoris
Vastus intermedius
Vastus lateralis
Vastus medialis

Range of Motion

0 to 135 degrees

May extend 10 degrees beyond 0 in those with hyperextension

Position of Client

Seated, with hips flexed and a small pillow under the thigh to maintain 90 degrees of hip flexion

Client grasps table edge for stabilization while examiner places one hand on the distal anterior thigh

Isolation and Assessment

Client extends the knee through the available range of motion as the examiner applies resistance to the distal end of the anterior leg to bend it at the knee. Do not allow the client to hyperextend the knee or lift the thigh off the table.

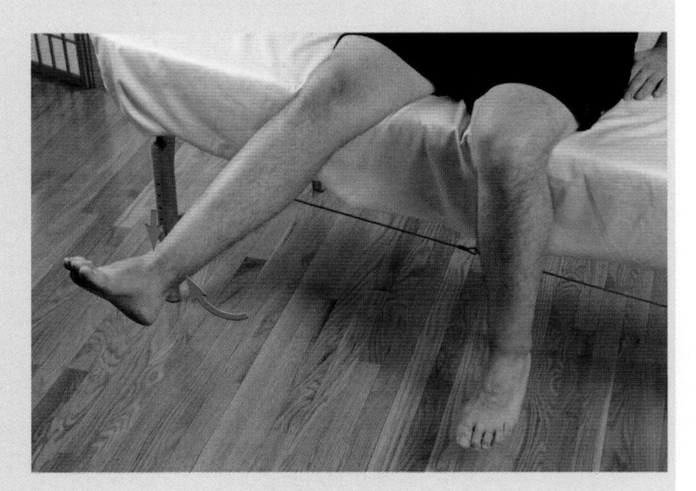

ACTIVITY 10.5—cont'd

Plantar Flexion

Assesses for strength and endurance in the isolation position and tension or shortening in the dorsiflexion pattern

Muscles Involved

Gastrocnemius
Soleus
Flexor digitorum longus
Flexor hallucis longus
Plantaris
Tibialis posterior

Range of Motion

0 to 50 degrees

Position of Client

Gastrocnemius: Prone, with the ankle dorsiflexed off the end of the table and knee extended

Soleus: Prone, with knee flexed and ankle dorsiflexed

Isolation and Assessment (Both Positions)

Client initiates plantar flexion of the ankle through the available range of motion while the examiner applies resistance to the posterior calcaneus or sole of the foot to push the foot into dorsiflexion.

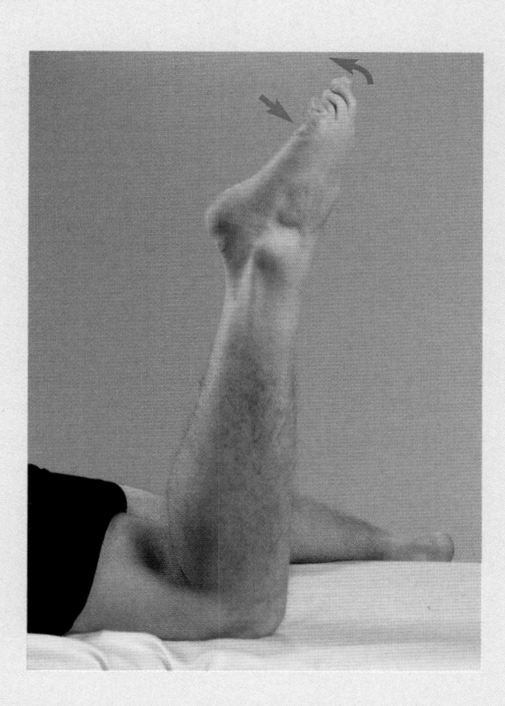

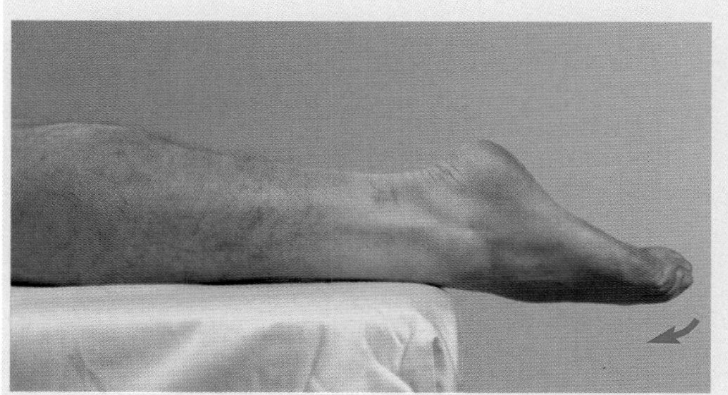

Foot Dorsiflexion

Assesses for strength and endurance in the isolation position and tension or shortening in the plantar flexion pattern

Muscles Involved

Tibialis anterior
Fibularis tertius
Extensor digitorum longus (extensor of lesser toes)
Extensor hallucis longus (greater toe extensor)

Range of Motion

0 to 20 degrees

Position of Client

Supine with leg straight

Isolation and Assessment

Client initiates dorsiflexion of the ankle, keeping toes relaxed, and examiner applies resistance to pull the foot into plantar flexion.

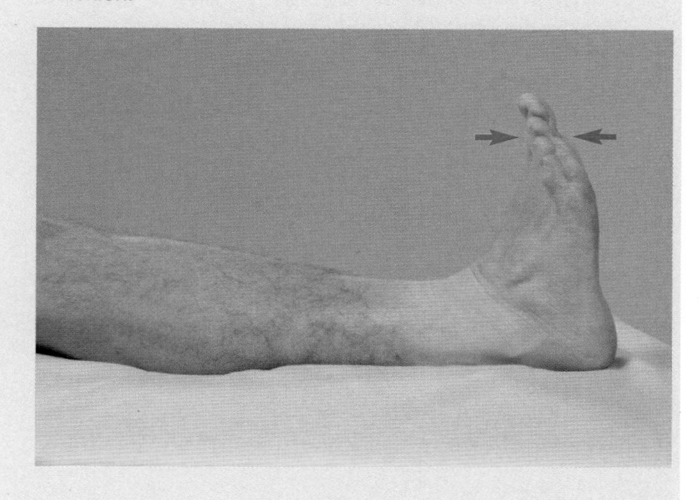

Continued

ACTIVITY 10.5—cont'd

Foot Inversion

Assesses for strength and endurance in the isolation position and tension or shortening in the eversion pattern

Muscles Involved

Tibialis anterior
Tibialis posterior
Flexor digitorum longus (flexor of lesser toes)
Flexor hallucis longus (great toe flexor)
Gastrocnemius (medial head)

Range of Motion

0 to 30 degrees

Position of Client

Supine or side-lying on the test side with the ankle in a neutral position

Isolation and Assessment

Client inverts foot through the available range of motion as examiner applies resistance to the medial edge of the forefoot to pull it into eversion. Client keeps toes relaxed.

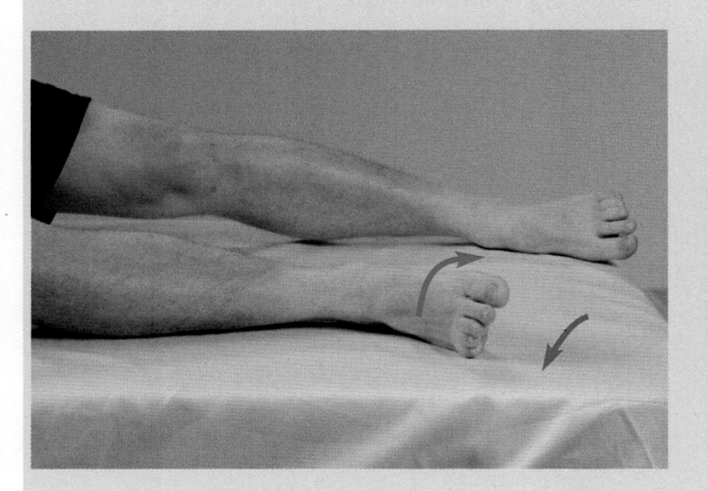

Foot Eversion

Assesses for strength and endurance in the isolation position and tension or shortening in the inversion pattern

Muscles Involved

Fibularis longus
Fibularis brevis
Fibularis tertius
Extensor digitorum longus

Range of Motion

0 to 15 degrees

Position of Client

Supine or side-lying on the nontest side with the ankle in a neutral position

Isolation and Assessment

Client everts foot through full range while examiner applies resistance to the lateral edge of the foot to pull it into inversion.

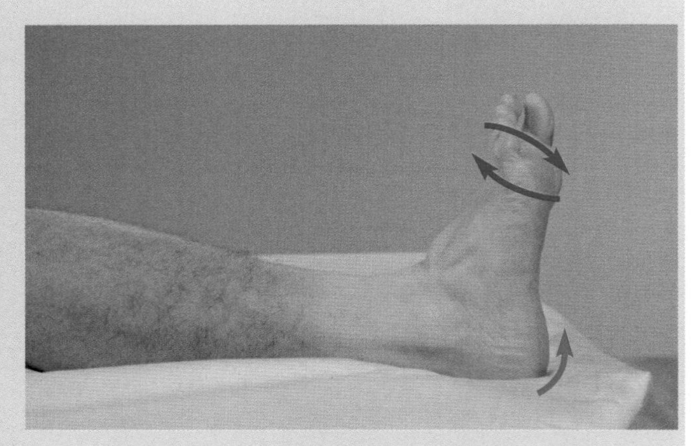

ACTIVITY 10.5—cont'd

Toe Flexion

Assesses for strength and endurance in the isolation position and tension or shortening in the extension pattern

Muscles Involved

Flexor digitorum longus
Flexor digitorum brevis
Flexor hallucis longus
Flexor hallucis brevis
Flexor digiti minimi brevis
Lumbricales
Interossei (dorsal and plantar)

Range of Motion

Great toe: 0 to 45 degrees
Lateral four toes: 0 to 40 degrees

Position of Client

Supine with foot and ankle in a neutral position
Examiner stabilizes metatarsals

Isolation and Assessment

Great toe is tested separately from the lateral four toes. Client flexes great toe while examiner applies light resistance to the plantar surface of proximal phalange to push it into extension. Client flexes four toes while the examiner applies light resistance to the plantar surface of proximal phalanges to push each toe into extension.

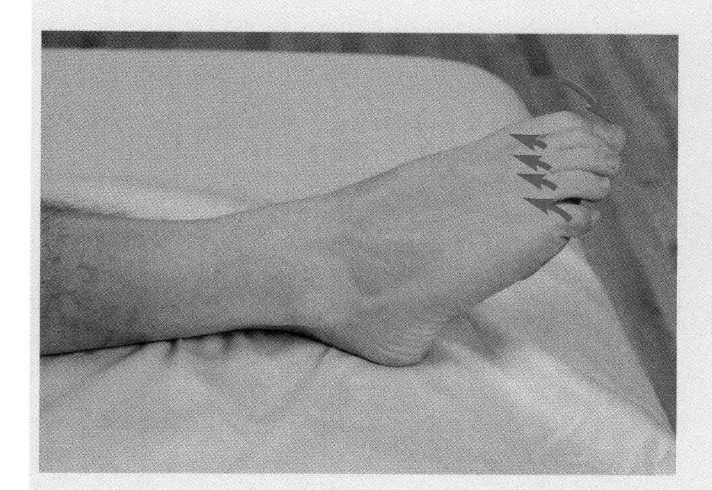

Toe Extension

Assesses for strength and endurance in the isolation position and tension or shortening in the flexion pattern

Muscles Involved

Extensor digitorum longus
Extensor digitorum brevis
Extensor hallucis longus

Range of Motion

Great toe: 0 to 70 degrees
Lateral four toes: 0 to 40 degrees

Position of Client

Supine with foot and ankle in a neutral position
Examiner stabilizes metatarsals

Isolation and Assessment

Great toe is tested separately from the lateral four toes. Client extends great toe while examiner applies light resistance to the dorsal surface of proximal phalange to pull it into flexion. Client extends four toes while examiner applies light resistance to the dorsal surface of proximal phalanges to pull each toe into flexion.

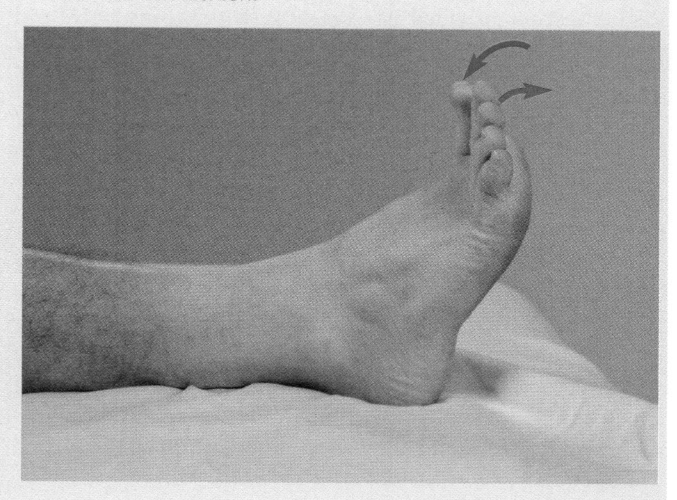

Continued

- Assess the body by region.
  - Study Biomechanics by Region (see Figs. 10.15–10.30, Activities 10.1–10.5, and Table 10.1).

PATHOLOGICAL CONDITIONS

SECTION OBJECTIVES

Chapter objective covered in this section:

7. Identify and describe the three main biomechanical dysfunctional patterns and the associated indications and contraindications for massage.

After completing this section, the learner will be able to:

- Categorize biomechanical dysfunction.
- Describe three degrees of postural imbalance.
- Describe three degrees of distorted motor function.
- Classify biomechanical dysfunction into three stages.

The Practical Application at the end of the chapter provides assessments and suggested treatments for kinetic chain function and dysfunction related to gait. The Biomechanics by Region section provided assessment activities using active and passive joint movement to assess for range of motion, in addition to providing body positioning for muscle strength testing. Together these assessments provide data to determine biomechanical dysfunction.

Biomechanical dysfunctions include local functional block, local hypermobility or hypomobility, altered firing patterns, and postural imbalance, which lead to changes in motor function. Differential diagnosis to determine the causal factors of biomechanical dysfunction is beyond the scope of this text. However, the modalities studied in the specific application of massage therapy have much to offer in the normalization of some types of movement dysfunction. The four areas most effectively addressed by these methods are postural, neuromuscular-related, myofascial-related, and joint-related dysfunction.

FOCUS ON PROFESSIONALISM

Recall that there are four main outcomes that clients request when they receive a massage: relaxation, stress management, pain management, and functional mobility. The content in this chapter provides the platform to address the goals of pain management and functional mobility. Clients want results from the massage and will pay for a massage that is relaxing and supports stress management, especially when this occurs at the same time physical assessment is occurring. The information in this chapter needs to be used to perfect assessment skills so that you are able to adapt massage to a particular client's goals. Clients pay for results.

There are multiple approaches and classifications for describing biomechanical dysfunction. It is helpful to simplify patterns of dysfunction and some models are presented. Predictable neuromuscular chain reactions can occur. As described by Vladimir Janda, these chain reactions can be divided into two patterns: the upper and lower crossed syndromes (Figs. 10.31 and 10.32) (Chaitow and DeLany, 2008). The upper and lower crossed syndromes may be related to dysfunction in the kinetic chain functions of stability and mobility, particularly involving myofascial slings described by Dr. Vleming. These concepts often appear together in the discussion of musculoskeletal pain syndromes (Page et al., 2010; Fernández-de-las-Peñas, 2015; Rutte and Patijn, 2015).

Dr. Shirley Sahrmann also has described functional movement system impairment syndromes based on the concepts of sustained alignment in a nonideal position; repeated movements in a specific direction are associated with several musculoskeletal conditions in various body regions. The model emphasizes the contribution of (1) the musculoskeletal system as the effector of movement, (2) the nervous system as the regulator of movement, and (3) the cardiovascular, pulmonary, and endocrine systems, which provide support for the other systems but also are affected by movement (Sahrmann et al., 2017).

The Four-Element Movement System Model describes primary elements (motion, force, motor control, and energy) essential to the performance of all movements.

- Motion: ability of a joint or tissue to be moved passively.
- Force: ability of the contractile (i.e., muscles) and non-contractile structures (i.e., tendons) to produce movement and provide dynamic stability around joints during static and dynamic tasks.
- Motor control: ability to plan, execute, and adapt goal-directed movements such that they are accurate, coordinated, and efficient.
- Energy: the ability to perform sustained or repeated movements and is dependent on the integrated functioning of the cardiovascular, pulmonary, and neuromuscular systems.

The 4-Element Model is a systematic observational assessment approach using five observation targets abbreviated as CASSS (control, amount, speed, symmetry, symptoms).

- Control: smoothness, coordination, and timing of movement
- Amount: amplitude (range, magnitude, or distance) of movement at each joint
- Symmetry: observed in bilateral tasks or comparing unilateral performance between limbs; speed is the length of time
- Symptoms: stiffness, pain, instability, or fatigue.

Potential impairments are identified to implement treatment strategies (Zarzycki et al., 2022).

There are other systems, but as massage therapists, we need to develop care plans that are within our scope of practice. The following information guides the critical thinking process relevant to massage therapy practice.

Common Postural Deviations

Because standing is a closed kinetic chain activity (see Chapter 8) and because of the tensegric nature of body form, the position or motion of one joint affects the positions or motions of other joints.

Generally, if a person tends to maintain a posture in which a curve is increased, the muscles on the concave side tend to shorten and tighten, whereas the muscles on the convex side tend to become long and weak but still feel tight. For example, a client with lumbar lordosis will likely have tight and short

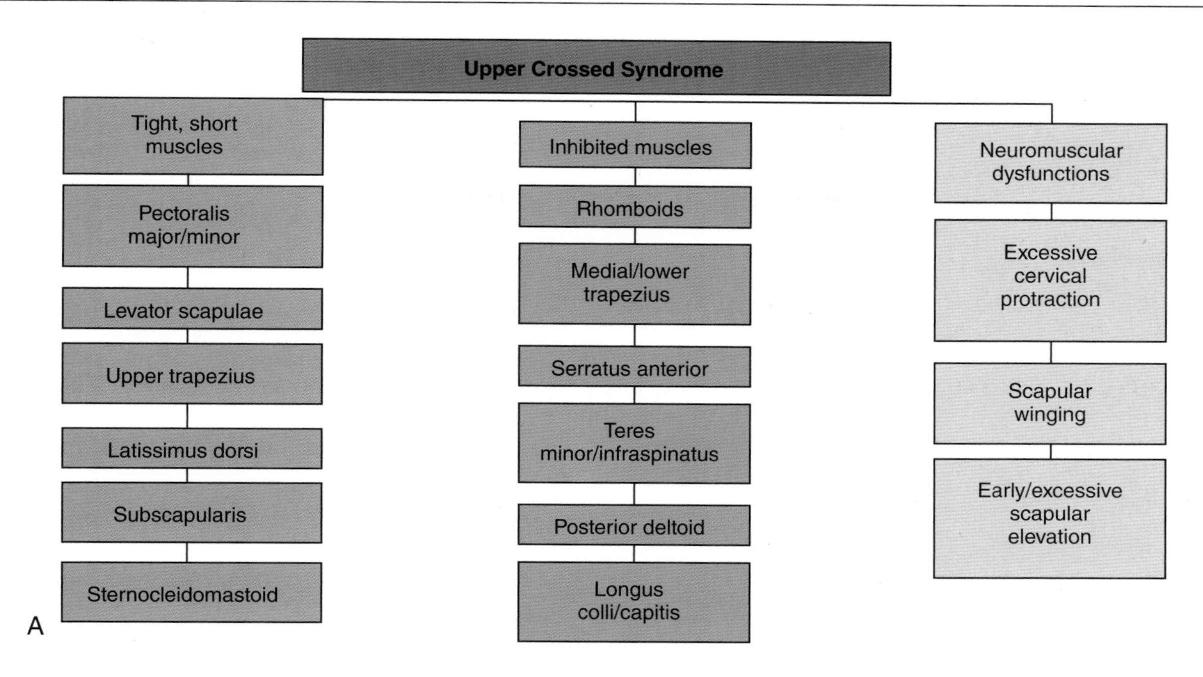

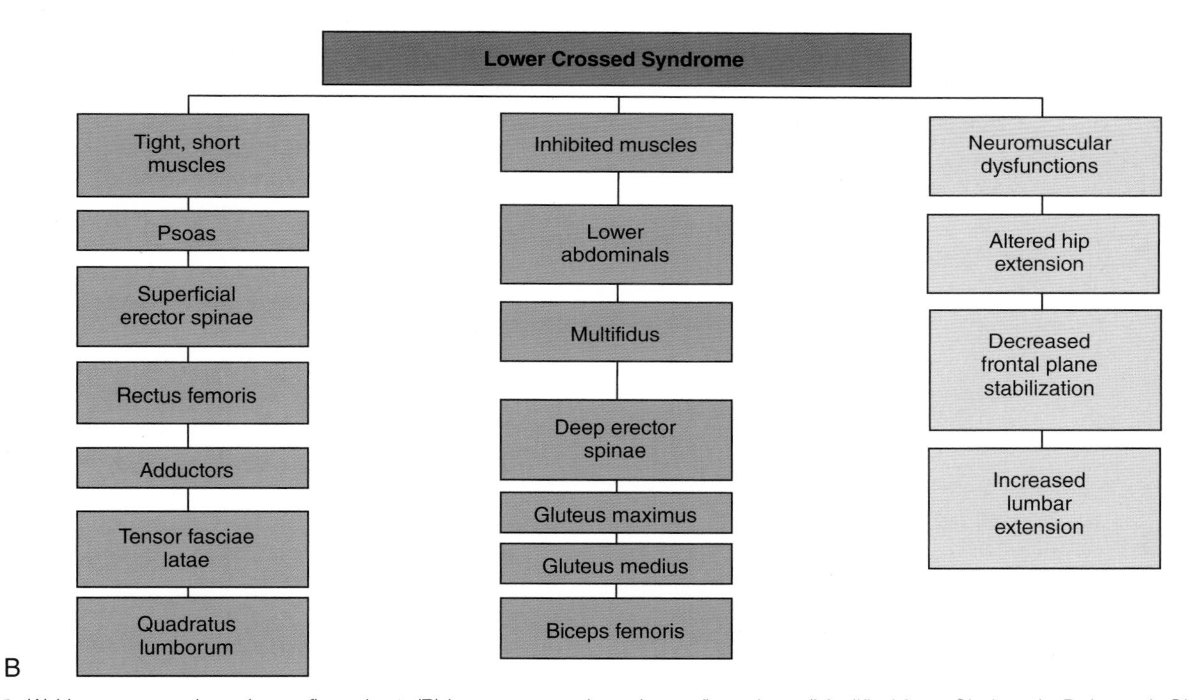

FIG. 10.31 (A) Upper crossed syndrome flow chart. (B) Lower crossed syndrome flow chart. (Modified from Chaitow L, DeLany J. *Clinical Applications of Neuromuscular Techniques. Vol. 1, The Upper Body*. 2nd ed. Churchill Livingstone/Elsevier; 2008.)

back extensors and weak and long abdominal muscles. Massage application helps reverse the functional strain by addressing the shortening on the concave side and stimulating the inhibited muscles on the convex side of the curve. Stretching is required for the short areas and appropriate exercise for the long areas (Fig. 10.33).

This book does not describe the individual causes and effects of postural problems. However, we can make some general statements regarding cause and effect:

- Poor posture can result from structural problems that may be caused by congenital malformation or acquired through trauma, such as a compression fracture.
- Postural deviations also may result from neurological conditions causing paralysis or spasticity.
- Most postural problems are functional, or nonstructural. For example, a person who sits or stands for lengthy periods tends to slouch, resulting in a muscle imbalance, which causes positional strain.

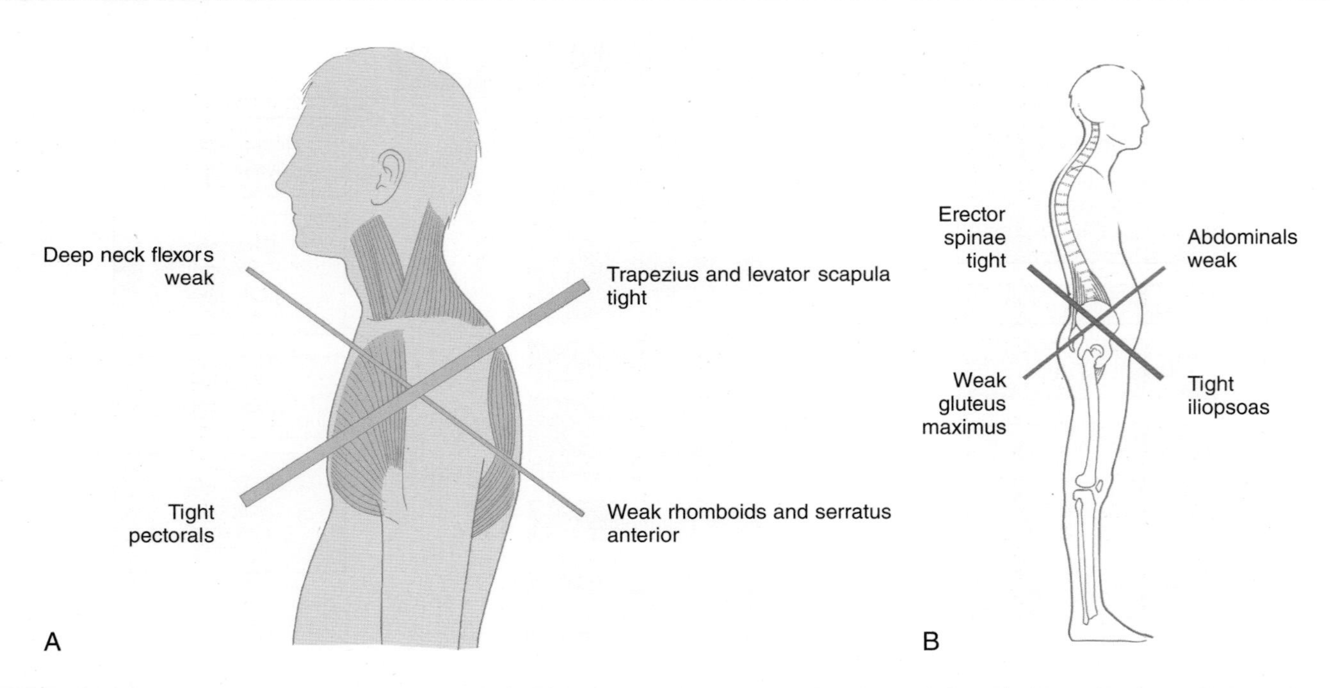

FIG. 10.32 (A) Upper crossed syndrome (after Janda). (B) Lower crossed syndrome (after Janda). (Modified from Chaitow L, DeLany J. *Clinical Applications of Neuromuscular Techniques. Vol. 1, The Upper Body*. 2nd ed. Churchill Livingstone/Elsevier; 2008.)

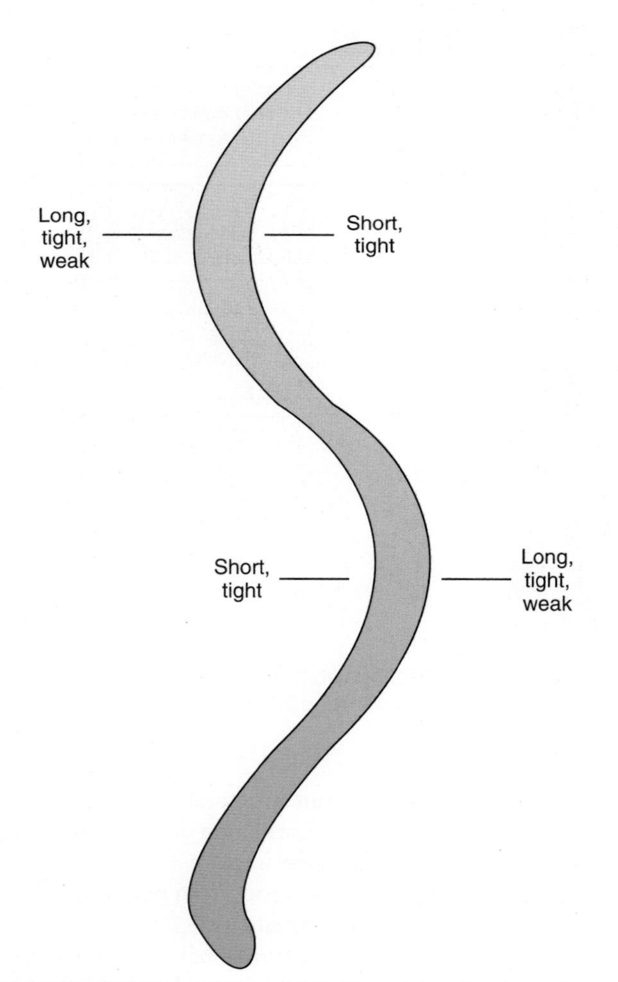

FIG. 10.33 First, massage application lengthens the short, tight areas. Coupled with therapeutic exercise, massage then stimulates the long, tight, and weak areas.

- Many postural problems are due to problems with core stability and distortion in normal vertebral curves.
- Postural problems can occur if the arches of the feet are abnormal or if the ankles are unstable.

Efficient posture can be achieved as follows:

- Head is lifted and the chin drawn back.
- Eyes are forward and level with the horizontal plane.
- Shoulders roll back and down, and the medial borders of the scapula move toward each other.
- Thorax at the sternum moves out and down.
- Core muscles engage as the abdomen is drawn in and the lumbar area moves back and flattens a bit, reducing lordosis.
- The pelvis tips slightly posteriorly as the lower back flattens and the symphysis pubis moves up.
- Sacrum moves down vertically.
- Thighs shift back; the leg (below the knee) shifts forward.
- Weight is distributed to the feet.
- Feet are flat with the weight distributed somewhat evenly but with a slight increase to the heel of the foot, which will act to lift the body vertically.

This pattern should be taught to clients with postural problems. When in this posture, the person will feel taller.

Regional Postural Muscular Imbalance

Muscles and muscle groups have a constant muscular tone that is regulated by the central nervous system. Some muscles have higher tone, such as those that support the vertical position of the body, and others are necessary for functions, such as eating and breathing. Postural stress, pattern overload, repetitive movement, lack of core stability, and lack of neuromuscular efficiency cause biomechanical neuromuscular imbalances. Most often, the tone of postural muscles, which have greater tone, to begin with, increases and thus the imbalance appears. The muscles tense and shorten, inhibiting muscles that function for movement and causing sensations of fatigue and heaviness in the limbs.

Nonoptimal Motor Function

All human beings create optimal carriage—how they uniquely hold and move their bodies—and optimal motor function. Optimal motor function defines the degree of mobility that the body needs to operate in the most economical way. When all goes well, movement usually proceeds efficiently. With pathological changes, however, motor function changes as well. Carriage is disturbed, joint mobility becomes limited, tissues and joints are altered, and the tone-strength balance in the tissues is altered. The person spends more energy performing normal movements, which causes fatigue more quickly. The change of the optimal motor function influences the work of the viscera, which in turn influences the condition of the muscles and joints and in turn, alters motor function and carriage even more. Thus a vicious cycle starts in which the worsening of different processes negatively contributes to each process.

Neuromuscular-Related Dysfunction

Neuromuscular-related dysfunction manifests as a breakdown or confusion in the nervous system's interaction with muscle activity. Neuromuscular dysfunction can develop in many forms, including:

- Neurotransmitter fluctuations
- Hypermuscular or hypomuscular activity and altered muscle activation sequences (firing patterns)
- Increased tension in individual motor units or the entire muscle
- Hypersensitivity or hyposensitivity in the proprioceptive feedback loop and reflex arcs
- Central nervous system processing difficulties
- Gait reflex and kinetic chain disturbance

The myotonic unit becomes disrupted, with patterns of overly tense muscles and corresponding weakened or reciprocally inhibited muscles. All these patterns can be reduced to two: regional postural muscular imbalance and nonoptimal motor function.

Myofascial-Related Dysfunction

Connective tissue changes occur as function is altered or as the result of trauma, including microtrauma caused by accumulated overuse. We have described and discussed connective tissue in previous chapters of this textbook; reviewing these sections, primarily in Chapters 8 and 9, would be prudent.

Practically speaking, most often connective tissue loses hydration, which affects the viscous and plastic qualities and results in shortening, reduced sliding, and reduced pliability.

Connective tissues also can become overstretched and lax, reducing their ability to stabilize the body. Joint hypermobility syndrome is a connective tissue disorder. Ligaments hold joints together and keep them from moving too much or too far out of range. In people with joint hypermobility syndrome, those ligaments are loose or weak. Symptomatic hypermobility can be due to:

- Disorders of connective tissue, like Ehlers-Danlos syndromes, Marfan syndrome, Stickler syndrome, osteogenesis imperfect, and others.
- Joint shape, looser ligaments, or poor muscle tone (without a connective tissue disorder)
- Injury or repeated stretching/training (e.g., in yoga enthusiasts and gymnasts)

Joint-Related Dysfunction

Joint-related dysfunction can be within the capsule itself or noncapsular. The most common noncapsular pattern is the *functional block*, which is the reversible limitation of the range of movement that occurs because of a change in connective tissue after long-term muscle spasms. The muscle spasm first appears as a reflex defense mechanism against painful movement in an affected jointed area. Immobility of the joint increases the stagnation of tissues, which leads to more pain, resulting in the development of the pain-spasm-pain cycle.

Contributing factors to functional block development include:

- Holding a weight that is too heavy for too long
- Constant loading on the spine, such as occurs during work situations that demand long-term sitting
- Powerful effort, such as that used in lifting during sport or work
- Passive overstretching, such as holding a heavy weight in the hand, which can cause the development of functional block in the shoulder joint
- Reflex influences on muscles near joints
- Long-term immobility, such as when wearing a cast or when bedridden

The appropriate medical professional needs to assess, diagnose, and treat specific joint dysfunction. Massage application can complement the intervention of professionals, such as orthopedic physicians, osteopathic physicians, chiropractors, physical therapists, and athletic trainers.

INDICATIONS/CONTRAINDICATIONS for Therapeutic Massage

In postural imbalance, some postural muscles are shortened and their antagonists are weakened. Motor function is altered as a result. Postural imbalance often manifests as lumbar and cervical hyperlordosis but also could lead to other changes in the spine and joints of the limbs. The four transitional areas where the myofascial diagrams are found are vulnerable areas because these locations allow rotation and therefore are common points for compensation. Consider the balance of function in a kinetic chain, including myofascial and neuromuscular muscle synergies, by assessing firing patterns/activation sequences and gait. Consider individual joint function in relation to whole body adaptation. These changes often play a pathogenic role in movement and add to the adaptive strain and nociceptive load experienced by clients.

When assessing the client's posture, recall that neutral posture is when joints are not bent and the spine is aligned and not twisted. No one has a consistent neutral posture in the standing position. Everyone is asymmetrical to some degree. However, alignment of body segments correlates with minimal amounts of stress to allow for ease of movement in all directions. Thus, functional posture and relative structural balance are important. It is logical that the more asymmetrical a person is in the standing position, the more strained their maintenance of posture and production of movement. The body has an amazing ability to adapt, and massage therapists need to understand resourceful compensation related to functional posture and movement. It is not necessary to change posture specifically or alter movement using massage therapy interventions. Instead, understand the adaptive responses and support the compensation and any corrective exercise programs the client may be participating in with other health care professionals (Henning et al., 2017).

The tender/trigger point phenomenon, whatever physiology is involved, is a consistent indicator of symptom patterns. If involved in the symptom pattern, these areas become nociceptive generators. The points are typically located in areas of neurovascular bundles and pressing hard on any of the areas will elicit a pain sensation. Only the points that create sensations similar to the client's symptoms should be addressed. Massage therapists can borrow the assessment process called STAR from osteopathic discipline (Kuchera, 2007). STAR is specific to palpation assessment. Massage applied mindfully *is* a palpation assessment and gathers the following information:

- **S**ensitivity to measured palpation
- **T**issue texture changes
- **A**symmetry
- **R**estricted motion

Interventions for tender points include a variety of methods to calm the nociceptive input. The intervention methods should be gentle, avoiding an increase in symptoms during and after method application. The most common is broad-based compression on the tender point with just enough pressure so the client begins to experience the symptoms. There should be no tensing or guarding, and the client should experience the sensation at the "right spot." Then the client slowly moves the adjacent joints within their easiest range of motion.

Functional block may be treated successfully by massage techniques for relaxation, stress, and pain management; mobilization techniques (e.g., repeated passive movement and traction); muscle energy techniques (e.g., various forms of active muscle contraction followed by muscle lengthening); and flexibility and stability programs to address outcomes of functional mobility.

Caution is required for hypermobility syndromes. Massage therapy can manage the soft tissue discomfort around the hypermobile joints but the joints should not be moved beyond normal range of motion.

Degrees and Stages of Dysfunction

It is common to categorize dysfunction as an aid for the development of treatment plans. There are generally three degrees of postural imbalance and distorted motor function. Depending on the combined dysfunctions, the client's condition can be categorized into three stages of severity.

Postural Imbalance

Three degrees of postural imbalance of muscles may occur:

- *First degree:* Shortening or weakening of some muscles or the formation of local changes in tension or connective tissue in these muscles
- *Second degree:* Moderately expressed shortening of postural muscles and weakening of antagonist muscles
- *Third degree:* Clearly expressed shortening of postural muscles and weakening of antagonist muscles with the appearance of specific, nonoptimal movement

Assessment defines mobility through active and passive movements of the affected parts and observation of distortion in these movements. In addition, muscle testing can show the functional relationships of the muscles. To determine the appropriate therapeutic intervention, defining which muscles are shortened and which are inhibited is important for chronic joint, muscular, and nervous system disorders.

Distorted Motor Function

There are three degrees of distorted motor function:

- *First degree:* For usual and simple movements, a person has to use additional muscles from different parts of the body. As a result, movement becomes uneconomical and labored.
- *Second degree:* Moderately peculiar postures and movements of some parts of the body are present. Postural and movement distortion, such as altered firing patterns, begins to occur.
- *Third degree:* Significantly expressed peculiarity in postures and movement occurs. Increased postural and movement distortions result.

Biomechanical Dysfunction

Pathobiomechanical disturbances may occur in all age groups. Based on the three degrees of distorted motor function, there are three stages in the development of postural and movement pathological conditions:

- *Stage 1, functional tension:* At this stage, a person tires more quickly than normal. This fatigue is accompanied by some functional block in the first- or second-degree limitation of mobility, painless local myodystonia (changes in the muscle tension/length relationship), postural imbalance in the first or second degree, and nonoptimal motor function of the first degree.
- *Stage 2, functional stress:* This stage is characterized by a feeling of fatigue after moderate activity; discomfort, slight pain, and the appearance of singular or multiple functional blocks; and any degree of limited mobility. Functional block may be painless or result in first-degree pain; it may be accompanied by local hypermobility. Functional stress also is characterized by fascial/connective tissue changes, regional postural imbalance, and distortion of motor function in the first or second degree.
- *Stage 3, connective tissue changes in the musculoskeletal system:* The reasons for connective tissue changes are overloading, tissue malnutrition, microtraumas, microhemorrhages, unresolved edema, and other endogenous and exogenous factors. Genetic predisposition is also a consideration. In stage 3, osteochondrosis of the spine and weight-bearing joints may appear as single or multiple functional blocks, local hypermobility and instability of several vertebral motion segments, hypomobility, widespread painful muscle tension and fascial and connective tissue changes in the muscles, regional postural imbalance in the second or third degree in many joints, and temporary nonoptimal motor function with second- or third-degree distortion. Visceral disturbances may be present (Gurevich, 1992) (Box 10.3).

Box 10.3 How Textbook Content Translates Into Practical Application

A client has arrived for a massage. Begin with an updated history and physical assessment.

A client tells you their shoulder hurts when they move it.

You ask them to show you what movement hurts.

They put their hands on their hips.

As soon as the client has demonstrated the position, you can identify that this is internal rotation of the shoulder.

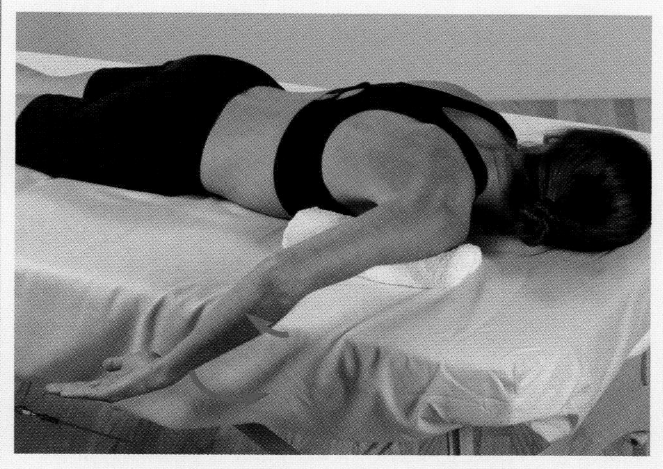

Shoulder internal (medial) rotation causes discomfort, and the opposite movement is shoulder external (lateral) rotation.

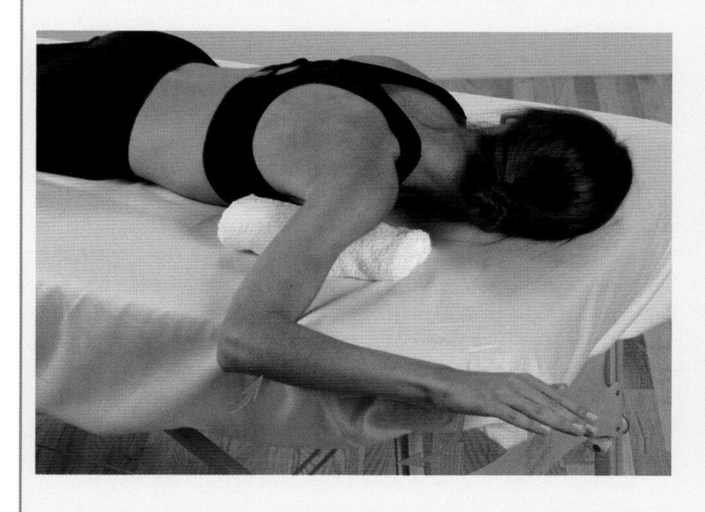

Textbook Investigation: Shoulder Internal or Medial Rotation

- Muscles involved (use Chapter 9 to identify more information about each muscle):
  - Subscapularis
  - Pectoralis major
  - Latissimus dorsi
  - Teres major
  - Deltoid (anterior)
- Range of motion (provides normal functional range):
  - 0 to 80 degrees

How to Assess

Position of client: Prone with shoulder abducted to 90 degrees, upper arm supported on a table, elbow flexed, and forearm hanging over the edge of the table. Examiner stabilizes the upper arm.

Isolation and Assessment

Client moves forearm through internal rotation (backward and upward) while examiner applies resistance to forearm above wrist to push it down.

Shoulder External or Lateral Rotation

Described functional assessment: Antagonist/opposite movement area strength and endurance in the isolation position and tension or shortening in the shoulder internal or medial rotation pattern.

Muscles involved (use Chapter 9 to identify more information about each muscle):

Infraspinatus

Teres minor

Deltoid (posterior)

Range of Motion

0 to 90 degrees

Position of Client

Prone, with head turned toward the test side

Shoulder is abducted to 90 degrees with upper arm fully supported on a table, elbow flexed, and forearm hanging over the edge of the table.

Isolation and Assessment

Client moves forearm upward toward the level of the table, keeping an upper arm on the table, while examiner applies resistance to distal forearm above the wrist to push it down.

NOTE: Notice that the movements in this section of the textbook are organized into pairs: flexions/extensions, adductions/abductions, and in this instance, external/internal rotation.

The blue arrow on the screen images indicates the direction of muscle isolation, and the red arrow indicates the direction of force used for muscle testing. You should recognize that this is an agonist-antagonist interaction.

The shoulder internal rotators and external rotators are agonist and antagonist pairs, which means that both actions will be involved as you work with the client—so you read about both movements and then begin the massage.

Joint Movement Assessment

During massage application, all of the joints should be moved through the client's easy range of motion and assessed to identify if they are within normal range or are hypermobile or hypomobile.

Assessment indicates 60 degrees of internal shoulder rotation.

During the massage, you assess the shoulder movement and find a limited internal rotation. From your textbook, you know that the range of motion for internal rotation should be 0 to 80 degrees. The client's internal rotation is about 60 degrees.

What are the Possibilities?

Now that you have some data, it is time to think about what might be involved in causing the client's symptoms and what is responsible for the limited range of motion. It is unrealistic to expect that you will remember all the details about individual muscles; that is why knowing how to look up information is so important.

Two situations may be occurring: The shoulder joint itself could be dysfunctional, or the muscles and soft tissue involved in external rotation are short and limiting the internal rotation.

A pattern is beginning to emerge as you think about the limited range of motion for internal rotation identified during

Box 10.3 How Textbook Content Translates Into Practical Application—cont'd

assessment of the client's shoulder. If for some reason the external shoulder rotators were short, they would restrict the ability of the shoulder to move into internal rotation. During massage, it is common to ask clarifying questions to help determine the best course of action.

You ask the client if they have recently done something that would have had them hold their arm in external rotation. Clients often do not know what the terminology means, so it is helpful to demonstrate external rotation.

They think awhile and then remember they had been doing some new exercises at the gym. You ask them to explain and show the position of the exercises.

Indications and Contraindications: Should I or Shouldn't I?

It is important to determine if the client should be referred for diagnosis or if the reason for the dysfunction is based on some sort of logical event that would explain the situation. To rule out specific joint dysfunction, have the client move the joint through the range of motion and determine if it hurts. Next, the therapist moves the joint with passive range of motion. If the pain occurs during passive range of motion, it may be a joint problem and should be referred. You now have a logical reason for the external rotators to be short and the condition is indicated for massage. This client was doing new exercise involving external rotation. The client is functioning fine except that their shoulders hurt when they put their hands on their hips. Massage with the proper methods would be appropriate. If the condition persists or becomes worse, then the referral would be indicated.

You know that if one group of muscles is short, it can inhibit its agonist/antagonist pair. In this situation, you are beginning to think that your client has short external rotators that are inhibiting the internal rotators, primarily subscapularis. So, you position the shoulder to isolate the subscapularis and then use a muscle test to determine if the muscle is able to hold against resistance and perform the concentric function. As you apply a steady moderate pressure to move the shoulder into external rotation, the client says ouch—that is what hurts. Additionally, the muscle cannot hold against the resistance and is considered weak.

Recreating the Symptom

- Tender/trigger point referred pain patterns

If you push on any part of the body hard enough, it will hurt. It is important to work only with a familiar pain sensation. It is a common error to massage everything that hurts, not realizing that often it is the pressure or location of the massage application that is causing the pain. Instead, the general massage is an assessment, finding the action or location of the structure causing the pain. Tender/trigger points in muscles might be a part of the cause of the symptoms. Even though there is controversy about the trigger point concept, it remains helpful during the critical thinking process. It is common for short muscles to develop a tender/trigger point in the belly of the muscle that results in the muscle remaining short. If you apply compression on the area that recreates the client's symptoms and lengthen the muscle, the condition should improve.

The client's problem is with short external shoulder rotators, so during the massage you use various methods to reduce the shortening and decrease the motor tone of the infraspinatus, teres minor, and posterior deltoid.

When you apply inhibitory pressure on the belly of the infraspinatus, the client says that they experienced pain in the shoulder. You ask the client if the pain sensation is the same as the one they have been experiencing. They say yes. You suspect a referred pain pattern and when you check your textbook, you find that a trigger point in the belly of the infraspinatus can refer pain into the posterior deltoid region. You use various methods to calm the sensitivity and lengthen the muscles involved in external rotation by moving the joint into internal rotation. When there is a limit to the motion, including discomfort, you have the client push or pull against your resistance (muscle energy techniques) and then lengthen just a little (¼–½ inch) further. You do this about three times and continue with the massage.

Assess–Intervention if Needed–Reassess

It is necessary to assess movement and muscle function before the massage. If the assessment is not complete, there will be no information with which to compare results after the massage. You have to know what the situation is before the massage to see if the benefit was achieved after the massage.

During the massage, the process of palpation is used to continue to gather information, as are active and passive movement incorporated into the massage. At some point, an intervention will be made to cause the body to shift toward more normal function. Intervention methods include inhibitory pressure in areas of increased tone, increased drag on short connective tissue structures to increase tissue pliability, lymphatic drain to reduce edema, muscle energy techniques followed by lengthening to normalize short structures, and so forth.

No intervention method is used without an assessment process to indicate the nature of the issue. This is another error during massage—intervention without assessment. Hopefully, by now you have come to realize that general full-body massage incorporating movement at each joint is an assessment process. The full body massage that takes about 45 minutes is assessment. Yes, it is relaxing and supports parasympathetic function, which reduces the stress response. If that is the client's goal for the massage; if you find areas during the massage that are tender, have reduced movement, or are binding, you should ignore them because specific intervention would interfere with the general relaxation outcome. There will likely be improvement just because of the general effects of massage. The postassessment would identify if the client is more relaxed.

Another error made during massage is not leaving things alone or knowing when to quit.

It is important to reassess during the massage to find out if the methods used have been effective. By moving the shoulder into internal rotation, you identify that the range of motion has increased by about 10 degrees. The client now has about 70 degrees of internal rotation.

Knowing better than to overwork an area and realizing that a 10-degree increase in range of motion is a good outcome for internal shoulder rotation, you finish the massage and reassess. The client again performs the assessment movement of putting their hands on their hips and there is no pain, just a little stiffness. The massage application was successful in achieving the client's goals.

Box 10.3 How Textbook Content Translates Into Practical Application—cont'd

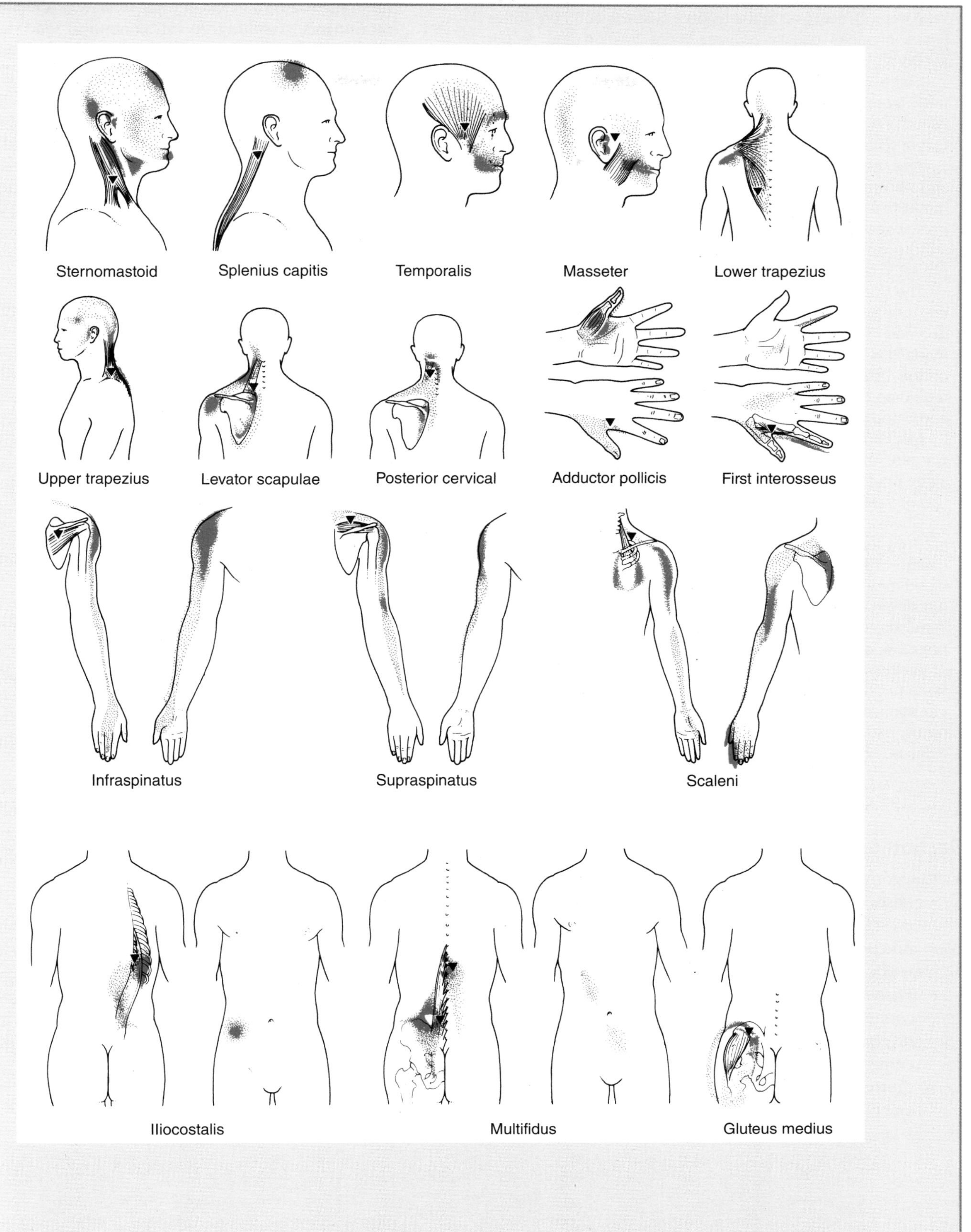

Continued

INDICATIONS/CONTRAINDICATIONS for Therapeutic Massage

Working with stages 2 and 3 functional stress and connective tissue changes usually requires more training and proper supervision using a multidisciplinary approach.

Stage 1 functional tension can often be managed effectively by massage modalities and with entry-level training that includes an understanding of the information presented in this text and technical training in the therapist's chosen modality.

Any massage modality influences the systems, tissues, and viscera of the body mechanically and reflexively. Massage modalities may improve local blood circulation, reduce chronic muscle tension, normalize the range of motion of the joint, and restore proprioceptive function. Following are biologically plausible responses to massage therapy.

The body perceives any technique first as a tactile sensation because the surface of the skin is altered by various degrees, depending on the methods used. Second, massage modalities alter the degree of muscle tension. Proprioceptors of the deep tissues report to the central nervous system regarding the condition of muscle tension, capillary pressure, and blood pressure of muscles and vessels.

Mechanical forces introduced into the tissues produce warmth. This heat acts as a thermal stimulant that signals the sympathetic and parasympathetic systems to cause vasodilation or vasoconstriction.

Chemical substances, such as histamine and acetylcholine, are formed in the tissues. Histamine stimulates the discharge of adrenaline. These substances are carried with the blood throughout the body, altering circulation, influencing the functions of inner organs (viscera), speeding up nerve impulses, mobilizing the immune system, normalizing blood pressure, and stimulating muscle activity.

All these signals create the reaction of the central nervous system. The goal is to generate, through massage methods, the stimulation required to generate self-regulating mechanisms, allowing the body to self-correct and restore dynamic balance, or homeostasis.

Section Summary

- Categorize biomechanical dysfunction.
  - Postural deviation, nonoptimal motor function, neuromuscular-related dysfunction, myofascial-related dysfunction, joint-related dysfunction.
- Describe three degrees of postural imbalance.
  - *First degree:* Shortening/weakening of some muscles/connective tissue tension in these muscles. *Second degree:* Moderate shortening of postural muscles/weakening of antagonist muscles. *Third degree:* Exaggerated shortening of postural muscles and weakening of antagonist muscles with nonoptimal movement.
- Describe three degrees of distorted motor function.
  - *First degree:* Recruitment of additional muscles for simple movements, resulting in uneconomical and labored movement. *Second degree:* Moderately peculiar postures/movements of some parts of the body, resulting in postural/movement distortion, such as altered firing patterns. *Third degree:* Exaggerated peculiarity in postures/movements, resulting in altered firing patterns and gait.
- Classify biomechanical dysfunction into three stages.
  - *Stage 1:* Functional tension. *Stage 2:* Functional stress. *Stage 3:* Connective tissue changes in the musculoskeletal system.

SUMMARY

This chapter has presented the basic principles of biomechanics. The kinetic chain describes three main biomechanical dysfunctional patterns, which we discussed with intervention suggestions and referral recommendations. A practice assessment protocol for the biomechanical function was provided.

The concepts in this chapter may seem complex and difficult to understand at times. Comprehending how all the aspects of the movement work together requires knowledge and an understanding of the relationship between the pieces and how they function. Many learners find themselves lost in the terminology of all the pieces: the bones, ligaments, names of the joints, actions of movement, names of the muscles, and directions for isolation. When this happens, the learner should slow down and perform the movement while saying the words. This entire unit has been about movement. Movement is best understood by moving. The learner should continue to look up the definitions of the words that are confusing. Persist in understanding biomechanical concepts. Competency in therapeutic massage is based on the integrated applications described in this chapter.

Balance and center may be the most important concepts of all. The learner should remember that the importance of being centered often is expressed as being present in the moment and responding resourcefully to each unfolding second of life.

Visit the Evolve website:
https://evolve.elsevier.com/Fritz/essential/

The Evolve website provides support for the review of the chapter content and chapter quizzes to help you prepare for the MBLEx or other massage therapy certification or licensing exams. End of chapter questions for discussion and review answer key and rationales and author's response to critical thinking and clinical reasoning scenarios.

PRACTICAL APPLICATION

Protocol for Gait Muscle Testing

The body has many gait-related kinetic chain patterns. The coordination between the upper and lower limbs allows for normal arm swing in relation to leg movements. The figures illustrate these patterns and how to assess for function. If assessment identifies altered function intervention may be indication.

Intervention

Use massage methods to inhibit muscles that test as too strong by remaining in concentric contraction patterns when they should be inhibited. Appropriate methods are slow compression, kneading, gliding, and shaking. Strengthen muscles that inhibit when they should hold strong. Appropriate methods are percussion and rhythmic contraction of inhibited muscles. Then retest the pattern; it should be normal.

This procedure is demonstrated in detail on the website.

To perform this assessment, you must understand two important definitions:

- Control group: For this particular purpose, the control group is the group of muscles that initiates the reflex response.
- Test group: Also in this case, the test group is the muscle group that responds to the stimulus from the control group.

Activate the control group first by having the client hold against resistance applied by the practitioner. Maintain the activation of the control group while accessing the response from the text group by applying resistance. The test group should remain strong or inhibit depending on the part of the gait being assessed.

For testing of the arm flexors and extensors, the humerus should be stabilized superior to the elbow joint, and the femur should be stabilized above the knee.

A to D are contralateral (opposite arm and leg) assessments
E to H are unilateral (same side arm and leg) assessments.

A

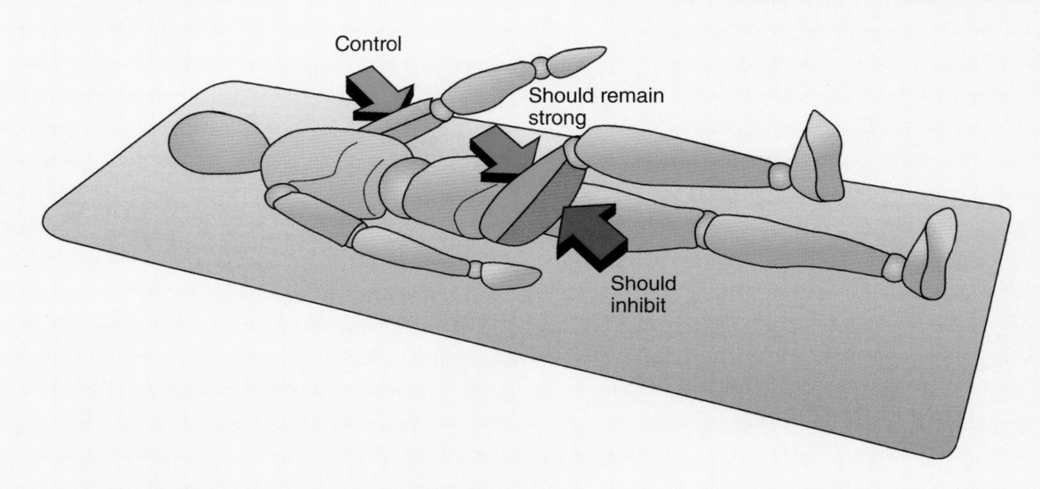

B

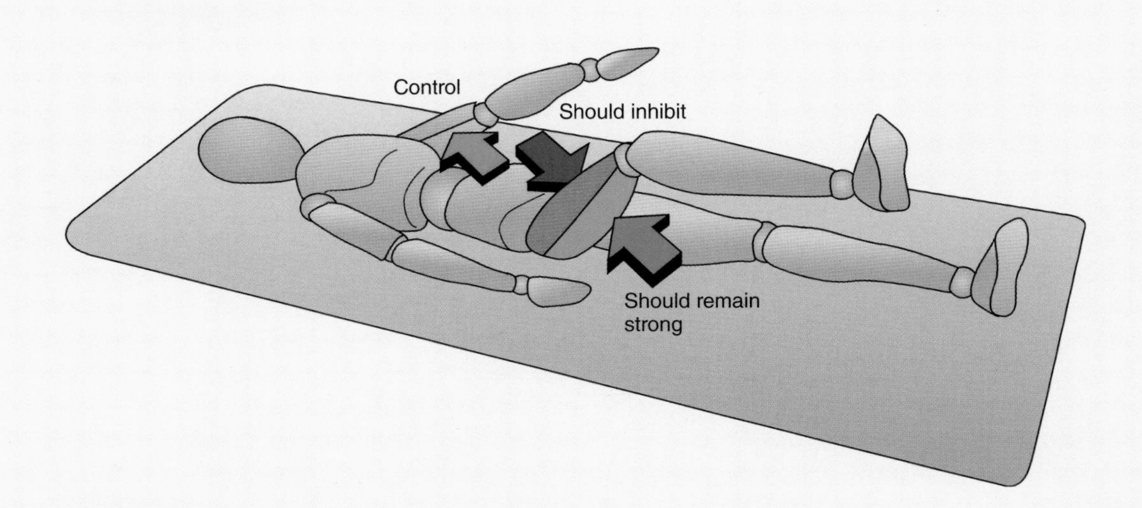

Practical application—cont'd

C

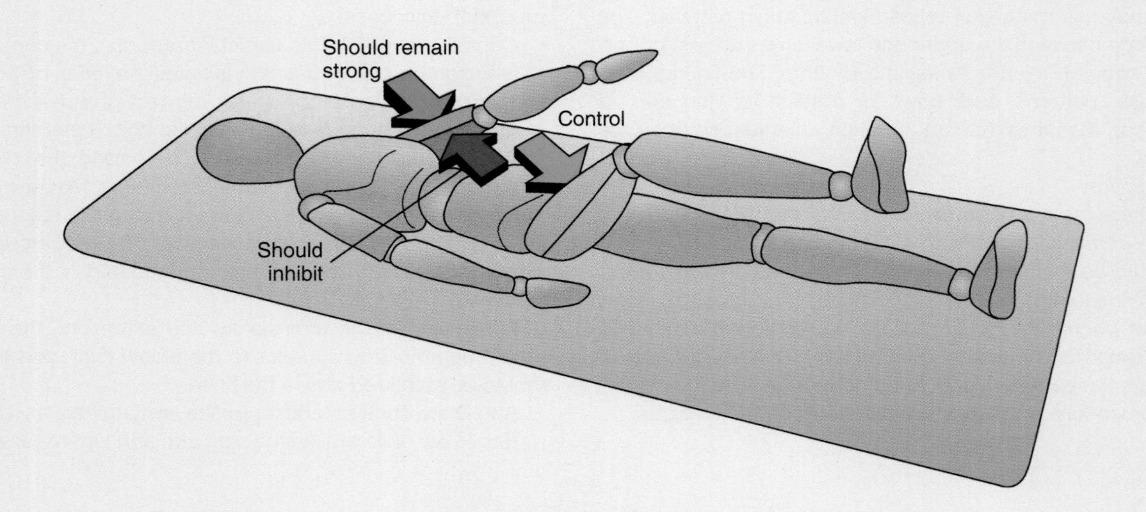

D

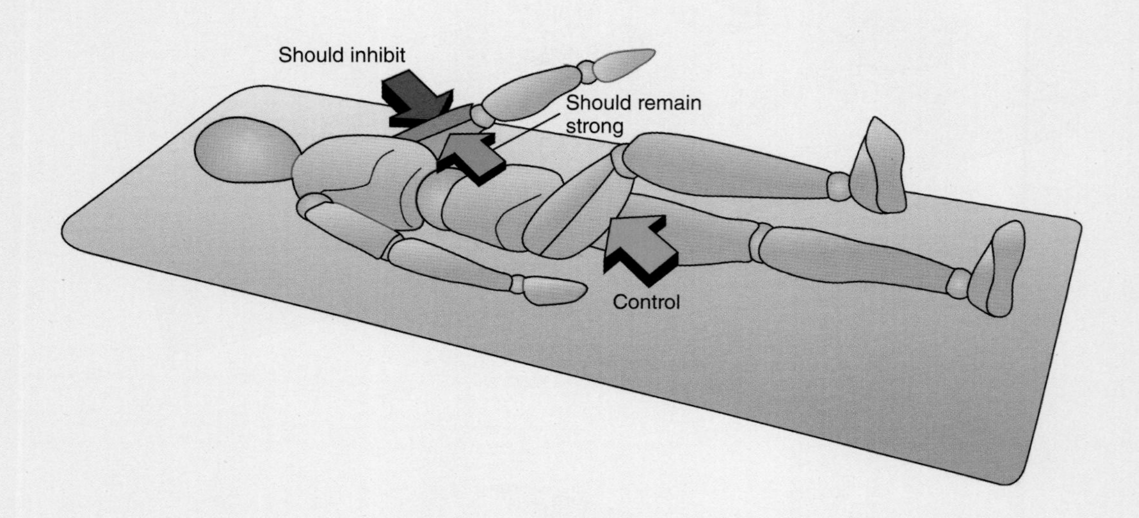

E

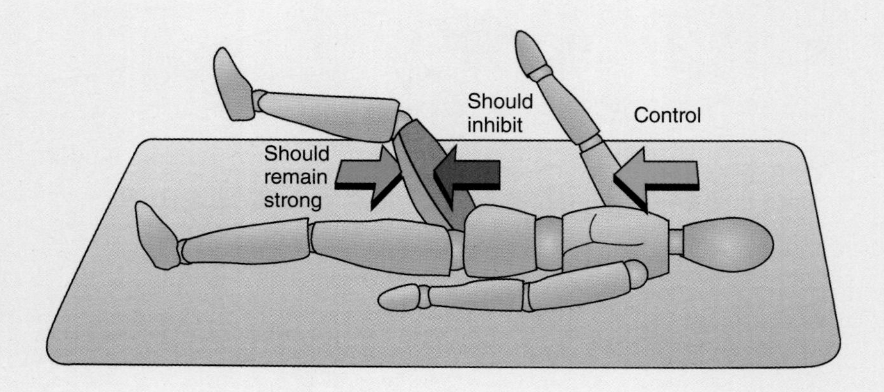

Practical application—cont'd

F

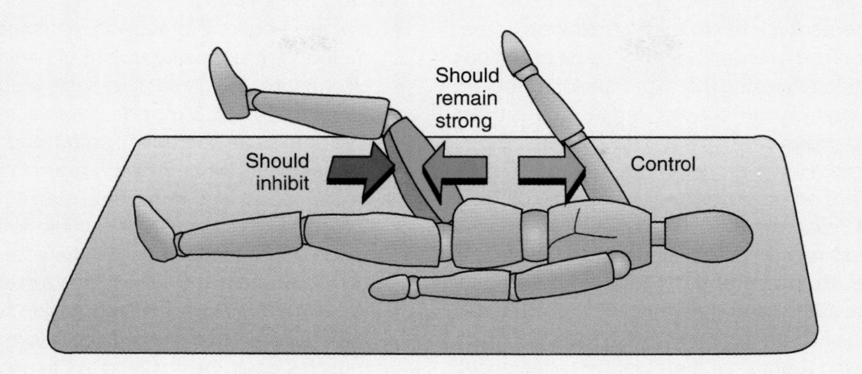

G

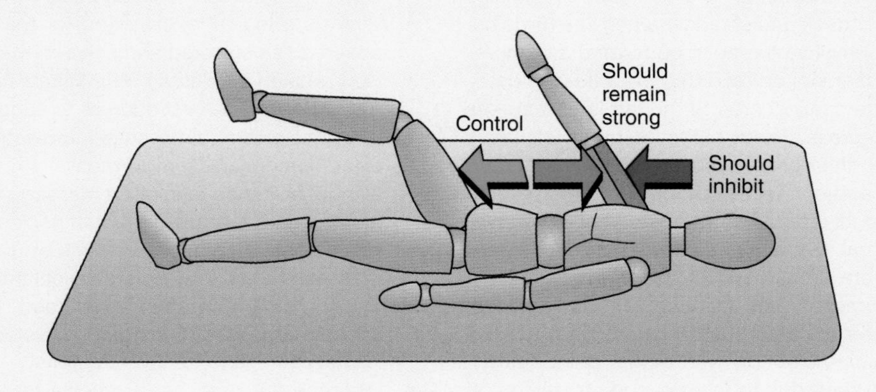

H

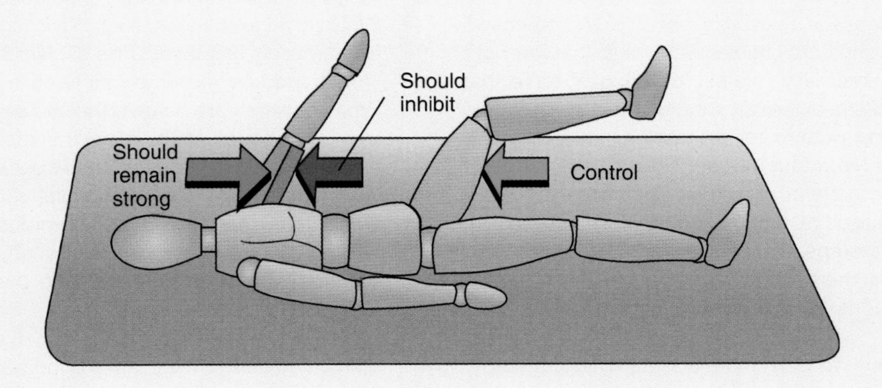

Continued

CRITICAL THINKING/CLINICAL REASONING

Each chapter will feature a critical thinking and clinical reasoning application of the content related to massage therapy practice. A client scenario will be presented with recommendations for additional research often using MedlinePlus or PubMed. Relevant questions based on the chapter content outline are provided to guide the discussion. There are no specific current answers to the questions. However, responses should be supportive of evidence-informed practices and based on biological plausibility if sufficient research is not available. The author's decision-making process related to the scenario and questions is on the EVOLVE site. Compare and contrast your thoughts and discussion with the author and determine where you agree or disagree.

Ms. Mathews is seeing a physical therapist for a decreased range of motion in her right shoulder and her neck. She is also experiencing pain in her neck and shoulder when she turns her head to the right. The physical therapist performed a comprehensive physical assessment and recorded the following data:

Lateral flexion of the cervical area to the left is 35 degrees and to the right is 20 degrees. Range of motion to the left within normal range. Limits to the right are related to pain at the end of the available range and connective tissue shortening on the left. Muscle testing of right lateral flexors is fair. Shoulder movement on the left is normal. On the right shoulder, flexion, extension, and abduction are limited to 90 degrees before pain occurs. Muscle assessment is only fair. Scapular movement is limited, especially in the abduction and upward rotation. The rhomboid muscles palpate as short with trigger point activity. The client's gait is disturbed due to the reduced arm swing on the right.

When you (the massage therapist) observe Ms. Mathews walk, you notice that she holds herself stiffly and that her right shoulder is high and internally rotates. You also observe that the left hip is high and she externally rotates the left leg. During the massage, the firing pattern for the abdominal muscles is weak and the client's hip adductors are short during range of motion as part of the general massage. The outcome of the massage is for generalized relaxation and increased soft tissue pliability to support therapeutic exercise and stretching performed by the physical therapist.

Explore: Medline Plus. Search terms. Neck pain Shoulder pain.

Do an internet search to learn more about physical therapy.

Research: Pubmed using search terms massage and neck pain, massage and shoulder pain.

Discuss These Points

- Is there evidence to support massage therapy as a beneficial method for the management of neck and shoulder pain?
- How might you present research evidence for the benefits of massage to Ms. Mathews physical therapist?
- The physical therapist performed the primary physical assessment. What findings are related to the sagittal plain, frontal plane, and transverse plane?
- Describe the process of muscle testing for the decreased range of motion in her right shoulder and her neck.
- How is scapular movement involved in shoulder dysfunction?
- What muscles are involved in the scapular movement that may be a scouse of the client's symptoms. Which of these muscles could be involved in the neck systems?
- How might the sternocleidomastoid muscle be involved?
- What is a logical explanation for the client's left hip being observed as elevated and she externally rotates the left leg?
- How would you classify Ms. Walters condition: Which would massage therapy best address to support physical therapy?
- List principles of a massage intervention plan based on efficient biomechanical movement.
- Is there evidence to support massage therapy as a beneficial method for the management of neck and shoulder pain?
- How might you present research evidence for the benefits of massage to Ms. Mathews physical therapist?
- The physical therapist performed the primary physical assessment. What findings are related to the sagittal plain, frontal plane, and transverse plane?
- Describe the process of muscle testing for the decreased range of motion in her right shoulder and her neck.
- What postural changes did the massage assessment identify? What muscle functional units explain the postural distortion?
- How is scapular movement involved in shoulder dysfunction?
- What muscles are involved in the scapular movement that may be a cause of the client's symptoms? Which of these muscles could be involved in the neck systems?
- How would you classify Ms. Walters' condition:
- Nonoptimal motor function, neuromuscular-related dysfunction, myofascial-related dysfunction, or joint-related dysfunction? Which would massage therapy best address to support physical therapy?
- Based on degrees and stages of dysfunction what is your opinion related to the client's conditions?
- Describe the principles of a massage intervention plan based on efficient biomechanical movement.

MULTIPLE CHOICE QUESTIONS FOR REVIEW AND DISCUSSION

The answers, with rationales, can be found on the Evolve site.

These questions are used for review and discussion. It is as important to understand why wrong answers are wrong as it is to know why the correct answer is correct. The answers to the questions, with rationales and explanations about why the correct answer is correct and why wrong answers are wrong, can be found on the Evolve site. Guidance also is provided on how questions are developed and how the textbook content can be presented in a multiple-choice question format. At the end of the question section here in the textbook, you will find an exercise that asks you to write more questions. Use the various questions in the chapter as examples. This is one of the best study strategies for test taking.

It is important to understand that the actual licensing exam you take may not contain any of the specific questions found in this textbook or the review material and practice tests on the Evolve site. Therefore, just because you can answer any of these questions correctly does not mean you will pass the licensing exam. The questions are content and style examples to help you prepare—this is why understanding why wrong answers are wrong is just as important as identifying the correct answer. Also, make sure you understand all the terminology used in the questions and possible answers in the review and discussion questions. Look up words you do not understand.

1. Which of the following is likely to result in joint-related dysfunction?
   a. Constant loading of a joint
   b. Generalized edema
   c. Closed kinematic chain
   d. Optimal firing pattern
2. An example of a core stabilization inner unit muscle would be?
   a. Latissimus dorsi
   b. Adductor longus
   c. Quadriceps
   d. Transversus abdominis
3. Which of the following most often would be considered the fulcrum?
   a. Quadriceps muscles
   b. Radius
   c. Deltoid ligament
   d. Glenohumeral joint
4. When one is carrying a massage table from the car to the office, what is the responsibility of the muscles?
   a. Create a lever to distribute the load
   b. Exert effort to move the load
   c. Provide a fulcrum for the lever
   d. Maintain static balance
5. During normal gait in the adult, the lumbar rotation is countered by a cervical spine rotation in the opposite direction for what reason?
   a. To keep the eyes on a level plane and the head oriented forward with the trunk
   b. To maintain the same-side counterbalance action of the arms and legs
   c. To coordinate the lever action of the elbows with the knees
   d. To activate the second-class lever system of the lift of the heel when moving onto the toes
6. After tripping down a stair, but not falling, a client describes a sudden onset of pain during twisting and reaching movements. Which type of biomechanical dysfunction is most likely occurring?
   a. Neuromuscular
   b. Myofascial
   c. Joint related
   d. Capsular pattern
7. A massage professional positions the client's body to assess the strength of the hip flexors. Which is the correct position for the hand applying resistance?
   a. Near the hip
   b. At the ankle
   c. At the distal end of the femur
   d. On the tibia
8. A client is experiencing an upper chest breathing pattern. Which of the following muscle(s) may test as short and too strong from this type of breathing?
   a. Diaphragm
   b. Suprahyoid muscles
   c. Scalene muscles
   d. Infraspinatus
9. A client complains of pain and tension in the lower back more to the left side. Physical assessment indicates that the pelvis is elevated on the left compared with the right. The client also indicates difficulty raising the left arm over the head. Which of the following muscles may be involved?
   a. Psoas
   b. Rectus abdominis
   c. Latissimus dorsi
   d. Semispinalis
10. If the scapula remains fixed and immobile, what will result at the glenohumeral joint?
    a. Range of motion would be limited.
    b. Internal and external rotation would be enhanced.
    c. Flexion would be unaffected.
    d. Horizontal abduction would be the only limitation.
11. The glenohumeral joint is a good example for describing which of the following correct biomechanical principles?
    a. When mobility increases, stability also increases.
    b. When stability is less, mobility also decreases.
    c. The more mobility, the less stability.
    d. Mobility is supported before stability.
12. A client is unable to turn the palm up past 45 degrees. Which of the following movements is hypomobile?
    a. Supination
    b. Pronation
    c. Flexion
    d. Extension
13. A client is lying supine, and observation indicates that the left leg is rotated internally. What should muscle testing reveal?
    a. Muscles that externally rotate the hip are short, and muscles that internally rotate the hip are inhibited.
    b. Muscles that externally rotate the hip are inhibited, and muscles that internally rotate the hip are overly strong.
    c. Gluteus medius should test weak.
    d. Adductor longus should test weak.
14. The knee is placed in 100 degrees of extension, and the client is asked to hold this position. Resistance is applied to the concentrically contracting muscles. Pain and weakness are felt. What is a logical explanation for this?
    a. The hamstring muscle group is weak.
    b. The Q angle is being altered in a lateral direction by the contraction of the vastus medialis.
    c. The popliteus muscle has been unable to unlock the screw-home mechanism.
    d. The quadriceps muscle group is unable effectively to hold a contraction against resistance.
15. A client experienced a second-degree ankle sprain when the foot was forced into inversion. Which of the following muscles would have experienced an extension injury?
    a. Fibularis longus
    b. Soleus
    c. Flexor digitorum longus
    d. Interossei
16. An individual was running up some stairs carrying a heavy briefcase in the left hand. Later that day the person felt increased tension in the left biceps muscle. Two days

later, during a regular massage session, the client described weakness and heaviness in one leg when walking upstairs or on a hill. If normal gait reflexes are functioning, where would assessment likely find an inhibited muscle pattern?
   a. Right arm extensors
   b. Left hip flexors
   c. Right hip flexors
   d. Left hip extensors
17. A client experienced an auto accident 4 years ago that resulted in compression at L4. The injury has since healed with minimal difficulties. During the assessment, palpation indicates a moderate decrease in pliability of the lumbar dorsal fascia and mild shortening in the lumbar muscles. Forward flexion and rotation of the lumbar area are impaired mildly. The massage was focused to reduce the muscle shortening in the lumbar area and increase connective tissue pliability. Immediately after the massage, the client reported increased mobility but within 15 minutes began to complain of lower back pain. What is the most likely explanation for this occurrence?
   a. A shift of the condition from second-degree functional stress to first-degree functional tension
   b. Increase in stability around the past injury
   c. Decrease in mobility in the area around the past injury
   d. Destabilization of resourceful compensation in the lumbar area around the past injury
18. A client complains of joint pain in the knee, and assessment indicates hypermobility with pain on passive movement. Which of the following would be the most appropriate treatment plan?
   a. General massage to the body with specific muscle energy work and lengthening of the extensors and flexors of the knee
   b. General massage with regional contraindications to the knee area and referral for a more appropriate diagnosis of possible capsular dysfunction
   c. Referral for diagnosis before any massage
   d. General massage with attention to friction methods at the joint capsule
19. A client is experiencing pain with any activity involving external or lateral rotation of the right shoulder. The range of motion is limited to 40 degrees. This condition has been coming on gradually. Muscle testing indicates weakness when resistance is applied to move the shoulder from external rotation to internal rotation. There is a shortening in the muscles of internal rotation. Which of the following would be the most logical treatment plan?
   a. Muscle energy methods to support the lengthening of the infraspinatus and methods to increase tone in the subscapularis
   b. Deep massage to the rhomboid muscles and stretching of the lumbar fascia
   c. Traction of the scapulothoracic junction
   d. Massage to reduce tension in the pectoralis major and latissimus dorsi with tapotement to increase tone in the infraspinatus and teres major
20. When a joint is moved so that the joint angle is decreased, what is occurring?
   a. Prime movers and synergists concentrically contract. The antagonist eccentrically functions while lengthening to allow the movement.
   b. Prime movers concentrically contract with the antagonist so that synergists lengthen to allow movement.
   c. Movement occurs as the antagonist contracts and prime movers eccentrically control the movement.
   d. Resistance is applied to the fixators, providing the movement and activating the prime movers.

CHAPTER 11

Integumentary, Cardiovascular, Lymphatic, and Immune Systems

https://evolve.elsevier.com/Fritz/essential/

CHAPTER OBJECTIVES

After completing this chapter, the learner will be able to:

1. Explain the physiology of touch.
2. List and describe the components and functions of the integumentary system.
3. Identify pathologies of the integumentary system and describe indications and contraindications for massage.
4. List and describe the components and functions of the cardiovascular system.
5. Identify pathologies of the cardiovascular system and describe indications and contraindications for massage.
6. List and describe the components and functions of the lymphatic system.
7. Identify pathologies of the lymphatic system and describe indications and contraindications for massage.
8. Define immunity.
9. List and describe nonspecific and specific immune responses of the body.
10. Explain how the mind/body connection affects immunity.
11. Identify pathologies of the immune system and describe indications and contraindications for massage.

CHAPTER OUTLINE

KEY TERMS

antibodies: (AN-ti-bod-eez) Serum proteins of the immunoglobulin class that are secreted by plasma cells.

arterioles: Small blood vessels that connect arteries to capillaries.

arteriosclerosis: (ar-tee-ree-o-skle-RO-sis) A term meaning "hardening of the arteries"; refers to arteries that have lost their elasticity.

artery: (AR-ter-ee) A blood vessel that transports oxygenated blood from the heart to the body or deoxygenated blood from the heart to the lungs.

atherosclerosis: (ath-er-o-skle-RO-sis) A condition in which fatty plaque is deposited in medium-sized and large arteries.

atrium: (AY-tree-um) One of the two small, thin-walled upper chambers of the heart.

blood: A thick, red fluid that provides oxygen, nourishment, and protection to the cells and carries away waste products.

blood pressure: The measurement of pressure exerted by the blood on the walls of the blood vessels. The highest pressure exerted is called systolic pressure, which results when the ventricles contract. *Diastolic pressure*, the lowest pressure, results when the ventricles relax.

capillary: (KAP-i-lair-ee) The smallest blood vessel; found between arteries and veins. Capillaries allow the exchange of gases, nutrients, and waste products.

coronary arteries: (KOR-o-nair-ee) The arteries that supply oxygenated blood to the heart muscle itself; located in grooves between the atria and ventricles and between the two ventricles.

dermatitis: (der-mah-TIE-tis) A general term for acute or chronic skin inflammation characterized by redness, eruptions, edema, scaling, and itching.

dermis: (DER-mis) The deep layer of skin that contains collagen and elastin fibers, which provide much of the structure and strength of the skin.

epidermis: (ep-i-DER-mis) The superficial layer of skin; composed of epithelial tissue in sublayers called strata.

heart: A hollow, cone-shaped, muscular organ responsible for pumping blood. It is about the size of a fist and is located in the mediastinum of the thoracic cavity.

heart valves: Four sets of valves that keep the blood flowing in the correct direction through the heart.

hemorrhage: (HEM-or-ej) The passage of blood outside of the cardiovascular system.
immunity: Resistance to disease; the immune system is a functional system rather than an organ system in the anatomical sense.
integument: (in-TEG-yoo-ment) The skin and its appendages: hair, sebaceous and sweat glands, nails, and breasts.
lymph: (limf) Fluid derived from interstitial fluid; contains lymphocytes, returns plasma proteins that have leaked out through capillary walls, and transports fats from the gastrointestinal system to the bloodstream.
lymph nodes: Small, round structures distributed along the network of lymph vessels; they filter wastes and pathogens out of lymph.
pericardium: (pair-i-KAR-dee-um) A double-membrane, serous sac that surrounds and protects the heart.
plasma: (PLAZ-mah) A thick, straw-colored fluid that makes up about 55% of the blood.
Standard Precautions: Safety measures established by the Centers for Disease Control and Prevention (CDC). The precautions were instituted to prevent the spread of bacterial and viral infections by setting up specific methods of dealing with human fluids and waste products.
superficial fascia: The subcutaneous tissue that comprises the third layer of skin; consists of loose connective tissue and contains fat or adipose tissue.
tumor: A growth of new tissues that may be benign or malignant; also referred to as a neoplasm.
veins: Blood vessels that collect blood from the capillaries and transport it back to the heart.
ventricles: (VEN-tri-kulz) The two large lower chambers of the heart; they are thick walled and are separated by a thick interventricular septum.
venules: (VEN-yoolz) Small blood vessels that connect capillaries to veins.

LEARNING HOW TO LEARN

Eight body systems are covered in these final two chapters. Visualizing is a valuable learning tool. When you are learning about each system, also think about the applications for massage. Ask yourself the following questions:

- How would I apply massage to this area?
- What would be the outcomes of massage for this system?

Visualize yourself massaging the area. Learn massage applications and the structure and function of each body system. Incorporate all you have learned about learning and remember to take brain breaks.

The title of this textbook, *Mosby's Essential Sciences for Therapeutic Massage*, closely reflects the content. The material in this textbook is essential for the successful practice of massage therapy. Previous chapters have provided an overview of anatomy and physiology, mechanisms of health and disease, and scientific language. This information set the stage for the complex study of the body systems that monitor and control physiology—namely, the nervous and endocrine systems. The information on kinesiology and biomechanics presented core content for the practice of massage.

This unit has two chapters. Chapter 11 covers four body systems: integumentary, cardiovascular, lymphatic, and immune systems. Chapter 12 also covers four body systems: respiratory, digestive, urinary, and reproductive systems.

The reason for the condensed coverage of these body systems is that massage therapy benefits these systems through secondary effects on the nervous system, primarily the autonomic nervous system (ANS), and the endocrine system. Massage benefits are considered systemic; that is, they generally influence a system. Additionally, the organs of these systems are primarily found in the thoracic, abdominal, and pelvic cavities of the torso. To some extent, massage can work mechanically to affect the connective tissue and membrane secretions and support normal sliding for the organs within the cavities, but specific direct massage application is unlikely. It is also possible that massage can directly influence some aspects of the blood, lymphatic, and digestive systems. These would be considered local effects. However, at the entry level, it is not necessary to provide in-depth coverage other than to support general learning and to provide a foundation for understanding a client's health history, making intelligent decisions about massage adaptation and referral, and designing a safe and beneficial massage for each client.

For massage therapy students in entry-level education, the basic study of the body systems presented in this chapter and Chapter 12 supports students' learning about the most pertinent information relative to massage. In essence, the content has been presorted based on relevance to massage therapy. It is not necessary to memorize all the content. Instead, the information can be used as a basis for asking questions and seeking appropriate answers.

If, in the future, you decide to specialize in an area related to one of the eight body systems presented, then a more in-depth study of the system is essential. For example:

- If you want to work with clients who have respiratory disorders (e.g., asthma), you will need to know more about the respiratory system.
- If you want to work with clients with various types of cancer (e.g., breast and gastrointestinal cancer), you will need to know more about the integumentary and digestive systems.
- If you want to work with a cosmetic surgeon, you will need to know more about the integumentary system.
- If you want to work with cardiac rehabilitation specialists, you will need to learn more about the cardiovascular system.
- If you want to work with clients who have autoimmune diseases (e.g., lupus and multiple sclerosis), you will need to know more about the immune system.
- If you want to work with clients who have diabetes, in addition to the endocrine system, you will need to know more about the digestive system, nutrition, and the urinary system (because diabetes affects the kidneys).
- If you want to perform prenatal and postnatal massage, you will need to know about the reproductive system.

- If you want to work with clients who have post-injury swelling (e.g., as occurs with various athletic injuries), you will need to learn more about the lymphatic system.

INTEGUMENTARY SYSTEM

SECTION OBJECTIVES

Chapter objectives covered in this section:

1. Explain the physiology of touch.
2. List and describe the components and functions of the integumentary system.
3. Identify pathologies of the integumentary system and describe indications and contraindications for massage.

After completing this section, the learner will be able to:

- Explain the importance of touch.
- Describe the function of the integumentary system.
- Describe two main concerns with integumentary pathological conditions.
- Describe the three types of skin cancer.

Physiology of Touch

The skin is the most sensitive of our organs. It is the home of the touch receptors of the nervous system. Touch is one of the five basic senses, along with taste, vision, smell, and hearing; it expands the ways in which we experience the world. Touch is the first sense to develop in the embryo, and the need for touch remains throughout our lives. As massage professionals, we touch our clients, and the skin is our contact point; therefore, we must understand the effects of skin stimulation.

We can survive without sight, hearing, taste, and smell, but without the ability to feel, we are in constant danger. In fact, a complete loss of the sense of touch can cause a psychotic breakdown. Not being touched can be life-threatening and can contribute to a condition called *marasmus* (wasting away), especially in infants, the elderly, and those with weakened immune systems. Sensory stimulation is essential to well-being at all stages of life, and touch is a necessary component. Deprivation of this sense leads to reduced production of the neuroendocrine chemicals necessary for well-being. It is common for touch-deprived individuals to develop inappropriate forms of sensory stimulation or abusive or addictive behavior (often food or drugs) in an attempt to stimulate the production of chemicals that the body needs.

As a survival mechanism, touch alerts us to danger through variations in temperature, vibration, and pressure received by millions of sensory receptors in the skin. Touch informs us of differences in texture, shape, resistance, and tension. About one-third of the 5 million or so sensory receptors are in the skin of our hands. The fingertips alone have more than 1,000 nerve endings per square inch, and the lips and tongue have even more.

Pressure applied to the skin is the primary stimulus for the sense of touch. Another stimulus, vibration, emerges with a rapid and regular change in pressure. Different types of touch are identified by different receptors in the skin. The degree of pressure in light touch as opposed to firm or heavy touch is sensed by specific sensory receptor mechanisms and can evoke entirely different responses. A slow, light touch can relay compassion or intimacy. A deeper slow touch can evoke relaxation or security, whereas an abrupt touch startles and alerts. Touch can evoke pleasure, which we seek, and pain or discomfort, which we avoid. Discriminative touch detects the physical properties of tactile stimuli such as location, shape, texture, and force. Affective touch conveys emotional value that is interpreted as safe or not safe by social context and experience. Pleasant affective touch provides emotional and psychological benefits by indirectly activating the endogenous reward/pleasure circuits. As described in Chapters 4 and 5, C tactile (CT) fibers innervate hairy skin. Gentle slow stroking on the hairy skin of humans decreases heart rate indicating a soothing state with a reduced level of stress (Liu et al., 2022). Each of these sensations triggers the manufacture and release of specific neurochemicals (see Chapters 4–6). One of these neurochemicals, oxytocin, has been the focus of research related to relationships. Known as the "feel good" hormone, oxytocin helps inspire positive thinking and maintain an optimistic outlook. The role of oxytocin for bonding also extends to helping generate feelings of compassion during interactions. This can contribute to an expansion of trust among individuals during social situations. Oxytocin helps humans connect to others and promotes feel-good sensations that foster a sense of well-being and happiness. Physical touch increases levels of dopamine and serotonin, two neurotransmitters that help regulate mood and relieve stress and anxiety. Dopamine is also known to regulate the pleasure center in the brain, reducing feelings of anxiety.

The human brain has evolved with two distinct but parallel pathways for processing touch information. The first pathway, which is part of the sensory pathway, is called the *primary somatosensory cortex*—this is the first region to be hit by the experience of touch, which gives us the facts about touch (e.g., vibration, pressure, location, and fine texture). The second pathway processes social and emotional information, determining the emotional content of mostly interpersonal touch using different sensors in the skin. This pathway activates brain regions associated with social bonding, pleasure, and pain centers.

Because of the separation of the two pathways used for processing touch, certain brain disorders cause the separation of the physical sensation of pain from its emotional impact. So, too, can the pleasurable aspect of touch be removed from the actual sensation.

Essentially touch is a bio-physio-social communication. What form of communication is more intimate than touch? Its importance is reflected even in the language: That was a touching experience; what you said touched me; you hurt my feelings; let's stay in touch. The various kinds of touch—nurturing, angry, parental, fearful, sexual, happy, comforting, and playful—are, in some amazing way, understood by the neuropathways of the skin. The experience of touch occurs through the nervous system and endocrine system. The experience of touch is much larger than the structure and function of the skin. Massage therapists know this both intuitively and scientifically. Every massage method involves some sort of touch and skin stimulation. Because we access all body structures during massage by first touching the skin, it is important to understand the basics of the structure and function of the integument.

Structure of the Integument

The word **integument** means "covering." The integumentary system, which covers our bodies, is made up of the skin and its appendages: hair, sebaceous glands, sweat glands, nails, and breasts (Fig. 11.1).

Some of the major functions of the integumentary system are:

- Protecting the internal organs and structures from trauma, sun exposure, chemicals, and water loss
- Assisting in **immunity** by preventing the entry of bacteria and viruses
- Synthesizing vitamin D when exposed to ultraviolet rays of the sun
- Detecting the stimuli sensed through touch, temperature, pain, and pressure
- Regulating body temperature
- Excreting sweat and salts and secreting sebum

Skin

The skin is the largest and heaviest organ of the body and is composed of two major layers: the epidermis and the dermis.

The **epidermis** is the outer layer of the skin. It contains no nerves or blood vessels and consists of sublayers called *strata*. Most areas have four layers, but areas subject to pressure or friction (e.g., the palms and the soles) have five layers. In all areas, the outermost layer is the stratum corneum. This layer is made up of 20 to 30 layers of flat, keratin-filled dead cells that are continuously shed and are replaced from the layer deep to it. The innermost layer is the stratum basale, which produces a continuous supply of new cells. As the new cells develop and mature, they move up through the other layers until they reach the top and are shed, a process that takes about 2 to 3 weeks. This lowest layer also contains melanocytes, which produce melanin, a pigment that colors the skin.

The melanin pigment protects the skin from the harmful effects of ultraviolet radiation. The cumulative effects of exposure to ultraviolet radiation can damage fibroblasts located in the dermis, leading to faulty manufacture of connective tissue and wrinkling of the skin. Also, damage to the chromosomes of multiplying cells in the stratum germinativum (basale) can cause skin cancer.

Keratin is produced in the epidermis by keratinocytes. Keratin is the fibrous protein that protects the skin and makes it waterproof.

The **dermis**, the layer of skin deep to the epidermis, is much thicker than the epidermis. The dermis is composed of dense connective tissue that contains collagen and elastin fibers, which provide much of the structure and strength of the skin. The fibers are arranged so that the skin can be moved in many directions. Stretch marks result when these fibers are overstretched. The top layer of the dermis forms into ridges and presses up into the epidermis to create our fingerprints. Hair, sebaceous and sweat glands, and nails originate in the dermis and also push upward through the epidermis. Blood vessels and nerves are found in the dermis as well.

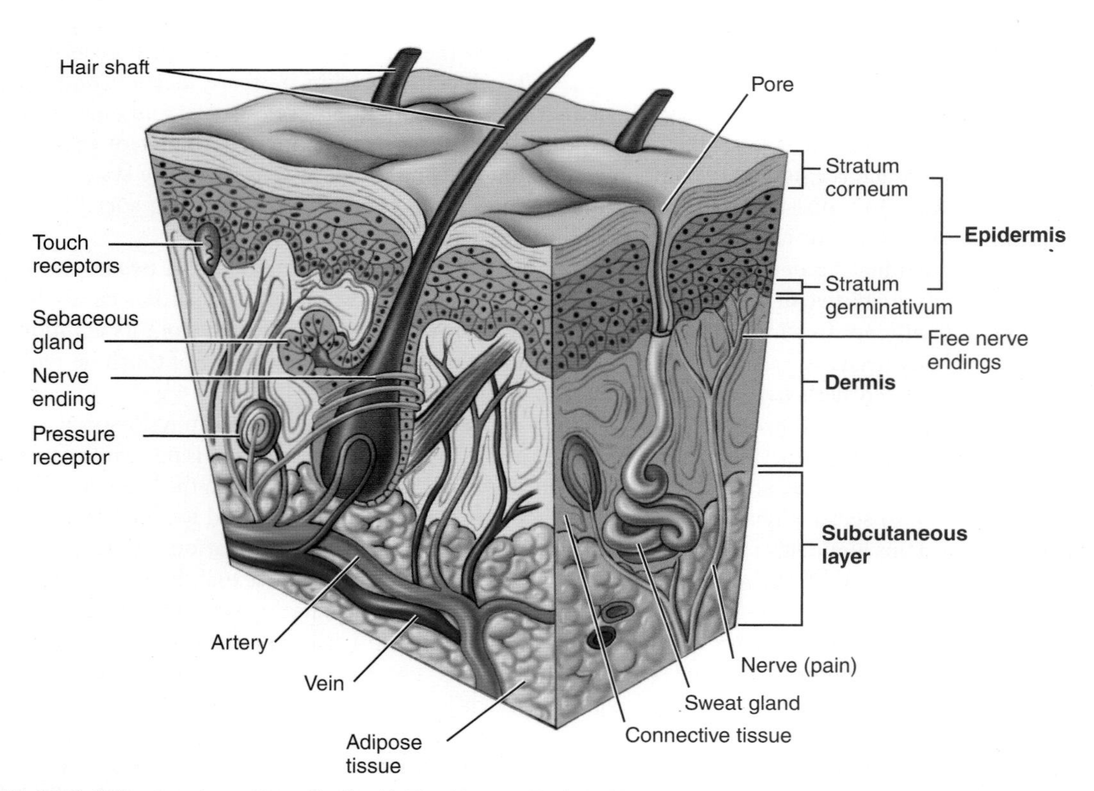

FIG. 11.1 Skin structure. From Herlihy H. *The Human Body in Health and Disease*. 4th ed. (Mosby/Elsevier; 2011.)

Fig. 11.2 shows lines of the cleavage of the skin. This pattern of collagen and elastin fiber bundles in the dermis follows the lines of tension in the skin. Injuries to the skin that are at right angles to the lines tend to gap because the cut elastin fibers recoil and pull the wound apart. Healing is slower, and more scarring occurs in these kinds of injuries than in injuries that are parallel to the lines. Surgeons attempt to make their incisions parallel to lines of cleavage to promote healing and reduce scarring.

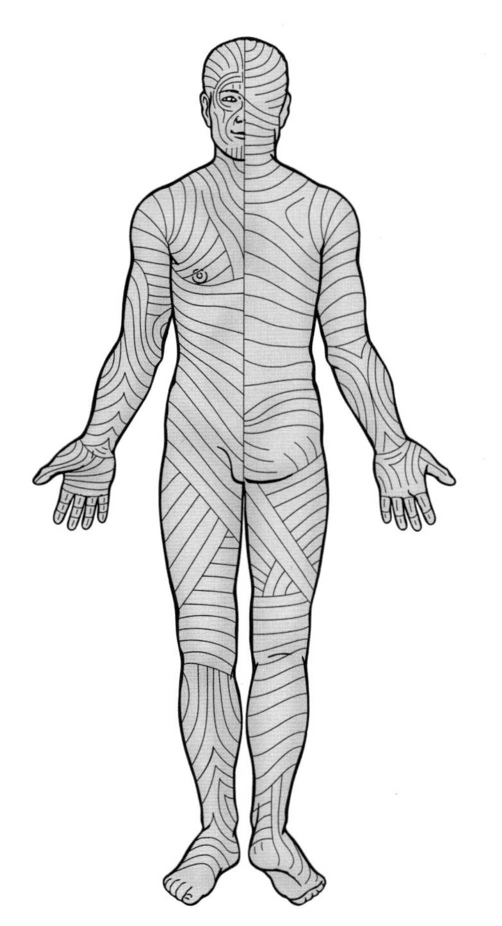

FIG. 11.2 Cleavage lines.

The subcutaneous layer, consisting of loose connective tissue and adipose tissue, is found below the dermis. This layer, also known as the **superficial fascia**, attaches to muscle and bone. The subcutaneous layer is not a part of the integument, but because it contains loose connective tissue that attaches to the dermis, it usually is described along with the integumentary system. The adipose tissue insulates and provides padding; its distribution varies in men and females and is affected by genetic factors.

The skin has an extensive blood supply. The volume of blood flowing in the vessels of the skin varies according to the need to replace heat lost from the body. A simple assessment of circulation is to apply pressure to the nail body for 2 to 3 seconds and then release. Watch the color change as the blood refills the area. If this refilling process is longer than 2 to 3 seconds, circulation is sluggish.

Interstitium

A layer of tissue below the surface of the skin was thought to be dense connective tissue. However, recent research using new technology has revealed that this layer of tissues is a body-wide interconnected system of fluid-filled compartments (Fig. 11.3). It appears that spaces containing interstitial fluid are present in dense connective tissue and exist in more areas of the body than previously realized. This network of fluid-filled spaces is located everywhere tissues expand or compress as part of normal function. The physical structure of this tissue consists of fluid-filled spaces supported by a lattice of collagen lined on one side by what appears to be a type of stem cell. These cells may help make collagen and could aid in wound healing. Similarly, they could contribute to conditions associated with inflammation and aging.

Although it was known that interstitial fluid is the major source of lymph fluid, which carries immune cells throughout

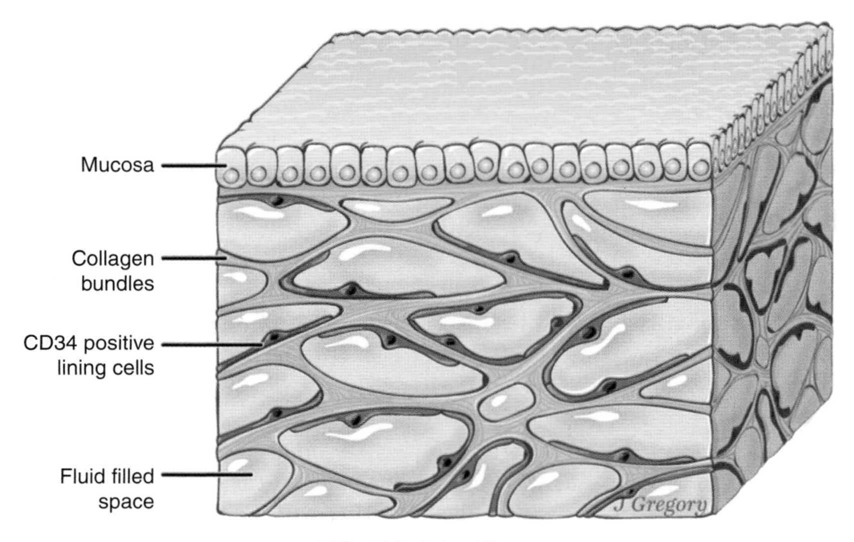

FIG. 11.3 Interstitium.

the body, just how it reaches the lymphatic system was unclear. The research shows that the Interstitium drains into the lymph vessels (Benias et al., 2018). Interestingly, it's the space where tattoo pigment resides. There is much more to learn and understand. It is logical and biologically plausible that the mechanical forces generated during massage compress and pull on the interstitium. What benefit this may have has yet to be discovered.

MENTORING TIP

This discovery of the Interstitium has generated excitement in the massage therapy community. There has been speculation for many years that this type of structure existed and that various bodywork methods affected its functions. The ability to see the Interstitium expanded our understanding of the thin layer of dense connective throughout the body, just under our skin and within the middle layer of visceral organs. What seemed to be a solid, dense, connective tissue layer is now being explored as a complex network of fluid-filled cavities that are strong and flexible, yet so tiny that they escaped detection until sufficient research technology evolved to find them. The Interstitium has always been there. Maybe an increased understanding of the Interstitium will help explain methods such as acupuncture, myofascial release therapy, lymphatic drainage, cranial sacral therapy, and other forms of bodywork that elude scientific mechanistic explanation. The potential is exciting, but caution is needed. Just because we hope for an explanation does not mean there is one.

Appendages of the Skin

The appendages of the skin are special structures that perform a variety of functions.

Hair

Hair protects the skin and orifices of the body, keeps us warm, and assists our sense of touch. It is found all over the body except on the palms of the hands, the soles of the feet, the palmar and plantar surfaces of the digits, the lips, the nipples, and portions of the external genitalia. Even though some parts of the body appear to be hairless, they have fine hair. Hair is composed of dead cells that have become keratinized or hardened. Follicles, including the hair root and connective tissues, hold the hair in place. A root hair plexus is a nerve that is stimulated each time the hair is moved. Tiny muscles called *erector pili* attach to hair follicles and cause the hair to stand on end at times. When this happens, the body is more sensitive to changes in air pressure and more alert to movements that may be possible signs of danger. One reason forms of near touch or light touch energy-based bodywork are thought to be effective is that the near touch and light touch and gentle movements stimulate the root hair plexuses, providing sensory stimulation.

Nails

Toenails and fingernails are hard, keratinized cells that protect the ends of the digits and assist us in grasping. The lunula is the crescent-shaped white area at the base of the nail. It is white because the blood vessels are covered with connective tissue and do not show. The nail grows from the lunula. The clear, visible portion of the nail is the nail body (Fig. 11.4).

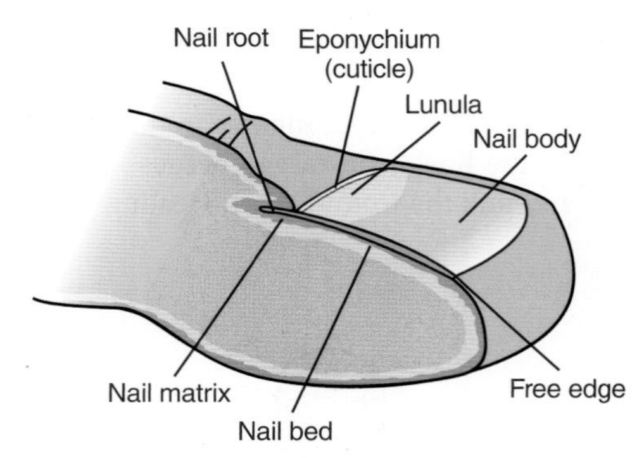

FIG. 11.4 Structure of the nail.

Sebaceous (Oil) Glands

Most oil glands are connected to hair follicles by small ducts. They can be found over most of the body except on the palms and soles. By secreting an oily substance known as *sebum*, the oil glands prevent dehydration, soften the skin and hair, and slow the growth of bacteria. Hormones, primarily androgens, stimulate the secretion of sebum. If the sebum builds up and blocks the oil gland, a whitehead can form. If the sebum dries and contacts oxygen, a blackhead can form. Acne is a bacterial inflammation of the sebaceous glands.

Sweat Glands

Also known as *sudoriferous glands*, sweat glands are found in most areas of the body, primarily on the forehead, palms, and soles. They are classified according to their structures and locations; the two main types are the eccrine glands and the apocrine glands.

The *eccrine glands*, which are the most common, are responsible for the moisture that appears on the surface of the body when the body temperature rises, particularly during physical activity. Eccrine glands cool the body and provide minor elimination of metabolic waste. Sweat is 99% water and 1% solutes in the water. The sympathetic division of the ANS regulates sweating. Heat-induced sweating tends to begin on the forehead and then spreads to the rest of the body, whereas emotion-induced sweating, stimulated by fright, embarrassment, or anxiety, begins on the palms and in the axillae (armpit) and then spreads to the rest of the body.

The *apocrine glands*, which are located in areas of body hair—primarily in the axillary and anogenital areas—begin to function during puberty. When a person is under stress, these glands produce secretions that are thicker and have a stronger odor than those of the eccrine glands. The exact function of these glands has yet to be determined, but because they are stimulated during sexual arousal and phases of the menstrual cycle, they may be similar to the sexual scent glands in other animals.

Ceruminous glands are modified apocrine glands found in the external ear canal. They secrete a sticky substance called *cerumen*, or earwax, that prevents foreign material from entering the ear and repels insects.

Mammary Glands

Mammary glands develop in the pectoral region of the chest, specifically the *breasts*. They are accessory reproductive structures in the female but are flat, nonfunctional organs in the male. Developmentally, the mammary glands are modified apocrine sweat glands. Each mammary gland is contained within a rounded, skin-covered breast anterior to the pectoral muscles of the thorax. A ring of pigmented skin called the *areola* surrounds the nipple. Internally, each mammary gland consists of 15 to 25 lobes located around the nipple. The lobes are padded and separated from each other by fibrous connective tissue and fat. Ligaments attach the breast to the underlying muscle fascia and the overlying skin, providing support. During lactation glandular alveoli produce milk, which collects in lobules within the lobes and passes through lactiferous ducts to the nipple.

Skin Color

Skin color is created by combinations of pigments in the skin and the blood flowing through the skin. These pigments are melanin, carotene, and hemoglobin.

Melanin, which is found in the epidermis, ranges in color from yellow to black. Melanin makes up most of our skin color. All of us have the same number of melanocytes, or melanin-producing cells, but the amount of melanin produced depends on genetic factors and exposure to ultraviolet light. Melanin is a natural sunscreen that protects us from ultraviolet rays by darkening our skin; this is an adaptive homeostatic function. Freckles, moles, age spots, and actinic keratoses (scaly patches that develop from sun exposure) result from increases in melanin concentration or from changes in melanocytes.

Carotene is a yellow pigment found in the dermis that naturally gives the skin of some individuals a yellow tint. If plant foods containing carotene make up a large part of a person's diet, carotene can accumulate in the skin and adipose tissue and give the skin a temporary yellow or orange color, especially on the face and the palms.

Hemoglobin is the oxygen-carrying red pigment molecule in the blood. In persons with light skin, the color of the hemoglobin shows as pink.

The color of the skin can indicate health or a pathological condition. For example, a blue tint to the skin is called *cyanosis*, a condition caused by defective or deficient oxygenation of the blood. In dark-skinned patients, cyanosis may present as gray or whitish (not bluish) skin around the mouth. A yellow-gold color of the skin may result from jaundice or liver disorders. A bronze or metallic hue often is a sign of Addison disease, a hypofunction of the adrenal cortex. Black-and-blue marks on the skin, or bruises, result when blood leaves the blood vessels and clots in the surrounding tissues. Most commonly caused by trauma or injury, constant bruising may indicate a vitamin C deficiency or a blood clotting disorder. Inflammation in tan, brown, or dark brown appears to be more gray or violet.

Pallor, or deficient in color or intensity of color of the skin, may be caused by emotional factors. Pallor may be difficult to detect in dark-toned skin and may present as ashen or grey. In brown-toned skin, the skin will present more yellowish. An alternative method for identifying pallor in darker skin tones can be assessing the palmer surface which can appear paler. The skin can contain as much as 5% of the blood in our bodies. During sympathetic autonomic activation, when the muscles need blood, the vessels of the skin contract to move the blood out. Sudden pallor may be caused by stressful situations, such as those provoking anger or fear. Anemia is a decrease in functioning red blood cells or hemoglobin; people with anemia appear pale. Some people, however, are naturally pale as a result of the opaqueness of the epidermis. Excessive redness may be caused by embarrassment resulting in blushing, an increase in body temperature or fever, hypertension, inflammation, allergy, rosacea, or hormonal fluctuations.

Practical Application

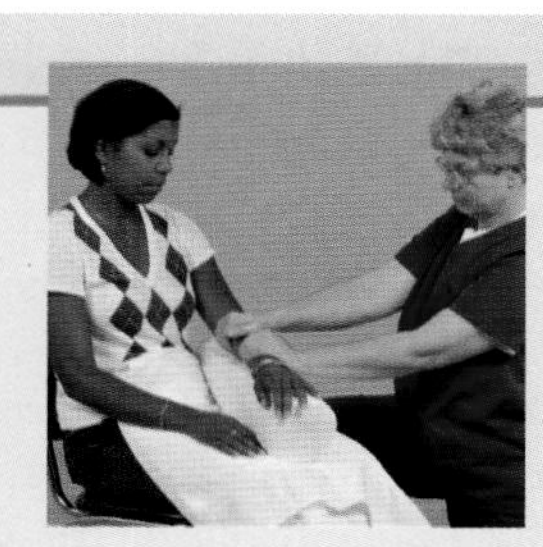

Observation of a person's skin color and changes in the appearance, texture, and suppleness of the skin and the appendages can provide information about changes in a person's health status. Because massage therapists are likely to touch the skin more than any other professional, they should be especially observant of the skin and its appendages, which can be indicators of dysfunction or improved health. Massage therapists need to be especially aware of any signs of skin cancer. Early detection is the key to successful treatment. Visit the MedlinePlus website and use the search terms skin cancer, and skin sun damage.

Stem Cells, Wound Healing, and Scar Tissue

Stem cells are cells that can become, or differentiate into, any of several types of cells. There are stem cells located within the skin. Stem cells are a major focus of medical research. One of the major obstacles to stem cell research is obtaining stem cells. Recently, researchers at Rockefeller University identified two proteins that enable skin stem cells to renew themselves. Scientists have created liver cells in a laboratory using these reprogrammed cells from human skin, paving the way for the potential development of new treatments for liver diseases that kill thousands each year.

Delayed healing of skin wounds is a major healthcare concern. The research on massage benefits for wound healing is scant, but there is some indication that massage is helpful. The majority of the research involves burn healing. Massage may reduce itching and pain related to wound healing, and although not related to skin, massage also reduces anxiety and improves mood. Massage may also support productive scar tissue development. A recent research study found that connective tissue growth factor (CTGF) was reduced after 24 hours of cell stretching. These findings suggest that cyclic stretching of fibroblasts contributes to antifibrotic processes by reducing CTGF production. Massage is a method of producing cell stretching. Whether massage produces a significant effect on scar development has not been substantiated, but it may be possible.

Pathological Conditions of the Integumentary System

Pathological conditions of the integument give rise to two main concerns related to impairment of the structural integrity of the skin. The first concern is the loss of the protection of internal structures. The second concern is the loss of the ability of the skin to prevent the pathogens of contagious diseases from entering the body. Observing the **Standard Precautions** guidelines established by the Centers for Disease Control and Prevention (CDC) and proper sanitation methods maintains the security of the skin and its protective barriers. Pathological conditions of the skin, especially sores, rashes, and changes in color and texture (Figs. 11.5 and 11.6), can indicate a more serious systemic disease and the practitioner should refer the client to a physician for diagnosis.

Bacterial Infections

Acne

Acne vulgaris, the common form of acne, is a chronic inflammation of the sebaceous glands and hair follicles caused by the interaction of bacteria, sebum, and sex hormones. Acne vulgaris is most common at puberty and may recur in females during menopause. The condition can produce blackheads, whiteheads, cysts, pustules, and inflamed nodules.

Boils

Boils are local staphylococcal infections similar to acne, but they are not caused by an interaction with sex hormones. Boils look like acne except that the lesions are bigger and more painful, and they usually occur singly rather than being spread over a large area. Sometimes they occur in a cluster called a *carbuncle*. The bacteria that cause boils are virulent and communicable. Local massage is contraindicated, and the therapist should take care to make sure that the infection is not systemic.

Impetigo

Impetigo is an acute, highly contagious bacterial skin infection usually found on the face. Impetigo is characterized by small red spots that develop into vesicles, which become filled with pus; burst; and develop a thick, yellow crust.

Cellulitis

Cellulitis is a rapidly spreading, acute bacterial infection of the skin usually found in the lower extremities. Bacteria enter through damaged skin or as a result of complications of diabetes or poor circulation. Symptoms include redness, heat, swelling, and pain.

Erysipelas

Erysipelas is a streptococcal infection that kills skin cells, leading to painful inflammation of the skin. Erysipelas usually occur on the face or lower legs. The bacterial infection can invade the **lymph** and circulatory systems. Massage is systemically contraindicated until the infection has passed completely.

Ecthyma

Ecthyma is a skin infection that is similar to impetigo but more deeply invasive. Usually caused by a streptococcal infection, ecthyma goes through the epidermis to the dermis of the skin, possibly causing scars.

Viral Skin Infections

Chickenpox

Chickenpox is a viral infection that causes a blister-like rash on the surface of the skin and mucous membranes. Chickenpox blisters usually appear first on the trunk and face and then spread to almost every other area of the body, including the scalp and penis, and inside the mouth, nose, ears, and vagina. Chickenpox blisters are about 0.2 to 0.4 inch (5–10 mm) wide, have a reddish base, and appear in crops over 2 to 4 days. Some people get only a few blisters, and others have several hundred. As blisters itch and break, scabs form and the blisters may become infected by bacteria, which is considered a secondary bacterial infection.

Some individuals may experience fever, abdominal pain, or a vague sick feeling along with skin blisters. These symptoms usually last 3 to 5 days, and the person's temperature stays in the range of 101° to 103°F (38.3°–39.4°C). Younger children often have milder symptoms and fewer blisters than older children or adults. Generally, chickenpox is a mild illness, but it can be deadly in people who have leukemia or other diseases that weaken the immune system.

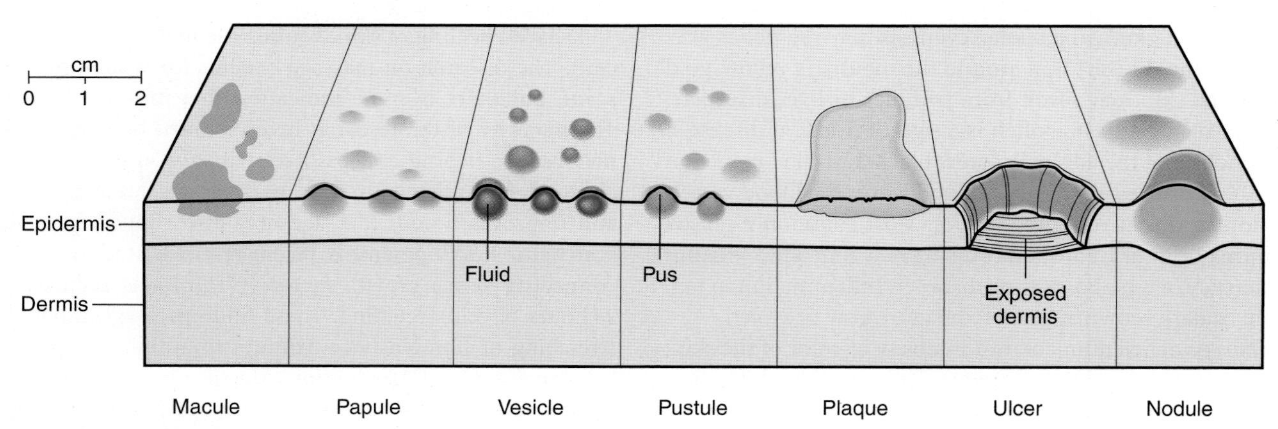

FIG. 11.5 Appearance of various skin lesions. (From Damjanov I. *Pathology for the Health-Related Professions*. 4th ed. Saunders/Elsevier; 2012.)

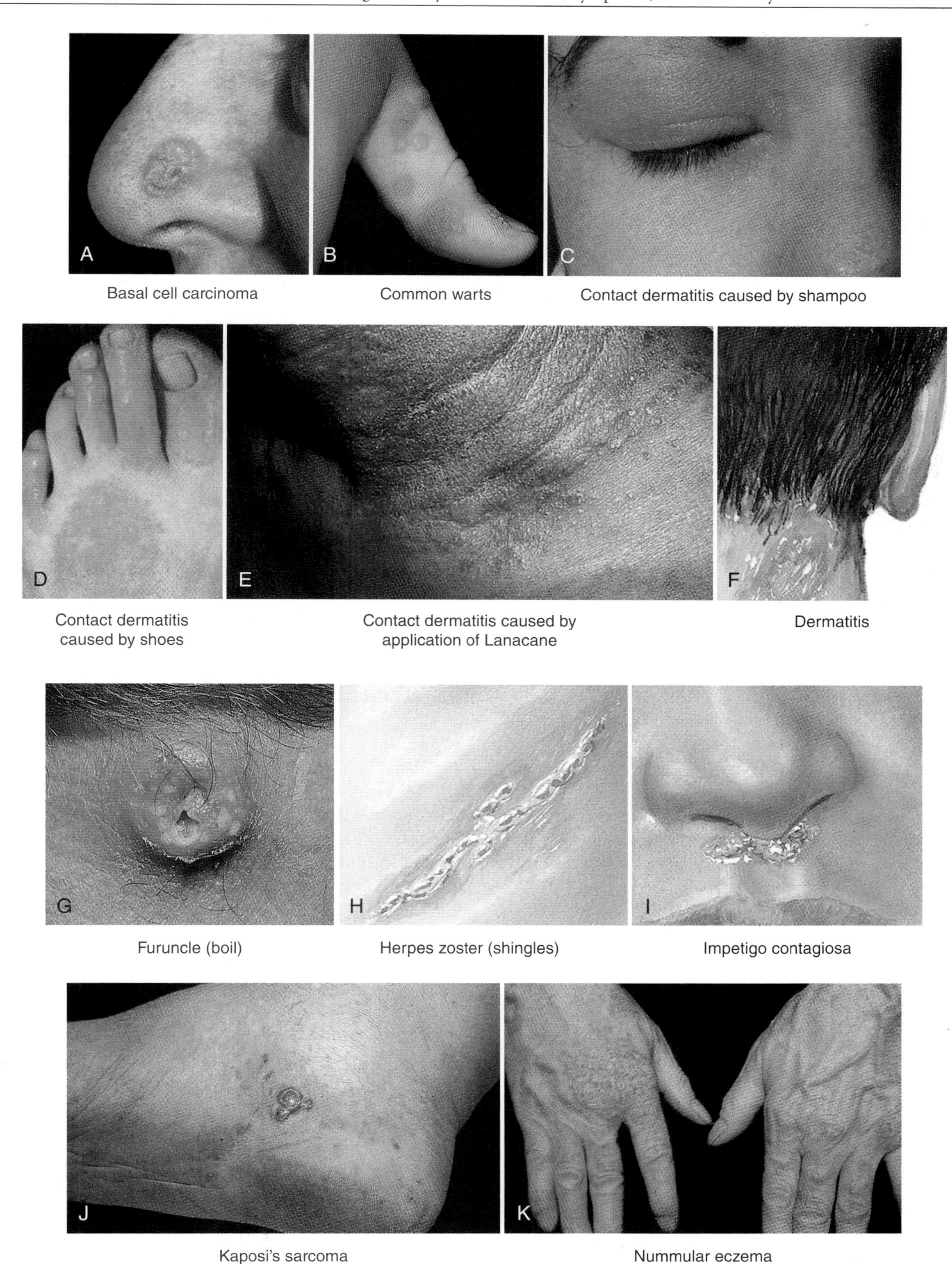

FIG. 11.6 (A–P) Common skin disorders. Skin problems may result from various causes, such as parasitic infestations; fungal, bacterial, or viral infections; reactions to substances encountered externally or taken internally; and new growths. Many of the skin manifestations have no known cause; others are hereditary. (A and M, From Habif TP. *Clinical Dermatology: A Color Guide to Diagnosis and Therapy*. 4th ed. Mosby; 2004; B, From Habif TP. *Clinical Dermatology*. 2nd ed. Mosby; 1990; C, D, K, L, and P, Reprinted with permission from the American Academy of Dermatology. Copyright 2012. All rights reserved; E, From Zitelli BJ, Davis HW. *Atlas of Pediatric Physical Diagnosis*. 5th ed. Mosby; 2007; F, H, I, N, and O, From Bork K, Brauninger W. *Skin Diseases in Clinical Practice*. 2nd ed. WB Saunders; 1998; G, From Jaime A Tschen, MD, Department of Dermatology, Baylor College of Medicine, Houston; J, From Habif TP. *Clinical Dermatology: A Color Guide to Diagnosis and Therapy*. 3rd ed. Mosby; 1996.)

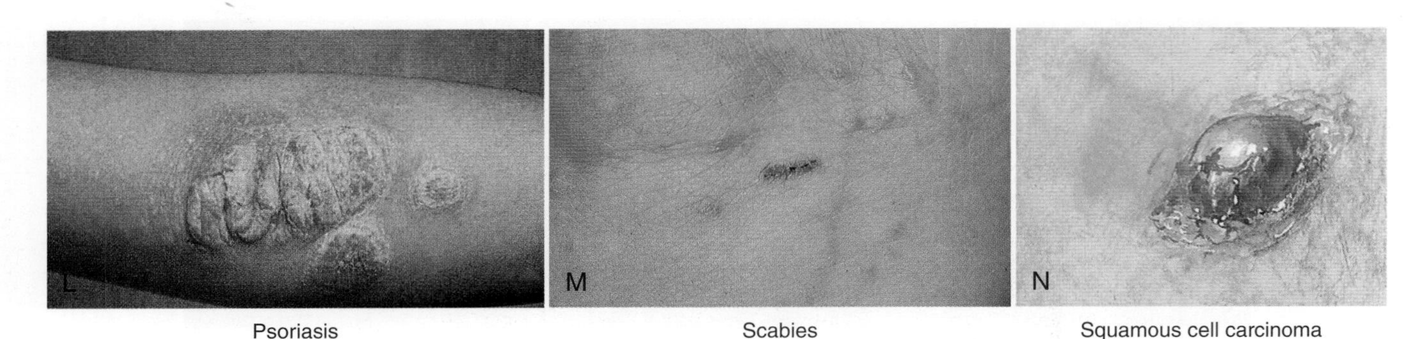

Psoriasis Scabies Squamous cell carcinoma

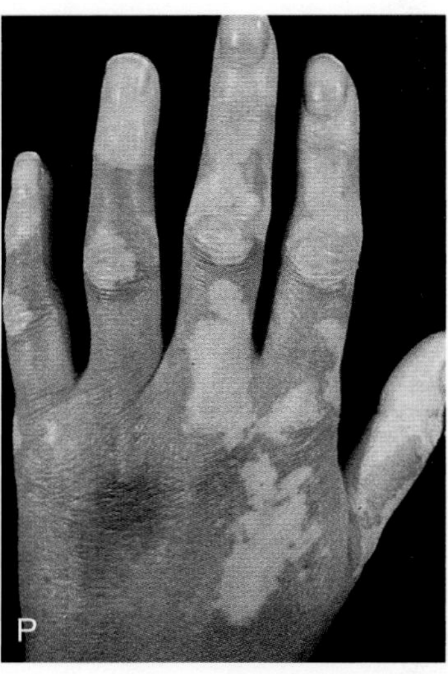

Tinea corporis (ringworm) Vitiligo

FIG. 11.6, cont'd

Usually, a person has only one attack of chickenpox in a lifetime. But the virus that causes chickenpox can stay dormant in the body and can cause a different type of skin eruption, called *shingles*, later in life.

Herpes Simplex

Herpes simplex is a viral infection resulting in cold sores or fever blisters on the face or in the mouth (type 1) or around the genitals, thighs, or buttocks (type 2). All the herpes viruses are contagious. As with all herpes viruses, herpes simplex remains dormant in the nerves of the body until resistance is low, at which time it travels down the nerve to cause the eruption. Herpes outbreaks often are preceded by 2 to 3 days of tingling, itching, or pain. Blisters then appear, gradually crust, and disappear, usually within 2 weeks.

Measles

Measles is a serious infection that spreads easily from person to person. It is caused by the measles virus. Symptoms begin 10 to 12 days after contact with an infected person and include fever (often high), fatigue, runny nose, cough, and watery red eyes. After 2 or 3 days, tiny white spots may appear in the mouth, and after 2 more days, a raised, red rash starts on the face and spreads down the body and out to the arms and legs. The rash usually lasts 4 to 7 days. Symptoms usually last 1 to 2 weeks, and measles is contagious for about 1 week before to 1 week after the rash begins. Serious complications of measles can occur. Those with measles should stay away from others until at least 4 full days have passed since the rash first appeared.

Measles is spread from person to person by the droplets issuing from the mouth, nose, and throat of an infected person. The infected droplets are spread through the air or directly onto another person's hands and face through coughing and sneezing.

German measles, or rubella, is a mild viral illness caused by the rubella virus. It involves fever and a rash, along with aches in the joints when it affects adults. Children usually are not affected seriously. Commonly, the first manifestation is a fine, pink rash spreading from the forehead and face downward. The rash may last 1 to 5 days. Glands (lymph nodes) are enlarged, especially those behind the ears and on the back of the head. Adults often feel more unwell before the rash appears and may have arthritis-type pain in the joints. The major reason to eradicate this virus is the serious effects it has on an unborn baby when a person who is pregnant contracts it in early pregnancy.

Molluscum Contagiosum

Molluscum contagiosum is a superficial skin infection. The virus invades the skin, causing the appearance of firm, flesh-colored, doughnut-shaped bumps 2 to 5 mm in diameter.

Their sunken centers contain a white, curd-like material. The bumps can occur almost anywhere on the body, including the buttocks, thighs, and external genitalia. They often remain unchanged for many months and then disappear.

Molluscum contagiosum is caused by a virus belonging to the poxvirus family. Close physical contact is usually necessary for transmission; indirect transmission through shared towels, swimming pools, and so forth also may be responsible for infection. The incubation period varies from several weeks to several months. Shaving or scratching may cause the infection to spread.

Warts

A wart is a benign growth of the keratin-producing cells of the epidermis and mucous membranes that is caused by the human papillomavirus. Warts are transmitted through direct contact. The common wart (*Verruca vulgaris*) has a rough, elevated surface and is found mainly on the hands and fingers of children and young adults. Filiform warts are longer, slender growths on the face, neck, and axillae. Periungual warts are found around the nails of the fingers and toes. Flat warts are flesh colored and form when several warts spread, through scratching or shaving. Plantar warts have rough surfaces and are located in the thickened skin of the sole. They may be mistaken for calluses but often have small, dark spots that calluses do not have. Normal skin lines stop at the edge of the wart.

Fungal Skin Infections

Candidiasis

Candidiasis is an infection of the skin or mucous membranes, most often caused by the organism *Candida albicans.* Red, scaly patches may appear in the creases of the axillae and groin and under the breasts, as well as between the fingers and toes. Associated infections can occur in the ear, vagina, and mouth. When it develops in the mouth, it is called *thrush. C. albicans* is a common cause of diaper rash in infants.

Dermatophytosis

More commonly known as *ringworm*, tinea is a group of common fungal infections contracted by touching contaminated items or an infected person's skin. The types of tinea are named by their location on the body. Tinea corporis appears on the nonhairy portions of the skin as fast-growing, reddish, elevated lesions surrounded by a dry and scaly or moist and crusty, raised, ringlike border, which gives it the ringworm appearance. Tinea pedis, or athlete's foot, is marked by blisters and cracking of the skin between the toes and on the ball of the foot. Tinea cruris, or jock itch, is a ringworm of the pubic area.

Parasitic Skin Infections

Lice

Lice are parasites, and three types affect human beings. Head lice (*Pediculosis capitis*) are the most common type. They are found mainly on the scalp and sometimes in the eyebrows and eyelashes, and they cause intense itching. Outbreaks generally occur among schoolchildren. The bite of the body louse (*Pediculosis corporis*) leaves visible, itchy red spots primarily on the shoulders, buttocks, and abdomen. Genital lice (*Pediculosis lpubis;* crab lice) usually are found in the pubic area and are transmitted during sexual activity or contact with contaminated bedding.

Scabies

Scabies is a contagious skin disease characterized by intense itching caused by a microscopic, parasitic mite that burrows under the epidermis. Scabies can attack any area of the body, but the parts most susceptible are the finger webs, anterior wrists, elbows, axillary regions, areolae of the breasts, genitals, and lower buttocks. The parasite is transmitted by skin-to-skin contact with human beings or pets or by direct contact with contaminated items.

(NOTE: Although bed bugs are not technically a skin infection, it might be useful to be familiar with the appearance of their bites.)

Ulcers

An ulcer is a round open sore of the skin or mucous membrane that results from the tissue damage that accompanies inflammation, infection, or malignancy.

Decubitus Ulcer

A decubitus ulcer is an open sore that develops primarily over the bony areas of the heels and hips of those who are immobile, bedridden, or in wheelchairs. Continuous pressure on the skin diminishes or stops circulation, and the tissue dies.

Neurotrophic Ulcer

Neurotrophic ulcers develop at pressure-point areas on the feet when pain sensation is diminished or absent, as in diabetic neuropathy. Although often deep and infected, these ulcers are painless. Callus formation around the ulcer, like the ulcer itself, results from chronic pressure.

Benign Tumors and Growths

A neoplasm, or **tumor**, is a growth of new tissues that may be benign or malignant. The following are considered benign.

Mole

A mole, or nevus, is a benign pigmented skin growth formed by melanocytes.

Callus

A callus is an area of thickened, hardened skin, like corn, which develops in an area of friction or a region of recurrent pressure. A callus involves skin that normally is thick, such as the sole or the palm, and usually is painless. If a callus is painful, an underlying plantar wart may be present.

Corn

A corn is a painful, conical thickening of the skin over bony prominences of the feet caused by continual pressure and friction on normally thin skin. Corns located in moist areas, such as between the toes, are called *soft corns.*

Lipoma
A lipoma is a benign tumor formed of mature fat cells. The tumor appears as a soft, movable subcutaneous nodule that is typically found on the trunk, forearms, or neck.

Sebaceous Cyst
A sebaceous cyst is a slow-growing, benign tumor caused by the blockage of a sebaceous gland. The cyst contains keratin, sebum, and hair follicle cells.

Seborrheic Keratosis
Seborrheic keratosis is a slightly raised skin lesion most commonly seen on the chest, back, neck, and face. These benign growths usually appear in middle-aged and elderly individuals as light brown or black flat areas. They may grow quickly and can be mistaken for moles or warts.

Skin Tag
A skin tag is a small, soft, flesh-colored, or pigmented benign growth found on the neck or in the axillary or groin region.

Angioma
An angioma is a benign tumor composed of blood or lymphatic vessels. Angiomas are common in newborns and usually disappear during childhood.

Malignant Skin Tumors
Skin cancer is the most common of all malignancies. Most skin cancers appear on the head, neck, and other areas frequently exposed to the sun. Too much sun exposure damages the skin by causing the elastin fibers to clump, leading to leathery skin and wrinkling. Immune function may be depressed temporarily, and deoxyribonucleic acid (DNA) is altered, leading to skin cancer. Three types of malignancy can occur.

Basal Cell Carcinoma
The most common form of skin cancer, basal cell carcinoma is associated with exposure to ultraviolet light. It grows slowly and is the easiest type to treat successfully when recognized early.

Squamous Cell Carcinoma
Also related to exposure to ultraviolet light, squamous cell carcinoma is responsible for one-third of all skin cancers. Like basal cell carcinoma, squamous cell carcinoma is best treated in the earlier stages before it metastasizes. People with fair skin, blond or red hair, and chronic skin inflammation, who are exposed to the sun or who suffered sun damage when young, are at greater risk for basal cell and squamous cell carcinomas.

Malignant Melanoma
Malignant melanoma is the least common and the most dangerous of the skin cancers. It is not connected directly to sun exposure. Because melanoma spreads rapidly, it must be identified and treated quickly.

The memory device that helps in identifying melanoma is "ABCD": *a*symmetry, *b*order irregularity, *c*olor change, and increase in *d*iameter. Most melanomas are not evenly round but have irregular borders with white, blue, or red edges turning brown or black. Moles are especially susceptible to transformation into melanomas.

Breast Disorders

Fibrocystic Disease
Fibrocystic disease is the most common disorder of the breast. The condition involves the growth of small, lumpy cysts that develop because of changes in the milk-producing glands. The disease affects about 50% of females. No treatment is necessary, but because the incidence of breast cancer is higher in these females, healthcare providers must address recommendations for breast self-examination and the frequency of mammograms for each person.

Breast Cancer
The peak incidence of breast cancer occurs in the early menopausal age group, when some females develop a painless, firm lump, often in the upper outer quadrant. In one form of breast cancer, no lump develops. The diagnosis is made by using low-voltage soft tissue radiographs called *mammograms* and by performing fine-needle biopsy. The standard medical treatment is based on many factors, including the size of the lump, the patient's age and physical condition, and the involvement of lymph nodes and other tissues. Muscle tissue and lymph nodes are removed when metastasis has occurred.

Surgical intervention consists of one of the following procedures: a lumpectomy (removal of the tumor), a simple mastectomy (removal of the affected breast only), a radical mastectomy (removal of the breast, pectoralis major and pectoralis minor muscles, and the axillary lymph nodes), an extended radical mastectomy (in addition to the aforementioned, removal of the internal mammary lymph nodes near the sternum), or a modified radical mastectomy (removal of the breast and axillary lymph nodes, preserving the pectoralis major muscle). Radiation therapy, chemical therapy (chemotherapy), and hormone therapy are other methods of intervention, which may be used alone or with surgery.

Although the number of males who develop breast cancer is small, lumps and changes in the tissues of the breast cannot be ignored, and such clients should be referred to a physician for examination.

Anatomical and Physiological Problems After a Mastectomy. With the removal of the pectoralis major muscle, some flexion and adduction of the arm are lost. The client may develop the anterior part of the deltoid, as well as the coracobrachialis and the long head of the biceps, to help with flexion.

Loss of lymphatic channels in the axillae causes obstruction of lymph flow from the arm, and localized edema develops. Elevation of the arm and the use of a special sleeve to provide compression are helpful. Massage may help in mild cases.

Burns
The term *burn* refers to cells that have been destroyed or inflamed because of heat, chemicals, radiation, or electricity. Fluid loss and secondary bacterial infection can occur as a consequence of the tissue damage. Burns are classified by the depth of damage and are identified by degree.

In a first-degree burn, only the epidermis sustains injury. Signs and symptoms include redness, mild stinging or pain, and mild swelling. These burns usually heal within a matter of days or weeks. A mild sunburn is a first-degree burn.

In a second-degree burn, the epidermis and the dermis are damaged. Along with redness and moderate to intense pain and swelling, blisters usually develop. In deeper burns, the tissues may be white because of damage to the vascular supply. Second-degree burns can take 6 weeks to a few months to heal and commonly leave scars.

In a third-degree burn, the epidermis and entire dermis are damaged severely or destroyed. Damage to nerves can interrupt pain signals in the actual area of the burn. The skin may appear white, black, or charred, and no blisters form. Dehydration and infection may occur because of the loss of the protective skin barrier. A third-degree burn develops scars and may require a skin graft and a long healing period.

Other Integumentary Disorders

Dermatitis and Eczema

Dermatitis is a general term for acute or chronic skin inflammation characterized by redness, eruptions, edema, scaling, and itching. The term *eczema* is used interchangeably with the term *dermatitis*, but many medical references limit the designation *dermatitis* to conditions caused by internal factors. Three major types of dermatitis have been recognized:

Atopic dermatitis: Caused by an allergy or hypersensitivity, most commonly pollens, cosmetics, or foods. The condition is commonly associated with other hypersensitivity disorders. Symptoms include inflammation, oozing and crusting, and intense itching.

Seborrheic dermatitis: A chronic condition that manifests in inflammation, scales, and crusting. The skin may be dry or greasy. The adult form of seborrheic dermatitis is a mild form of dandruff, most commonly seen at the eyebrows and on the scalp as a dry or greasy scaling. Cradle cap is the associated childhood form. Genetic predisposition, weather, stress, and some neurological diseases may be risk factors.

Contact dermatitis: Caused by sensitivity to a substance that damages or irritates the skin, such as poison ivy, a medication, cosmetics, or rubber. The condition may be marked by blisters or itchy, flaky skin.

Pseudofolliculitis barbae

Pseudofolliculitis barbae (razor bumps) is a common condition of the beard area that occurs in people with curly hair. The problem results when highly curved hairs grow back into the skin, causing inflammation and a foreign-body reaction. Over time, this can cause keloidal scarring, which looks like hard bumps on the beard area and neck.

Psoriasis

Psoriasis is a common, noncontagious autoimmune chronic skin disease characterized by reddened skin covered by dry, silvery scales. It is found most commonly on the scalp, elbows, knees, back, or buttocks.

Rosacea

Rosacea is a noncontagious chronic skin problem in which the small blood vessels of the forehead, cheeks, and nose become dilated. Rosacea may affect a small area or the entire face. Eye inflammation (conjunctivitis) may develop. Rosacea may lie dormant for a time and then be activated by stress, infection, hot or spicy food, sunlight, or physical activity.

Urticaria (Hives)

Urticaria, or hives, is a condition of localized skin eruptions, called *wheals*, in the dermis. Hives are caused by allergy, exposure to heat or cold, or an emotional reaction. Urticaria may be accompanied by local pruritus (itching).

Alopecia

Alopecia is hair loss or baldness on parts or all of the body. Alopecia can be caused by aging, genetic predisposition, local diseases, chemotherapy, stress, or nutritional imbalances. Androgens seem to play a part in hair loss. Male-pattern baldness features hair loss on the forehead and top of the head, whereas female-pattern baldness involves thinning of the hair in the frontal and parietal regions.

Scleroderma

Scleroderma (systemic sclerosis) is an autoimmune disorder of the connective tissue that is characterized by inflammation and overproduction of collagen. The resulting scarring causes the tissues to stiffen and compress the capillaries, thus diminishing or halting blood flow. The disease usually appears in persons between 30 and 50 years of age and affects females more often than males. Characteristics include increased joint stiffness, muscle weakness, swelling of the fingers, and skin-thickening collagen deposits. Collagen deposits can invade not only the integument but also many of the body systems, such as the gastrointestinal tract, reducing the absorption of nutrients, and the lungs, diminishing respiratory effectiveness. Hypersensitivity to cold in the fingers, toes, ears, and nose, as occurs in Raynaud syndrome, may be present. In the most serious cases, heart and lung failure may occur.

Vitiligo

Vitiligo is a disease marked by loss of skin pigmentation in irregular patches. Vitiligo usually affects exposed areas of the skin in persons under 30 years of age who have a family history of the disease.

Section Summary

- Explain the importance of touch.
- Touch involves variations in temperature, vibration, and pressure while informing differences in texture, shape, resistance, and tension. Touch is the first sense to develop in the embryo. Not being touched leads to reduced neuroendocrine chemicals related to well-being and can contribute to *marasmus* (wasting away), especially in infants, the elderly, and those with weakened immune systems.

INDICATIONS/CONTRAINDICATIONS for Therapeutic Massage

Integumentary System

Therapeutic massage is not typically contraindicated with localized skin conditions, but local (regional) avoidance of the affected area is necessary. Localized touch can irritate most skin disorders. Massage is contraindicated if the skin is inflamed or if the condition is contagious or transmissible through touch.

A wound is any injury to the skin that has not healed and that is vulnerable to infection if exposed to bacteria or other microorganisms. Skin injuries are vulnerable as long as a visible crust or scab remains. Massage is contraindicated locally for any unhealed skin injury in which bleeding has occurred. When the underlying epidermis has been replaced completely, the scab falls off and the wound is no longer at risk for infection. Massage may be contraindicated systemically if the skin injury is connected to a contraindicated underlying condition, such as diabetes. Standard Precautions are indicated for all skin pathologies. Skin cancers are not a general contraindication, and local avoidance of the area is indicated. More importantly, the massage professional needs to be able to recognize skin changes related to possible skin cancers and refer the client for a diagnosis.

- Describe the function of the integumentary system.
  Protect internal structures and organs, prevent entry of bacteria and viruses, synthesize vitamin D, detect touch/temperature/pain/pressure, regulate body temperature, excrete sweat and salts, and secrete sebum.
- Describe two main concerns with integumentary pathological conditions.
  Loss of protection for internal structures and loss of ability to prevent pathogens from entering the body.
- Describe the three types of skin cancer.
  Basal cell carcinoma: Most common. Associated with exposure to ultraviolet light. Grows slowly. The easiest type to treat upon early detection. *Squamous cell carcinoma:* Responsible for one-third of all skin cancers. Related to ultraviolet light exposure. Best treated in earlier stages, before metastasis. (People with fair skin/blond or red hair/chronic skin inflammation are at greater risk for basal and squamous cell carcinoma.) *Malignant melanoma:* Least common but most dangerous. Not connected directly to sun exposure. Spreads rapidly. Must be identified and treated quickly. Most have irregular borders with white/blue/red edges turning to brown/black. Moles are especially susceptible to transforming into melanomas. Mnemonic is ABCD: *A*symmetry, *B*order irregularity, *C*olor change, *D*iameter increase.

CARDIOVASCULAR SYSTEM

SECTION OBJECTIVES

Chapter objectives covered in this section:

4. List and describe the components and functions of the cardiovascular system.
5. Identify pathologies of the cardiovascular system and describe indications and contraindications for massage.

After completing this section, the learner will be able to:

- List the components of the cardiovascular system.
- List the components of blood.

The cardiovascular system is a transport system composed of the heart, blood vessels, and blood (Fig. 11.7). The **heart** is the pump that sends the oxygen and nutrient-rich blood out to the body by way of the arteries and **arterioles**. The oxygen and nutrients in the blood leave the capillaries and enter the tissues. Carbon dioxide and metabolic wastes leave the tissues, reenter the capillaries, and pass through the **venules** and **veins** on their way back to the heart. The heart then pumps the blood to the lungs, where carbon dioxide diffuses out of the blood so that it can be eliminated from the body. The blood also picks up oxygen and travels back to the heart, where the cycle starts all over again.

FOCUS ON PROFESSIONALISM

Much of the outdated information and many of the myths about massage therapy are related to the eight body systems described in this chapter and Chapter 12. It is important to learn to examine the evidence of any massage claim. Even when textbooks are revised on a regular basis, some of the content can become outdated. Your critical thinking skills will help you keep current on the latest information about massage therapy. Massage therapy is moving to a practice based on research and the consensus of groups of experts. In the past, massage therapy benefits, mechanisms of action, and the underlying physiology of the effects of massage methods were often mistakenly based on opinion, perpetuating myths, and outdated information. With an increase in scholarly research and greater scrutiny of massage claims, this situation is changing. The Massage Therapy Foundation is committed to supporting the development of best practices for massage therapy. Best practices are methods and techniques that have consistently shown results superior to those achieved by other means.

Heart

The heart is the major organ of the cardiovascular system (see Fig. 11.7). It is a hollow, muscular pump about the size of a clenched fist located in the mediastinum (the space between the lungs). The heart rests on the diaphragm. The **pericardium** is a sac that surrounds the heart and secretes a lubricating fluid that prevents friction resulting from the movement of the heart. The pericardium also secures the heart within the thoracic cavity.

The myocardium is the heart muscle that makes up the thickest part of the heart. Contractions of the myocardium perform the pumping action of the heart. The outer membrane of the heart is called the *epicardium* and is continuous with the pericardium. The endocardium is the smooth, thin inner lining of the heart. The blood slides along the endocardium as it flows through the heart.

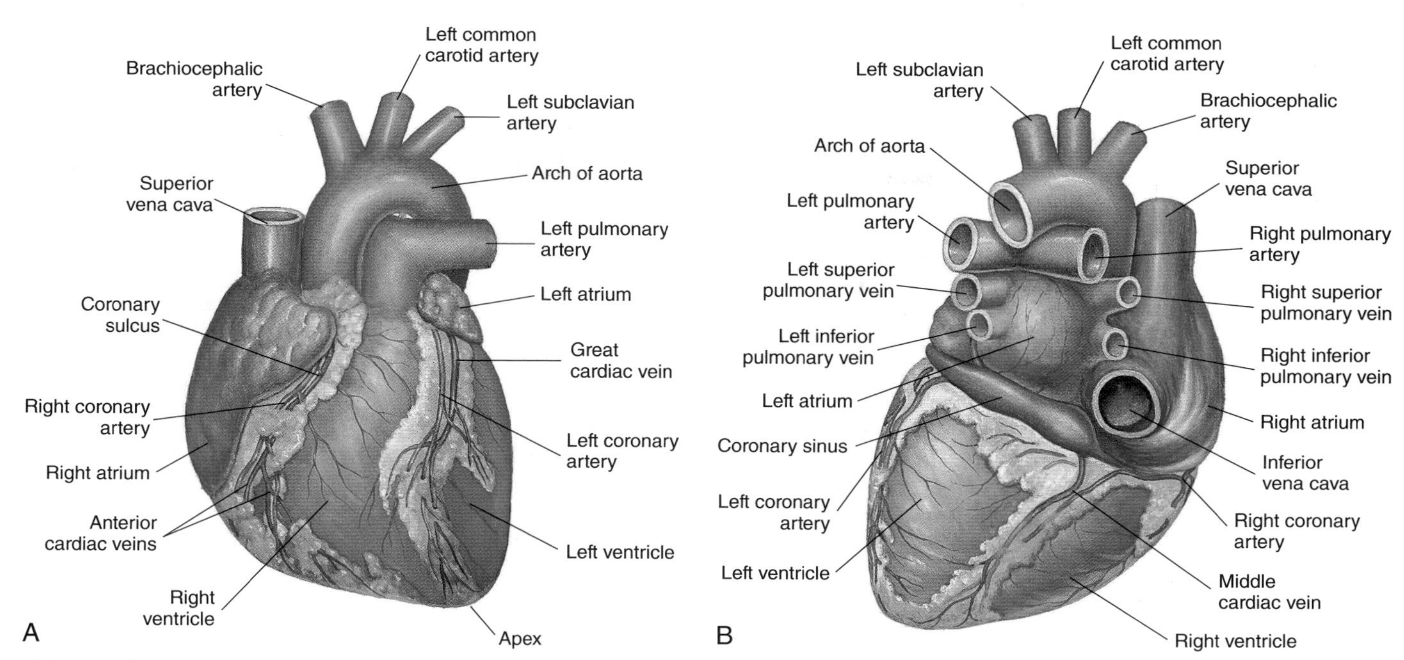

FIG. 11.7 Cardiovascular system. (A) Anterior view of the heart. (B) Posterior view of the heart. (From Seidel HM, et al. *Mosby's Guide to Physical Examination*. 7th ed. Mosby/Elsevier; 2011.)

The heart is divided into four chambers. The two small, thin-walled superior chambers are the atria, known separately as the left atrium and the right atrium; they are separated by the interatrial septum. The two larger, inferior chambers are the left and right ventricles; their thick walls are separated by the interventricular septum. The atria and ventricles are separated by a fibrous structure called the *skeleton of the heart*.

MENTORING TIP

The heart is often used to symbolize moral, emotional, spiritual, and even intellectual qualities. Massage therapists are typically warm, kind, empathetic, and compassionate people. Massage is provided in a heartfelt and wholehearted manner. We offer an open-hearted and sincere professional touch. Professional touch is based on empathy and compassion. Empathy is the ability to understand the emotional state of another person or oneself, and compassion includes the desire to alleviate or reduce the suffering of another. Clients can have broken hearts, physically and emotionally. So can we. Healing a broken heart takes time. Massage therapy provided by professional massage therapists who understand the ethics and boundaries of a heart-to-heart massage relationship can be part of heart healing.

Heart Valves

Created from the folds of the endocardium and maintained within the skeleton of the heart are the heart valves. This set of four valves regulates the flow of blood through the heart. Atrioventricular valves allow blood to flow from the atria into the ventricles and keep it from returning into the atria when the ventricles contract. The ventricles contract quite forcefully, shooting blood upward. Strings of connective tissue known as *chordae tendineae cordis* connect between the ventricle wall and the valves. They keep the cusps, or flaps, of the valve closed when the ventricle contracts to keep the force of the blood from pushing open the valve. This ensures that the blood moves forward into the aorta and pulmonary arteries, not back into the atria. The bicuspid, or mitral (left atrioventricular), valve is located between the left atrium and the left ventricle; the tricuspid (right atrioventricular) valve is located between the right atrium and the right ventricle.

Semilunar valves control the blood flow out of the ventricles into the aorta and pulmonary arteries. They prevent backflow of blood into the ventricles. The aortic valve is between the left ventricle and the aorta, and the pulmonary valve is between the pulmonary artery and the right ventricle. These valves open in response to pressure generated when the blood leaves the ventricle. They close when blood pools in small pockets of the cusps of the valves and pushes the valves closed (Fig. 11.8).

Blood Vessels

Arteries carry oxygenated blood away from the heart. The only exceptions are the pulmonary arteries. They carry blood away from the heart to the lungs, but it is deoxygenated blood. Veins carry deoxygenated blood from the body to the heart. The only exceptions are the pulmonary veins. They carry blood to the heart from the lungs, but it is oxygenated blood.

Arteries branch into small vessels called *arterioles*. These enter the tissues and branch into capillaries. Capillaries are the smallest blood vessels. They allow the exchange of gases, nutrients, and waste products between the blood and tissue cells. Capillaries join into venules, which in turn join into veins. Arteries, arterioles, capillaries, venules, and veins are discussed in more detail in the section on the vascular system.

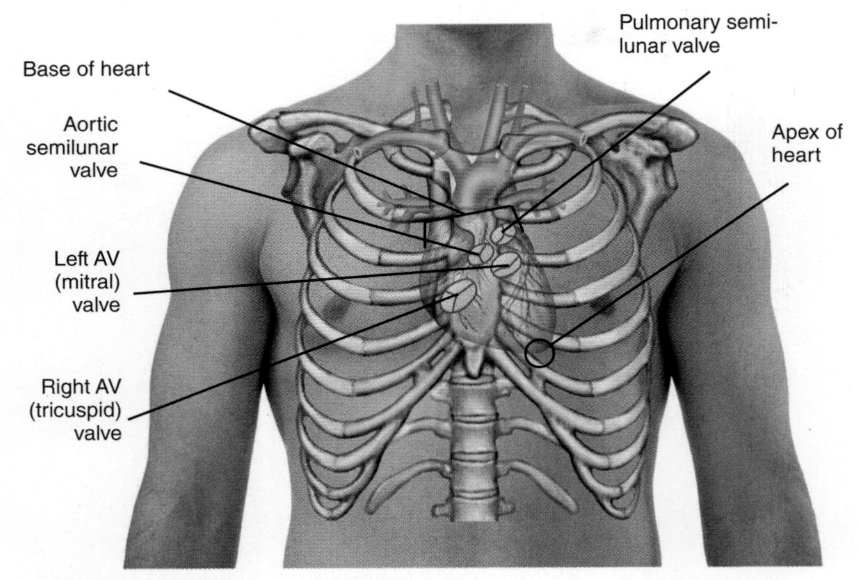

FIG. 11.8 Relation of the heart to the anterior wall of the thorax. Valves of the heart are projected on the anterior thoracic wall. *AV*, atrioventricular. (From Seidel HM, et al. *Mosby's Guide to Physical Examination*. 7th ed. Mosby/Elsevier; 2011.)

The term *great vessels* refers to the large blood vessels entering or leaving the heart that transport blood to the lungs and the rest of the body. The three great vessels are the:

- *Aorta:* The artery that carries oxygen and nutrients away from the heart to the body
- *Pulmonary trunk:* The artery that carries blood to the lungs to release carbon dioxide and take in oxygen
- *Superior vena cava:* The vein that returns deoxygenated blood to the right atrium from the upper venous circulation

Other major blood vessels include the:

- *Inferior vena cava:* The vein that returns deoxygenated blood from the lower venous circulation to the right atrium
- *Pulmonary veins*: The four veins, two from each lung, that take oxygenated blood to the left atrium

Blood Supply to and from the Heart

The two **coronary arteries**, which originate from the base of the aorta, supply oxygenated blood to the heart muscle. Coronary veins follow parallel to the arteries and return the blood to the right atrium by way of the coronary sinus. Both types of coronary vessels run in grooves between the atria and ventricles and between the two ventricles. All the veins of the heart drain into the coronary sinus, which drains the deoxygenated blood from the heart tissues into the right atrium.

Blood Flow through the Heart

Blood moves into and out of the heart in a well-coordinated and precisely timed rhythm. The rhythm can be divided into the following stages (Fig. 11.9):

Stage 1: Deoxygenated blood from the body enters the superior and inferior venae cavae. Deoxygenated blood from the heart drains into the coronary sinus. All three empty into the right atrium. When the blood reaches a certain volume, it pushes open the tricuspid valve, and blood empties into the right ventricle. The right atrium then contracts to squeeze a little more blood into the right ventricle.

Stage 2: The right ventricle contracts and pushes blood through the pulmonary valve into the pulmonary artery. This artery divides into the left and right pulmonary arteries and takes the blood to each lung.

Stage 3: This process takes place at the same time as the process described in stage 1. Four pulmonary veins leave the lungs, carrying oxygenated blood back to the left atrium. When the blood reaches a certain volume, it pushes open the bicuspid (mitral) valve, and blood empties into the left ventricle. The left atrium then contracts to squeeze a little more blood into the left ventricle.

Stage 4: This process takes place at the same time as the process described in stage 2. The left ventricle contracts and pushes blood through the aortic valve into the aorta. Arteries branch off the aorta and the descending aorta to carry oxygenated blood to all parts of the body. The myocardium of the left ventricle is much thicker than the myocardium of the right ventricle to provide the extra strength needed to pump blood out into the entire body.

The heart has built-in rhythm. Not only can each cardiac cell contract without nerve stimulus, but the heart can contract (for a short time) even if removed from the body. However, the ANS does affect the rate of the rhythm and the force of contraction through sympathetic and parasympathetic activation.

As seen in the previous section, both atria contract while both ventricles are relaxed, and when the atria relax, the ventricles contract. This synchronization leads to the sequence of events known as the *cardiac cycle*, which consists of one heartbeat. *Diastole* is the term for relaxation, and *systole* is the term for contraction. Therefore, the ventricles are in diastole when the atria are in systole, and the atria are in diastole when the ventricles are in systole. Because the myocardium of the

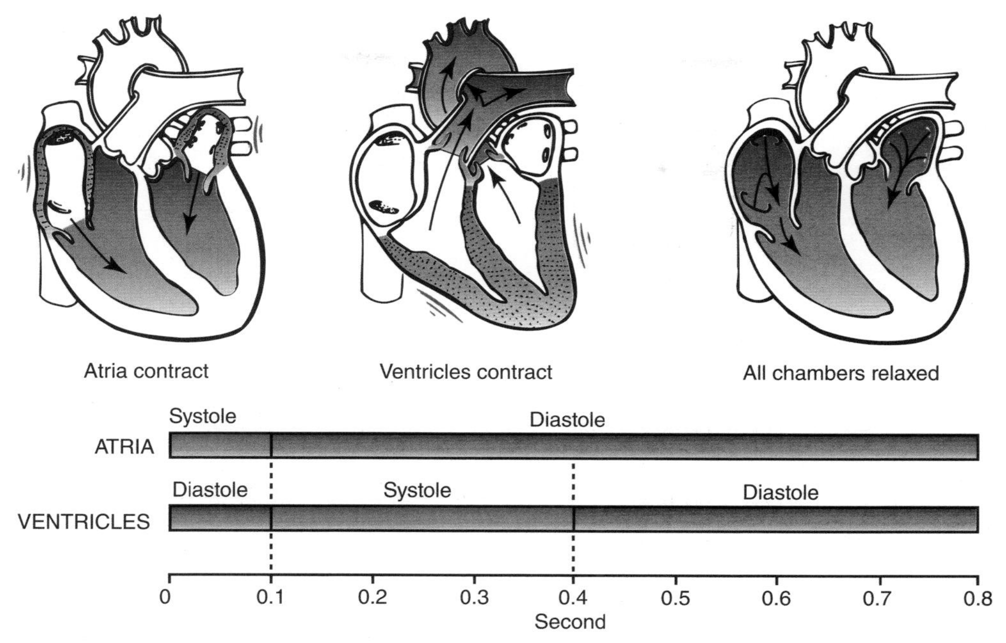

FIG. 11.9 Heart and blood flow patterns. (Modified from Applegate E. *The Anatomy and Physiology Learning System*. 4th ed. Saunders/Elsevier; 2011.)

ventricles is much thicker than the myocardium of the atria, the heartbeat felt is ventricular systole.

The heart rate is identified by the number of cardiac cycles that occur in 1 minute. The average healthy person has 60 to 70 cycles, or beats, per minute.

Conduction System of the Heart

The coordinated rhythm of the heart is initiated by a built-in electrical system called the *conduction system of the heart*. The sinoatrial node, located in the right atrium, sets the pace of the heart rate. A nerve impulse originates in the sinoatrial node and travels to the left atrium, causing the atria to contract. At the precise moment that the atria have completed their contraction, the signal travels through the atrioventricular bundle, located in the interventricular septum, to the right ventricle and into the left ventricle, causing the ventricles to contract. The rhythm can be checked by an electrocardiogram (ECG), which monitors the electrical changes in the heart. A portable ECG machine, known as a *Holter monitor*, can measure heart signals over 24 hours. If difficulty with the electrical system develops in the sinoatrial node, physicians can implant a device known as a *pacemaker* to assist or take over the initiation of the signal.

Heart Sounds

Heart sounds can be heard through a stethoscope. These heart sounds are caused by the closure of the heart valves. Valves usually are quiet as they open. Closure of the valves produces two main sounds. The first is a low-pitched "lubb" generated by blood turbulence as the mitral and tricuspid valves close. The second is a higher pitched "dubb" caused by blood turbulence as the aortic and pulmonary valves close. Extra sounds, such as those resulting from faulty valves, are referred to as *murmurs*.

Blood Volume and Flow

Cardiac output is the amount of blood pumped by the left ventricle in 1 minute. The average output under normal conditions is 5 to 6 L of blood. To pump more oxygen and nutrients to the cells during exercise and in times of stress, output may rise to 20 L or more. The output increases because the heart beats faster and stronger. The speed of the blood flow is fastest in arteries and moderate in veins. The slowest blood movement is in the capillaries to allow for the exchange of nutrients and waste products between tissues and blood.

Vascular System

The vascular system is the other part of the cardiovascular system. It consists of blood vessels that carry blood from the heart to the lungs and body tissues and back to the heart in a continuous cycle. As discussed previously in the section on blood vessels, a blood vessel that transports blood from the heart is called an *artery*. Arteries eventually branch off into smaller and smaller arteries, the smallest of which are called *arterioles*. A **capillary** is one of the tiny blood vessels located between the arterioles and the venules, the smallest of the veins. The veins get larger and larger as they get closer to the heart. The largest veins return blood to the right atrium of the heart (Fig. 11.10). The endothelium maintains the proper dilation and constriction of the blood vessels. This function determines on a moment-to-moment basis how much blood is received by the body's various tissues. Endothelial "tone" also largely determines a person's blood pressure, and how much work the heart must do to pump blood out to the body.

Endothelium

The endothelium is a thin membrane that lines the inside of the heart and blood vessels and lymphatic vessels. It consists of a thin layer of simple, or single-layered, squamous cells called

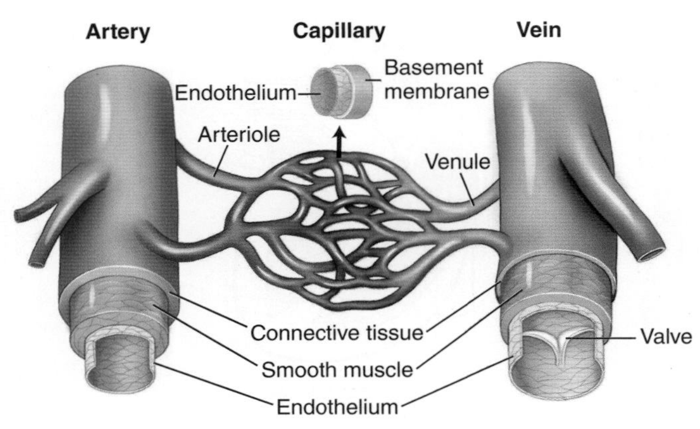

FIG. 11.10 The peripheral vascular system consists of arteries, which carry oxygenated blood (*red*), and capillaries and veins, which carry deoxygenated blood (*blue*). The thick wall of the arteries is composed of distinct layers of smooth muscle cells and elastic laminae that separate these layers. In comparison, the veins have much thinner walls. The walls of the capillaries consist of a single layer of endothelium. The cross-section of the heart tissue is included for comparison. (From VanMeter K, Hubert R. *Microbiology for the Healthcare Professional*. Elsevier; 2010.)

endothelial cells. The endothelium is responsive to levels of nitric oxide (NO) in blood vessel walls. NO is produced by nearly every type of cell in the human body and is one of the most important molecules for blood vessel health. It's a vasodilator, meaning it relaxes the inner muscles of blood vessels, causing the vessels to widen. In this way, nitric oxide increases blood flow and lowers blood pressure. The endothelium protects tissues from various toxic substances; regulates the blood clotting mechanism; controls the fluid, the electrolytes, and the numerous other substances that pass back and forth between the blood and the tissues; and regulates inflammation in the tissues.

Arteries

The body has three types of arteries:

- *Elastic arteries* are large arteries capable of undergoing passive stretching. They have thick walls that contain a great deal of elastic tissue. They recoil when the ventricles relax, which maintains the pressure necessary to move the blood. The aorta and pulmonary artery are elastic arteries.
- *Muscular arteries* constitute most of the arteries in the body. These are small to medium-sized arteries that distribute blood to all tissues by contracting or dilating to control blood flow. Located between the elastic layers are many smooth muscle cells and some collagen. Although the walls of muscular arteries are distensible to a certain extent, as they become smaller and smaller with each successive branching, the amount of elastic tissue decreases, and the number of smooth muscles increases. Muscular arteries vary in size from about 1 cm in diameter close to their origin at the elastic arteries to about 0.5 mm in diameter. Muscular arteries are composed almost entirely of smooth muscle. The larger arteries may have 30 or more layers of smooth muscle cells, whereas the smallest peripheral arteries have only two or three layers. These arteries are highly contractile; the degree of their contraction and relaxation is controlled by the autonomic nervous system and by endothelium-derived vasoactive substances. A few fine elastic fibers are scattered among the smooth muscle cells but are not organized into sheets. These are most numerous in the large muscular arteries, which are a direct continuation of the distal end of the elastic arteries.
- *Arterioles* are the smallest branches of the arterial tree. Arterioles vary in diameter ranging from 30 μm (0.03 mm) to 400 μm (0.4 mm). Any artery smaller than 0.5 mm in diameter is considered an arteriole. The arterioles offer considerable resistance to blood flow because of their small radius. This resistance has several functions. First, together with the elastic arteries, the resistance converts the pulsing ejection of blood from the heart into a steady flow through the capillaries; the arterioles constrict and dilate to control the amount of blood entering the capillaries. Second, if no resistance was present and high pressure persisted in the capillaries, a considerable loss of blood volume into the tissue would occur through the movement of the fluid across the capillary wall and around the cells. The arterioles are also important in determining the blood supply to various tissues and regions.

Capillaries (Microvasculature)

Capillaries are small-diameter blood vessels with thin, partially permeable walls that permit the diffusion of substances through them. This is how nutrients, oxygen, ions, and other molecules move from the blood into tissue cells, and how wastes, carbon dioxide, cell products (e.g., hormones), and other molecules move from the cells into the blood.

The smallest vessels of the circulatory system, capillaries form a complex interlinking network. Specialized regions near the junctions between the terminal (smallest) arterioles and the capillaries, known as *precapillary sphincters*, consist of a few smooth muscle cells arranged circularly. Relaxed sphincters allow the capillary beds distal to the sphincters to be open and full of blood, partially constricted sphincters reduce blood flow to the capillaries, and fully contracted sphincters allow no blood flow.

The efficient exchange between capillary blood and the surrounding tissue fluid occurs because the capillaries are so numerous and so small that the blood within them flows at its slowest rate, which ensures the maximum contact time between blood and tissue. This flow of blood through the capillary bed is referred to as the *microcirculation*.

Some tissues have a much more abundant network of capillaries than others. For example, dense connective tissue has a poor capillary network compared with cardiac tissue or that of the kidneys and liver.

Capillary networks drain into a series of venules and veins that have increasingly larger diameters.

Arteriovenous shunts, or arteriovenous anastomoses, are direct connections between the arterial and venous systems that bypass the capillary beds. These short connecting vessels have strongly developed muscular control and are directed by the sympathetic nervous system. They are found in many tissues and organs; for example, in the skin, these connections

Practical Application

The massage therapist may be able to affect arterial blood flow in two ways. First by affecting the autonomic nervous system (ANS) balance. Stimulating sympathetic autonomic functions increases the heart rate, providing more push to the blood in the arteries. The action is a reflexive, indirect method that involves the use of homeostatic mechanisms to maintain balance. It may be that massage modulates the ANS and down-regulates the sympathetic nervous system response affecting endothelial function. Autonomic regulation of vascular function only receives sympathetic innervation, whereas capillaries receive no innervation. Vessels at different locations may react differently to sympathetic stimulation. For example, during the "fight or flight" response the sympathetic nervous system causes vasodilation in skeletal muscle, but vasoconstriction in the skin. Massage can be structured so that it is stimulating to the sympathetic autonomic nervous system. In general, the methods used are brisk and involve active contraction of the muscles, which increases the client's respiratory rate. Massage can also be structured to reduce sympathetic ANS output. This approach is what is considered the relaxation style of massage.

Second, the massage therapist may be able to affect arterial blood flow mechanically through the pump-and-tube mechanism of the cardiovascular system, which functions in the same way as the fluid dynamics of hydraulics. Arteries are pliable muscular tubes that carry blood (a fluid) under pressure from the heart pump. Crimping or closing causes pressure to build up between the pump (the heart) and the barrier, like water behind a dam. With the removal of the barrier, the buildup of pressure provides an initial extra push to the fluid. Compression over more superficial arteries to close off the flow of blood temporarily results in the same phenomenon. Back pressure builds, and on release of the compression, the blood pushes forward with more force than would have been available from the heart action alone. The massage therapist applies compression against the arteries in the legs and arms to assist peripheral circulation. The rhythm of compression and release is a rate of approximately 60 beats per minute, to coincide with the heart rhythm. The increase in blood flow is temporary, and in healthy individuals with adequate blood flow, the effect may be negligible (Figs. 11.11 and 1.12).

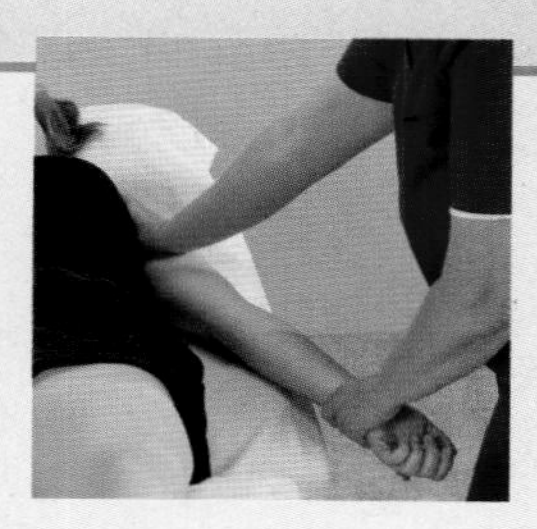

enable cutaneous blood flow to increase to allow the dissipation of heat from the body surfaces.

Veins

The venous system acts as a collecting system, returning blood from the capillary networks to the heart passively, as blood flows down a pressure gradient (Fig. 11.13). The capillaries merge to form venules, which in turn unite to form larger but fewer veins, which eventually converge into the venae cavae. Some of the superficial veins in the hands and arms are visible, but they all empty into the deeper veins that usually are found near arteries.

The walls of veins consist of the same three layers found in the arteries, but with less smooth muscle. In general, the walls of veins are thinner and more expandable than those of arteries. Veins have a relatively large diameter (the venae cavae are 2 to 3 cm in diameter) and thus offer low resistance to blood flow. Some veins, especially in the arms and legs, have internal folds in the endothelial lining that form valves. These valves prevent the backflow of blood, allowing it to flow only *toward* the heart. The veins of the legs contain more valves than the veins of the arms because they must fight the effects of gravity and prevent blood from pooling in the feet. Long periods of high venous pressure can damage these valves by overstretching them; this occurs during pregnancy and in people who stand for extended periods. The valves become weak and lose their ability to function; varicose veins develop and may lead to edema and varicose ulcers.

As much as 75% of the body's total blood volume is contained in the venous system, so veins sometimes are referred to as *capacity vessels*. The capacity of the venous system can be modified by altering the lumen size of the venules and veins, which is accomplished by changing the venomotor tone (the degree of smooth muscle contraction in the vein). Venomotor

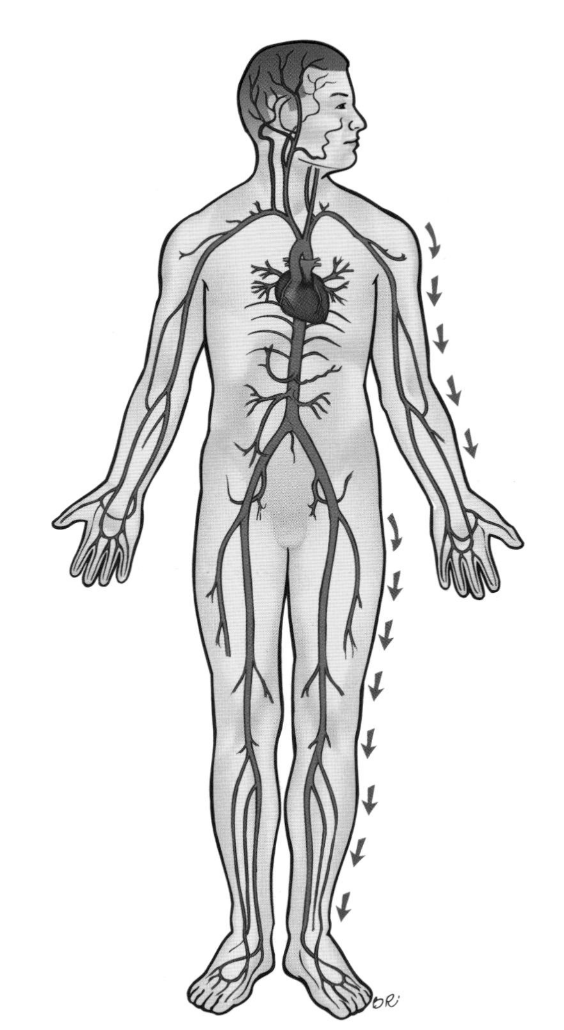

FIG. 11.11 Direction of compression over arteries to increase arterial flow. (From Fritz S. *Mosby's Fundamentals of Therapeutic Massage*. 6th ed. Mosby/Elsevier; 2016.)

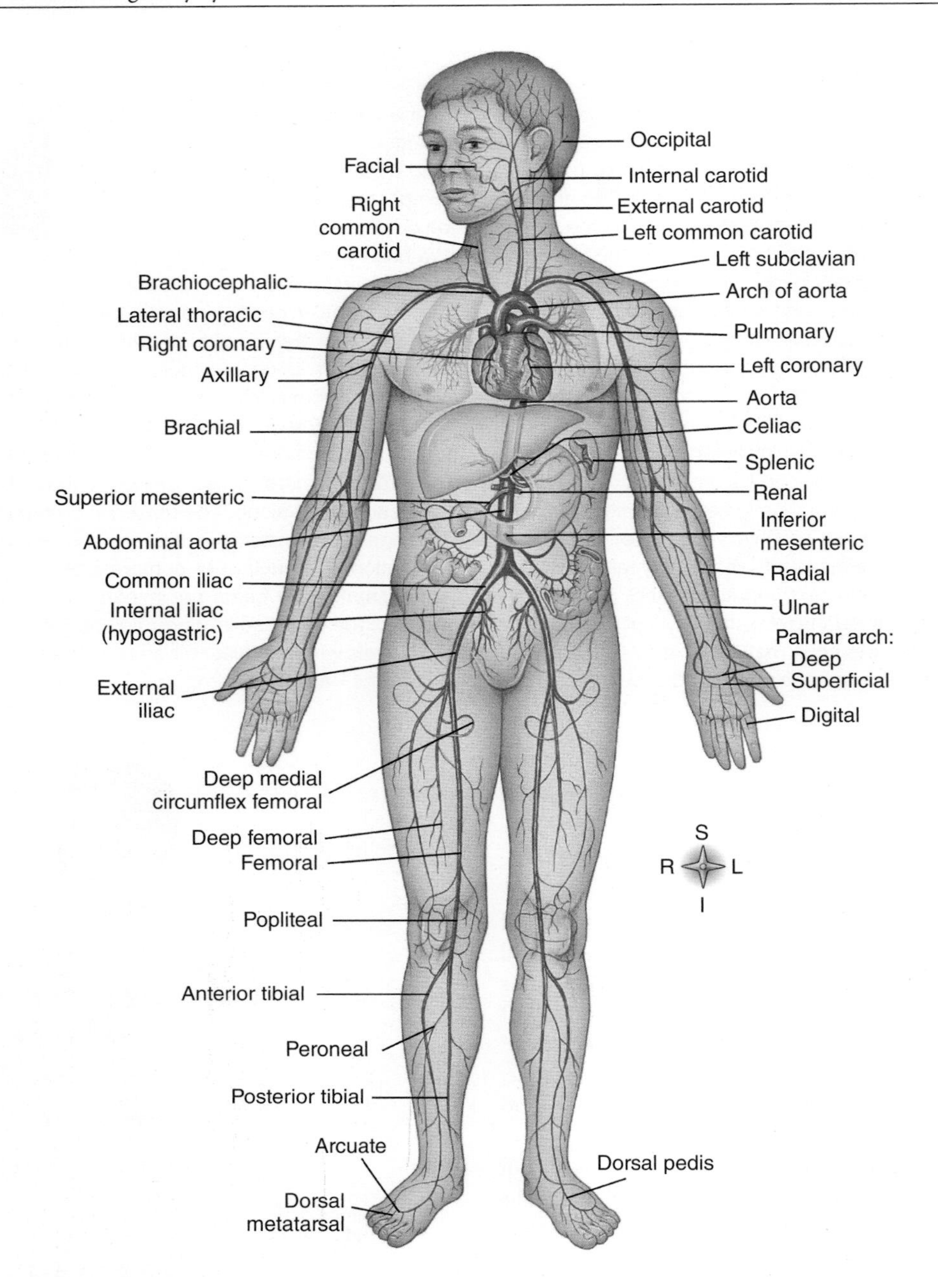

FIG. 11.12 Principal arteries of the body. (From Thibodeau GA, Patton KT. *Anatomy and Physiology*. 6th ed. Mosby/Elsevier; 2006.)

Practical Application

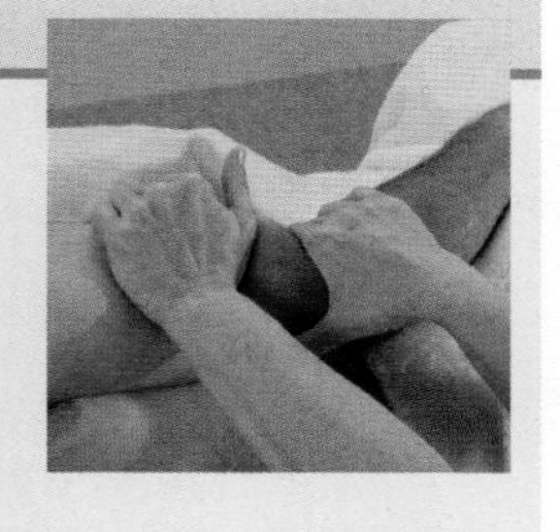

The massage practitioner can use compression and kneading to encourage the movement of blood through the capillaries. Research evidence supports the effect of massage on local capillary circulation. The mechanical forces created by massage support the exchange between capillary blood and the surrounding tissue fluid, somewhat like what happens when a sponge is squeezed.

tone is controlled predominantly by the sympathetic nervous system, and changes in the venomotor tone increase or reduce the capacity of the venous circulation. Therefore, they can compensate partially for variations in the effective circulating blood volume.

Venous Return

Venous blood flow occurs along pressure gradients, and even small variations in resistance and vessel size affect the flow.

The effect of gravity slows venous return. When a person is upright, blood tends to collect in the feet and legs because the veins are more distended and because of the hydrostatic

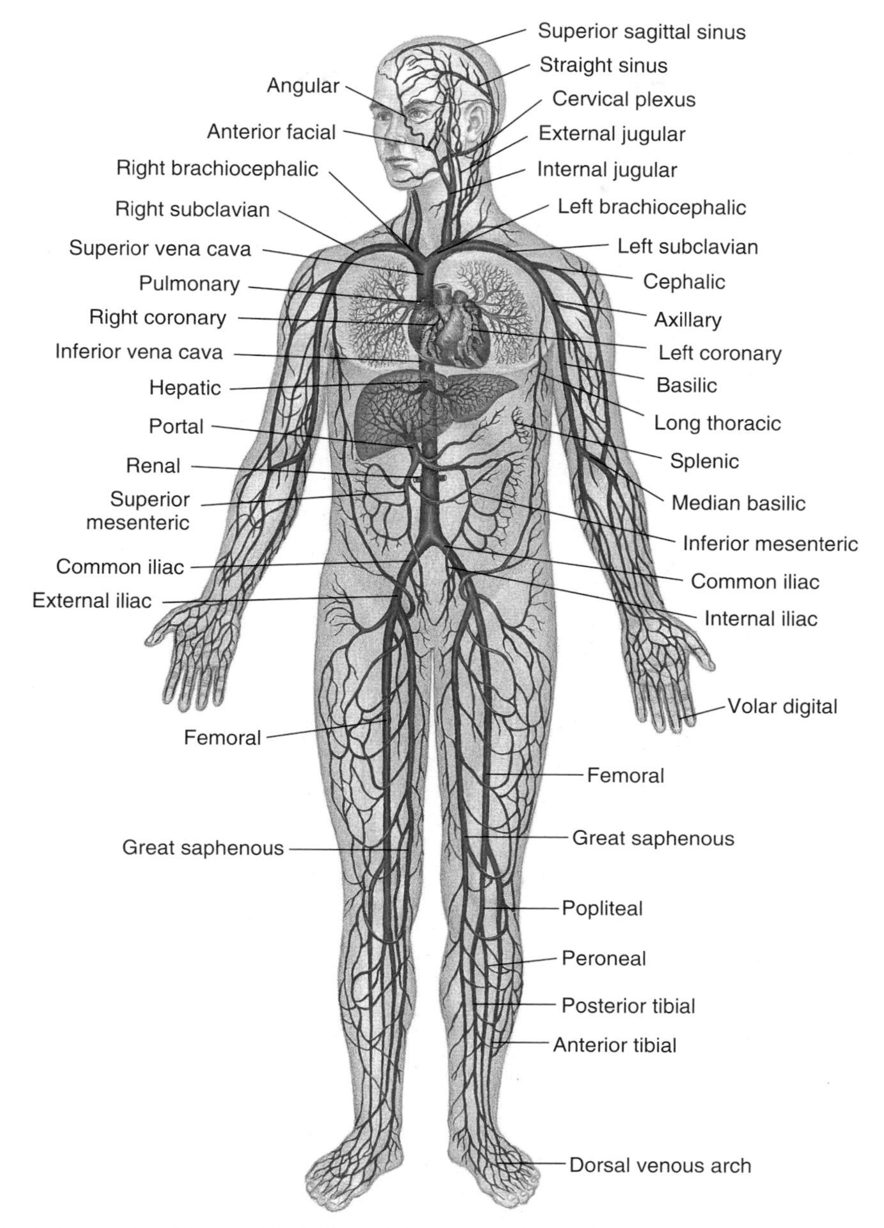

FIG. 11.13 Systemic circulation: veins. (From Seidel HM, et al. *Mosby's Guide to Physical Examination*. 7th ed. Mosby/Elsevier; 2011.)

pressure of blood in the veins below the level of the heart. The leg veins take on a more circular diameter that provides greater capacity. When a person is horizontal, the veins take on a more elliptical diameter that provides less capacity. Increasing the venomotor tone, which reduces the diameter and hence the capacity of the veins, helps reduce venous pooling. This pooling is not blood stagnation; rather, it indicates that the veins are accommodating a greater volume of blood.

Maintaining adequate venous return to the heart at all times is vital because cardiac output is determined by venous return, which is considered cardiac input. In most instances, the cardiac output equals the venous return. If the venous return falls, cardiac output and blood pressure also may drop. There are several mechanisms that help maintain the venous return at all times. Increasing the venomotor tone is an important mechanism because it reduces the capacity of the venous system and so aids in increasing venous return. After a long period of bed rest when the veins have not had to compensate, venomotor tone is reduced, and this method of reducing the effects of gravity is temporarily less efficient. The massage practitioner should remember to have the client slowly and steadily and support the person in case they become dizzy or feel faint.

Two additional systems, sometimes referred to as the *skeletal muscle pump* and the *respiratory pump*, also assist venous return. Skeletal muscle contraction, especially in the limbs, squeezes the veins and pushes blood in the extremities toward the heart; the numerous valves prevent backflow. Many communicating channels also allow the emptying of blood from the superficial veins of the limbs into the deep veins when rhythmic muscular contractions occur. Consequently, every time a person moves the legs or tenses the muscles, these actions push a certain amount of blood toward the heart. The more frequent and powerful such rhythmic contractions are the more efficient their action. Sustained continuous muscle contractions, unlike rhythmic contractions, impede blood flow because of continuous blocking of the veins. When an individual stands still for long periods, muscle pumping and venous return decrease; this results in fainting because of inadequate cerebral blood flow. When one is standing still for long periods, it is advisable to contract the muscles of the legs and buttocks periodically to encourage venous return.

Respiration produces variations in intrapleural and intrathoracic pressure. Each inspiration lowers the pressure in the thorax and the right atrium of the heart. It also increases the pressure gradient, helping blood to flow back to the heart. At the same time, the movement of the diaphragm into the abdomen raises the intraabdominal pressure and increases the gradient to the thorax, again promoting venous return. With expiration the pressure gradients reverse, and blood tends to flow in the opposite direction; the valves in the medium-sized veins prevent this.

Maintaining adequate circulating blood volume also is necessary. If the blood volume is depleted for some reason (e.g., dehydration or hemorrhage), the body increases the effective circulating volume in the short term by venoconstriction and vasoconstriction in the blood reservoirs of the body, such as the skin, liver, lungs, and spleen. More blood is then available to flow to the other organs. However, fluid replacement is eventually necessary to restore blood volume. The pressures in the central regions of the venous system directly reflect the blood volume (Fig. 11.14).

Practical Application

The massage application can incorporate the principles affecting venous return by mimicking normal venous return flow:

- *Muscular pump:* Rhythmic contraction and relaxation of the muscles during movement encourage venous return flow. Restoring normal muscle function and reducing muscle tension supports venous return flow.
- *Gravity:* Positioning the limbs higher than the heart passively assists venous return flow.
- *Respiratory pump:* Slow, deep diaphragmatic breathing enhances venous return flow.
- *Massage application:* Stroking over the veins toward the heart passively moves the blood in the veins. This method is particularly effective in the limbs. The practitioner can encourage rhythmic contraction of the muscles by having the person move their limbs through a complete range of motion against resistance in a contract-and-relax rhythm of approximately 60 cycles per minute. The therapist then applies short strokes (1 or 2 inches long) over the veins, stroking toward the heart with sufficient pressure to move the blood in the superficial veins (Fig. 11.15). At the same time, the therapist places the client's limbs in a supported position above the heart so that gravity can help the return flow. The client should be encouraged to relax and breathe deeply.

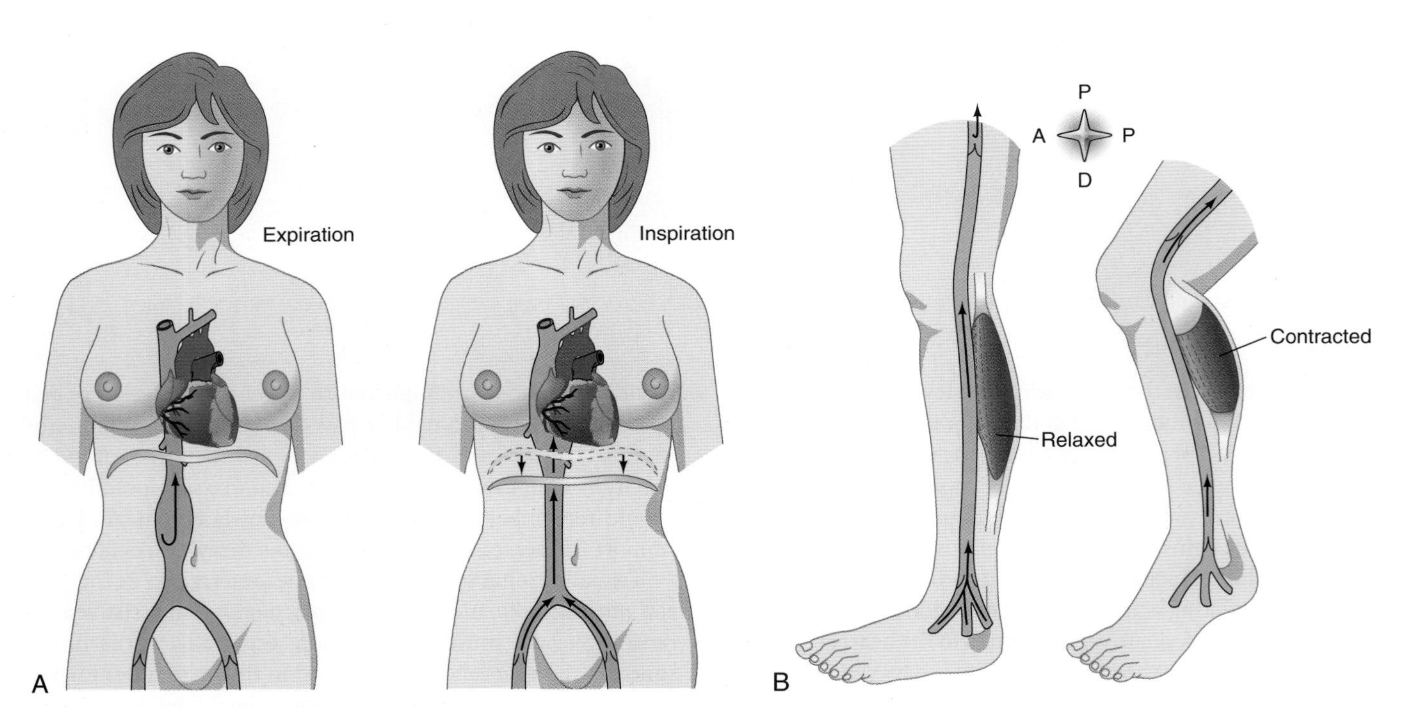

FIG. 11.14 Venous pumping mechanisms. (A) The respiratory pump operates by alternately reducing thoracic pressure during inspiration (thus pulling venous blood into the central veins) and increasing pressure in the thorax during expiration (thus pushing central venous blood into the heart). (B) The skeletal muscle pump operates by the alternate increase and decrease in peripheral venous pressure that normally occurs when the skeletal muscles are used for the activities of daily living. Both pumping mechanisms rely on the presence of semilunar valves in the veins to prevent backflow during the low-pressure points in the pumping cycle. (From Thibodeau GA, Patton KT. *Anatomy and Physiology*. 6th ed. Mosby/Elsevier; 2006.)

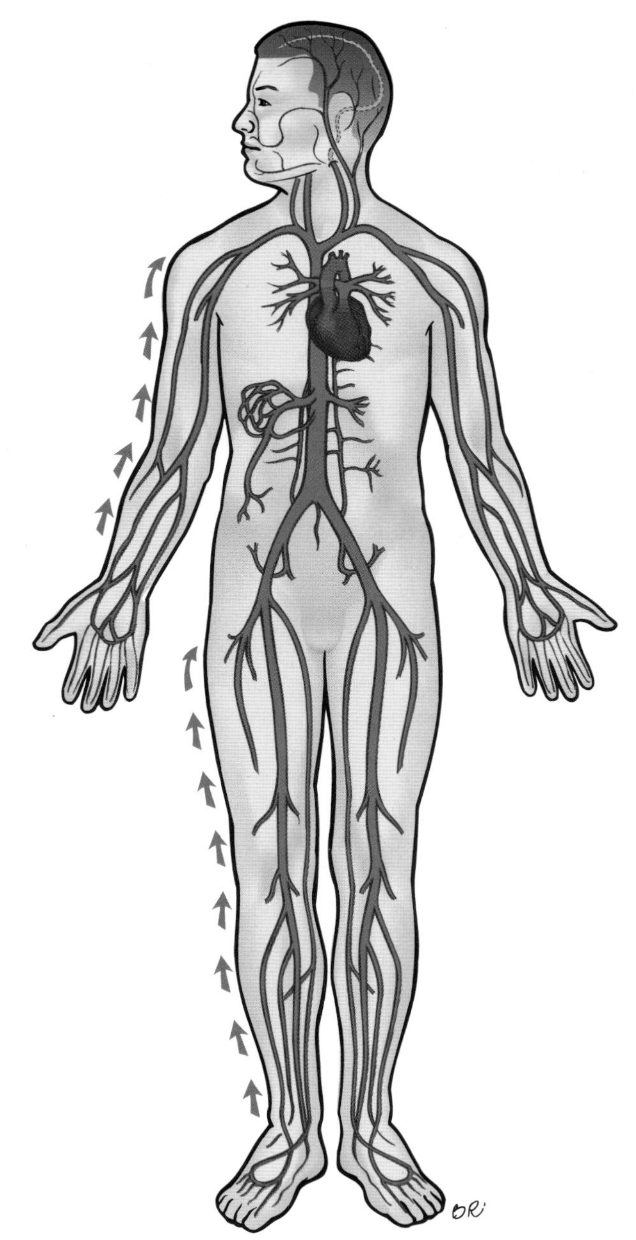

FIG. 11.15 Direction of gliding strokes to facilitate venous flow. (From Fritz S. *Mosby's Fundamentals of Therapeutic Massage*. 5th ed. Mosby/Elsevier; 2013.)

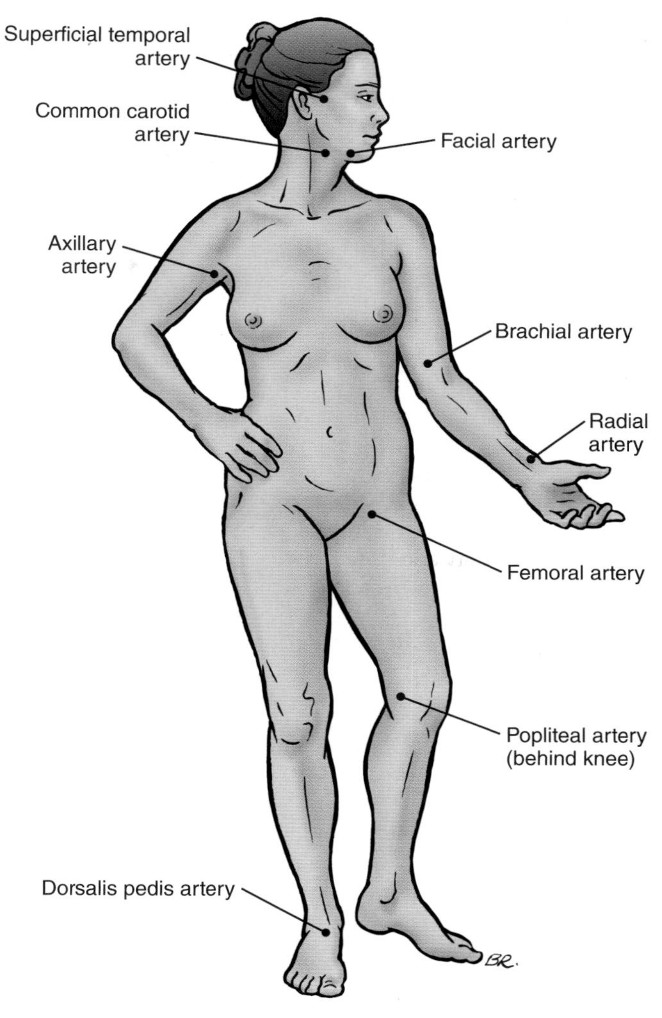

FIG. 11.16 Pulse points. Each pulse point is named after the artery with which it is associated.

Pulse and Blood Pressure

Blood forced into the aorta during systole sets up a pressure wave that travels along the arteries and expands the arterial wall. This expansion can be palpated by pressing the artery against tissue. The number of waves is known as the *pulse*, which is a direct reflection of the heart rate. The pulse rate, measured when a person is at rest, may be regular or irregular, strong or weak. An irregular pulse occurs commonly with atrial fibrillation and premature contractions. A strong pulse occurs with hyperthyroidism; a weak one with shock and myocardial infarction. A resting heart rate greater than 100 beats per minute is known as *tachycardia;* a heart rate less than 50 or 60 beats per minute is known as *bradycardia* (Fig. 11.16).

The amount of pressure exerted by the blood on the walls of the blood vessels is called **blood pressure**. The higher pressure, called *systolic pressure*, occurs when the ventricles contract. The lower pressure, called *diastolic pressure*, occurs when the ventricles relax. Blood pressure is measured with a sphygmomanometer, a cloth-covered rubber bag that is wrapped around the arm over the brachial artery.

Sympathetic nerves in the arterioles regulate blood pressure. Normally, arterioles are in a state of partial constriction called *arteriole tone*. Stimulation of the sympathetic system causes further arteriolar constriction and an increase in blood pressure. Nonstimulation results in a decrease in blood pressure. With hypertension the sympathetic system is in a state of continuous stimulation, resulting in constant high blood pressure.

As the vessels become increasingly remote from the heart, the systolic and diastolic pressures equalize. As the vessels change from arteries to arterioles to capillaries to venules to veins, the pressure decreases until, in the large veins, the pressure may be zero or negative. For this reason, it is necessary to pull back on the syringe when drawing venous blood. A blood

Box 11.1 Facts About Blood Pressure

- Blood pressure depends on the person's size.
- The average newborn has a blood pressure of 90/60.
- At 15 years of age, the average blood pressure is approximately 120/60.
- An average, healthy young adult has a blood pressure of less than 120/80.
- A blood pressure with a systolic reading of less than 90 is considered hypotension.
- A pressure of 120/80 or higher is considered prehypertension.
- A pressure of 140/90 or higher is considered stage I, or mild, hypertension.
- A pressure of 160/100 or higher is considered stage II, or moderate to severe, hypertension.
- The blood pressure changes under various conditions and a single reading should never be used as a final determinant.
- A systolic increase occurs under temporary conditions, such as anxiety and exercise.
- Hypertension involves an increase in the systolic and diastolic pressures.
- Hypotension is a decrease in the systolic and diastolic pressures and is an important manifestation of shock, which results from an inadequate blood supply to vital organs.

pressure reading is the number of millimeters of mercury (mm Hg) displaced by the changes in pressure. The first number is the systolic pressure, and the second number is the diastolic pressure. When recording the pressure, only the numbers are written; "mm Hg" usually is dropped (Box 11.1).

Practical Application

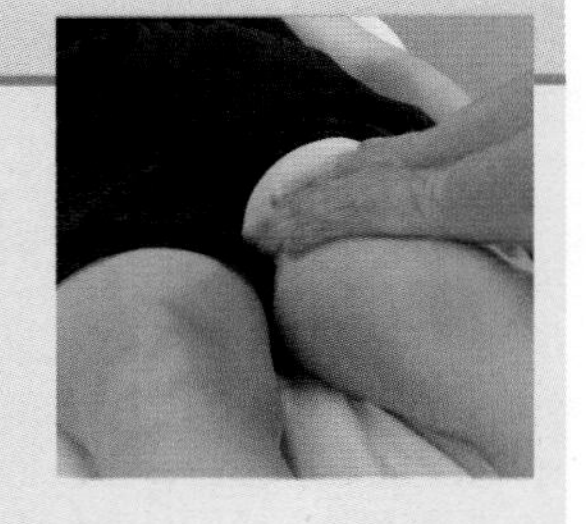

The massage therapist can monitor the pulse during the assessment of the client. In general, the pulses should feel bilaterally equal. Should the practitioner note differences, they should refer the client for diagnosis. The pulse rate ranges from 50 to 70 beats per minute at rest. A rate much slower or faster indicates the need for referral. If the general intent of the therapy session is stress management focused on relaxation and parasympathetic predomination, the pulse rate should slow somewhat throughout the session. The opposite is true if the goal is increased arousal of the sympathetic system to energize the client

Hydrostatic Pressure

All fluids in a confined space exert pressure. The term *hydrostatic pressure* refers to the force a liquid exerts against the walls of its container, as in the pressure blood exerts in the vascular system (the blood pressure). Pascal's principle states that if pressure is exerted on a confined fluid, the pressure is transmitted equally in all directions. The flexibility of the container, as with veins, influences the hydrostatic pressure. If the container is flexible, the pressure in the fluid is lower than it is in a rigid container. If a weak point exists in the wall of the container and the pressure exerted is great enough, the container wall may break. This is what happens when an aneurysm bursts. In a hypertensive individual, the blood vessels harden (undergo sclerotic changes called **arteriosclerosis**), which prevents the vessels from bursting as a result of the increased pressure of the blood.

The flow of a fluid through a vessel is determined by the pressure difference between the two ends of the vessel and also by the resistance to flow. For any fluid to flow along a vessel, a pressure difference must exist; otherwise, the fluid will not move. In the cardiovascular system, the pumping of the heart generates the pressure head, or force, and a continuous drop in pressure occurs, starting in the left ventricle of the heart and going to the tissues and from the tissues back to the right atrium of the heart. Without this drop in blood pressure, no blood would flow through the circulatory system. Resistance is a measure of the ease with which a fluid flows through a tube—the easier the flow, the less the resistance to flow, and vice versa. In the cardiovascular system, the resistance usually is described as *vascular resistance because* it originates mainly in the peripheral blood vessels; it also is known simply as the *peripheral resistance.*

Resistance is essentially a measure of the friction between the molecules of the fluid and between the tube wall and the fluid. The resistance is determined by the viscosity of the fluid and the radius and length of the tube. The smaller the radius of a vessel, the greater the resistance to the movement of particles. This increased resistance results from a greater probability that the particles of the fluid will collide with the vessel wall. When a particle collides with the wall, some of the kinetic energy (energy of movement) of the particle is lost on impact, resulting in the slowing of the particle. Thus, in a vessel that has a smaller diameter, a greater number of collisions occur, reducing the energy content and speed of the particles moving through the vessel. The result is a decrease in the hydrostatic pressure.

Small alterations in the radius of the blood vessels, particularly of the more peripheral vessels, can influence the flow of blood. Changes in the walls of large and medium-sized arteries cause narrowing of the lumen of the vessels and result in increased vascular resistance. The nature of the endothelial lining of the tube or vessel also influences the way fluids flow. If the lining of the blood vessel is smooth, the fluid flows evenly because there is less friction; this is known as *streamlined*, or *laminar, flow*. However, if the lining is rough or uneven, friction increases. The fluid itself can flow irregularly. In both cases, the fluid flows turbulently. Laminar flow is characteristic of most parts of the vascular system and is silent, whereas turbulent flow is audible, such as during blood pressure measurements with a sphygmomanometer.

Viscosity of the Fluid

Viscosity is a measure of the tendency of a liquid to resist flow. The greater the viscosity (thickness) of a fluid, the greater the force required to move that liquid. For example, water has less viscosity than a milkshake.

Normally, the viscosity of blood remains constant, but in polycythemia, in which the red cell content is high, the viscosity of the blood can be considerably greater, reducing the blood flow. Severe dehydration (in which loss of plasma occurs) and cooling of the blood also can lead to increased viscosity.

Medulla and Baroreceptors

In the medulla of the brain, the cells of the reticular formation regulate three vital signs: heart rate, blood pressure, and respiration. They work with signals from the various nerve centers in the body. One type of nerve center in the cardiovascular system is the baroreceptor.

Baroreceptors are stretch receptors in the carotid arteries, the aorta, and nearly every large artery of the neck and thorax. When blood pressure increases, arteries stretch. The baroreceptors transmit signals about sudden, brief changes in blood pressure, such as when we change position. When blood pressure is elevated for a long period, the baroreceptor reflex resets to the new blood pressure level.

When blood pressure suddenly drops, the frequency of signals from the baroreceptors declines. This change sets off a response in the cardioregulatory center of the medulla that increases sympathetic stimulation and decreases parasympathetic stimulation, resulting in an increase in the heart rate and blood pressure. Conversely, when blood pressure increases, the signal increases, and the medulla changes its output to slow the heart rate and blood pressure by increasing parasympathetic signals. This is another example of how a negative feedback system works in the body.

Practical Application

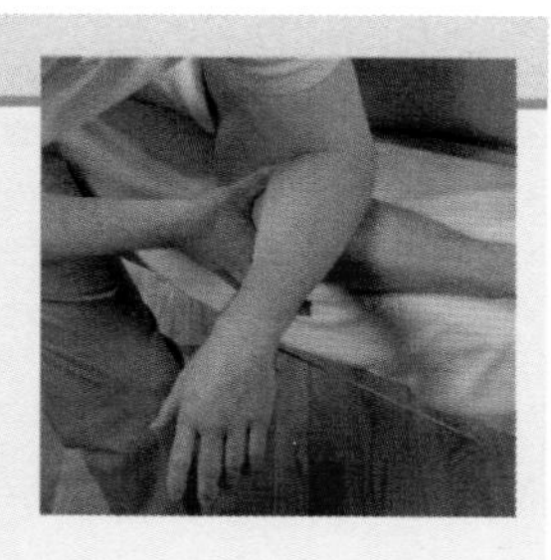

Stress management programs include methods of movement and moderate aerobic exercise, flexibility programs, massage, and other forms of soft tissue methods. Although these approaches initially elevate blood pressure, when continued, they activate parasympathetic quieting responses, such as slow, deep breathing and progressive relaxation. Therefore, they tend to have a normalizing effect on the blood pressure. These methods are classified as nonspecific constitutional approaches; they allow the homeostatic mechanisms to reset to a more effective pattern after disruption.

Practical Application

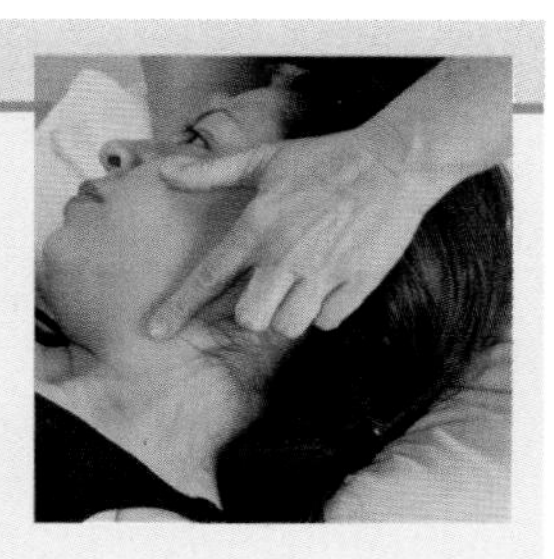

Stimulation of baroreceptors during therapeutic massage could affect blood pressure. The blood pressure could drop, and the client may be lightheaded and show other signs of low blood pressure. It is important to monitor the client for signs of being lightheaded, dizzy, or faint. You may be able to reduce the potential of dizziness and lightheadedness that occurs with low blood pressure by instructing the client to move slowly when changing position. After a massage, instruct the client to breathe deeply for a few minutes and then slowly sit up before standing. Should a client become dizzy while standing, have them cross the thighs in a scissors fashion and squeeze them together or put one foot on a ledge or chair and lean as far forward as possible. These maneuvers encourage blood to flow from the legs to the heart.

Names of Specific Arteries and Veins

The names of most arteries and veins are derived from the anatomical structures they serve. The femoral artery and the femoral vein, for example, are found close to the femur, where these blood vessels serve the tissues of the upper and lower legs. The renal artery is so named because it exits the abdominal aorta and enters the kidney. The renal vein exits the kidney and enters the inferior vena cava. Arteries and veins are found on both sides of the body and are identified as right or left (e.g., the right common carotid artery, the left common carotid artery).

The following is a list of the main arteries and veins. Many of them change names as they enter into and pass through certain areas of the body. Use the illustrations to trace the locations of these vessels (see Figs. 11.12 and 11.13).

Arteries

Main Arteries of the Head and Neck

The arch of the aorta gives rise to three arteries; from right to left, they are the brachiocephalic (or innominate) artery, the left common carotid artery, and the left subclavian artery. The subclavian artery supplies the upper extremities.

The brachiocephalic artery, a short artery, becomes the right common carotid artery and the right subclavian artery.

The common carotid arteries branch at the level of the upper part of the thyroid cartilage to become the external and internal carotid arteries. The common carotid artery is an important pulse-taking artery; damage to this artery may result in a transient ischemic attack. The internal carotid artery supplies the brain; the external carotid artery supplies the face, head, and neck.

The superficial temporal artery is the cranial termination of the external carotid artery. The superficial temporal artery is a pulse-taking artery located superior and anterior to the ear.

The two vertebral arteries become the basilar artery, which helps supply the brain.

Main Arteries of the Upper Extremities

The subclavian artery becomes the axillary artery at the clavicle.

Near the head of the humerus, the axillary artery becomes the brachial artery. The brachial artery is the main artery for measuring blood pressure and is also a pulse-taking artery.

The brachial artery divides at the elbow region into the ulnar and radial arteries.

The ulnar artery lies deep and medial. The radial artery lies more superficial and lateral. Both arteries communicate in the hand by way of two deep interconnected vessels, called *anastomoses*, and a superficial and deep palmar arch.

Main Arteries of the Trunk

After supplying the head, neck, and upper extremities, the aorta descends posteriorly as the thoracic aorta, sending branches to the intercostal muscles as the right and left intercostal arteries.

The intercostal arteries anastomose anteriorly with the left and right internal thoracic arteries. If the aorta is damaged, the intercostal muscles, which are important for breathing, may still receive a blood supply by way of the internal thoracic arteries.

Main Arteries of the Abdomen

When the thoracic aorta penetrates the diaphragm, it is known as the *abdominal aorta*, which supplies the abdominal organs. The following structures, listed in a cranial to caudal direction, are the main branches of the abdominal aorta:

- Celiac trunk: Supplies the stomach, spleen, and liver by way of the gastric, splenic, and hepatic arteries
- Superior mesenteric artery: Supplies the small intestine, part of the pancreas, and half of the colon
- Renal arteries: Supply the kidneys
- Testicular or ovarian arteries: Supply the gonads
- Inferior mesenteric artery: Supplies the remaining half of the colon to the rectum

The abdominal aorta then divides into the left and right common iliac arteries. The common iliac artery divides into the internal iliac artery, which supplies the pelvic organs, and the external iliac artery.

Main Arteries of the Lower Extremities

After passing under the inguinal ligament, the external iliac artery becomes the femoral artery. The femoral artery lies superficially at the femoral triangle and then descends posteriorly through the adductor muscles. The femoral artery is an important pulse-taking artery. When the femoral artery emerges behind the knee in the popliteal region, it becomes the popliteal artery. The popliteal artery then divides to become the anterior and posterior tibial arteries.

The anterior tibial artery becomes the dorsalis pedis artery on the dorsal aspect of the foot. The dorsalis pedis is an important pulse-taking artery.

The posterior tibial artery descends behind the medial malleolus and is also a pulse-taking artery but usually is more difficult to find than the dorsalis pedis.

Veins

Main Veins of the Head and Neck

The following are veins of the head and neck:

- Superficial: The right and left external jugular veins drain blood from the face, head, and neck. Each external jugular vein empties into a subclavian vein.
- Deep: Venous drainage from the brain is accomplished by the internal jugular veins. Each internal jugular vein joins a subclavian vein to form a brachiocephalic vein.

Main Veins of the Upper Extremities

Superficial veins originate on the dorsum of the hand as the dorsal venous plexus. They curve around the wrist to the ventral side as the cephalic vein, which runs along the lateral aspect of the forearm and arm, goes deep at the deltoid muscle; the basilic vein, which runs along the medial aspect of the forearm and arm, goes deep at the biceps muscle. The medial cubital vein is an anastomosis between the basilic and cephalic veins.

The deep veins form from branches in the hand and forearm. Although sometimes an individual has a short brachial vein, most often the first main deep vein is the axillary vein. The axillary vein becomes the subclavian vein when it passes under the clavicle.

Main Veins of the Trunk

The subclavian vein joins the internal jugular vein to become the brachiocephalic vein. The subclavian vein is an important central vein for intravenous infusion.

Two brachiocephalic veins join to become the superior vena cava, which empties into the right atrium.

The azygos system, which lies on the posterior body wall, drains the intercostal veins. The azygos vein empties into the superior vena cava.

The inferior vena cava drains blood from the abdominal viscera into the right atrium. The digestive organs and spleen first drain into the portal vein, which empties into the liver. The following veins, listed from cranial to caudal, are branches of the inferior vena cava:

- Hepatic veins from the liver
- Right and left renal veins from the kidneys
- Right and left testicular or ovarian veins from the gonads
- Two common iliac veins (the continuation of the femoral veins)

Main Veins of the Lower Extremities

The veins of the lower extremity can be divided into three systems: superficial, deep, and their mutual interconnections (perforating veins). These systems are situated in different compartments formed by the arrangement of the deep fascia.

Superficial veins of the leg begin as a dorsal venous arch on top of the foot. The great saphenous vein ascends medially from the foot up the leg to the thigh and drains into the femoral vein. The great saphenous veins may become chronically dilated in some persons and develop into varicose veins. They then may become inflamed and form blood clots, a condition known as *thrombophlebitis*.

The small saphenous vein runs laterally from the foot along the gastrocnemius muscle and drains into the popliteal vein.

The anterior tibial vein and posterior tibial vein drain into the popliteal vein.

The popliteal vein becomes the femoral vein after it passes the knee. The deep veins of the leg may become inflamed, a condition referred to as *deep vein thrombosis* (DVT), which is a more serious condition than superficial thrombophlebitis. The clot may break off and travel to the heart and then lodge in the lung as a pulmonary embolism (see Fig. 11.13).

Hepatic Portal System

A portal system is one in which blood drains from one venous system into another without arteries in between. This occurs between the hypothalamus and the pituitary gland, which is how hormones from the hypothalamus travel to the pituitary gland. Another portal system is in the abdomen between the digestive tract and the liver.

The hepatic portal system begins in the capillaries of organs of the digestive tract and ends in the portal vein. The splenic vein and the superior mesenteric vein anastomose to form the portal vein. The inferior mesenteric vein typically joins with the splenic vein at some point along its course deep to the pancreas. The portal vein is deep to the proper hepatic artery and common bile duct and runs within the free right edge of the lesser omentum. This set of three structures—the hepatic artery, bile duct, and portal vein—is called the *hepatic triad.* The portal veins enter the liver and become smaller and smaller until reaching the second venous capillary bed, called the *sinusoids* of the liver. Portal blood contains substances absorbed by the stomach and intestines. As this blood passes through the liver, the liver cells absorb, excrete, or convert nutrients and toxins.

Once filtered, the blood passes into the central vein, which is the beginning of the second venous system. This venous system is filled with progressively larger veins known as *hepatic veins.* The hepatic veins eventually drain the filtered blood through the three large hepatic veins. Restriction of outflow through the hepatic portal system can lead to portal hypertension. Portal hypertension most often is associated with cirrhosis.

The liver receives approximately 30% of resting cardiac output and is therefore a vascular organ. The hepatic vascular system has a considerable ability to store and release blood, and it functions as a reservoir within the general circulation. Normally, 10% to 15% of the total blood volume is in the liver, with roughly 60% of that in the sinusoids. With loss of blood, the liver dynamically adjusts its blood volume and can eject enough blood to compensate for a moderate amount of hemorrhage. Conversely, when vascular volume increases acutely, as with rapid infusion of fluids, the hepatic blood volume expands, providing a buffer against acute increases in systemic blood volume.

Blood

Blood is a thick red liquid form of connective tissue. Blood transports nutrients to the individual cells and removes waste products. Whole blood consists of solid, formed elements and the liquid matrix, or plasma.

Red blood cells, white blood cells, and platelets are the formed elements of blood that float in the plasma, a thick, straw-colored fluid. Amino acids, carbohydrates, electrolytes, hormones, lipids, proteins, vitamins, and waste materials are the other constituents of blood. A person who weighs 140 to 150 pounds has about 5 quarts of blood.

In an adult, blood cells form mainly in the red marrow of the bones of the chest, vertebrae, and pelvis. Yellow marrow can convert to red marrow if the body requires increased production of blood cells. *Hematopoiesis* is the term for the stages of blood cell development in red marrow. All blood cells, whether they are red, white, or platelets, originate from a common precursor cell called the *stem cell.* Immature blood cells are blast cells. When the cells are mature, they move into the bloodstream. In certain types of leukemia, blast cells may be seen in peripheral blood because the body sends them out before they are mature.

Red Blood Cells

Red blood cells, also known as *erythrocytes* or *red blood corpuscles*, make up more than 90% of the formed elements. They are round with raised edges and a flattened middle. Their function is to transport oxygen to the cells and carbon dioxide away from the cells. Inside red blood cells, oxygen and carbon dioxide bind to an iron and protein molecule called *hemoglobin*, but not at the same time. A red blood cell loses its nucleus and most of its organelles during development so that a great deal of hemoglobin can fit inside it. Because it does not have organelles necessary for cell division, red blood cells cannot divide.

Males have slightly more red blood cells than females, and the cells live slightly longer in males (about 120 days) than in females (110 days). The body recycles dead red blood cells, using their hemoglobin in new red blood cells and their proteins either in new red blood cells or other body cells. Because red blood cells cannot divide, they must be produced frequently to replace dead cells. Red bone marrow produces enough red blood cells daily to replace dead blood cells. The body needs a proper intake and assimilation of iron, vitamin B_{12}, and folic acid to produce new red blood cells. An abnormal increase in red blood cells is known as *polycythemia;* an abnormal decrease is called *anemia.*

A variety of chemical markers, or antigens, are present in red blood cells. Some of these chemical markers commonly are called *factors* and are used to identify the type of blood. The best-known grouping method is the ABO system. This system has four blood groups: A, B, AB, and O. These are commonly called the *blood types.* The Rh system, the most complex of all the blood grouping methods, has 42 different groups. The most commonly known fact about the Rh system is whether the red blood cells have it or not. If a person's red blood cells have it the blood type is positive. If a person's blood cells do not have it, the blood type is negative.

White Blood Cells

White blood cells also are called *leukocytes* or *white blood corpuscles*. Their white color results from their lack of hemoglobin. The usual ratio of white to red blood cells is 1 to 500. The main function of the white blood cells is to protect the body from pathogens and remove dead cells and substances. White blood cells are divided into the following five groups:

- *Neutrophils:* Neutrophils are granular leukocytes; more than half of all white blood cells are neutrophils. These cells fight disease by phagocytizing pathogens. The buildup of neutrophils and the debris that they collect is called *pus.*
- *Lymphocytes:* Lymphocytes account for about 30% of the total number of white blood cells in the body. They produce **antibodies** and chemicals that are active in regulating disease and allergic reactions and controlling tumors.
- *Monocytes:* Monocytes are the largest of the white blood cells, yet they account for only about 6% of the total number. They also protect the body through phagocytosis. Monocytes are unique because when they leave the blood and enter the tissues, they can develop into large phagocytic cells called *macrophages.*

- *Eosinophils:* About 3% of the total white blood cell count is made up of eosinophils. However, the number increases greatly with parasitic infections or allergic reactions (e.g., hay fever). Eosinophils are capable of phagocytic activity, and they release chemicals during the inflammatory process.
- *Basophils:* Basophils are also granular white blood cells, and they make up about 1% of the total white blood cell count. Their exact function is not yet understood clearly.

Platelets

Thrombocytes, also called *platelets*, are the smallest cellular elements of the blood. They are involved in blood clotting, which prevents blood loss when blood vessels are damaged.

Damage to a blood vessel causes the release of chemicals. Special proteins, called *clotting factors*, are activated and then form additional clotting factors. A special protein called *fibrin* forms and seals the damaged blood vessels by trapping red blood cells, platelets, and fluid to form a clot, or thrombus. Fibrin then anchors the clot. The clotting process starts the instant the blood vessel is damaged and takes only a few minutes to complete. Calcium and vitamin K are important to the success and speed of the clotting process.

Pregnancy is a state of hypercoagulation, which is likely an adaptive mechanism to reduce the risk of hemorrhage during and after the birth. Normal pregnancy is accompanied by changes in the coagulation and fibrin action that include increases in a number of clotting factors, resulting in an increased risk of thromboembolism during pregnancy and the postpartum period.

Plasma

Plasma, the straw-colored liquid found in blood and lymph, is about 90% water; the rest comprises nutrients, gases, and waste products. Plasma constitutes about 55% of blood and plays a major role in the movement of water between the tissues and the blood.

Pathological Conditions of the Cardiovascular System

Cardiovascular disease is a major cause of death. Many risk factors are associated with cardiovascular disease. The aging process and hereditary predisposition are risk factors that cannot be altered. Many people with cardiovascular disease have elevated or high cholesterol levels. Low levels of high-density lipoprotein (HDL) cholesterol (known as *good cholesterol*) and high levels of low-density lipoprotein (LDL) cholesterol (known as *bad cholesterol*) are more specifically linked to cardiovascular disease than total cholesterol. A blood test, administered by most health care professionals, is used to determine cholesterol levels. Hypertension is a major risk factor for cardiovascular disease. Abdominal fat, especially brown fat inside the abdomen, as opposed to fat that accumulates on the hips, is associated with an increased risk of cardiovascular disease and heart attack. Overweight individuals are more likely to have additional risk factors related to heart disease, specifically hypertension, high blood sugar levels, high cholesterol, high triglycerides, and diabetes. People with cardiovascular disease may not have any distinct symptoms but may experience difficulty breathing during exertion or when lying down, fatigue, lightheadedness, dizziness, fainting, depression, memory problems, confusion, frequent waking during sleep, chest pain, an awareness of the heartbeat, sensations of fluttering or pounding in the chest, swelling around the ankles, or a large abdomen. All of these symptoms can be attributed to other conditions, especially generalized stress, which is why many with cardiovascular disease go undiagnosed.

Vital Signs

Vital signs show how well the body is functioning. Vital signs include blood pressure and heart rate as well as respiratory rate and body temperature.

- A normal blood pressure reading for adults is lower than 120/80 and higher than 90/60.
- The heart rate, or pulse, measures how fast your heart is beating. A normal heart rate is between 60 and 100 beats per minute.
- The respiratory rate is the number of breaths taken per minute. The normal respiratory rate for an adult at rest is 12 to 20 breaths per minute.
- Temperature measures how hot your body is. A body temperature higher than normal (over 98.6°F) is called a *fever*.

Cardiac Disorders

Bradycardia

In bradycardia, the resting heart rate is less than 60 beats per minute. However, healthy athletes often have heart rates between 50 and 60 beats per minute, which in these individuals is not necessarily a pathological condition. Primary treatment, when necessary, involves the administration of atropine, a parasympathetic blocking agent.

Tachycardia

In most healthy people the heart rate increases in response to extra demands on it, such as those imposed by exercise. In tachycardia, the heartbeat increases suddenly without any increase in physical or emotional stress. Treatment ranges from no intervention to administration of sympathetic blocking agents. Interventions for people with paroxysmal supraventricular tachycardia include interrupting the sympathetic signals by methods such as holding the breath or rinsing the face with cool water. Because stimulation of the vagus nerve slows the heart rate, the Valsalva maneuver (forced expiration against a closed airway) may help. A physician may massage the carotid baroreceptor or inject medication to reduce the heart rate.

Arrhythmia

In arrhythmias, the rhythm of the heart may be partly or completely irregular, or it may be regular but with a frequency that is too slow or too fast. Treatment may include medication, installation of a pacemaker to initiate the heartbeat, or use of a defibrillator to restore normal heart rhythm.

Mitral Valve Dysfunction

Although all valves may undergo some changes in structure or function, the mitral valve is the one most commonly affected. This is because the left ventricle contracts so forcefully that pressure of the blood against the mitral valve may damage it. Mitral valve prolapse is a deformity that may be congenital or may result from rheumatic fever or some other heart disease. The valve does not close completely, and blood leaks back into the left atrium. Although many people do not notice any symptoms, others may experience chest pain, palpitation, fatigue, or shortness of breath. This condition may be a factor in anxiety-related disorders.

Mitral valve stenosis is scarring that causes the parts of the valve to stick together and gradually narrow. Blood backs up in the left atrium and pressure increases, which causes blood to back up into the pulmonary veins.

Angina Pectoris

Angina pectoris is chest pain or discomfort that results when the amount of oxygen supplied to the heart declines. However, there is no lasting tissue damage to the heart. Angina pectoris is caused mainly by coronary artery disease but also can be a sign of heart disease, anemia, or hyperthyroidism. Symptoms most often occur during exertion, emotional upset, or cold weather. The pain begins in the center of the chest and often spreads to the arms, neck, or jaw. In severe cases, pain may occur when the person is at rest. Rest or the use of nitroglycerin usually relieves the symptoms.

Myocardial Infarction (Heart Attack)

An infarct is an area of dead tissue that results when the blood supply to that area is cut off. Most heart attacks occur because of blockage of a coronary artery by a blood clot, especially in arteries narrowed by coronary artery disease. The blocking of blood flow damages or destroys the heart muscle. The first symptom is usually a crushing pain in the center of the chest over the sternum (Fig. 11.17 and Box 11.2). Pain also may occur in the arms, neck, jaw, and upper abdomen and occasionally in the back. The person also may perspire heavily and complain of dizziness, chills, or nausea. Immediate treatment is essential.

Congestive Heart Failure

Heart failure occurs when the heart muscle weakens and cannot pump sufficient blood; when the heart valves are damaged; or when hypertension exists or excessive demands are made on the heart. Blood pools in the veins, and not enough of it reaches the heart. The heart compensates by

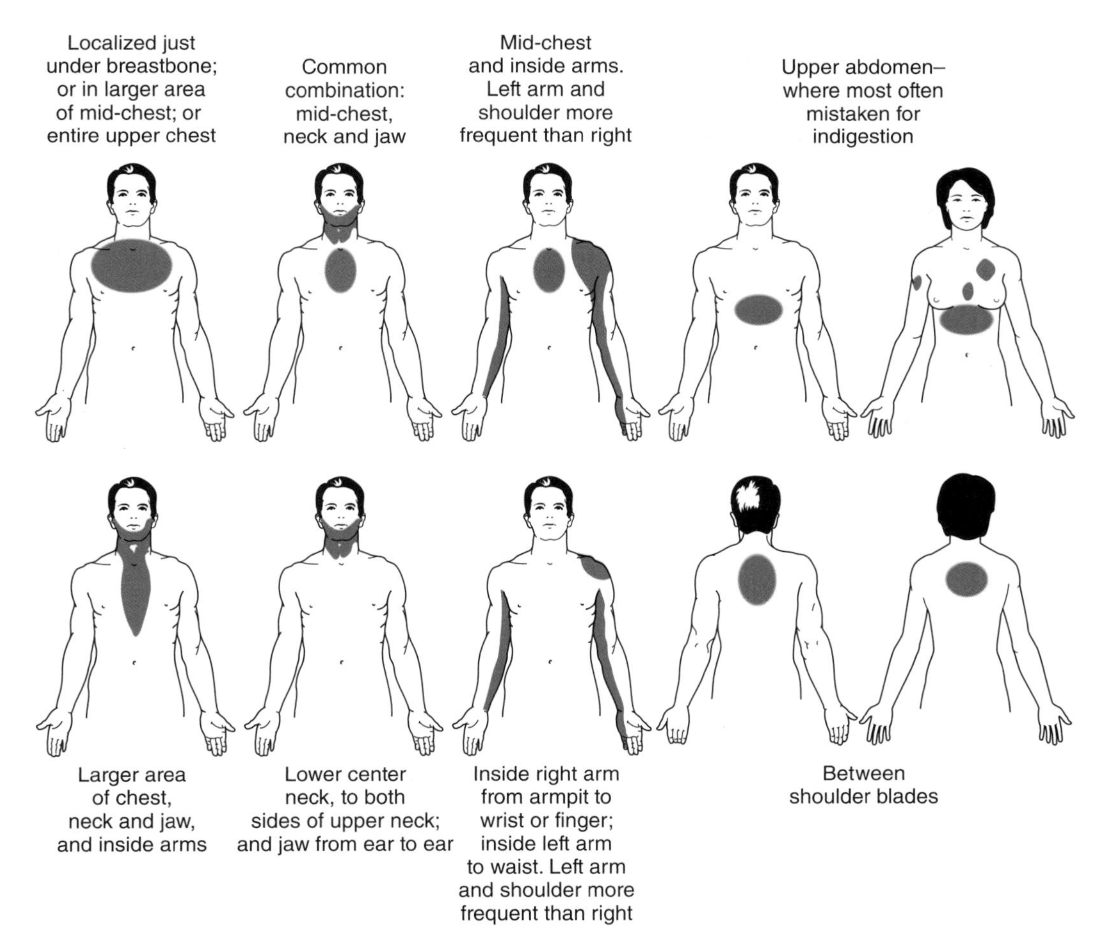

FIG. 11.17 Early warning signs of a heart attack. (From Goodman CG. *Differential Diagnosis for Physical Therapists: Screening for Referral*. 5th ed. Saunders/Elsevier; 2013.)

Box 11.2 Warning Signs of a Heart Attack

Most Common Warning Signs of Heart Attack

- Uncomfortable pressure, fullness, squeezing, or pain in the center of the chest (prolonged)
- Pain that spreads to the throat, neck, back, jaw, shoulders, or arms
- Chest discomfort with lightheadedness, dizziness, sweating, pallor, nausea, or shortness of breath
- Prolonged symptoms unrelieved by antacids, nitroglycerin, or rest

Atypical, Less Common Warning Signs (Especially in Females)

- Unusual chest pain: quality (e.g., burning, heaviness), location (e.g., left chest, stomach, or abdominal pain)
- Continuous midthoracic or interscapular pain
- Continuous neck or shoulder pain
- Isolated right biceps pain
- Pain unrelieved by antacids; pain unrelieved by nitroglycerin
- Nausea and vomiting; flulike manifestation without chest pain or discomfort
- Unexplained intense anxiety, weakness, or fatigue
- Breathlessness, dizziness

From Goodman CG. *Differential Diagnosis for Physical Therapists: Screening for Referral.* 5th ed. Saunders/Elsevier; 2013.

pumping out more blood, causing even more pooling in the veins and organs. This buildup of fluid is called *congestion*, and the condition is called *congestive heart failure.* Treatment usually includes the use of a diuretic, such as furosemide (Lasix), to eliminate excess fluid and reduce blood pressure (Fig. 11.18).

Rheumatic Heart Disease

Rheumatic fever may occur in young children after an untreated streptococcal throat infection; it is an immunological response to bacterial substances remaining in the body. Besides its signature rash, other signs and symptoms include joint pain, swelling, fever, and endocarditis. If left untreated, the endocarditis may cause rheumatic heart disease, in which the inflamed heart valves, particularly the mitral valve, become deformed.

Heart and Pericardial Inflammation

Inflammation that affects the heart and pericardial sac is uncommon. Pericarditis is an inflammation of the pericardium; myocarditis is an inflammation of the heart muscle. Endocarditis may affect the endocardium, heart valves, or both. Inflammation usually follows acute or chronic viral or bacterial infections or accompanies alcohol abuse or radiation therapy. The symptoms usually are mild but can lead to heart failure or arterial blockage if the condition is not treated early.

Vascular Disorders

Ischemia

Ischemia is a temporary deficiency or a diminished supply of blood to a tissue.

Arteriosclerosis and Atherosclerosis

Often the two terms are used interchangeably, but that is incorrect. *Arteriosclerosis* is a general term that means "hardening of the arteries" and refers to arteries that have lost their elasticity. In **atherosclerosis**, the most common type of arteriosclerosis, small fat deposits from cholesterol in the blood build up at stress points in the arteries. These stress points occur when the arteries branch out or incur damage. The fat combines with connective tissue sent to repair the damage and forms plaque. As this process continues, the arterial walls harden and blood flow diminishes. Symptoms do not usually appear until a major blockage occurs. The body compensates by enlarging the artery, if possible. Sometimes the artery enlarges, forms an aneurysm, and ruptures. Problems also occur when the plaque breaks off and travels elsewhere in the body. It can lodge in a vessel smaller in diameter than it is and completely block the vessel. In the brain, it can cause a stroke.

People in countries where it is common to consume high-fat diets (particularly diets high in saturated fatty acids and cholesterol) have higher incidences of atherosclerosis. Nonsurgical interventions, such as modifying the diet and taking part in aerobic exercise, may be able to enlarge an artery, increasing the blood flow. Also, collateral circulation may develop around the blockage as new vessels develop. Surgical interventions may include creating a bypass out of blood vessels transferred from other parts of the body, excising the blockage, or enlarging the vessel (Fig. 11.19).

Coronary Artery Disease

Coronary artery disease is commonly caused by arteriosclerosis, atherosclerosis, and thrombus formation in one or more of the coronary arteries. Occlusion, or blockage, of the artery, diminishes the amount of oxygen and nutrients reaching the heart tissues. Partial occlusion causes the transient chest and arm pain of angina pectoris. Total occlusion causes the crushing or squeezing pain of myocardial infarction and heart tissue death. Some of the many risk factors that contribute to coronary artery disease can be controlled, such as diet, weight, and avoidance of smoking. Treatment commonly includes the use of beta blockers and calcium channel blockers to slow the heart rate and reduce the strength of the contraction. In addition to lowering blood pressure, calcium channel blockers dilate the coronary arteries.

Hypertension

Most authorities consider hypertension to be a sustained blood pressure greater than 140/90 mm Hg or higher. Hypertension is graded as mild, moderate, borderline high, or severe, depending on the diastolic reading. In most cases, the cause is unknown (called *essential hypertension*), although kidney disease and arteriosclerosis may play roles. With hypertension, continuous sympathetic stimulation constricts arterioles. Chronic untreated hypertension leads to hypertensive heart disease. The heart becomes enlarged because of the increased work of the left ventricle against arteriolar resistance, and heart

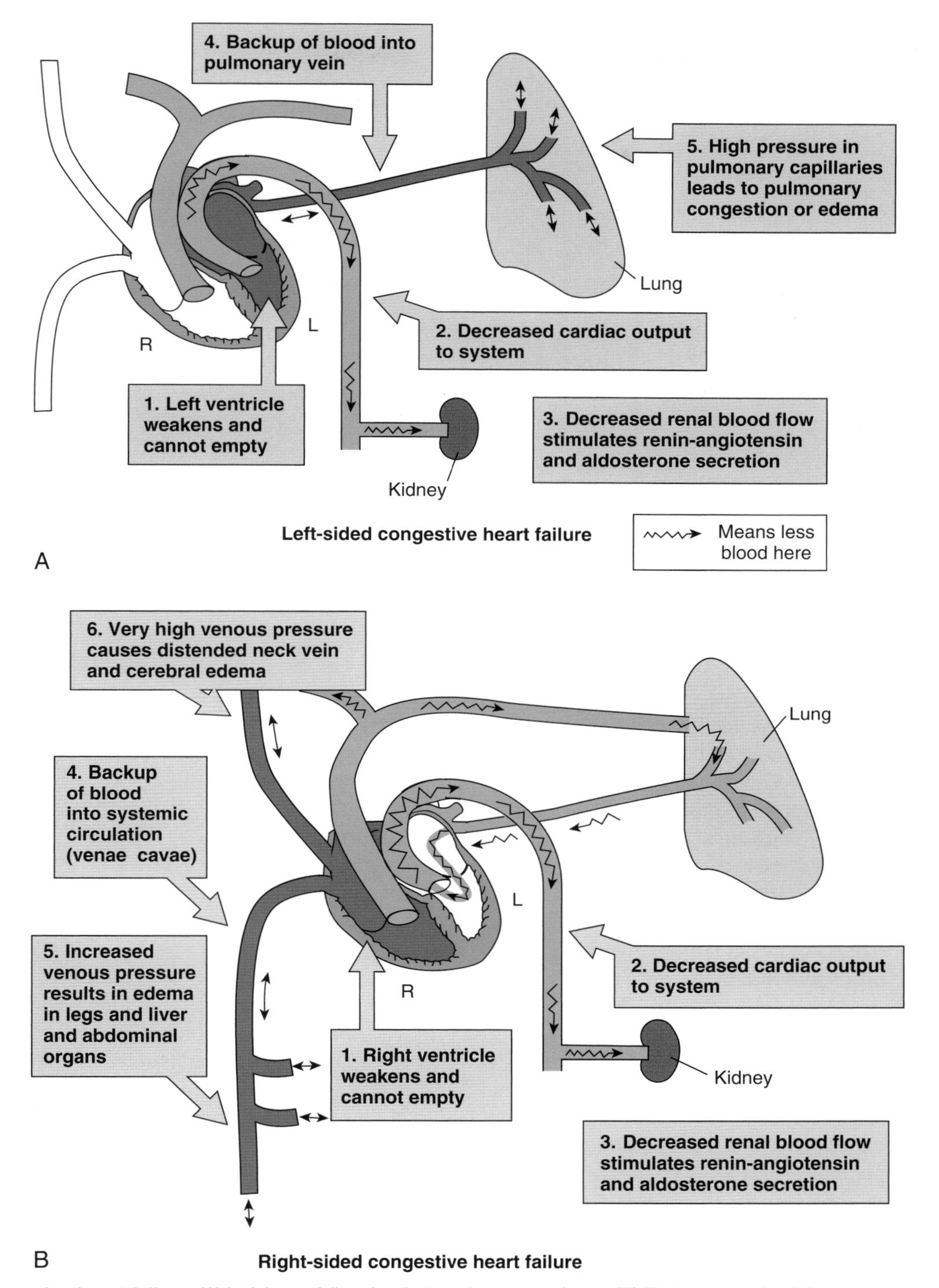

FIG. 11.18 Congestive heart failure. (A) Left heart failure leads to pulmonary edema. (B) Right ventricular failure causes peripheral edema that is most prominent in the lower extremities. (From VanMeter KC, Hubert RJ. *Gould's Pathophysiology for the Health Professions*. 5th ed. Elsevier; 2014.)

failure or infarction may result. Other important complications of untreated hypertension are stroke and kidney disease.

Nondrug therapy consists of restricting salt (which reduces fluid retention), losing weight (which reduces the resistance against which the heart must pump), reducing the consumption of alcohol, avoiding smoking, and participating in stress management and aerobic exercise programs.

Medical treatment may include a diuretic, a beta blocker, a calcium channel blocker, an angiotensin-converting enzyme inhibitor, or a combination of these medications as needed.

Varicose Veins

Varicose veins result when veins stretch so much that the valves cannot close sufficiently. More females than males are affected

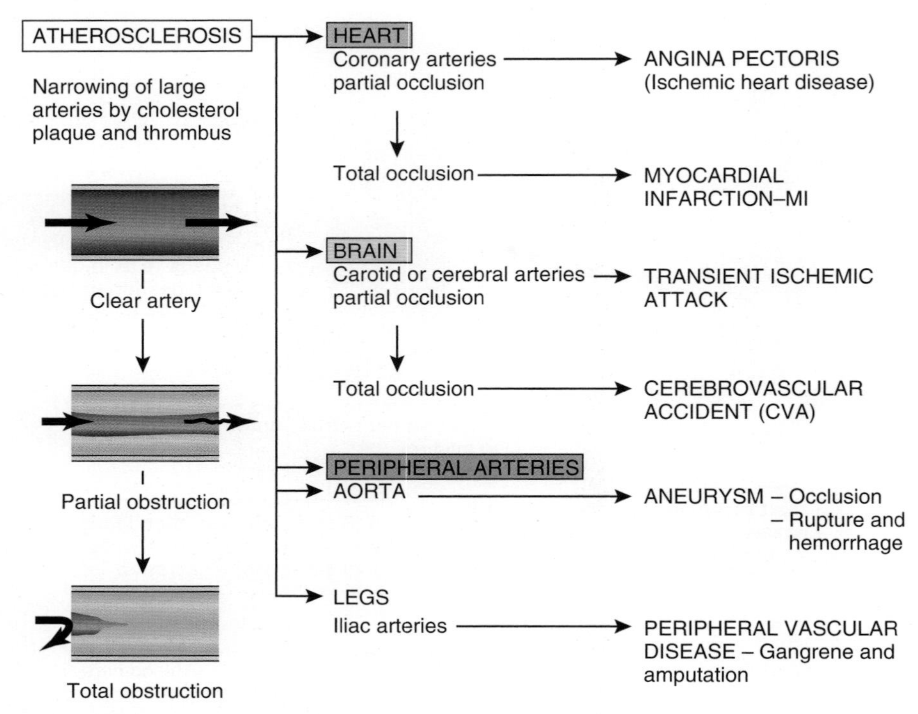

FIG. 11.19 The four major forms of atherosclerosis are classified as coronary, cerebral, aortic, and peripheral vascular. (From VanMeter KC, Hubert RJ. *Gould's Pathophysiology for the Health Professions*. 5th ed. Elsevier; 2014.)

because estrogen makes the connective tissue, including that in veins, in females more pliable than in males. This means that venous walls can become more easily distended. The condition may be congenital and may result from remaining in one position, especially standing, too long or may be caused by obesity, pregnancy, or menopause. The great and small saphenous veins are affected most commonly. Hemorrhoids are another common type of varicose vein.

Treatment includes rest, elevating the legs, wearing compression stockings, surgical removal of the vein, or sclerotherapy (injection of a saline solution into the vein) (Fig. 11.20).

Aneurysm

An aneurysm is a permanent bulge in the wall of a vessel because of weakness or damage to its structure. Although the usual result of arteriosclerosis is an aneurysm, the condition also may be congenital or may result from inflammation. The most common sites are the aorta and the arteries of the brain. Aneurysms are dangerous because they may rupture and hemorrhage.

Shock

Shock is a condition that results when the blood supply to vital organs becomes inadequate, causing diminished function by these organs. The blood vessels dilate rapidly, and blood pressure drops. The brain receives insufficient oxygen and can be damaged. Treatment usually consists of administering intravenous fluids until the person's condition stabilizes and the cause can be determined.

The four main types of shock are (1) hypovolemic shock, which results from a loss of blood or other bodily fluids; (2) cardiogenic shock, which occurs when the heart does not pump sufficient blood; (3) septic shock, which is caused by a bacterial infection (e.g., toxic shock syndrome); and (4) anaphylactic shock, which results from an allergy or overreaction by the immune system.

Arterial Inflammation

Endarteritis obliterans is a defect in which the artery walls become inflamed, blocking the opening of the vessel and blocking the smaller vessels.

Raynaud Disease and Phenomenon

Raynaud disease, a primary condition, and Raynaud phenomenon, a secondary condition, are primarily disorders that affect the blood supply to the fingers and toes and occasionally to the nose. Temporary spasms in the small arteries reduce or stop blood flow to the area, and the skin turns pale and then blue. Tissue damage, ulceration, or both may follow. The Raynaud disorders are aggravated by cold and emotional disturbances and often occur in individuals with connective tissue disorders or other systemic disorders.

Temporal Arteritis

Temporal arteritis is an inflammation of the temporal arteries, which causes pain, swelling, and tenderness. The condition also can cause a decrease in or a loss of vision and, in severe cases, stroke.

Blood Disorders

Anemia

Anemia is a decrease in the normal number of red blood cells or the amount of hemoglobin or iron in the blood. The various anemias are classified according to whether the cause is

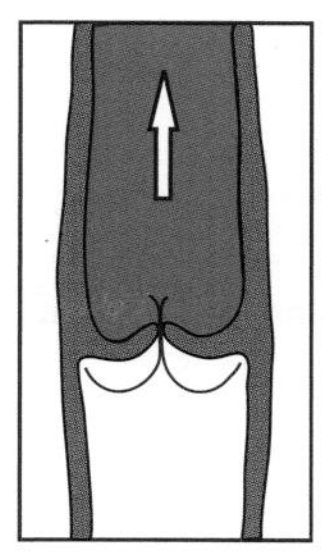

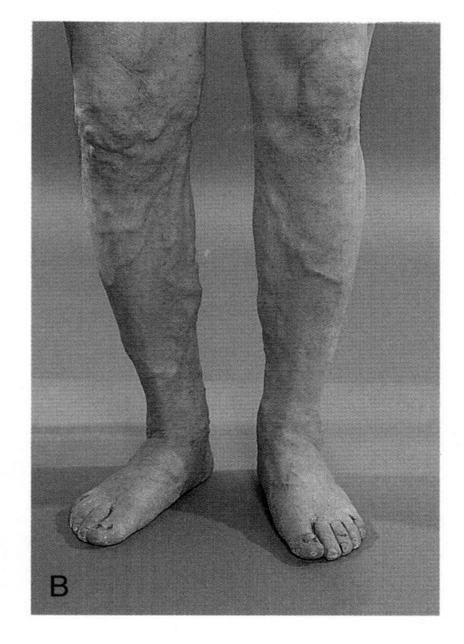

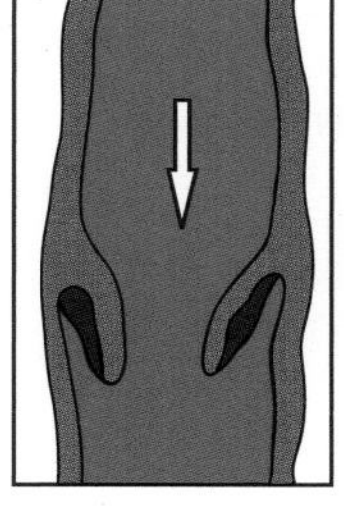

FIG. 11.20 (A) Varicose veins of the calf. (B) The inset shows venous valvular insufficiency, which accounts for the reflux of blood. (A, From O'Toole M, ed. *Miller-Keane Encyclopedia and Dictionary of Medicine, Nursing, and Allied Health*. 6th ed. Saunders; 1997; B From, Forbes CD, Jackson WF. *Color Atlas and Text of Clinical Medicine*. 3rd ed. Mosby; 2003.)

a loss in the number a change in the operation of red cells or whether it involves a decline in the production of red cells.

Nutritional Anemias

Iron deficiency anemia may result from the inability to absorb sufficient iron in the small intestine or maintain iron levels in the blood. Pernicious anemia usually results from the lack of intrinsic factors in the stomach, which leads to the inability to absorb vitamin B_{12}. Other nutritional anemias may result from deficiencies in nutrients, such as folic acid. Folic acid is necessary for the production of red blood cells. Intrinsic factor is needed to absorb vitamin B_{12} from the digestive tract.

Bone Marrow Suppression Anemia

Various types of anemia result from bone marrow suppression. Marrow suppression may occur in individuals undergoing chemotherapy or taking certain antibiotics, as a complication of radiation therapy, or in those with chronic diseases. The red blood cells may be damaged or destroyed, and the body often tries to compensate by producing new ones and sending them out before they mature. Severe cases require blood transfusions, along with bone marrow transplantation.

Thrombosis

A thrombosis is clotting in an unbroken blood vessel. If it breaks loose, it becomes an embolus (Figs. 11.21 and 11.22).

Phlebitis, Thrombophlebitis, and Deep Vein Thrombosis

The term *phlebitis* refers to the inflammation of a vein caused by injury, infection, or swelling. These diminish blood flow, which may cause thromboses to develop. If the thrombosis becomes inflamed, a condition known as *thrombophlebitis* develops. The superficial leg veins are the most common sites, primarily the saphenous veins. Clots also may form in the deep veins, especially in the legs and abdomen, a condition known as *deep vein thrombosis* (DVT). The clot can break off and travel in the bloodstream as an embolus.

Embolus

An embolus is a blood clot (thrombus), plaque, air or gas, fat, tumor cells, tissue, or clumps of bacteria in the bloodstream. If the embolus lodges in a blood vessel smaller in diameter than it is, it can block blood flow.

In pulmonary embolism, a clot detaches from a deep vein in the leg or pelvis and travels to the right atrium, then to the right ventricle, and on to the pulmonary artery. Predisposing factors for clot formation are obesity, heart failure, surgery and immobilization, and a history of thrombophlebitis. A clot that lodges at the junction of the pulmonary trunk and the pulmonary arteries may cause death. A clot that moves into a pulmonary artery and lodges there destroys lung tissue and is called a *pulmonary infarction*. The person suddenly becomes short of breath. Other signs and symptoms are chest pain, fever, and wheezing. The diagnosis is made by means of a lung scan and pulmonary angiogram. Treatment consists of intravenous anticoagulant (heparin) therapy to prevent further clotting and the use of a clot-dissolving medication. Subsequent therapy often involves orally administered warfarin (Coumadin).

Hemorrhage

Hemorrhage refers to the passage of blood outside of the cardiovascular system. Depending on the source, hemorrhage may be classified as cardiac, aortic, arterial, capillary, or venous. Clinically, hemorrhage may be of sudden onset, such as from an acute puncture wound; may be chronic, such as

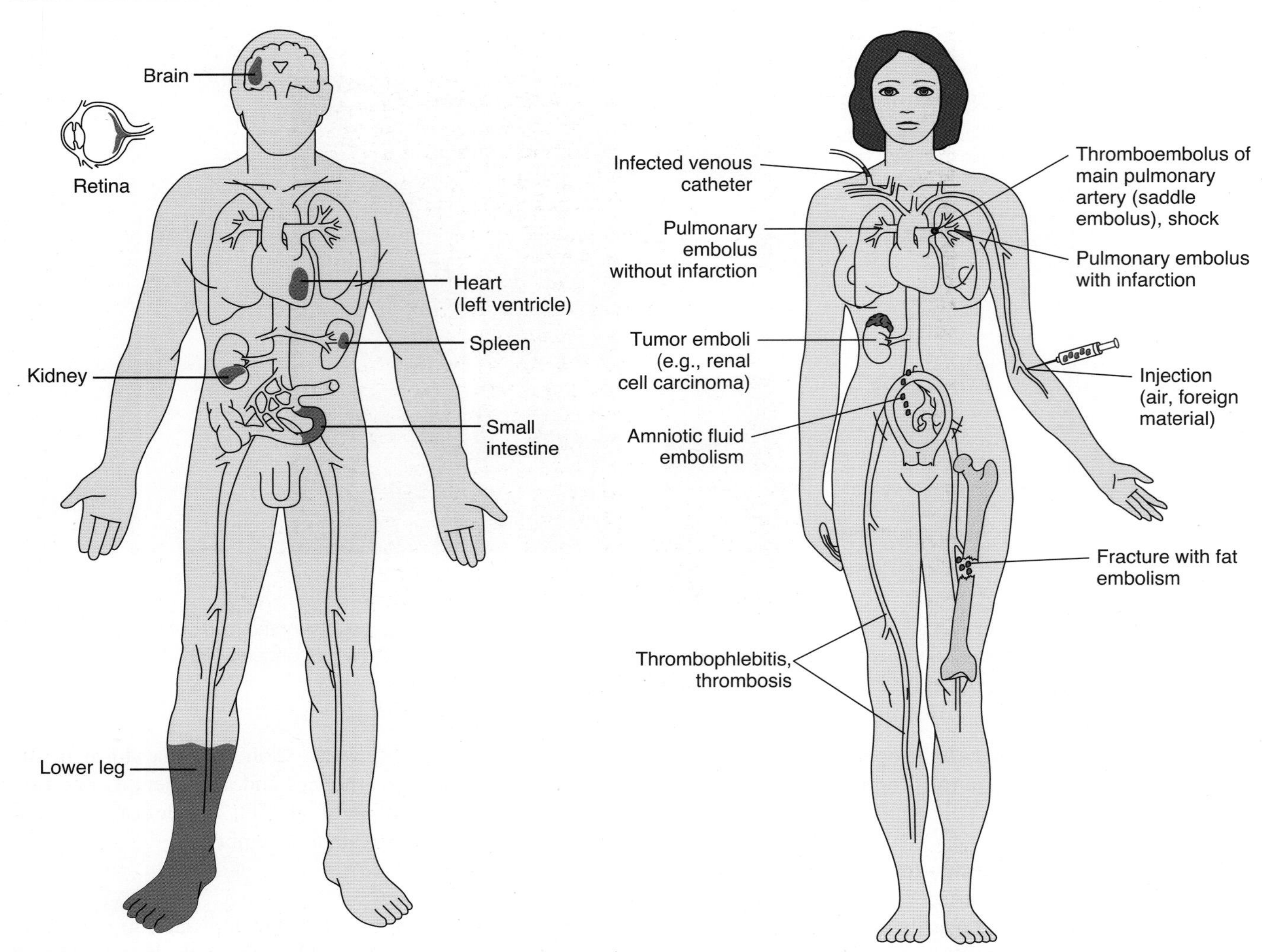

FIG. 11.21 Common sites of thrombus formation. (From Goodman CC, Fuller KS. *Pathology for the Physical Therapist Assistant*. Elsevier; 2012.)

from an ulcer; or may be recurrent and marked by repeated episodes of blood loss. The following are clinical terms that describe various forms of hemorrhage:

- *Hemoptysis:* Respiratory tract bleeding with expectoration, which means expelling from the lungs or throat by coughing and spitting
- *Hematemesis:* Vomiting of blood
- *Melena:* Passage of black, discolored blood in the stool (This represents upper gastrointestinal tract bleeding in which the blood is exposed to hydrochloric acid, which produces the color change.)
- *Hematuria:* Blood in the urine
- *Metrorrhagia:* Uterovaginal bleeding (Heavy menstrual bleeding is called *menorrhagia.*)

Sickle Cell Disease

Sickle cell disease causes premature destruction of red blood cells. These blood cells contain hemoglobin S because of an amino acid substitution in the hemoglobin molecules. These cells collapse and form a sickle or crescent shape. Because of their abnormal shape, they do not flow smoothly through the vessels and can block them. When the sickle cells block small blood vessels, multiple infarctions can result throughout the body. Common signs and symptoms are jaundice, diminished growth and development, and pain in the arms, legs, and abdomen resulting from the lack of oxygen. Infection or a cerebrovascular accident causes death. The primary treatment is symptomatic and includes the administration of oxygen, blood transfusions, and the use of analgesics.

Sickle cell disease is a genetic disease that affects mainly those who live or are descendants of those who lived, in the malaria belt around the world. The malaria belt includes parts of the Mediterranean region, sub-Saharan Africa, and tropical Asia. People with two sickle cell genes have severe anemia; those with only one defective gene have minor problems. The gene that causes the red blood cells to sickle also changes the permeability of the cell membranes of sickled cells, causing potassium ions to leak out. Low levels of potassium kill the malaria parasites that may infect sickled cells. Because of this, a person with one normal gene and one sickled gene has a higher-than-average resistance to malaria. Thus the single sickle cell gene gives a survival advantage.

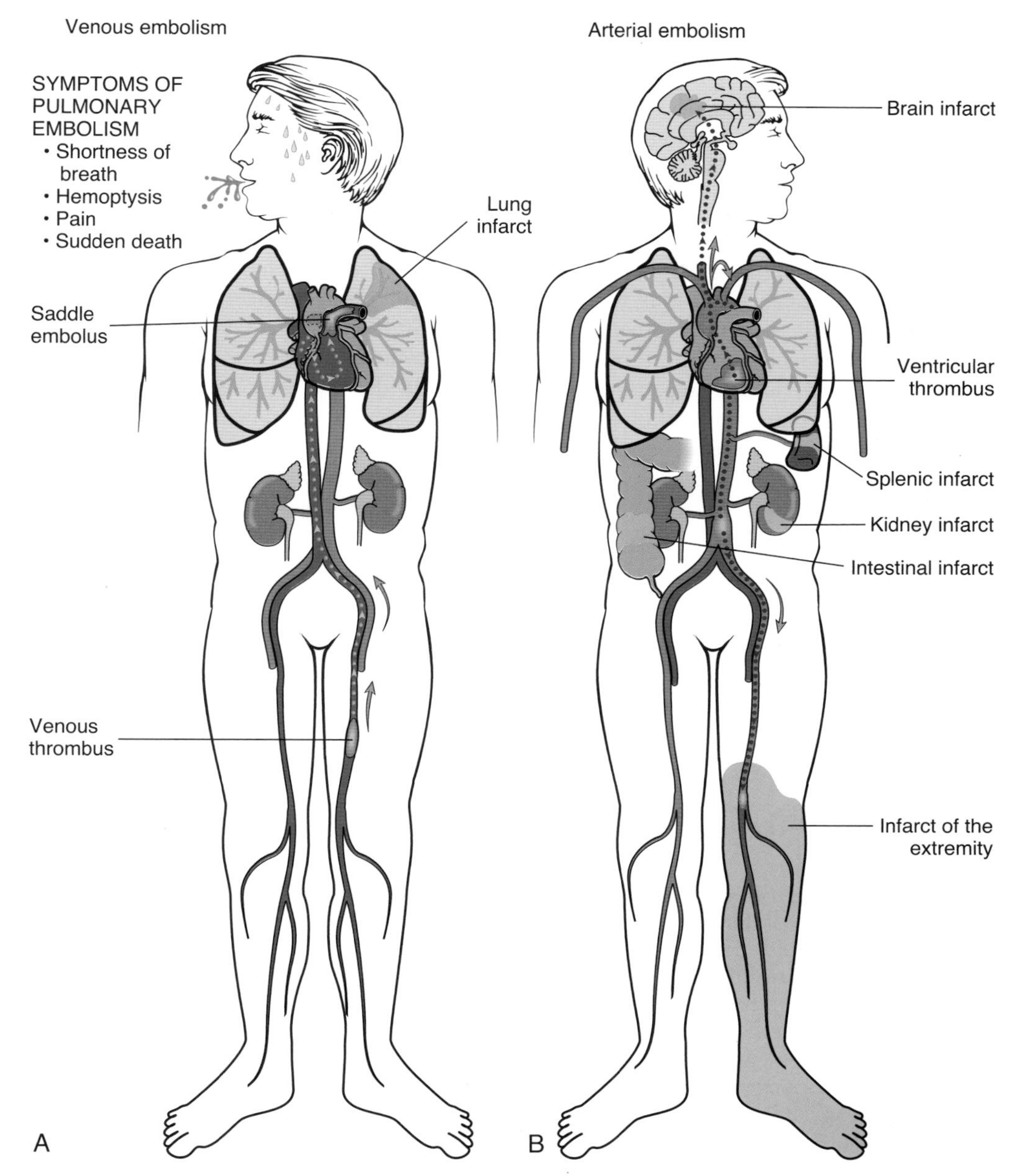

FIG. 11.22 Venous and arterial emboli. (A) Venous emboli can lodge in the lung, causing a variety of symptoms and conditions. (B) Arterial emboli may occlude arteries in many organs. (From Damjanov I. *Pathology for the Health-Related Professions*. 4th ed. Saunders/Elsevier; 2012.)

Hemophilia

Hemophilia is a genetic disorder in which factor VIII, a vital clotting factor in the blood, is greatly diminished or absent, resulting in the blood's inability to clot. It is recessively sex linked. This means that it is carried on the X chromosome. Therefore, a female can carry the gene but will not develop severe symptoms because a corresponding nondefective gene on her other X chromosome prevents the gene from becoming fully active. A male with the hemophilia gene on his X chromosome, however, does not have a corresponding, nondefective gene on his Y chromosome, so the gene becomes fully active. Although hemophilia is passed on by females, they usually have only minor bleeding problems or no symptoms. Males with hemophilia may experience extended episodes of bleeding and may be susceptible to internal bleeding caused by minor trauma.

Polycythemia

Polycythemia is an abnormally high amount of red blood cells. This raises the viscosity of blood and makes blood more difficult for the heart to pump. Increased viscosity also contributes to high blood pressure and an increased risk of stroke. Causes of polycythemia include abnormal increases in red blood cell production, low amounts of oxygen in the tissues, dehydration, blood doping, or the use of erythropoietin (EPO) in athletes. EPO increases red blood cell production. Blood doping involves using transfusions to boost the number of red blood cells in the bloodstream to enhance athletic ability. The increased red blood cells mean more oxygen can be carried to tissues.

Thrombocytopenia

Thrombocytopenia is a decrease in platelets, which diminishes the ability of the blood to clot. Common causes include blood loss, infection, cancer (especially Hodgkin disease and leukemia), and lupus. The condition also may result from radiation therapy or chemotherapy. Idiopathic thrombocytopenic purpura is an autoimmune disease in which antiplatelet antibodies are present. Common signs include easy bruising, nosebleeds, bleeding gums, and blood in the urine. Complications include cerebral hemorrhage and bleeding into nerve tissue, which can cause paralysis.

Coronavirus Disease

Coronavirus disease (COVID-19), caused by the severe acute respiratory syndrome coronavirus 2 (SARS-CoV-2) and all the mutations causing variants, is a global public health concern and is characterized by an exaggerated inflammatory response. The exaggerated inflammatory response can lead to a hypercoagulable state indicating a potential risk for deep vein thrombosis and pulmonary thromboembolism.

INDICATIONS/CONTRAINDICATIONS for Therapeutic Massage

Cardiovascular System

In general, cardiovascular disease presents contraindications for therapeutic massage. If the contraindication does not arise from the disease itself, the medication taken to control the disease may pose problems. Blood thinners, for example, increase the possibility of bruising and hemorrhage. Nonetheless, therapeutic massage often is indicated as part of a supervised treatment program. The key is supervision by a qualified healthcare provider because cardiovascular diseases can be complex in the presenting pathological conditions and the treatment protocols. The general stress management and homeostatic normalization effects of therapeutic massage treatments are desirable for most cardiovascular difficulties as long as the treatments are supervised as part of a total therapeutic program.

Take care to refrain from performing any type of therapeutic massage over sites of thrombophlebitis or deep vein thrombosis (DVT). Systemic contraindications also may be present. The practitioner should refer for diagnosis any client with unexplained leg pain, a cardinal sign of thrombophlebitis or DVT.

Section Summary

- List the components of the cardiovascular system.
  Heart, blood vessels, and blood. The heart pumps oxygenated and nutrient-rich blood to body tissues via the arteries and arterioles. Oxygen and nutrients leave the blood and enter tissues via the capillaries. The venules and veins then transport the unoxygenated blood (now carrying carbon dioxide and metabolic wastes) back to the heart, which pumps it to the lungs, which diffuse the carbon dioxide and resupply oxygen.
- List the components of blood.
  Plasma is a straw-colored liquid composed of 90% water and 10% nutrients, gases, and waste products. Its function is to transport water, nutrients, hormones, proteins, red blood cells, white blood cells, and platelets. Red blood cells (erythrocytes) contain an iron and protein molecule called hemoglobin, to which oxygen and carbon dioxide bind. Their function is to transport oxygen to cells and to take away carbon dioxide. White blood cells (leukocytes) lack hemoglobin. They are divided into neutrophils, lymphocytes, monocytes, eosinophils, and basophils. Their function is to protect the body from pathogens and remove dead cells/substances. Platelets (thrombocytes) are involved in clotting to prevent blood loss.

THE LYMPHATIC SYSTEM

SECTION OBJECTIVES

Chapter objectives covered in this section:

6. List and describe the components and functions of the lymphatic system.
7. Identify pathologies of the lymphatic system and describe indications and contraindications for massage.

After completing this section, the learner will be able to:

- List the components of the lymphatic system.
- List the components of lymph.
- Describe how lymph moves through the body.

Overview of the Lymphatic System

The lymphatic system is a specialized component of the circulatory system that is responsible for waste disposal and immune response. The lymphatic system transports fluid from around the cells through a system of filters. Lymph and blood are similar, except that lymph does not have red blood cells or platelets. Lymph has slightly higher protein content than blood, and it carries large molecules, such as proteins, lipids, bacteria, and other debris.

The lymphatic system permeates the entire tissue structure of the body in a one-way drainage network of vessels, ducts, nodes, lacteals, and lymphoid organs, such as the spleen, tonsils, and thymus. It is a one-way system that begins in the tissues and ends when it reaches the blood vessels. The system helps the body maintain homeostasis by collecting accumulated tissue fluid around the cells and returning it to blood circulation. The lymph nodes play an active part in the immune defenses of the body by filtering out and destroying foreign substances and microorganisms. Special lymph capillaries called *lacteals* absorb lipids from the small intestine so the lymph can transport them to the bloodstream (Fig. 11.23).

To get an idea of the extensive lymph network, visualize the roots of a plant. Tiny lymph vessels, known as *lymph capillaries*, are distributed throughout the body, except in the eyes, brain, and spinal cord. Fluid collects in the lymph capillaries in a manner somewhat similar to the way water is drawn up

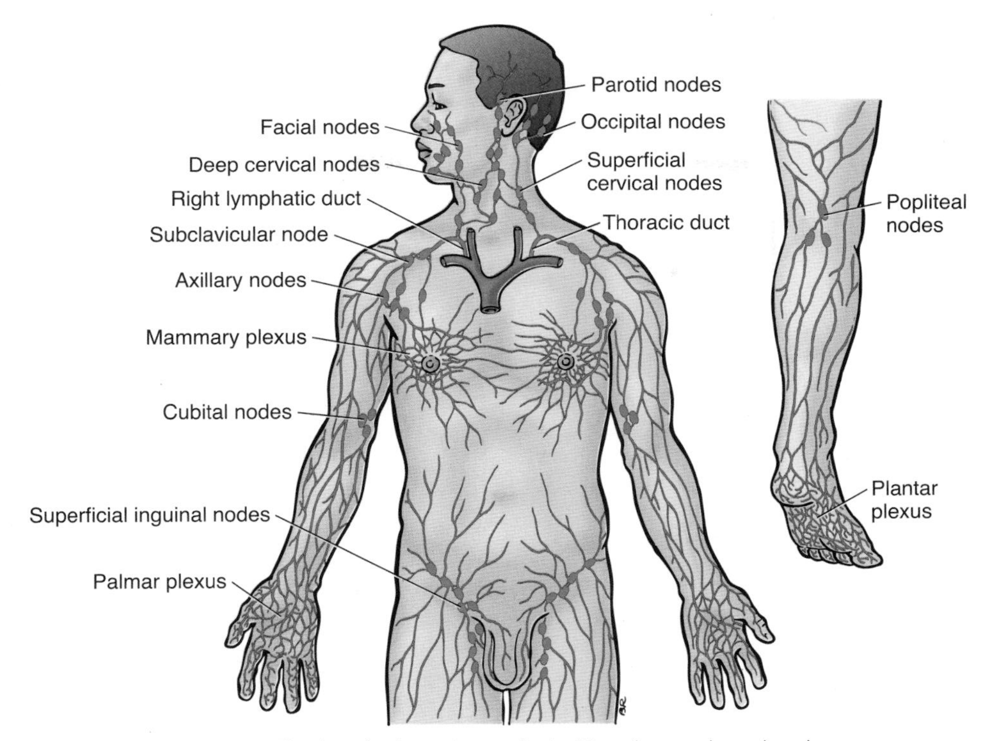

FIG. 11.23 The lymphatic system: principal lymph vessels and nodes.

into a plant's roots. Segments of lymph capillaries are divided by one-way valves and a spiral set of smooth muscles called *lymphangions*. This system moves fluid against gravity in a peristalsis-type undulation.

The lymphatic tubes merge until major channels and vessels are formed. These vessels run from the distal parts of the body toward the neck, usually alongside veins and arteries. Valves in the vessels prevent the backflow of lymph.

Lymph nodes are enlarged portions of the lymph vessels that generally cluster at the joints. This arrangement assists the movement of the lymph through the nodes by means of the pumping action from joint movement. These nodes filter the fluid and produce lymphocytes.

All of the body's lymph vessels converge into two main channels, the thoracic duct and the right lymphatic duct. Vessels from the entire left side of the body and the right side of the body below the chest converge into the thoracic duct, which in turn empties into the left subclavian vein, situated beneath the left clavicle. The right lymphatic duct collects lymph from the vessels on the right side of the head, neck, upper chest, and right arm. It empties into the right subclavian vein beneath the right clavicle. Waste products then are carried by the bloodstream to the spleen, intestines, and kidneys for detoxification.

Lymph moves along a pressure gradient from areas of high pressure to areas of low pressure. It moves from the interstitial space (high pressure) into the lymph capillaries (low pressure) through a pressure mechanism exerted by respiration, peristalsis of the large intestine, the compression of muscles, and the pull of the skin and fascia during movement. This action is especially prominent at the plexuses in the hands and feet. Major lymph plexuses are found on the soles of the feet and the palms of the hands. The rhythmic pumping of walking and grasping probably facilitates lymphatic flow. There is also a primary intrinsic pumping mechanism in the lymphatic system.

Lymph circulation involves two steps:

- First, plasma is forced out of blood capillaries into the space around the cells. The fluid now located around the cells is called *interstitial fluid*. As fluid pressure increases between the cells, the cells move apart, pulling on the microfilaments that connect the endothelial cells of the lymph capillaries to tissue cells. The pull on the microfilaments causes the lymph capillaries to open like flaps, allowing interstitial fluid to enter the lymph capillaries. Once the fluid is in the lymph capillaries, it is called *lymph*.
- Next, the lymph moves through the network of contractile lymphatic vessels. The lymphatic system does not have a central pump like the heart. Various factors assist the transport of lymph through the lymphatic vessels.

The "lymphatic pump" is the spontaneous contraction of lymphatic vessels as a result of the increased pressure of lymphatic fluid. These contractions usually start in the lymphangions adjacent to the terminal end of the lymph capillaries and spread progressively from one lymphangion to the next, toward the thoracic duct or the right lymphatic duct. The contractions are similar to abdominal peristalsis and are stimulated by increases in pressure inside lymphatic vessels. Contractions of the lymphatic vessels are not coordinated with the heart or breath rate. If the pressure inside the lymphatic vessels exceeds or falls below certain levels, lymphatic contractions stop.

Breathing is an essential part of lymphatic movement. During inhalation, the thoracic duct is squeezed, which pushes fluid forward and creates a vacuum in the duct. During exhalation, fluid is pulled from the lymphatics into the thoracic duct to fill the partial vacuum.

Practical Application

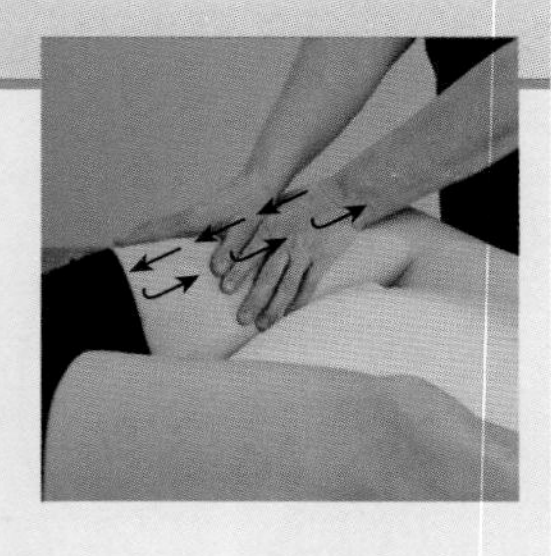

Manual lymphatic drainage (MLD) methods use a very gentle skin/superficial fascia stretching technique or massage designed to move the skin/superficial fascia in specific directions based on the underlying structure and physiology of the lymphatic system. The intent of the various interventions is to drain lymph already in the lymph vessels (collectors) and stimulate the formation of lymph by increasing the flow of interstitial fluid to the lymphatic capillaries (initial lymphatics). The working hypothesis (educated guess) for the manual methods is to support more normal fluid flow by creating spaces in the tissues and then massaging fluid into these spaces by external tissue compression.

The massage-like skin stretching used in MLD and the rhythmic rocking and compression described in the osteopathic approach are also part of therapeutic massage. The management of simple edema as part of a general massage seems to be within the scope of practice; however, if pathology does exist, focused treatment by a massage therapist without direct supervision of a physician, nurse, or physical therapist may be outside the scope of practice.

Lymphatic System of the Brain

The discovery of the central nervous system's lymphatic system adds to the understanding of the importance of the lymphatic system. Researchers first identified what is called the *glymphatic system* functioning as a waste-clearance system and circulating glucose, lipids, amino acids, and neurotransmitters. The lymphatic system (discussed in Chapter 4) uses a unique system of tunnels around blood vessels formed by astroglial cells to transport fluid. The glymphatic system is the analog of the lymphatic system in the CNS. The glymphatic network serves as the initial collector for waste clearance and is connected to the lymphatic network within the dura covering the brain, as well as cranial nerves and large vessels at the skull exits. The meningeal lymphatic vessels are embedded in the dura mater and located alongside blood vessels. The anatomical and functional interconnections between the glymphatic and meningeal lymphatic vessels are not completely understood (Sun et al., 2017; Nistal and Mocco, 2018; Benveniste et al., 2018).

The glymphatic system functions primarily when we are sleeping. The restorative function of sleep may be related to the enhanced removal of potentially neurotoxic waste products that accumulate in the awake central nervous system. This is relevant to the massage therapist because the evidence supports massage therapy as beneficial for sleep quality (Nerbass et al., 2010; Kashani and Kashani, 2014; Pinar and Afsar, 2015; Owais et al., 2018; Hablitz and Nedergaard, 2021).

Lymph

Interstitial fluid comes from blood plasma that seeps through capillaries. The interstitial fluid becomes lymph when it moves into the lymph capillaries. Lymph contains proteins and other cell products as well as pathogens and cell debris. As lymph travels through lymph vessels, it is filtered by lymph nodes that remove pathogens and cell debris. Lymph then travels to the bloodstream and once again becomes plasma.

Lymph Vessels, Nodes, and Organs

Lymph Vessels

The lymph capillaries are tiny open-ended channels located in tissue spaces throughout the entire body except for the cornea (Fig. 11.24). A lymphatic capillary network of vessels slightly larger than blood capillaries drains tissue fluid from nearly all tissues and organs that have blood vascularization. The cardiovascular system is a closed system, whereas the lymphatic system is open ended, beginning in the interstitial spaces.

The moment that interstitial fluid enters a lymph capillary, a flap valve prevents it from returning to the interstitial space. Lymph capillaries join to form larger lymph vessels that resemble veins but have thinner, more transparent walls. Like veins, they have valves to prevent backflow. The large vessels continue to merge and eventually become two main ducts called the *right lymphatic duct* and the *thoracic duct* (left lymphatic duct). The right lymphatic duct drains the upper right half of the body and empties into the right subclavian vein. The thoracic duct drains the rest of the body and empties into the left subclavian vein.

Lymph Nodes

Lymph nodes are small, round structures located along the lymph vessels. For the most part, they are clustered at the joints; movement of the joints helps pump lymph through the nodes. The superficial lymph nodes are most numerous in the groin, axillae, and neck, whereas most of the deep lymph nodes are found alongside blood vessels in the pelvic, abdominal, and thoracic cavities. All lymph passes through one or more nodes before it enters the bloodstream. Lymph nodes contain mature lymphocytes, white blood cells that destroy bacteria, virus-infected cells, pathogens, foreign matter, and waste materials. During periods of infection, an immune response occurs (discussed in more detail in the Specific Immunity section) in which the number of lymphocytes increases. The additional activity in the nodes and the buildup of the lymphocytes can make the nodes swollen and painful. The nodes also provide a filtering system that removes waste products and transfers them for detoxification in the other systems of the body.

The locations of the lymph nodes are as follows:

- Preauricular lymph nodes are located just in front of the ear and drain the superficial tissues and skin on the lateral side of the head and face.
- Submental and submaxillary nodes are located on the floor of the mouth and drain lymph from the nose, lips, and teeth.
- Cervical lymph nodes are located at the neck.
- Superficial cubital or supratrochlear nodes are located just above the bend of the elbow and drain lymph from the forearm.

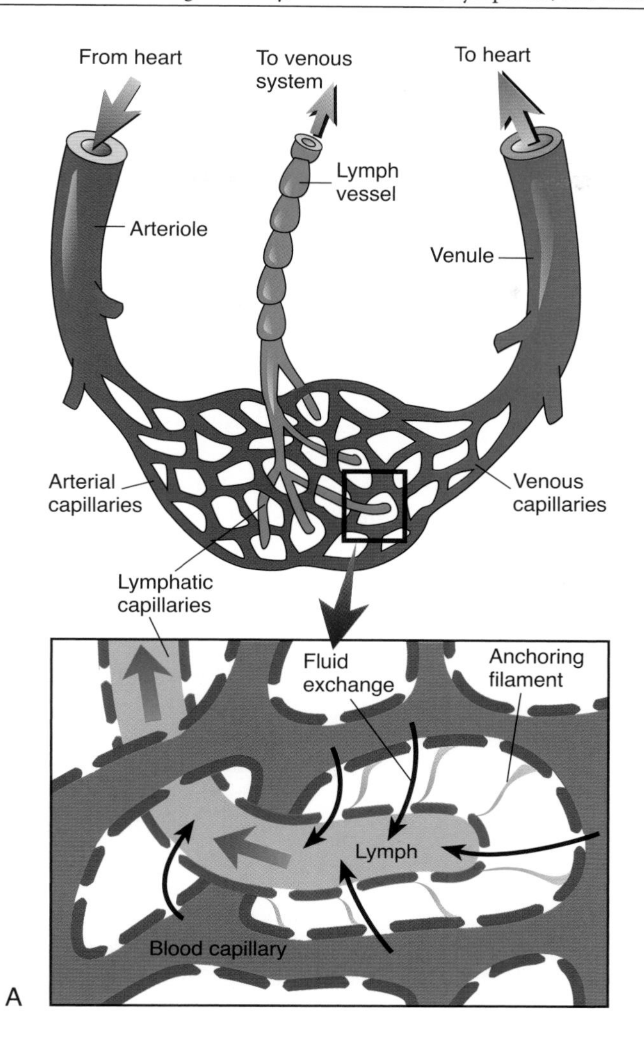

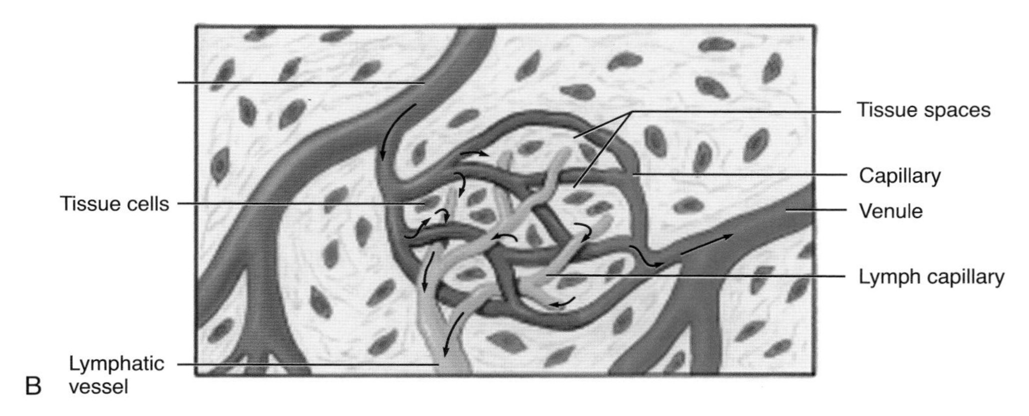

FIG. 11.24 (A) Structure of a typical lymphatic capillary. The interstitial fluid enters through clefts between overlapping endothelial cells that form the wall of the vessel. Semilunar valves ensure a one-way flow of lymph out of the tissue. (B) Distribution on lymphatic capillaries in the tissue. (A, From Huether SE, McCance KL. *Understanding Pathophysiology*. 5th ed. Mosby; 2014; B, From Applegate E. *The Anatomy and Physiology Learning System*. 4th ed. Saunders/Elsevier; 2011.)

- Axillary lymph nodes located deep in the underarm and upper chest drain lymph from the arm and upper part of the thoracic wall, including the breast.
- Inguinal lymph nodes located in the groin drain lymph from the leg and external genitals.
- Popliteal lymph nodes are located behind the knee.

Spleen

The spleen, the largest of the lymphatic organs, is located near the stomach under the diaphragm. Macrophages in the spleen filter out worn-out red blood cells and destroy microorganisms in the blood. The spleen serves as a blood reservoir and can release small amounts of blood into the circulation during times of emergency or blood loss. The spleen functions with the lymphatic system by storing lymphocytes and releasing them as part of the immune response.

Thymus

The thymus is a triangular gland composed of lymphatic tissue. It is located in the upper chest, superior to the superior vena cava, and inferior to the thyroid gland. This gland is most prominent in the newborn and begins to atrophy after puberty, becoming only a small remnant in the adult. The thymus is important in the development and maturation of certain lymphocytes and in programming them to become T cells in the immune system.

Lymph Nodules

Lymph nodules are small masses of lymph tissue (up to approximately 1 mm in diameter) that contain lymphocytes enmeshed within reticular fibers. Collectively, this tissue is referred to as *mucosa-associated lymph tissue*, and along with the spleen and thymus, it is involved in the development of immunity. This tissue does not filter lymph but is positioned strategically to protect the respiratory and gastrointestinal tracts from microbes and other foreign materials. Lymph nodules are scattered throughout loose connective tissue, especially in the mucous membrane lining the upper respiratory tract, digestive tract, reproductive tract, and urinary tract. Lymph nodules appear to be distributed strategically to defend the body against disease-causing organisms that could penetrate the linings of passageways that open outside the body.

Most lymphatic nodules are small and solitary. However, some are found in large clusters. For example, large aggregates of lymph nodules occur in the wall of the lower portion (ileum) of the small intestine. These masses of lymph nodules are known as *Peyer patches*. Tonsils, strategically located under the epithelial lining of the oral cavity and pharynx so that they can defend against invading bacteria, are also aggregates of lymph nodules. The lingual tonsils are located at the base of the tongue. The single pharyngeal tonsil is located in the posterior wall of the nasal portion of the pharynx above the soft palate and often is referred to as the *adenoid*.

Lymph nodules include the following:

- Palatine and lingual tonsils located between the mouth and the oral part of the pharynx
- Pharyngeal tonsil located on the wall of the nasal part of the pharynx
- Solitary lymphatic follicles dispersed throughout the body
- Aggregated lymphatic follicles (Peyer patches) located in the wall of the small intestine
- Vermiform appendix, an outgrowth from the cecum (the first part of the large intestine)

Lymphatic Pump and Drainage

Although the lymph system has no muscular pumping organ such as the heart, the movement of joints provides some pumping action, and lymph moves along slowly and steadily. It flows through the thoracic duct and reenters the general circulation at the rate of about 3 L per day, despite the fact that most of the flow is against gravity. Lymph moves through the system in the correct direction because of the large number of valves that permit fluid to flow only toward the center of the body.

The movement of lymph is known as *lymphatic drainage*. It begins when lymph moves out of the interstitial spaces and into the lymph capillaries, a movement that is assisted by the pressure exerted by the compression of skeletal muscles against the vessels during movement; by changes in internal pressure during respiration; and by the opening of lymph vessels resulting from the pull of the skin and fascia during movement. Major lymph plexuses are found on the soles and the palms, possibly because the rhythmic pumping of walking and grasping facilitates lymphatic flow. Current research suggests that the lymph vessels themselves may have an intrinsic pumping action. Every 6 to 20 mm, there is a valve that lies directly between two or three layers of spiral smooth muscle. The unit is called a *lymphangion*. The rhythmic smooth muscle contraction causes the lymph vessels to undulate, almost in the manner of intestinal tract peristalsis. Some researchers think that this contraction is the sensation felt by those who sense a rhythmic pulsation in the human body.

Specialized application of massage may be effective in increasing lymph removal from stagnant or edematous tissue. Massage that uses light pressure to drag the skin has the potential to increase superficial lymph movement. Crosswise and lengthwise stretching of the lymph vessels' anchoring filaments opens the lymph capillaries, thus allowing the interstitial fluid to enter the lymphatic system. The practitioner applies the massage strokes in the direction of normal lymphatic drainage, thus speeding up lymph movement.

The lymph in the left arm flows from the fingers toward the axilla and from there to the neck, where it joins the thoracic duct. Lymph from the right arm does the same, except that it drains into the smaller right lymphatic duct. Both ducts empty at the junction of the subclavian and internal jugular veins. The lymph from the right side of the chest, face, and scalp also flows toward the right axilla and into the right lymphatic duct. The lymph from the left side of the face and scalp flows into the thoracic duct.

The lymph from the feet and legs drains upward toward the groin and into the abdomen and empties into the lower end of the thoracic duct, called the *cisterna chyli*.

1. Of the lymph flow from the chest, 85% drains into the respective axillary nodes. The remaining lymph drains into nodes located behind the sternum and into lymph vessels located in the pectoralis muscle. In general, lymph moves toward the groin and the axillae.
2. The alteration of valves and smooth muscles gives a characteristic moniliform shape to these vessels, like pearls on a string. Lymphatic circulation is separated into two layers:
   - The superficial circulation, which constitutes 60%–70% of lymph circulation, is located just under the skin in the junction between the superficial fascia and the dermoepidermal junction. The superficial circulation is not stimulated directly by exercise but is influenced by the stretching and pulling of the skin and superficial fascia during movement.
   - The deep muscular and visceral circulation, below the fascia, is activated by muscular contraction.

Practical Application

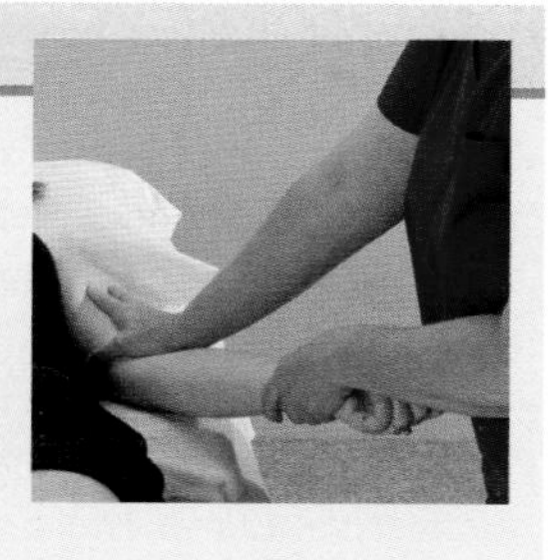

Simple muscle tension and binding by connective tissues put pressure on the lymph vessels and may block them, interfering with efficient drainage. Therapeutic massage can relax muscle tension and improve connective tissue pliability. As the muscles relax and the connective tissue has more space, the lymph vessels open. The relationship between the fluid-filled pockets of the interstitium and the lymphatic vessels presents interesting possibilities for fluid movement as the tissue is compressed and pulled. Lymphatic massage mechanically stimulates the flow of lymph by tracing the lymphatic routes with light pressure (Fig. 11.25). This pull on the skin and superficial connective tissues affects the anchoring filaments of the lymph capillaries, ultimately opening the capillaries. The focus of the pressure is on the dermis. Little pressure is required to reach the area; too much pressure is thought to squeeze the capillaries closed and nullify any effect. Rhythmic, gentle, passive, and active joint movement and rhythmic muscle contraction reproduce the way the body normally pumps lymph, especially in the deep lymphatic circulation. During massage, the practitioner can stimulate this process by using rhythmic compression with enough depth to compress the muscles. The client helps the process by breathing slowly and deeply, which stimulates lymph flow. When possible, position the area being massaged above the heart so that gravity can assist the lymph flow. Because lymph capillary plexuses are present on the bottoms of the feet, rhythmic compression on the soles also enhances lymph flow. When applying lymph drainage techniques, the practitioner must take care not to promote excessive increases in the volume of lymph flow in people who have heart and kidney conditions, because the venous system must accommodate the load once the fluid has been delivered to the subclavian veins. Significantly increasing the load could place excessive strain on the heart and kidneys. Caution is required for massage applied to edematous tissue especially when skin changes and fibrous and adipose deposits have occurred.

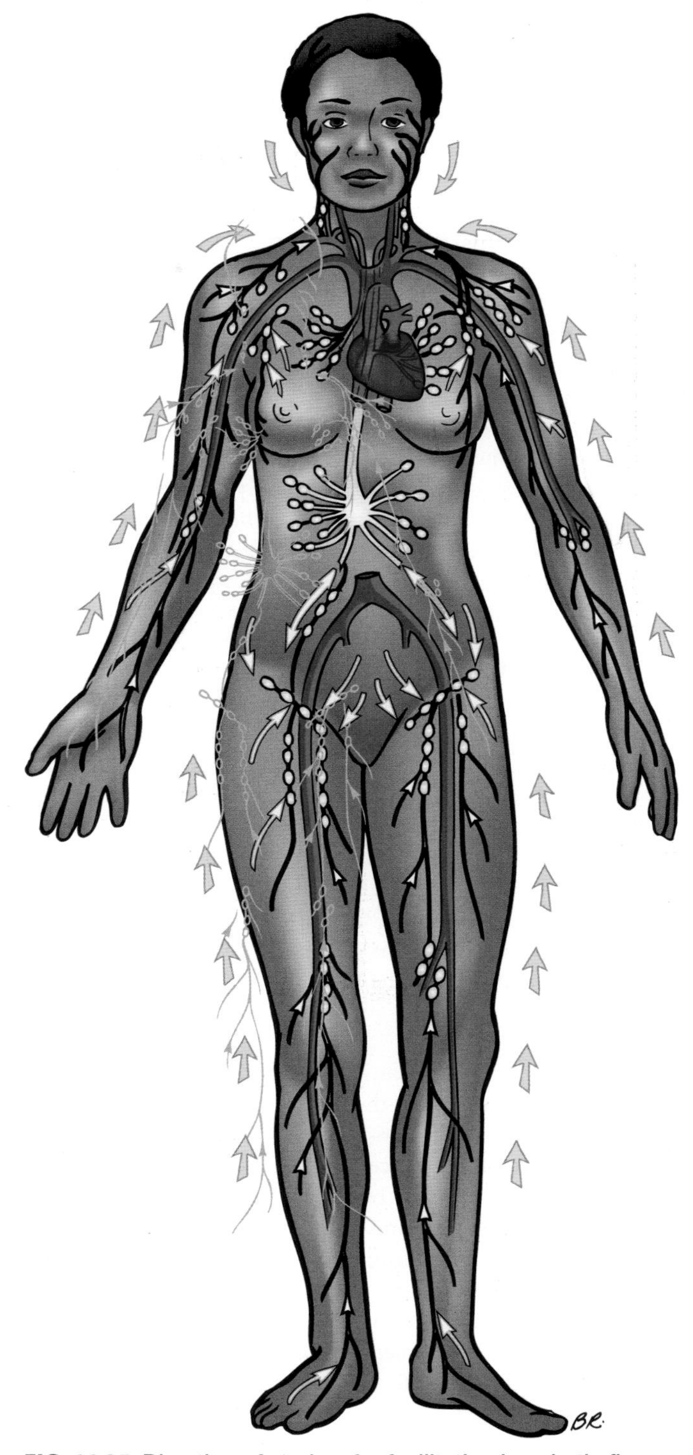

FIG. 11.25 Direction of strokes for facilitating lymphatic flow. (From Fritz S. *Mosby's Fundamentals of Therapeutic Massage*. 5th ed. Mosby/Elsevier; 2013.)

Pathological Conditions of the Lymphatic System

The lymphatic system clears away infection and keeps body fluids in balance. When it is not working properly, fluid builds in the tissues and causes swelling, called *lymphedema*. Other lymphatic system problems can include blockage infections, cancer, and lymphatic malformation (LM).

Edema

Edema is the accumulation of abnormal amounts of fluid in tissue spaces and often accompanies congestion, which is an increase in the volume of blood in dilated vessels. Common causes of edema are heart failure, kidney disease, and liver disease. Localized edema occurs with inflammation and lymphatic obstruction.

Lymphedema

Lymphedema is an increase in tissue fluid caused by inflammation or obstruction by scar tissue, parasites, or trauma. For example, after a radical mastectomy in which axillary lymph channels are removed, arm drainage may be partially blocked, causing the arm to swell. The primary treatment for generalized edema is the cautious use of diuretics to remove the fluid.

Stage 1 is early edema which improves when the limb is elevated. Stage 2 involves pitting edema. Stage 3 includes fibroadipose and skin changes. Some forms of massage are effective for managing stage 1 lymphedema. External pumping sleeves that rhythmically compress the area are beneficial in chronic cases. The practitioner should refer a client with any form of edema for diagnosis because edema is symptomatic of many disease processes, particularly cardiovascular disease.

Lymphatic Filariasis

Lymphatic filariasis is a tropical parasitic disease caused by microscopic threadlike worms. The adult worms live only in the human lymph system. Lymphatic filariasis is spread from person to person by mosquitoes. People with the disease can suffer from lymphedema and elephantiasis, which is a condition caused by long-term obstruction of lymphatic vessels that leads to engorgement and thickened skin. It causes disfigurement, often of the leg. Lymphatic filariasis is a leading cause of permanent disability worldwide. The condition is treated with antiparasitic medication.

Infectious Mononucleosis

Infectious mononucleosis is a contagious viral infection that occurs most commonly in teenagers and young adults. Mononucleosis affects the lymphocytes, causing an increase in the number and a change in the structure of some of these cells. The infection is transmitted primarily by kissing, hence its nickname, the "kissing disease." Common signs and symptoms are fever, sore throat, enlarged cervical lymph nodes, a rash, and, in some, anemia. Complications include ruptured spleen, hepatitis, encephalitis, meningitis, and depression. The primary treatment is bed rest for several weeks or months.

Leukemia

Leukemia is the term for any of a number of cancers of the white blood cells in which the body produces abnormal cells at a faster rate than normal or the cells live longer than normal (or both). Because the cancerous cells do not have the same structure as healthy white blood cells, they do not function properly. They build up and invade the organs of the body, interfering with organ function. The increased abnormal white blood cells crowd out functioning red blood cells and platelets. Leukemia may also affect red blood cell and platelet production, resulting in anemia or diminished clotting ability. Brain hemorrhage and infection may follow.

Acute leukemia progresses rapidly; chronic leukemia progresses slowly. Usually, the acute forms show mostly immature blast cells, and the chronic forms show mostly mature cells. Two categories of leukemia are described by the white blood cells they affect. Lymphocytic leukemia affects the cells that become lymphocytes; myelocytic leukemia affects the cells that develop into granulocytes or monocytes. The myelocytic leukemias also may be identified by the terms *granulocytic* or *monocytic leukemia*.

Common leukemias are:

- Acute myelogenous leukemia: Develops rapidly and demonstrates such symptoms as an increase in infections, sores in the mouth, and a greater tendency to bruise or bleed.
- Chronic myelogenous leukemia: Found in young adults and most often associated with a chromosome abnormality.
- Acute lymphoblastic (acute lymphocytic) leukemia: Affects children; incidence peaks at 5 years of age; commonly can be cured by chemotherapy, and complete remission often occurs.
- Chronic lymphocytic leukemia: Affects older persons; the increase in abnormal white cells reduces the number and effectiveness of the normal white blood cells, sometimes resulting in anemia and an increase in infections. Often, no therapy is required unless symptoms are evident.

Lymphomas

A lymphoma is a tumor of the lymphatic system that is almost always malignant. Most lymphomas, or lymphomata, are first felt as enlarged, painless lymph nodes or lymphoid tissues. Lymphomata generally are divided into two categories: Hodgkin disease and non-Hodgkin lymphoma.

Hodgkin Disease

Hodgkin disease is a cancer that involves painless swelling of the lymph nodes, primarily in the neck and groin, caused by enlarged, mutated lymphocytes. Radiation and chemotherapy are the primary treatment methods, and this disease has one of the highest cure rates of any form of cancer. Some individuals may require bone marrow transplantation.

Non-Hodgkin Lymphoma

Non-Hodgkin lymphoma is any cancer of lymphatic tissue that is not classified as Hodgkin disease. Most non-Hodgkin lymphomas involve mutation of lymphocytes, correlation with retroviruses, or T-cell leukemia. As with Hodgkin disease, the first symptom is swollen lymph nodes, most often in the neck, axilla, or groin. But unlike Hodgkin disease, non-Hodgkin lymphoma is a group of diverse lymphomas that may manifest different primary and secondary symptoms, such as enlarged lymph nodes, swollen abdomen (belly), feeling full after eating small amounts of food, chest pain or pressure, shortness of breath or cough, fever, weight loss, night sweats, and fatigue. Non-Hodgkin lymphoma often is subcategorized by grade and area of tumor involvement.

Some forms of leukemia may be classified as lymphomas because they involve lymphocytes. However, not all types of leukemia are disorders of lymphatic tissue; instead, some could be classified as blood disorders.

Lymphatic Malformation

LM is a sponge-like collection of abnormal channels and cystic spaces that contain clear fluid. They occur as localized swelling and sometimes more extensive enlargement of soft tissues and bones. LM in the superficial skin presents as tiny clear bubbles (vesicles) that often become dark red as a result of bleeding. LM is a common basis for enlargement of any structure (e.g., lip, cheek, ear, tongue, limb, finger, or toe). Generalized swelling caused by trapped tissue fluid, called *lymphedema*, can also be caused by a type of LM. Old terms for LM are "cystic hygroma" and "lymphangioma." Lymphatic channels sprout from veins in early embryonic life. Although the precise cause is unknown, LMs are believed to be caused by an error in the formation of these tiny thin-walled sacs and tubes in the embryonic period. Two ways to manage LMs are sclerotherapy (direct injection of an irritating solution) and surgical removal.

INDICATIONS/CONTRAINDICATIONS for Therapeutic Massage

Massage may be locally or generally contraindicated in the presence of malignant and infectious conditions. Consultation with the client's healthcare professional may be indicated. Do not specifically massage a lymphatic malformation. Modification of massage application is necessary according to the type of treatment the client is receiving and their stress and fatigue levels. Massage that relaxes the client supports well-being and is helpful.

The massage practitioner can manage simple edema by using a massage application focused on supporting the lymphatic system. The appropriate health professional must supervise massage in clients with more complicated lymphedema.

Section Summary

- List the components of the lymphatic system.
  Lymph capillaries collect interstitial fluid, join into larger lymph vessels, and merge into two main ducts: the right lymphatic duct (which empties into the right subclavian vein and drains the upper right half of the body) and the thoracic duct (left lymphatic duct), which empties into the left subclavian vein and drains the remainder of the body. Lymph nodes (predominantly clustered at joints) contain mature lymphocytes (white blood cells). which destroy bacteria, viruses, and pathogens and filter foreign matter and waste materials. The spleen stores lymphocytes and releases them during the immune response. The thymus gland helps develop and program certain lymphocytes into T cells. Lymph nodules protect the respiratory and gastrointestinal tracts.
- List the components of lymph.
  Lymph contains white blood cells, proteins, salts, fats, pathogens, and cell debris. Lymph starts as interstitial fluid. Interstitial fluid comes from blood plasma seeping through capillaries. The interstitial fluid becomes lymph when it enters the lymph capillaries.
- Describe how lymph moves through the body.
  Lymphatic drainage is the movement of lymph. Interstitial fluid movement into lymph capillaries is assisted by skeletal muscle contraction, respiration, and stretching of skin and superficial fascia. Lymph is pumped by joint movement (location of lymph nodes), and compression of the soles of the feet and palms of the hands (location of lymph plexuses). Layers of smooth muscle contract around valves called *lymphangions* to help move fluid through lymph vessels. Manual lymphatic drainage mimics these processes via movement of the skin and superficial fascia in the direction of drainage, joint movement, muscle contraction, and rhythmic rocking and compression.

IMMUNE SYSTEM

SECTION OBJECTIVES

Chapter objectives covered in this section:

8. Define immunity.
9. List and describe nonspecific and specific immune responses of the body.
10. Explain how the mind/body connection affects immunity.
11. Identify pathologies of the immune system and describe indications and contraindications for massage.

After completing this chapter, the learner will be able to:

- Define immunity and the immune system.
- Define nonspecific immunity and specific immunity.

Immunity is a complex response that involves all the systems of the body as they join together to eliminate any pathogen, foreign substance, or toxic material that could damage the body. The immune system is not a specific structural organ system, but rather a functional system (Figs. 11.26 and 11.27) that draws on the structures and processes of each organ, tissue, and cell and the chemicals produced in them. The immune system responds in one of two ways. In a nonspecific (innate) immune response, the body responds the same way to all substances that are not identified as part of the body. People are born with nonspecific immunity. Specific immunity involves particular responses to each foreign substance identified. Special memory cells are called upon to identify a pathogen if it reappears. Specific immunity can be acquired in two ways: (1) through natural immunity, which is the result of exposure; and (2) through artificial immunity, in which a substance, such as a vaccine, is introduced into the body to stimulate the immune response.

The key to immunity is the ability of the body to recognize self and nonself. The recognition of self begins during fetal development and continues throughout life. The body must be able to identify the substances capable of causing a threat before it initiates any response; such recognition is immunological. An antigen (i.e., any substance that causes the body to produce antibodies) is usually something that has been identified as harmful or potentially dangerous to the body. A foreign antigen comes from outside the body; a self-antigen comes from within. An antibody is a specific protein produced to destroy or suppress antigens.

Microorganisms are minute life forms that may be damaging to the body or may interfere with its function. All microorganisms are microscopic. Many microorganisms do not normally cause disease in human beings but exist either in a state of commensalism, in which they give little or no benefit or harm to human beings, or in a state of mutualism, in which both gain some benefit. This nonharmful balance exists when the immune system works well, but these same organisms can cause infection if the immune system does not function properly. Many other microorganisms can cause infectious diseases and are called *pathogens*. Pathogens, as explained in Chapter 2, fall into five main groups:

- Viruses
- Bacteria
- Fungi
- Protozoa
- Pathogenic animals

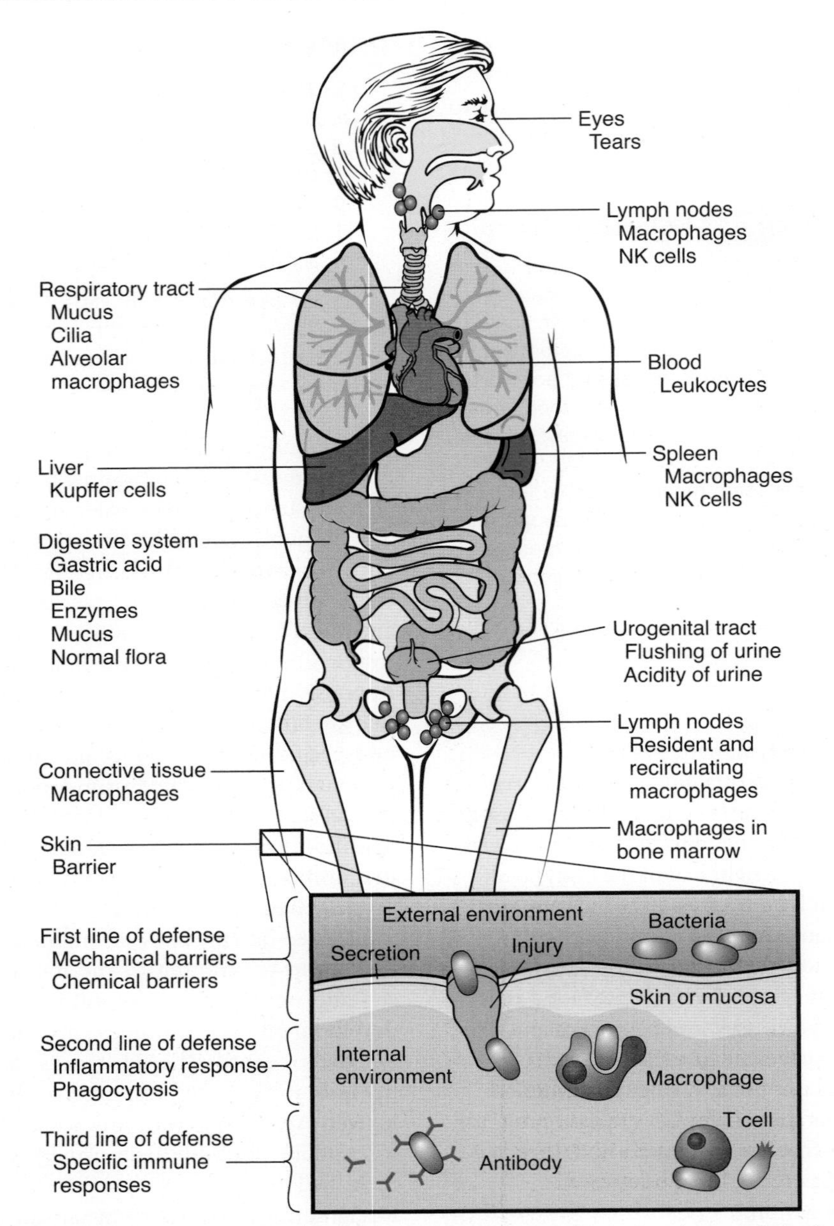

FIG. 11.26 Natural protective mechanisms of the human body. *NK*, Natural killer. (From Damjanov I. *Pathology for the Health-Related Professions*. 4th ed. Saunders/Elsevier; 2012.)

In addition, two other classes of small agents can cause disease:

- Ticks and mites
- Mesozoa and leeches

These organisms live in and on the body, causing infestations rather than the infectious disease caused by bacteria or viruses.

Infectious disease is by far the greatest cause of disease and death worldwide. Respiratory infections and gastrointestinal infections cause more deaths worldwide than all other diseases added together. General symptoms of infectious diseases are:

- Fever
- Increased catabolism
- Malaise

Opportunistic infections occur when the normal human defenses are so weak that they allow infection by organisms that generally would not cause infection in a healthy human being. Nosocomial infections are transmitted in hospitals; some of these may be opportunistic infections, or they may occur because of the special nature of the hospital environment.

The time between exposure to a pathogen and the first appearance of symptoms is called the *incubation period*, and although no symptoms are apparent, the organism may be causing substantial damage during this time. There may follow a period known as the *prodrome*, in which nonspecific signs and symptoms, such as headache, fever, and lethargy, appear before the development of the acute phase and specific symptoms. Once the acute stage has passed, there is a period

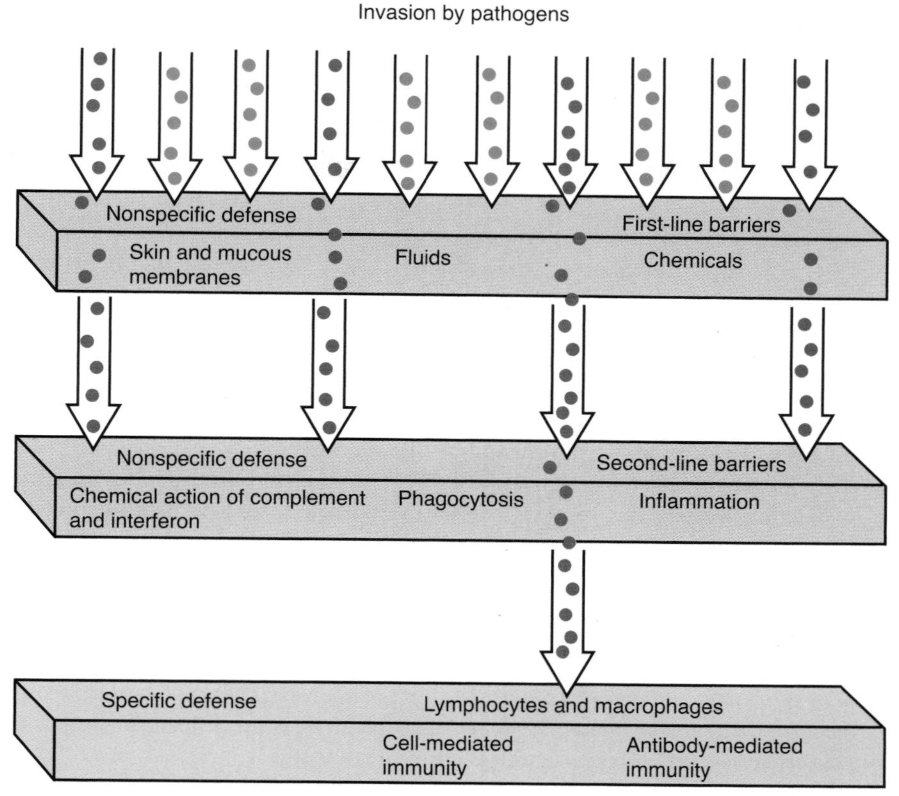

FIG. 11.27 Overview of defense mechanisms. (From Applegate E. *The Anatomy and Physiology Learning System*. 4th ed. Saunders/ Elsevier; 2011.)

of resolution, in which the severity of the symptoms gradually decreases. Finally, during convalescence, the symptoms have largely disappeared, but the body is still recovering.

The time, course, and severity of the disease are determined by the balance between the virulence (strength) of the infecting agent and the success with which the immune system combats the organism. Infections that are not sufficiently severe to produce clinical symptoms are called *asymptomatic* or *subclinical infections*. Clinical infections have a number of outcomes, ranging from death to complete recovery. The term *latency* refers to a situation in which a pathogen persists in a dormant, inactive form without causing damage but could reactivate to cause problems at a later date. An example is the herpes simplex virus, which lies dormant within the dorsal root ganglia after the primary infection but may reactivate periodically to cause cold sores.

Microorganisms are everywhere. They are in the air we breathe and in or on the food we eat. Thus our epithelial surfaces (skin, respiratory tract, gastrointestinal tract, and genitourinary tract) are exposed to microorganisms continuously. Disease occurs when microorganisms invade epithelial surfaces. However, given our constant exposure to microorganisms, it is surprising that we enjoy such long infection-free periods and that infections are the exception rather than the rule.

When the immune system is operating effectively, it protects the body from infectious microorganisms and any of the cells of the body that have turned against it (i.e., cells that have overreacted in their response or that have begun to develop and grow at an unhealthy rate or have mutated into cancer). The immune system performs this protection directly by attacking the cells and indirectly by releasing mobilizing chemicals and protective antibodies.

FOCUS ON PROFESSIONALISM

The COVID-19 pandemic created increased public awareness of the immune system's response to the infection. It is now understood that SARS-CoV-2, both the infection and the excessive inflammation response of the immune system, affects a person's disease experience from mild to severe and susceptibility to lingering symptoms. Researchers are beginning to understand how the human immune system contributes to the varied responses to COVID-19. When people get severely ill from COVID-19 it is not only from the viral infection but in the case of COVID-19 an exaggerated immune response to that infection. It is flawed to think that the immune response always needs to be increased when illness is present. As learned during the pandemic "too much" immune response is as detrimental as "not enough" immune response.

Nonspecific Defenses

Nonspecific (innate or natural) immunity involves mechanical barriers (e.g., intact skin and mucous membranes) and chemical barriers (e.g., stomach acid). No matter what the invading substance is, the body responds in the same manner, with the same chemicals and cells mediating the actions. This general response is a preventive measure and the first reaction to pathogenic invasion.

Sanitary practices, such as hand washing, disinfecting, and sterilizing, support immunity by preventing exposure to pathogens.

Each body area has mechanical and chemical aspects of innate immunity.

Skin

Just as the husk of a fruit or berry protects it from drying up in drought or swelling in rain, the skin protects the body from undue entry or loss of water. When intact, the skin is virtually impermeable to microorganisms and also protects from chemicals (e.g., weak acids, alkalis) and most gases (although some gases developed for use in chemical warfare can be absorbed through the skin). The integument provides some protection from physical trauma. Sebum from sebaceous glands is composed of triglycerides, waxes, and cholesterol. The main function of the sebum is to waterproof the skin, but sebum is also antibacterial.

Each square centimeter of skin may contain as many as 3 million microorganisms, most of which are harmless. The skin does not provide a hospitable environment for bacteria unless they have adapted through evolution to live there. The application of deodorants and the use of strong soaps that change the skin pH from acid to alkaline upset the fine balance that exists between our parasites and us. These agents tend to kill or inhibit the normal flora, leaving the area open to potential colonization by pathogens.

Arms and legs have the fewest microorganisms (only 1,000 to 10,000 per square centimeter), whereas the forehead may contain as many as 1 million per square centimeter and the area between the toes may have as many as 1 billion per square centimeter.

Microorganisms thrive in moist conditions, so the axillae (armpits) and groin provide favorable areas for their growth. The skin can never be sterilized completely. The topical application of alcohol and iodine-based lotions may cause the death of a large percentage of resident organisms, but such applications do not remove those bacteria that inhabit the hair follicles and make up at least 20% of the resident bacteria.

Eye

Tears produced by the lacrimal glands constantly irrigate the surface of the eyeball. Tears contain high levels of lysozyme—in fact, the highest levels of any of the body's secretions—so they form an effective barrier against infection. If the diet is lacking in vitamin A, the production of lysozyme in the tears decreases and can predispose a person to eye infection. Blinking is a defense reflex that eliminates irritants and ensures even distribution of the tears.

In some conditions, such as facial paralysis and stroke, this reflex is lost, and preventing the eye from drying up by keeping it closed or covered and performing regular irrigation becomes necessary.

Ear

Ceruminous glands located in the outer ear canal are modified sweat glands that produce cerumen, or earwax. Cerumen provides a sticky barrier to foreign agents entering the ear canal.

Mouth

The mouth is lined with a mucous membrane that is constantly irrigated by saliva. This flow is directed toward the throat and has the dual purpose of preventing microorganisms from infecting the salivary glands and trapping the organisms so that they can be swallowed and disposed of in the digestive tract.

Saliva contains an enzyme called *lysozyme* that is antibacterial and mucus that contains immunoglobulin A. Dehydrated people have a reduced flow of saliva and are at a higher risk for mouth infections.

The resident bacteria in the mouth are generally harmless. Indeed some, such as alpha-hemolytic streptococcus, are of benefit because they produce hydrogen peroxide, which helps keep the mouth clean.

Individuals who are on prolonged courses of oral antibiotics run the risk of having their normal flora (bacteria) wiped out, which can result in opportunistic infection of the mouth by other microorganisms. A common organism that can become problematic is the unicellular fungus *Candida albicans*, which causes thrush.

The tonsils also assist in protecting the oral cavity.

Stomach

The hydrochloric acid present in the gastric juices produced by the stomach lining is of a sufficiently low pH to kill most organisms entering the body with food or drink or by being swallowed. Some organisms, however, can resist this strong acid. Examples include the tubercle bacillus, enteroviruses, salmonella, and the eggs of parasitic worms.

Milk and proteins are effective buffers against stomach acid, and organisms that enter the stomach accompanied by this type of food stand a greater chance of escaping the damaging effects of hydrochloric acid. Thus contaminated meat and dairy products tend to be more dangerous in terms of an infection.

Vomiting may be considered a defense mechanism because it rids the body of irritants and toxins (e.g., alcohol, drugs, and bacterial toxins in some instances), although this protection is by no means fully effective.

Intestines

The small and large intestines rely to a great extent on the bactericidal action of the stomach. In addition, the normal beneficial flora of the area, such as *Escherichia coli*, nonhemolytic streptococci, and anaerobic bacteroides, contribute to the normal functioning of the intestines. Their importance becomes more evident when the administration of broad-spectrum antibiotics or indiscriminate use of laxatives removes them. The intestines then are open to colonization by pathogenic bacteria, such as *Staphylococcus pyogenes*, that may be resistant to antibiotics.

In addition, the small and large intestines are supplied liberally with lymphatic tissue throughout their length. The lymph participates in the nonspecific and acquired immune defense systems of the body.

Like vomiting, diarrhea can be considered a defense mechanism, although in most instances it occurs far too late in the course of an infection to be of much benefit.

Respiratory Tract

Upper Respiratory Tract

Hairs in the nose prevent insects and large particles from entering the upper respiratory tract. The ciliated nasal mucosa secretes a backward-flowing stream of mucus that is sticky and traps smaller particles. It also has bactericidal and virucidal properties. Lysozyme is also present in nasal secretions.

The epithelium of the upper respiratory tract is thin and unfortunately is prone to infections by rhinoviruses and adenoviruses, which are not affected by the nasal secretions. Sneezing is a protective reflex that expels irritants.

Trachea and Lungs

The trachea and bronchi are lined with a ciliated mucous membrane that traps any organisms in debris that may have escaped from the upper tract. The cilia beat upward and shift a stream of mucus away from the lungs and toward the pharynx to be swallowed. Should any organisms reach the alveoli, alveolar macrophages phagocytize them. The lung is well supplied with lymph nodes that function as another filter.

Coughing is a defensive reflex that removes particulate matter or excessive mucus from the lower tract.

Genitourinary Tract

The constant downward flow of urine through the ureter and bladder tends to protect against ascending infections. Urination irrigates the urethra. Urination is an effective response in the long male urethra but is less so in the female. The adult female urethra is only 2 to 3 cm long and forms a short and readily available entry point for organisms to invade the bladder.

Sexual activity in the female may predispose the occurrence of urethritis (an inflammation of the urethra) and cystitis (a bladder infection). The most common offending organism is a coliform bacillus from the perineal area.

The beneficial resident florae of the vagina, especially lactobacillus, help maintain an acidic environment, creating an inhospitable habitat for invading pathogens. Some vaginal deodorants disturb the pH balance of the vaginal area and can result in infection, often by the opportunistic *C. albicans*.

Inflammatory Response

Complements are proteins found in blood that combine to create substances that phagocytize bacteria. Interferon, a protein produced by cells infected by viruses, forms antiviral proteins to help protect uninfected cells.

Cellular response is the action of the blood cells (primarily white blood cells) that deal with pathogens. Natural killer cells are a subset of lymphocytes that can eliminate virus-infected cells. Cells such as macrophages and neutrophils begin to phagocytize, or to surround and destroy, pathogens. Basophils and mast cells (from connective tissue) release chemicals that initiate inflammation. Eosinophils release chemicals that slow or stop the inflammatory response.

Inflammatory response is a sequence of events involving chemical and cellular activation that destroys pathogens and aids in the repair of tissues (see Chapter 2). For example, when damage occurs to tissue, basophils and mast cells release chemicals that increase the blood flow, which brings neutrophils and macrophages to the area. The phagocytic white cells, mainly macrophages, enter the tissues to destroy any bacteria. At the same time, the chemical response changes the permeability of the blood vessel wall so that fibrin can enter the tissues to repair the damage. This process continues until the damage has been repaired and all bacteria have been removed (Fig. 11.28).

Specific Immunity

Specific immunity is the ability to recognize certain antigens and destroy them (Table 11.1).

Lymphocytes are the cells of specific immunity because they can recognize and destroy specific molecules. When a person has a disease (e.g., measles), memory cells set up a lymphocyte pattern at the time of the first infection that can respond to a second exposure and prevent reinfection. Lymphocytes develop in three ways:

- All lymphocytes form in the red bone marrow. T cells mature in the thymus and then travel to lymphatic tissue, such as is found in the spleen, lymph nodules, and lymph nodes. They can recognize antigens and respond by releasing inflammatory and toxic substances. Specialized T cells also regulate immune responses. These cells release molecules that amplify the response, whereas other T cells suppress the response of the body when the infection has been contained. Some T cells develop into memory cells and handle secondary responses on reexposure to antigens that have already produced a primary response.
- B cells stay in the bone marrow to mature and then travel to lymphatic tissue. They differentiate into plasma cells, which produce antibodies. Antibodies are in the immunoglobulin class of proteins. They circulate in body fluids and destroy specific antigens. Some B cells modify and become antigen nonspecific, which provides them with a greater ability to respond to bacterial and viral pathogens. Some B cells, like T cells, become memory cells and handle reexposure to antigens.
- A few lymphocytes do not develop the same structural or functional characteristics as the T cells and B cells. These cells are known as natural killer cells. They too develop in the bone marrow and, when mature, can attack and kill tumor cells and virus-infected cells during their initial developmental stage before the immune system is activated.

Specific defense responses can develop quickly. Because lymph capillaries pick up proteins and pathogens from nearly all body tissues, immune cells in lymph nodes are in a strategic position to encounter a large variety of antigens. Lymphocytes and macrophages in the tonsils act primarily against microorganisms that invade the oral and nasal cavities, and the spleen acts as a filter to trap blood antigens.

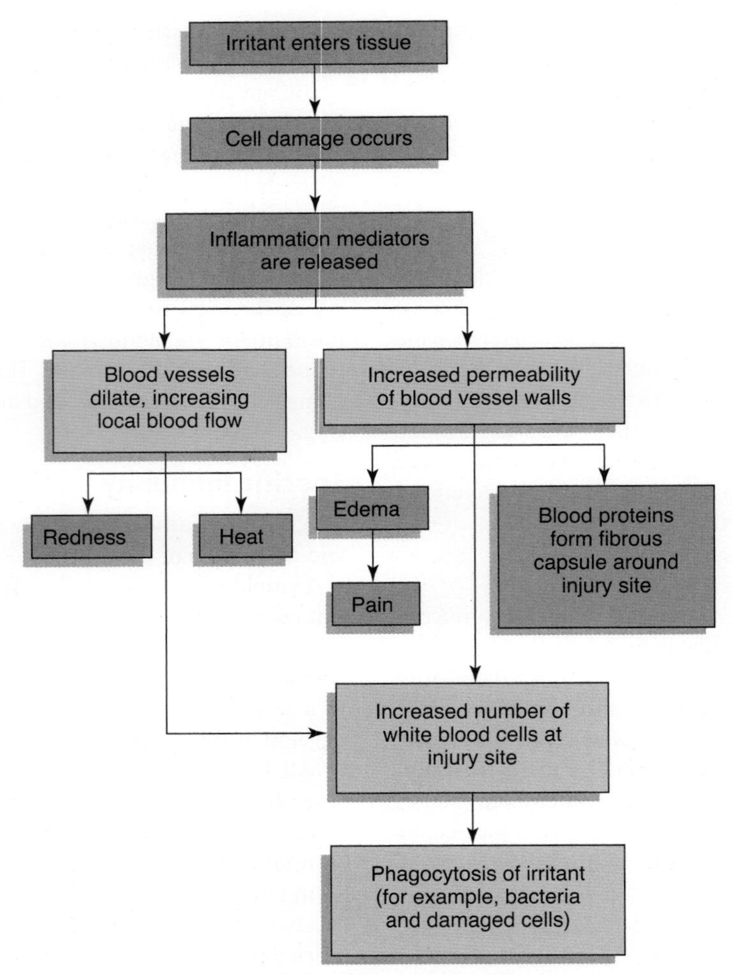

FIG. 11.28 Inflammatory response. Tissue damage caused by bacteria triggers a series of events that produce an inflammatory response and promote phagocytosis at the site of injury. These responses tend to inhibit or destroy the bacteria.

Table 11.1 Types of Adaptive Immunity

Type	Description or Example
Natural immunity	Exposure to the causative agent is not deliberate.
Active (exposure)	A child develops measles and acquires immunity to a subsequent infection.
Passive (exposure)	A fetus receives protection from the mother through the placenta, or an infant receives protection through the mother's milk.
Artificial immunity	Exposure to the causative agent is deliberate.
Active (exposure)	Injection of the causative agent (e.g., vaccination against polio) confers immunity.
Passive (exposure)	Injection of protective material (antibodies) developed by another individual's immune system.

From Patton KT, Thibodeau GA. *Anatomy and Physiology*. 7th ed. Mosby/Elsevier; 2010.

Lymphocytes fight infection in three ways:

1. Elimination of extracellular microorganisms
   - In response to infection, B cells mature into plasma cells that secrete antibodies. B cells recognize microbes because they have a protein in their cell membrane that acts as an antigen receptor. An antibody recognizes structures on the surfaces of microorganisms, as well as proteins, carbohydrates, and lipids. Thus each person's plasma contains many different types of antibodies, each of which recognizes different microorganisms. As discussed previously, antibodies circulate in body fluids to target extracellular microorganisms. When the antibody binds to a microorganism, it activates mechanisms that eliminate the microorganism.
   - In the primary response, at the time of the first infection, no antibody exists in the blood, and the level of antibody does not begin to increase until 7 to 10 days later. The level of antibody rises slowly to a low peak and then gradually declines toward baseline.
   - In the secondary response, on subsequent exposure to the same microorganisms, the level of antibody begins to increase within 24 hours and reaches and sustains a high level.
2. Production of local hormones to stimulate T cells
   - Helper T cells, also known as *CD4 T cells*, secrete local hormones called cytokines. Cytokines stimulate another type of T cell, called *killer T cells, CD8 T cells*, or *cytotoxic T cells*, to multiply and lymphatic tissue to search for microorganisms inside body cells.

3. Elimination of microorganisms that have infected body cells
   - The most common type of microorganism that infects body cells is viruses. During intracellular replication, virus proteins appear on the surface of the infected cell. CD8 T cells recognize these viral antigens as foreign and secrete cytotoxic molecules that kill the infected cells.

Mind/Body Connection

The sheer power of the mind to affect the body as a whole and the general state of health is amazing.

Studies of neuroimmunomodulation have discovered that left-handed people are more likely to suffer from immune system disorders than right-handed people. These studies indicate that the left hemisphere most directly controls the immune cells through the T-cell response but that the right hemisphere enhances and modulates the response. Other investigations have shown that although the nervous and immune systems have different chemical languages, they seem to share a few of the more important chemical signals, such as those of the opiate neuropeptides. Like neurons, many cells involved with the immune response have receptors for the opiate neuropeptides, which have long been known to influence mood and behavior. Many scientists are convinced that macrophages have receptors for these neuropeptides, which are released by pain-sensing neurons and lymphocytes. Why these cells, which are active in immunity, should respond to or react to chemicals used by the nervous system to deal with pain is not understood fully. This process is thought to be an important link in the communication between the brain and body.

High levels of natural opiates (which act like heroin) suppress the activity of natural killer cells. During times of stress and severe depression, the number of T cells is lower, which weakens the immune system and increases susceptibility to physical illness. Hormones (e.g., corticosteroids and epinephrine) also provide chemical links between the two systems.

Immune function gradually declines as humans age. Scientists do not understand this process, but studies of longevity have found a link between living vitally in the advanced years and a balanced life that includes physical activity, a simple diet, a moderate lifestyle, regular sleep and wake cycles, loving relationships, a sense of purpose or reason for being, and spiritual strength. These same factors have been shown to support the immune response and the regeneration and healing capacities of the body.

Immunity is a body-wide process. The integumentary system, especially the keratinized epithelial cells, provides a mechanical barrier, and these same cells function as an alarm system, triggering responses when the integument is breached. The skeletal system provides the bone marrow as the developmental home for the lymphocytes and macrophages. The heat from the muscle system actively initiates fever-like effects. The nervous and endocrine systems interact directly, linking the mind/body effects of the immune response through a shared chemical language. The cardiovascular system provides the travel network, lymphatic system, and filtering system. The respiratory system provides oxygen needed by immune cells, and the digestive system nourishes the immune cells and secretes acids hostile to pathogens. The urinary system eliminates waste and maintains the protective acid balance. The reproductive system works with the endocrine system to influence the process through hormone function.

The immune system is the best example of teamwork, or a multidisciplinary approach, in the body, and a lesson can be learned here. When any one of us does not do our job, others are overtasked; in the body, this is an immune deficiency. When we overreact, our hypersensitivities are unproductive and we feel miserable, wasting energy that could be better used in other ways. When we are unaware of ourselves (autoimmunity), we not only attack ourselves but also fail to combine efforts to support others. Energy for the common good is wasted, and the lack of self-recognition destroys us, little by little. The amazing multidimensional links of the immune system support the idea that we truly are what we think, eat, do, hate, love, breathe, support, and become. Living well in our bodies and sharing space with all forms of life on this planet reflects the ancient spiritual wisdom of living in a balanced way with cooperation and respect.

Pathological Conditions of the Immune System

The organizational structures and responses of the immune system can break down. The imbalances that occur in that circumstance are immune deficiencies, hypersensitivities (Box 11.3), and autoimmune diseases.

Immune deficiency is a condition in which the body is unable to mount the proper immune response to a pathogen. An analogy is an office that has too much work and not enough workers to get the job done. The work piles up, the workers get further and further behind, and eventually, the office system breaks down. Some immune deficiencies are present at birth. These congenital problems affect the development of lymphocytes and result in a severe inability to respond to disease. Other immune deficiencies can arise later in life, such as acquired immunodeficiency syndrome (AIDS). Chronic stress also suppresses the immune system. Stress can be caused by physical mechanisms (e.g., chronic pain), other forms of chronic disease, and unresolved emotional or spiritual disturbances. When immunosuppressed, the body is more likely to be susceptible to a variety of bacterial, viral, and toxic pathogenic activities.

Hypersensitivity

The immune system also can become overactive, a condition called *hypersensitivity* or *allergy*. Few people die of allergies, but the symptoms can make life miserable. Allergies are an overblown immune response to an allergen, something that causes an allergic reaction. Anaphylactic shock is the exception, and although rare, it is life-threatening. Anaphylactic shock is a severe, usually immediate reaction to a substance that causes respiratory distress, anxiety, and weakness. In extreme cases, anaphylactic shock also can involve arrhythmia and can result in death if not treated immediately (see Box 11.3).

Box 11.3 Four Classes of Immune Hypersensitivity Malfunction

Type I: Immediate Anaphylactic Hypersensitivity

Type I hypersensitivity is best exemplified by allergic asthma, atopic dermatitis (eczema), allergic rhinitis (hay fever), and acute urticaria (hives).

- Type I hypersensitivity is considered one of the most powerful effector mechanisms of the immune system. This reaction begins rapidly. The most serious and extreme systemic form is anaphylaxis.
- Allergies now are recognized as common, affecting 20% of people in the United States. Allergies are considered the most common immune disorder in the world.

Type II: Antibody-Dependent Cytotoxic Hypersensitivity

Type II hypersensitivity, which involves antibody responses against antigens on cells, is also an immediate reaction (e.g., the reaction that occurs when incompatible blood is given during a transfusion).

- Exposure to certain medications can cause a similar process; the drug molecules probably combine with a protein in the blood before being misidentified as an antigen.
- Penicillin and its derivatives are responsible for most of the recorded allergic reactions to drugs and 97% of the deaths caused each year by drug allergies.
- Symptoms are typically mild: hives, some fever, chills, swelling of lymph nodes, and sometimes arthritis-like discomfort.

Type III: Immune Complex-Mediated Hypersensitivity

In type III hypersensitivity the immune system misidentifies a protein in antiserum as potentially harmful and develops a response against the antiserum.

- Type III response is similar to a type I response in that some of the same effects occur: blood vessel dilation, sneezing, coughing, and itching.

Type IV: Cell-Mediated (Delayed Type) Hypersensitivity

Type IV hypersensitivity involves T cells and macrophages, not antibodies.

- This type of reaction is an important part of the process of immune reactions to many intracellular infectious agents, and this response also is involved in graft rejection and tumor immunity.

Acquired Immunodeficiency Syndrome and Human Immunodeficiency Virus Infection

AIDS is caused by a dysfunction in the immune system of the body. The diseases of AIDS are caused by pathogens encountered in everyday life. Some of these pathogens live permanently in small numbers inside the human body. When the immune system weakens, these pathogens have the opportunity to multiply freely; thus the diseases these pathogens cause are called *opportunistic diseases*.

The human immunodeficiency virus (HIV) is a ribonucleic acid (RNA) virus. In most RNA viruses, the viral RNA directly hijacks the host cell. However, HIV is different. After the virus enters the host cell, the RNA strand "writes" dual strands of viral DNA. This backward writing is called *reverse transcription*. The newly written DNA strands then hijack the cell and oversee the production of new RNA replicas. Reverse-writing viruses, such as HIV, are called *retroviruses*.

As a group, retroviruses can live in their hosts for a long time without causing any sign of illness. In most animals, such infections last for life. Retroviruses are not tough; they die when exposed to heat, are killed by many common disinfectants, and usually do not survive if the tissue or blood they are in dries. However, they have a high rate of mutation, and as a result, they tend to evolve quickly into new strains or varieties. HIV seems to share this trait and others with other known retroviruses.

HIV replicates in T cells and macrophages. The favorite target of the virus is the CD4 T cell. HIV infection of the CD4 T cells creates a defect in the immune system that eventually may cause AIDS. After HIV hijacks a T cell, the lymphocyte stops functioning normally, although this change is not immediately apparent. Little or no viral replication takes place for an indefinite period. The HIV takeover is a quiet event. When the CD4 T cell does become active, rather than functioning normally, it manufactures viral RNA strands. An infected CD4 T cell no longer detects invaders and triggers alarms. Eventually, the infected CD4 T cells begin to die, gradually reducing the CD4 T cell alarm network and allowing opportunistic diseases to enter and grow within the body.

HIV must travel from the inside of one person to the inside of another person, arriving with its RNA strands intact. Then the virus, or its intact RNA strands, must get into the bloodstream of the new host and find and enter a T cell. Once inside a host cell, HIV can prepare for replication. After replication, replica viruses infect other host cells, probably attaching to new host cells when the infected host cell collides with other cells in the bloodstream.

Viruses generally are not able to enter the body through intact skin. Therefore viruses must enter the body through an open wound or one of a number of possible body openings. Most of these openings contain mucous membranes that protect the body. These membranes secrete mucus, which contains germicidal chemicals and keeps the surrounding tissues moist. Mucous membranes are found in the mouth, inside the eyelids, in the nose and air passages leading to the lungs, in the stomach, along the digestive tract, in the vagina, in the anus, and inside the opening of the penis. Many viruses, if placed on the surface of a mucous membrane, can travel through the membrane and enter the tiny blood vessels inside.

The danger with HIV is different; the major infection sites are the bloodstream and the central nervous system. Although HIV-carrying macrophages (roving white blood cells that engulf invaders but are susceptible to HIV infection) are found in the connective tissues of the lungs and oral and mucous membranes, the number of viral organisms present does not appear to be great. This means that HIV is present in low concentrations, if at all, in saliva and sputum, so coughing should not expel a large quantity of HIV, if any. HIV cannot easily cross the mucous membrane, and large concentrations of HIV probably are necessary for it to do so.

HIV can be found in any bodily fluid or substance that contains lymphocytes—blood, semen, vaginal and cervical secretions, breast milk, saliva, tears, urine, and feces—but the presence of HIV in a substance does not necessarily mean that it is capable of transmitting infection. All of these substances are, in theory, able to transmit disease, but in reality, the most dangerous substances seem to be blood, semen, cervical and vaginal secretions, and perhaps feces. Despite an extensive search, no one has been able to find a clear-cut case in which saliva caused transmission, although kissing theoretically could.

The concentration of HIV in these substances is important when it comes to infection. The higher the concentration of viral organisms in a substance, the more likely it is to transmit HIV. Below a certain concentration, the substance cannot effectively transmit infection.

Hepatitis

Hepatitis is an inflammatory process and an infection of the liver caused by a virus. Hepatitis A, the least serious form, usually is transmitted by fecal contamination of food and water and does not become chronic. Once infected, a person becomes immune to future hepatitis A infections.

Hepatitis B, transmitted by routes similar to those of HIV, may be acute or chronic. The acute symptoms are similar to those of hepatitis A, but hepatitis B is much more severe in the chronic and acute stages. As liver cells die, liver function is impaired and death can result. Two types of vaccines are available for preventing hepatitis B, but more than 1 million people in the United States are estimated to be carriers of the hepatitis B virus, which is 100 times more contagious than HIV.

Hepatitis C accounts for 85% of the new cases of hepatitis each year. This form is transmitted mostly by blood transfusions or when intravenous drug users share needles, and it usually becomes chronic.

Hepatitis D infects only those who have hepatitis B, and the symptoms are more severe than other forms of hepatitis. Vaccines do not appear to be effective for hepatitis D.

Hepatitis E is transmitted by food and water contaminated with feces and is usually a self-limited type of hepatitis that may occur after a natural disaster if sanitation is not maintained.

The treatment for all forms of hepatitis is rest and antiviral medications. Observance of the Standard Precautions can prevent the spread of hepatitis. People must avoid all behaviors that could transmit HIV and hepatitis.

Autoimmune Disease

Autoimmune diseases occur when the body cannot distinguish self from nonself; self-antigens are treated as foreign antigens. When the recognition of self breaks down, the immune cells begin to attack the self. Some of the autoimmune diseases are multiple sclerosis, Graves disease, rheumatoid arthritis, and juvenile diabetes.

The inflammatory response triggered by the immune complex is the pathogenic mechanism of tissue injury in a number of autoimmune diseases, including arthritis, vasculitis, and glomerulonephritis (Table 11.2). Immune complex injury may result from the activation of resident inflammatory cells and the recruitment of circulating monocytes or neutrophils at various sites. A growing consensus among scientists is that common disorders (e.g., atherosclerosis, colon cancer, and Alzheimer disease) are caused in part by a chronic inflammatory syndrome.

INDICATIONS/CONTRAINDICATIONS for Therapeutic Massage

Immune System

Therapeutic massage approaches help immune function by supporting balanced homeostatic functions. No specific methods are used for the immune system, yet any behavior that supports wellness, including regular massage, supports immunity. Any modality that normalizes autonomic nervous system functions supports immunity.

Any activity, including therapeutic massage, which causes the body to adapt puts stress on the system. If the client is healthy, they will be able to adapt without overstressing the body. However, if a client's immunity is suppressed, the reserves needed for adaptation are already at the breakdown point. The massage practitioner must gauge the intensity and duration of bodywork methods against the ability of the body to adapt so that the stress introduced supports a return to balance and is not "the straw that breaks the camel's back." The premise of "less is more" is a wise approach for individuals with immune dysfunction. Massage professionals should follow Standard Precautions to prevent the spread of contagious diseases.

Section Summary

- Define immunity and the immune system.
  Immunity is a complex response involving all body systems to eliminate potentially harmful substances and pathogens. Antigens are substances that cause the production of antibodies. Antibodies are proteins produced to destroy or suppress antigens. The immune system is a functional system (not an organ system) that relies on the structures and processes of organs and tissues to protect the body.
- Define nonspecific immunity and specific immunity.
  With nonspecific (innate) immunity, the body responds the same way to all antigens. People are born with nonspecific immunity. With specific immunity, the body responds to identified antigens using special memory cells. Specific immunity can be acquired through natural immunity (the result of exposure) or artificial immunity (introduction of a substance such as a vaccine).

SUMMARY

This chapter began with a discussion of touch, an important topic that certainly could be explored in greater depth because massage therapy depends on touch not only for therapeutic benefit but also for the compassionate, nurturing connection that is established between practitioner and client.

We presented basic anatomy, physiology, and pathological conditions of the integumentary, cardiovascular, lymphatic, and immune systems.

Table 11.2 Examples of Autoimmune Diseases

Disease	Possible Self-Antigen	Description
Addison disease	Surface antigens on adrenal cells	Hyposecretion of adrenal hormones, resulting in weakness, reduced blood sugar, nausea, loss of appetite, and weight loss
Cardiomyopathy	Cardiac muscle	Disease of cardiac muscle (i.e., the myocardium), resulting in loss of pumping efficiency (heart failure)
Diabetes mellitus (type 1)	Pancreatic islet cells, insulin, insulin receptors	Hyposecretion of insulin by the pancreas, resulting in extremely elevated blood glucose levels (in turn causing a host of metabolic problems, even death if untreated)
Glomerulonephritis	Blood antigens that form immune complexes that are deposited in the kidney	Disease of the filtration apparatus of the kidney (renal corpuscle), resulting in fluid and electrolyte imbalance and possibly total kidney failure and death
Graves disease (type of hyperthyroidism)	TSH receptors on thyroid cells	Hypersecretion of thyroid hormone and resulting increase in metabolic rate
Hemolytic anemia	Surface antigens on RBCs	Condition of low RBC count in the blood resulting from excessive destruction of mature RBCs (hemolysis)
Hypothyroidism	Antigens in thyroid cells	Hyposecretion of thyroid hormone in adulthood, causing decreased metabolic rate and characterized by reduced mental and physical vigor, weight gain, hair loss, and edema
MS	Antigens in myelin sheaths of nervous tissue	Progressive degeneration of myelin sheaths, resulting in widespread impairment of nerve function (especially muscle control)
Myasthenia gravis	Antigens at the neuromuscular junction	Muscle disorder characterized by progressive weakness and chronic fatigue
Pernicious anemia	Antigens on parietal cells; intrinsic factor	Abnormally low RBC count resulting from the inability to absorb vitamin B_{12}, a substance critical to RBC production
Reproductive infertility	Antigens on sperm or tissue surrounding ovum (egg)	Inability to produce offspring (in this case, resulting from the destruction of gametes)
Rheumatic fever	Cardiac cell membranes (cross-reaction with group A streptococcal antigen)	Rheumatic heart disease; inflammatory cardiac damage (especially to the endocardium valves)
RA	Collagen	Inflammatory joint disease is characterized by synovial inflammation that spreads to other fibrous tissues
SLE	Numerous	Chronic inflammatory disease with widespread effects, characterized by arthritis, a red rash on the face, and other signs
Ulcerative colitis	Mucous cells of the colon	Chronic inflammatory disease of the colon, characterized by watery diarrhea containing blood, mucus, and pus

From Patton KT, Thibodeau GA. *Anatomy and Physiology*. 7th ed. Mosby/Elsevier; 2010.

MS, Multiple sclerosis; *RA*, rheumatoid arthritis; *RBCs*, red blood cells; *SLE*, systemic lupus erythematosus; *TSH*, thyroid-stimulating hormone.

The justification activity at the end of this chapter (provided again at the end of Chapter 12) represents the outcomes of competency-based education. All the problem-solving activities support competency. Being a competent massage therapist requires much more than recalling factual data, and competence is based on how you use that data in the professional application of massage. Clinical reasoning is necessary if you are to use information in professional practice. How do you plan and organize an effective massage session? How do you provide an assessment to determine indications for and contraindications to massage? How do you choose a massage application based on physiological effects? How do you collect and analyze data to develop appropriate treatment plans and then obtain informed consent? How do you know whether you are functioning within your scope of practice? How do you identify the most logical approach to massage application, including time management, body mechanics, and ergonomic practice, and the type of equipment needed? How do you evaluate the behaviors, feelings, and outcomes of the professional relationship as measured against the outcomes of the massage? All these issues are relevant to ethical, professional practice, as are the principles of respect and the provision of benefits that outweigh the burden of treatment and do no harm.

The justification exercises began the process of explaining and validating therapeutic massage. Being able to justify the effectiveness of therapeutic massage in supporting health maintenance or as part of a multidisciplinary approach to pathological conditions will become increasingly important as more people use these methods. The ability to explain the benefits of therapeutic massage and the skills each professional has to offer, based on a solid foundation of anatomy and physiology, adds to professional development and supports the use of these important treatments.

It is common for the student to find the justification activities difficult. Rising above the discomfort to achieve an integrated practice is necessary. The student should go back and do the activities repeatedly, using different scenarios and conditions. The student should remember that in professional practice, clinical reasoning, problem-solving, and the integration of knowledge with the application are the measures of a competent massage therapist (Activity 11.1).

ACTIVITY 11.1

We must be able to explain and justify the therapeutic value of the work we do. The following activity assists you in developing the skills to explain the effectiveness of therapeutic massage to clients and other healthcare professionals. Use the clinical reasoning model that follows to accomplish this task. Choose a pathology from this chapter and develop a care plan or describe how massage therapy supports the normal function of one of the systems from this chapter.

Methods/Applications

1. What are the facts?
   a. Which system is involved, and which structures of that system can be reached directly or indirectly?
   b. Which of these structures are most affected by this massage?
   c. Which physiological functions are affected by this approach?
   d. When the treatment is applied, what changes in function will occur in the following:
      (1) This system?
      (2) The whole body?
   e. What is considered normal or balanced function?
   f. How are the functions of this system related to the homeostasis of the body?
   g. What has worked or has not worked?
   h. Where could you find information that would support the use of this modality as a therapeutic intervention?
   i. What research is available to support the use of the therapeutic intervention?
   j. How does the intervention support a healthy state?
   k. Under which pathological or dysfunctional conditions is the therapeutic massage most likely to be beneficial?
2. What are the possibilities?
   a. What do the data suggest?
   b. What are the reasons for using the proposed method?
   c. What are the possible interventions?
   d. List at least three applications of massage that would affect the structure and function of the system involved.
   e. What are other ways to look at the situation?
   f. What other methods could provide similar benefits?
3. What is the logical outcome of therapeutic intervention?
   a. What would be the logical progression of the symptom pattern, contributing factors, and current behaviors?
   b. What are the benefits and drawbacks of each intervention suggested?
   c. What are the costs in terms of time, resources, and finances?
   d. What is likely to happen if the modality is not used?
   e. What is likely to happen if the modality is used?
4. For the intervention proposed, what would be the effect on the persons involved, specifically the client, practitioner, and other professionals working with the client?
   a. How does each person involved (including, besides the aforementioned, the client's family and support system) feel about the possible interventions?
   b. Does the practitioner feel qualified to work with the situation and apply the identified modality to the particular person?
   c. Does a feeling of cooperation and agreement exist among all those involved, and how would the practitioner recognize this feeling?

Justification

Using the information developed in the clinical reasoning model, present a clear, concise statement of how the particular soft-tissue or movement modality would be beneficial in supporting the particular body system in a healthy condition or as part of a treatment plan for a pathological or dysfunctional condition. On the basis of the preceding information, give a summary of the effectiveness of the modality for this system.

CRITICAL THINKING/CLINICAL REASONING

Each chapter will feature a critical thinking and clinical reasoning application of the content related to massage therapy practice. A client scenario will be presented with recommendations for additional research often using MedlinePlus or PubMed. Relevant questions based on the chapter content outline are provided to guide the discussion. There are no specific current answers to the questions. However, responses should be supportive of evidence-informed practices and based on biological plausibility if sufficient research is not available. The author's decision-making process related to the scenario and questions is on the Evolve site. Compare and contrast your thoughts and discussion to those of the author and determine where you agree or disagree.

Scenario

The client has been referred to a new massage therapist because their long-time massage therapist has moved to a different state. During the review of the client's history, the client indicates that they were diagnosed with a hepatitis C virus (HCV) infection and successfully treated with an antiviral regimen. Fortunately, the client does not have liver complications related to the HCV. However, there is concern about the development of atherosclerosis. It is unclear if the cardiac risks are related to HCV infection, but the risk for stroke and heart attack decreases when HCV is treated. The client has embarked on a heart-healthy lifestyle, which includes exercise, a healthy diet, and stress management. The client explains that they have the Raynaud phenomenon, which has improved since being treated for HCV. The client did not realize it, but their doctor explained that they have cryoglobulinemia, which is an immune response to chronic HCV infection. The client also explains that this whole diagnosis and treatment process began 3 years ago when their massage therapist found some swollen lymph nodes and skin changes and referred them to the doctor. The client has received regular weekly massages for years because of work-related common aches and stiffness. Since learning more about HCV, they now wonder if the muscle and joint aching are more related to the symptoms of the virus. During the first massage, the massage therapist identifies a small lump on the back. The client is aware of it and that it is a sebaceous cyst. Because it doesn't bother them, their doctor decided to just watch for any changes.

Continued

CRITICAL THINKING/CLINICAL REASONING—CONT'D

Explore

MedlinePlus, using these search terms: *hepatitis C, atherosclerosis, Raynaud phenomenon, cryoglobulinemia, swollen lymph* nodes, and *sebaceous cyst*.

The Centers for Disease Control and Prevention website for information about hepatitis: https://www.cdc.gov.

Discuss

- What is hepatitis and are there risks to the massage therapist?
- Of the conditions listed in this case study, which are primarily related to the cardiovascular system?
- Are the concerns about increased risk for stroke or heart attack related to the hepatitis C infection?
- How does the immune system relate to the client's past and current condition?
- What condition in the history is primarily integumentary and how does it affect the massage session?
- Is it possible that the client's observation is correct that the muscle and joint aching is a symptom of hepatitis C?
- What prompted the client's previous massage therapist to refer him to the doctor, and was this the correct action?
- In justifying massage therapy to benefit the client's current health situation, what are the most biologically plausible reasons for continued massage therapy?

Visit the Evolve website: https://evolve.elsevier.com/Fritz/essential/

The Evolve website provides support for the review of the chapter content and chapter quizzes to help you prepare for the MBLEx or other massage therapy certification or licensing exams. End of chapter questions for discussion and review answer key and rationales and author's response to critical thinking and clinical reasoning scenarios.

MULTIPLE CHOICE QUESTIONS FOR REVIEW AND DISCUSSION

The answers, with rationales, can be found on the Evolve site.

These questions are used for review and discussion. It is as important to understand why wrong answers are wrong as it is to know why the correct answer is correct. The answers to the questions, with rationales and explanations about why the correct answer is correct and why wrong answers are wrong, can be found on the Evolve site. Guidance also is provided on how questions are developed and how the textbook content can be presented in a multiple-choice question format. At the end of the question section here in the textbook, you will find an exercise that asks you to write more questions. Use the various questions in the chapter as examples. This is one of the best study strategies for test-taking.

It is important to understand that the actual licensing exam you take may not contain any of the specific questions found in this textbook or the review material and practice tests on the Evolve site. Therefore, just because you can answer any of these questions correctly does not mean you will pass the licensing exam. The questions are content and style examples to help you prepare—this is why understanding why wrong answers are wrong is just as important as identifying the correct answer. Also, make sure you understand all the terminology used in the questions and possible answers in the review and discussion questions. Look up words you do not understand.

The answers, with rationales, can be found on the Evolve site.

1. Which of the following is a contagious skin disease?
   a. Impetigo
   b. Alopecia
   c. Scleroderma
   d. Vitiligo
2. A massage professional identifies a few small lumps in the axillary area of a female client. What might be a pathological concern?
   a. Basal cell carcinoma
   b. Candidiasis
   c. Psoriasis
   d. Fibrocystic disease
3. During a general massage, the massage practitioner notices that the dorsalis pedis pulse is weaker on the left. Where is the practitioner palpating?
   a. Upper arm
   b. Wrist
   c. Knee
   d. Ankle
4. A client reports commonly having a blood pressure of 90/50 mm Hg. What would this condition be called?
   a. Tachycardia
   b. Hypertension
   c. Hypotension
   d. Bradycardia
5. Applying deep pressure during massage to the neck near the sternocleidomastoid muscles could compress which artery?
   a. Basilar
   b. External carotid
   c. Axillary
   d. Mesenteric
6. Which of the following is considered contagious?
   a. Hodgkin disease
   b. Mononucleosis
   c. Leukemia
   d. Lymphoma
7. Which of the following is considered sterilization for aseptic pathogen control?
   a. Iodine
   b. Chlorine
   c. Alcohol
   d. Extreme heat

8. Which of the following is an autoimmune disorder?
a. Callus
b. Stress fracture
c. Ganglion
d. Rheumatoid arthritis

9. What is a substance used to stimulate the production of antibodies and provide immunity against one or several diseases such as SARS-CoV-2
a. antibiotic
b. antiviral
c. vaccine
d. antihistamine

10. What is the condition called when the immune system produces too many inflammatory signals, sometimes leading to organ failure and death?
a. Cytokine storm
b. Fungal infection
c. Congestive heart failure
d. Acquired immunity

11. A medical emergency caused by the body's response to an infection is
a. Sepsis
b. Primary immune response
c. Cellulitis
d. Innate immunity

12. Which of the following are aspects of the venous pump?
a. Capillaries and arteries
b. Breathing and muscle contraction
c. Entrainment and pulses
d. Bradycardia and arrhythmia

13. Which of the following functions of the integumentary system is supported by maintaining sanitary procedures?
a. Protecting against water loss
b. Detecting sensory stimuli
c. Preventing the entry of bacteria and viruses
d. Excreting sweat and salts

14. A massage practitioner notices that a client's skin has a yellowish-gold color. This would be an indication of ______.
a. Cyanosis
b. Anemia
c. Fever
d. Jaundice

15. A client has a history of heart attack and has reduced blood flow to the heart. Which of the following vessels is most involved?
a. Coronary
b. Left external carotid
c. Celiac
d. Renal

16. Which of the following would be an indication for referral?
a. A radial pulse of 85 beats per minute
b. A femoral pulse of 55 beats per minute
c. A carotid pulse of 70 beats per minute
d. A dorsalis pedis pulse of 52 beats per minute

17. Which of the following would be an indication for referral?
a. Blueish skin color and slow capillary refill
b. Bilateral dorsalis pedis pulse of 62 beats per minute
c. Local tenderness at a vaccination site
d. Patchy loss of skin color

18. A client has been experiencing ongoing work and family stress and cannot seem to recover from an upper respiratory infection. What is the most logical cause?
a. Ongoing stress increases natural killer cells.
b. Ongoing stress supports the development of autoimmune disease.
c. Ongoing stress suppresses T-cell activity.
d. Decrease in cortisol suppresses the immune system.

19. A client is immune suppressed. The physician has provided approval for the massage. What would be the best massage treatment plan?
a. General massage with specific use of stimulation techniques to encourage sympathetic dominance
b. General massage with a focus on aggressive lymphatic drainage
c. General massage with active stretching to encourage parasympathetic dominance
d. General massage to support nonspecific homeostatic regulation and restorative sleep

20. The most likely transmission route for the human deficiency virus and hepatitis is
a. handshaking
b. body fluids
c. environmental contact
d. droplets in the air.

Write Your Own Test Questions

Create at least three more multiple-choice questions. Make sure to develop plausible wrong answers and double-check that the correct answer is correct. Then write a rationale for each question. The more questions you write, the better you will understand the material.

CHAPTER

12 Respiratory, Digestive, Urinary, and Reproductive Systems

https://evolve.elsevier.com/Fritz/essential/

CHAPTER OBJECTIVES

After completing this chapter, the student will be able to perform the following:

1. List and describe the components and function of the respiratory system.
2. Explain the mechanics of breathing.
3. Describe the pathological conditions of the respiratory system and the associated indications and contraindications for massage.
4. Explain the interlinked physiology of the digestive system, gut microbiota, nervous system, and endocrine system.
5. List and describe the components of the digestive system.
6. Describe the process of digestion.
7. Explain the importance of nutrition.
8. List and describe the main food groups.
9. Explain metabolic rate, energy balance, and body weight.
10. Describe the pathological conditions of the digestive system and the associated indications and contraindications for massage.
11. List the functions of the urinary system.
12. List and describe the components of the urinary system.
13. Describe urinary function and the processes of fluid electrolyte balances.
14. Describe the pathological conditions of the urinary system and the associated indications and contraindications for massage.
15. List and describe the components and functions of the male reproductive system.
16. List and describe the components and functions of the female reproductive system.
17. Explain the three stages of pregnancy and the process of lactation.
18. Describe the pathological conditions of the reproductive system and the associated indications and contraindications for massage.

CHAPTER OUTLINE

Key Terms

absorption: The movement of food molecules from the digestive tract to the cardiovascular and lymphatic systems so that they can be transported to the cells of the body.

basal metabolic rate (BMR): (BA-sal) The rate of energy expenditure of the body in a quiet, resting, fasting state.

breathing pattern disorder: A complex set of behaviors that leads to overbreathing without the presence of a pathological condition.

diaphragm: A dome-shaped sheet of muscle attached to the thoracic wall that separates the lungs and thoracic cavity from the abdominal cavity. As the chest cavity enlarges, the diaphragm moves downward and flattens to create a vacuum that allows air to flow into the lungs. As the chest contracts and the diaphragm relaxes, the diaphragm arches upward, helping air to flow out of the lungs.

digestion: The mechanical and chemical breakdown of food from its complex form into simple molecules.

elimination (egestion): The removal and release of undigested and unabsorbed food as solid waste products.

external respiration: The exchange of oxygen and carbon dioxide between the lungs and the bloodstream.

gestation: (jes-TAY-shun) The period of fetal growth from conception until birth.

hyperventilation (hye-per-ven-ti-LAY-shun): Abnormally deep or rapid breathing in excess of physical demands.

ingestion: (in-JEST-chun) Taking food into the mouth.

internal respiration: The exchange of gases between the tissues and the blood.
lower respiratory tract: The larynx, trachea, bronchi, and alveoli.
lungs: The primary organs of respiration. The lungs are soft, spongy, highly vascular structures that are separated into the left and right lungs by the mediastinum. Each lung is separated into lobes. The right lung has three lobes: upper, middle, and lower; the left lung has two lobes: upper and lower.
microbiome: (mi·cro·BI·ome) All of the genes inside of microbial cells.
microbiota: (mi·cro·BI·o·ta) A wide variety of bacteria, viruses, fungi, and other single-celled animals that live in the body.
peristalsis: (pair-ih-STAL-sis) The rhythmic contraction of smooth muscles that propels products of digestion along the tract from the esophagus to the anus.
respiration: The movement of air in and out of the lungs, the exchange of oxygen and carbon dioxide between the lungs and the blood, and the exchange between the blood and the body tissues.
sinuses: (SYE-nus-ez) Four groups of air-filled spaces that open into the internal nose. They are located in the frontal, ethmoid, sphenoid, and maxillary bones of the skull. They lighten the weight of the skull and play a role in sound production.
thorax: (THOR-aks) Also known as the ***chest cavity***, the thorax is the upper region of the torso. It is enclosed by the sternum, ribs, and thoracic vertebrae and contains the lungs, heart, and great blood vessels.
upper respiratory tract: The nasal cavity and all its structures and the pharynx.

LEARNING HOW TO LEARN

It helps to have a focus and some direction about the depth of detail needed when studying. The information in Chapter 11 and this chapter is important, but for the massage therapist, the detail does not have to be as comprehensive as it is for other health professionals such as a nurse. All of the body systems discussed in this chapter are indirectly affected by massage through the nervous system and endocrine system. This is considered a systemic effect. Massage therapy can have a more direct effect on the respiratory and digestive systems because techniques can mechanically address anatomy related to these systems. This is considered a local effect. Massage supports the mechanics of breathing, which include muscle and connective tissue function and mobility of the ribs and entire thorax. The large intestine of the digestive system in particular can be addressed by massage to support waste movement in the body. One of the functions of the urinary system is to control blood pressure. Massage can support this function by affecting the autonomic nervous systems and the cardiovascular system. The study of the reproductive system supports a massage population specialty of prenatal and postnatal massage.

RESPIRATORY SYSTEM

SECTION OBJECTIVES

Chapter objectives covered in this section:

1. List and describe the components and functions of the respiratory system.
2. Explain the mechanics of breathing.
3. Describe pathological conditions of the respiratory system and the associated indications and contraindications for massage.

After completing this section, the student will be able to perform the following:

- Define *respiration*.
- List the organs of the respiratory system.
- List the muscles involved in respiration.
- Define *lung volume*.
- Describe breathing pattern disorder.

Of all the basic life support systems in the body, the respiratory system is the only one under voluntary and automatic control. The respiratory system obtains the oxygen necessary to create energy for body functions and eliminate the carbon dioxide produced during cellular metabolism. Respiratory movements are under voluntary control, most often in connection with speech. This voluntary control of breathing helps regulate the autonomic nervous system. Therefore, control of breathing becomes important in many relaxation and meditation practices. Respiration and breath are intimately connected to the expression of emotion, such as laughing, crying, exploding in anger, holding one's breath in fear, and sighing with relief.

The respiratory system may have one of the most vital functions because the heart and brain require a continuous supply of oxygen to function. Apnea, the lack of spontaneous breathing, can cause irreversible brain damage if it continues for more than 3 or 4 minutes.

Respiration is the movement of air in and out of the lungs. Breathing is a mechanical action of inhalation and exhalation that draws oxygen into the lungs and releases carbon dioxide into the atmosphere.

Respiration is also the exchange of oxygen and carbon dioxide between the lungs and the blood and between the blood and the body tissues. **External respiration** is the exchange of oxygen and carbon dioxide between the lungs and the bloodstream. The exchange of gases between the body cells and the blood is called **internal respiration**.

On average, we breathe 12 to 16 times per minute. Each breath contains approximately 500 mL of air (about 2 cups), so in 1 hour we breathe about 360 L, or 82 gallons, of air.

The organs of the respiratory system are divided into upper and lower regions. The **upper respiratory tract** consists of the nasal cavity, all its structures, and the pharynx; the **lower respiratory tract** consists of the larynx, trachea, bronchi, and alveoli in the lungs (Fig. 12.1).

Organs of the Respiratory System

Nose and Nasal Cavity

The nose is divided into two parts, the external and internal portions. The lower two-thirds of the external nose is composed mostly of cartilage. The upper third, or bridge of the nose, is formed by two small, hard nasal bones. The tip of the nose is the apex, and the nostrils are the nares. Air enters the external nares and passes across internal nasal hairs that trap particles of dirt and other foreign material; the air then flows into the nasal cavity.

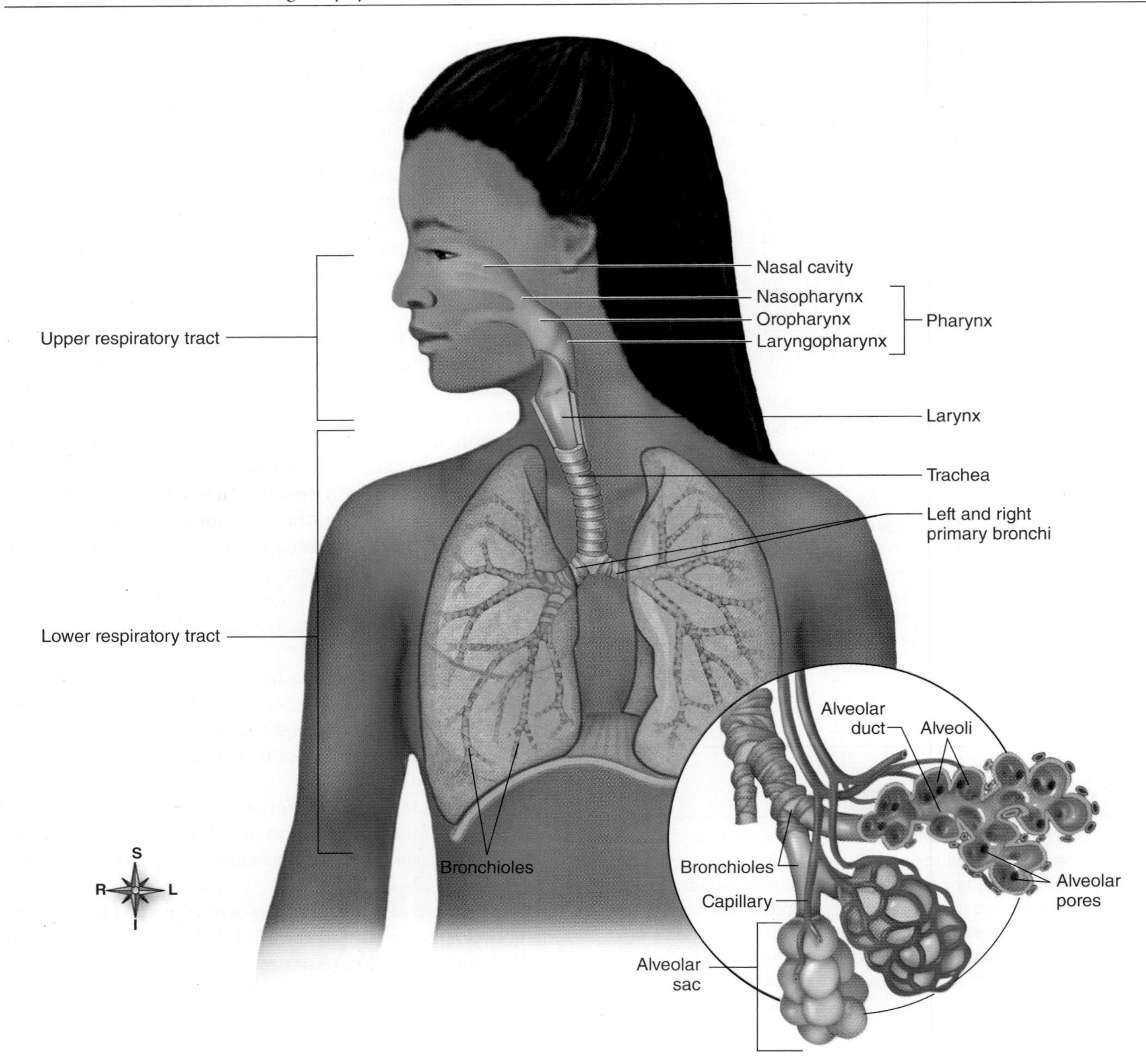

FIG. 12.1 The organs and structures of the respiratory system.

The internal nose is the continuation of the nose inside the skull and above the mouth and includes the sinuses. The roof is formed by a small portion of the frontal bone and the ethmoid and sphenoid bones, and the floor is formed by the hard palate, consisting of the maxillae and palatine bones. The internal nares are the portion of the internal nose that communicates with the throat. The nasal cavity is the actual space inside the external and internal nose structures and is separated into left and right sides by the septum, a partition composed of cartilage and bone. At the upper portion of the nasal cavity, three thin, curled bones, the turbinates, or conchae, project inward from the two outer walls. These turbinates separate into small, grooved passageways, each called a *meatus*, that continue to move the air.

Mucous membranes line the entire respiratory tract, starting in the nasal cavity. Deep in the mucous membrane are small blood vessels. Air that passes through the upper respiratory tract is warmed by blood in the blood vessels and moistened by the mucous membranes. Sticky mucus traps smaller inhaled particles, which helps prevent infection. Small hairs that line the nasal cavity and cilia that line the throat and air passageways in the lungs transport these foreign particles upward, where they are either swallowed (and destroyed in the digestive tract) or expelled from the body through coughing or sneezing.

The ends of the olfactory nerve lie in the upper third of both sides of the nasal septum, the olfactory region, and are stimulated by odor particles. Olfactory nerve fibers pass through small holes in the ethmoid bone to the olfactory bulb and then to the cortex, which interprets the impulses as smell.

Venous areas called *swell bodies* are located on the turbinates. About every half hour, the swell bodies on one side of the nasal cavity engorge with blood, resulting in decreased airflow on that side, with good flow on the other side. Then the process reverses. These periodic changes permit the inside of the nose to recover from drying. This same mechanism becomes important during sleep. When a person lies with their head to one side, the swell bodies of the lower nostril become congested. The chamber narrows, and the lumen closes. Therefore, a person breathes through only one nostril at a time while sleeping. The closure of the nostril then initiates movement of the head from one side to the other, which in turn causes a major movement and turning of the body. This head-body moving cycle, initiated by the nose, ensures maximal rest during sleep. A poorly functioning nose may allow the body and head to remain in one position and can cause symptoms, such as backaches, numbness, cramps, and circulatory dysfunction.

The nasal septum is supplied with sensory nerves and blood vessels. Nasal reflex responses and referred phenomena are well established among the nose, ears, throat, larynx, heart, lungs, diaphragm, nervous system, and body temperature. Contained in the coordination of these various reflex patterns is the mechanism of entrainment among heart rate, breathing rate, and synchronization of other body rhythms. Most relaxation methods and the methods of ritual, meditation, and many healing practices incorporate a form of structured breathing. This practical application of coordinating body rhythms seems to be accomplished through the coordination of airflow through the nose.

A deviated septum is a condition in which the cartilage is bent, usually as the result of a blow to the nose. It results in difficulty in breathing through one side of the nose. As simple as this seems, because of reflex patterns, any disruption of airflow through the nose can lead to body-wide effects, such as disturbed sleep patterns.

Sinuses

The **sinuses** are four groups of air-filled spaces that open into the internal nose. They are located in the frontal, ethmoid, sphenoid, and maxillary bones of the skull. Sinuses are lined with mucosa and lighten the weight of the skull, making it easier to hold up the head. They also help with the production of sound, also known as *phonation*. Because the sinus mucosa communicates with the nasal cavity, sinuses are prone to the same infections as the nasal cavity.

Pharynx

The pharynx, or throat, is divided into three areas. The nasopharynx is the continuation of the nasal cavity into the throat; it transports air. The auditory or eustachian tubes from the inner ear open into the nasopharynx; they help equalize pressure in the head, nose, and pharynx. The oropharynx is the portion of the throat that you can see; it contains the tonsils and functions as a passageway for food between the mouth and the esophagus and as a passageway for air between the nose, mouth, and trachea. The laryngopharynx begins at the hyoid bone and separates into the esophagus and larynx; it is a pathway for both air and food. At the entrance to the larynx is a small cartilaginous flap, the epiglottis. As food is swallowed, the epiglottis closes over the glottis, preventing food and fluids from entering the lungs.

Larynx

The larynx, or voice box, connects the pharynx to the trachea and consists of cartilage, ligaments, connective tissue, muscles, and the vocal cords. The cartilage provides a rigid structural framework for the larynx and trachea below, ensuring that the airway is open at all times. The thyroid cartilage, known as the *Adam's apple*, is located on the anterior portion of the larynx and is larger in males than in females. The vocal cords and the spaces between the cords are located inside the glottis.

The function of the larynx, in addition to permitting air passage to and from the lungs, is to produce sound. As we exhale, the vocal cords vibrate to produce high or low sounds, or pitch. In high-pitched sounds, the glottis is narrower and the vocal cords are more tense, whereas in low-pitched sounds, the glottis is more open and the vocal cords are more relaxed. The lips and the tongue create speech.

Laryngitis is an inflammation of the vocal cords caused by overuse, infection, or irritation by cigarette smoke or a tumor. Laryngitis can cause hoarseness or loss of the voice. Obstruction of the glottis (e.g., by food) can be fatal. Bacterial infection of the epiglottis (epiglottitis) in children is a life-threatening but rare cause of obstruction.

Trachea

The trachea, or windpipe, is the main airway to the lungs and is a 4- to 5-inch tube that begins at the glottis and ends at the junction of the two main bronchi near the level of the sternal angle. The trachea consists of 16 to 20 horseshoe-shaped rings of cartilage that have connective tissue between them. When a foreign particle enters the trachea, mucus, and cilia trap it and initiate the cough reflex.

The trachea branches off into two bronchi, which have the same structural framework as the trachea except that they have more smooth muscle. The first branches of the bronchial tubes are the right and left primary bronchi. Each main bronchus divides into two (left lung) or three (right lung) lobar bronchi.

Lungs

The two **lungs** are the primary organs of respiration. These soft, spongy, highly vascular structures are separated into the left and right lungs by the mediastinum. Each lung is separated into lobes. The right lung has three lobes: upper, middle, and lower; the left has two lobes: upper and lower.

Each of the lobar bronchi, which extend from the trachea, divides into 10 segmental bronchi, which then divide further. The amount of cartilage in each tube gradually decreases until the tubes lack cartilage. At that point, the tubes are about 1 mm in diameter and are known as the *bronchioles*, which terminate in the air sacs, or alveoli. The alveoli are surrounded by capillaries, and this is where external respiration takes place.

The lungs are enclosed in a pleural cavity lined by two pleural membranes. One connects directly to the surface of the lung, and the other attaches to the mediastinum and inside the chest wall. This cavity created by the membranes contains approximately a half teaspoon of lubricating fluid that reduces friction between the two layers as we breathe. Increases in the amount of fluid often occur with diseases (such as lung cancer and pulmonary edema) and can make breathing difficult. Pneumothorax is a condition in which air enters the pleural cavity as a result of trauma or rupture of part of the lung. This can be caused by a penetrating injury, such as from a bullet or knife, or in a disease process, such as emphysema. A chest tube, called a *thoracotomy tube*, is inserted between the ribs and connected to a pump to remove the air. In hemothorax, blood is in the pleural cavity; physicians can drain blood from the pleural space in a manner similar to how air is drained.

Diaphragm

The **diaphragm** is a dome-shaped sheet of muscle attached to the thoracic wall that separates the lungs and thoracic cavity from the abdominal cavity. As the chest cavity enlarges, the diaphragm moves downward and creates a vacuum that allows air to flow into the lungs. As the chest contracts and the diaphragm relaxes, the diaphragm arches upward, which helps push air out of the lungs. The diaphragm is part of a larger muscle synergy pattern and myofascial chain. It is one of the structures that is oriented in the transverse plane. As described in Chapter 10, seldom does any muscle function independently. The optimal function of the diaphragm requires coordinated and integrated soft tissue function.

Thorax

The **thorax**, or chest cavity, is the upper region of the torso. It is enclosed by the sternum, ribs, and thoracic vertebrae and contains the lungs, heart, and great vessels.

Nerves and Vessels of the Lungs and Respiratory Muscles

The autonomic nervous system supplies the bronchi and bronchioles. Stimulation of the vagus nerve, a major parasympathetic nerve, causes contraction of the smooth muscles and narrows the diameter of the tubes; this is called *bronchoconstriction*. Stimulation of sympathetic nerves initiates smooth muscle relaxation, resulting in the widening of the tubes; this is called *bronchodilation*.

The nerve supply to the intercostal muscles extends from spinal nerves T1–T11. The phrenic nerve originates at C3–C5 and innervates the diaphragm. The reason the nerve supply originates in such a distant location is that during fetal development, the diaphragm actually begins its growth in the neck and then descends from the neck to the abdomen. A broken neck that injures the spinal cord below C5 allows the person to continue breathing because the diaphragm does most of the breathing. Injury to both phrenic nerves or a spinal cord injury above C3–C5 severely compromises breathing. A person with such an injury needs to be on a ventilator, which essentially does the breathing.

The pulmonary arteries and veins participate in the exchange of oxygen and carbon dioxide between the capillaries and alveoli. Branches of the aorta and upper intercostal arteries supply blood to most of the lung tissue. Venous drainage takes place from the azygos vein on the right side of the thorax and from the first intercostal vein on the left.

Mechanics of Breathing

During the moments before we take a breath, the pressure inside the lungs and outside the body is equal, whereas the pressure inside the pleural space is slightly lower. When we begin to inhale, the external intercostal muscles between the ribs contract, lifting the lower ribs up and out. This creates a vacuum that expands the lungs, causing the pressure inside the lungs to decrease. The diaphragm moves down, increasing the volume of the pleural cavities and decreasing lung pressure even more. Elastic fibers in the alveolar walls stretch, permitting expansion of the air sacs. The lungs draw in air until the pressure is equal again.

Exhalation mainly results from the elastic recoil of the alveoli. Additionally, as we exhale, the pressure inside the pleural cavity increases; the external intercostals, diaphragm, and alveolar walls relax; the volume inside the lungs decreases; and the pressure in the lungs increases until it again equals the atmospheric pressure.

In diseases such as asthma, bronchitis, and emphysema, the accessory muscles of respiration are often used. Contraction of the sternocleidomastoid and other muscles of the neck aid inspiration, whereas the use of the internal intercostals and abdominal muscles aids expiration (Figs. 12.2–12.4).

Practical Application

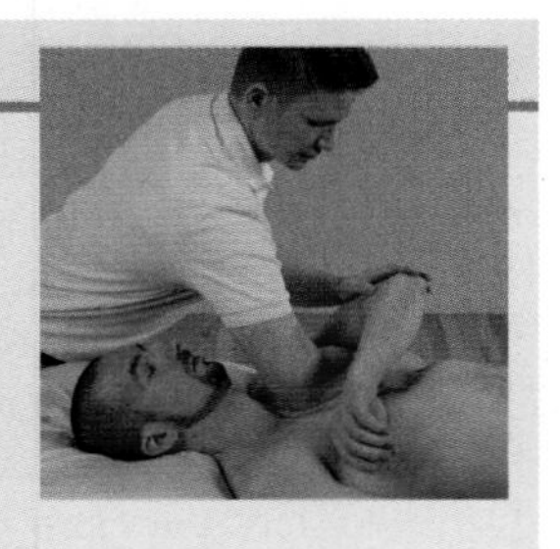

Massage therapy that targets the trunk, including the back, chest, and abdomen, can be applied to support normal breathing. The main goal is for the soft tissues to be sufficiently pliable so that the ribs can move efficiently during inspiration and expiration. Also, recall from Chapter 10 that the superficial erector spinae, psoas, deep erector spinae, transverse abdominis, abdominal obliques, diaphragm, lumbar multifidus, and muscles of the pelvic floor provide intersegmental stabilization of the trunk during functional movement. Also called the intrinsic stabilization subsystem, dysfunction in any of these structures can lead to sacroiliac joint instability and low back pain. It is logical to expect that breathing function is also a factor in low back dysfunction and blowback issues affect breathing.

Lung Volumes

There are various volumes of air that can be breathed in and out. It is possible to measure four different pulmonary volumes that may be used as guidelines in health assessments. The tidal volume is the amount of air taken in or exhaled in a single breath during normal breathing, usually while the person is resting. It is about half a liter. Inspiratory reserve volume is the amount of air that can be inhaled forcefully after normal tidal volume inspiration; it is about 3 L in the average male and almost 2 L in the average female (the difference is because males usually have larger body sizes, so they have larger lungs).

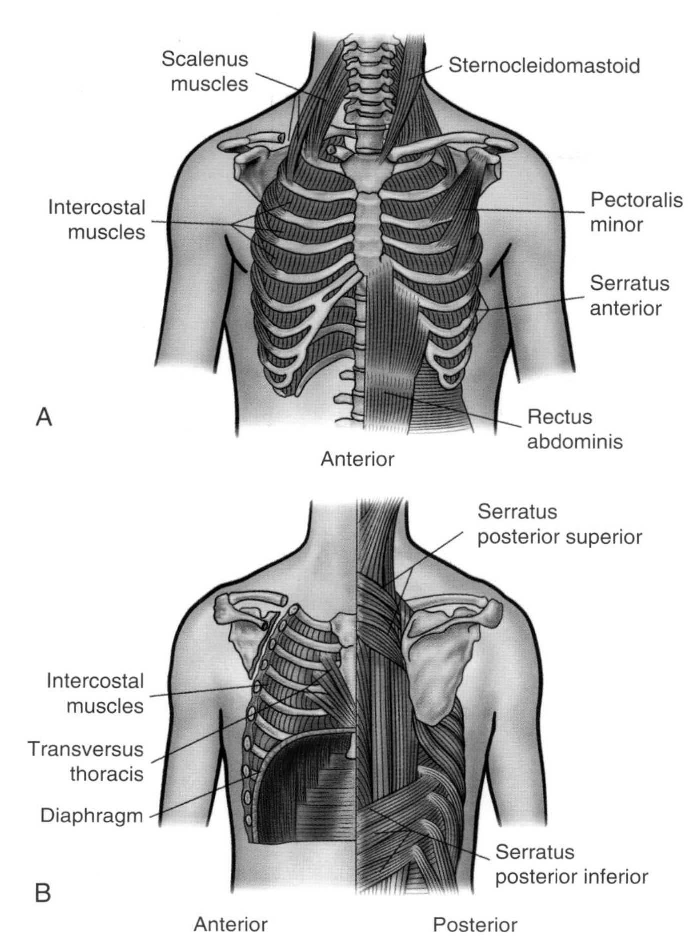

FIG. 12.2 Muscles of respiration: (A) anterior view and (B) posterior view. (Modified from Seidel HM, et al. *Mosby's Guide to Physical Examination.* 5th ed. Mosby/Elsevier; 2003.)

Expiratory reserve volume is the amount of air that can be exhaled forcefully after a normal exhalation; it is a little more than a liter in males and a little less than a liter in females. Reserve volume is the amount of air that remains in the lungs and passageways after a maximal expiration. Vital capacity is the total of the tidal volume, inspiratory reserve volume, and expiratory reserve volume. In the normal, healthy adult lung, vital capacity usually is about 5.5 L of air for males and 3.5 L of air for females.

In diseased lungs, such as those affected by asthma or emphysema, the vital capacity and expiratory reserve volumes are abnormal. A person with asthma, for example, may have a normal tidal volume and vital capacity but decreased expiratory reserve volume, whereas a person with emphysema may have a normal (but often decreased) tidal volume and decreased vital capacity and expiratory reserve volume. Ultimately, because of the pathological condition of the lung tissues, the person cannot exhale effectively.

Transport of Oxygen and Carbon Dioxide

The pulmonary arteries bring oxygen-deficient blood from the right ventricle of the heart to the lungs. Carbon dioxide diffuses from the bloodstream through the capillary and alveolar membranes into the alveoli. Oxygen diffuses in the opposite direction, from the alveoli through both membranes and into the bloodstream. The carbon dioxide is then exhaled from the lungs while the pulmonary veins return oxygen-rich blood to the left atrium of the heart.

The amount of oxygen in the blood depends on the amount of oxygen available in the atmosphere. The air in the average room is composed of the following:

- Nitrogen (N_2): 79%
- Oxygen (O_2): 20.96%
- Carbon dioxide (CO_2): 0.04%

Red blood cells transport oxygen in the blood as oxyhemoglobin. Red blood cells move into the capillaries. At the arteriole end of the capillary, oxygen leaves the red blood cell and then diffuses through the capillary membrane into the tissue fluid. Oxygen then diffuses into cell membranes to be used for cellular metabolism.

Carbon dioxide moves out of the tissue cell in the reverse direction, through the same membranes, into the red blood cells, where most of it is converted into a bicarbonate ion (HCO_3). The plasma transports bicarbonate to the lungs, where the bicarbonate ion is converted back into carbon dioxide in the alveolar membrane so that it can be exhaled.

Control of Breathing

The respiratory center is a group of nerve cells in the medulla and pons of the brain. A variety of stimuli affect the center. Impulses from the cerebral cortex under voluntary control modify respiration, as do changes in the carbon dioxide content and acidity of blood and cerebrospinal fluid. Chemoreceptors, nerve cells found near the baroreceptors, are sensitive to the oxygen level and to a lesser extent to carbon dioxide and pH (acid/base balance) levels in the bloodstream. Two chemoreceptors, called *aortic bodies*, are located near the arch of the aorta. There is also one in each carotid artery; these are called *carotid bodies*. The aortic bodies transmit impulses to the respiratory center in the medulla through the vagus nerve; the carotid bodies transmit by way of the glossopharyngeal nerve. A low concentration of oxygen in the body stimulates these chemoreceptors, and the respiratory rate increases as a result.

Respiratory Rate

The respiratory rate in an adult is about 12 to 20 breaths per minute, and in a newborn about 35 breaths per minute, which gradually decreases to adult values at about age 20. A respiration rate under 12 or more than 25 breaths per minute while resting is considered abnormal. Emotions are powerful stimuli for respiratory changes. Fear, grief, and shock slow the rate, whereas excitement, anger, and sexual arousal increase the respiratory rate.

Besides the effects of emotions, changes in breathing rates can occur as a result of increased oxygen requirements induced by exercise; in obesity as a result of increased vessel resistance; during infections and fever because of increased energy requirements; in heart failure as a result of decreased oxygen flow; during pain because of increased nervous stimulation; with anemia because of decreased oxygen

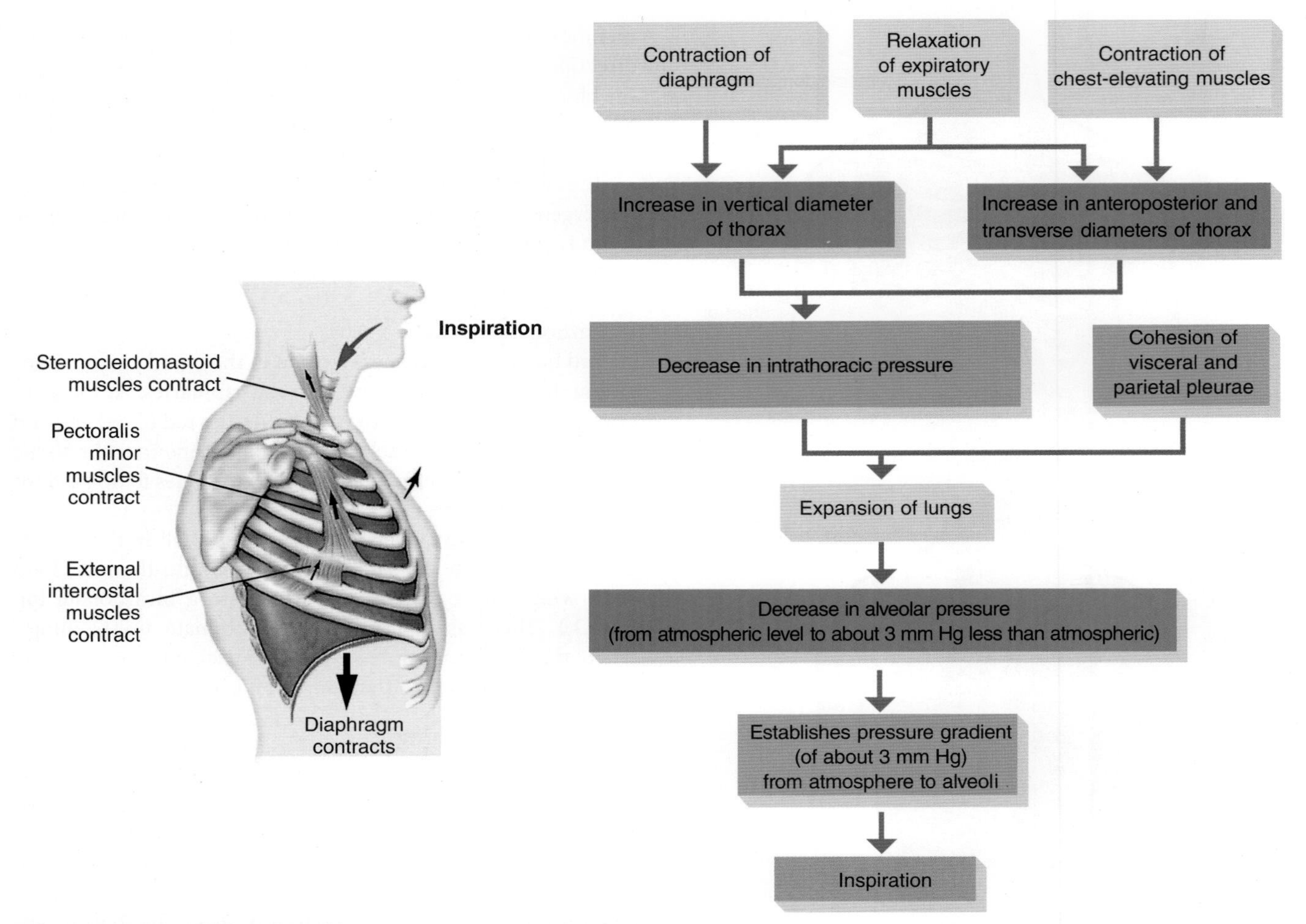

FIG. 12.3 Mechanism of inspiration. (From Patton KT, Thibodeau GA. *Anatomy and Physiology.* 5th ed. Mosby/Elsevier; 2003.)

transport; in hyperthyroidism because of an increase in metabolic rate; and during emphysema because of blockage of oxygen. Hyperpnea is fast breathing, and tachypnea is rapid, shallow breathing. These types of breathing can lead to acute **hyperventilation** or chronic overbreathing, called **breathing pattern disorder**, which causes a variety of signs and symptoms, as discussed later in this section. Bradypnea, or slow breathing, occurs in intoxication by alcohol and other depressant drugs because of the action of these substances in the brain. Bradypnea also occurs in cases of increased intracranial pressure on account of pressure on the respiratory center and in diabetic coma. Periods of hyperpnea alternating with periods of apnea (no breathing) sometimes occur in the sleep of infants, particularly premature ones. These patterns also appear in those with brain injury and in the terminally ill.

Reflexes that Affect Breathing

Foreign matter or other irritants in the trachea or bronchi stimulate the cough reflex. The epiglottis and glottis reflexively close, and contraction of the expiratory muscles causes air pressure in the lungs to increase. The epiglottis and glottis open suddenly, resulting in an upward force of air in a cough that removes the irritant from the throat.

The sneeze reflex is similar to the cough reflex, except that contaminants or irritants in the nasal cavity provide the stimulus. A burst of air moves through the nose and mouth, forcing the contaminant out of the respiratory tract.

A hiccup is an involuntary, spasmodic contraction of the diaphragm that causes the glottis to close suddenly, producing the characteristic sound. A yawn is a slow, deep inspiration through the open mouth. Scientists still have not found the actual physiological mechanism of yawning.

Pathological Conditions of the Respiratory System

Respiratory diseases can arise from a number of causes. Infections, genetic predisposition, inhalation of toxic substances, accidents, and lifestyle choices (such as smoking) can cause respiratory pathology. People with lung disease have difficulty breathing. The term *lung disease* refers to many disorders affecting the lungs, such as asthma, chronic obstructive pulmonary disease (COPD), and cancer.

Common Cold

More than 200 viruses can cause the common cold; these viruses are easily spread. Usually affecting the nasal mucosa, the viruses may spread to the sinuses and pharynx and down

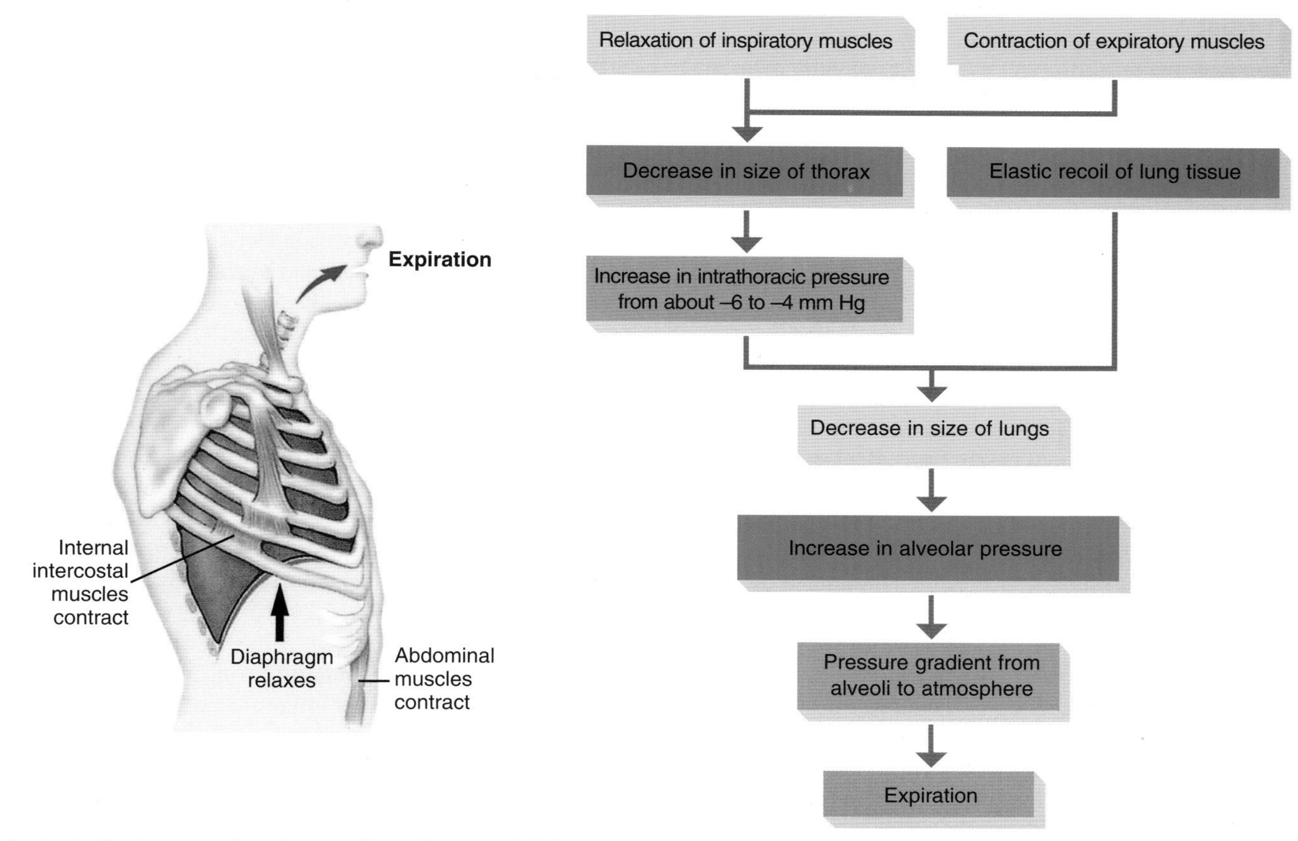

FIG. 12.4 Mechanism of expiration. (From Patton KT, Thibodeau GA. *Anatomy and Physiology.* 5th ed. Mosby/Elsevier; 2003.)

the respiratory tract. The person's temperature rises to eliminate the virus. Irritation in the nose and pharynx causes coughing and sneezing. Fluids and bed rest are recommended.

Influenza

Influenza is commonly called the *flu*. It is a common viral infection of the entire body, resulting in fever, muscle aches and weakness, backache, and cough. The primary treatment, as with most viral infections, is bed rest and fluids.

Coronaviruses

Commonly human coronaviruses cause mild respiratory illnesses like the common cold. Four types of human coronaviruses cause 10 to 30 percent of upper respiratory tract infections in adults. Like many other respiratory viruses, coronaviruses spread quickly through droplets that you project out of the mouth or nose when an individual breathes, coughs, sneezes, or speaks. The seven coronaviruses that can infect people are:

229E (alpha coronavirus)

NL63 (alpha coronavirus)

OC43 (beta coronavirus)

HKU1 (beta coronavirus)

MERS-CoV (the beta coronavirus that causes Middle East respiratory syndrome, or MERS)

SARS-CoV (the beta coronavirus that causes severe acute respiratory syndrome, or SARS)

SARS-CoV-2 (the novel coronavirus that causes coronavirus disease 2019, or COVID-19)

Possible symptoms include:

- Fever or chills
- Cough
- Shortness of breath or difficulty breathing
- Fatigue
- Muscle or body aches
- Headache
- New loss of taste or smell
- Sore throat
- Congestion or runny nose
- Nausea or vomiting
- Diarrhea

This list does not include all possible symptoms. Post–COVID-19 conditions are new, returning, or ongoing health problems people can experience 4 or more weeks after initial infection with the SARS-CoV-2 virus, the virus that causes COVID-19.

Sinusitis

Sinusitis is inflammation of the sinuses; most commonly, it accompanies a nasal infection. Congestion, edema, and pain are present because of irritation of the sensory nerve endings in the periosteum. Pain takes the form of a headache, particularly if the frontal sinus is involved. Congestion blocks drainage into the nasal cavity. The maxillary sinus lies over the upper teeth, and sometimes a person has difficulty telling whether the problem is a sinus attack or a toothache because of the similarity of the pain pattern. Treatment often consists of an antibiotic and a decongestant.

Sore Throat

Sore throat, or pharyngitis, is an inflammation of the pharynx. If the tonsils are involved, the condition is tonsillitis. The cause is usually viral, but a throat culture may show a *Streptococcus* species, the organism that causes rheumatic fever, rheumatic heart disease, or glomerulonephritis as complications in certain individuals. Common signs and symptoms are a red, tender throat; enlarged cervical lymph nodes; and fever. Treatment consists of rest, an analgesic, saline gargles, and an antibiotic if the culture is positive for *Streptococcus* species.

Croup

Croup is a viral infection in children that most commonly affects boys between 3 months and 5 years of age. The larynx, trachea, and bronchi are red and swollen and may block the glottis. A "seal bark" cough is usually present. A high-pitched whistling inhalation is sometimes present and affected children must use their neck and abdominal muscles to breathe. Humidified air often eases the symptoms; if not, oxygen therapy may help.

Pneumonia

Pneumonia is an acute infection of the lungs caused by bacteria or viruses, fungi, exposure to certain chemicals, or inhaled substances. Symptoms include fever, chills, chest pain, difficulty breathing, headache, loss of appetite, muscle and joint pain, a cough usually accompanied by yellow or green sputum, and rales (the sound of the movement of air and fluid in the bronchial tree). The diagnosis is usually made by reviewing the patient's history and test results, most often a chest radiograph showing an abnormal white area. Evaluation of sputum and blood tests commonly show an elevated white count. The primary treatment for bacterial pneumonia is an antibiotic, bed rest, and fluids. In serious cases, the person must be hospitalized and given oxygen and antibiotics.

Asthma

Asthma is the reversible narrowing of the small airways for reasons other than cardiovascular disease. Asthma manifests as acute attacks that constrict and obstruct these airways. Asthma attacks may be triggered by allergic reactions, air pollutants, exercise, hypersensitivity to substances (such as wood and flour, chemicals, viral infections), and emotional upsets. During an episode, the smooth muscle layer of the bronchi and bronchioles goes into bronchoconstricting spasms, and the glands of the bronchi hypersecrete mucus. The airways fill with thick mucus, and air cannot leave the lungs. Breathlessness, coughing, chest tightness, and wheezing occur as the person tries to force air out of the lungs. Arterial blood gases may initially show a low amount of carbon dioxide, leading to a condition called *respiratory alkalosis*. Long-term therapy may include the use of a bronchodilator, a mast cell stabilizer, or corticosteroids. Antibiotics may benefit the person if the trigger is a respiratory infection.

Chronic Obstructive Pulmonary Disease

Although the processes involved in the evolution of emphysema and bronchitis are different, the result is irreversible respiratory insufficiency, sometimes called *chronic obstructive pulmonary disease (COPD)*. In emphysema, the obstruction is in the alveoli; in bronchitis, the obstruction is in the bronchi. A component of each appears in heavy smokers. The lung tissue changes, and the person becomes less able to tolerate exercise and activity.

Acute bronchitis often occurs along with an upper respiratory infection, measles, or the flu. A virus usually causes infection, but the cause also may be bacterial. Symptoms include a mild fever, an increase in secreted mucus, and coughing in an attempt to loosen and remove the phlegm, which may be yellow or green. Prolonged irritation by cigarette smoke is the usual cause of chronic bronchitis. Sputum production increases in response to the constant irritation of the tissues. The smoke damages the cilia such that excessive mucus cannot be moved out of the airway, and the person usually has a chronic cough. The person may also make wheezing noises. The evidence suggests that the condition does not reverse, but further deterioration can be halted after quitting smoking. Treatment involves the use of bronchodilators and oxygen therapy.

Pleurisy

Pleurisy (pleuritis) is an inflammation of the pleural membrane, usually the result of a lung infection, such as pneumonia. The inflamed membranes rub against each other, causing stabbing pain that is worse during inhalation.

Lung Cancer

About 90% of all cases of lung cancer are caused by smoking tobacco. Primary tumors usually develop in the bronchi and block air passages. Cancer in the lung can spread to other parts of the body. Symptoms commonly begin with cough, blood in the phlegm, wheezing, chest pain, and fever. A large tumor may cause problems in swallowing. Diagnosis is by physical examination, radiographs, and computed tomography (CT) scans.

Pulmonary Edema

Pulmonary edema is the accumulation of fluid in the lungs. The most common cause is heart failure, although kidney disease, pneumonia, and other disorders may also cause pulmonary edema. Treatment usually involves diuretics and oxygen therapy.

Tuberculosis

Tuberculosis is an infection that develops as chronic inflammatory lesions caused by the bacillus *Mycobacterium tuberculosis*. It is contagious and is contracted by inhaling or ingesting infected droplets dispersed by infected persons by way of coughing and nasal discharge. Once thought to occur rarely, tuberculosis is on the rise again in adults who are immunosuppressed. Although any site of the body may be affected, pulmonary tuberculosis is by far the most common. In rare cases, tuberculosis may also affect the bones and kidneys. Early symptoms include listlessness and fatigue, chest pain, fever, and weight loss. The disease progresses to impair respiratory function severely and spreads to involve other body sites. Treatment includes rest, nutritional support, and a medication regimen that may last more than 1 year. The disease is no longer infectious once sputum tests are free of bacteria, although the bacteria may lie dormant.

Cystic Fibrosis

Cystic fibrosis is a genetic disorder that causes abnormally thick and sticky mucus to be produced throughout the body. In the lungs, the mucus cannot be moved out by the cilia, so bacteria and viruses are held in instead of being released by the body. Infections develop, causing obstruction of the smaller airways. (See the Pathological Conditions of the Digestive System section for more information.)

Choking

Choking commonly occurs when a person is talking while eating and inhales at the same time as swallowing. The piece of food, usually meat, obstructs the larynx. The person coughs, which often dislodges the object. If not, the airway can become completely blocked. The person usually appears distressed, grasps their neck, and cannot inhale or exhale. The term *café coronary* has been used because it is common for choking to occur in a restaurant, and it superficially resembles a heart attack. Other objects, such as chewing gum or balloons, are frequently the cause of obstructions in children. First aid for choking is the Heimlich maneuver. Being able to correctly perform this life-saving procedure is one of the important reasons that all massage therapists need to be trained in emergency first aid.

Sleep Apnea

Persons with sleep apnea stop breathing while sleeping. The breathing is interrupted for a few seconds at least a few times per hour. Each time breathing stops, oxygen levels fall and cause the person to wake up. Sleep apnea commonly occurs because of obstructed breathing, which is identified as obstructive sleep apnea (OSA). It is more common in men, especially those who are overweight. Persons taking medications (such as sleeping pills) can suffer from OSA because the upper airway muscles can relax too much and the tongue falls back, obstructing the airway.

Infant apnea is associated with infections that obstruct the airway. Sudden infant death syndrome (SIDS) may be related to infant apnea.

Carbon Monoxide Poisoning

Carbon monoxide poisoning is the leading cause of gas-related deaths in this country. Carbon monoxide is odorless and binds to hemoglobin 210 times more readily than oxygen, forming the molecule carboxyhemoglobin.

Red blood cells are able to carry very little oxygen. Most deaths occur as a result of smoke inhalation during fires. Some deaths are caused by automobile exhaust fumes and poorly ventilated or defective gasoline heaters and charcoal stoves. Poisonings also occur in machine shops in which ventilation is poor. The symptoms are headache, dizziness, weakness, and nausea; they occur when the blood has approximately 6% to 7% carboxyhemoglobin.

Emphysema

Emphysema can result from long-term irritation of the bronchi and bronchioles. Mucus and pus accumulate, and the air in the alveoli becomes trapped. When the pressure exceeds the elastic limit, the alveoli become permanently ballooned, making exhalation difficult. The person typically develops a barrel chest from using the internal intercostals as well as the abdominal and neck muscles to breathe. Inflammation brings in more white blood cells, which break down the walls of the alveoli, which merge to form larger sacs. Alveolar destruction results in less surface area for the internal exchange of gases, so oxygen in the blood decreases. As emphysema progresses, the person becomes breathless with minor exertion. Emphysema is the most common cause of respiratory failure. Bronchodilators and oxygen therapy may help.

Breathing Pattern Disorder

Physiologists define *hyperventilation* as abnormally deep or rapid breathing in excess of physical demands. Now called *breathing pattern disorder*, it is a complex set of behaviors that leads to overbreathing in the absence of a pathological condition. Hyperventilation is a functional condition in which all the parts are working effectively, so a pathological condition does not exist, but the breathing pattern is inappropriate for the situation, resulting in confused signals to the central nervous system, setting up a whole chain of events. Persons experiencing this difficulty often are told that nothing is wrong, which may add to their anxiety, or they are told to take a few deep breaths, which increases their symptoms. One review indicates that as many as 28% of patients in various medical populations may experience functional breathing pattern disorder.

Increased ventilation is a common component of fight-or-flight responses, but when breathing increases while actions and movements are restricted, a person is breathing in excess of metabolic need. Blood levels of carbon dioxide fall, and symptoms may occur. As a person exhales too much carbon dioxide too quickly, the blood becomes more alkaline. These biochemical changes can cause many of the following signs and symptoms:

- *Respiratory:* Symptoms include shortness of breath, typically after exertion; irritable cough; tightness or oppression in the chest; difficulty breathing; asthma; air hunger; inability to take a satisfying breath; excessive sighing, yawning, and sniffing.
- *Cardiovascular:* Symptoms include palpitations; missed beats; tachycardia; sharp or dull atypical chest pain; angina; vasomotor instability; cold extremities; Raynaud phenomenon; blotchy flushing of blush area; and capillary vasoconstriction in the face, arms, and hands.
- *Neurological:* Cerebrovascular blood vessel constriction, a primary response to breathing pattern disorder, can reduce the oxygen available to the brain by about one-half. Symptoms include dizziness, unsteadiness, or instability; feelings of fainting but rarely actual fainting; visual disturbance, such as blurred or tunnel vision; headache (often migraine); paresthesia (i.e., numbness, heaviness, "pins and needles," burning, limbs feeling out of proportion or "not belonging," commonly of hands, feet, or face, sometimes scalp or whole body); intolerance of light or noise; enlarged pupils; and sensation of giddiness.

- *Psychological*: Symptoms include tension; anxiety; tearfulness; emotional instability; feelings of unreality; depersonalization; feeling "out of one's body"; hallucinations; impaired concentration, memory, and performance; disturbed sleep, including nightmares; emotional sweating in the axillae, palms, and sometimes the whole body; fear of insanity; panic; phobias; and agoraphobia. A fear of not getting enough air is a core factor in the cause of panic attacks.
- *Gastrointestinal:* Symptoms include difficulty in swallowing, dry mouth and throat, acid regurgitation, heartburn, hiatal hernia, nausea, flatulence, belching, air swallowing, abdominal discomfort, and bloating.
- *Muscular:* Symptoms include cramps; muscle pains, particularly in the occipital region, neck, shoulders, and between scapulae and less commonly in the lower back and limbs; tremors, twitching, weakness, stiffness, or tetany (seizing up) in muscles involved in the attack posture. Affected persons hunch their shoulders, thrust their heads and necks forward, scowl, and clench their teeth. There can also be generalized body tension, feelings of weakness, and a chronic inability to relax.

All the aforementioned symptoms can lead to exhaustion.

INDICATIONS/CONTRAINDICATIONS for Therapeutic Massage

Respiratory System

In any of the disorders of the respiratory system that are of viral or bacterial origin, massage is usually contraindicated until the disease has run its course. Whenever the body is under stress (as with respiratory infection), further stress on the system can worsen the condition. Simple palliative measures to provide comfort and encourage sleep are appropriate. The practitioner should follow all sanitary procedures and standard precautions.

In chronic conditions such as asthma and emphysema, general stress management and maintenance of normal function of the muscles of respiration are beneficial as long as the appropriate added stress levels caused by the stimulation of massage are considered. In cystic fibrosis, percussion helps loosen the phlegm but should not be attempted without medical supervision and training.

Therapeutic massage approaches and moderate application of movement therapies, such as tai chi, yoga, or aerobic exercise, often help with breathing pattern disorders. Almost every meditation and relaxation system uses breathing patterns because they are a direct link to altering autonomic nervous system patterns, which in turn alters mood, feelings, and behavior. Other ways to modulate breathing are through singing and chanting.

Constant activation of the accessory muscles of respiration when these muscles are not needed during normal activity results in dysfunctional muscle patterns. The accessory breathing muscles (such as the scalenes, sternocleidomastoid, serratus posterior superior, levator scapulae, rhomboids, abdominals, and quadratus lumborum) should only be activated for forced inhalation and expiration during heavy exertion, such as running. Therapeutic massage can bring balance into these areas to encourage a more effective breathing pattern. General stress management reduces anxiety and helps normalize the breathing pattern.

Although a detailed discussion of the many forms of meditation, breathing modulation, and retraining measures is beyond the scope of this text, two basic types of systems exist: one leads to physiological hyperarousal, and one leads to hypoarousal. Both processes facilitate the reestablishment of homeostasis, just as a muscle can be encouraged to relax by tensing it first and then releasing it or by using the antagonist pattern to initiate reciprocal inhibition, thus allowing the muscle to relax. Hyperarousal systems increase sympathetic activity and elicit a secondary parasympathetic balance. Aerobic exercise is an example. Hypoarousal systems directly activate parasympathetic responses. Examples are quiet reflection or meditation-type activity combined with vocalization to promote exhalation. Many resources use retraining programs to improve breathing patterns, and the recommendation is to find one that is comfortable and use it regularly.

Section Summary

- Define *respiration. Respiration* refers to the movement of air in and out of the lungs. *External respiration* is the exchange of oxygen and carbon dioxide between the lungs and the bloodstream. *Internal respiration* is the exchange of gases between the blood and body cells.
- List the organs of the respiratory system. The organs consist of the nose/nasal cavity, sinuses, pharynx (throat), larynx (voice box), trachea (windpipe), bronchi, and lungs.
- List the muscles involved in respiration. Dominant muscles of inhalation include the diaphragm and external intercostals. Accessory muscles of inhalation include the serratus posterior superior, sternocleidomastoid, scalenes, levator scapulae, rhomboids, and pectorals. Exhalation mainly results from the elastic recoil of the alveoli. Accessory muscles of exhalation include the internal intercostals, serratus posterior inferior, quadratus lumborum, and abdominals.
- Define *lung volumes. Tidal volume* refers to the amount of air taken in or exhaled in a single breath during normal breathing. *Inspiratory reserve volume* is the amount of air that can be inhaled forcefully after normal tidal volume inspiration. *Expiratory reserve volume* is the amount of air that can be exhaled forcefully after a normal exhalation. *Reserve volume* is the amount of air that remains in the lungs and passageways after a maximal expiration. *Vital capacity* is the total of the tidal volume, inspiratory reserve volume, and expiratory reserve volume.
- Describe breathing pattern disorder. Also known as *hyperventilation* or *chronic overbreathing. Breathing pattern disorder is disorder* is a complex set of behaviors that leads to abnormally deep or rapid breathing in excess of physical demands, causing a variety of system-wide symptoms. Massage helps by reducing the tone of accessory breathing muscles and stimulating parasympathetic dominance.

DIGESTIVE SYSTEM

SECTION OBJECTIVES

Chapter objectives covered in this section:

4. Explain the interlinked physiology of the digestive system, gut microbiota, nervous system, and endocrine system.
5. List and describe the components of the digestive system.
6. Describe the process of digestion.
7. Explain the importance of nutrition.
8. List and describe the main food groups.
9. Explain metabolic rate, energy balance, and body weight.
10. Describe the pathological conditions of the digestive system and the associated indications and contraindications for massage.

After completing this section, the student will be able to perform the following:

- Explain gut microbiota and the microbiome.
- Define *digestion*.
- Describe the effects of the autonomic nervous system on digestion.
- Describe the sequence of the digestive process.
- Define the *citric acid cycle*.
- Define *metabolic rate*.

Digestion is a physiological process that involves the intake and assimilation of nutrients and the **elimination (egestion)** of waste.

The intake of food is much more than a means of obtaining nutrients for the growth, repair, and maintenance of the body. Eating is a pleasurable activity and a social event that involves many neurochemical interactions. Food choices can have effects on health risks. Biological drives for food, especially foods high in fat and simple carbohydrates or sugars, played an important part in early human survival. These foods, which are rare in nature, supply quick and sustaining energy sources. An overabundance of fat and sugar, which are no longer rare in our society, feeds the biological cravings that we still have even though the energy required to acquire these food sources has decreased.

Overview of the Functional Digestive System

Feeding behavior is regulated by many hormones. Ghrelin and leptin are the best-known of these hormones. *Ghrelin* and *leptin* are stomach hormones associated with feeding behavior and energy. When the stomach is empty, ghrelin is secreted. When the stomach is stretched, secretion stops. It acts on hypothalamic brain cells both to increase hunger and to increase gastric acid secretion and gastrointestinal motility to prepare the body for food. Leptin has a significant role in food consumption and energy balance regulation as it reduces appetite and increases energy consumption. Ghrelin is an appetite stimulant. Leptin is an appetite suppressant.

Ghrelin and leptin not only regulate hunger but also help to regulate many hormonal axes such as growth hormone, thyroid hormones, follicle-stimulating hormone, and luteinizing hormone. Ghrelin reduces leptin's effect of reducing food consumption and body weight by modulating the release of several hypothalamic peptide hormones. Peptide hormones act as neurotransmitters in neurological systems. Along with neuromodulator effects, ghrelin appears to be involved in neurodegenerative diseases, addiction, schizophrenia, mood disorders, anxiety disorders, depression, and eating disorders. Studies indicate that ghrelin also targets the brain to regulate a diverse number of functions, including learning, memory, motivation, stress responses, anxiety, and mood. Ghrelin regulates the hypothalamic-pituitary-adrenal axis and affects anxiety and mood disorders, such as depression and fear, as well as obesity and eating disorders. Wasting syndromes called cachexia or marasmus may involve ghrelin imbalance. Sleep restriction compared with normal sleep significantly increases ghrelin levels. The levels of several hormones fluctuate according to the light and dark cycle and are also affected by sleep, feeding, and general behavior. Sleep disturbance is also associated with obesity, insulin insensitivity, diabetes, hormonal imbalance, and appetite dysregulation. Elevated ghrelin may be a mechanism by which sleep loss leads to increased food intake and the development of obesity. Leptin hormone influences the release of steroid hormones by acting on the hypothalamic-pituitary-adrenal axis, which modulates the stress response, and the hypothalamic-pituitary-thyroid axis, which is responsible for the regulation of metabolism. Leptin is also involved in brain development and neuroplasticity. The complex interactions of these gut-based hormones provide another example of how our body is interconnected, and even when studied as separate structures and systems, everything influences everything (Kim et al., 2015; Kara, 2018).

Because of all the neurochemical influences on the gut, it is logical that emotional eating is one type of substitution for touch and loving relationships because it stimulates similar chemicals. Foods such as chocolate and other fat-carbohydrate combinations, along with some forms of protein, generate serotonin and other feel-good neurochemicals as effectively as a hug does. Food behaviors can become as addictive as any other pleasurable activity. Exercise also produces these neurochemicals, so moderate exercise programs are good for mood as well as weight management. Because biological tendencies favor energy conservation, and our biological patterns are designed for survival in a more primitive environment, the internal drive toward movement and activity was originally used to provide shelter, food, and protection. In modern times, we find ourselves needing to move for the sake of movement, not because it is directly critical to our survival. This is a physiologically confusing process and may be part of the reason that many people are not motivated to exercise.

MENTORING TIP

Food sensations and biological responses to food ingestion are actually similar to touch sensations and biological responses to touch, pressure, and movement. Wasting syndromes (cachexia or marasmus) can involve touch deprivation. Wasting syndrome may occur during cancer treatment and dementia, and in those who are isolated from human contact, such as elder adults living alone. As massage therapists, we need to remember that touch provided during a massage is as important to well-being as a satisfying meal.

Gut Microbiome

The digestive system, the location in the abdomen, and various associated structures can be considered the gut. Within the gut is an entire ecosystem called the **microbiota**. The microbiota consists of a wide variety of bacteria, viruses, fungi, and other single-celled animals that live in the body. The **microbiome** is the name given to all of the genes inside these microbial cells. Numerous microorganisms colonize the human gastrointestinal tract and are essential to digestion and absorption of dietary components. The human mouth has one of the most diverse microbiomes in the human body. The microorganisms living inside the gastrointestinal tract amount to around 4 pounds of biomass. There are ongoing investigations of how interactions between food components and gut microbiota may influence or even determine human health and disease. The gut microbiota plays an important role in our lives and in the way our bodies function. Our gut microbiota contains tens of trillions of bacteria—10 times more cells than in our body. These commensal bacteria live in a benedictional relationship with their host. The composition of gut microbiota is unique to each individual, just like fingerprints.

Gut microbes are associated with many psychophysiological functions, including neurodevelopment, neurotransmission, emotional experience, stress response, anxiety, depression, learning and memory, social behavior, and aging. Studies have shown that chronic fatigue, schizophrenia, blood pressure, Alzheimer's disease, and Parkinson's disease can all be affected by the condition and health of our gut (Burnet et al., 2018).

The helpful gut bacteria are known as symbiotic bacteria. These bacteria support a well-functioning digestive system where food is efficiently digested and assimilated. These bacteria also produce vitamins, digestive enzymes, and hormones. There are also parasitic bacteria that can inhabit the gut. These organisms can damage the intestinal lining, contribute to chronic systemic inflammation, and are connected to many age-related diseases (Marques et al., 2018; Sarkar et al., 2018; Spychala et al., 2018).

The gut-brain axis is the bidirectional communication between gut microbes and the brain. The vagus nerve, as well as the entire enteric division of the autonomic nervous system, transfers information between the gastrointestinal tract and the central nervous system (CNS) to modulate intestinal motility, release of neurotransmitters, and guide intestinal immune function. The sympathetic branch of the autonomic nervous system is also involved in intestinal homeostasis and gut immune regulation. The sympathetic autonomic nervous system (ANS) can stimulate both pro- and antiinflammatory effects contributing to both immune protection and inflammatory disease of the gut. Gut microbiota may also synthesize (or modulate the synthesis of) a number of neurotransmitters, including dopamine, serotonin, and noradrenaline. The neuroimmune-endocrine and the microbiome-gut-brain axes may directly or indirectly affect chronic pain (Liu et al. 2023).

Healthy adult gut microbiota has more than 1000 different bacteria. The two most studied types of bacteria are Firmicutes and Bacteroidetes. Researchers now believe that the ratio of these bacteria within the human gut might moderate whether we are obese or lean. Firmicutes as part of the gut flora have been shown to be involved in energy resorption, and they are potentially related to the development of diabetes and obesity. Researchers observe a higher ratio of Firmicutes to Bacteroidetes in obese humans, whereas in leaner humans, a higher ratio of Bacteroidetes to Firmicutes can be found (Fig. 12.5).

The digestive system is functionally complex involving intricate communication among multiple systems, especially the nervous system, endocrine system, and immune system. The gut hosts an entire ecosystem of microbes, making us superorganisms.

Organs and Structures of the Digestive System

The digestive system is one long tube with accessory organs (Fig. 12.6). It starts at the mouth, extends through the body, and ends at the anus. This tube is known as the *gastrointestinal tract* and is also referred to as the *alimentary canal*. The gastrointestinal tract is about 30 feet long and contains several special structures in its length. The entire lining is a mucous membrane made up of three layers of tissues: epithelium, connective tissue, and smooth muscle.

The digestive tract consists of the mouth, pharynx, esophagus, stomach, small intestine, large intestine, rectum, and anus. Accessory structures include the salivary glands, pancreas, liver, and gallbladder. The enteric nervous system (ENS) is responsible for orchestrating and maintaining gastrointestinal (GI) homeostasis.

Mesentery, Omentum, and Peritoneum

The mesentery is a continuous set of tissues located in the abdominal cavity. The mesentery was recently classified as an organ. Structurally it attaches the intestines to the abdominal wall and holds them in place. Functionally the mesentery is involved in inflammation regulation and dysfunction, including the development of local and systemic inflammatory diseases, potentially having a role in Crohn's disease (Coffey and O'Leary, 2016; Rivera et al., 2018).

The omentum is a fat-derived, tissue-support structure present in the abdominal cavity surrounding the gastrointestinal organs. The omentum plays a protective role during inflammation or infection, and it hangs in front of the intestines. The omentum could be categorized into two parts: the greater omentum and the lesser omentum. The greater omentum contains accumulated adipose tissue. The omentum is a layer of the peritoneum.

The peritoneum is a two-layered serous membrane lining the abdominal cavity. The parietal peritoneum lies against the abdominal wall, and the visceral peritoneum surrounds the organs of the abdomen. It is generally described as a protective barrier and secretes slippery serous fluid to provide a frictionless interphase that covers abdominal viscera.

The mesentery, omentum, and peritoneum all have multiple roles other than structure and protection. These structures contain blood vessels, nerves, lymph nodes, fat, elastic fibers for stretching, and collagen fibers for strength. All are involved in immune function, including inflammatory regulation (Isaza-Restrepo et al., 2018).

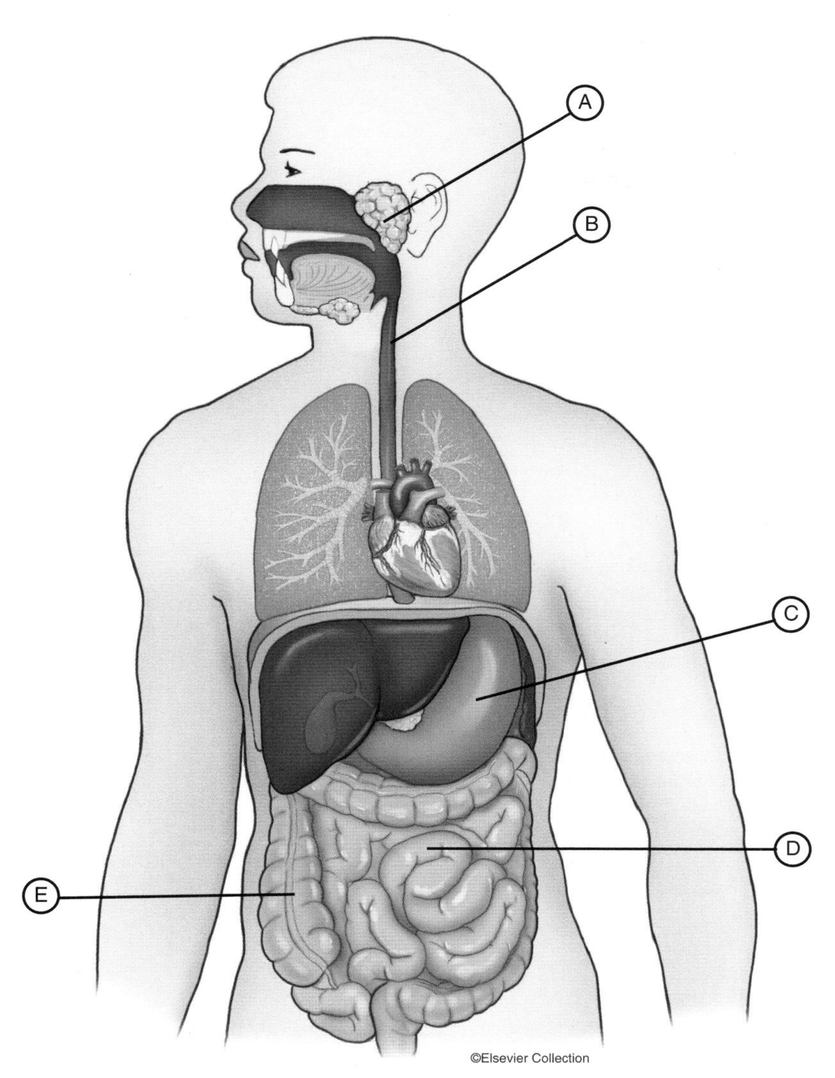

FIG. 12.5 Distribution of the normal human microbiota related to the digestive system. (A) Oral cavity—*Gemella*, *Granulicatella*, *Streptococcus*, and *Veillonella*. (B) Esophagus—*Bacteroides*, *Gemella*, *Megasphaera*, *Pseudomonas*, *Prevotella*, *Streptococcus*, *Veillonella*. (C) Stomach—*Streptococcus*, *Lactobacillus*, *Prevotella*, *Enterococcus*, *Helicobacter pylori*. (D) Small intestine—*Bacteroides*, *Clostridium*, *Streptococcus*, *Lactobacillus*, *Proteobacteria*, *Enterococcus.* (E) Cecum and colon—*Lachnospira*, *Roseburia*, *Butyrivibrio*, *Ruminococcus*, Fecalibacterium, Fusobacteria. *Streptococcus*, Enterobacterium, *Enterococcus*, *Lactobacillus*, *Peptostreptococcus*.

Adipose Tissue

The adipose tissue found in the mesentery and omentum has endocrine functions. Adipose tissue is responsible for the synthesis and secretion of several hormones. It is active in a range of processes, such as control of nutritional intake (leptin, angiotensin), control of sensitivity to insulin, and inflammatory process mediation. Adipose tissue can be classified into white adipose tissue, brown adipose tissue, and beige adipose tissue:

- White adipose tissue is the most abundant; it stores energy and secretes hormones. Subcutaneous white fat is energy storage. This is the fat removed during liposuction procedures. White visceral adipose tissue accumulates in the abdominal cavity. Visceral fat is metabolically active. The visceral fat secretes chemicals that can increase the risk of cardiovascular disease by promoting insulin resistance and chronic inflammation.
- Brown adipose tissue's major function is heat production, which is called thermogenesis. Brown fat is limited to small deposits. Adult humans have almost no brown fat, but infants do have brown fat deposits. Brown adipose tissue also regulates glucose and lipid metabolism.
- Beige adipose tissues consist of fat cells scattered throughout white fat tissue. Beige adipose tissue performs a thermoregulatory function when exposed to extreme cold. Cold, sensed by various mechanisms (including thermoreceptors in the skin), elicits sympathetic outflow, which activates beige fat. Also, during exercise muscle tissue releases the hormone *irisin*, which stimulates beige fat and converts white fat into brown fat. Irisin is released during moderate aerobic endurance activity when the cardiorespiratory system is engaged and muscles are active. Irisin appears to inhibit the formation of fatty tissue, providing another reason for the benefits of moderate exercise.

Mouth

The mouth is the oral cavity and makes up the first portion of the gastrointestinal tract. It includes the lips, cheeks, tongue, hard and soft palates, teeth, and salivary glands.

The tongue is a large, strong muscle that mixes the food particles with saliva and helps us swallow. It is the location of the taste buds.

The palate forms the roof of the mouth. The anterior hard part is the partition between the oral and nasal cavities and

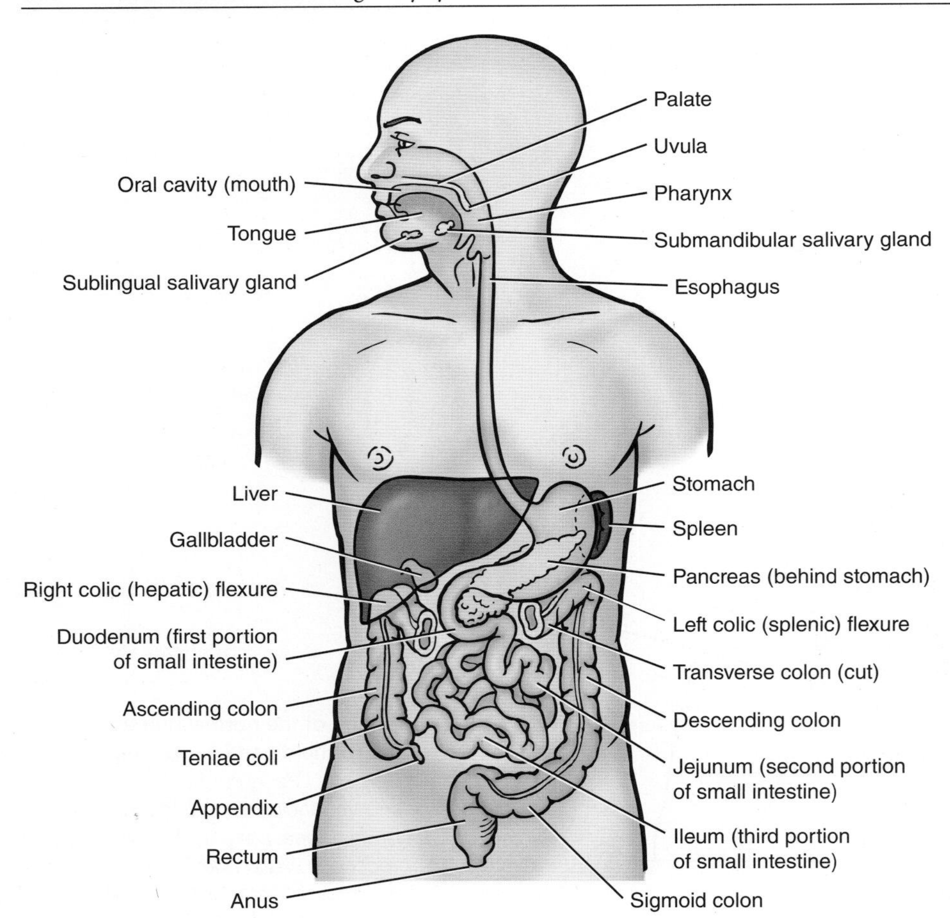

FIG. 12.6 Organs of the digestive system and some associated structures.

consists of the palatine and maxillae bones. The posterior soft portion is the partition between the oropharynx and nasopharynx.

Teeth are accessory structures used to bite off and mechanically break large pieces of food into smaller ones that can be swallowed. These bonelike structures are calcified connective tissue covered with enamel.

Salivary glands are located inside the mouth. They provide secretions that keep the mucous membrane of the mouth moist and lubricate food so that it is easier to swallow. Saliva is mainly water mixed with small amounts of salts and organic substances. One of these is the enzyme amylase, which breaks down carbohydrates. Another enzyme is lingual lipase, which begins lipid digestion. Smell, sight, taste, and the thought of food stimulate parasympathetic nerve fibers to increase the secretion of saliva. Food that has been mechanically chewed and mixed with saliva is referred to as a *bolus*.

Pharynx

The pharynx is a cavity located at the back of the mouth. It receives the bolus from the mouth.

Esophagus

The esophagus is a 10-inch muscular, collapsible tube directly behind the trachea. It extends from the pharynx to the stomach. The opening into the stomach is the esophageal hiatus, and at the point of attachment is a thickened region called the *cardiac sphincter*, which keeps the entrance to the stomach closed and prevents gastric regurgitation.

Stomach

The stomach is a J-shaped saclike organ that is an enlargement of the gastrointestinal tract. Its widest part is located beneath the diaphragm. The narrow distal end lies under the liver and empties into the duodenum. The stomach receives the bolus from the esophagus and continues the digestion process. With the addition of more liquids, the bolus breaks down and becomes a semiliquid known as *chyme*. The stomach contains folds called *rugae* that enable it to expand as food is ingested. The walls of the stomach contain gastric glands that secrete the hormone gastrin and gastric juices, including hydrochloric acid, protein-digesting enzymes, mucus, and water. The digestion of proteins begins in the stomach.

The pylorus is the part of the stomach that narrows to connect with the duodenum. The stomach ends at the pyloric sphincter, a muscle that regulates the flow of chyme into the small intestine. Some gastric cells have histamine receptors. Irritation of the stomach appears to liberate histamine, a potent stimulator of gastric acid secretion. Cimetidine (Tagamet) competes with histamine for receptor sites, thus blocking the secretion of acid and making it an effective medication for treating ulcers.

Small Intestine

The small intestine is a coiled muscular tube that is approximately 24 to 30 feet long. It consists of three parts:

- The duodenum (du-o-DE-num) is the shortest portion, making up the first 10 inches of the small intestine. The duodenum forms a C-shaped curve, circling the head of the pancreas, at which point it becomes the jejunum. Ducts from the liver, gallbladder, and pancreas enter this structure.
- The jejunum (je-JU-num) continues from the duodenum for the next 7 to 8 feet.
- The ileum (IL-e-um) makes up the final 12 feet of the small intestine. The ileum connects the small intestine to the large intestine at the ileocecal valve or sphincter.

Numerous glands located in the walls of the small intestine provide secretions for the digestive process, the primary function of the jejunum. The small intestine receives the chyme from the stomach. It continues the digestive process using intestinal juices containing enzymes secreted by the small intestine as well as secretions from the pancreas, liver, and gallbladder. The complete chemical digestion of carbohydrates, lipids, and proteins is finished in the small intestine.

Ninety percent of the absorption of food takes place in the small intestine; the other 10% occurs in the stomach and large intestine. Absorption is the movement of food molecules from the digestive tract to the cardiovascular and lymphatic systems so that they can be transported to the cells of the body.

Practical Application

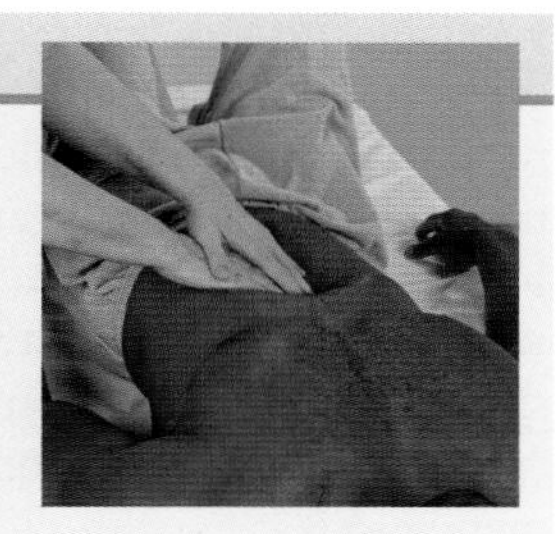

A general and non-specific massage application that targets digestive support involves a firm but nonpainful broad-based kneading and rolling of the abdomen. The goal is to support normal sliding of the internal organs and peristalsis. Deep prodding and poking of the abdomen should be avoided.

Pancreas

The pancreas is about 5 inches long and 1 inch wide. It lies behind the stomach and is connected to the duodenum by two pancreatic ducts. Most of the pancreas functions as an exocrine gland, producing pancreatic juices containing digestive enzymes. About 1% of the cells of the pancreas, the islets of Langerhans, are scattered throughout the pancreas and secrete the hormones insulin, glucagon, and somatostatin.

Liver

The largest gland of the body, weighing about 3 pounds, the liver lies under the diaphragm in the upper right quadrant. The liver has many functions, including the following:

- It is active in protein metabolism.
- It breaks down fatty acids and stores the fat we need for fuel.
- It removes glucose from the blood and stores it as glycogen when blood sugar levels are high, converting it back to glucose when blood sugar levels are low.
- It secretes bile, which is important in the digestion of lipids.
- It stores vitamins A, B_{12}, D, E, K, iron, and copper.
- It detoxifies the blood by removing drugs and hormones.
- It converts amino acids into glucose or fatty acids, depending on the needs of the body.
- It destroys old red blood cells.

Gallbladder

The gallbladder is a small 3- to 4-inch sac that lies on the undersurface of the liver; its function is to store and concentrate bile. The gallbladder releases bile into the small intestine by way of the cystic duct.

Large Intestine

The large intestine is a muscular tube, about 4 to 5 feet long and 2½ inches in diameter. The large intestine has few digestive functions but does reabsorb water and electrolytes, manufacture vitamins, and form and store the feces until defecation occurs. The large intestine, also called the *colon*, consists of eight parts:

- The cecum begins as a blind pouch about 3 inches long; it receives the digested matter from the ileum of the small intestine.
- The appendix is a narrow, twisted, close-ended tube attached to the cecum. The appendix contains lymphatic tissue, but its function has not been defined clearly.
- The ascending colon goes up on the right side of the abdomen to the underside of the liver, where it curves toward the left. This curve is known as the *hepatic flexure*.
- The transverse colon goes across the abdomen from the hepatic flexure to the spleen, where it turns downward at the splenic flexure.
- The descending colon extends down the left side of the abdomen from the splenic flexure to about the top of the iliac crest.
- The sigmoid colon forms an S-shaped curve beginning at the left iliac crest and continuing to the middle of the abdomen, where it connects the descending colon to the rectum.
- The rectum is a straight, 5- to 6-inch continuation of the sigmoid colon, beginning at about the level of S3.
- The anal canal is the last inch of the rectum, and it ends at the anus, a sphincter muscle of smooth and skeletal muscle that controls the involuntary and voluntary elimination of feces.

The colon contains large numbers of bacteria. They break down bile pigments, which results in the brown color of feces, and they produce some B vitamins and vitamin K.

Medicines often are given as rectal suppositories because the colon has great absorptive capacity. Feces are undigested matter that is eliminated from the body.

A colostomy is an artificial opening between the colon and the skin of the abdomen for the evacuation of feces. Usually done to relieve tumor obstruction, physicians can perform a colostomy as a temporary measure when inflammation or trauma is present.

Nerves

Parasympathetic stimulation by the vagus and pelvic nerves (from the sacral part of the spinal cord) increases peristalsis and the secretion of mucus, which protects the intestinal wall. Sympathetic stimulation has the opposite effect.

Digestion

The function of the digestive system is to break down foods so that they can be assimilated by the body. Digestion begins in the mouth and ends in the small intestine (Fig. 12.7), and it is accompanied by digestive enzymes that split large food particles into substances small enough to pass through the wall of the digestive tract into the blood and lymph capillaries. The gastrointestinal tract contains glands that secrete mucus and digestive enzymes (Table 12.1).

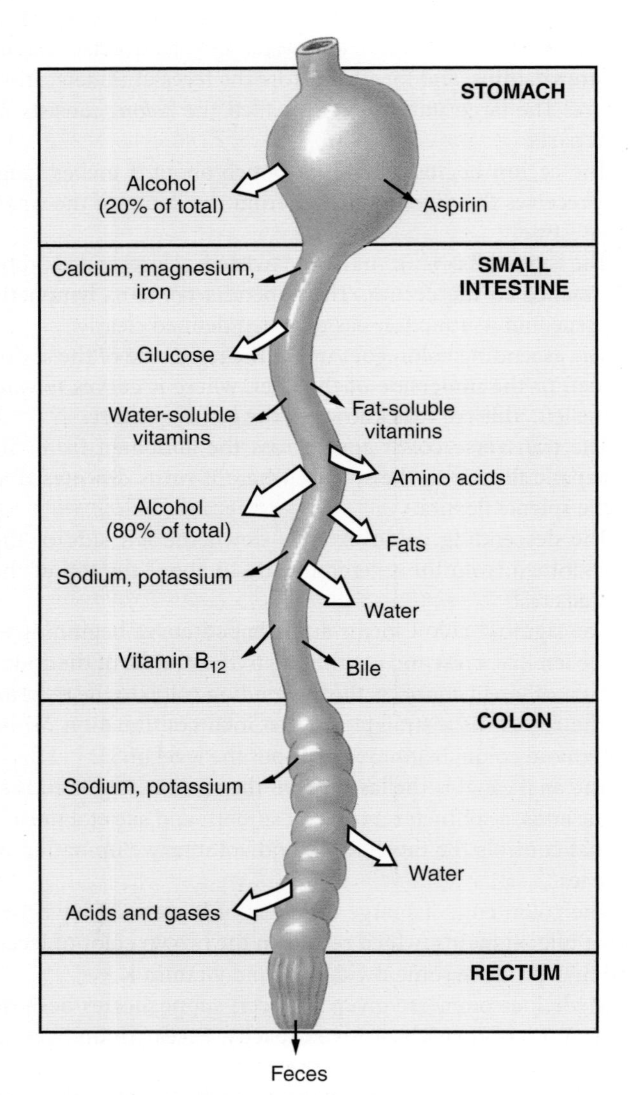

FIG. 12.7 Absorption sites in the digestive tract. The size of the arrow at each site indicates the amount of absorption of a particular substance at that site. Most absorption occurs in the intestines, particularly the small intestine. (From Patton KT, Thibodeau GA. *Anatomy and Physiology.* 6th ed. Mosby/Elsevier; 2007.)

The rhythmic contraction of smooth muscle, called **peristalsis**, propels products of digestion along the tract from the esophagus to the anus (Fig. 12.8). This is a form of mechanical digestion.

Box 12.1 shows the four essential steps in the process of digestion. *Digestion secretion* generally refers to the release of various substances from the exocrine glands that serve the digestive system (Table 12.2). Digestive secretion includes the release of saliva, gastric juice, pancreatic juice, bile, and intestinal enzymes.

Citric Acid Cycle

The citric acid cycle (Krebs cycle) is the main pathway by which food energy is released by cells to manufacture energy-rich adenosine triphosphate (ATP). The citric acid cycle is a complex transformation process. The result of many chemical reactions is energy for cellular function (Fig. 12.9).

Nutrition

Nutrition is the use of food for the growth and maintenance of the body. Poor nutrition has an effect on general health, stress responses, and sleeping. For most people, nutritional problems result from not following dietary recommendations. In elder adults, a decreased ability to digest and assimilate food may result in poor nutrition. Others may have diseases that can cause nutritional deficiencies. Food affects mood. Mood influences feelings. Behavior supports feelings, and the whole issue of food is often an emotional topic.

The basics of good nutrition include eating a diet high in vegetables, grains, legumes, and fruits that are fresh, clean, and grown in nutrient-rich soil. Human protein requirements are moderate and may be met by food from animal or non-animal sources. Fat and sugar requirements in the diet are small, but human beings have a strong urge for fats and sweets. An ideal diet is low to moderate in natural fats (hydrogenated fats should be avoided), sugars, and protein, with the bulk of the calories coming from complex carbohydrates. These recommendations vary with differing genetic predispositions, ages, and states of health, which influence the ratio of fats, proteins, and carbohydrates that best suit an individual.

The food we eat is only as good as the soil in which it is grown or the food the animals are fed. Many suggest that much of the soil used in agriculture is worn out, depleted, and toxic because of the continuous use of artificial fertilizers and pesticides and that the land has been overused and denied rest time to replenish itself. If this is the condition of the soil, what is the nutritional value of the food grown in it? Food is most nutritious when freshly harvested and ripe. Food eaten a day after harvest has already lost a substantial number of nutrients. Food, mostly fruit, picked green is not as nutritious as fruit allowed to ripen on the vine. All food-preservation methods result in a loss of the food's nutritional value. Under ideal conditions, we would harvest all of our food an hour before we eat it, but this is not possible for most of us. We have to make a trade-off between convenience and nutrition.

Many people take nutritional supplements, and many opinions exist on this topic. It must be remembered that these are supplements to our diet and should not be expected to replace

Table 12.1 Chemical Digestion

Digestive Juices and Enzymes	Substance Digested (or Hydrolyzed)	Resulting Product[a]
Saliva		
Amylase	Starch (polysaccharide)	Maltose (a double sugar, or disaccharide)
Gastric juice		
Protease (pepsin) plus hydrochloric acid	Proteins	Partially digested proteins
Pancreatic juice		
Proteases (e.g., trypsin)[b]	Proteins (intact or partially digested)	Peptides and *amino acids*
Lipases	Fats emulsified by bile	Fatty acids, monoglycerides, and glycerol
Amylase	Starch	Maltose
Nucleases	Nucleic acids (DNA, RNA)	Nucleotides
Intestinal enzymes[c]		
Peptidases	Peptides	Amino acids
Sucrase	Sucrose (cane sugar)	*Glucose* and *fructose*[d] (simple sugars, or monosaccharides)
Lactase	Lactose (milk sugar)	*Glucose* and *galactose* (simple sugars)
Maltase	Maltose (malt sugar)	Glucose
Nucleotidases and phosphatases	Nucleotides	Nucleosides

Modified from Patton KT, Thibodeau GA. *Anatomy and Physiology.* 7th ed. Mosby/Elsevier; 2010.
DNA, Deoxyribonucleic acid; *RNA*, ribonucleic acid.
[a]Substances in italic type are end products of digestion (i.e., completely digested nutrients ready for absorption).
[b]Secreted in an inactive form (trypsinogen); activated by enterokinase, an enzyme in the intestinal brush border.
[c]Brush-border enzymes.
[d]Glucose is also called *dextrose;* fructose is also called *levulose*.

proper food intake. The closer a supplement is to real food, the better the body is able to use it. Supplements usually are best taken with food to maximize absorption and use.

For the intestinal tract to function effectively, it is necessary to eat dietary fiber. Fiber is especially important for colon health. When combined with water, fiber expands or bulks in the colon, making the stool easier to pass.

Drinking a sufficient quantity of pure water is important for optimal body function. Recommendations are for at least 64 ounces of water per day for efficient body function.

Main Food Groups

Proteins

Proteins are large, high-molecular-weight substances containing carbon, hydrogen, oxygen, nitrogen, and small amounts of other elements. Proteins break down into amino acids, which the body then absorbs. The body's metabolic requirements include 24 amino acids. Most can be manufactured in the liver from other amino acids, but eight cannot. These eight are referred to as *essential amino acids:* phenylalanine, valine, threonine, leucine, isoleucine, methionine, tryptophan, and lysine. In addition, histidine and arginine are required for growth and development. Dietary proteins include animal products and bean and grain combinations.

Proteins are the chief structural components of the body. Enzymes, some hormones, muscle tissue, and a substantial portion of chromosomes are proteins. Proteins are essential components of the cell membrane. Important compounds (such as epinephrine and acetylcholine) are derived from amino acids.

Carbohydrates

Carbohydrates have basic components—carbon, hydrogen, and oxygen—in precise proportions. Complex carbohydrates are long chains of sugar molecules found in rice, vegetables, and so on. These long chains are called *polysaccharides*. Simple carbohydrates are sugars and consist of single sugar molecules, called *monosaccharides*, or double sugar molecules, called *disaccharides*. Animal starch, or glycogen, is the form glucose takes for storage in the liver and muscle. All carbohydrates are digested into one of several types of monosaccharides. All types of monosaccharides are converted into glucose by the liver because glucose is the main fuel for the manufacture of ATP in the cells.

Lipids

Lipids, or triglycerides, are broken down into fatty acids and glycerol by the digestive system. A fatty acid is a molecule consisting of a chain of carbons with no double bonds (saturated) or several double bonds (unsaturated). The unsaturated fats most closely resemble body fat and are more easily assimilated and used. Saturation (the addition of hydrogen molecules)

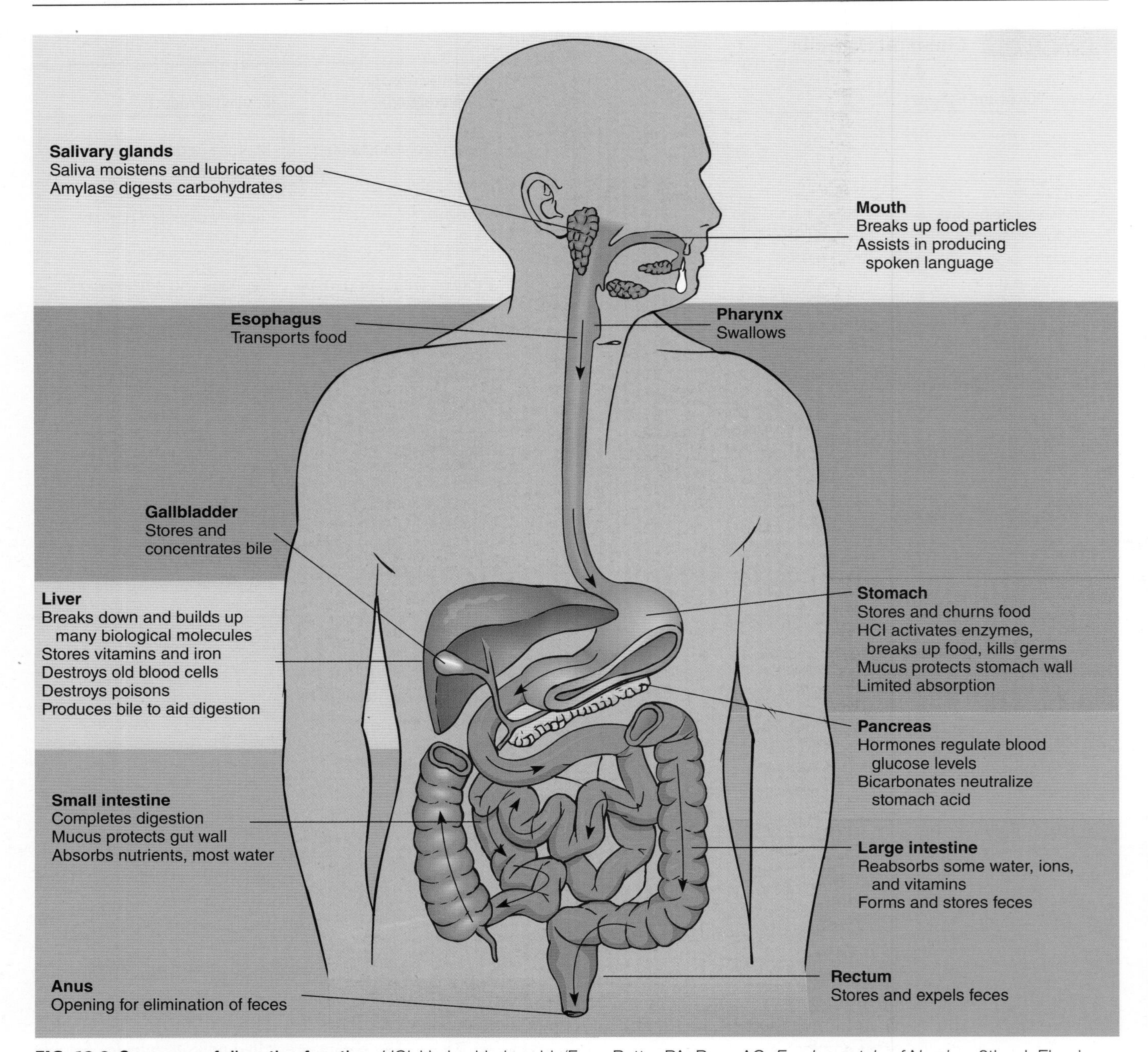

FIG. 12.8 Summary of digestive function. *HCl*, Hydrochloric acid. (From Potter PA, Perry AG. *Fundamentals of Nursing.* 8th ed. Elsevier; 2013.)

Box 12.1 Steps in the Digestion Process

Step 1
Ingestion: Food enters the mouth (i.e., eating).

Step 2
Digestion: The mechanical and chemical breakdown of food from its complex form into simple molecules.

Step 3
Absorption: The movement of the simple molecules from the digestive tract into the cardiovascular or lymphatic systems; vitamins and minerals are absorbed in the small intestine; amino acids, simple sugars, and small fatty acids pass through the intestinal villi into the bloodstream; larger fatty acids are reconstituted to fats in the intestinal wall and pass into the specialized lymphatic capillaries; capillaries of the intestinal villi become venules and then veins, and finally the large portal vein carries absorbed foodstuffs to the liver; and the liver converts these substances into compounds required for body functions.

Step 4
Elimination (egestion): Removal and release by defecation of solid waste products (feces) from food that cannot be digested or absorbed.

Table 12.2 Digestive Secretions

Secretion	Source	Substance	Functional Role
Saliva	Salivary glands	Mucus	Lubricates bolus of food; facilitates mixing of food
		Amylase	Enzyme; begins digestion of starches
		Sodium bicarbonate	Increases pH (for optimum amylase function)
		Water	Dilutes food and other substances; facilitates mixing
Gastric juice	Gastric glands	Pepsin	Enzyme; digests proteins
		Hydrochloric acid	Denatures proteins; decreases pH (for optimum pepsin function)
		Intrinsic factor	Protects and allows later absorption of vitamin B_{12}
		Mucus	Lubricates chyme; protects the stomach lining
		Water	Dilutes food and other substances; facilitates mixing
Pancreatic juice	Pancreas (exocrine portion)	Proteases (trypsin, chymotrypsin, collagenase, elastase)	Enzymes; digest proteins and polypeptides
		Lipases (lipase, phospholipase)	Enzymes; digest lipids
		Colipase	Coenzyme; helps lipase digest fats
		Nucleases	Enzymes; digest nucleic acids (RNA and DNA)
		Amylase	Enzyme; digests starches
		Water	Dilutes food and other substances; facilitates mixing
		Mucus	Lubricates
		Sodium bicarbonate	Increases pH (for optimum enzyme function)
Bile	Liver (stored and concentrated in the gallbladder)	Lecithin and bile salts	Emulsify lipids
		Sodium bicarbonate	Increases pH (for optimum enzyme function)
		Cholesterol	Excess cholesterol from body cells, to be excreted with feces
		Products of detoxification	From detoxification of harmful substances by hepatic cells, to be excreted with feces
		Bile pigments (mainly bilirubin)	Products of breakdown of heme groups during hemolysis, to be excreted with feces
		Mucus	Lubrication
		Water	Dilutes food and other substances; facilitates mixing
Intestinal juice	Mucosa of small and large intestine	Mucus	Lubrication
		Sodium bicarbonate	Increases pH (for optimum enzyme factor)
		Water	Small amount to carry mucus and sodium bicarbonate

From Thibodeau GA, Patton KT. *Anatomy and Physiology.* 7th ed. Mosby/Elsevier; 2010.
DNA, Deoxyribonucleic acid; *RNA*, ribonucleic acid.

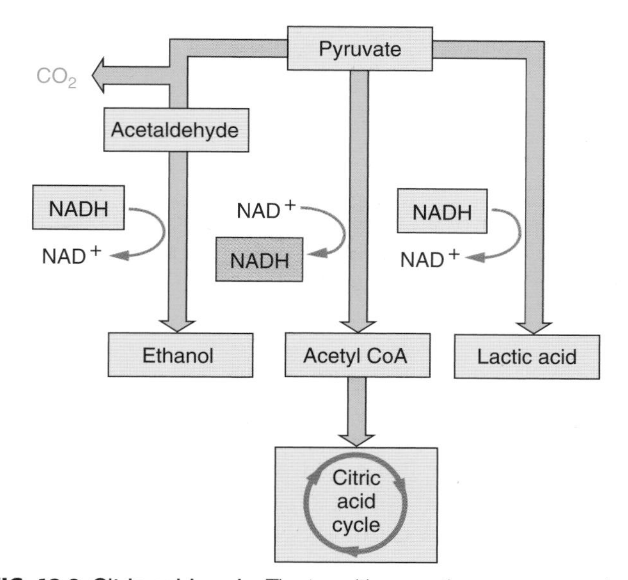

FIG. 12.9 Citric acid cycle. The transition reaction prepares each pyruvic acid molecule to enter the citric acid cycle, yielding a pair of high-energy electrons and a carbon dioxide (CO_2) molecule. Coenzyme A (*CoA*) picks up the acetyl group thus formed and takes it into the citric acid cycle proper, which is described here as a recurring series of eight steps. *ATP*, Adenosine triphosphate; *FADH₂*, hydroquinone form of flavin adenine dinucleotide; *NADH*, nicotinamide adenine dinucleotide (NAD) + hydrogen (H). (From Huether SE, McCance, KL. *Understanding Pathophysiology.* 5th ed. Mosby; 2012.)

makes fat more solid and less desirable in the diet. Linoleic acid is an example of a fatty acid essential to human nutrition. In addition to serving as a reservoir of stored energy, fats are essential components of many hormones, the cell membrane, and the myelin sheath of the nerve fiber. Dietary fats are found in nuts, seeds, oils, and animal products.

Vitamins

Vitamins are growth factors needed in small amounts for daily body metabolism. They are classified as fat soluble or water soluble. Many vitamins act as enzyme activators and are called *coenzymes.* The fat-soluble vitamins are more toxic because excess amounts are stored in the fat tissue and are not excreted readily. Water-soluble vitamins, however, are absorbed and excreted more easily (Table 12.3).

Minerals

Minerals are important for the formation of bones and teeth and the function of muscle, blood, and nerve cells. They are vital to overall mental and physical well-being. Minerals act as catalysts for many biological reactions within the body, including muscle response, the transmission of messages through the nervous system, and the utilization of nutrients in food.

Vitamins cannot be assimilated without the aid of minerals. Although the body can manufacture a few vitamins, it

Table 12.3 Functions and Sources of Vitamins

Vitamin	Function	Food Source	Adult Recommended Daily Allowance
Fat-soluble			
Vitamin A	Healthy mucous membranes, skin, and hair; essential for bone development and growth; component for the pigments in the retina needed for night vision	Milk and cheese; yellow, orange, and green vegetables	800–1000 µg
Vitamin D	Formation and development of bones and teeth; assists in absorption of calcium	Fortified milk, fish oils; made in the skin when exposed to sunlight	5–10 µg
Vitamin E	Conserves certain fatty acids; aids in protection against cell membrane damage	Whole grains, wheat germ, vegetable oils, nuts, green leafy vegetables	8–10 µg
Vitamin K	Needed for synthesis of factors essential in blood clotting	Green leafy vegetables, cabbage; synthesized by bacteria in the intestine	65–80 µg
Water soluble			
Thiamine (B_1)	Release of energy from carbohydrates and amino acids; growth; proper functioning of the nervous system	Whole grains, legumes, nuts	1.5 mg
Riboflavin (B_2)	Helps transform nutrients into energy; involved in the citric acid cycle	Whole grains, milk, green vegetables, nuts	1.7 mg
Niacin (B_3)	Helps transform nutrients into energy; involved in glycolysis and citric acid cycle	Whole grains, nuts, legumes, fish, liver	20 mg
Pyridoxine (B_6)	Involved in amino acid metabolism	Legumes, poultry, nuts, dried fruit, green vegetables	2 mg
Cyanocobalamin (B_{12})	Aids in the formation of red blood cells; helps in nervous system function	Dairy products, eggs, fish, poultry	2 µg
Pantothenic acid	Part of coenzyme A; functions in steroid synthesis; helps in nutrient metabolism	Legumes, nuts, green vegetables, milk, poultry	7 mg
Folic acid	Aids in the formation of hemoglobin and nucleic acids	Green vegetables, legumes, nuts, fruit juices, whole grains	200 µg
Biotin	Fatty acid synthesis; movement of pyruvic acid into the citric acid cycle	Eggs; made by intestinal bacteria	0.3 mg
Ascorbic acid (C)	Important in collagen synthesis; helps maintain capillaries; aids in absorption of iron	Citrus fruits, tomatoes, green vegetables, berries	60 mg

From Applegate E. *The Anatomy and Physiology Learning System.* 4th ed. Saunders/Elsevier; 2011.
µg, Microgram; *mg*, milligram.

cannot manufacture a single mineral. All tissue and internal fluids contain varying quantities of minerals (Table 12.4 and Box 12.2).

Metabolic Rate

The metabolic rate is the catabolic rate or rate of energy release. The basal metabolic rate (BMR) is not the minimum metabolic rate and does not indicate the smallest amount of energy that must be expended to sustain life. The BMR does indicate, however, the smallest amount of energy expenditure that can sustain life and also maintain the waking state and a normal body temperature in a comfortably warm environment. The BMR is the rate of energy expenditure under basal conditions, such as the following:

- When an individual is awake but lying down and not moving
- When an individual has not eaten for 18 to 23 hours
- When an individual is in a comfortably warm environment

The BMR is not identical for all individuals because of the influence of the following factors.

Size

BMR is calculated on the basis of the individual's height and weight. A large individual has more surface area and a greater BMR than a small individual.

Sex

Males oxidize their food approximately 5% to 7% faster than females, so a male has a BMR greater than a female of the same size. This sex difference in BMR results from the difference in the proportion of body fat, which is determined by sex hormones. Females tend to have a higher percentage of body fat (and thus a lower total lean mass) than males. Fat tissue is less metabolically active than lean tissues, such as muscle. Also, testosterone, found in much higher levels in males, increases metabolic rate. People who are pregnant or lactating, however, have a greatly increased BMR.

Age

The younger the individual, the higher the BMR for a given size and sex.

Table 12.4 Functions and Sources of Selected Minerals

Mineral	Function	Food Source	Adult Recommended Daily Allowance
Calcium	Component of bones and teeth; muscle contraction; blood clotting	Dairy products, green vegetables, legumes, nuts	800–1000 μg
Chloride	Acid-base balance of the blood; component of hydrochloric acid in the stomach	Table salt, milk, eggs, meat	750 mg
Phosphorus	Component of bones and teeth; component of ATP and nucleic acids; component of cell membranes	Legumes, dairy products, nuts, poultry, lean meats	800 mg
Sodium	Regulates body fluid volume; nerve impulse conduction	Table salt is the biggest source of sodium in the diet	500 mg
Potassium	Body fluid balance; muscle contraction; nerve impulse conduction	Fruits, legumes, nuts, vegetables; widely distributed	2000 mg
Magnesium	Component of some active enzymes; releases energy from nutrients	Whole grains, legumes, green vegetables, nuts	280–350 mg
Iron	Component of hemoglobin and myoglobin; releases energy from nutrients	Whole grains, nuts, legumes, poultry, fish, lean meats	10–15 mg
Iodine	Component of thyroid hormones	Iodized table salt, dairy products, fish	150 μg
Zinc	Component of several enzymes; formation of proteins; wound healing	Legumes, poultry, nuts, whole grains, fish, lean meats	12–15 mg
Fluoride	Healthy bones and teeth	Fluoridated water is the best source	1.5–4 mg

From Applegate E. *The Anatomy and Physiology Learning System.* 4th ed. Saunders/Elsevier; 2011.
ATP, Adenosine triphosphate; *μg*, microgram; *mg*, milligram.

Box 12.2 Nutritional Databases

The National Institutes of Health sponsors the Office of Dietary Supplements (http://ods.od.nih.gov) to provide safety and effectiveness information about supplements that are free of commercial influence. Medline Plus provides information about herbs and supplements.

The basics of balanced nutrition are explained in the Department of Agriculture's guide to good eating. These newer recommendations have reconfigured the previous six-section MyPyramid guide into MyPlate (www.ChooseMyPlate.gov). MyPlate illustrates the five food groups that are the building blocks for a healthy diet by using a place setting for a meal. The idea is to think about what goes on your plate or in your cup or bowl before you eat. The segmented place setting provides the proper proportions for how much of each food group you should be eating at each meal. A list of suggestions for each food group is also provided, as well as how much is needed, what constitutes a serving size, the health benefits and nutrients, and tips to help you eat from that food group. Daily food plans based on demographical (e.g., moms, preschoolers), sample menus and recipes, and a SuperTracker to help you plan, analyze, and track your diet and physical activity are all also included.

The United States Department of Agriculture (USDA), in conjunction with the U.S. Department of Health and Human Services (HHS), also publishes *The Dietary Guidelines for Americans*, which describes a healthy diet as one that does the following:

- Emphasizes fruits, vegetables, whole grains, and fat-free or low-fat milk and milk products
- Includes lean meats, poultry, fish, beans, eggs, and nuts
- Is low in saturated fats, trans fats, cholesterol, salt (sodium), and added sugars

The recommendations in the *Dietary Guidelines* and in MyPlate are for the general public over 2 years of age. MyPlate helps individuals use the *Dietary Guidelines* to do the following:

- Make smart choices from every food group
- Find a balance between food and physical activity
- Get the most nutrition out of calories
- Stay within daily caloric needs

Thyroid Hormones

Thyroid hormones (triiodothyronine [T_3] and thyroxine [T_4]) stimulate basal metabolism. Homeostasis depends on having thyroid hormones within normal ranges.

Body Temperature

An increase in body temperature increases BMR. A decrease in body temperature (hypothermia) has the opposite effect.

Drugs

Stimulants increase the BMR, and depressants decrease the BMR. The total metabolic rate is the amount of energy used or expended by the body in a given time. The BMR usually constitutes about 55% to 60% of the total metabolic rate. The energy used to do all kinds of skeletal muscle work contributes to the total metabolic rate. The metabolic rate increases for several hours after a meal, apparently because of the energy needed to metabolize foods.

The body attempts to maintain a state of energy balance; its energy input should equal its energy output. Energy input per day equals the total calories (kilocalories) in the food ingested per day. Energy output equals the total metabolic rate expressed in kilocalories. Energy intake versus output determines body weight.

Body weight remains constant (except for possible variations in water content) when the body maintains energy balance. Weight increases when energy input exceeds energy output, and the body synthesizes and stores fat. It decreases when energy input is less than energy output.

Pathological Conditions of the Digestive System

Digestive diseases can affect all organs and functions of the digestive system. These disorders have many causes, including acute and chronic infections, cancer, adverse effects of drugs and toxins, genetic predisposition, birth defects, and lifestyle choices. In many cases the cause of the disease is unknown.

Obesity

Obesity is defined as an abnormal or excessive accumulation of fat that may impair health, and it is a chronic disease. Excessive intake of calories that are not used is stored as fat. Obesity occurs with increases in fat cell number, fat cell size, or a combination of the two. There is evidence that low-grade inflammation within the adipose tissue predisposes one to obesity. Obesity is an epidemic affecting children and adults. The etiology of obesity is a complex interaction among genetics, hormones, and the environment. Obesity is associated with an increased risk of comorbidities or the simultaneous presence of two chronic diseases or conditions. Comorbid with obesity are type 2 diabetes mellitus, cardiovascular diseases, respiratory disorders, infertility, some forms of cancers, psychological and social problems, and functional limitations, which can have a substantial, negative impact on quality of life. The treatment of obesity and associated comorbidity is straining the healthcare system.

Obesity is now viewed as a state of systemic, chronic low-grade inflammation. In obesity, proinflammatory macrophages accumulate in adipose tissue and trigger chronic low-grade inflammation. The endocannabinoid system is a key player in adipose tissue regulation (van Eenige et al., 2018). The inflammatory process and endocannabinoid involvement may support a biologically plausible justification for the value of massage therapy in a multidisciplinary intervention for obesity.

Weight-Loss Surgery

There are three types of bariatric operations used most often: gastric band, gastric bypass, and gastric sleeve. Bariatric surgery can improve many health problems related to obesity, such as type 2 diabetes, high blood pressure, unhealthy cholesterol levels, and sleep apnea. Surgery also may lead to improved physical function and mood, and better quality of life. Bariatric surgery may cause side effects right after surgery or later. Side effects may include infection, diarrhea, nutritional shortages, gallstones, and hernias. *Dumping syndrome* is a condition that can develop after weight-loss surgery Also called rapid gastric emptying, dumping syndrome occurs when food, especially sugar, moves from the stomach into the small bowel too quickly. Most people with dumping syndrome develop signs and symptoms, such as abdominal cramps and diarrhea, 10 to 30 minutes after eating. Other people have symptoms 1 to 3 hours after eating, and still others have both early and late symptoms. Dumping syndrome can be managed by dietary changes including eating smaller meals and limiting high-sugar foods. People with more serious cases of dumping syndrome may need medications or surgery.

Prescription Medications to Treat Obesity

The Federal Drug Administration FDA has approved medications for long-term use for weight loss. Researchers are working to identify safer and more effective medications to help people lose weight and maintain a healthy weight for a long time. The medications mimic hormones that target areas of the brain that regulate appetite and food intake. Side effects include diarrhea, upset stomach (nausea or vomiting), heartburn, gas, or constipation.

Eating Disorders

Eating disorders are caused by a complex interaction of genetic, biological, behavioral, psychological, and social factors. Eating disorders are serious and often fatal illnesses that cause severe disturbances to a person's eating behaviors. Obsessions with food, body weight, and shape may be indications of an eating disorder.

Common eating disorders include anorexia nervosa, bulimia nervosa, and binge-eating disorder. People with anorexia nervosa may see themselves as overweight, even when they are dangerously underweight. People with anorexia nervosa severely restrict the amount of food they eat and eat small quantities of only certain foods. Anorexia nervosa has the highest mortality rate of any mental disorder. Although many young people with this disorder die from complications associated with starvation, others die from suicide.

People with bulimia nervosa have frequent episodes of eating unusually large amounts of food and feeling a lack of control over these episodes. This binge eating is followed by behavior that compensates for the overeating, such as forced vomiting, excessive use of laxatives or diuretics, fasting, excessive exercise, or a combination of these behaviors. People with bulimia nervosa usually maintain what is considered relatively normal weight, so the condition can go undetected. People with binge-eating disorder lose control over their eating behaviors. Binge-eating disorder is likely the most common eating disorder. Unlike bulimia nervosa, periods of binge eating are not followed by purging, excessive exercise, or fasting. As a result, people with binge-eating disorder often are overweight or obese.

Treatment for an eating disorder requires a multidisciplinary approach involving medical care, medications, and ongoing monitoring. Nutritional guidance and various forms of psychological counseling are necessary. It is important for the massage therapist to be supportive of the integrated treatment process. Massage therapy is useful as a stress management approach.

Constipation

Constipation is difficulty passing stools or an incomplete or infrequent passage of hard stool. Among the causes are dehydration, insufficient dietary fiber intake, intestinal obstruction, diverticulitis, and tumors. Functional impairment of the colon may occur in elder adults or bedridden clients who fail to respond to the urge to defecate. Backache and headache may be present. Constipation and diarrhea are common side effects of many medications. Increasing fluid, dietary fiber, and exercise may be helpful. Stool softeners may be prescribed for constipation. Education about regular bowel habits may be necessary.

Hemorrhoids

Hemorrhoids are dilated varicose veins of the anus. They can be due to constipation; straining to defecate causes the anal veins to become varicose. Hemorrhoids also often appear during pregnancy and delivery. External hemorrhoids lie distal to the anorectal margin; internal hemorrhoids lie proximal. Occasionally, a thrombus or clot forms, resulting in a painful, bluish mass. Hemorrhoids may cause pain, but the usual symptom is bleeding and itching caused by the drying up of the protective mucus. The primary treatment is sitz baths, steroid creams or suppositories, and stool softeners. The clot may be removed surgically under local anesthesia. Hemorrhoids also are treatable by laser to seal the blood vessels, cryosurgery, or surgical removal.

Gastroenteritis

Gastroenteritis is a general term for irritation, inflammation, or infection of the gastrointestinal tract. If the stomach is involved, the condition is called *gastritis*. Hemorrhagic gastritis is characterized by bleeding erosions and is also called *acute erosive gastritis* or *multiple gastric erosions*. It can occur without any apparent reason. It is associated, however, with aspirin ingestion, burns, traumatic injury, surgery, shock, liver disease, respiratory problems, and septicemia and can cause vomiting and diarrhea and lead to dehydration.

If the intestine is affected, the condition is called *enteritis*. Usually, the stomach and intestine are involved, so the term *gastroenteritis* applies. The most common cause is a virus, which can be passed from person to person. This stomach flu usually lasts 24 to 36 hours. If the cause is a bacterial toxin, the condition is food poisoning. Occasionally, bacterial infection or, rarely, protozoal infection, such as that involved in dysentery, causes enteritis. Food poisoning, caused by toxic foods, poisonous mushrooms, and so on, is implicated in many cases. Gastroenteritis can become dangerous if infectious organisms or toxic substances enter the bloodstream. The inflammation also may result from illness or dietary changes, especially when food and water are ingested in foreign countries, or may result from an extended use of antibiotics.

Diarrhea and generalized cramping abdominal pain are symptoms of the condition. The primary treatment is rehydration and relaxing the hyperactive bowel. Ingesting only fluids for 24 hours relaxes the intestine because food stimulates gastrointestinal hormone release and peristalsis. Several compounds slow the bowel; they include bismuth subsalicylate (Pepto-Bismol), diphenoxylate with atropine (Lomotil), and anticholinergic antispasmodics, such as dicyclomine (Bentyl). If a stool culture shows a bacterial or protozoal infection, an antibiotic or antiprotozoal is given.

Gut Microbiota Dysfunction

The intestinal bacteria prevent infection by interfering with pathogens. If, however, there is disruption in the microbiota, potentially pathogenic organisms such as *Clostridium difficile* can become active. Antibiotics that upset the normal bacterial balance can favor both infection by exogenous pathogens and overgrowth by endogenous pathogens. If the bowel wall is breached, enteric bacteria can escape into the peritoneum and cause peritonitis and abscesses.

Bacterial Diarrheas

Enterotoxin-Mediated Diarrheas

Enterotoxigenic bacteria, such as *Vibrio cholerae* and enterotoxigenic *Escherichia coli* strains, colonize the upper bowel and cause watery diarrhea by producing an enterotoxin that stimulates mucosal cells to secrete.

Invasive Diarrheas

Invasive bacteria, such as *Shigella* and *Campylobacter*, penetrate the intestinal mucosa. A bloody, mucoid diarrheal stool with inflammatory exudate is produced.

Viral Diarrheas

Rotavirus and Calicivirus (formerly Norwalk virus) are major causes of diarrheal disease. Rotavirus diarrhea affects mostly young children; Calicivirus causes disease in all age groups.

Norovirus infection can cause the sudden onset of severe vomiting and diarrhea. The virus is highly contagious and commonly spread through food or water that is contaminated during preparation or contaminated surfaces.

Parasitic Diarrheas

Some protozoa (especially *Entamoeba histolytica* and *Giardia lamblia*) as well as some intestinal helminths can cause diarrheal disease.

Irritable Bowel Syndrome

Irritable bowel syndrome is also known as spastic, or irritable, colon. Symptoms include abdominal pain, alternating constipation and diarrhea, nausea, and gas. Poor diet, tension, and emotional problems can induce irritable bowel syndrome. The condition is considered a microbiota-related condition. Peristaltic action is not well coordinated and results in changes in the pattern of bowel movements. Primary treatment includes a diet high in fiber, restriction of alcohol and tobacco, a psyllium laxative (such as Metamucil), and perhaps an anticholinergic medication (such as dicyclomine). A comprehensive stress management program is beneficial.

Inflammatory Bowel Disease

Two inflammatory diseases of the gastrointestinal tract affect mainly young people between the ages of 20 and 40, causing ulcerative lesions and thickening of the intestinal wall. The cause of both is unknown, but autoimmunity may be a factor. Ulcerative colitis affects primarily the sigmoid colon, with symptoms of lower abdominal pain and bloody diarrhea. Ulcers develop inside the large intestine. Regional enteritis is a chronic inflammation of the intestine, most commonly the ileum, and is known as Crohn's disease. It presents symptoms of cramping, right lower quadrant pain, and intermittent diarrhea. One or two attacks may occur, or they may occur regularly. The body does not absorb nutrients and loses weight. Some experts suggest that changes in the gut microbiome may play a role. Certain types of bacteria taking over the gut may contribute to inflammatory bowel disease, including Crohn's disease. Doctors treat Crohn's disease with medicines, bowel rest, and surgery. The goal of treatment is to decrease the inflammation, prevent flare-ups, and support remission.

Reflux Esophagitis/Gastroesophageal Reflux Disease

Reflux esophagitis, also known as gastroesophageal reflux disease (GERD), is the regurgitation of gastric acid up through an open esophageal sphincter, causing heartburn. This is usually caused by problems with control of the esophageal sphincter that may be due to a hiatal hernia or another, less common pathological condition. However, reflux esophagitis also may be caused by physical corrosion resulting from components in the diet, such as tobacco, alcohol, and acidic food. Lying flat or bending over often aggravates the discomfort and sitting upright relieves it. Reflux esophagitis commonly occurs in obese persons. Inflammation or ulceration of the esophagus is present. The primary treatment is weight loss if the person is overweight, which decreases the pressure on the abdominal structures and relieves the hiatal hernia, and the use of an antacid.

Peptic Ulcer Disease

A peptic ulcer is a gastric or duodenal ulcer that affects the lining of the esophagus, stomach, or duodenum. The sore can perforate the wall of the digestive tract. The term *peptic* means that pepsin is involved. Risk factors include being male, smoking, genetic predisposition, alcohol use, and stress. There is also a correlation with a bacterial infection caused by the organism *Helicobacter pylori*. Increased secretion of hydrochloric acid and pepsin and decreased tissue resistance contribute to the process. The normal protective mechanisms of the duodenal and gastric mucosa against hydrochloric acid and pepsin are blocked, and excessive vagal stimulation is present. The ulcer causes pain and may erode a vessel and cause bleeding. The ulcer may perforate the intestinal or stomach wall, causing peritonitis and shock. Studies indicate that a bacterial infection may cause many ulcers, and treatment involves the use of antibiotics.

Common signs and symptoms of peptic ulcer disease include the following:

- Heartburn or burning pain a ½ to 2 hours after a meal, relieved by antacids
- Vomiting of brownish-black material (the color of coffee grounds) or the passage of dark stools, indicating the presence of blood after perforation
- Tenderness on palpation of the epigastric region of the abdomen
- Nausea, weight loss, and decreased appetite, which may also indicate gastric cancer

Antacids, such as magnesium-aluminum hydroxide mixtures (Maalox, Mylanta), are useful. Cimetidine (Tagamet) or ranitidine (Zantac) inhibit gastric acid secretion. Stopping smoking, decreasing or stopping alcohol consumption, and using stress-management techniques also are indicated.

Appendicitis

Appendicitis is an inflammation of the appendix, usually caused by bacterial infection. Signs and symptoms often begin with discomfort in the umbilical region that becomes painful and localized in the lower right quadrant, with fever, nausea, and vomiting. The appendix may be inflamed or abscessed and may burst. If the appendix bursts, the pain initially decreases because of the pressure release, but the bacteria spread to the abdominal cavity, resulting in peritonitis, which is an infection of the peritoneal membrane and potentially fatal.

Hernia

A hernia is the protrusion of soft tissues through a tear or weak spot in the abdominal muscle wall. Hernias can occur anywhere but are most common in the abdomen. In a hiatal hernia, the intestines bulge through an opening in the diaphragm. A more common type is inguinal hernia, which produces a bulging of the abdominal organs down the inguinal canal, often into the scrotum or labia. Males experience this most often, and herniation can occur at any age. Females may experience a femoral hernia below the groin, often caused by changes that occur during pregnancy. A reducible hernia is one in which the protruding organ can be manipulated back into the abdominal cavity naturally by lying down or by manual reduction through a surgical opening in the abdomen. A strangulated hernia is one in which the hernia is not reducible, and blood flow to the affected organ (e.g., the intestine) is blocked, which may result in obstruction and gangrene. The individual usually experiences pain and vomiting, and immediate surgical repair is required.

Malabsorption and Intolerance Syndromes

Malabsorption syndromes involve poor absorption of nutrients and can be caused by a deficiency of digestive enzymes, inadequate transport of nutrients, abnormalities in the structure of the intestine because of disease or surgery, or a hypersensitivity reaction to a particular food. Wheat, corn, and dairy products are the most common foods to cause malabsorption syndrome, and elimination diets may be beneficial. Malabsorption can result from cystic fibrosis, diabetes mellitus, dietary intolerance (such as celiac disease), reaction to dietary gluten, or lactose intolerance as a result of lactase deficiency.

Diverticular Disease

Diverticula are small, saclike outpouchings of the intestinal wall found in weak areas of the colon near the locations of vessels. Most occur in the sigmoid colon. When multiple diverticula are present, the condition is called *diverticulosis*. If they become inflamed and infected, the condition is called *diverticulitis*. Perforation of a diverticular sac may cause peritonitis. Symptoms are similar to those of irritable bowel syndrome, except that patients with peritonitis may have a fever and acute onset of symptoms. Primary treatment consists of a high-fiber diet, increased intake of fluids, a bulk-forming laxative such as psyllium (Metamucil), and an antibiotic. Severe cases may require hospitalization.

Cirrhosis

Cirrhosis is the infiltration of connective tissue into the functioning cells of the liver that causes slow deterioration of the liver (Fig. 12.10). End-stage signs and symptoms include jaundice, portal hypertension, and fluid accumulation in the peritoneal cavity. The most common cause is alcoholism, although

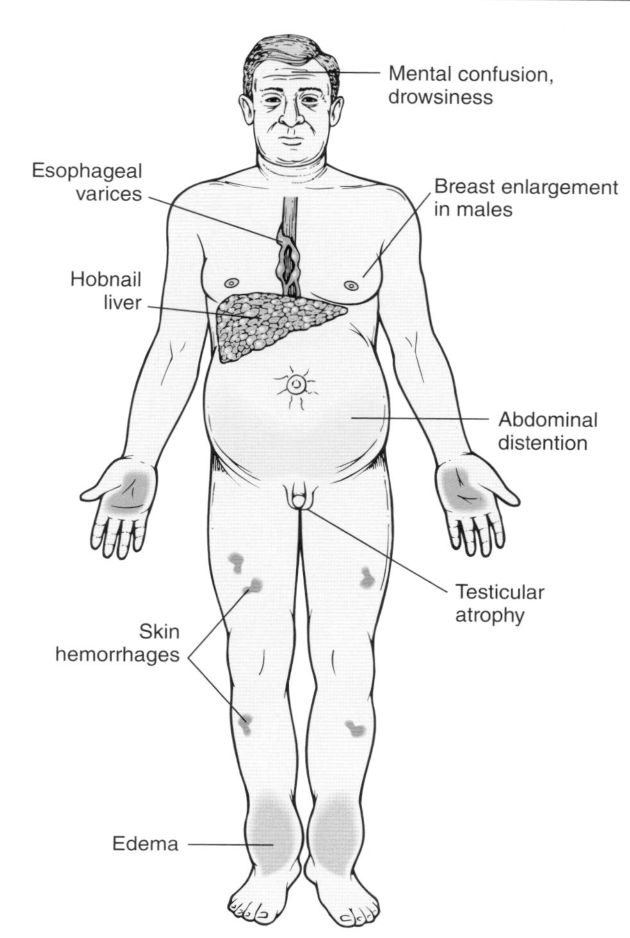

FIG. 12.10 Symptoms of cirrhosis. (From Frazier MS, Drzymkowski J. *Essentials of Human Disease and Conditions.* 4th ed. Saunders/Elsevier; 2008.)

cirrhosis also occurs in hepatitis. Cirrhosis interrupts many systemic functions. If the disease is not too far advanced and causal factors can be eliminated, liver regeneration capacity is good.

Gallbladder Disease

Gallbladder disease (cholelithiasis) is almost always the result of a gallstone composed of bile salts and cholesterol lodged in the cystic duct. A fatty meal often precedes an attack because the presence of fat stimulates the contraction of the gallbladder. Signs and symptoms are as follows:

- Pain in the right upper quadrant of the abdomen, often radiating to the right scapula or upper back
- Nausea and vomiting
- Fever

Gallbladder colic is pain caused by a stone that temporarily obstructs the cystic duct or common bile duct. Cholecystitis is inflammation of the gallbladder caused by obstruction of the cystic duct or common bile duct (choledocholithiasis or common bile duct stone). Cholangitis is infection.

Treatment of mild cases of gallbladder disease involves using an analgesic and eliminating fatty foods from the diet. If infection is present, antibiotics are used. Surgical removal of the gallbladder may be necessary.

Obstructions

An obstruction is a partial or complete closure of the small or large intestine. As a result, chyme backs up, the intestinal walls expand, local arteries may be compressed, and ischemic bowel disease can result. Obstructions may be caused by any of the following:

- *Adhesion*: Bands of fibrous tissue resulting from previous inflammation or surgical scars that grow between and around the loops of the intestine can cause strangulation.
- *Hernia:* The intestine protrudes through a weakness in the abdominal wall; if the loop of the intestine becomes trapped or strangulated, a medical emergency exists.
- *Tumors:* Growths, such as those seen in colon cancer, can obstruct the intestine.
- *Volvulus:* A knotting or twisting can cause strangulation in the intestine.

Gastroparesis

Gastroparesis, also called delayed gastric emptying, is a disorder that slows or stops the movement of food from the stomach into the small intestine, even though there is no blockage in the stomach or intestines. The symptoms of gastroparesis may include feeling full shortly after starting a meal, feeling full long after eating a meal, nausea, and vomiting. Diabetes is the most common known cause of gastroparesis.

Cystic Fibrosis

Cystic fibrosis is a genetic disease involving exocrine gland dysfunction. Secretions from the pancreas, mucous glands of the respiratory tract, and sweat glands are affected. Without the production of pancreatic enzymes, the digestive tract cannot break down food and absorb fats and nutrients. Treatment is a high-protein, high-calorie diet accompanied by the replacement of pancreatic enzymes. Antibiotics and inhalation and physical therapies are useful. Continuous home pulmonary care is often necessary.

Pancreatitis

Most cases of acute pancreatitis involve alcoholism and gallstones. Lipase, amylase, and trypsin (digestive enzymes) back up in the pancreas and are released into the surrounding tissue. This causes autodigestion of the pancreas and necrosis of tissues, including the peritoneum. Massive destruction of tissue accompanied by fluid and blood loss may lead to shock and death. Signs and symptoms include the following:

- Intense pain in the center of the upper abdomen radiating to the back
- Nausea and vomiting
- Distended, tender abdomen, with the seated position more comfortable than the supine position
- Elevated amylase and lipase levels in the bloodstream

Acute pancreatitis is a medical emergency. If the condition is suspected, immediate referral is necessary.

Chronic pancreatitis may occur after acute pancreatitis, gallstones, or alcohol abuse. Pancreatic function decreases and ultimately stops, and insulin and other pancreatic enzymes and hormones are no longer produced. Pain may be intense, although some patients with chronic pancreatitis do not experience any pain. A drastic treatment is the removal of a portion of the pancreas.

Colon Cancer

Colon cancer is the most common cancer and usually affects the lowest part of the rectum. Males and females are equally susceptible. Tumors in the ascending colon usually cause rectal bleeding; those in the descending colon cause constipation and obstructive symptoms. Polyps and ulcerative colitis are important risk factors. Screening for blood in the stool and sigmoidoscopy detect most lesions; 70% are located in the sigmoid colon and rectum. Treatment usually involves surgical removal of the bowel or removal of a section of the bowel, with the ends reattached to maintain a passageway.

Stomach Cancer

Stomach cancer is one of the more common causes of cancer death. Causal factors include chronic gastritis and exposure to environmental chemicals. Onset is slow and insidious, with little advanced warning or detection mechanisms. Indigestion appears; other signs and symptoms are unexplained weight loss, epigastric pain, a palpable upper abdominal mass, and iron-deficiency anemia resulting from gastric bleeding.

INDICATIONS/CONTRAINDICATIONS for Therapeutic Massage

A client with shoulder pain (referred), abdominal pain, or referred back pain may have one of several gastrointestinal disorders. In such cases, a referral is necessary for proper diagnosis. Many gastrointestinal diseases are bacterial or viral and are contagious. The practitioner should take appropriate precautions to maintain sanitary practice. Most chronic gastrointestinal diseases have a strong correlation with stress. The intestinal tract is highly responsive to changes in autonomic function and endocrine patterns. The influence of the vagus nerve is extensive, and research indicates that therapeutic massage influences vagal function. Sympathetic arousal changes peristaltic action and can send the intestinal tract into all kinds of dysfunction. Comprehensive stress management programs, including therapeutic massage methods, are often effective in managing these conditions.

Weight-loss surgery is becoming common and a massage therapist will likely work with clients who have had various types of surgical intervention. Those who have lost extreme amounts of weight may also need skin removal surgery. Massage is indicated to support healing and comfort. Cautions include surgical sites. Folds of excess skin can become irritated and infected. The massage therapist must be aware of local avoidance of the area if the skin is compromised. Indication of an eating disorder requires referral.

A specific type of massage to the large intestine can assist in managing constipation. The practitioner can teach this method to the client for self-care. Such massage is contraindicated in inflammatory bowel disease, and the practitioner should obtain permission from the physician to treat any other conditions. The massage consists of short, scooping strokes firmly against the abdomen beginning on the left, always directed toward the rectum. Progress continues along the length of the large intestine to the cecum in a fashion of two steps forward and one step back because the direction of the force is down and back toward the rectum. Beginning at the cecum on the right may push fecal material into a large mass, especially at the flexure (Fig. 12.11).

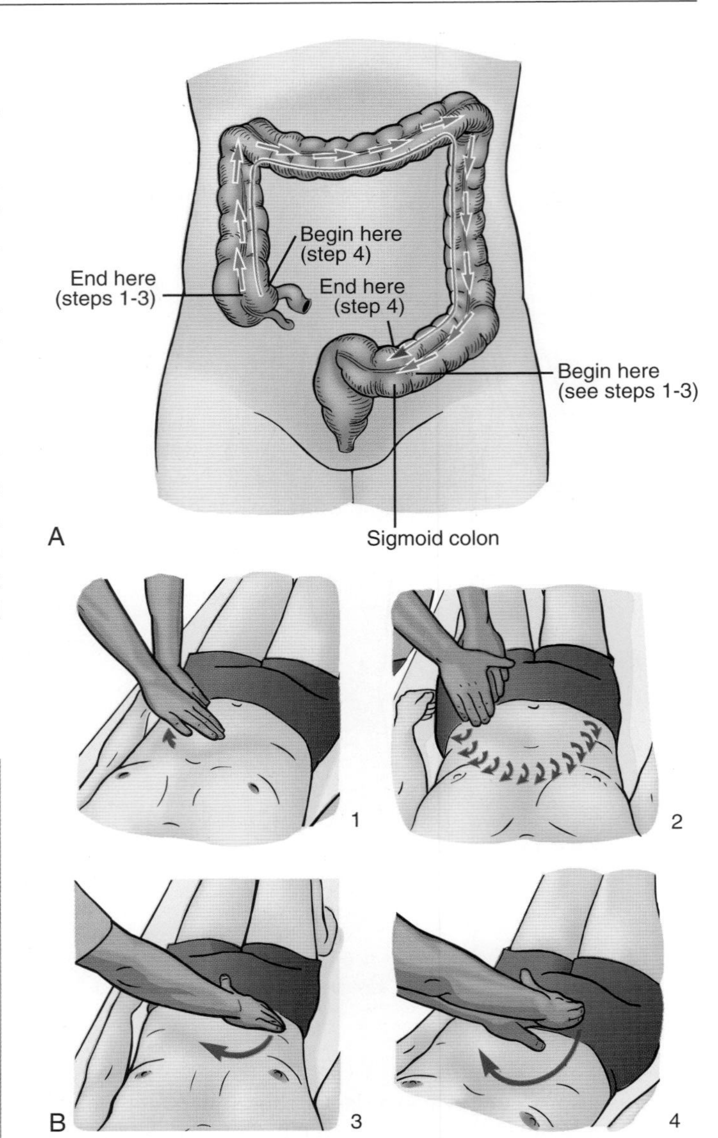

FIG. 12.11 (A) Colon with flow pattern arrows. All massage manipulations are directed in a clockwise fashion. The manipulations begin in the lower left-hand quadrant (on the left side of the illustration) at the sigmoid colon. The methods progressively contact all of the large intestines because they eventually end up encompassing the entire colon area. (B) Abdominal sequence. The direction of flow for emptying of the large intestine and colon is as follows: (1) Massage down the left side of the descending colon using short strokes directed to the sigmoid colon. (2) Massage across the transverse colon to the left side using short strokes directed to the sigmoid colon. (3) Massage up the ascending colon on the right side of the body using short strokes directed to the sigmoid colon. End at the right side ileocecal valve located in the lower right-hand quadrant of the abdomen. (4) Massage the entire flow pattern using long, light to moderate strokes from the ileocecal valve to the sigmoid colon. Repeat sequence.

Section Summary

- Explain gut microbiota and the microbiome. *Microbiota* refers to the entire ecosystem within the gut, consisting of various bacteria, viruses, fungi, and single-celled animals. *Microbiome* is the term given to all the genes inside these microbial cells. Numerous microorganisms colonize the human gastrointestinal tract and are essential to the digestion and absorption of dietary components.

- Define *digestion*. *Digestion* is the physiological process of intaking/assimilating nutrients and eliminating of waste.
- Describe the effects of the autonomic nervous system on digestion. The *enteric nervous system* (a division of the ANS) is responsible for maintaining gastrointestinal homeostasis. The sympathetic ANS can stimulate both inflammatory and antiinflammatory effects, contributing to both immune protection and disease of the gut.
- Describe the sequence of the digestive process. (1) Food is chewed/mixed with saliva (referred to as a *bolus*). (2) The bolus enters the stomach via the esophagus. (3) Gastric glands on the walls of the stomach secrete hormones and gastric juices to break down bolus into a semiliquid called *chyme*. Protein digestion starts in the stomach. (4) Chyme leaves the stomach and enters the small intestine. (5) The small intestine continues the digestive process using intestinal juices containing enzymes secreted by the small intestine as well as secretions from the pancreas, liver, and gallbladder. Protein, carbohydrate, and lipid digestion finishes in the small intestine; 99% of food *absorption* occurs in the small intestine; 10% occurs in the stomach and large intestine. (6) The large intestine receives the remaining chyme, reabsorbs water/electrolytes, forms/stores the undigested matter (called feces), then eliminates the feces via the anus.
- Define the *citric acid cycle*. The *citric acid cycle* (Krebs cycle) is the main transformative process by which food energy is released by cells to manufacture energy-rich adenosine triphosphate (ATP).
- Define *metabolic rate*. The *metabolic rate* is the rate of energy release (catabolic rate). The *basal metabolic rate (BMR)* is the smallest amount of energy expenditure needed to sustain life while also maintaining the waking state and normal body temperature. The *total metabolic rate* is the amount of energy used or expended by the body in a given time. The BMR usually constitutes about 55% to 60% of the total metabolic rate. Energy input equals total calories (kilocalories) ingested. Energy output equals the total metabolic rate expressed in kilocalories. Energy intake versus output determines body weight.

URINARY SYSTEM AND FLUID ELECTROLYTE BALANCES

SECTION OBJECTIVES

Chapter objectives covered in this section:

11. List the functions of the urinary system.
12. List and describe the components of the urinary system.
13. Describe urinary function and the processes of fluid electrolyte balances.
14. Describe the pathological conditions of the urinary system and the associated indications and contraindications for massage.

After completing this section, the student will be able to perform the following:

- List the organs of the urinary system.
- Describe electrolyte balance.
- Explain the relationship of pH to homeostasis.
- Describe how to test for edema.

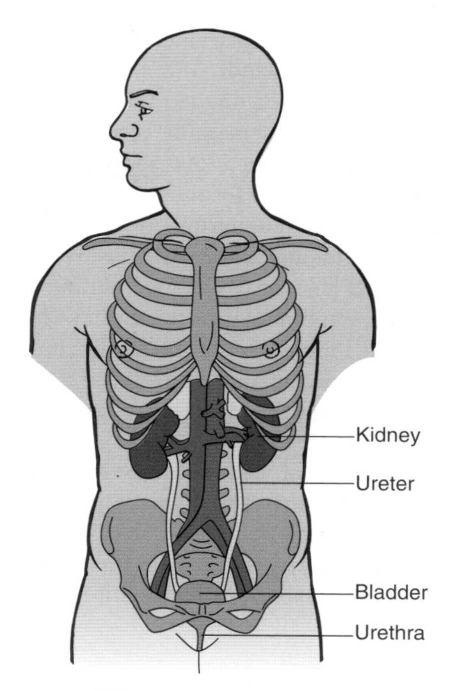

FIG. 12.12 Urinary system.

The urinary system consists of two kidneys, two ureters, one bladder, and one urethra (Fig. 12.12). The kidneys maintain homeostasis by filtering waste products from the blood and keeping the proper amount of water and electrolytes in the blood. Urine passes out of the kidneys and down through the ureters to the bladder for storage. When the bladder reaches a certain volume, it triggers the urge to void. The bladder expels urine through the urethra.

Functions of the Urinary System

The urinary system has the following important functions:

- Conservation of water
- Maintenance of the normal concentration of electrolytes
- Regulation of the acid-base balance
- Regulation of blood pressure
- Activation of vitamin D

The kidneys filter and eliminate most waste. In the average person, the kidneys filter about 100 L of blood per day, reabsorbing 99 L of filtrate and leaving about 1 L of urine. Substances secreted from the capillaries into the tubular filtrate include hydrogen, potassium, and ammonia.

Micturition (voiding, urination) is a parasympathetic action modified by voluntary control. It is initiated when afferent impulses from stretch receptors in the bladder stimulate the sacral portion of the spinal cord. The detrusor muscle contracts and the sphincter relaxes.

Organs of the Urinary System

Kidneys

The kidneys are two reddish-brown, bean-shaped organs located on the posterior wall of the abdomen against the back of the body wall musculature, just above the waist. They are embedded in fat and located at about the spinal level of T11–L3 on each side of the vertebral column. The right kidney is lower than the left because of its displacement by the liver. On top of each kidney is an adrenal gland.

The inside of a kidney is divided into a cortex, medulla, and pelvis. The cortex and medulla contain approximately 1 million nephrons, specialized tube-shaped filters that reabsorb or excrete substances to form urine. A nephron consists of a Bowman capsule; a glomerulus, which is composed of a group of capillaries; and a renal tubule. Water and small solids in the blood pass across the membrane of the capillaries and enter the tubule. From there, they travel through smaller loops and tubules to the collecting cups. Necessary substances (such as water and electrolytes) are returned to the blood, whereas the urine drains through ducts and eventually reaches the ureters.

The renal artery, renal vein, and ureters enter or exit the kidneys at the renal hilus. Although sympathetic and parasympathetic nerve fibers are present in the kidneys, the important component is sympathetic, causing vasoconstriction and the release of renin, a substance important in blood pressure control.

Kidneys and Homeostasis

Although we think of the kidneys as organs of excretion, they are more than that. The kidneys do remove wastes, but they also remove normal components of the blood that are present in greater-than-normal concentrations. When excessive water, sodium ions, calcium ions, and so on are present, the excess quickly passes out in the urine. Moreover, the kidneys step up their reclamation of these same substances when they are present in the blood in less-than-normal amounts. Thus, the kidneys continuously regulate the chemical composition of the blood within narrow limits. The kidneys are one of the major homeostatic devices of the body.

The kidneys produce erythropoietin, a hormone released in response to lowered levels of oxygen in the blood, and calcitriol (vitamin D_3), the active form of vitamin D that is involved in calcium assimilation. The kidneys also contribute to the acid-base balance.

Practical Application

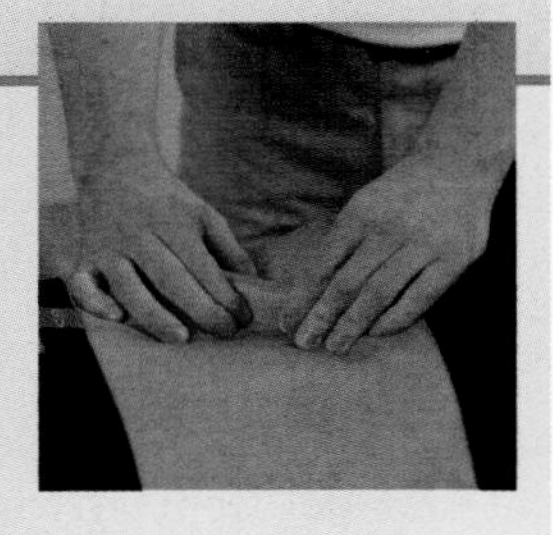

Massage therapy does not interact as directly with the urinary system as specifically as it does with the respiratory and digestive systems. Indirectly, massage influences the autonomic nervous system, which in turn regulates aspects of blood pressure. The influence of massage on the autonomic nervous system also affects the endocrine system, which in turn influences urinary function.

Ureters

The ureters are two narrow tubes extending from the kidney and connecting to the bladder. The two ureters lie on top of the psoas muscles. Each is a tube about 12 inches long, ¼ inch in diameter, and abundantly supplied with nerves. Peristalsis moves urine down into the bladder. Ureter walls contain muscle cells that help move the urine into the bladder. As the bladder fills, it presses against the ureters, compressing them and thus preventing a reverse flow of urine.

Urinary Bladder

The bladder is a muscular, baglike organ that lies in the pelvis and is a reservoir of urine. Urine flows continuously into the bladder from the ureters until a sufficient quantity of urine is collected for disposal through the urethra. When the bladder is distended by about 1 cup of urine, the signal to empty the bladder occurs, and the detrusor muscle causes the bladder to contract.

Urethra

The urethra is the tube that carries urine away from the bladder. The male urethra is about 8 inches long and serves to pass urine and semen. The female urethra is about 1½ inches long, lies anterior to the vagina, and functions only to pass urine. The opening at the end of the urethra is called the *meatus*. The proximity of the female urethra to the anus allows anal bacteria to migrate up the urethra to the bladder, ureters, and kidneys, predisposing females to ascending urinary tract infections.

Urinary Function

For the body to maintain homeostasis, the input of water and electrolytes must be balanced by output. The fluid, or water, content of the human body ranges from 40% to 60% of its total weight. The total body water can be subdivided into two major fluid compartments: the extracellular and the intracellular (Fig. 12.13). The extracellular fluid consists mainly of the plasma found in the blood vessels, the interstitial fluid that surrounds the cells, the lymph, the cerebrospinal fluid, and the specialized joint fluids. *Intracellular fluid* refers to the water inside the cells (see Fig. 12.13).

Extracellular fluid constitutes the internal environment of the body and serves the dual functions of providing a constant

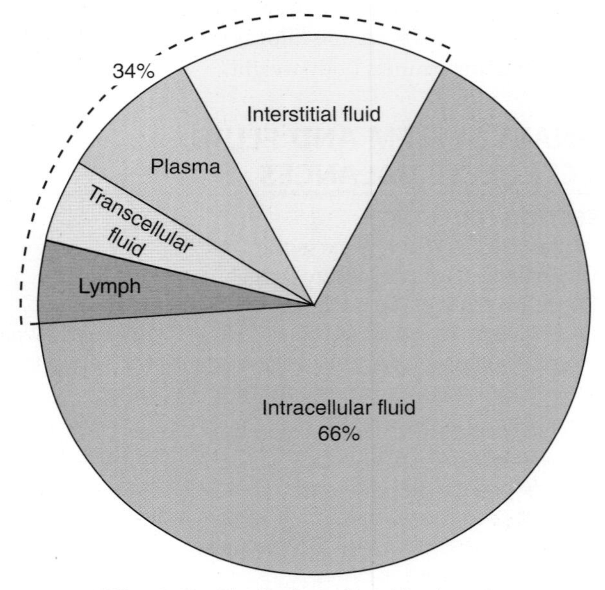

FIG. 12.13 Distribution of total body water.

environment for cells and transporting substances to and from them. Intracellular fluid facilitates intracellular chemical reactions that maintain life. With the exception of plasma, fluid volumes are proportionately larger in infants and children than in adults. The function of the urinary system is to maintain the fluid environment of the body.

Fluid regulation is essential to homeostasis. If water or electrolyte levels rise or fall beyond normal limits, many bodily functions are impaired. Dehydration is the most common imbalance. Maintaining normal pH levels is also important for normal body functioning because small changes in pH can produce major disruptions in metabolism.

Water Balance

Water is a component of all living things and often is referred to as the universal biological solvent. Only liquid ammonia can dissolve more substances than water.

Water acts to minimize temperature changes throughout the body because of its high specific heat. A considerable amount of energy is needed to break the hydrogen bonds between water molecules to make the water molecules move faster (i.e., increase the temperature of water). Therefore, water can absorb a great deal of heat without rapidly changing its temperature. Box 12.3 lists the many important functions of water in the body.

The water content of the body tissues varies. Adipose tissue (fat) has the lowest percentage of water; the skeleton has the second lowest water content. Skeletal muscle, skin, and blood are among the tissues that have the highest content of water in the body (Table 12.5).

Box 12.3 Functions of Water in Human Physiology

- Water provides a medium for chemical reactions.
- Water is crucial for the regulation of chemical and bioelectric distributions within cells.
- Water transports substances, such as hormones and nutrients.
- Water aids in oxygen transport from the lungs to body cells.
- Water aids in carbon dioxide transport from body cells to the lungs.
- Water dilutes toxic substances and waste products and transports them to the kidneys and the liver.
- Water distributes heat around the body.

Table 12.5 Percentage of Water in the Body Tissues

Tissue	Percentage of Water
Blood	83.0
Kidneys	82.7
Heart	79.2
Lungs	79.0
Spleen	75.8
Muscle	75.6
Brain	74.8
Intestine	74.5
Skin	72.0
Liver	68.3
Skeleton	22.0
Adipose tissue	10.0

Table 12.6 Where Water is Lost from the Body (Healthy Adult)

Organ	Mode of Water Loss	Percentage of Loss
Kidneys	Urine	62
Skin	Diffusion and sweat	19
Lungs	Water vapor	13
Gastrointestinal tract	Feces	6

The total water content of the body decreases most dramatically during the first 10 years of life and continues to decline through old age, at which time water content may be only 45% of the total body weight. Males tend to have higher percentages of water (about 65%) than Females (about 55%), mainly because of their increased muscle mass and smaller amount of subcutaneous fat.

The water in the body is in a constant state of motion, shifting between the two major fluid compartments and being continuously lost from and taken into the body. In a normal, healthy human being, water input equals water output. Maintaining this ratio is of prime importance in maintaining health. Approximately 90% of the water is taken in by the gastrointestinal tract in the form of food and liquids. The remaining 10% is called *metabolic water* and is produced as the result of various chemical reactions in the cells of the tissues. Table 12.6 shows the routes by which the healthy adult loses water.

The amount of water lost by way of the kidneys is under hormonal control. The average amount of water lost and consumed per day is approximately 2.5 L in a healthy adult.

The walls of the blood vessels form barriers to the free passage of fluid between interstitial fluid and blood plasma. At the capillaries, these walls are only one cell thick. These capillary walls are generally permeable to water and small solutes but impermeable to large organic molecules, such as proteins. Thus, the blood plasma tends to have a higher concentration of such molecules than the interstitial fluid. Much of this interstitial fluid becomes lymph, which eventually finds its way back into the bloodstream (see Chapter 11). Because water and small solutes (such as sodium, potassium, and calcium) can be exchanged freely between the blood plasma and the interstitial fluid, the action of the kidneys on the blood regulates these electrolytes. This exchange depends mainly on the hydrostatic and osmotic forces of these fluid compartments.

Hydrostatic Forces

Liquid exerts force by pushing against a surface, such as a dam in a river or the wall of a blood vessel. The pressure of blood in the capillaries is a major hydrostatic force in the human body, and it functions as a filter because the pressure of the fluid is higher at the arterial end of the capillary than at the venous end. The pressure of the interstitial fluid is negative (−5 mm Hg) because the lymphatic system is continuously taking up the excess fluid forced out of the capillaries.

Osmotic Pressure

Osmotic pressure is the attraction of water to large molecules, such as proteins. Because proteins are more abundant within the blood vessels than outside of them, the concentration of proteins in the blood tends to attract water from the interstitial space.

Overall, near equilibrium exists between the fluids forced out of the capillaries and the fluids reabsorbed, because the lymphatic system collects the excess fluid forced out at the artery end and eventually drains it back into the veins at the base of the neck.

A similar situation exists between the interstitial fluid and the intracellular fluid, although ion pumps and carriers complicate the process. Generally, water movement is substantial in both directions, but ion movement is restricted and depends on active transport by way of the pumps. Nutrients and oxygen, because they are dissolved in water, move passively into cells; waste products and carbon dioxide move out of cells.

The mechanisms that regulate body fluids are centered in the hypothalamus, which also receives input from the digestive tract that helps to control thirst. Antidiuretic hormone (ADH) regulates body fluid volume, extracellular osmosis, and many other areas. Primary among them is increasing the permeability of the collecting tubules in the kidneys, thus allowing more water to be reabsorbed by the kidneys. If the body is short of fluid intake (as during sleep), the urine is concentrated, so it is darker and low in volume. When an individual is overhydrated, the urine is diluted, so it is pale or colorless and high in volume, and ADH is absent.

The production of ADH is triggered primarily by osmoreceptors and baroreceptors (pressure receptors). Secondary triggers include stress, pain, hypoxia, and extreme exercise.

Osmoreceptors

Osmoreceptors are stimulated by dehydration. This may occur because of fluid loss or lack of fluid intake, or it may be relative dehydration in which the body loses no overall water content but gains sodium ions. The precise location of the osmoreceptors is as yet unclear, but they appear to be in the hypothalamus or the third ventricle of the brain.

The thirst response is connected to the activity of the osmoreceptors, but the actual mechanism is not understood completely. The moistening of the mucosal linings of the mouth and pharynx seems to initiate some sort of neurological response that sends a message to the thirst center of the hypothalamus. Perhaps more importantly, stretch receptors in the gastrointestinal tract appear to transmit nerve messages to the thirst center of the hypothalamus that inhibits the thirst response.

Baroreceptors

Changes in the circulating volume of body fluid also stimulate ADH secretion. The result is an increase or decrease in internal pressure, which is monitored by baroreceptors. If the normal volume of water in the body is reduced by 8% to 10% because of hemorrhage or excessive perspiration, ADH is secreted. Pressure receptors located in the atria of the heart and the pulmonary artery and vein relay their messages to the hypothalamus by way of the vagus nerve.

Electrolyte Balance

An electrolyte is any chemical that dissociates into ions when dissolved in a solution. Ions can be positively charged (cations) or negatively charged (anions). The major electrolytes found in the human body are as follows:

- Sodium (Na^+)
- Potassium (K^+)
- Calcium (Ca^{2+})
- Magnesium (Mg^{2+})
- Chloride (Cl^-)
- Phosphate (HPO_4^{2-})
- Sulfate (SO_4^-)
- Bicarbonate (HCO_3^-)

Sodium and chloride are the major electrolytes in the interstitial fluid and blood plasma. Potassium and phosphate are the major electrolytes in the intracellular fluid.

Sodium Balance

Sodium balance plays an important role in the excitability of muscles and neurons and is also crucial in regulating fluid balance in the body. The kidneys closely regulate sodium levels.

Potassium Balance

Potassium is the major electrolyte in intracellular fluid, where its level of concentration is 28 times that in extracellular fluid. Like sodium, potassium is important to the correct functioning of excitable cells, such as muscles, neurons, and sensory receptors. Potassium is also involved in the regulation of fluid levels within the cell and in maintaining the correct pH balance of the body. The pH balance of the body also affects potassium levels. In acidosis, potassium excretion decreases, whereas the opposite occurs in alkalosis.

Calcium and Phosphorus Balance

Calcium is found mainly in the extracellular fluids, whereas phosphorus is found mainly in the intracellular fluids. Both are important in the maintenance of healthy bones and teeth.

Calcium is important in the transmission of nerve impulses across synapses, the clotting of blood, and the contraction of muscles. If calcium levels fall below normal, muscles and nerves become more excitable.

Recall from Chapter 6 that decreased levels of calcium in the body stimulate the parathyroid gland to secrete parathyroid hormone, which increases the calcium and phosphate levels in the interstitial fluids by releasing these minerals from reservoirs lodged in the bones and the teeth. Parathyroid hormone also decreases calcium excretion by the kidneys. If the levels of calcium in the body become too high, the thyroid gland releases calcitonin, which inhibits the release of calcium and potassium from the bones. Calcitonin also inhibits the absorption of calcium from the gastrointestinal tract and increases calcium excretion by the kidneys.

Phosphorus is required for the synthesis of nucleic acids and high-energy compounds, such as ATP. Phosphorus is also important in the maintenance of pH balance.

Magnesium Balance

Most magnesium is found in the intracellular fluid and bone. Within cells, magnesium functions in the sodium-potassium pump and as an aid to enzyme action. It plays a role in muscle contraction, action potential conduction, and bone and teeth production. Aldosterone controls magnesium concentrations in the extracellular fluid. Low magnesium levels result in the secretion of more aldosterone, which increases magnesium reabsorption by the kidneys.

Chloride Balance

Chloride is the most plentiful extracellular electrolyte. Its extracellular concentration is 26 times that of its intracellular concentration. Chloride ions can diffuse easily across plasma membranes, and their transport is linked closely to sodium movement, which also explains the indirect role of aldosterone in chloride regulation. When sodium is reabsorbed, chloride follows passively. Chloride helps to regulate osmotic pressure differences between fluid compartments and is essential in pH balance. The chloride shift within the blood helps to move bicarbonate ions out of the red blood cells and into the plasma for transport. In the gastric system, chlorine and hydrogen combine to form hydrochloric acid.

pH Balance

Recall from Chapter 1 that pH level is a measurement of the hydrogen concentration of a solution. Lower pH values indicate higher hydrogen concentration or higher acidity. Higher pH values indicate lower hydrogen concentration or higher alkalinity. The relative number of hydrogen ions is referred to as *pH balance* or *acid-base balance*. Hydrogen ion regulation in the fluid compartments of the body is critical to health. Even a slight change in hydrogen ion concentration can significantly alter the rates of chemical reactions and can affect the distribution of sodium, potassium, and calcium ions and the structure and function of proteins.

The normal pH of the arterial blood is 7.4, whereas that of the venous blood is 7.35. The venous blood has a lower pH because it has a higher concentration of carbon dioxide, which dissolves in water to make a weak acid called *carbonic acid*. When the pH in the arterial blood changes, one of two conditions may result: acidosis or alkalosis. Acidosis occurs when the hydrogen ion concentration in the arterial blood increases and the pH therefore decreases. Alkalosis occurs when the hydrogen ion concentration in the arterial blood decreases and the pH therefore increases.

Sources of hydrogen ions in the body include the carbonic acid previously mentioned, sulfuric acid (a by-product in the breakdown of proteins), phosphoric acid (a by-product of protein and phospholipid metabolism), ketone bodies produced by the metabolism of fat, and lactic acid (a product formed in skeletal muscle during exercise).

Of all the acids formed by or introduced into the body, about half of them are neutralized by the ingestion of alkaline foods. The remaining acid is neutralized by three major systems: chemical buffers, the respiratory system, and the kidneys. Chemical buffers have an instantaneous effect on pH changes. They are effective in minimizing pH changes but do not eliminate them. Within cells, chemical buffers generally take about 2 to 4 hours to minimize changes in pH. The respiratory system also helps minimize pH changes; therefore, the effects occur within minutes. Renal regulation can return the pH to absolute normal but requires hours or several days.

Pathological Conditions of the Urinary System

The disease of the urinary system primarily affects the kidneys and bladder. Because the kidneys maintain homeostasis by filtering waste products from the blood and keeping the proper amount of water and electrolytes in the blood, any pathology of the kidneys has body-wide effects. Bladder infections are common. One function of the urinary system is to allow urine to leave the body. If the structures that carry the urine become blocked, bladder and kidney damage can occur.

Clinical Problems With Fluid Balance

The fluid balance in the body can be upset in many ways, all of which can cause severe problems and even death.

Dehydration

Dehydration occurs when water is unavailable (Fig. 12.14). However, conditions such as diarrhea, severe vomiting, excessive sweating, bleeding, and surgical removal of body fluids also can result in dehydration. There are three types. *Hypertonic dehydration* occurs when the fluid loss results in an increase in electrolyte levels, causing the blood pressure to fall and the blood to become thicker, which can result in heart failure. *Isotonic dehydration* results in no perceptible difference from the normal electrolyte balance and may lead to *hypotonic dehydration*, in which the fluid and electrolyte losses keep pace with each other. Any intake of pure water alters the fluid-electrolyte balance because this results in too much water and not enough electrolytes. Replacing the body fluid with a balanced

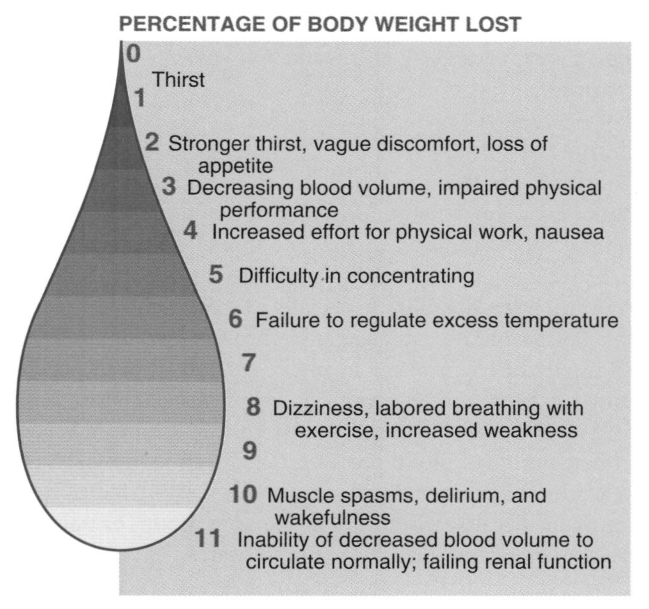

FIG. 12.14 The effects of dehydration. (From Mahan K, Escott-Stump S, Raymond JL. *Krause's Food and the Nutrition Care Process.* 13th ed. Saunders; 2012.)

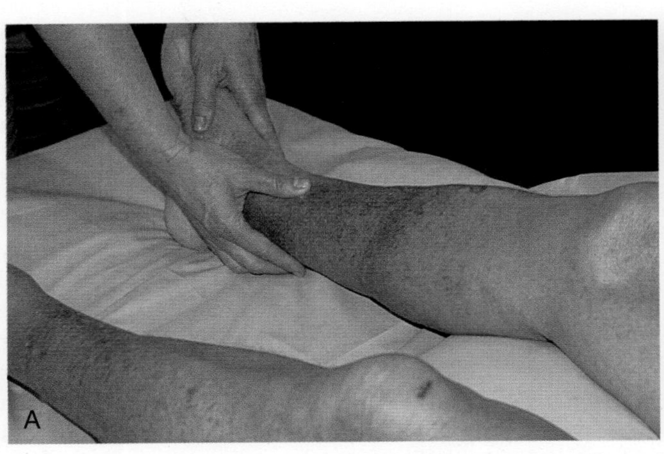

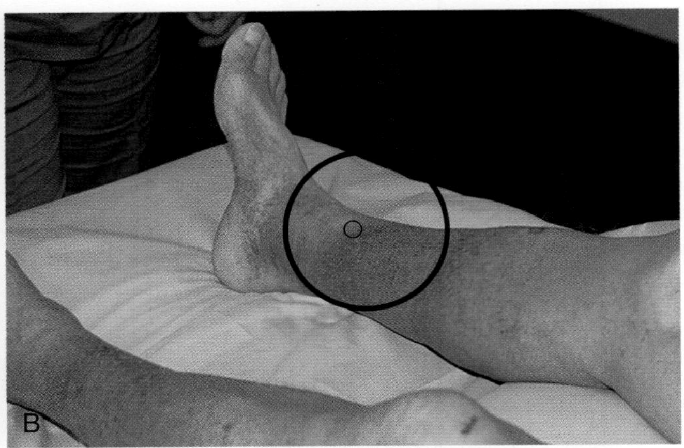

FIG. 12.15 (A) Test for edema. (B) Identification of pitting edema.

preparation of electrolytes and water is important in cases of severe diarrhea.

Problems in the production of urine also can lead to dehydration. Impaired ability to concentrate urine can be caused by the following:

- *Damage to the medulla of the kidneys:* Inadequate water reabsorption occurs, and the urine is too dilute, resulting in fluid loss.
- *Inadequate ADH production:* Inadequate ADH production occurs in diabetes insipidus. Individuals suffering from this disorder may eliminate as much as 5 to 20 L (8½ to 34 pints) of urine per day. In the psychological disorder known as *polydipsia*, the sufferer is obsessed with drinking (usually water), which results in dilution of the plasma, causing artificial lowering of the osmolarity and decreasing ADH secretion.
- *Solute diuresis in individuals suffering from diabetes mellitus:* Elevated blood sugar levels can make the kidneys unable to reabsorb water, which results in excess fluid loss.

In any of the aforementioned conditions, fluid balance must be maintained; otherwise, dehydration or even hypovolemic shock, caused by an insufficient volume of body fluid, may occur.

Edema

Edema is a condition in which an excess of fluid exists in the interstitial compartment. The condition often results in tissue swelling and is common whenever lymphatic blockage occurs. It is also caused by an impaired ability of the body to dilute the urine and by renal failure, especially in the early stages of acute renal failure and the later stages of chronic renal failure.

Liver failure can result in inefficient metabolism of aldosterone, a hormone that controls sodium levels. Heart failure means that the production of aldosterone is enhanced because of the lowering of blood pressure. The result is the same as in liver failure. Excessive ADH secretion is a rare condition that may occur because of tumors in the lung, brain, or pancreas, resulting in increased reabsorption of water.

To test for edema, apply steady pressure with the thumb on the lower leg for 10 to 20 seconds. If a depression remains after removal of the pressure, fluid retention is indicated (Fig. 12.15).

Urinary Tract Infections

The following symptoms are warning signs of urinary tract infection:

- Increased urge and frequency of urination (usually small amounts of urine)
- Pain or burning sensation with urination
- Pain in the lower abdomen or back
- Blood visible in the urine
- Fever and chills
- Rapid heart rate
- Nausea and vomiting

The following suggestions decrease the risk of urinary tract infections:

- Drink plenty of fluids.
- Lie on the left side to increase kidney efficiency and output.
- Wear cotton underwear.
- Avoid tight-fitting clothes.
- Keep the vaginal area clean: Always wipe from front to back after urinating or having a bowel movement.
- Avoid perfumed soaps and panty liners.

Bladder Infections (Cystitis)

Bladder infections (cystitis) are common, particularly in females. The infection usually is caused by bacteria that have spread from the perineal region into the bladder. Symptoms include pain in the lower abdomen, stinging or burning during urination, and frequent urination of only small amounts (frequency). Another symptom is a continuous, sometimes uncontrollable urge to urinate (urgency). Antibiotics (such as nitrofurantoin [Macrodantin]), sulfa-containing agents (such as trimethoprim/sulfamethoxazole [Bactrim, Septra]), and synthetic penicillins (ampicillin or amoxicillin) are effective. Cranberry juice also seems to be beneficial in managing bladder infection, because it prevents the *Escherichia coli* organism from adhering to bladder walls.

Pyelonephritis

Pyelonephritis is an infection of the kidney that affects the nephrons or filtering units. Bacteria may reach the kidney from the bladder or by spreading through the bloodstream from another infected site, such as the tonsils, middle ear, sinuses, or prostate. Common symptoms are flank and back pain, usually on one side; abdominal pain that moves into the groin; and fever, sometimes with chills and nausea. Treatment includes the use of an appropriate antibiotic. If not treated, pyelonephritis may become chronic and lead to kidney failure.

Incontinence

Urinary incontinence is the inability to control urination. Commonly caused by weak pelvic floor muscles or nerve damage, factors include age, infection, obesity, brain or spinal cord lesion, damage to the nerves to the bladder, or injury to the sphincter (which usually occurs during childbirth). Stress incontinence is urine leakage during coughing, straining, sneezing, and so on, when stress is placed on the muscles. Urge incontinence is feeling the need to void frequently; it may be caused by irritation or infection or may result from the decrease in the amount of estrogen in a female body during and after menopause, which can weaken pelvic floor muscles and reduce the size of the mucous membranes, resulting in both stress and urge incontinence.

Kidney Stones

Kidney stones are small crystalline substances that develop in the kidney. Most kidney stones, also called *calculi*, consist of calcium, but some contain amino acids, uric acids, and other excretory products. The most common cause of stone formation is dehydration; most kidney stones occur during the summer. Other factors are urinary tract infection, impaired tubular reabsorption of calcium, gout, family history, medications (such as diuretics), dietary imbalances, and immobilization. Excessive intake of calcium does not lead to kidney stones. Kidney stones are usually undiscovered until one passes into a ureter, causing sudden, excruciating flank pain. Nausea and vomiting may occur. Treatment includes increasing fluid intake to help pass the stone if it is small enough to pass through the ureter. If the stone is too large, surgical removal may be necessary, or the stone may be crushed by an ultrasonic beam or shock wave.

Obstruction

Obstruction of the urethra, causing retention of urine, is most common in older males who have prostate problems. (The Reproductive System section of this chapter discusses the topic in further detail.)

Glomerulonephritis

Glomerulonephritis is a group of diseases involving antigen-antibody reactions affecting the glomeruli. The antigen may be an external one, such as beta-hemolytic streptococci, or may involve an autoimmune reaction. The most common type occurs after a streptococcal infection, such as pharyngitis, tonsillitis, or impetigo, when antibodies react with streptococci. Immune complexes are deposited in the glomeruli. For mild cases without bacterial infections, treatment is bed rest and salt restriction. Streptococcal infections require antibiotic treatment, whereas autoimmune reactions require treatment with immunosuppressant medications or steroids.

Kidney Failure

Kidney failure, also known as *renal failure*, is the inability to excrete waste products and retain electrolytes. In acute kidney failure, the kidneys suddenly stop working, commonly because of acute glomerulonephritis, allergic reactions to medications, shock, or obstruction. Waste products back up in the blood. Kidney failure may cause hypertension, edema, dehydration, and itching of the skin because of the accumulation of waste products in the blood vessels of the skin. The buildup of excessive amounts of nitrogen wastes in the blood is known as *uremia*. Chronic kidney failure is caused by a gradual decrease in kidney function, often as a result of inflammation, glomerulonephritis, or diabetes mellitus. As in the acute stage, the kidneys are unable to excrete waste products or water, and these substances back up in the blood and tissues. In the chronic stage, scar tissue builds up in the kidneys, and they are unable to function. Scarring leads to end-stage kidney failure in which the kidneys are unable to function at all—a life-threatening situation.

Signs and symptoms include the following:

- Weakness and fatigue resulting from sodium, potassium, and calcium abnormalities, such as anemia and acidosis
- Hypertension
- Itching caused by the accumulation of waste products in skin vessels
- Dehydration caused by water loss
- Generalized edema

Treatment includes cautious administration of amino acids, adequate calories, sodium, and calcium, as well as antihypertensive medication. Severe anemia caused by kidney failure may require blood transfusions. The body can survive with only one functioning kidney. If both kidneys fail, however, hemodialysis, the filtering of wastes from blood using a machine, is required. A kidney transplant may be necessary. Of organ transplant procedures, kidney transplants are among the most successful. Careful matching of blood and genetic types, as well as up-to-date immunosuppressive drug therapy, may result in long-term survival rates.

INDICATIONS/CONTRAINDICATIONS for Therapeutic Massage

Urinary System

Therapeutic massage may slightly increase blood volume flow in general through the kidneys by way of mechanical and reflexive processes. In healthy individuals, massage therapy supports the filtration process of blood by potentially increasing blood flow in general. However, in those with kidney disease, the increased volume can strain the kidneys' functioning. Therefore, cautions exist for anyone with kidney disease. Therapeutic massage modalities may be useful for pain and stress management, but only with the careful supervision of the treating physician.

Acute infectious processes contraindicate massage until the infection has run its course. Massage therapy may be used in chronic infection as part of a supervised treatment plan. Stress contributes to incontinence, so any form of stress management helps somewhat with both stress and urge incontinence. Remember that incontinent clients require easy access to the restroom.

Section Summary

- List the organs of the urinary system. *Kidneys* filter waste products from the blood and maintain proper amounts of water/electrolytes in the blood. *Ureters* transfer urine from the kidneys to the bladder. The *bladder*, upon reaching a certain volume, triggers the urge to void the urine through the *urethra*.
- Describe electrolyte balance. *Electrolytes* are any chemical that dissociates into ions when dissolved in a solution. Ions can be positively charged (cations) or negatively charged (anions). Major body electrolytes include sodium, potassium, calcium, magnesium, chloride, phosphate, sulfate, and bicarbonate. *Electrolyte balance* (the proper ratios of these electrolytes) is essential for many important homeostatic functions such as muscle/nerve excitability, bone health, and pH balance.
- Explain the relationship of *pH* to homeostasis. Lower pH values indicate higher hydrogen concentration or higher acidity. Higher pH values indicate lower hydrogen concentration or higher alkalinity. pH balance affects electrolyte balance and protein function. Acids introduced to the body are neutralized by ingestion of alkaline foods, chemical buffers, the respiratory system, and the kidneys.
- Describe how to test for *edema*. Apply pressure with the thumb on the lower leg for 10 to 20 seconds. If a depression remains after pressure removal, fluid retention is indicated.

REPRODUCTIVE SYSTEM

Note: This content targets the anatomy and physiology of the reproductive system. Sexual anatomy and physiology is a continuum including female, male, and intersexed characteristics. Gender may or may not align with an individual's sex anatomy/physiology. Gender identity is a person's internal sense of being female, male, some combination of male and female, or neither male nor female. Sexual orientation is about emotional and sexual attraction. Sexual orientation, gender identity, and congruence need to be respected.

SECTION OBJECTIVES

Chapter objectives covered in this section:

15. List and describe the components and functions of the male reproductive system.
16. List and describe the components and functions of the female reproductive system.
17. Explain the three stages of pregnancy and the process of lactation.
18. Describe the pathological conditions of the reproductive system and the associated indications and contraindications for massage.

After completing this chapter, the student will be able to perform the following:

- List the organs of the male reproductive system.
- List the organs of the female reproductive system.
- Describe the stages of pregnancy.
- Explain the birth process.
- Describe the best sleeping/massage position for most during pregnancy.
- Describe indications/contraindications for massage therapy related to pregnancy

The continuation of the species is the biological function of the reproductive system, yet sexuality is more than reproduction and more than genitals. This last section, the reproductive system, connects the study of the body to the beginning, the cell.

The most obvious differences between male and female bodies are in the construction and functions of the reproductive systems, but even in the differentiation, continuity exists. The same hormones from the hypothalamus stimulate the ovaries and testes. The musculature is similar, as is nervous system distribution. The main difference lies in the development of the sex cells (ovum and sperm), the anatomy required to deliver the sperm to the ovum, and the organs to house the developing infant. The difference is not so prevalent in young children before puberty or in those in their mature years (i.e., after 60 or so), but during the reproductive years, the differences are more evident.

Male Reproductive System

The male reproductive system consists of the testicles, epididymis, vas deferens, ejaculatory duct, urethra, penis, and scrotum (Fig. 12.16). The two testicles are enclosed in an external sac called the *scrotum*.

Tiny seminiferous tubules in the testicles produce sperm. The production of sperm is called *spermatogenesis*. Sperm cells travel from the testicles into the epididymis, where they mature. Sperm then moves into the vas deferens, which extends upward into the body cavity, over the symphysis pubis, and around the urinary bladder to connect with the two seminal vesicles.

The seminal vesicles produce and secrete a viscous fluid that makes up most of the semen and joins with the sperm to pass from the vas deferens into the ejaculatory duct. The ejaculatory duct passes through the prostate gland and joins with the urethra. The prostate gland is a group of small glands that surround the urethra as it exits the bladder; it produces a milky alkaline fluid that becomes a component of semen.

The duct of the bulbourethral, or Cowper, glands connects to the urethra below the prostate. These two small glands secrete a thick lubricating fluid, which is also a component of semen. On ejaculation, semen flows through the urethra to the outside of the body.

The penis is composed of a meshwork of erectile tissue, meaning it can become firm by engorgement with blood. It consists of a shaft, the end of which is covered with a loose flap of skin called the *prepuce*, or *foreskin*. This foreskin often is removed in a surgical process called *circumcision*. The end of the penis is called the *glans penis*. The penis functions to deposit sperm cells into the vagina.

Hormonal and Nervous System Control

Follicle-stimulating hormone (FSH) and luteinizing hormone (LH) from the pituitary gland control testicular function. FSH stimulates sperm production, whereas LH stimulates the secretion of testosterone from interstitial cells. Gonadotropin-releasing hormone from the hypothalamus stimulates the production of FSH and LH.

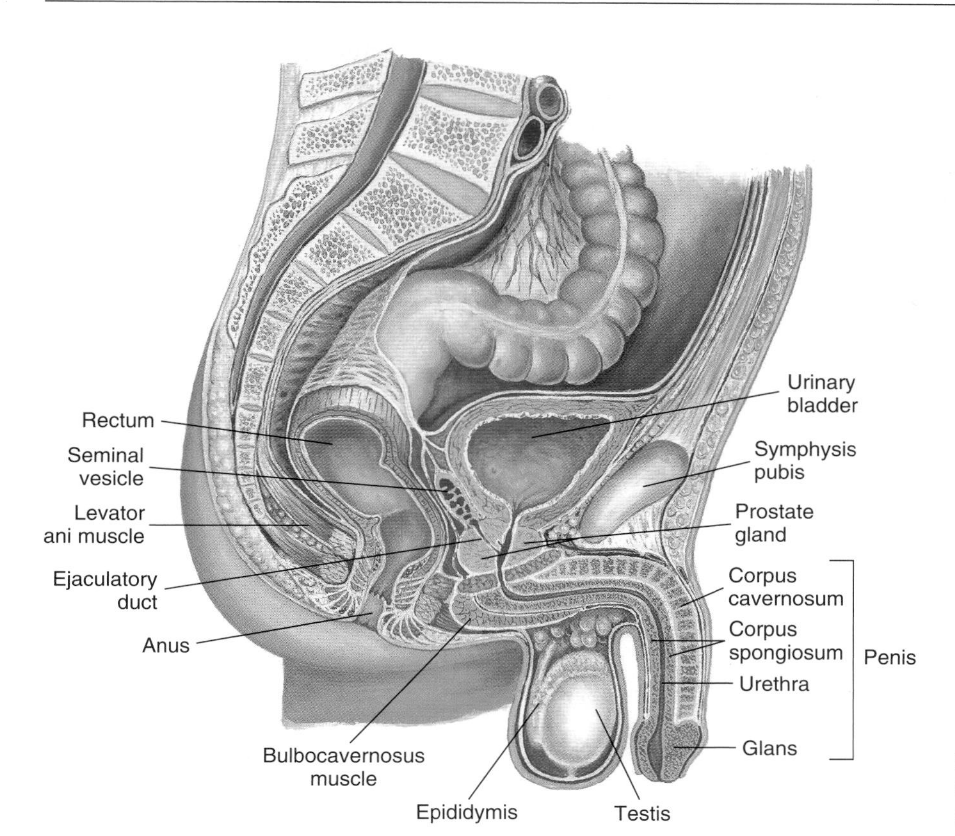

FIG. 12.16 Male pelvic organs. (From Seidel HM, et al. *Mosby's Guide to Physical Examination.* 7th ed. Mosby/Elsevier; 2011.)

Before puberty, males produce little testosterone because no releasing hormone is secreted. During adolescence the hypothalamus matures, and gonadotropin-releasing hormone stimulates the production of FSH and LH. The number of interstitial cells is increased by LH, and acceleration occurs in the production of testosterone, which increases the synthesis of protein in cells, creating an anabolic effect. Male secondary sex characteristics appear. Body growth accelerates; muscle and bone mass increase; the penis and scrotum enlarge; the larynx develops and the voice deepens; and hair appears on the face, chest, axillae, abdomen, and pubis.

Hormones stimulate the sebaceous glands of the skin, increasing the likelihood of acne. Testosterone stimulates the male sexual drive or libido, and boys may begin to exhibit more aggressive social behavior. The production of sperm accelerates. Testosterone and sperm are produced throughout life, but levels gradually diminish after age 40. Spermatogenesis takes place at a temperature lower than body temperature, so the testes are located in the scrotal sac, where the temperature is cooler, although during cold weather the cremaster muscle contracts and elevates the testes closer to the body.

Erection is a parasympathetic response in which arteries of the penis dilate and veins constrict, allowing blood flow into the erectile tissue but blocking venous outflow. A variety of stimuli cause an erection. Emission involves the contraction of the epididymis, the vas deferens, the prostate, and the seminal vesicles. Semen moves into the urethra. Ejaculation consists of contraction of the muscles at the base of the penis (bulbocavernosus, ischiocavernosus), which propels approximately 3 mL of semen through the penile urethra at high pressure.

Male Contraceptive Methods

Several contraceptive methods are available for males: abstinence, the condom, the condom with spermicidal jelly or foam, withdrawal, and vasectomy. The condom alone and the withdrawal method are not reliable. The condom with a spermicide is a fairly reliable method. In addition, the condom protects against some, but not all, sexually transmitted infections. Vasectomy is performed in a physician's office with the area under local anesthesia; the procedure involves removing a 2 cm piece of the vas deferens and tying the remaining ends. A vasectomy is considered a permanent method of sterilization, even though the cut ends can be rejoined; reattainment of fertility occurs in fewer than 50% of cases after rejoining.

Female Reproductive System

The female reproductive system is designed for childbearing. The system consists of two ovaries, two fallopian tubes, a uterus, and a vagina. Also included in the system are the external genitalia and the mammary glands (Fig. 12.17).

Internal Organs

The two ovaries are held in position, one on each side of the uterus, by several ligaments. The largest of these ligaments is called the *broad ligament;* it holds the ovaries in close proximity to the fallopian tubes.

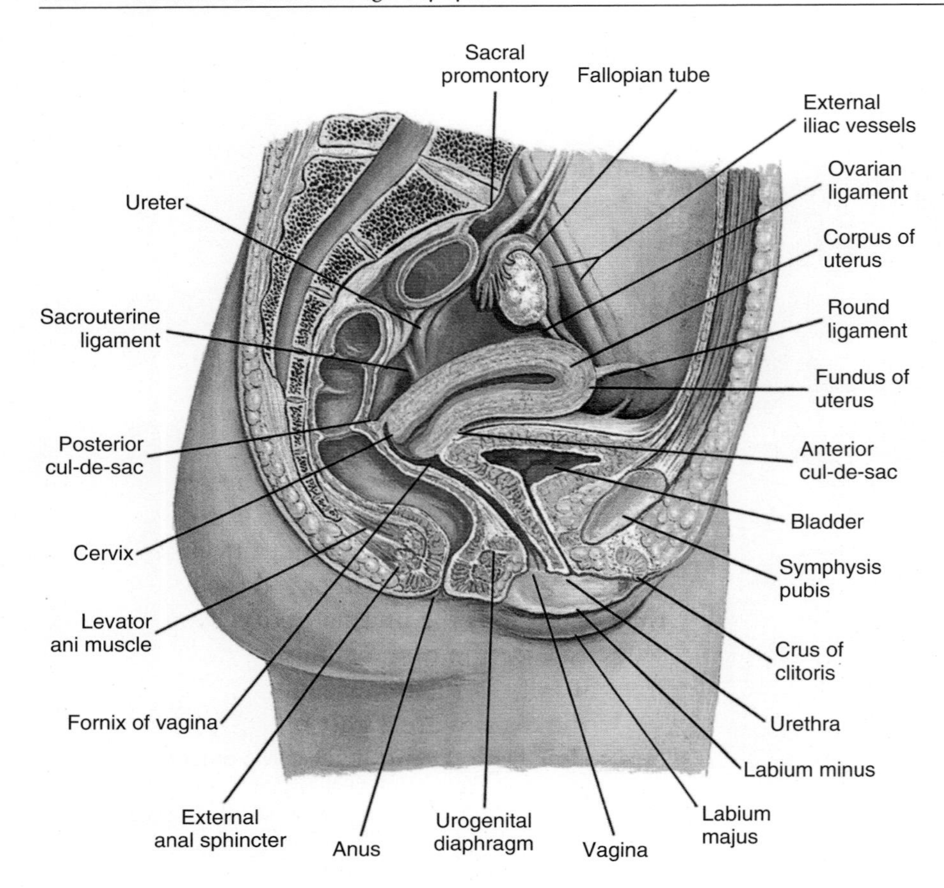

FIG. 12.17 Female pelvic floor, midsagittal view. (From Seidel HM, et al. *Mosby's Guide to Physical Examination.* 7th ed. Mosby/Elsevier; 2011.)

The ovaries are solid glands that produce the hormones estrogen and progesterone. The cortex of the ovaries contains numerous small masses of cells called ovarian (graafian) follicles. Each follicle contains an ovum.

Each funnel-shaped fallopian tube is about 4 inches long and serves as a duct to transport the ovum to the uterus, or womb, a hollow, muscular organ in the shape of an inverted pear. It lies between the urinary bladder and the rectum. The upper part of the uterus is the fundus; the middle part is the corpus; the lower, narrow portion is the cervix, which opens into the vagina. The uterus receives the ovum and allows the embryo to grow and develop into a fetus. The inner lining is a soft, spongy layer, the endometrium, the surface of which is shed each month during menstruation. Uterine contractions at the end of the **gestation** period push the fetus into the vagina.

The vagina is a flexible, fibromuscular tube about 0 to 3½ inches long that receives the sperm from the male and serves as the birth canal. The region between the vagina and anus is the clinical perineum and may tear during the birth process because of overstretching.

The vagina has a dual function: sexual intercourse and the delivery of a baby. The mucus in the vagina during nonsexual times comes from uterine glands. During sexual arousal, Bartholin glands secrete mucus into the vagina. During orgasm, the muscular layer of the vagina contracts, moving semen into the cervix. Changes in the vaginal mucosa reflect cyclic endocrine changes that may be used to determine times of increased fertility.

External Organs

The external organs of the female reproductive system include the labia majora, labia minora, clitoris, mons pubis, vestibule, vaginal orifice, and Bartholin (vestibular) glands. The aforementioned external genitalia are known collectively as the *vulva*. The mons pubis, located over the symphysis pubis, becomes covered with hair during puberty.

Each Bartholin gland opens into the mucosal surface near the superior portion of the labia minora. The gland discharges a clear secretion during sexual arousal. Cysts and abscesses are common in these glands.

The mammary glands (breasts) are accessory organs that produce and secrete milk after pregnancy. They are included in the integument and are discussed in Chapter 11.

Beginning with puberty and for the next 35 to 40 years, the ovaries undergo cyclic changes in which a certain number of ovarian follicles develop. When one ovum completes the developmental process, it is released into one of the fallopian tubes. If fertilization does not occur, the developed ovum disintegrates and a new cycle begins.

A series of hormonal events takes place approximately every 28 days. Known as the *menstrual cycle*, day number 1 begins with the first day of uterine bleeding, called *menses* or *menstruation*. Cyclic hormonal changes occur in the pituitary, uterus, ovaries, and vagina. As in the male, FSH and LH from the pituitary gland affect the gonads. FSH stimulates the growth of the follicle containing the egg and the secretion of female hormones called *estrogens* and *progesterone*. The main estrogen is estradiol, responsible for female secondary sex characteristics, growth of the maturing follicle, growth of the uterine lining (endometrium), and negative feedback control of FSH. LH has two main functions: (1) ovulation and (2) formation of the corpus luteum (from the old follicle). The corpus luteum secretes estrogen and another group of hormones, the progestins. The main progestin, progesterone, is responsible for the secretory phase of the uterine cycle, glandular growth in the breast, and negative feedback control of LH.

In the female, as in the male, almost no gonadal hormones are formed before age 9 or 10. As the hypothalamus matures, gonadotropin-releasing hormone stimulates the production of FSH and LH. In response, the ovaries produce estradiol and then progesterone. Breast buds and pubic hair appear at about age 11. The breasts grow, and axillary hair appears; the adrenal cortex is responsible for initial axillary and pubic hair growth in both sexes. The uterus and vagina enlarge. Uterine bleeding (the menarche) begins about 2 years after breast bud development and is often sporadic for several months. Ovulation takes place after the menarche.

As puberty progresses, the hips broaden, the forearms diverge more at the elbows, and scant body hair but much head hair is evident. The voice retains a high-pitched quality. Estradiol is not as anabolic as testosterone, so muscular development, bone size, and general body growth are not as great as in the male. Estrogens cause the skin to have a smooth texture. Prepubertal characteristics, such as voice pitch, head hairline, sparse body hair (compared with that of the male), and distribution of body fat are retained and accentuated. Estradiol and testosterones are responsible for the female libido. In mammals, estrogens induce mating behavior, receptiveness of the female for the male, and nesting and maternal characteristics. As in the male, libido is influenced by cerebral control. Libido increases at ovulation and sometimes during menstruation.

At about the age of 40 or 50, a decrease in the responsiveness of the ovaries to FSH and LH occurs and is accompanied by irregular menstrual cycles. This is menopause. Although levels of estradiol and progesterone decrease, it is common for there to be little change in libido.

The autonomic nervous system exerts influence over the female reproductive system; as in the male, sexual arousal is a parasympathetic function, and orgasm is a sympathetic activation. Sympathetic deviances can interfere with ovulation and menstruation and thus are implicated in menstrual disorders and infertility.

Female Contraceptive Methods

In contrast to males, females have available a multitude of contraceptive methods. Tying or cauterizing the fallopian tubes, known as *tubal ligation*, is a permanent procedure. As with the vasectomy, even though the ends of the cut and tied fallopian tubes may be rejoined later, fertility decreases. Tubal ligation by cauterization is almost impossible to reverse. Currently used methods of birth control are the birth control pill, injections of hormones, implanted hormone-releasing devices, the intrauterine device, the diaphragm, spermicidal agents, abstinence, and the rhythm method. The most reliable methods are the pill, injections and implants, the condom plus a spermicidal agent, the intrauterine device, and the diaphragm with a spermicidal agent, in decreasing order of effectiveness. In some, especially smokers older than 35, the pill contributes to venous thromboembolism. In others, the pill may cause weight gain. The condom with a spermicidal agent has the added benefit of protection from some, but not all, sexually transmitted infections.

Pregnancy

Fertilization is the penetration of the egg by a sperm, restoring the diploid number (46) of chromosomes. Fertilization usually occurs as the egg moves down the fallopian tube. The ovum contains one X chromosome. A sperm contains an X or a Y chromosome, so the male determines the sex of the baby. If a male sperm (Y) reaches the egg, a male baby results; if a female sperm (X) reaches the egg, a female baby is produced. After the head of the sperm enters the egg, the tail detaches, and the ovum prohibits the entrance of other sperm. The chromosomes of egg and sperm nuclei arrange themselves at the two poles of the fertilized egg, and it begins to divide. Gestation is measured in the following ways: 280 days, 40 weeks, 10 lunar months, or 9 calendar months, and is divided into trimesters. The first trimester of pregnancy is week 1 through week 12, or about 3 months. The second trimester is week 13 through week 27. The third trimester of pregnancy spans from week 28 to the birth.

FOCUS ON PROFESSIONALISM

Massage therapists can specialize. This means that additional education targets a specific group of people with similar needs. Massage specialties can include pain management, stress management and breathing pattern disorders, oncology care, and prenatal and postnatal care. Most pregnancies are normal events with appropriate alterations in homeostasis. Adaption during massage primarily involves position for comfort, avoidance of aggressive stretching, and using only gentle massage methods on the abdomen. If there are increased risks related to pregnancy, then the learning curve increases substantially because the pregnancy is no longer normal. There is no special massage protocol related to specialization. There is increased information, experience, and possibly supervision to balance benefits and risks. As a professional, you understand the difference between entry-level practice and more advanced practice, which may include specialization, and the commitment needed to earn the right to claim the designation of an experienced and educated massage therapist.

First Trimester

Various physiological changes occur during the first trimester, along with radical hormonal changes. The changes influence mood, digestion, sleep, and energy levels.

Early pregnancy is a different experience for each individual. Actual menstruation stops, but slight bleeding may occur throughout the first trimester, which is why some often do not realize they are pregnant until about 3 months into the pregnancy. About 7 days after conception, implantation bleeding may occur. This bleeding is rare but normal; the formation of new blood vessels causes vaginal spotting. The urge to urinate occurs more frequently because the uterus begins to enlarge and press down on the bladder. Hormonal changes, such as mega bursts of progesterone, result in the retention and release of more water.

Most feel changes in their breasts. The breasts may swell, tingle, throb, or hurt because of the developing milk glands and the increased blood supply to the breasts. The veins become more pronounced and visible. The nipples enlarge and become more erect, and the areolae darken and become broader. Some notice early on that their nipples feel sensitive and sore.

Fatigue is another major symptom at this stage. It begins after the first missed period and persists until the 14th to 20th week of pregnancy. The need for sleep increases. About 10 hours of sleep per night is suggested during the first trimester.

Increased levels of progesterone also may cause the person who is pregnant to feel faint and constipated. The progesterone dilates the smooth muscle of the blood vessels and causes blood to pool in the legs, and more blood begins to flow to the uterus, which can cause low blood pressure and may result in fainting. Standing or sitting for long periods tends to trigger faintness. Lying flat and doing exercises that get the blood circulating prevent this.

Progesterone also relaxes the smooth muscles of the small and large intestines, slowing down the digestive process and leading to constipation. Lower back pain also occurs because the expanding uterus might put pressure on the sciatic nerve.

Between 60% and 80% of all pregnant people suffer nausea and vomiting in the first trimester. Discomfort that begins in the morning, often called *morning sickness*, can persist 24 hours a day for the first few weeks of pregnancy. Sometimes the nausea is not bad enough to cause vomiting but is an ever-present condition that can be controlled by eating dry crackers or drinking juice.

Numerous other symptoms accompany morning sickness, including an aversion to certain tastes or smells. Changes in hormone levels somehow affect the stomach lining and stomach acids, causing nausea. An empty stomach aggravates the nausea. Also, a strong connection exists between nausea and low blood sugar levels. Eating well is important during pregnancy. Some require a vitamin supplement; some must discontinue taking vitamin supplements to relieve or prevent other symptoms.

Fitness and exercise are important but in moderation.

Second Trimester

In the second trimester, the individual settles into the pregnant state and often has a general sense of well-being. Appetite increases, blood volume increases, and the body places an additional workload on all physiological functions.

Increased blood in the vaginal area causes more vaginal secretions and discharge. Progesterone depresses the central nervous system and may cause moodiness or depression. The hormones that slow down the intestinal tract also relax the sphincter between the stomach and esophagus, allowing stomach juices to flow up into the esophagus. Reflux of stomach juices into the esophagus causes a burning sensation in the middle of the chest that is called *heartburn*. As the uterus grows, it crowds the intestines, and heartburn may get much worse.

Table 12.7 Weight Gain During Pregnancy

Area of Gain	Amount of Gain (pounds)
(At term)	
Uterus	2–3
Breasts	1–3
Blood volume	3–5
Body fluid	1–3
Fat, protein, and so on	5–8
Baby (at 9 months)	
Baby	7–8
Amniotic fluid	2–4 2½
Placenta	1–5 1½
Total	**22–32**

By week 15, the baby weighs almost 2 ounces. The bones are growing, and the muscle movement is increasing. The person who is pregnant probably does not feel the baby moving yet, and the first movements feel like flutters. A soft, fine hair called *lanugo* covers the baby. The neck of the baby becomes longer, and the head can move. The arms move freely in front of the body, and the hands can grasp each other. Ultrasound has picked up babies sucking their thumbs by this time.

Table 12.7 provides an approximation of weight distribution during pregnancy. This distribution varies with each person and increases with twins, triplets, and quadruplets. With multiple babies, the weight of each baby is lower.

The amount of blood circulating throughout the body, especially in the areas of the vagina and rectum, continues to increase. New vessels form, but they are not strong and often bulge or swelling in the vaginal area, rectum, and legs, and varicose veins may form around the labia, vagina, and legs. When the vessels in the rectum swell, hemorrhoids develop and may protrude out of the rectum with strenuous bowel movements.

By 21 weeks, the baby weighs almost 1 pound and is nearly 10 to 11 inches long. Every system is progressing in development. The primitive structures of the brain have been developed for some time. Now the fine details of the nerve pathways in the brain are forming. Nerve cells that allow the baby's brain to receive and transmit messages are forming layers in the brain. This process continues at a much slower rate for another 3 months.

The baby can hear sounds from outside of the body and is aware of the constant rhythm created by the beating heart as well as the swishing and gurgling of fluids inside the body. The baby's eyes remain fused shut. By the end of week 21, the layers of the retina have developed and the skin is forming a white coating called *vernix caseosa*, a fatty film that protects the baby's skin from breakdown in the amniotic fluid. Vernix also prevents the loss of water and electrolytes from the baby into the amniotic fluid. The permanent ridges that form the fingers, hands, and feet are now developed, and the fingernails and toenails are getting harder.

The baby is swallowing more than 2 teaspoons of amniotic fluid per day, and by the end of the pregnancy may be swallowing nearly 2 cups of amniotic fluid per day. The digestive system has developed, and the digestive processes are beginning. A stool called *meconium* forms in the bowel. The air sacs in the lungs, called *alveoli*, are beginning to emerge.

During pregnancy, the progesterone that has slowed the digestive system affects the gallbladder in much the same way. The gallbladder takes a longer time to empty, allowing bile salts to accumulate in the system and absorb through the skin. This causes significant itching that is particularly noticeable around the navel, entire belly, chest, neck, face, and sometimes hands.

The growing uterus and baby put a lot of pressure on the two main blood vessels that lead into and out of the heart, the vena cava and the aorta. Pressure occurs when lying flat on the back. The side-lying position is best.

As the pregnancy progresses, the capillaries become more permeable and tend to leak water. When the capillaries leak water, the result is an increase in water retention or edema. Some edema is normal in pregnancy, but edema that increases all over the body, particularly in the legs, arms, lower back, and face, could indicate a serious problem requiring immediate referral to a physician.

Following are suggestions and cautions to ease the discomforts of swelling:

- Drink plenty of fluids to stimulate the kidneys.
- Avoid tight-fitting clothing, especially socks, hose, pant legs, and waistbands.
- Avoid standing or sitting in one place for long periods.
- Rest with the legs elevated on a chair or pillow.
- Lie down on the left side to increase kidney function.
- Increase protein intake to pull the fluid back into the vessels.
- Exercise (such as walking and swimming) increases circulation and lymphatic movement of water back into the vessels.
- Do not take diuretics for water retention in pregnancy.

The renal system changes during pregnancy. The kidneys produce more urine, and the bladder has decreased tone. The same progesterone that alters other systems influences the urinary system and makes it less efficient. As a result, many pregnant persons may develop urinary tract infections, which can become serious and cause not only pain and discomfort but also preterm labor. If untreated, a mild urinary tract infection can lead to a serious bladder or kidney infection that could require hospitalization and treatment with intravenous antibiotics.

At the end of the second trimester, the baby is at a milestone in development. The eyes are no longer fused shut; the fine details of optic nerve development, peripheral vision, and focus are present. Hearing has completely developed. The brain is functioning at a higher level, as are all of the baby's senses: sight, hearing, taste, touch, and smell. The baby has developed a schedule of sorts, moving while awake and being still while asleep. An early sucking reflex is present, although the ability to suck and swallow will not be present until about 34 weeks. The baby is also practicing the motions needed for breathing.

Third Trimester

The last trimester finds the heavy with the baby, and postural changes are evident. Internal organs are crowded. Physiological systems are strained by the need to sustain the person who is pregnant and the baby. The connective tissue structure softens to permit the expansion needed for the birth. This is a time of rest and waiting (Fig. 12.18).

The third trimester begins after about 26 weeks of pregnancy. During these last 3 months, the baby continues to grow and develop. Although a baby might survive if born during the early to middle part of the last trimester, these months are critical to the development of organs, such as the lungs and the brain.

The baby is now about 15 inches long and weighs around 3 pounds. The baby may suck the thumb, hiccup, and respond to stimuli, such as light, pain, and sounds.

The lower abdomen may hurt from time to time, and they may have an occasional brief contraction in which the uterus hardens and then returns to normal. Vaginal discharge may become heavier, and they may feel breathless for no apparent reason and have difficulty sleeping. Colostrum, the early form of milk, may leak from the breasts and they may feel apprehensive or excited about the coming labor and delivery.

By the eighth month, the baby has grown to about 18 inches, weighs approximately 5 pounds, and can see and hear. The lungs are still immature, but many other organs are well developed. Brain growth is especially rapid during this time. At some point during the eighth month, the baby shifts into a position until birth.

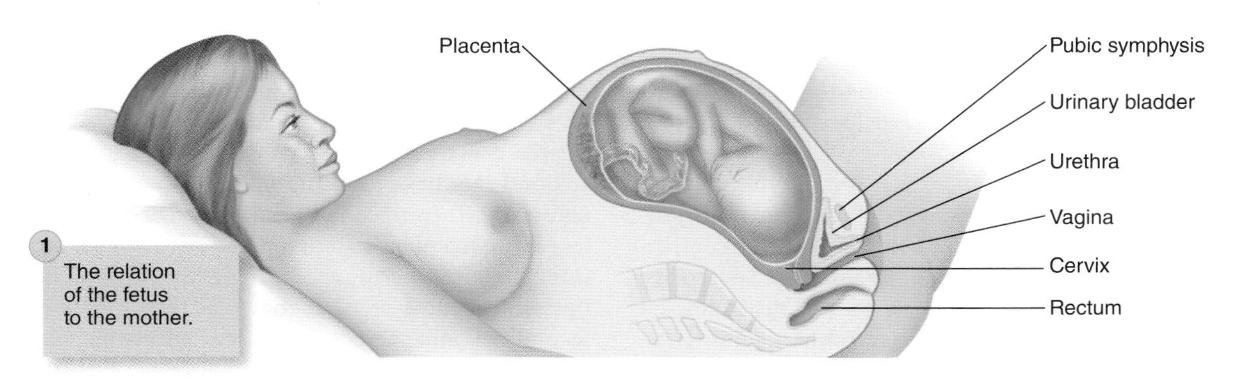

FIG. 12.18 Fetus in utero. (From Thibodeau GA, Patton KT. *Structure and Function of the Body.* 4th ed. Mosby/Elsevier; 2012.)

By 36 weeks, the baby is about 20 inches long, weighs 6 to 7 pounds, and will gain about ½ pound a week until delivery. The baby's lungs are mature. Movement often slows down because of the cramped space and head-down position in the pelvis.

During this stage of pregnancy backache and heaviness increase, the abdomen may itch, and the pelvis may be uncomfortable. After the baby drops, breathing and eating become easier, but urinary urge increases. Uterine contractions may increase and feel more intense.

Birth

The exact stimulus for birth is unknown, but increased fetal activity seems to play a role. Oxytocin stimulates the contraction of the uterus, causes delivery of the placenta after the expulsion of the fetus, and promotes parental bonding with the baby.

Prelabor

Prelabor can begin any time during the last few weeks or last days of pregnancy. They also may get diarrhea and possibly a severe backache, both precursors to early labor. Diarrhea empties the intestinal tract before actual labor begins, and painless Braxton Hicks contractions may begin to be more frequent.

At this stage, the cervix softens and may start to thin out a little, which allows it to dilate slightly. A bloody discharge called *bloody show*, may occur which means that the mucus plug sealing the cervical opening is now pink, or blood-streaked, and is leaking discharge.

As the baby's head presses down against the amniotic membranes containing fluid, the membranes may break in what is known as "breaking the water," the classic prelabor symptom. People expect this event to be like a flood of water suddenly rushing out of their vaginas, and it commonly happens that way, but the fluid also may just trickle out. The fluid normally is clear and odorless. Some think that they have wet their pants when this happens. If the water has not broken at this point, it probably will during more active labor.

Early Labor

Prelabor slowly unfolds into early labor. This phase lasts about 7 or 8 hours. Early labor and active labor also are known as the first stages of labor. Early labor is characterized by contractions that cause the cervix to dilate 3 to 4 cm. These contractions can feel wavelike. They build up and then recede. They are mildly intense and begin in the lower back. They also can feel like heavy menstrual cramps. The contractions occur between 5 and 20 minutes apart, become more intense each time they occur, last anywhere from 30 to 45 seconds, get longer each time they occur, and occur more closely together.

Active Labor

Active labor is similar to early labor but is far more pronounced. This phase lasts from 3 to 5 hours. Now the contractions occur every 2 to 4 minutes and last as long as 60 seconds. They may be moderately or extremely painful, depending on the person. At this point, the physician could administer an epidural, a painkiller that numbs from the breasts down. In natural childbirth, this type of procedure is not used. Whether or not they receive an epidural, there will be a strong urge to push, much like the urge to push during a bowel movement. They may start to feel warm or get chills.

Transition Phase

The transition phase proceeds to delivery and lasts anywhere from 30 to 90 minutes. Active labor has been in progress for approximately 3 hours and is likely tired and frustrated; may have no idea what time it is; may be shaking, hiccupping, vomiting, or having chills; may have cold feet and dry mouth and lips; and may be hyperventilating, moaning, crying, or screaming. They may have a tremendous urge to push and experience rectal pressure. Contractions are intense, occurring every 30 seconds and lasting 90 seconds. The cervix is almost fully dilated. Some individuals may want to use the bathroom, which will help them to relax and encourage pushing.

Delivery: Bearing Down

Instead of holding back the urge to push, pushing begins. At this phase, the hardest part is pushing out the head. As the head emerges, there may be intense burning and stinging sensations. The vagina is like a huge elastic band that stretches for this event.

Episiotomy

An episiotomy is a minor surgical procedure in which the physician makes an incision in the perineum, the area between the rectum and vagina. The episiotomy enlarges the opening for vaginal births, making it easier for the baby's head to come out.

A routine episiotomy cuts through skin, vaginal mucosa, and three layers of muscle in an otherwise sensitive area. The side effects include pain, bleeding, a breakdown of stitches, and delayed healing. Many doctors believe that a little natural tearing, which often takes place without the episiotomy, not only heals much more quickly than a surgical procedure but is less painful.

Any medical emergency during delivery can be a reason for an episiotomy. For example, an episiotomy might be deemed necessary when the baby's heartbeat becomes abnormal during pushing, when delivery must be facilitated because the baby is premature or breech, and whenever forceps are necessary (e.g., if the head is in an awkward position). The procedure is also necessary when the delivery of the baby's head is progressing at a rate or manner that will badly tear the perineum or when the vagina is not stretching. But for the majority of normal, vaginal deliveries, episiotomy is not necessary.

Cesarean Birth

A cesarean section, or C-section, is a surgical procedure that is essentially an abdominal delivery. Cesarean section is considered major pelvic surgery that usually involves a spinal or epidural anesthetic (only in some cases is a general anesthetic necessary). The surgeon makes a vertical or horizontal incision just above the pubic hair and then (usually) cuts horizontally through the uterine muscle and eases the baby out. Sometimes this second cut is vertical, known as the *classic incision*. The second cut, into the uterine muscle, affects the viability of a vaginal birth after a prior cesarean delivery. With a horizontal cut, some have gone on to have normal second vaginal births.

In some instances, there is a scheduled cesarean section. The pelvis may be too small; or the cervix may have irreparable scarring, because of previous pelvic surgery, that prevents dilation; or an emergency may be detected in utero (in the womb) that requires immediate removal of the fetus. In these cases, the problem usually does not appear until labor.

Placenta

The placenta is known as the *afterbirth, birth of placenta*, or just the *third stage of labor*. In a vaginal delivery, whether or not an episiotomy has been performed, the uterus contracts enough to loosen the placenta from the uterine wall after the birth of the baby. These contractions may be painful, but they are mild compared with the previous contractions. The placenta then slips out with one or two pushes. The uterus then continues to contract against exposed blood vessels where the placenta used to be as a natural way to control bleeding.

Hormones secreted by the placenta, including chorionic gonadotropin and other substances having estrogenic, progestational, or adrenocorticoid activity, play important roles during pregnancy. Parental bonding with the infant immediately after birth is important. The touch, sound, and smell of parents and infants in the first hours of birth establish biological and emotional bonds. The hormone oxytocin seems to play a role in this bonding process for both parents.

Lactation

The main physiological function of the mammary glands is to provide proper nutrition for the baby, as well as to protect the infant from infections during the first few months of life by transferring antibodies to the baby. The breasts enlarge substantially after the second month of pregnancy because of increased amounts of estrogen and progesterone. Prolactin causes the production and secretion of milk. The actual ejection (letdown) of milk from the nipple requires suckling and the release of oxytocin from the posterior pituitary gland. The cry of the infant, and in some cases emotional responses, may cause oxytocin release and lactation. Because milk production is based on demand, lactation persists for months, even years, if suckling continues. The breasts secrete a yellow fluid, colostrum, during the last part of pregnancy and for the first day or two after delivery. Colostrum has a high protein content and contains antibodies. The breasts start to secrete milk 1 to 3 days after delivery (Fig. 12.19).

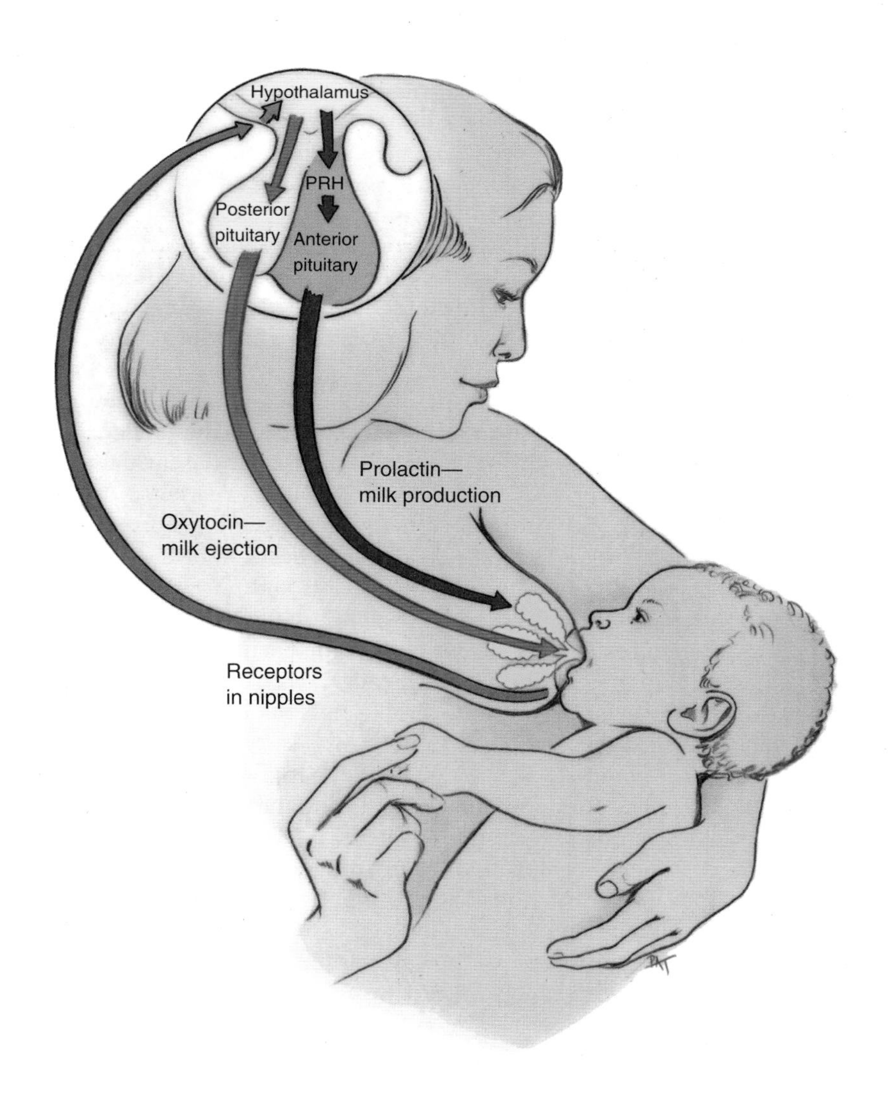

FIG. 12.19 Stimulus for lactation. *PRH*, Prolactin releasing hormone. (From Applegate E. *The Anatomy and Physiology Learning System*. 4th ed. Saunders/Elsevier; 2011.)

Postpartum

A postpartum (or postnatal) period begins immediately after the birth of a child as the body, including hormone levels and uterus size, returns to a non-pregnant state. The initial or acute period involves the first 6 to 12 hours postpartum. The person needs to be monitored for crises such as postpartum hemorrhage, uterine inversion, amniotic fluid embolism, and eclampsia.

The second phase is the subacute postpartum period, which lasts 2 to 6 weeks. During this phase, the body is undergoing major changes in terms of hemodynamics, genitourinary recovery, metabolism, and emotional status.

The third phase is the delayed postpartum period, which can last up to 6 months. Changes during this phase are extremely gradual, and pathology is rare. This is the time of restoration of muscle tone and connective tissue to the pre-pregnant state. Although change is subtle during this phase, the body is not fully restored to prepregnant physiology until about 6 months post-delivery.

Pelvic floor dysfunction after childbirth is common and includes stress urinary incontinence, incontinence of flatus or feces, uterine prolapse, cystocele, and rectocele. A cystocele happens when the bladder pushes against weakened tissue in the vagina and drops down into the vagina. A rectocele happens when the rectum bulges into the vagina. These problems can cause discomfort, leaking of urine or bowel movements, bladder infections, constipation, and pain during sex. Postpartum pelvic pain is extremely common. It can occur after childbirth due to the loosening of ligaments and joints during pregnancy, which occurs as the body works to strengthen the pelvic floor and hip rotators. Pelvic rehabilitation is a type of physical therapy that can be helpful for postpartum moms. Pregnancy and childbirth can damage the muscles and connective tissue of the pelvic floor, causing all kinds of inconvenient and uncomfortable symptoms after giving birth.

The World Health Organization (WHO) describes the postpartum period as the most critical and yet the most neglected phase in the lives of parents and babies. During the subacute postpartum period, psychological disorders may emerge. Among these are postpartum depression, post-traumatic stress disorder, and in rare cases, postpartum anxiety or psychosis. Postpartum depression is moderate to severe depression experienced after giving birth. It may occur soon after delivery or up to a year later. Most of the time, it occurs within the first 3 months after delivery. Feelings of anxiety, irritation, tearfulness, and restlessness are common in the week or two after pregnancy. These feelings are often called the postpartum or "baby blues." They almost always go away soon, without the need for treatment.

Postpartum depression may occur when the baby blues *do not* fade away or when signs of depression start 1 or more months after childbirth. A new birth parent who has any symptoms of postpartum depression should contact their provider right away to get help. Postpartum anxiety (PPA) can involve physical symptoms, including changes in eating and sleeping habits, dizziness, hot flashes, rapid heartbeat, and nausea. Postpartum anxiety may feel like being constantly on edge and typically manifests in the form of worry. Of the people who develop postpartum psychosis, research has suggested that there is approximately a 5% suicide rate and a 4% infanticide rate associated with the illness. This is because experiencing psychosis is undergoing a break from reality. This is a medical emergency.

Practical Application

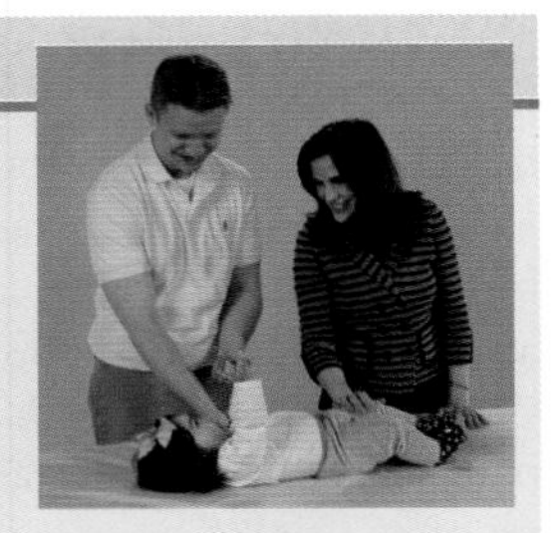

Massage therapy can be supportive during pregnancy, labor, delivery, lactation, and the eventual return of the body to a non-pregnant state. During the pregnancy, the main goal is stress management, sleep support, and management of some of the muscular and skeletal discomforts of pregnancy.

Recommendations for Massage During Pregnancy

Unless specific circumstances or complications are involved, massage for those who are pregnant should be a general massage. Massage therapy is indicated during all pregnancy-related stages, from conception to postpartum, in a normal pregnancy. Do not massage vigorously or extremely deep, do not overstretch, and do not massage the abdomen other than with gentle superficial pressure. Watch for fever, edema, varicose veins, and severe mood swings. Pregnancy is typically considered a hypercoagulable state—meaning that blood clots more readily than normal and is predisposed to deep-vein thrombosis or other clot-related conditions. Keep in mind that blood clots during pregnancy are rare, but if they occur they are serious conditions that may become life-threatening when the blood clot is dislodged from the site of formation. The blood clot can become stuck in smaller blood vessels in the lung, a condition known as pulmonary embolism. If the thrombus or blood clot goes to the heart, one will experience a heart attack, and a thrombus that reaches the brain may result in a stroke. The massage therapist needs to be aware of the signs and symptoms of blood clots and refer the client for proper care. These blood clots usually produce swelling, redness, or pain in one part of the client's body, especially in the legs. The pain typically increases during walking. The veins may be more visible and look larger than normal. During massage, it is important to screen for the potential for blood clots as the pregnancy progresses. The tendency for clot formation increases during the third trimester and early postpartum period. Because of the normal increase in blood coagulation during pregnancy, it is important to make sure that massage does not cause tissue damage and that any methods that are aggressive and invasive, such as deep transverse friction or sustained compression over a small area, are avoided. During massage on the legs, caution is necessary and the massage application should be adapted using a light to moderate broad-based contact. Do not apply deep stripping methods. After birth, postpartum depression, anxiety, and psychosis can become serious problems for some. Refer a client with these conditions to their physician immediately.

Pathological Conditions of the Reproductive System

Abnormal Pregnancy

Bleeding

Not all bleeding means that a miscarriage is imminent. Nevertheless, although some bleeding during early pregnancy is fairly common, it is still not normal. An individual with bleeding that requires heavy-duty pads that need to be changed frequently should report the condition immediately. Other signs and symptoms, including cramps, pain in the abdomen, fever, weakness, and possibly vomiting, are serious. The blood may have clumps of tissue in it and have an unusual odor. Another kind of bleeding is brown, intermittent, or continuous vaginal spotting or light bleeding accompanied by severe abdominal or shoulder pain. Finally, light bleeding that continues for more than 3 days may also indicate an intrauterine problem requiring evaluation.

Miscarriage

Heavy bleeding and cramping at any time between the end of the second month to the end of the third month are classic signs of miscarriage. Cramps without any bleeding are also a dangerous sign of miscarriage. The bleeding may be heavy enough to soak several pads in an hour, or it may be manageable and more like a heavy period. Cramping may occur with passing clots, which are dark red clumps that look like small pieces of raw beef liver. Sometimes grayish or pinkish tissue is passed. A miscarriage also can take place with persistent, light bleeding and milder cramping at this stage.

Several kinds of spontaneous abortions can occur:

- *Threatened abortion:* The cervix still is closed, but there are cramps, bleeding, or staining. The doctor performs a physical examination, checks the fetal heartbeat, and may prescribe bed rest. In some cases, the bleeding stops, and the pregnancy continues normally.
- *Inevitable abortion:* In this case, nature has taken its course already and the process of miscarriage has started. Bleeding is heavy, cramps increase, and the cervix begins to dilate, expelling everything still intact: the fetus, amniotic sac, and placenta, accompanied by a great deal of blood.
- *Incomplete abortion:* In this condition, the uterus has spontaneously expelled some, but not all, pregnancy tissue. Usually what remains are fragments of the placenta. The condition is correctable with a dilation and curettage procedure to clean out the uterus and help it heal.
- *Complete abortion:* Complete abortion occurs when all pregnancy tissue passes spontaneously. Although dilation and curettage may be indicated, the procedure usually is not necessary.
- *Missed abortion:* The fetus dies in the uterus but is not expelled. Symptoms that something is wrong may not be apparent. Instead, all of the pregnancy symptoms gradually disappear. It is common for the physician to diagnose missed abortion during a routine examination when the fetal heartbeat is no longer audible. Treatment depends on the duration of the pregnancy.

The reason for miscarriage usually has to do with a fetus self-terminating because of improper development or genetic problems.

Ectopic Pregnancy

An ectopic pregnancy occurs when the fetus fails to implant itself in the uterus and starts to develop in the fallopian tube. Ectopic pregnancies are dangerous. The rupture of the tube could be a life-threatening situation. The classic symptoms of ectopic pregnancy are sharp abdominal cramps or pains on one side. The pains may start out as dull aches that get more severe. Neck pains and shoulder pains are also common. The person also may experience a menstrual type of bleeding along with the pain, but the pain is the most obvious sign. The problem with an ectopic pregnancy is that they may not realize they are pregnant.

Individuals in groups at high risk for ectopic pregnancy generally have the following characteristics:

- They are users of intrauterine devices.
- They have histories of pelvic inflammatory disease.
- They have histories of pelvic surgery resulting in scarring that may block the tube and prevent the fertilized egg from traveling to the uterus.
- They have histories of ectopic pregnancies.
- Their pregnancies result from assisted contraception techniques in which gametes or embryos have been injected into the fallopian tubes.

Preeclampsia, Toxemia, and Pregnancy-Induced Hypertension

Preeclampsia is a disease that occurs only during pregnancy. The terms *preeclampsia, pregnancy-induced hypertension*, and *toxemia* are essentially interchangeable. The complications of preeclampsia are swelling, high blood pressure, poor kidney function, poor liver function, pulmonary edema, the presence of protein in the urine, and possible seizure. A poor blood supply to the baby decreases the baby's nutrients, interfering with development. Preeclampsia occurs in 5% to 10% of all pregnancies and can appear without warning at any time during pregnancy or labor or in the early postpartum period. This disease also can be chronic, gradually becoming worse over time. Preeclampsia may be mild or severe, but the only cure is the delivery of the baby.

Hyperemesis Gravidarum

Hyperemesis gravidarum is severe nausea and vomiting during pregnancy, which results in dehydration and the loss of at least 10 pounds. Individuals in this state may be unable to eat or drink anything for days. They may require intravenous hydration and may have abnormalities in blood chemical levels. Hyperemesis gravidarum is exhausting and emotionally distressing but usually has no effect on the developing fetus.

Bartholin Cyst

Bartholin glands are located on each side of the vaginal opening. Obstruction of a duct sometimes occurs because of a bacterial infection that makes the area painful and swollen. Treatment may require drainage.

Breast Lumps

Most breast lumps are not cancerous, although the incidence of cancer increases with age (see Chapter 11). However, clients should be referred to their physician for evaluation of any new lumps or masses, either in the axillae or breasts.

Cervical Cancer

Cervical cancer is the third most common malignancy in females after breast and colon cancer. Cervical dysplasia is a change in the cells of the cervix. Some of these abnormal cells can develop into cancerous cells. Early detection and treatment by removing or destroying the cells may prevent cancer. Factors contributing to the development of cervical cancer are as follows: becoming sexually active at an early age; having multiple sexual partners; having genital herpes; and, possibly, previous infection with human papillomavirus (HPV). Cervical cancer that is not treated in the early stages can spread into other tissues, especially lymph nodes and the uterus. Vaccines are now available that may prevent infection with various strains of HPV and prevent some forms of cervical cancer.

Cervicitis

Cervicitis is inflammation of the cervix. Acute cervicitis usually is caused by the same organisms that cause vaginitis (fungus, bacteria, or protozoa). Symptoms vary and may include redness, bleeding, pelvic pain, and discharge.

Chronic cervicitis is a recurrent inflammation of the cervix, commonly causing pelvic pain, often with a heavy discharge. Treatment of cervicitis is medication if it is caused by organisms or cauterization if the condition becomes chronic.

Endometriosis

Endometriosis is a disease in which endometrial tissue is present in non-uterine locations, such as on the intestines or ovaries or even in the fallopian tubes. Endometriosis occurs most often in females between the ages of 25 and 50, especially if they have borne no children. Although symptoms may be mild, common symptoms are heavy menstrual periods, intense back or pelvic pain, painful menstruation (dysmenorrhea), and painful intercourse (dyspareunia). Pregnancy often eliminates the problem. Birth control pills may help because they cause a change in the endometrial tissue. Sometimes surgical intervention is necessary.

Infertility

Infertility is a decrease in the ability to conceive, whereas sterility is a total loss of the ability to conceive. Infertility may be temporary and can result from structural or functional problems in the male, female, or both. Common causes in males are impotence (the inability to have an erection), a decrease in sperm number, or abnormalities in sperm anatomy and motility. In females, common causes include lack of ovulation; disorders of the fallopian tubes (often the result of a previous infection); and abnormal mucus secretion by the cervix, which creates an environment hostile to sperm. A low sperm count may be caused by excessive use of alcohol, tobacco, and caffeine; poor nutrition; and fatigue. Males should not wear tight underwear because it pulls the testes close to the body, increasing the temperature and decreasing the sperm count. Drugs are available that are effective in inducing ovulation. Surgery may help to correct tubal scarring. The administration of estrogen may restore normal cervical mucus. Generalized stress can be a cause of infertility.

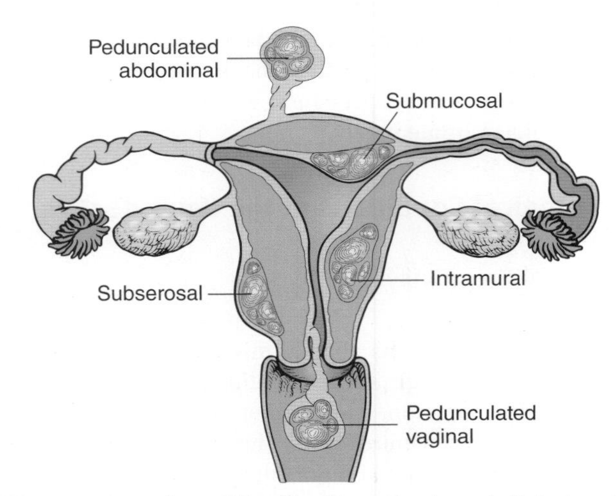

FIG. 12.20 Location of fibroids. (From Damjanov I. *Pathology for Health Professions.* 3rd ed. Saunders/Elsevier; 2006.)

Uterine Disorders

A myoma, or fibroid, is a benign tumor in the uterus that grows inside the uterine muscle wall or attaches to the wall (Fig. 12.20). Also called a leiomyoma, this tumor may be small, grow slowly, and cause no symptoms. Tumors that grow large or rapidly cause heavy bleeding. If blood loss is extensive, anemia may occur. Fibroids are the most common disorder of the uterus. Occurring in late reproductive years, these tumors are estrogen dependent. Prolonged or abnormal menstrual bleeding is usually the first sign. Treatment may be dietary for the anemia. In the rare cases in which the tumor grows large enough to cause severe bleeding, a hysterectomy is required.

Polyps are small growths of the endometrium extending into the body of the uterus. They are common in all age groups, especially in females with no pregnancies. The main symptom is increased menstrual bleeding between periods or post-menopausal bleeding. Removal of the polyps by a uterine curet (curettage) is indicated if symptoms are problematic. Cervical polyps occur when the lining of the cervix develops growths that hang outside the cervix.

Dysfunctional uterine bleeding is abnormal bleeding throughout much of the 28-day cycle. The main form of diagnosis and treatment is dilation and curettage.

Vaginitis

Vaginitis is inflammation of the vagina. Signs and symptoms are vaginal discharge, itching (pruritus), and irritation. A foul odor or itching or a yellow or green discharge may indicate a vaginal infection. A curd-like white discharge with itching probably indicates a yeast infection, which is treatable. A foul-smelling discharge or one that is yellow or green could indicate a more serious infection.

Yeast vaginitis (candidiasis, moniliasis) is a common infection caused by the fungus *Candida albicans*. The infection responds to an antifungal ointment, such as miconazole (Monistat) or nystatin or tablets of fluconazole (Diflucan).

Trichomonas vaginitis (trichomoniasis) is caused by a protozoal parasite that may infect the urinary tract of both sexes and is a sexually transmitted organism. Metronidazole (Flagyl) is effective. The sexual partner also may require treatment.

Vaginitis caused by species of the *Gardnerella* genus (formerly called *Haemophilus*) is a bacterial infection of the vagina. It responds to metronidazole or clindamycin.

Prostate Disorders

Prostatitis is an infection of the prostate, usually resulting from a urinary tract infection. Perineal pain, fever, chills, painful urination, and a tender prostate on rectal examination are common signs. If bacteria are causing the prostatitis, treatment with an antibiotic is indicated. Chronic prostatitis commonly occurs in older males with enlarged prostate glands.

Benign prostatic hypertrophy is the enlargement of the prostate, a disorder that occurs in males 45 years and older; it may be caused by a decrease in the ratio of testosterone to estrogen. As testosterone declines, estrogen produced by the adrenal cortex seems to stimulate the central portion of the prostate, causing an overgrowth of prostate tissue. The amount of enlargement is not as important as its ability to compress the urethra, which causes problems with urination, such as straining, dribbling, and sometimes urinary retention. Medical treatment, including catheterization and surgery, is indicated in the most severe cases. The herb saw palmetto has been shown to be beneficial in decreasing hypertrophy.

Prostatic cancer is the most common malignancy in males after skin cancer. It grows slowly, is commonly asymptomatic, and is usually found during a physical checkup. Early-stage cancer is usually slow growing, whereas in later stages metastasis to bone commonly occurs, particularly in the thoracic and lumbar vertebrae and the sacrum. Symptoms include urinary retention if obstruction has taken place and lower back pain if metastasis has occurred. Primary treatment depends on the age of the person and the stage of the cancer; it may focus on relieving symptoms or removing the cancer by prostatectomy, radiation therapy, or removal of the testes because testosterone stimulates cancer cells.

Sexually Transmitted Infections

Sexually transmitted infections include vaginal infections, hepatitis B infection, non-gonococcal urethritis or chlamydia, genital warts, herpes genitalis, acquired immunodeficiency syndrome, gonorrhea, syphilis, and body lice. Most of these diseases have been discussed elsewhere in the text.

Gonorrhea is an infectious disease caused by a bacterium. It is becoming more resistant to antibiotics because mutant strains have developed. Gonorrhea infects the urethra of both sexes, producing urethritis several days after exposure. The person may show no signs or mild symptoms, which the person ignores while the bacteria spread.

In males, gonorrhea affects primarily the urethra, where it can cause scarring. If untreated, the bacteria can infect and inflame the prostate or the epididymis. Symptoms include difficult urination and a cloudy discharge.

In females gonorrhea usually infects the cervix, causing cervicitis. Untreated gonorrhea may infect the uterus or fallopian tubes, causing scarring that may result in infertility. Involvement of the tubes and surrounding pelvic area is called *pelvic inflammatory disease*. If gonorrhea travels to the abdominal cavity, it can cause peritonitis. Signs and symptoms of gonorrhea in females include fever, abnormal bleeding, cloudy vaginal discharge, bilateral pelvic pain (usually during the menses), and tenderness on the movement of the cervix (stretching the broad ligament).

Untreated gonorrhea in both sexes can infect the bloodstream, causing blood poisoning, and can spread to the skin, bones, joints, and tendons.

Syphilis is a bacterial infection transmitted sexually or during birth to the fetus. The frequency of infections declined with the discovery of penicillin but, as with gonorrhea, resistant strains are appearing. Syphilis appears in three stages:

Stage 1: Painless sores appear on the skin and are treated primarily with antibiotics.

Stage 2: A skin rash, which may be helped by antibiotics (stages 1 and 2 are highly contagious), appears.

Stage 3: Referred to as *late syphilis*, stage 3 is not as contagious, except when blood is exchanged between two persons. If the person does not recognize the symptoms of stages 1 or 2, the third stage can flare at any time and affect the brain, nervous system, aorta, and other organs of the body. Syphilis cannot be reversed in the third stage.

Herpes simplex is a virus that causes painful blisters and small ulcers in and around the mouth and the genital area. Type 1 usually infects the upper body, and type 2 affects the genital area. Type 2 is a common sexually transmitted disease. The primary infection lasts about 1 to 4 weeks. Recurrent lesions are less painful and debilitating, often emerging every month or two and lasting 7 to 10 days. The blisters form and then break open, remaining open for 2 to 3 weeks. The open blisters are painful. Herpes is transmitted when it is active—that is, when the lesions are present and up to 7 days afterward. Lesions recur in some affected persons. In others, recurrence takes place once or twice and never again.

Fever, emotional stress, menses, sunlight, infections, and trauma may activate herpes lesions. Genital lesions in females consist of painful vesicles and erosions on the labia, vagina, or cervix. In males, the lesions are commonly located on the penis.

ACTIVITY 12.1

We must be able to explain and justify the therapeutic value of the work we do. The following activity assists you in developing the skills to explain the effectiveness of therapeutic massage to clients and other healthcare professionals. Use the clinical reasoning model that follows to accomplish this task. Choose a pathology from this chapter and develop a care plan or describe how massage therapy supports the normal function of one of the systems from this chapter.

Methods/Applications

1. What are the facts?
   a. Which system is involved, and which structures of that system can be reached directly or indirectly?
   b. Which of these structures is most affected by this massage?
   c. Which physiological functions are affected by this approach?
   d. When the treatment is applied, what changes in function will occur in the following:
      (1) This system?
      (2) The whole body?
   e. What is considered normal or balanced function?
   f. How are the functions of this system related to the homeostasis of the body?
   g. What has worked or has not worked?
   h. Where could you find information that would support the use of this modality as a therapeutic intervention?
   i. What research is available to support the use of the therapeutic intervention?
   j. How does the intervention support a healthy state?
   k. Under which pathological or dysfunctional conditions is the therapeutic massage most likely to be beneficial?
2. What are the possibilities?
   a. What do the data suggest?
   b. What are the reasons for using the proposed method?
   c. What are the possible interventions?
   d. List at least three applications of massage that would affect the structure and function of the system involved.
   e. What are other ways to look at the situation?
   f. What other methods could provide similar benefits?
3. What is the logical outcome of therapeutic intervention?
   a. What would be the logical progression of the symptom pattern, contributing factors, and current behaviors?
   b. What are the benefits and drawbacks of each intervention suggested?
   c. What are the costs in terms of time, resources, and finances?
   d. What is likely to happen if the modality is not used?
   e. What is likely to happen if the modality is used?
4. For the intervention proposed, what would be the effect on the persons involved, specifically the client, practitioner, and other professionals working with the client?
   a. How does each person involved (including, besides the aforementioned, the client's family and support system) feel about the possible interventions?
   b. Does the practitioner feel qualified to work with the situation and apply the identified modality to the particular person?
   c. Does a feeling of cooperation and agreement exist among all those involved, and how would the practitioner recognize this feeling?

Justification

Using the information developed in the clinical reasoning model, present a clear, concise statement of how the ways in which the particular soft-tissue or movement modality would be beneficial in supporting the particular body system in a healthy condition or as part of a treatment plan for a pathological or dysfunctional condition. On the basis of the preceding information, give a brief summary of the effectiveness of the modality for this system.

INDICATIONS/CONTRAINDICATIONS for Therapeutic Massage

Reproductive System

As with all acute infections, massage is contraindicated until any infectious diseases of the reproductive system have run their course. Massage in clients with malignancies should occur as part of a comprehensive treatment plan developed by the health care team.

Therapeutic massage during a normal pregnancy is part of a wellness program, with accommodation for the changes that occur during pregnancy. Certainly, anyone working with people who are pregnant should learn more about pregnancy and fetal development than is provided in this text. Massage in the first trimester is fine if the client is generally healthy. Most reproductive system conditions present regional contraindications. As it does with most chronic illnesses and pain, therapeutic massage offers generalized support for homeostasis and can offer palliative or comfort care for the maintenance of these conditions (Activity 12.1).

Section Summary

- List the organs of the male reproductive system. The male reproductive organs are the testicles, epididymis, vas deferens, ejaculatory duct, urethra, penis, and scrotum.
- List the organs of the female reproductive system. The female reproductive organs are the ovaries, fallopian tubes, uterus, vagina, external genitalia, and mammary glands (breasts).
- Describe the stages of pregnancy. The ovum contains one X chromosome. A sperm contains an X or a Y chromosome, so the male determines the sex of the baby. If a male sperm (Y) reaches the egg, a male baby results; if a female sperm (X) reaches the egg, a female baby is produced. Gestation is measured in the following ways: 280 days, 40 weeks, 10 lunar months, or 9 calendar months divided into trimesters:
  - *First trimester*—Duration: week 1 to week 12. Baby development: from the zygote to the fetus, the baby grows to about 2.5 inches long, and facial features/arms/legs/fingers/toes/organs/external genitals begin to form. Common characteristics are breast changes/discomfort, fatigue, faintness (particularly after sitting/standing for long periods), morning sickness, and aversion to certain smells/tastes.
  - *Second trimester*—Duration: week 13 to week 27. Baby development: the baby grows to about 9 to 10 inches, responds to sound, lungs develop, and sex becomes apparent (usually by week 14). Common characteristics: may begin to feel baby movement, increased vaginal secretions/discharge, emotional changes related to CNS

depression, heartburn, swollen blood vessels (potentially causing varicose veins/hemorrhoids), itchiness, more frequent urination, edema (some edema is normal—body-wide edema requires immediate referral).
 - *Third trimester*—Duration: week 28 to week 40/until birth. Baby development: the baby fully develops (average 14 inches/7.5 pounds), kicks and stretches, grows hair, begins breathing, responds to light, and may turn its head down. Common characteristics: exaggerated postural changes (due to the size/weight of the baby), occasional abdomen pain/contractions, backache, breathlessness, sleep difficulties, and leakage of colostrum (the early form of milk) (see Table 12.7).
- Explain the birth process. *Prelabor* begins the last weeks/days of pregnancy. "Breaking the water" occurs in this stage. *Early labor* lasts 7 to 8 hours. Characterized by contractions occurring every 5 to 20 minutes causing cervix dilation to 3 to 4 cm. *Active labor* lasts 3 to 5 hours. Characterized by contractions occurring every 2 to 4 minutes. The *transition phase* precedes delivery and lasts 30 to 90 minutes. Characterized by contractions occurring every 30 seconds causing nearly complete cervix dilation. During *delivery*, pushing/bearing down occurs and the baby is born.
- Describe the best sleeping/massage position for most during pregnancy. Generally, the best position is side-lying, particularly on the left side.
- Describe indications/contraindications for massage therapy related to pregnancy. Massage therapy is indicated during all pregnancy stages from conception to postpartum in a normal pregnancy. Side-lying position should be used, particularly after the second trimester. Limit time in the supine position, particularly after the third trimester. Screen for signs/symptoms of a blood clot. Contraindications include overstretching, and vigorous/deep pressure (especially over the abdomen—only light superficial touch should be applied to/near the abdomen).

SUMMARY

On completion of the last set of justification exercises, you, the learner, should be familiar with a logical model of reasoning that honors intuition as well as the emotions and perceptions of the persons involved. As with all knowledge, you must question the process, make it your own, and improve it. This model is only a framework; however, the model helps you become more objective and addresses questions and issues that you may not think of on your own. It is good to consider various perspectives and then make your own best decisions.

The respiratory, digestive, urinary, and reproductive systems contribute to the complete function of the body as a whole. These systems concern the movement of energy, water, and air and the creation of new life inside and outside of the body. They reveal the interconnectedness involved in being alive and, with these systems, the need for interaction outside of yourself as you breathe in air, take in food and water, and connect with one another to produce life.

CRITICAL THINKING/CLINICAL REASONING

Each chapter will feature a critical thinking and clinical reasoning application of the content related to massage therapy practice. A client scenario will be presented with recommendations for additional research, often using MedlinePlus or PubMed. Relevant questions based on the chapter content outline are provided to guide the discussion. There are no specific correct answers to the questions. However, responses should be supportive of evidence-informed practices and based on biological plausibility if sufficient research is not available. The author's decision-making process related to the scenario and questions is on the Evolve site. Compare and contrast your thoughts and discussion with the authors and determine where you agree or disagree.

SCENARIO

The client is a 31-year-old person who is pregnant. The client works part-time at a coffee house and takes care of their 4-year-old child while managing household chores. The client has been receiving massage sessions weekly during this pregnancy. Today, the client has entered week number 34. Their back is beginning to feel achy, and their feet are swollen slightly. The client has been short of breath for the last month and has had heartburn and increased intestinal gas. During the massage, the client asked to use the restroom. When they got up from the table, they passed gas but just chuckled saying that they just can't control it these days. When the client returned, they mentioned that it burned a little when urinating and mentioned they had been leaking urine when coughing or sneezing.

Explore

MedlinePlus

Search Terms: Pregnancy, heartburn, backache, urinary tract infection, incontinence, edema, miscarriage, postpartum depression.

Discuss

See the author's response on the Evolve website.

What is the most logical reason for the client to be short of breath? What accessory muscles are being used to counter the shortness of breath? What muscle-related aching may occur with the activation of these accessory breathing muscles?

What predisposes pregnant people to heartburn, and how might this be related to shortness of breath and intestinal gas?

Is there a relationship between the burning sensation during urination, incontinence, and backache that would indicate a recommendation for referral?

What is the likely cause of lower extremity swelling? Is edema an indication for referral?

During the massage session, the client disclosed that they had had a miscarriage scare at about 10 weeks into the pregnancy and had heard that massaging the legs and ankles could cause miscarriage. How would you respond?

The client also comments that their sibling experienced postpartum depression. What would you need to research to best understand what the client is discussing? How might you respond if the client showed signs of postpartum depression?

Visit the Evolve website: https://evolve.elsevier.com/Fritz/essential/

The Evolve website provides support for the review of the chapter content and chapter quizzes to help you prepare for the MBLEx or other massage therapy certification or licensing exams. End of chapter questions for discussion and review answer key and rationales and author's response to critical thinking and clinical reasoning scenarios.

MULTIPLE CHOICE QUESTIONS FOR REVIEW AND DISCUSSION

The answers, with rationales, can be found on the Evolve site.

These questions are used for review and discussion. It is as important to understand why wrong answers are wrong as it is to know why the correct answer is correct. The answers to the questions, with rationales and explanations about why the correct answer is correct and why wrong answers are wrong, can be found on the Evolve site. Guidance also is provided on how questions are developed and how the textbook content can be presented in a multiple-choice question format. At the end of the question section here in the textbook, you will find an exercise that asks you to write more questions. Use the various questions in the chapter as examples. This is one of the best study strategies for test-taking.

It is important to understand that the actual licensing exam you take may not contain any of the specific questions found in this textbook or in the review material and practice tests on the Evolve site. Therefore, just because you can answer any of these questions correctly does not mean you will pass the licensing exam. The questions are content and style examples to help you prepare—this is why understanding why wrong answers are wrong is just as important as identifying the correct answer. Also, make sure you understand all the terminology used in the questions and possible answers in the review and discussion questions. Look up words you do not understand.

1. During the first trimester, there is an increase in progesterone. Which of the following results can therapeutic massage directly and mechanically influence?
   a. Increased urination
   b. Constipation
   c. Nausea
   d. Lymphatic stagnation

2. A client has been vaccinated for SARS-CoV-2. What body system is better protected from infection?
   a. Respiratory
   b. Digestive
   c. Integumentary
   d. Nervous

3. During assessment, a client is observed with mild tachypnea, tension in the muscles of the neck and shoulder, and nervousness. Which of the following is most true?
   a. Nitrogen levels have risen and oxygen levels have decreased, creating a decrease in tidal volume.
   b. Oxyhemoglobin is saturated with carbon dioxide, and the muscles display tetany.
   c. An increase in carbon dioxide in the blood triggers sympathetic activation.
   d. Oxygen levels have increased and carbon dioxide levels have dropped, predisposing to breathing pattern disorder.

4. Massage methods that modulate the breathing rhythm also ______.
   a. Predispose a person to pulmonary embolism
   b. Interfere with treatment for sleep apnea
   c. Interact with the autonomic nervous system
   d. Interfere with most meditation methods

5. A client has severely limited all dietary fat. Which of the following might occur?
   a. Inability to digest protein
   b. Difficulty with hormone production
   c. Interference with the absorption of water-soluble vitamins
   d. Decreased conversion of galactose

6. Appropriate massage for the colon ______.
   a. Begins at the ascending colon, ends at the rectum, and moves toward the cecum
   b. Begins at the sigmoid colon and ends at the cecum, with directional flow toward the rectum
   c. Begins at the rectum and ends at the cecum, with a directional flow toward the cecum
   d. Begins at the splenic flexure and ends at the hepatic flexure, with directional flow toward the sigmoid colon

7. Why might massage be contraindicated for those with renal insufficiency?
   a. Massage causes an increase in blood pressure.
   b. Massage increases blood volume through the kidneys.
   c. Massage spreads bacteria through the urinary system.
   d. Massage increases the difficulty with incontinence.

8. Thirty minutes into a relaxation massage, a client has an erection. What is the most logical reason for this response?
   a. The client has been "sexualizing" the massage.
   b. Erection is a parasympathetic response.
   c. Stimulation of the skin shifts blood flow.
   d. Activation of sympathetic reflexes triggers the response.

9. If a client is in the second trimester of pregnancy, which of the following would most apply?
   a. Massage will be most comfortable if it is given with the client prone.
   b. Massage will be most comfortable if the client is positioned on the side.
   c. Massage of the feet is contraindicated.
   d. Massage should focus most on lymphatic drainage.

10. During the massage, a lactating client experiences a let-down response. What would be the most likely cause?
   a. Massage stimulates the release of oxytocin.
   b. Massage stimulates the production of testosterone.
   c. Massage decreases colostrum.
   d. Massage decreases libido.

11. A client with a diagnosis of asthma is referred for massage. What would be the most likely benefits of massage?
    a. Activation of the sympathetic nervous system that would support bronchoconstriction
    b. Reduction in anxiety and increased mobility of the ribs
    c. Stimulation of the client's ability to inhale but inhibition of excessive exhalation
    d. Increase in tone of respiratory muscles, supporting effective exhalation
12. A regular client reports various digestive upsets including dry mouth and constipation. The physician, who wants a treatment plan and justification, has cleared the client for massage. Which of the following would be the best plan to submit to the physician?
    a. Stimulating massage coupled with teaching self-help breathing support an increase in oxygen and a decrease in carbon dioxide to support ongoing autonomic nervous system sympathetic dominance
    b. General massage combined with deep massage to the colon to suppress peristalsis and break down concentrated fecal matter
    c. General massage focuses on generating relaxation with diaphragmatic breathing and rhythmic stroking of the colon to stimulate peristalsis
    d. General massage to create parasympathetic dominance and lymphatic drainage, with visceral massage to the liver to increase detoxification and support upper chest breathing
13. A client is experiencing weakness and exhaustion; impaired concentration, memory, and performance; disturbed sleep; and emotional sweating. A complete physical has ruled out any existing pathological condition. Stress is indicated as a probable cause. Which of the following treatment plans would best reverse the stress response?
    a. Massage to promote lymphatic drainage and stimulate arterial circulation
    b. Massage to support proper breathing function and reverse breathing pattern disorder
    c. Massage to reduce scar tissue and prevent adhesions
    d. Massage to stimulate an increase in heart rate and blood pressure
14. A couple has experienced difficulties conceiving a third child. The doctors can find no reason for the difficulties. What is the best response for how massage may help this couple conceive?
    a. Massage can assist in the success of sexual intercourse by encouraging adrenaline secretion.
    b. Massage can increase the rate of ovulation by stimulating the hypothalamus to secrete follicle-stimulating hormone.
    c. Massage can encourage more efficient homeostatic mechanisms in the body, promoting general health, including fertility.
    d. Massage can increase the levels of testosterone, prolactin, and progesterone, promoting ovulation.
15. Which of the following is a mechanical action of inhalation and exhalation that draws oxygen into the lungs and releases carbon dioxide into the atmosphere?
    a. Breathing
    b. External respiration
    c. Internal respiration
    d. Egestion
16. Which of the following is contagious?
    a. Tuberculosis
    b. Hay fever
    c. Emphysema
    d. Cystic fibrosis
17. The abdominal cavity is lined with a mucous membrane called the _______.
    a. Peritoneum
    b. Gastrointestinal tract
    c. Omentum
    d. Mesentery
18. Which portion of the small intestine contains ducts from the liver, gallbladder, and pancreas?
    a. Ileum
    b. Jejunum
    c. Duodenum
    d. Mesentery
19. Which of the following pathological conditions of the digestive system affects the liver?
    a. Cystic fibrosis
    b. Diverticular disease
    c. Cirrhosis
20. Which of the following sexually transmitted diseases has a bacterial origin?
    a. Genital warts
    b. Herpes genitalis
    c. Gonorrhea

Exercise

Using the foregoing questions as examples, now write at least three more questions. Develop plausible wrong answers and be sure that the correct answer is correct. Then write a rationale for each question. The more questions you write, the better you will understand the material.

Glossary

A

Abduction: Lateral movement away from the midline of the trunk.

Absorption: The movement of food molecules from the digestive tract to the cardiovascular and lymphatic systems so they can be transported to the cells of the body.

Acceleration: The rate of change in speed.

Acetylcholine: A neurotransmitter that stimulates the parasympathetic nervous system and the skeletal muscles and is involved in memory.

Acne: A chronic inflammation of the sebaceous glands and hair follicles caused by interactions among bacteria, sebum, and sex hormones.

Active transport: The transport of substances into or out of a cell using energy.

Activities of daily living (ADLs): Normal daily living activity, such as eating, bathing, dressing, grooming, going to work, performing housekeeping duties, and engaging in leisure activities.

Acupuncture: The practice of inserting needles at specific points on meridians, or channels, to stimulate or sedate energy flow to regulate or alter body function. A branch of Chinese medicine, acupuncture is the art and science of manipulating the flow of qi, the basic life force, and of xue, the blood, body fluids, and nourishing essences. Western medicine uses acupuncture primarily to reduce pain. Acupressure, which uses digital pressure, follows the same Asian principles.

Acute diseases: Disease that has a specific beginning and signs and symptoms that develop quickly, last a short time, and then disappear.

Acute pain: Pain that is usually temporary, of sudden onset, and easily localized. Acute pain can be a symptom of a disease process or a temporary aspect of medical treatment. Acting as a warning signal, acute pain activates the sympathetic nervous system.

Adduction: A medial movement toward the midline of the body.

Adenosine triphosphate (ATP): A compound that stores energy in the muscles. When ATP is broken down during catabolic reactions, it releases energy.

Adrenergic: Stimulation of the sympathetic nervous system causing a release of epinephrine and similar neurotransmitters and hormones.

Afferent: Toward a center or point of reference.

Afferent nerves: Sensory nerves that link sensory receptors with the central nervous system (CNS) and transmit sensory information.

Agonist: A muscle that causes or controls joint motion through a specified plane of motion; also known as a *mover*.

Alimentary canal: The tube-shaped portion of the digestive system known as the *gastrointestinal tract*, the alimentary canal is about 30 feet long and contains several special structures throughout its length.

Allodynia: Pain, generally on the skin, caused by something that would not normally cause pain.

All-or-none response: The property of a muscle fiber (cell) which, when stimulated to contract, contracts to its full ability or does not contract at all.

Alopecia: Hair loss or baldness on parts or all of the body.

Amphiarthrosis: A slightly movable joint that connects bone to bone with fibrocartilage or hyaline growth cartilage. The two types in the human body are symphyses and synchondroses.

Amyotrophic lateral sclerosis: Also called *Lou Gehrig's disease*. A progressive disease that begins in the CNS and involves the degeneration of motor neurons and the subsequent atrophy of voluntary muscle.

Anabolism: Chemical processes in the body that join simple compounds to form more complex compounds of carbohydrates, lipids, proteins, and nucleic acids. The processes require energy supplied from adenosine triphosphate.

Anaplasia: Meaning "without shape," the term describes abnormal or undifferentiated cells that fail to mature into specialized cell types. Anaplasia is a characteristic of malignant cells.

Anatomical position: A standard position in which the person stands upright with the feet slightly apart, arms hanging at the sides, and palms facing forward with thumbs outward.

Anatomical range of motion: The amount of motion available to a joint based on the structure of the joint and determined by the shape of the joint surfaces, joint capsule, ligaments, muscle bulk, and surrounding musculotendinous and bony structures. The anatomical range of motion (ROM) is the limit of passive ROM.

Anatomy: The study of the structures of the body and the relationship of its parts.

Androgens: Male sex hormones.

Anemia: A decrease in the normal number of red blood cells or in the amount of hemoglobin or iron in the blood.

Aneurysm: A permanent dilation of part of a blood vessel caused by weakness or damage to its structure. The most common sites of aneurysms are the aorta and the arteries of the brain.

Antagonist: A muscle usually located on the opposite side of a joint from the mover (agonist) and having the opposite action. The antagonist must lengthen when the mover contracts and shortens.

Anterior pelvic rotation: Anterior movement of the upper pelvis; the iliac crest tilts forward in a sagittal plane.

Antibodies: Serum proteins of the immunoglobulin class that are secreted by plasma cells.

Antigen: Any substance that causes the body to produce antibodies.

Aorta: The large artery that carries oxygen and nutrients out of the heart.

Apical surface: The surface of epithelial cells that is exposed to the external environment.

Apocrine: A type of sweat gland that discharges a thicker and more odoriferous form of sweat.

Aponeurosis: A broad, flat sheet of fibrous connective tissue.

Appendicular skeleton: The part of the skeleton composed of the limbs and their attachments.

Arterioles: The smallest arteries.

Arteriosclerosis: A term meaning "hardening of the arteries"; refers to arteries that have lost their elasticity.

Artery: A blood vessel that transports oxygenated blood from the heart to the body or deoxygenated blood from the heart to the lungs.

Arthritis: The most common type of joint disorder, *arthritis* literally means "inflammation of the joint."

Arthrokinematics: Movement of bone surface in the joint capsule including roll, spin, and slide.

Articulation: A place where two or more bones meet to connect parts and allow for movement in the body. Also called a *joint*.

Ascending tracts: Tracts in the spinal cord that carry sensory information to the brain.

Atherosclerosis: A condition in which fatty plaque is deposited in medium-sized and large arteries.

Atom: The smallest particle of an element that retains and exhibits the properties of that element. Atoms are made up of protons, neutrons, and electrons.

Atrium: One of the two small, thin-walled upper chambers of the heart.

Atrophy: A decrease in the size of a body part or organ caused by a decrease in the size of the cells.

Attachments: Connections of skeletal muscles to bones; often referred to as the *origin* and *insertion*.

Autonomic nervous system (ANS): A division of the peripheral nervous system (PNS) composed of nerves that connect the CNS to the glands, heart, and smooth muscles to maintain the internal body environment.

Avulsion: Injury to a ligament or tendon involving tearing off of its attachment.

Axial skeleton: The axis of the body; the axial skeleton consists of the head, vertebral column, ribs, and sternum.

Axis: Series of glands that signal each other in a sequence.

Axon: A single elongated projection from the nerve cell body that transmits impulses away from the cell body.

B

Balance: The ability to control equilibrium. Two types of balance are static, or still, balance and dynamic, or moving, balance.

Ball-and-socket joint: A joint that allows movement in many directions around a central point. Ball-and-socket joints are ball-shaped convex surfaces fitted into concave sockets. This type of joint gives the greatest freedom of movement but also is the most easily dislocated.

Basal metabolic rate (BMR): The rate of energy expenditure of the body in a quiet, resting, fasting state.

Basal surface: The tissue surface that faces the inside of the body.

Basement membrane: A permeable membrane that attaches epithelial tissues to the underlying connective tissues.

Benign: Usually describes a non-cancerous tumor that is contained and does not spread. More broadly, it can also be defined by a term such as *nonthreatening* to cover instances when the tumor is not associated with cancer.

Biologically plausible: A therapy is sufficiently scientifically plausible when the biological rationale fits plausibly within the current understanding of anatomy and physiology even if proof of its efficacy is lacking—it "makes biological sense." Plausibility is not proof of validity of a method and because biological knowledge is ever expanding, lack of biological plausibility does not necessarily disprove a theory about affect.

Biological rhythm: The internal, periodic timing component of an organism, also known as a *biorhythm*.

Biomechanics: The principles and methods of mechanics applied to the structure and function of the human body.

Biotensegrity: A concept that the bones of the skeletal system are held together by tension forces produced from interrelated muscular and fascial chains.

Blood: A thick red fluid that provides oxygen, nourishment, and protection to the cells and carries away waste products.

Blood pressure: The measurement of pressure exerted by the blood on the walls of the blood vessels. The highest pressure exerted is called *systolic pressure*, which results when the ventricles contract. Diastolic pressure, the lowest pressure, results when the ventricles relax.

Brain: The largest and most complex unit of the nervous system, the brain is responsible for perception, sensation, emotion, intellect, and action.

Brainstem: The inferior, primitive portion of the brain that contains centers for vital functions and reflex actions, such as vomiting, coughing, sneezing, posture, and basic movement patterns.

Breathing pattern disorder: A complex set of behaviors that lead to overbreathing without the presence of a pathological condition.

Buffers: Compounds that prevent the hydrogen ion concentration from fluctuating too much and too rapidly to alter the pH.

Bursa: A flat sac of synovial membrane in which the inner sides of the sac are separated by a fluid film. Bursae are located where moving structures rub over each other and are considered high-friction areas.

Bursitis: Inflammation of a bursa.

C

Callus: An area of thickened, hardened skin that develops in an area of friction or region of recurrent pressure.

Cancer: Malignant, nonencapsulated cells that invade surrounding tissue. They often break away, or metastasize, from the primary tumor and form secondary cancer masses.

Capillary: The smallest blood vessel; found between arteries and veins. Capillaries allow the exchange of gases, nutrients, and waste products.

Carbohydrates: Sugars, starches, and cellulose composed of carbon, hydrogen, and oxygen.

Cardiac cycle: A synchronized sequence of events that takes place during one full heartbeat.

Cardiac muscle fibers: Smaller, striated, involuntary muscle fibers (cells) in the heart that contract to pump blood.

Cardiac output: The amount of blood pumped by the left ventricle in 1 minute.

Carotene: A yellow pigment found in the dermis that provides a natural yellow tint to the skin of some individuals.

Cartilage: A form of flexible connective tissue. Types of cartilage include hyaline, fibrocartilage, and elastic cartilage.

Catabolism: Chemical processes in the body that release energy as complex compounds are broken down into simpler ones.

Catecholamines: A group of neurotransmitters involved in sleep, mood, pleasure, and motor function.

Causation: One event is the result of the occurrence of the other event. This is also referred to as cause and effect.

Cell: The basic structural unit of a living organism. A cell contains a nucleus and cytoplasm and is surrounded by a membrane.

Center of gravity: An imaginary midpoint or center of the weight of a body or object, where the body or object could balance on a point.

Central nervous system (CNS): The brain and spinal cord and their coverings.

Cerebellum: The second largest part of the brain, the cerebellum is involved with balance, posture, coordination, and movement.

Cerebrospinal fluid (CSF): A clear, colorless fluid that flows throughout the brain and around the spinal cord, cushioning and protecting these structures and maintaining proper pH balance.

Cerebrum: The largest of the brain divisions, the cerebrum consists of two hemispheres that occupy the uppermost region of the cranium. The cerebrum receives, interprets, and associates incoming information with past memories and then transmits the appropriate motor response.

Cerumen: A sticky substance released by glands in the ear. Also known as *earwax*, cerumen protects the ear from the entry of foreign material and repels insects.

Ceruminous gland: Modified apocrine glands found in the external ear canal that secrete cerumen.

Chakra: A wheel-like energy center believed to receive, assimilate, and express life force energy.

Charting: The process of keeping a written record of the treatment received by a client or patient. The most effective charting methods follow clinical reasoning, which emphasizes a problem-solving approach. Many systems of charting are used, but they all have similar components based on the problem-oriented medical record and subjective, objective, analysis/assessment, and plan (SOAP).

Chemical properties: Properties that demonstrate how a substance reacts with other substances or responds to a change in the environment.

Chronic diseases: Conditions that have a vague onset, develop slowly, and last for a long time, sometimes for life. Some chronic disorders are initiated by an acute injury/disease.

Chronic pain: Pain that continues or recurs over a prolonged time, usually for more than 6 months. The onset may be obscure, and the character and quality of the pain may change over time. Chronic pain usually is poorly localized and not as intense as acute pain, although for some the pain is exhausting and depressing. May involve central sensitization of the CNS.

Circadian rhythms: Biological rhythms that work in a 24-hour period to coordinate internal functions, such as sleep.

Circumduction: Circular movement of a limb, combining the movements of flexion, extension, abduction, and adduction, to create a cone shape.

Clinical plausibility: Clinical data from epidemiological studies, case reports, case series, and small, formal open or controlled clinical trials are used to support clinical plausibility.

Closed kinematic chain: The positioning of joints in such a way that motion at one of the joints is accompanied by motion at an adjacent joint.

Close-packed position: The position of a synovial joint in which the surfaces fit precisely together and maximal contact between the opposing surfaces occurs. The compression of joint surfaces permits no movement, and the joint possesses its greatest stability.

Collagen: A protein substance composed of small fibrils that combine to create the connective tissue of fasciae, tendons, and ligaments. Collagen constitutes approximately one-fourth of the protein in the body.

Collagenous fibers: Strong fibers with little capacity for stretch. They have a high degree of tensile strength, which allows them to withstand longitudinal stress.

Collaterals: Branches from an axon that allow communication among neurons.

Combining vowel: A vowel added between two roots or a root and a suffix to make pronunciation of the word easier.

Communicable diseases: Infectious diseases that spread through contact with infected individuals; also called *contagious diseases*.

Compact (dense) bone: The hard portion of bone that protects spongy bone and provides the firm framework of the bone and the body.

Compounds: Substances made up of different kinds of atoms.

Concentric action: A contraction in which the muscle shortens with tone because its contractile force is greater than the opposing force at the attachments of the muscle. Concentric contractions are contractions of a mover (agonist) wherein it creates the movement of a body part.

Concentric contraction: The action of a prime mover or agonist by which a muscle develops tension as it shortens to provide enough force to overcome resistance, described as *positive contraction*.

Concentric function: A contraction in which the muscle shortens with tone because its contractile force is greater than the opposing force at the attachments of the muscle. Concentric contractions are contractions of a mover (i.e., an agonist) wherein it creates the movement of a body part.

Condyle: A rounded projection at the end of a bone.

Condyloid (condylar) joint: A joint that allows movement in two planes, but one motion predominates. The joint resembles a condyle, which is a rounded protuberance at the end of a bone forming an articulation.

Congenital diseases: Condition present at birth, not acquired during life.

Connective tissue: The most abundant type of tissue in the body. It supports and holds together the body and its parts, protects the body from foreign matter, and is organized to transport substances throughout the body.

Contractility: The ability of a muscle to shorten forcibly with adequate stimulation. This property sets muscle apart from all other types of tissue.

Contracture: The chronic shortening of a muscle, especially the connective tissue component.

Contusion: A bruise.

Corn: A painful, conical thickening of skin over bony prominences of the feet caused by continued pressure and friction on normally thin skin. Soft corns are those located in moist areas, such as between the toes.

Coronary arteries: The arteries that supply oxygenated blood to the heart muscle itself; they are located in grooves between the atria and ventricles and between the two ventricles.

Coronary veins: Veins that return the deoxygenated blood from the heart to the right atrium.

Correlation: A relationship between two or more events that appear to be related but are not.

Cortisol: A glucocorticoid also known as *hydrocortisone*. Levels of stress often are measured by cortisol levels.

Cramps: Painful muscle spasms or involuntary twitches that involve the whole muscle.

Cranial nerves: Twelve pairs of nerves that originate from the olfactory bulbs, thalamus, visual cortex, and brainstem. They transmit information to and from the sensory organs of the face and the muscles of the face, neck, and upper shoulders as well as organs of the thorax and abdomen.

Creep: The slow movement of viscoelastic materials back to their original state and tissue structure after release of a deforming force.

Cytoplasm: Material enclosed by the cell membrane.

Cytoskeleton: A framework of proteins inside the cell providing flexibility and strength.

Cytosol: The fluid that surrounds the nucleus or organelles inside the cell membrane.

D

Deep fascia: A coarse sheet of fibrous connective tissue that binds muscles into functional groups and forms partitions, called *intermuscular septa*, between muscle groups.

Degenerative joint disease: Osteoarthritis.

Dendrites: Branching projections from the nerve cell body that carry signals to the cell body.

Deoxyribonucleic acid (DNA): Genetic material of the cell that carries the chemical "blueprint" of the body.

Depression: Downward or inferior movement.

Dermatitis: A general term for acute or chronic skin inflammation characterized by redness, eruptions, edema, scaling, and itching.

Dermatome: A cutaneous (skin) section supplied by a single spinal nerve.

Dermis: The deep layer of skin that contains collagen and elastin fibers, which provide much of the structure and strength of the skin.

Descending tracts: Tracts in the spinal cord that carry motor information from the brain to the spinal cord.

Developmental anatomy: How anatomy changes over the life cycle.

Diagnosis: When a licensed medical professional categorizes a disease by identifying its signs and symptoms.

Diagonal abduction: Movement of a limb through a diagonal plane directly across and away from the midline of the body.

Diagonal adduction: Movement of a limb through a diagonal plane toward and across the midline of the body.

Diaphragm: A dome-shaped sheet of muscle attached to the thoracic wall that separates the lungs and thoracic cavity from the abdominal cavity. As the chest cavity enlarges, the diaphragm moves downward and flattens to create a vacuum that allows air to flow into the lungs. As the chest contracts and the diaphragm relaxes, the diaphragm arches upward, helping air to flow out of the lungs.

Diarthrosis: A freely movable synovial joint.

Diffusion: Movement of ions and molecules from an area of higher concentration to that of a lower concentration.

Digestion: The mechanical and chemical breakdown of food from its complex form into simple molecules.

Disease: An abnormality in functions of the body, especially when the abnormality threatens well-being.

Disharmony: Distortions in health that result when the functions or systems are neither balanced nor working optimally. In Chinese medicine, disharmony can be created by the imbalance of the *six pernicious influences* or the *seven emotions*.

Disk herniation: A pathological condition that occurs when the fibrocartilage that surrounds the intervertebral disk ruptures, releasing the nucleus pulposus that cushions the vertebrae above and below. The resultant pressure on spinal nerve roots may cause pain and damage the surrounding nerves.

Dopamine: A catecholamine found in the brain and autonomic system. Generally a stimulant, dopamine is involved in emotions and moods and in regulating motor control and the executive functioning of the brain.

Dorsal root: Also called the *posterior root*. Posterior attachment of a spinal nerve to the spinal cord. Transmits sensory information into the spinal cord.

Dorsiflexion (dorsal flexion): Movement of the ankle that results in the top of the foot moving toward the anterior tibia.

Dosha: Physiological function; described in Ayurveda.

Dynamic force: Force applied to an object that produces movement in or of the object.

E

Eccentric action: A contraction in which the muscle lengthens with tone because its contractile force is less than the opposing force at the attachments of the muscle. Eccentric contractions are contractions of an antagonist that usually restrain or control the action of the prime mover. Eccentric contractions sometimes are described as *negative contractions*.

Eccentric contraction: The action of an antagonist by which a muscle lengthens while under tension and changes in tension to control the descent of the resistance. Eccentric contractions may be thought of as controlling movement against gravity or resistance and are described as *negative contractions*.

Eccrine: A type of sweat gland that releases a watery fluid known as *sweat*, which cools the body and provides minor elimination of metabolic waste.

Edema: The accumulation of abnormal amounts of fluid in tissue spaces.

Efferent: Away from a center or point of reference.

Efferent nerves: Motor nerves that transmit motor impulses; they link the CNS to the effectors outside it.

Effort: The force applied to overcome resistance.

Elastic fibers: Connective tissue fibers that are extensible and elastic. They are made of a protein called *elastin*, which returns to its original length after being stretched.

Elasticity: The ability of a muscle to recoil and resume its original resting length after being stretched.

Elastin: A connective tissue fiber type that has elastic properties and allows flexibility of connective tissue structures.

Element: Substance containing only a single kind of atom.

Elevation: Upward or superior movement.

Elimination (egestion): The removal and release of undigested and unabsorbed food as solid waste products.

Endocrine glands: Ductless glands that secrete hormones directly into the bloodstream.

Endocytosis: The cellular process of engulfing particles located outside the cell membrane into a cell by forming vesicles.

Endoplasmic reticulum: A network of intracellular membranes in the form of tubes that is connected to the nuclear membrane.

Endorphins: Peptide hormones that mainly work like morphine to suppress pain. They influence mood, producing a mild euphoric feeling, such as is seen in runner's high.

Endoskeleton: The bony support structure found inside the human body that accommodates growth.

Endosteum: A thin membrane of connective tissue that lines the marrow cavity of a bone.

Energy: The capacity to work; work is the movement of or a change in the physical structure of matter.

Enteric nervous system (ENS): A subdivision of the PNS that controls the digestive system.

Entrainment: A coordination or synchronization to an internal or external rhythm, especially when a person responds to certain patterns by moving in a manner that is coordinated with those patterns.

Enzyme: A protein that speeds up chemical reactions but is not consumed or altered in the process.

Epicondyle: A bony projection above a condyle.

Epidemiology: The field of science that studies the frequency, transmission, occurrence, and distribution of disease in human beings.

Epidermis: The superficial layer of skin; composed of epithelial tissue in sublayers called *strata*.

Epilepticus: A continuous seizure.

Epinephrine: A catecholamine released by the nervous system and involved in fight-or-flight responses, such as dilation of blood vessels to the skeletal muscles. Epinephrine is classified as a hormone when secreted by the adrenal gland.

Epithelial tissues: A specialized group of tissues that cover and protect the surface of the body and its parts, line body cavities, and form glands. Epithelial tissue usually is found in areas that move substances into and out of the body during secretion, absorption, and excretion.

Equilibrium: All forces acting on an object are equal. Equilibrium may be static or dynamic. A body at rest or completely motionless is in static equilibrium. Dynamic equilibrium occurs when all of the applied and internal forces acting on the moving body are in balance, resulting in movement with no change in speed or direction.

Erythrocytes: Red blood cells that contain hemoglobin and function to transport oxygen to the cells and carbon dioxide away from the cells.

Essential tremor: A chronic tremor that does not result from any other pathological condition.

Etiology: The study of the factors involved in the development of disease, including the nature of the disease and the susceptibility of the person.

Eversion: Movement of the sole of the foot outward away from the midline.

Excitability: The ability of a muscle to receive and respond to a stimulus.

Exocrine glands: Glands that secrete hormones through ducts directly into specific areas. Exocrine glands are part of the endocrine system.

Exocytosis: The movement of substances out of a cell.

Extensibility: The ability of a muscle to be stretched or extended.

Extension: A movement that increases the angle between two bones, usually moving the body part back toward the anatomical position.

External respiration: The exchange of oxygen and carbon dioxide between the lungs and the bloodstream.

External rotation: Rotary movement around the longitudinal axis of a bone away from the midline of the body. Also known as *rotation laterally, outward rotation*, and *lateral rotation*.

F

Facet: A smooth, flat surface on a bone.

Facilitated diffusion: The transport of substances by carriers to which the substance binds to move the substance into a cell along the concentration gradient without energy.

Fascia: A fibrous or loose type of connective tissue; a fibrous membrane covering, supporting, and separating muscles; the subcutaneous tissue that connects the skin to the muscles.

Feedback loop: A self-regulating control system in the body that receives information, integrates that information, and provides a response to maintain homeostasis. Negative feedback reverses the original stimulus, whereas positive feedback enhances and maintains the stimulus.

Fibrocartilage: A connective tissue that permits little motion in joints and structures. It is found in places such as the intervertebral disks and the menisci of the knees.

Fibromyalgia: A syndrome with symptoms of widespread pain or aching, persistent fatigue, generalized morning stiffness, non-restorative sleep, and multiple tender points. A disrupted sleep pattern, coupled with the dysfunction of myofascial repair mechanisms, seems to be a factor.

Fibrous joint: An articulation in which fibrous tissue connects bone directly to bone.

Fistula: A tract that is open at both ends, through which abnormal connections occur between two surfaces.

Fixator: A stabilizing muscle located at a joint or body part that contracts to fix, or stabilize, the area, enabling another limb or body segment to exert force and move. The fixator also may be described as a muscle (or other force) that stops one attachment of a muscle from moving so that the other attachment of the muscle must move.

Flaccid: A term used to describe a muscle with decreased or absent tone.

Flexion: A movement that decreases the angle between two bones as the body part moves out of the anatomical position.

Fontanels: Areas of the skull of an infant in which the bone formation is incomplete. The fontanels allow for compression of the skull as the infant travels through the birth canal and expansion as the brain grows.

Foramen: An opening in a bone, such as the foramen magnum of the skull.

Force: Push or pull on an object in an attempt to affect motion or shape.

Fossa: A depression in the surface or at the end of a bone.

Free nerve endings: Sensory receptors that detect itch and tickle sensations.

Frontal (coronal) plane: A vertical plane that divides the body into anterior and posterior (front and back) parts.

G

Gait: The rhythmic and alternating motions of the legs, trunk, and arms resulting in the propulsion of the body.

Gait cycle: Subdivided into the stance phase and swing phase, this cycle begins when the heel of one foot strikes the floor and continues until the same heel strikes the floor again.

Gallbladder: A small 3- to 4-inch sac that stores and concentrates bile.

Ganglion: Cystic, round, usually non-tender swellings located along tendon sheaths or joint capsules.

General adaptation syndrome: The method the body uses to mobilize different defense mechanisms when threatened by actual or perceived harmful stimuli.

Gestation: The period of fetal growth from conception until birth.

Gibbus: An angular deformity of a collapsed vertebra, the causes of which include metastatic cancer and tuberculosis of the spine.

Gliding joints: Known also as *synovial planes*, gliding joints allow only a gliding motion in various planes.

Gray matter: Unmyelinated nervous tissue in the CNS.

Gross anatomy: The study of body structures visible to the naked eye.

Ground substance: The medium in which the cells and protein fibers are suspended. Ground substance is usually clear and colorless and has the consistency of thick syrup.

H

Half-life: The amount of time required for half of a drug or hormone to be eliminated from the bloodstream.

Health: A condition of homeostasis resulting in a state of physical, emotional, social, and spiritual well-being; the opposite of disease.

Heart: A hollow, cone-shaped, muscular organ responsible for pumping blood. It is about the size of a fist and is located in the mediastinum of the thoracic cavity.

Heart rate: The number of cardiac cycles in 1 minute. In the average, healthy person the rate works out to be 60 to 70 cycles or beats per minute.

Heart sounds: The two main sounds resulting from the closure of the valves. Murmurs are extra sounds, such as those resulting from faulty valves.

Heart valves: Four sets of valves that keep the blood flowing in the correct direction through the heart.

Hemoglobin: The oxygen-carrying, red-colored molecule in the blood.

Hemorrhage: The passage of blood outside of the cardiovascular system.

Hernia: Weakness in a muscle or structure that allows for protrusion of a muscle, organ, or structure through the resulting opening.

Herpes simplex: A DNA virus that causes painful blisters and small ulcers in and around the mouth and on the genital area.

High-energy bonds: Covalent bonds created in specific organic substrates in the presence of enzymes.

Hinge joint: A joint that allows flexion and extension in one plane, changing the angle of the bones at the joint, like a door hinge.

Histamine: A neurotransmitter that is considered a stimulant. Histamine is released by the mast cells as part of the inflammatory process and can cause itching.

Homeostasis: The relatively constant state of the internal environment of the body that is maintained by adaptive responses. Specific control and feedback mechanisms are responsible for adjusting body systems to maintain this state.

Horizontal abduction: Movement of the humerus in the horizontal plane away from the midline of the body. Also known as *horizontal extension* or *transverse abduction*.

Horizontal adduction: Movement of the humerus in the horizontal plane toward the midline of the body. Also known as *horizontal flexion* or *transverse adduction*.

Hyaline cartilage: The thin covering of articular connective tissue on the ends of the bones in freely movable joints in the adult skeleton. Hyaline cartilage forms a smooth, resilient, low-friction surface for the articulation of one bone with another, distributes forces, and helps absorb some of the pressure imposed on the joint surfaces.

Hyperalgesia: An increased sensitivity to pain.

Hyperextension: A movement that takes the body part further in the direction of the extension, further out of anatomical position.

Hypermobility: A ROM of a joint greater than would be permitted normally by the structure. Hypermobility may result, leading to instability. Some hypermobility may be present without instability if sufficient dynamic stabilization is present.

Hyperplasia: An uncontrolled increase in the number of cells of a body part.

Hypersecretion: The excessive release of a hormone.

Hypertension: An increase in systolic and diastolic pressures.

Hypertrophy: An increase in the size of a cell, which results in an increase in the size of a body part or organ.

Hyperventilation: Abnormally deep or rapid breathing in excess of physical demands.

Hypomobility: A ROM of a joint less than what would be permitted normally by the structure. Hypomobility results in restricted ROM.

Hyposecretion: The insufficient release of a hormone.

Hypotension: A decrease in systolic and diastolic pressures. Hypotension is an important manifestation of shock, which causes inadequate blood supply to vital organs.

Hypothalamic-pituitary-adrenal (HPA) axis: A complex set of direct influences and feedback interactions among the hypothalamus, the pituitary gland, and the adrenal glands.

I

Idiopathic: Refers to diseases with undetermined causes.

Immunity: Resistance to disease; the immune system is a functional system rather than an organ system in the anatomical sense.

Impermeable: The quality of not permitting entry of a substance.

Incontinence: The inability to control urination or defecation, most often because of weak pelvic floor muscles or nerve damage.

Inertia: The property of matter in which it remains at rest or in uniform motion in the same straight line unless acted on by some external force.

Inflammation: A protective response of the tissues to irritation or injury that may be chronic or acute. The four primary signs are redness, heat, swelling, and pain.

Inflammatory response: A sequence of events that involves chemical and cellular activation that destroys pathogens and aids in repairing tissues.

Ingestion: Taking food into the mouth.

Inherited disease: Conditions due to genetics.

Inorganic compounds: Chemical structures that do not have carbon and hydrogen atoms as the primary structure.

Insertion: The attachment of a muscle that moves (or usually moves) when the muscle contracts. The insertion of a muscle is usually the distal attachment of the muscle. For muscles located on the axial body, the insertion is usually the superior attachment of the muscle or the part of the muscle that attaches farthest from the midline, or center, of the body.

Integument: The skin and its appendages: hair, sebaceous and sweat glands, nails, and breasts.

Internal respiration: The exchange of gases between the tissues and blood.

Internal rotation: Medial rotary movement of a bone. Also known as *rotation medially, inward rotation*, and *medial rotation*.

Interoception: The body's ability to recognize and interpret its own internal cues.

Interphase: The period during which a cell grows and carries on its internal activities but is not yet dividing.

Intractable pain: The continuation of chronic pain without active disease present or when chronic pain persists even with treatment.

Inversion: Movement of the sole of the foot inward toward the midline.

Ion pumps: Carriers that transport charged particles into or out of a cell using energy.

Ischemia: A temporary deficiency or decreased supply of blood to a tissue.

Isometric action: A contraction in which the muscle stays the same length with tone because its contractile force equals that of the opposing force at the attachments of the muscle. The muscle tenses but does not produce movement. Isometric contractions are usually contractions of a fixator/stabilizer muscle (or neutralizer muscle) that acts to stabilize or fix a body part in position while another joint action is occurring.

Isometric contraction: The action of the prime mover that occurs when tension develops within the muscle but no appreciable change occurs in the joint angle or the length of the muscle. Movement does not occur.

Isometric function: A contraction in which the muscle stays the same length with tone because its contractile force equals that of the opposing force at the attachments of the muscle. The muscle tenses but does not produce movement. Isometric contractions are usually contractions of a fixator/stabilizer muscle (or neutralizer muscle) that acts to hold (i.e., stabilize or fix) a body part in position while another joint action is occurring.

Isotonic action: The action of the muscle that occurs when tension develops in the muscle while it shortens or lengthens.

Isotonic contraction: The action of the prime mover that occurs when tension develops in the muscle while it shortens or lengthens.

J

Joint capsule: A connective tissue structure that connects the bony components of a joint.

Joint play: The involuntary movement that occurs between articular surfaces that is separate from the axial ROM of a joint produced by muscles. Joint play is an essential component of joint motion and must occur for normal functioning of the joint.

K

Kapha dosha: Physiological function that blends the water and earth elements.

Keratin: The fibrous protein produced in the epidermis that protects our skin and makes it waterproof.

Kinematics: A branch of mechanics that involves the aspects of time, space, and mass in a moving system.

Kinesiology: The study of movement that combines the fields of anatomy, physiology, physics, and geometry and relates them to human movement.

Kinesthesia: The sense of movement of body parts.

Kinetic chain: An integrated functional unit. The kinetic chain is made up of the myofascial system (muscle, ligament, tendon, and fascia), articular (joint) system, and nervous system. Each of these systems works interdependently to allow structural and functional efficiency in all three planes of motion: sagittal, frontal, and transverse.

Kinetics: Those forces causing movement in a system.

Kyphosis: A condition of exaggeration of the thoracic curve.

L

Lateral flexion (side bending): Movement of the head or trunk laterally away from the midline. Abduction of the spine.

Lateral recumbency (side-lying): Lying horizontally on the right or left side.

Least-packed position: Joint capsule is at its most lax. Joints assume least-packed position when they are inflamed.

Leukocytes: White blood cells that protect the body from pathogens and remove dead cells and substances.

Lever: A solid mass, such as a crowbar or a person's arm, that rotates around a fixed point called the *fulcrum*. The rotation is produced by a force applied to a lever at some distance from the fulcrum.

Ligaments: Dense bundles of parallel connective tissue fibers, primarily collagen, that connect bones and strengthen and stabilize the joint.

Lipids: Organic compounds that have carbon, hydrogen, and oxygen atoms but in a different proportion than that of carbohydrates.

List: A lateral tilt of the spine.

Locomotion: Moving from one place to another; walking.

Loose-packed position: The position of a synovial joint in which the joint capsule is most lax and the joint is least stable. Joints tend to assume this position to accommodate the increased volume of synovial fluid when inflammation occurs.

Lordosis: A condition of exaggeration of the normal lumbar curve.

Lower respiratory tract: The larynx, trachea, bronchi, and alveoli.

Lungs: The primary organs of respiration. The lungs are soft, spongy, highly vascular structures separated into the left and right lungs by the mediastinum. Each lung is separated into lobes. The right lung has three lobes: upper, middle, and lower; the left lung has two lobes: upper and lower.

Lymph: Fluid derived from interstitial fluid; contains lymphocytes, returns plasma proteins that have leaked out through capillary walls, and transports fats from the gastrointestinal system to the bloodstream.

Lymph nodes: Small, round structures distributed along the network of lymph vessels; they filter wastes and pathogens out of lymph.

Lysosome: A cell organelle that is part of the intracellular digestive system.

M

Matrix: The basic substance between the cells of a tissue. Matrix is composed of amorphous ground substance consisting of molecules that expand when water molecules and electrolytes bind to them. As much as 90% of connective tissue is ground substance. Fibers make up the other component of matrix.

Maximal stimulus: The point at which all motor units of a muscle have been recruited and the muscle is unable to increase in strength.

Mechanical receptors: Sensory receptors that detect changes in pressure, movement, temperature, or other mechanical forces.

Mechanics: The branch of physics dealing with the study of forces and the motion produced by their actions.

Mechanotransduction: The ability to convert mechanical force into neurochemical signals forming a body-wide communication network.

Medical terminology: Terms used to accurately describe the human body, medical treatments and conditions, and processes of health care in a science-based manner.

Meiosis: A type of cell division in which each daughter cell receives half the normal number of chromosomes from the parent cell, forming two reproductive cells.

Melanin: The pigment that colors our skin and works as a natural sunscreen to protect us from ultraviolet rays by darkening our skin.

Membrane: A thin, sheetlike layer of tissue that covers a cell, an organ, or some other structure; that lines a tube or a cavity; or that divides or separates one part from another.

Metabolism: Chemical processes in the body that convert food and air into energy to support growth, distribution of nutrients, and elimination of waste.

Metabolites: Molecules synthesized or broken down inside the body by chemical reactions.

Microbial endocrinology: The study of the ability of microorganisms to both produce and recognize neurochemicals that originate either within the microorganisms themselves or within the host they inhabit.

Microbiome: The genetic material within a microbiota that is the entire collection of microorganisms in a specific area of the body such as the human gut.

Microbiota: A wide variety of bacteria, viruses, fungi, and other single-celled animals that live in the body.

Microorganisms: Small life forms that may be damaging to the body or interfere with its function.

Microvilli: Small projections of the cell membrane that increase the surface area of the cell.

Micturition: The clinical term for urination or voiding.

Mitochondria: Rod- or oval-shaped cell organelles that provide energy for cellular activity.

Mitosis: Cell division in which the cell duplicates its deoxyribonucleic acid (DNA) and divides into two identical daughter cells.

Mixed nerves: Nerves that contain sensory and motor axons.

Mole: Also known as a *nevus*, a mole is a benign pigmented skin growth formed of melanocytes.

Molecule: A combination of two or more atoms. A molecule is the smallest portion of a substance that can exist separately without losing the physical and chemical properties of that substance.

Monoplegia: Paralysis of a single limb or a single group of muscles.

Motion: A change in position with respect to some reference frame or starting point.

Motor point: The location where the motor neuron enters the muscle and where a visible contraction can be elicited with a minimal amount of stimulation. Motor points most often are located in the belly of the muscle.

Motor unit: A motor neuron and all of the muscle fibers it controls.

Muscle synergies: The coordinated recruitment of a group of muscles.

Muscle tissue: A specialized form of tissue that contracts and shortens to provide movement, maintain posture, and produce heat.

Myasthenia gravis: A disease that usually affects muscles in the face, lips, tongue, neck, and throat but can affect any muscle group.

Myelin: A white, fatty insulating substance formed by the Schwann cells that surrounds some axons. Also produced in the CNS by oligodendrocytes.

Myoglobin: A red pigment similar to hemoglobin that stores oxygen within the muscle cells.

Myotome: A skeletal muscle or group of skeletal muscles that receives motor axons from a particular spinal nerve.

N

Negative feedback system: A control mechanism that provides a stimulus to decrease a function, such as a fire alarm, which causes a series of reactions that work to reduce the fire.

Neoplasm: The abnormal growth of new tissue. Also called a *tumor*, a neoplasm may be benign or malignant.

Nerve: A bundle of axons or dendrites or both.

Nervous tissue: A specialized tissue that coordinates and regulates body activity. It can develop more excitability and conductivity than other types of tissue.

Neuroendocrine system: Interactions between the nervous system and the endocrine system.

Neuroglia: Specialized connective tissue cells that support, protect, and hold neurons together.

Neurolemma: Also called *Schwann's membrane, sheath of Schwann*, and *endoneural membrane*. The outer cell membrane of a Schwann cell that encloses the myelin sheath found on certain peripheral nerves. It is essential in the regeneration of injured axons.

Neurons: Nerve cells that conduct impulses.

Neuropathic pain: Pain caused by a lesion or disease of the somatosensory nervous system.

Neuroplastic pain: Pain symptoms caused by learned neuropathways in the brain, and are not due to structural damage or disease in the body.

Neurotransmitters: Chemical compounds that generate action potentials when released in the synapses from presynaptic cells.

Neurovascular bundle: A spinal nerve, artery, deep vein, and deep lymphatic vessel bound together by connective tissue, traveling the same pathway in the body.

Nociceptive pain: Pain as a result of the activation of type C and Aδ nociceptive neurons. The receptors of these neurons have high stimulation thresholds, making them sensitive to stimuli that are damaging to normal tissues or may become damaging if prolonged.

Nociceptors: Sensory receptors that detect the potential for tissue damage; painful or intense stimuli.

Norepinephrine: A catecholamine primarily involved in emotional responses. Norepinephrine is found in the CNS and the sympathetic division of the autonomic nervous system and causes constriction of blood vessels in the skeletal muscles.

Nucleic acids: The two types of nucleic acid are DNA and ribonucleic acid (RNA).

Nutrients: Essential elements and molecules obtained from the diet that are required for normal body function.

Nutrition: The use of food for growth and maintenance of the body.

O

Open kinematic chain: A position in which the ends of the limbs or parts of the body are free to move without causing motion at another joint.

Opportunistic pathogens: Organisms that cause disease only when the immunity is low in a host.

Opposition: Movement of the thumb across the palmar aspect to make contact with the fingers.

Organelles: The basic components of a cell that perform specific functions within the cell.

Organic compounds: Substances that have carbon and hydrogen as part of their basic structure.

Origin: The attachment of a muscle that does not move (or usually does not move) when the muscle contracts. The origin of a muscle is usually the proximal attachment of the muscle. For muscles located on the axial body, the origin is usually the inferior attachment of the muscle or the part of the muscle that attaches closest to the midline, or center, of the body.

Osmosis: Diffusion of water from a region of lower concentration of solution to a region of higher concentration of solution across the semipermeable membrane of a cell.

Osteokinematics: The movement of bones as opposed to the movement of articular surfaces; also known as *range of motion*.

Osteoporosis: A disorder of the bones in which a lack of calcium and other minerals and a decrease in bone protein leaves the bones soft, fragile, and more likely to break.

Oxygen debt: The extra amount of oxygen that must be taken in to remove the buildup of lactic acid from anaerobic respiration of glucose (to convert lactic acid to glucose or glycogen).

P

Pain: An unpleasant sensation. Pain is a complex, personal, subjective experience with physiological, psychological, and social aspects. Because pain is subjective, it is often difficult to explain or describe.

Paraplegia: Paralysis of the lower portion of the body and of both legs.

Parasympathetic nervous system: The energy conservation and restorative system associated with what commonly is called the *relaxation response*.

Passive transport: Transportation of a substance across the cell membrane without the use of energy.

Pathogen: Disease-causing organism; a type of infectious agent.

Pathogenesis: The development of a disease.

Pathogenicity: The ability of the infectious agent to cause disease.

Pathological range of motion (ROM): The amount of motion at a joint that fails to reach the normal physiological range or exceeds normal anatomical limits of motion of that joint.

Pathology: The study of disease as observed in the structure and function of the body.

Pericardium: A double-membrane, serous sac that surrounds and protects the heart.

Periosteum: The thin membrane of connective tissue that covers bones except at articulations.

Peripheral nervous system (PNS): The system of somatic and autonomic neurons outside the CNS. The PNS comprises the afferent (sensory) division and the efferent (motor) division.

Peristalsis: The rhythmic contraction of smooth muscles that propel products of digestion along the tract from the esophagus to the anus.

Peritoneum: The mucous membrane that lines the abdominal cavity to prevent friction from the organs.

Phagocytosis: The process of endocytosis followed by digestion of the vesicle contents by enzymes present in the cytoplasm.

Phantom pain: A form of pain or other sensation experienced in the missing extremity after a limb amputation.

Pharmacology: The study of medications and their uses in treating or preventing a disease.

Pharynx: The throat.

Phospholipid bilayer: A cell membrane made up of lipids, carbohydrates, and proteins.

Physiological range of motion (ROM): The amount of motion available to a joint determined by the nervous system from information provided by joint sensory receptors. This information usually prevents a joint from being positioned such that injury could occur.

Physiology: The study of the processes and functions of the body involved in supporting life.

Piezoelectric: The ability to produce electrical current when deformed or compressed, especially in a crystalline substance, such as bone matrix. Also means that when electric currents pass through them, these substances deform slightly and vibrate.

Pitta dosha: The physiological function that combines fire and water.

Pivot join: A bony projection from one bone fits into a ring formed by another bone and ligament structure to allow rotation around its own axis in one plane.

Plantar flexion: An extension movement of the ankle that results in the foot and toes moving away from the body.

Plasma: A thick, straw-colored fluid that makes up about 55% of the blood.

Plastic range: The range of movement of connective tissue that is taken beyond the elastic limits. In this range, the tissue permanently deforms and cannot return to its original state.

Plexus: A network of intertwining nerves that innervates a particular region of the body.

Polio: A viral infection first of the intestines and then (for about 1% of exposed persons) the anterior horn cells of the spinal cord.

Posterior pelvic rotation: Posterior movement of the upper pelvis; the iliac crest tilts backward in a sagittal plane.

Prefix: A word element added to the beginning of a root to change the meaning of the word.

Pressure: The amount of force on a specific area.

Process: Any prominent bony growth that projects out from the bone.

Prognosis: The expected outcome in a client who has a disease.

Pronation: Internal rotary movement of the radius on the ulna that results in the hand moving from the palm-up to the palm-down position.

Prone: Lying horizontal with the face down.

Proprioceptors: Sensory receptors that provide the body with information about position, movement, muscle tension, joint activity, and equilibrium.

Proteins: Substances formed from amino acids.

Protraction: Forward movement remaining in a horizontal plane.

Psoriasis: A common, chronic skin disease characterized by reddened skin covered by dry, silvery scales. Psoriasis most often is found on the scalp, elbows, knees, back, or buttocks.

Pulmonary trunk: The large artery that carries blood to the lungs to release carbon dioxide and take in oxygen.

Pulmonary veins: The four veins from the lungs that bring oxygen-rich blood to the left atrium.

Q

Qi: Also spelled *chi, qi* refers to the life force.

Quadriplegia: Paralysis or loss of movement of all four limbs.

Quality of life: An individual's perceptions of his or her position in life in the context of the culture and value systems in which the person lives and in relation to his or her goals, expectations, standards, and concerns.

R

Reciprocal inhibition: Stimulation of an antagonist muscle to inhibit action in the prime mover.

Reciprocal innervation: The circuitry of neurons that allows reciprocal inhibition to take place. The massage therapist can use reciprocal innervation therapeutically to assist in muscle relaxation.

Reduction: Return of the spinal column to the anatomical position from lateral flexion. Adduction of the spine.

Referred pain: Pain felt in a surface area far from the stimulated organ.

Reflex: An automatic, involuntary reaction to a stimulus.

Reflex arc: The pathway that a nerve impulse follows in a reflex action.

Regional anatomy: The study of the structures of a particular area of the body.

Remission: The reversal of signs and symptoms that may occur in clients who have chronic diseases. Remission can be temporary or permanent.

Resilience: The capacity to recover quickly from difficulties; toughness.

Resistance: Resistance opposes force.

Respiration: The movement of air in and out of the lungs, the exchange of oxygen and carbon dioxide between the lungs and blood, and the exchange between blood and body tissues.

Respiratory rate: The number of breaths in 1 minute.

Resting tone: The state of tension in resting muscles.

Reticular fibers: Delicate connective tissue fibers that occur in networks and support small structures, such as capillaries, nerve fibers, and the basement membrane. Reticular fibers are made of a specialized type of collagen called *reticulin*.

Retraction: Backward movement in a horizontal plane.

Reverse action: When a muscle contracts and the attachment that normally stays fixed (the origin) moves, and the attachment that usually moves (the insertion) stays fixed.

Ribonucleic acid (RNA): RNA is a type of nucleic acid. It is transcribed (copied) from DNA by enzymes. RNA carries information from DNA to ribosomes, where it is read and translated so that cells can make the proteins necessary for body functions.

Root: A word element that contains the basic meaning of the word.

Rotation: Partial turning or pivoting in an arc around a central axis.

Rupture: The tearing or disruption of connective tissue fibers that takes place when they exceed the limits of the plastic range.

S

Saddle joint: A joint that is convex in one plane and concave in the other with the surfaces fitting together like a rider on a saddle.

Salutogenic: The process of healing, recovery, and repair. The term was first used by Aaron Antonovsky to contrast with *pathogenesis*.

Schwann cell: A specialized cell that forms myelin.

Scoliosis: A lateral curvature of the spine.

Sebaceous glands: The oil glands found in the skin.

Sebum: The oily substance secreted by sebaceous glands that prevents dehydration, softens skin and hair, and slows the growth of bacteria.

Sensitization: An increased responsiveness to stimuli.

Serotonin: A neurotransmitter that works primarily as an inhibitor in the CNS, is synthesized into melatonin, and affects our sleep and moods.

Sesamoid bones: Round bones that often are embedded in tendons and joint capsules. The largest of these is the patella.

Seven emotion: The Asian concept that joy, anger, fear, fright, sadness, worry, and grief are emotional responses that may trigger disharmony in the body, mind, or spirit under certain conditions.

Shock: An inadequate blood supply to vital organs, causing reduced function in these organs.

Signs: Objective changes that can be seen or measured by someone other than the client.

Sinus: A tract leading from a cavity to the surface.

Sinuses: Four groups of air-filled spaces that open into the internal nose. They are located in the frontal, ethmoid, sphenoid, and maxillary bones of the skull. They lighten the weight of the skull and play a role in sound production.

Six pernicious influences: The Asian concept that heat, cold, wind, dampness, dryness, and summer heat, which are natural climate changes, may induce disease under certain conditions.

Skeletal muscle fibers: Large, cross-striated cells that make up muscles connected to the skeleton; under voluntary control of the nervous system.

Sliding filament mechanism: The process describing skeletal muscle contraction in which the thick and thin filaments slide past one another.

Smooth muscle fibers: Muscle fibers that are neither striated nor voluntary. These muscle cells help regulate blood flow through the cardiovascular system, propel food through the digestive tract, and squeeze secretions from glands.

SOAP notes: The acronym refers to Subjective, Objective, Analysis or assessment, and Plan, the four parts of the written account of record keeping.

Somatic nervous system: A system of nerves that keeps the body in balance with its external environment by transmitting impulses among the CNS, skeletal muscles, and skin.

Somatic pain: Pain that arises from the body wall. Superficial somatic pain comes from the stimulation of receptors in the skin, whereas deep somatic pain arises from stimulation of receptors in skeletal muscles, joints, tendons, and fasciae.

Spastic: Term used to describe a muscle with excessive tone.

Spinal cord: The portion of the CNS that exits the skull and extends into the vertebral column. The two major functions of the spinal cord are to conduct nerve impulses and to be a center for spinal reflexes.

Spinal nerves: Thirty-one pairs of mixed nerves, originating in the spinal cord and emerging from the vertebral column; they are part of the PNS.

Spongy (cancellous) bone: The lighter-weight portion of bone, which is made up of trabeculae.

Stability: The resistance to change in the acceleration of the body or the resistance to the disturbance of the equilibrium of the body.

Stabilizer: A force or an object that helps maintain a position. Stabilization is essential to assess movement patterns accurately.

Standard Precautions: Safety measures established by the Centers for Disease Control and Prevention (CDC). The precautions were instituted to prevent the spread of bacterial and viral infections by setting up specific methods of dealing with human fluids and waste products.

Static force: Force applied to an object in such a way that it does not produce movement.

Status epilepticus: A medical emergency characterized by a continuous seizure lasting longer than 30 minutes.

Stress: Any external or internal stimulus that requires a change or response to prevent an imbalance in the internal environment of the body, mind, or emotions. Stress may be any activity that makes demands on mental and emotional resources. Some responses to stress may stimulate neurons of the hypothalamus to release corticotropin-releasing hormone.

Subacute: Diseases that have characteristics that fall between those described as acute or chronic.

Suffix: A word element added to the end of a root to change the meaning of the word.

Superficial fascia: The subcutaneous tissue that make up the third layer of skin; consists of loose connective tissue and contains fat or adipose tissue.

Supination: External rotary movement of the radius on the ulna that results in the hand moving from the palm-down to the palm-up position.

Supine: Lying horizontal with the face up.

Surface anatomy: The study of internal organs and structures as they can be recognized and related to external features.

Suture: A synarthrotic joint in which two bony components are united by a thin layer of dense, fibrous tissue.

Sweat glands: The sudoriferous glands in the skin; they are classified as apocrine or eccrine depending on their location and structure.

Sympathetic nervous system: The part of the autonomic nervous system that provides for most of the active function of the body; when the body is under stress, the sympathetic nervous system predominates with fight-or-flight responses.

Symphysis: A cartilaginous joint in which the two bony components are joined directly by fibrocartilage in the form of a disk or plate.

Symptoms: The subjective changes noticed or felt only by the client or patient.

Synapse: A space between neurons or between a neuron and an effector organ.

Synarthrosis: A limited-movement, non-synovial joint.

Synchondrosis: A joint in which the material used for connecting the two components is hyaline cartilage.

Syndesmosis: A fibrous joint in which two bony components are joined directly by a ligament, cord, or aponeurotic membrane.

Syndrome: A group of different signs and symptoms that identify a pathological condition, especially when they have a common cause.

Synergist: Movers of a joint other than the prime mover(s)—that is, assistant, secondary, or emergency movers. *Synergists* may be more broadly defined as any muscle that helps the action occur (i.e., also may be fixator, neutralizer, or support muscles, as well as other movers).

Synovial fluid: A thick, colorless lubricating fluid secreted by the joint cavity membrane.

Synovial joints: Freely moving joints allowing motion in one or more planes of action.

Systemic anatomy: The study of the structure of a particular body system.

T

Tao: An ancient philosophical concept that represents the whole and its parts as one and the same.

Tendinitis: Inflammation of a tendon.

Tenosynovitis: Inflammation of a tendon sheath.

Terminology: A vocabulary used by people involved in a specialized activity or field of work. Also, the study of the meaning of words used in a language.

Thermal receptors (thermoreceptors): Sensory receptors that detect changes in temperature.

Thorax: Also known as the *chest cavity*. The thorax is the upper region of the torso. It is enclosed by the sternum, ribs, and thoracic vertebrae and contains the lungs, heart, and great blood vessels.

Threshold stimulus: The stimulus at which the first observable muscle contraction occurs.

Tissue: A group of similar cells combined to perform a common function.

Tone: The state of tension in resting muscles.

Trabeculae: An irregular meshing of small, bony plates that makes up spongy bone; its spaces are filled with red marrow.

Tracts: Collections of nerve fibers in the brain and spinal cord that have a common function.

Trigger points: A hyperirritable locus within a taut band of skeletal muscle, located in the muscular tissue or its associated fascia. The spot is painful on compression and can evoke characteristic referred pain and autonomic phenomena.

Trochanter: One of two large bony processes found only on the femur.

Tropic (or trophic) hormones: Hormones produced by the endocrine glands that affect other endocrine glands.

Tubercle: A small rounded process on a bone.

Tuberosity: A large rounded protuberance on a bone.

Tumor: Also referred to as a *neoplasm*, a tumor is a growth of new tissues that may be benign or malignant.

U

Ulcer: A round, open sore of the skin or mucous membrane.

Ultradian rhythms: Biological rhythms that repeat themselves at a rate that ranges from 90 minutes to every few hours.

Upper respiratory tract: The nasal cavity and all its structures and the pharynx.

Upward rotation: Scapular motion that turns the glenoid fossa upward and moves the inferior angle superiorly and laterally away from the spinal column.

V

Vata dosha: Physiological function formed from ether and air.

Vector: The direction of the force.

Veins: Blood vessels that collect blood from the capillaries and transport it back to the heart.

Vena cava: One of two large arteries that returns poorly oxygenated blood to the right atrium of the heart.

Ventral root: Also called the *anterior root*. Anterior attachment of a spinal nerve to the spinal cord. Transmits motor information away from the spinal cord.

Ventricles: The two large lower chambers of the heart; they are thick walled and are separated by a thick interventricular septum.

Venules: Small blood vessels that connect capillaries to veins.

Virulent: A quality of organisms that readily cause disease.

Visceral pain: Pain that results from the stimulation of receptors or an abnormal condition in the viscera (internal organs).

Viscoelasticity: The combination of resistance offered by a fluid to a change of form and the ability of material to return to its original state after deformation.

W

Whiplash: An injury to the soft tissues of the neck caused by sudden hyperextension or flexion of the neck (or both).

White matter: Myelinated nerve tissue in the CNS.

Word elements: The parts of a word; the prefix, root, and suffix.

Y

Yellow elastic cartilage: Cartilage that is more opaque, flexible, and elastic than hyaline cartilage and is distinguished further by its yellow color. The ground substance is penetrated in all directions by frequently branching fibers.

Yin/yang: *Yin* and *yang* are terms used to describe polar relationships. Yin/yang refers to the dynamic balance between opposing forces and the continual process of creation and destruction. Yin/yang reflects the natural order and duality of the whole universe and everything in it, including the individual.

Bibliography

Abbott NJ, et al. The role of brain barriers in fluid movement in the CNS: is there a glymphatic system? *Acta Neuropathol.* 2018:1–21.

Adeel M, Lin BS, Chaudhary MA, Chen HC, Peng CW. Effects of Strengthening Exercises on Human Kinetic Chains Based on a Systematic Review. *J Funct Morphol Kinesiol.* 2024;9(1):22.

Adstrum S, et al. Defining the fascial system. *J Bodyw Mov Ther.* 2017;21(1):173–177.

Adstrum S, Hedley G, Schleip R, Stecco C, Yucesoy CA. Defining the fascial system. *J Bodyw Mov Ther.* 2017;21(1):173–177.

Ajimsha MS, Shenoy PD, Gampawar N. Role of fascial connectivity in musculoskeletal dysfunctions: a narrative review. *J Bodyw Mov Ther.* 2020;24(4):423–431.

Akhu-Zaheya L, Al-Maaitah R, Bany Hani S. Quality of nursing documentation: paper-based health records versus electronic-based health records. *J Clin Nurs.* 2018;27(3–4):e578–e589.

Albert WJ, Currie-Jackson N, Duncan CA. A survey of musculoskeletal injuries amongst Canadian massage therapists. *J Bodyw Mov Ther.* 2008;12:86.

Albert WJ, Duncan C, Currie-Jackson N, et al. Biomechanical assessment of massage therapists. *Occup Ergon.* 2006:61.

Alfaro-LeFevre R. *Critical Thinking and Clinical Judgment: A Practical Approach to Outcome-Focused Thinking.* 4th ed. Elsevier; 2009.

American Massage Therapy Association. *2014 Massage Therapy Industry Fact Sheet. 2014 Massage Therapy Industry Fact Sheet.* American Massage Therapy Association; 2014. Retrieved from http://www.amtamassage.org/uploads/cms/documents/2014industryfactsheet.

Anderson SK. *The Practice of Shiatsu.* Mosby/Elsevier; 2008.

Kennedy AB. *"A Qualitative Study of the Massage Therapy Foundation's Best Practices Symposium: Clarifying Definitions and Creating a Framework for Practice." PhD Diss.* University of South Carolina; 2015.

Applegate E, Thomas P. *The Anatomy and Physiology Learning System.* 4th ed. Saunders/Elsevier; 2011.

Argubi-Wollesen A, et al. Human body mechanics of pushing and pulling: analyzing the factors of task-related strain on the musculoskeletal system. *Saf Health Work.* 2017;8(1):11–18.

Arnheim DD, Prentice WE. *Principles of Athletic Training.* 12th ed. McGraw-Hill; 2006.

Anyfantis ID, Biska A. Musculoskeletal disorders among Greek physiotherapists: traditional and emerging risk factors. *Saf Health Work.* 2017.

Ault P, Plaza A, Paratz J. Scar massage for hypertrophic burns scarring—a systematic review. *Burns.* 2017.

Barbosa F, Ferreira FC, Silva JC. Piezoelectric electrospun fibrous scaffolds for bone, articular cartilage and osteochondral tissue engineering. *Int J Mol Sci.* 2022;23(6):2907.

Barnett RL, Liber T. Human push capability. *Ergonomics.* 2006;49:293.

Baron KG, Reid KJ. Circadian misalignment and health. *Inter Rev Psych.* 2014;26(2):139–154.

Basmajian JV, DeLuca CJ. *Muscles Alive: Their Functions Revealed by Electromyography.* 5th ed. Williams & Wilkins; 1985.

Basmajian JV, Nyberg R. *Rational Manual Therapies.* Williams & Wilkins; 1993.

Bates B. *Bates' Guide to Physical Examination and History Taking.* 9th ed. Lippincott, Williams & Wilkins; 2005.

Benias PC, et al. Structure and distribution of an unrecognized interstitium in human tissues. *Sci Rep.* 2018;8(1):4947.

Benveniste H, et al. The glymphatic system and waste clearance with brain aging: a review. *Gerontology.* 2018:1–14.

Berryman N, Lovelace-Chandler V, Soderberg GL, et al. *Muscle and sensory. Testing.* 2nd ed. Elsevier; 2005.

Bergmark A. Stability of the lumbar spine: a study in mechanical engineering. *Acta Orthop Scand.* 1989;60(suppl 230):1–54.

Bhargava A, Arnold AP, Bangasser DA, Denton KM, Gupta A, Hilliard Krause LM, Mayer EA, et al. Considering sex as a biological variable in basic and clinical studies: an endocrine society scientific statement. *Endocr Rev.* 2021;42(3):219–258.

Bïrch SJ, Felt RL. *Understanding Acupuncture.* Churchill Livingstone; 1999.

Birnbaum JS. *The Musculoskeletal Manual.* 3rd ed. Academic Press; 1982.

Bisiacchi DW, Huber LL. Physical injury assessment of male versus female chiropractic students when learning and performing various adjustive techniques: a preliminary investigative study. *Chiropract Osteopath.* 2006;14(1):17.

Blau G, Monos C, Boyer E, et al. Correlates of injury-forced work reduction for massage therapists and bodywork practitioners. *J Ther Massage Bodywork.* 2013;6(3):6.

Bobba-Alves N, Juster R-P, Picard M. The energetic cost of allostasis and allostatic load. *Psychoneuroendocrinology.* 2022;146:105951. T.

Bordoni B, Zanier E. Clinical and symptomatological reflections: the fascial system. *J Multidiscip Health.* 2014;7:401–411.

Boulanger K, Campo S. Are personal characteristics of massage therapists associated with their clinical, educational, and interpersonal behaviors? *Int J Ther Massage Bodywork.* 2013;6(3):325–334.

Brennan R. *The Alexander Technique Workbook: Your Personal System for Health, Poise and Fitness.* Vega Books; 2003.

Broncel A, Bocian R, Kłos-Wojtczak P, Kulbat-Warycha K, Konopacki J. Vagal nerve stimulation as a promising tool in the improvement of cognitive disorders. *Brain Res Bull.* 2020;155:37–47.

Buck FA, Kuruganti U, Albert WJ, et al. Muscular and postural demands of using a massage chair and massage table. *J Manip Physiol Ther.* 2007;30:357–364.

Buckingham G, Das R, Trott P. Position of undergraduate learners' thumbs during mobilisation is poor: an observational study. *Aust J Physiother.* 2007;53:55.

Bullock BL, Rosendahl PP. *Pathophysiology: Adaptations and Alterations in Function.* 4th ed. JB Lippincott; 1996.

Burnet PW. The microbiome in psychology and cognitive neuroscience. *Trends Cogn Sci.* 2018.

Butler DS. *Mobilization of the Nervous System.* Churchill Livingstone; 1991.

Cailliet R. *Neck and Arm Pain.* 3rd ed. FA Davis; 1991.

Cailliet R. *Shoulder Pain.* 3rd ed. FA Davis; 1991.

Cailliet R. *Knee Pain and Disability.* 3rd ed. FA Davis; 1992.

Cailliet R. *Hand Pain and Impairment.* 4th ed. FA Davis; 1994.

Cailliet R. *Low Back Pain Syndrome.* 5th ed. FA Davis; 1995.

Cailliet R. *Soft Tissue Pain and Disability.* FA Davis; 1996.

Cailliet R. *Foot and Ankle Pain.* 3rd ed. FA Davis; 1997.

Campo M, Weiser S, Koenig KL, et al. Work-related musculoskeletal disorders in physical therapists: a prospective cohort study with 1-year follow-up. *Phys Ther.* 2008;88:608.

Cassar M-P. *Handbook of Massage Therapy: A Complete Guide for the Student and Professional Massage Therapist.* Butterworth-Heinemann; 1999.

Cavallaro Goodman C, Fuller KS. *Pathology: Implications for the Physical Therapist*. 3rd ed. Elsevier; 2005.

Chaitow L. *The Acupuncture Treatment of Pain*. Healing Arts Press; 1990.

Chaitow L. *The Book of Natural Pain Relief*. Harper Paperbacks; 1995.

Chaitow L. The amazing fascial web, part I. *Massage Today*. 2005;5(5).

Chaitow L. *Modern Neuromuscular Techniques*. 2nd ed. Churchill Livingstone; 2003.

Chaitow L, DeLany J. *Clinical Applications of Neuromuscular Techniques: Volume 1—The Upper Body*. Churchill Livingstone/Elsevier; 2008. 2nd ed.

Chaitow L, Delany J. *The lower body. Clinical Application of Neuromuscular Techniques*. Churchill Livingstone; 2011. vol. 2.

Chaitow L. *Muscle Energy Techniques*. 4th ed. Churchill Livingstone; 2013.

Chaitow L, Bradley D. *Gilbert C. Recognizing and Treating Breathing Disorders: A Multidisciplinary Approach*. 2nd ed. Churchill Livingstone/Elsevier; 2014.

Chaitow L, Gilbert C, Morrison D. *Recognizing and Treating Breathing Disorders (e-Book)*. Elsevier Health Sciences; 2014.

Chen WG, Schloesser D, Arensdorf AM, Simmons JM, Cui C, Valentino R, Gnadt JW, et al. The emerging science of interoception: sensing, integrating, interpreting, and regulating signals within the self. *Trends Neurosci*. 2021;44(1):3–16.

Choi BK, et al. The hyaluronic acid-rich node and duct system is a structure organized for innate immunity and mediates the local inflammation. *Cytokine*. 2018;113.

Chompoopan W, Eungpinichpong W, Chompoopan W, Sujimongkol C. The effect of traditional thai massage on quality of sleep in adults with sleep problem. *Trends Sci*. 2022;19(7): 3063-3063.

Chow AY, La Delfa NJ, Dickerson CR. Muscular exposures during standardized two-handed maximal pushing and pulling tasks. *Trans Occup Ergon Hum Factors*. 2017;5(3–4):136–147.

Chumnanya M, Perngparn U, Sayorwan W. Health problems from working as Thai traditional massage therapists in Thailand. *J Health Res*. 2013;27(2):119–122.

Chung HS, Choi KM. Adipokines and myokines: a pivotal role in metabolic and cardiovascular disorders. *Current Med Chem*. 2018;25(20):2401–2415.

Clarke G, et al. Minireview: gut microbiota: the neglected endocrine organ. *Mol Endocrinol*. 2014;28(8):1221–1238.

Clayton BD, Stock YN. *Basic Pharmacology for Nurses*. 16th ed. Mosby; 2012.

Coffey JC, O'Leary DP. The mesentery: structure, function, and role in disease. *Lancet*. 2016;1(3):238–247.

Coleman E, Radix AE, Bouman WP, Brown GR, De Vries ALC, Deutsch MB, Ettner R, et al. Standards of care for the health of transgender and gender diverse people, version 8. *Int J Transgend Health*. 2022;23(sup1):S1–S259.

Cromie JE, Robertson VJ, Best MO. Work-related musculoskeletal disorders in physical therapists: prevalence, severity, risks, and responses. *Phys Ther*. 2000;80:336.

Cross S. *Underwood's Pathology: A Clinical Approach*. 6th ed. Churchill Livingstone/Elsevier; 2013.

Croy I, Fairhurst MT, McGlone F. The role of C-tactile nerve fibers in human social development. *Curr Opin Behav Sci*. 2022;43:20–26.

Cummings NH, Stanley-Green S, Higgs P. *Perspectives in Athletic Training*. Elsevier; 2009.

Cuppet M, Walsh K. *General Medical Conditions in the Athlete*. 2nd ed. Mosby/Elsevier; 2012.

Dalamaga M, Kounatidis D, Tsilingiris D, et al. The Role of Endocrine Disruptors Bisphenols and Phthalates in Obesity: Current Evidence, Perspectives and Controversies. *Int J Mol Sci*. 2024;25(1):675.

Damjanov I. *Pathology for the Health Professions*. 5th ed. Saunders/Elsevier; 2016.

DeStefano L. *Greenman's Principles of Manual Medicine*. 4th ed. Lippincott Williams & Wilkins; 2011.

Di Lima SN, Painter SJ, Johns LT, eds. *Orthopaedic Patient Education Resource Manual. Gaithersburg*. Aspen (three-ring binder with CD ROM); 2001.

Dischiavi SL, et al. Biotensegrity and myofascial chains: a global approach to an integrated kinetic chain. *Med Hypotheses*. 2018;110:90–96.

Dowell D, Ragan KR, Jones CM, Baldwin GT, Chou R. CDC Clinical Practice Guideline for Prescribing Opioids for Pain—United States, 2022. *MMWR Recomm Rep*. 2022;71(RR-3):1–95. https://doi.org/10.15585/mmwr.rr7103a1. https://www.cdc.gov/mmwr/volumes/71/rr/rr7103a1.htm?s_cid=rr7103a1_w.

Drake R, Vogl AW, Mitchell AWM. *Gray's Anatomy for Students*. 2nd ed. Churchill Livingstone/Elsevier; 2010.

Drake R, Vogl AW, Mitchell AWM, et al. *Gray's Atlas of Anatomy*. 2nd ed. Churchill Livingstone/Elsevier; 2015.

Drake R, Vogl AW, Mitchell AWM. *Gray's Anatomy for Students*. 3rd ed. Churchill Livingstone/Elsevier; 2015.

Dommerholt J, Fernández-de-las-Peñas C, eds. *Trigger Point Dry Needling: An Evidenced and Clinical-Based Approach*. 1st ed. Churchill Livingstone/Elsevier; 2013.

Donatelli R. *Sport-Specific Rehabilitation*. Churchill Livingstone/Elsevier; 2007.

Do K, Kim J, Yim J. Acute effect of self-myofascial release using a foam roller on the plantar fascia on hamstring and lumbar spine superficial back line flexibility. *Phys Ther Rehab Sci*. 2018;7(1):35–40.

Engelhardt B, et al. Vascular, glial, and lymphatic immune gateways of the central nervous system. *Acta Neuropathol*. 2016;132(3):317–338.

Evans, JM, Laura SM, Julian RM. The gut microbiome: the role of a virtual organ in the endocrinology of the host. *J Endocrinol*. 2013;218(3):R37–47.

Fedak K, et al. Applying the bradford hill criteria in the 21st century: how data integration has changed causal inference in molecular epidemiology. *Emerg Themes Epidemol*. 2015;12 14.

Federation of State Massage Therapy Boards. https://www.fsmtb.org https://www.fsmtb.org/media/1126/model_massage_therapy_practice_act.pdf. Retrieved 14.09.19.

Feelisch M, Cortese-Krott MM, Santolini J, Wootton SA, Jackson AA. Systems redox biology in health and disease. *EXCLI J*. 2022;21:623.

Fernández-de-las-Peñas C. *Manual Therapy for Musculoskeletal Pain Syndromes: An Evidence-and Clinical-Informed Approach*. Elsevier Health Sciences; 2015.

Field T. Pain and massage therapy: a narrative review. *Curr Res Complementary Altern Med*. 2018. https://doi.org/10.29011/2577-2201/100025.

Finlay S, Rudd D, McDermott B, Sarnyai Z. Allostatic load and systemic comorbidities in psychiatric disorders. *Psychoneuroendocrinology*. 2022;140:105726.

Finlay S, Roth C, Zimsen T, Bridson TL, Sarnyai Z, McDermott B. Adverse childhood experiences and allostatic load: a systematic review. *Neurosci Biobehav Rev*. 2022;136:104605.

FIPAT. *Terminologia Anato mica*. 2nd ed. Federative International Programme for Anatomical Terminology; 2019. FIPAT.library.dal.ca.

Freeman LW, Lawlis GF. *Mosby's Complementary and Alternative Medicine: A Research-Based Approach*. 3rd ed. Mosby; 2008.

Furlan AD, Imamura M, Dryden T, et al. Massage for low back pain: an updated systematic review within the framework of the Cochrane Back Review Group. *Spine*. 2009;34(16):1669–1684.

Gomes AC, Hoffmann C, Mota JF. The human gut microbiota: metabolism and perspective in obesity. *Gut Microbes*. 2018;9:1–18.

Goodman CC, Snyder TEK. *Differential Diagnosis for Physical Therapists: Screening for Referral*. 5th ed. Saunders/Elsevier; 2013.

Green AE, DeChants JP, Price MN, Davis CK. Association of gender-affirming hormone therapy with depression, thoughts of suicide, and attempted suicide among transgender and nonbinary youth. *J Adolesc Health*. 2022;70(no. 4):643–649.

Greene DP, Roberts SL. *Kinesiology: Movement in the Context of Activity*. Elsevier; 1999.

Greene D, Roberts S. *Kinesiology: Movement in the Context of Activity*. 2nd ed. Mosby; 2004.

Greene DP, Roberts SL. *Kinesiology: Movement in the Context of Activity*. 2nd ed. Mosby; 2005.

Gunn C. *Bones and Joints*. 5th ed. Churchill Livingstone; 2007.

Guntur A, Rosen C. Bone as an endocrine organ. *Endocrin Pract*. 2012;18(5):758–762.

Gurevich D. *Russian Medical Massage*. (self-published); 1992.

Guruprasad S, Ramakrishnan KS, Gowda H. Prevalence of musculoskeletal problems in masseuse. *Inter J Ther Rehab Res*. 2016;5(5):140–148.

Hablitz LM, Nedergaard M. The glymphatic system: a novel component of fundamental neurobiology. *J Neurosci*. 2021;41(37):7698–7711.

Hairani IHM, et al. *Adv Res Occup Safety Health*. 2018;1(1):1.

Hansen JT. *Netter's Clinical Anatomy*. 3rd ed. Saunders/Elsevier; 2014.

Han Y, et al. Paracrine and endocrine actions of bone—the functions of secretory proteins from osteoblasts, osteocytes, and osteoclasts. *Bone Res*. 2018;6

Hassan S, Thacharodi A, Priya A, et al. Endocrine disruptors: Unravelling the link between chemical exposure and Women's reproductive health. *Environ Res*. 2024;241:117385.

Heinerman J. *Healing Powers of Herbs*. 2nd ed. Globe Communications; 2004.

Henning S, Mangino LC, Massé J. *Postural restoration: A Tri-planar asymmetrical framework for understanding, assessing, and treating scoliosis and other spinal dysfunctions*. Innovations in Spinal Deformities and Postural Disorders. 2017.

Hislop HJ, Avers D, Brown M. *Daniel and Worthingham's Muscle Testing: Techniques of Manual Examination and Performance Testing*. 9th ed. Saunders/Elsevier; 2013.

Hislop HJ, Montgomery J. *Daniels & Worthingham's Muscle Testing: Techniques of Manual Examination*. 9th ed. Saunders/Elsevier; 2014.

Hooper J, Teresi D. *The Three-Pound Universe*. Dell; 1986.

Howick J, Glasziou P, Aronson JK. The evolution of evidence hierarchies: what can Bradford Hill's *guidelines for causation* contribute? *J Royal Soc Med*. 2009;102(5):186–194.

Howland RH. Vagus nerve stimulation. *Curr Behav Neurosci Rep*. 2014;1(2):64–73. https://doi.org/10.1007/s40473-014-0010-5.

Huan Z, Rose K. *Who Can Ride the Dragon?*. Paradigm Publications; 1999.

Huber FE, Wells CL. *Therapeutic Exercise: Treatment Planning for Progression*. Saunders/Elsevier; 2006.

Hu MT, Hsu AT, Lin SW, et al. Effect of general flexibility on thumb-tip force generation: implication for mobilization and manipulation. *Man Ther*. 2009;14:490.

Huber FE, Wells CL. *Therapeutic Exercise: Treatment Planning for Progression*. Saunders/Elsevier; 2006.

Howick J, Glasziou P, Aronson JK. The evolution of evidence hierarchies: what can Bradford Hill's *guidelines for causation* contribute? *J Royal Soc Med*. 2009;102(5):186–194.

Howland RH. Vagus nerve stimulation. *Curr Behav Neurosci Rep*. 2014;1(2):64–73. https://doi.org/10.1007/s40473-014-0010-5.

Hu MT, Hsu AT, Lin SW, et al. Effect of general flexibility on thumb-tip force generation: implication for mobilization and manipulation. *Man Ther*. 2009;14:490.

Isaza-Restrepo A, Martin-Saavedra JS, Velez-Leal JL, Vargas-Barato F, Riveros-Dueñas R. The peritoneum: beyond the tissue. *Front Physiol*. 2018;9:738.

Jacobs PH, Anhalt TS. *Handbook of Skin Clues of Systemic Diseases*. 2nd ed. Lea & Febiger; 1992.

Jacobs K. *Ergonomics for Therapists*. 3rd ed. Mosby/Elsevier; 2007.

Jacobs, et al. Marked for life: epigenetic effects of endocrine disrupting chemicals. *Ann Rev Environ Res*. 2017;42:105–160.

Jang Y, Chi CF, Tsauo JY, et al. Prevalence and risk factors of work-related musculoskeletal disorders in massage practitioners. *J Occup Rehabil*. 2006;16:425.

Janssen MM, Drevelle X, Humbert L, et al. Differences in male and female spino-pelvic alignment in asymptomatic young adults: a three-dimensional analysis using upright low-dose digital biplanar x-rays. *Spine*. 2009;34:E826.

Jane SW, et al. Effects of massage on pain, mood status, relaxation, and sleep in Taiwanese patients with metastatic bone pain: a randomized clinical trial. *Pain*. 2011;152(10):2432–2442.

Jerath R, Beveridge C, Jensen M. Central pain syndrome: etiological perspectives from the 3D default space model of consciousness. *World J Neurosci*. 2018;8(2):277.

Jessen NA, Anne SFM, Iben L, Maiken N. The glymphatic system: a beginner's guide. *Neurochem Res*. 2015;40:2583–2599.

Jiménez A, Lu Y, Jambhekar A, Lahav G. Principles, mechanisms and functions of entrainment in biological oscillators. *Interface Focus*. 2022;12(3):20210088.

Jyothish U, Karthika Das S. Effect of left nostril breathing on postexercise recovery time. *J Curr Res Sci Med*. 2021;7(2):70.

Kageyama K, Nemoto T. Molecular mechanisms underlying stress response and resilience. *Int J Mol Sci*. 2022;23(16):9007.

Kara H. Leptin, ghrelin, and other peptide hormones: an overview of their structures and functions. *Klin Psikofarmakol Bul*. 2018;28:323–324.

Karsenty G. Update on the biology of osteocalcin. *Endo Pract*. 2017;23(10):1270–1274.

Kashani F, Kashani P. The effect of massage therapy on the quality of sleep in breast cancer patients. *Iran J Nurs Midwif Res*. 2014;19(2):113.

Kasper DL, Fauci AS, Hauser SL, et al. *Harrison's Principles of Internal Medicine*. 19th ed. McGraw-Hill; 2015.

Katsumi Y, Theriault JE, Quigley KS, Barrett LF. Allostasis as a core feature of hierarchical gradients in the human brain. *Netw Neurosci*. 2022:1–56.

Kemmerer David. What modulates the Mirror Neuron System during action observation?: Multiple factors involving the action, the actor, the observer, the relationship between actor and observer, and the context. *Prog Neurobiol*. 2021;205:102128.

Kendall FP. *Florence Kendall's Muscle Testing Video Library*. Williams & Wilkins; 1987: Vols 1–5.

Kennedy AB, et al. Advancing health promotion through massage therapy practice: a cross-sectional survey study. *Prevent Med Rep*. 2018.

Kennedy AB, et al. *J Bodywork Move Ther*. 2018;20(3):484–496.

Kim TW, Jeong JH, Hong SC. The impact of sleep and circadian disturbance on hormones and metabolism. *Int J Endocrin*. 2015.

Kisner C, Colby LA. *Therapeutic Exercise: Foundations and Techniques*. 5th ed. FA Davis; 2007.

Koning Bjorn Bde, Mok Katrina, Marcus Nadine, Ayres Paul. Investigating the role of hand perspective in learning from procedural animations. *Br J Educ Psychol*. 2022.

Koul A, et al. Action observation areas represent intentions from subtle kinematic features. *Cerebr Cort*. 2018;28(7):2647–2654.

Kruger H, Khumalo V, Houreld NN. The prevalence of osteoarthritic symptoms of the hands amongst female massage therapists. *Health SA Gesondheid*. 2017;22(1):184–193.

Kuhn T, et al. Medical Informatics Committee of the American College of Physicians. Clinical documentation in the 21st century: executive summary of a policy position paper from the American College of Physicians. *Ann Intern Med*. 2015;162:301–303. https://doi.org/10.7326/M14-2128.

Kumar V, Abbas AK, Aster JC. *Robbins Basic Pathology*. 9th ed. Saunders/Elsevier; 2013.

Kumar SS, Kumar Mishra A, Ghosh AR. *Endocrine role of adipose tissue in obesity and related disorders. Cellular and Biochemical Mechanisms of Obesity*. Springer; 2021:23–42.

Kwong EH, Findley TW. Fascia—Current knowledge and future directions in physiatry: narrative review. *J Rehab Res Devel*. 2014;51(6).

Laimi K, et al. Effectiveness of myofascial release in treatment of chronic musculoskeletal pain: a systematic review. *Clin Rehab*. 2018;32(4).

Langevin HM, et al. Effect of stretching on thoracolumbar fascia injury and movement restriction in a porcine model. *Am J Phys Med Rehab*. 2018;97(3):187–191.

Leadbeater CW. *The Chakras*. Theosophical Publishing House; 1927.

Le Blanc-Louvry I, Costaglioli B, Boulon C, et al. Does mechanical massage of the abdominal wall after colectomy reduce postoperative pain and shorten the duration of ileus? Results of a randomized study. *J Gastrointest Surg*. 2002;6(1):43–49.

Lei Y, Hongbin H, Fan Y, Aqeel J, Yong Z. The brain interstitial system: anatomy, modeling, in vivo measurement, and applications. *Prog Neurobiol*. 2017;157:230–246. https://www.sciencedirect.com/science/article/pii/S0301008215300691.

Levine D, Richards J, Whittle MW. *Whittle's Gait Analysis*. 5th ed. Churchill Livingstone/Elsevier; 2012.

Lim CJ, Yoo JH, Kim Y, et al. Gross morphological features of the organ surface primo-vascular system revealed by hemacolor staining. *Evid Based Complement Alternat Med*. 2013. https://doi.org/10.1155/2013/350815.

Liu PY, Irwin MR, Krueger JM, Gaddameedhi S, Van Dongen HPA. Night shift schedule alters endogenous regulation of circulating cytokines. *Neurobiol Sleep Circadian Rhythms*. 2021;10:100063.

Liu B, Qiao L, Liu K, Liu J, Piccinni-Ash TJ, Chen ZF. Molecular and neural basis of pleasant touch sensation. *Science*. 2022;376(6592):483–491. https://doi.org/10.1126/science.abn2479.

Liu L, Wu Q, Chen Y, Ren H, Zhang Q, Yang H, Zhang W, et al. Gut microbiota in chronic pain: Novel insights into mechanisms and promising therapeutic strategies. *Int Immunopharmacol*. 2023;115:109685.

Lombardi, et al. What is evidence-based about myofascial chains: a systematic review. *Arch Phys Med Rehab*. 2016;97(3):454–461.

Lombardi G, et al. Implications of exercise-induced adipo-myokines in bone metabolism. *Endocrine*. 2016;54(2):284–305.

Lorme KJ, Naqvi SA. Comparative analysis of low-back loading on chiropractors using various workstation table heights and performing various tasks. *J Manip Physiol Ther*. 2003;26(1):25–33.

Louveau I, et al. Structural and functional features of central nervous system lymphatic vessels. *Nature*. 2015;523(7560):337–341.

Louveau A, Igor S, Keyes T, et al. Structural and functional features of central nervous system lymphatic vessels. *Nature*. 2015. http://www.nature.com/nature/journal/v523/n7560/full/nature14432.html.

Louw A, et al. The efficacy of pain neuroscience education on musculoskeletal pain: a systematic review of the literature. *Phys Theory Pract*. 2016;32(5):332–355.

Louw A, et al. The effect of neuroscience education on pain, disability, anxiety, and stress in chronic musculoskeletal pain. *Arch Phys Med Rehabil*. 2018;92(12):2041–2056.

Lu WA, Chen GY, Kuo CD. Foot reflexology can increase vagal modulation, decrease sympathetic modulation, and lower blood pressure in healthy subjects and patients with coronary artery disease. *Altern Ther Health Med*. 2011;17(4):8–14.

Lowe DT. Cupping therapy: an analysis of the effects of suction on skin and the possible influence on human health. *Compl Ther Clin Pract*. 2017.

Maciocia G. *The Foundations of Chinese Medicine: A Comprehensive Text*. 3rd ed. Churchill Livingstone/Elsevier; 2015.

Magee DJ, Zachazewski JE. *Scientific Foundations and Principles of Practice in Musculoskeletal Rehabilitation*. Mosby; 2007.

Magee DJ. *Orthopedic Physical Assessment*. 6th ed. Saunders/Elsevier; 2014.

Mahan LK, Escott-Stump S. *Krause's Food & Nutrition Therapy*. 12th ed. Elsevier; 2010.

Malfliet A, et al. Effect of pain neuroscience education combined with cognition-targeted motor control training on chronic spinal pain: a randomized clinical trial. *JAMA Neurology*. 2018.

Mansfield PJ, Neumann DA. *Essentials of Kinesiology for the Physical Therapist Assistant*. 2nd ed. Mosby/Elsevier; 2014.

Marieb EN. *Human Anatomy and Physiology*. 7th ed. Benjamin/Cummings; 2006.

Martinez de Castillo SL. *Strategies, Techniques, & Approaches to Critical Thinking: A Clinical Reasoning Workbook for Nurses*. 5th ed. Saunders/Elsevier; 2014.

Marques FZ, Mackay CR, Kaye DM. Beyond gut feelings: how the gut microbiota regulates blood pressure. *Nat Rev Cardiol*. 2018;15(1):20.

Masunaga S, Ohashi W. *Zen Shiatsu: How to Harmonize Yin and Yang for Better Health*. Japan Publications; 1977.

Mazurek KA, Rouse AG, Schieber MH. Mirror neuron populations represent sequences of behavioral epochs during both execution and observation. *J Neurosci*. 2018;38(18):4441–4455.

McCance KL, Huether SE, Brashers VL. *Pathophysiology, the Biologic Basis for Disease in Adults and Children*. 6th ed. Elsevier; 2010.

McEwen BS, Nicole PB, Jason DG, Matthew NH, Richard GH, Ilia NK, Carla N. Mechanisms of stress in the brain. Nat Neurosci. 2015;18(10):1353–1363.

McEwen BS, Gray JD, Nasca C. Recognizing resilience: learning from the effects of stress on the brain. *Neurobiol Stress*. 2015;1(1).

Mennell JM. *The Musculoskeletal System: Differential Diagnosis from Symptoms and Physical Signs*. Aspen; 1992.

Mohr EG. Proper body mechanics from an engineering perspective. *J Body Mov Ther*. 2010;14:139.

Morhenn V, Beavin LE, Zak PJ. Massage increases oxytocin and reduces adrenocorticotropin hormone in humans. *Alt Ther Health Med*. 2012;18(6):11.

Moseley GL, Butler DS. Fifteen years of explaining pain: the past, present, and future. *J Pain*. 2015;16(9):807–813.

Myers TW. *Anatomy Trains: Myofascial Meridians for Manual and Movement Therapists*. 3rd ed. Churchill Livingstone/Elsevier; 2014.

Micozzi MS. *Fundamentals of Complementary and Alternative Medicine*. 5th ed. Saunders/Elsevier; 2015.

Mosby's. *Drug Reference for Health Professions*. 6th ed. Mosby/Elsevier; 2017.

Muscolino JE. *The Muscular System Manual, the Skeletal Muscles of the Human Body*. 3rd ed. Mosby/Elsevier; 2010.

Muscolino JE. *Kinesiology: The Skeletal System and Muscle Function*. 2nd ed. Mosby/Elsevier; 2011.

Muscolino JE. *The Muscle and Bone Palpation Manual With Trigger Points, Referral Patterns and Stretching*. 2nd ed. Mosby/Elsevier; 2016.

Myers TW. *Anatomy Trains: Myofascial Meridians for Manual and Movement Therapists*. 2nd ed. Churchill Livingstone; 2009.

Nedelec B, et al. 103 Randomized controlled trial of the immediate and long-term effect of massage on adult postburn scar. *J Burn Care Res*. 2018;39(suppl 1): S57–S57.

Nielsen A, Dusek JA, Taylor-Swanson L, Tick H. Acupuncture therapy as an evidence-based nonpharmacologic strategy for comprehensive acute pain care: the academic consortium pain task force white paper update. *Pain Med*. 2022;23(9):1582–1612.

Nerbass FB, et al. Effects of massage therapy on sleep quality after coronary artery bypass graft surgery. *Clinics*. 2010;65(11):1105–1110.

Netter FH. *The Ciba Collection of Medical Illustrations*. Ciba-Geigy Corporation; 1991.

Netter FH. *The Ciba Collection of Medical Illustrations*. 2nd ed. Ciba-Geigy Corporation; 1992.

Netter FH. *Atlas of Human Anatomy*. 6th ed. Saunders/Elsevier; 2014.

Neuhuber WL, Berthoud H-R. "Functional anatomy of the vagus system: how does the polyvagal theory comply?.". *Biol Psychol*. 2022:108425.

Neumann DA. *Foundations for Rehabilitation*. 2nd ed. Elsevier; 2010.

Neumann DA. *Kinesiology of the Musculoskeletal System, Foundations for Rehabilitation*. 3rd ed. Elsevier; 2016.

Nikola RJ. *Creatures of Water: Hydrotherapy Textbook*. Europa Therapeutic; 1995.

Nistal D, Mocco J. Central nervous system lymphatics and impact on neurologic disease. *World Neurosurg*. 2018;109:449–450.

Nix S. *Williams' Basic Nutrition and Diet Therapy*. 14th ed. Elsevier/Mosby; 2013.

Nord CL, Garfinkel SN. Interoceptive pathways to understand and treat mental health conditions. *Trends Cogn Sci*. 2022.

Norkin CC, Levangie PK. *Joint Structure and Function*. 2nd ed. FA Davis; 1992.

Norkin CC, Levangie PK. *Joint Structure and Function: A Comprehensive Analysis*. 2nd ed. FA Davis; 2005.

Nunes HC, et al. Bisphenol a and mesenchymal stem cells: recent insights. *Life Sci*. 2018.

O'Reilly D, Delis I. Dissecting muscle synergies in the task space. *Elife*. 2024;12:RP87651.

Oschman JL. What is healing energy? III. Silent pulses. *J Bodyw Mov Ther*. 1997;1(3):179.

Olson KA. *Manual Physical Therapy of the Spine*. 2nd ed. Saunders/Elsevier; 2016.

Onder Y, Green CB. Rhythms of metabolism in adipose tissue and mitochondria. *Neurobiol Sleep Circadian Rhythms*. 2018;4:57–63.

Owais S, Chow CH, Furtado M, Frey BN, Van Lieshout RJ. Non-pharmacological interventions for improving postpartum maternal sleep: a systematic review and meta-analysis. *Sleep Med Rev*. 2018.

Page LT. *Licensed massage therapist strain index scores Proceedings of the Human Factors and Ergonomics Society Annual Meeting*. 56. SAGE Publications; 2012:1163–1167 1.

Page P, Frank C, Lardner R. *Assessment and Treatment of Muscle Imbalance: The Janda Approach*. Human Kinetics; 2010.

Palomeque-del-Cerro L, et al. A systematic review of the soft-tissue connections between neck muscles and dura mater: the myodural bridge. *Spine*. 2017;42(1):49–54.

Parameswaran G, Ray DW. Sleep, circadian rhythms, and type 2 diabetes mellitus. *Clin Endocrin*. 2022;96(1):12–20.

Patin A, Scheele D, Hurlemann R. Oxytocin and interpersonal relationships. *Curr Top Behav Neurosci*. 2017;35:389–420.

Patton KT, Thibodeau GA. *Anatomy & Physiology*. 9th ed. Mosby/Elsevier; 2016.

Pavan B, Bianchi A, Botti G. In vitro cell models merging circadian rhythm and brain waves for personalized neuromedicine. *Iscience*. 2022:105477.

Pavan PG, Stecco A, Stern R, et al. Painful connections: densification versus fibrosis of fascia. *Curr Pain Headache Rep*. 2014;18(8):441.

Peckenpaugh NJ. *Nutrition Essentials and Diet Therapy*. 10th ed. Elsevier; 2008.

Pinar R, Afsar F. Back massage to decrease state anxiety, cortisol level, blood pressure, heart rate and increase sleep quality in family caregivers of patients with cancer: a randomized controlled trial. *Asian Pacific J Cancer Prevention*. 2015;16(18):8127–8133.

Pizzorno JE, Murray MT. *Textbook of Natural Medicine*. 4th ed. Churchill Livingstone/Elsevier; 2013.

Porges SW. Polyvagal theory: a science of safety. *Front Integr Neurosci*. 2022;16.

Pollack GH, Cameron IL, Wheatley DN, eds. *Water and the Cell*. Springer; 2006.

Pope RE. The common compensatory pattern: its origin and relationship to the postural model. *Am Acad Osteopath J*. 2003;14(4):19–40.

Pratesi A, Tarantini F, Di Bari M. Skeletal muscle: an endocrine organ. *Clin Cases Miner Bone Metab*. 2013;10(1):11–14. PMC. Web. 6 July 2018.

Premkumar K. *Pathology A to Z: A Handbook for Massage Therapists*. VanPub Books; 1996.

Premkumar K. *The Massage Connection: Anatomy, Physiology & Pathology*. VanPub Books; 1997.

Price SA, Wilson LM. *Pathophysiology, Clinical Concepts of Disease Processes*. 6th ed. Mosby/Elsevier; 2003.

Punnett L, Fine LJ, Keyserling M, et al. Back disorders and nonneutral trunk postures of automobile assembly workers. *Scan J Work Environ Health*. 1991;17:337.

Quinn L, Gordon J. *Documentation for Rehabilitation: A Guide to Clinical Decision Making*. 2nd ed. Elsevier; 2010.

Rai R, Chandra V, Kwon BS. A hyaluronic acid-rich node and duct system in which pluripotent adult stem cells circulate. *Stem Cells Develop*. 2015;24(19):2243–2258.

Rattray F, Ludwig L. *Clinical Massage Therapy: Understanding, Assessing, and Treating Over 70 Conditions*. Talus; 2000.

Reese NB, Bandy WD. *Joint Range of Motion and Muscle Length Testing*. 2nd ed. Saunders/Elsevier; 2010.

Reese NB. *Muscle and Sensory Testing*. 3rd ed. Saunders/Elsevier; 2012.

Romm MJ, Ahn S, Fiebert I, Cahalin LP. A meta-analysis of therapeutic pain neuroscience education, using dosage and treatment format as moderator variables. *Pain Pract*. 2021;21(no. 3):366–380.

Rossettini G, et al. Prevalence and risk factors of thumb pain in Italian manual therapists: an observational cross-sectional study. *Work*. 2016;54(1):159–169.

Sahrmann SA. *Diagnosis and Treatment of Movement Impairment Syndromes*. Mosby/Elsevier; 2002.

Sahrmann S, Azevedo DC, Van Dillen L. Diagnosis and treatment of movement system impairment syndromes. *Braz J Phys Ther*. 2017

Schuenke A, et al. The sacroiliac joint: an overview of its anatomy, function and potential clinical implications. *J Anat*. 2012;221(6):537–567.

Schwartz, et al. Toward a reasoned classification of diseases using physico-chemical based phenotypes. *Front Physiol*. 2018;9:94.

Salvo SG. *Mosby's Pathology for Massage Therapists*. 3rd ed. Mosby/Elsevier; 2014.

Sarkar A, et al. The microbiome in psychology and cognitive neuroscience. *Trends Cogn Sci*. 2018

Schwerdtfeger AR, Paul L, Rominger C. Momentary feelings of safety are associated with attenuated cardiac activity in daily life: preliminary evidence from an ecological momentary assessment study. *Int J Psychophysiol*. 2022;182:231–239.

Seidel HM, Ball JW, Dains JE, et al. *Mosby's Physical Examination Handbook*. 7th ed. Mosby/Elsevier; 2011.

Selye H. *The Stress of Life*. McGraw-Hill; 1978.

Seeley RR, Stephens TD, Tate P. *Essentials of Anatomy and Physiology*. 6th ed. McGraw-Hill; 2006.

Shiland BJ. *Mastering Healthcare Terminology*. 5th ed. Mosby/Elsevier; 2016.

Simons K, et al. Innervation of the thoracolumbar fascia and its relationship to lower back pain. *Spine Scholar*. 2018;10392018(1):3669.

Sieg K, Adams S. *Illustrated Essentials of Musculoskeletal Anatomy*. 4th ed. Megabooks; 2002.

Simons DG. Understanding effective treatments of myofascial trigger points. *J Bodyw Mov Ther*. 2006;10(3):176–177.

Smith LK, Weiss E, Lehmkuhl L. *Brunnstrom's Clinical Kinesiology*. 5th ed. FA Davis; 1996.

Smith BH. SP0073 Opioid prescribing: what's the problem? *Ann. Rheum Dis*. 2018;77(2):19–20.

Smith SM, Wylie WV. The role of the hypothalamic-pituitary-adrenal axis in neuroendocrine responses to stress. *Dialogues Clin Neurosci*. 2022.

Snodgrass SJ, Rivett DA, Chiarelli P, et al. Factors related to thumb pain in physiotherapists. *Aust J Physiother*. 2003;49:243.

Soh KS, Kang KA, Ryu YH. 50 years of bong-han theory and 10 years of primo vascular system. *Evid Based Complement Alternat Med*. 2013. https://doi.org/10.1155/2013/587827.

Sorrentino SA. *Mosby's Textbook for Nursing Assistants*. 8th ed. Mosby/Elsevier; 2012.

Spychala MS, et al. Age-related changes in the gut microbiota influence systemic inflammation and stroke outcome. *Ann Neurol*. 2018.

Standen C, ed. *Textbook of Osteopathic Medicine*. Elsevier Health Sciences; 2017.

Standring S. *Gray's Anatomy: The Anatomical Basis of Medicine and Surgery*. 39th ed. Churchill Livingstone; 2005.

Stefanov M, Potroz M, Kim J, et al. The primo vascular system as a new anatomical system. *J Acupunct Meridian Stud*. 2013;6(6):331–338.

Stevens A, Lowe JS, Young B. *Wheater's Basic Histopathology*. 4th ed. Churchill Livingstone; 2003.

Sturgeon JA, Cooley C, Minhas D. Practical approaches for clinicians in chronic pain management: Strategies and solutions. *Best Pract Res Clin Rheumatol*. 2024:101934.

Sun BL, et al. Lymphatic drainage system of the brain: a novel target for intervention of neurological diseases. *Prog Neurobiol*. 2017.

Swanson RL. Biotensegrity: a unifying theory of biological architecture with applications to osteopathic practice, education, and research—a review and analysis. *J Am Osteopath Assoc*. 2013;113(1):34–52.

T'Sjoen G, Arcelus J, Gooren L, Klink DT, Tangpricha V. Endocrinology of transgender medicine. *Endocr Rev*. 2019;40(no. 1): 97–117.

Takahashi I, Kikuchi S, Sato K, et al. Mechanical load of the lumbar spine during forward bending motion of the trunk—a biomechanical study. *Spine*. 2006;31:18.

Takayanagi Y, Onaka T. Roles of oxytocin in stress responses, allostasis and resilience. *Int J Mol Sci*. 2021;23(1):150.

Thompson GW, Floyd RT. *Manual of Structural Kinesiology with Dynamic Movement*. 14th ed. Mosby/Elsevier; 2000.

Thibodeau GA, Patton KT. *Anatomy and Physiology*. 7th ed. Mosby/Elsevier; 2010.

Thibodeau GA, Patton KT. *Structure & Function of the Body*. 14th ed. Mosby/Elsevier; 2012.

Thibodeau GA, Patton KT. *The Human Body in Health & Disease*. 6th ed. Mosby/Elsevier; 2014.

Tick H, Arya N, Kenneth RP, Robert B, Samantha S, Ronald G, et al. Evidence-Based Nonpharmacologic Strategies for Comprehensive Pain Care: The Consortium Pain Task Force White Paper. *Explore*. 2018;14(3):177–211.

Timmons BH, Ley R, eds. *Behavioral and Psychological Approaches to Breathing Disorders*. Plenum Press; 1994.

Treede RD, Rief W, Barke A, Aziz Q, Bennett MI, Benoliel R, Cohen M, et al. Chronic pain as a symptom or a disease: the IASP Classification of Chronic Pain for the: International Classification of Diseases (ICD-11). *Pain*. 2019;160(1):19–27.

Trew M, Everett T. *Human Movement: An Introductory Text*. 5th ed. Churchill Livingstone; 2006.

Tortora GJ, Grabowski SR. *Principles of Anatomy and Physiology*. 11th ed. Wiley; 2005.

Tian JJ, Levy M, Zhang X, Sinnott R, Maddela R. Counteracting health risks by modulating homeostatic signaling. *Pharmacol Res*. 2022:106281.

van Eenige R, van der Stelt M, Rensen PC, Kooijman S. Regulation of adipose tissue metabolism by the endocannabinoid system. *Trends Endocrinol Metab*. 2018.

van Griensven H, Strong J, Unruh AM, eds. *Pain: A Textbook for Health Professionals*. 2nd ed. Churchill Livingstone/Elsevier; 2014.

VanMeter K, Hubert R. *Gould's Pathophysiology for the Health Professions*. 5th ed. Saunders; 2014.

Vaughn-Coaxum RA, Wang Y, Kiely J, Weisz JR, Dunn EC. Associations between trauma type, timing, and accumulation on current coping behaviors in adolescents: results from a large, population-based sample. *J Youth Adolesc*. 2018;47(4):842–858.

Viseux FJF. The sensory role of the sole of the foot: review and update on clinical perspectives. *Neurophysiol Clin*. 2020;50(1):55–68.

Vleeming A, et al. The sacroiliac joint: an overview of its anatomy, function and potential clinical implications. *J Anat*. 2012;221(6):537–567.

Wang L, He JL, Zhang XH. The efficacy of massage on preterm infants: a meta-analysis. *Am J Perinatol*. 2013;30(9):731–738.

Wei YC, Hsu CH, Huang WY, et al. Vascular risk factors and astrocytic marker for the glymphatic system activity. *Radiol Med*. 2023;128(9):1148–1161.

Whittle MW. *Gait Analysis: An Introduction*. 4th ed. Butterworth-Heinemann/Elsevier; 2007.

Whitney EN, Rolfes SR. *Understanding Nutrition*. 13th ed. Wadsworth Publishing; 2012.

WHO. *WHOQOL: Measuring Quality of Life*. https://www.who.int/healthinfo/survey/whoqol-qualityoflife/en/. Retrieved 15.09.19.

Winter M, Tyree K. *Polyvagal theory. Encyclopedia of Evolutionary Psychological Science*. Springer International Publishing; 2021:6062–6066.

Wiseman N, Feng Y. *A Practical Dictionary of Chinese Medicine*. 2nd ed. Paradigm; 1998.

Yamashita T, Kazuhiko Y, Mitsuru S, Shingo A. Improvement of postural control in the frail older adults through foot care: a pre- and post-intervention study. *Med Eng Phy*. 2024:104115.

Yang M, Luo S, Yang J, Chen W, He L, Liu D, Zhao L, Wang X. Myokines: novel therapeutic targets for diabetic nephropathy. *Front Endocrin*. 2022;13.

Yates J. *A physician's Guide to Therapeutic Massage: Its Physiological Effects and their Application to Treatment*. Massage Therapist Association of British Columbia; 1990.

Young B, Woodford P, O'Dowd G. *Wheater's Functional Histology: A Text and Colour Atlas*. 6th ed. Churchill Livingstone/Elsevier; 2013.

Zaccaro A, Perrucci MG, Parrotta E, Costantini M, Ferri F. Brain-heart interactions are modulated across the respiratory cycle via interoceptive attention. *NeuroImage*. 2022;262:119548.

Zahourek J. *Myologik: An Atlas of Human Musculature in Clay*. Zahourek Systems, Inc. Rochester, VT, 1990: Healing Arts Press; 1996: Vols 1–5.

Mohammad-Reza Z, Khakpai F. State-dependent memory and its modulation by different brain areas and neurotransmitters. *EXCLI J*. 2020;19:1081.

Zarzycki R, Malloy P, Eckenrode BJ, Fagan J, Malloy M, Mangione KK. Application of the 4-element movement system model to sports physical therapy practice and education. *Int J Sports Phys Ther*. 2022;17(1):18.

Zelano C, et al. Nasal respiration entrains human limbic oscillations and modulates cognitive function. *J Neurosci*. 2016;36(49):12448–12467.

Zhao K, Zhang Z, Wen H, Liu B, Li J, Andrea d'Avella, et al. Muscle synergies for evaluating upper limb in clinical applications: A systematic review. *Heliyon*. 2023;9(5):e16202.

Zheng N, et al. Orientation and property of fibers of the myodural bridge in humans. *Spine J*. 2018;18(6):1081–1087.

Zi N. *The Art of Breathing*. Vivi; 1997.

Zink JG, Lawson WB. An osteopathic structural examination and functional interpretation of the soma at four regional transition zones of the body. *Osteopath Ann*. 1979;7(12):433–440.

Zukav G. *The Dancing Wu Li Masters*. Bantam Books; 1980.

Index

Note: Page numbers followed by "*f*" indicate figures "*t*" indicate tables and "*b*" indicate boxes.

C